HEMATOLOGY
A Problem-Oriented Approach

HEMATOLOGY
A Problem-Oriented Approach

Samuel Gross, M.D.

Professor and Chairman Emeritus
Pediatric Hematology-Oncology
University of Florida College of Medicine
Gainesville, Florida

Distinguished Professor of Chemistry
University of Central Florida
Orlando, Florida

Stuart Roath, M.D., FRCPath, FIBiol

Professor of Pathology (Courtesy)
University of Florida College of Medicine
Gainesville, Florida

Professor of Chemistry (Courtesy)
University of Central Florida
Orlando, Florida

Honorary Consultant (Emeritus)
Southampton University Hospitals
UNITED KINGDOM

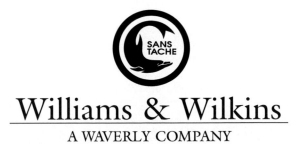

Williams & Wilkins
A WAVERLY COMPANY

BALTIMORE • PHILADELPHIA • LONDON • PARIS • BANGKOK
BUENOS AIRES • HONG KONG • MUNICH • SYDNEY • TOKYO • WROCLAW

Acquisitions Editor: Jonathan W. Pine, Jr.
Managing Editor: Molly L. Mullen
Production Coordinator: Linda C. Carlson
Copy Editors: Anne Schwartz, Carol Zimmerman
Designer: Julie Burris
Illustration Planner: Lorraine Wrzosek
Cover Designer: Dan Pfisterer
Typesetter: Graphic World, Inc.
Printer: R.R. Donnelley & Sons Co., Crawfordsville, IN

Copyright © 1996 Williams & Wilkins

351 West Camden Street
Baltimore, Maryland 21201-2436 USA

Rose Tree Corporate Center
1400 North Providence Road
Building II, Suite 5025
Media, Pennsylvania 19063-2043 USA

Accurate indications, adverse reactions and dosage schedules for drugs are provided in this book, but it is possible that they may change. The reader is urged to review the package information data of the manufacturers of the medications mentioned.

Printed in the United States of America

Library of Congress Cataloging-in-Publication Data

Problem solving in hematology   /   [edited by] Samuel Gross, Stuart Roath.
      p.   cm.
   Includes bibliographical references and index.
   ISBN 0-683-03636-X
   1. Hematology.   2. Hematology—Case studies.   3. Blood—Diseases.
   4. Blood—Diseases—Case studies.   I. Gross, Samuel.   II. Roath, Stuart.
   [DNLM: 1. Hematologic Diseases—case studies.   WH   120   P962   1996]
   RC633.P76   1996
   616.1′5—dc20
   DNLM/DLC
   for Library of Congress   95-42903
                                                                              CIP

The publishers have made every effort to trace the copyright holders for borrowed material. If they have inadvertently overlooked any, they will be pleased to make the necessary arrangements at the first opportunity.

To purchase additional copies of this book, call our customer service department at **(800)638-0672** or fax orders to **(800)447-8438.** For other book services, including chapter reprints and large quantity sales, ask for the Special Sales department.

Canadian customers should call **(800)268-4178,** or fax **(905)470-6780.** For all other calls originating outside of the United States, please call **(410)528-4223** or fax us at **(410)528-8550.**

***Visit Williams & Wilkins on the Internet:* http://www.wwilkins.com** or contact our customer service department at **custserv@wwilkins.com.** Williams & Wilkins customer service representatives are available from 8:30 am to 6:00 pm, EST, Monday through Friday, for telephone access.

                                                     96   97   98   99   00
                                        1   2   3   4   5   6   7   8   9   10

To my parents, Albert and Rose, long gone, who left the dark December of their homeland so that their children could live free and be educated; to my wonderful wife, Ina, and no less wonderful children, Tom, Abby, Sara, and Ellen, who added further dimensions of love and inspiration; and to all of my colleagues and all of my patients, past and present, who won even when they lost.
—SG

To my wife, Jo, for her tolerance with this process.
—SR

Foreword

In the era before Abraham Flexner's report on the teaching of the art and science of medicine in the United States, most medicine was taught in the clinic, at the bedside, and in the surgery by senior physicians who had devoted their careers to physical diagnosis and applied therapeutics, much of which was empiric but traditional. Following Flexner's landmark report, medical education underwent a transformation, since enough preclinical science was then known to justify formal instruction in anatomy, biochemistry, bacteriology, pharmacology, physiology, etc. Medical education evolved to include two years of lectures and laboratories in the preclinical sciences followed thereafter by two years of lectures and clinical experience in the major medical and surgical specialties of the day.

Most U.S. medical schools divided the curriculum between the preclinical department, which commanded the students' time during the first two years of medical school, and the clinical department, which gradually evolved into an increasing number of specialties and subspecialties. Laboratory research by the faculty in the preclinical departments has a long tradition; however, state-of-the-art, controlled clinical investigation is a new and extraordinarily more challenging development.

Although logical for their day, these educational trends led to an unwholesome separation between the preclinical and clinical sciences. The curriculum became stereotyped and students did not encounter real clinical problems for much of the first two years—in essence, compartmentalized learning.

Fortunately, a few educators had the vision to restructure curricula at selected schools by introducing students to real patients and real problems during the initial medical school year. This major, innovative effort to integrate preclinical and clinical sciences was spearheaded at Case Western Reserve University School of Medicine where one of the authors (SG) participated in this experiment. It was subsequently emulated by most of the medical schools in the United States.

The authors have applied the principles of that successful experiment to this text, which presents synopses of clinical problems and illustrates the synthesis of information, deductive reasoning, acceptance or rejection of clues—all of which lead students to conclusions and management decisions that are most likely to be correct.

The text illustrates so well the processes that should be followed to integrate didactic knowledge with diagnostic and therapeutic skills: to make judgments based upon the evaluation and synthesis of findings, and, hopefully, after years of experience, to gain wisdom in their application.

G. Denman Hammond, M.D.
Associate Vice President, Health Affairs
Professor of Pediatrics
University of Southern California
School of Medicine

Foreword

The appalling complexities and confounding elements inherent in problems encountered by physicians resulted, in the past, in near stagnation of clinical medicine at an empiric level. Applications of classic physiology, bacteriology, and biochemistry made slow but notable inroads by unravelling some clinical problems, especially by defining underlying mechanisms and, sometimes, by providing solutions. But the enormous expansion in basic sciences led inevitably to such specialization that individuals who could master clinical medicine no longer could be expected to have the additional capacity to master even one basic science area: in the time allotted the mass of requisite information was just too great. Now add to this the great salutary advances achieved and being made by a diversity of basic science areas through application of contemporary molecular biology and newer biologies. Indeed, physiological and biochemical processes have been revealed for which clinical disorders have yet to be discerned—mechanisms in search of diseases. The growing distance between clinical medicine and basic sciences threatens both areas: the proven, more valuable cross fertilization process should instead be fostered.

Drs. Gross and Roath have here contributed a text in which carefully selected, illustrative hematologic case presentations lure the reader on to closely coupled patho-physiologic and basic science data pertinent for solution (or explication) of the patient's problem. The skillful, sometimes nearly imperceptible, transition to sound *biomedical* data presented in the problem solving mode weld into a coherent whole what might otherwise be apparently disparate approaches. Moreover, an appropriate and comprehensive survey of the general area of the specific problem is provided.

As clearly demonstrated here, hematologic problems lend themselves exceptionally well to: (*a*) definition in the patient; (*b*) transfer to the laboratory or clinic for analysis, generation of generalized data, and resolution; and (*c*) the all-important return to the patient.

For the beginning student of medicine, for the emerging resident and fellow, and for the practicing physician, the authors have done all a service by employing an effective instructional mode that exemplifies how valuable and inextricable basic science can be to medicine, how stimulating clinically defined problems can be to basic science, and how clinical problems may be approached, resolved, and brought back to benefit the patient.

John W. Harris, M.D.
Professor of Medicine
Case Western Reserve University
Director of Hematology Research
MetroHealth Medical Center

Preface

Medical education is not completed at the medical school.
—William H. Welch, M.D., 1892, Bulletin of Harvard Medical School Association

When one of us (SG) joined the faculty at Western Reserve University (now Case Western Reserve University), he became a member of a dramatically new educational experience: a four-year curriculum dedicated to an early introduction to clinical problems within the fabric of an integrated systems approach to the study of medicine. The traditional blocks of proscribed time in Anatomy, Pharmacology, Biochemistry, Physiology and the like were replaced by integrated studies within a systems framework, i.e., cardiovascular, neurological, musculoskeletal, hematopoietic, etc. A similar approach was followed at the University of Southampton (SR) from its founding in 1971. For many students and faculty, this approach entailed a difficult, albeit fortunately short-lived, adjustment. Yet for most of our medical lives, we trained ourselves to digest traditionally presented pedagogical material and laboriously meld its en bloc components into an integrated product. It was the *presentation* of integrated material that appeared to be so formidable. Once the apprenticeship approach to medical education was abandoned, block education in medicine held sway until the mid-1950s, because, like so many other educational endeavors, it was considered disciplined and efficient, and thus pedagogically sound. The teaching of a science, for example, as part of a foreign language course was considered impractical and wasteful, but that approach, ironically, was the only method available for many students who found themselves in a strange new land studying new subjects in a foreign tongue. It was, in fact, the first example of (unintended) integrated learning.

The key to integrated education is the stepwise accumulation of data rather than the constant sorting out of past information for subsequent integration. It is not sufficient, for example, to note that one has attained an education if, at the very least, one understands how to use a library. More than teaching us to use a library or on-line information, medical education needs *inter alia* to teach us to learn. The library and the laboratory are essential parts of the educational process, but only as tools to examine information or seek out new avenues of exploration. This philosophy was key both to the establishment and maintenance of the Integrated Systems Approach in medicine, wherein the traditional block components disappeared only to re-emerge as an integrated entity in every aspect of the education process, from pluripotent stem cells to fully organized, mature systems.

This textbook, conceived in the mid-1960s and nourished intellectually for over 20 years prior to its birth in the 1990s, stands as a paradigm for the broad, integrated approach that lends itself so well to the study of medicine. It was not designed to serve as a compendium text, replete with carefully indexed information, of which there are many outstanding examples. Its intent, rather, is to introduce the process of integrating basic sciences with clinical expressions to learners at all levels. Well-organized and efficient medical care mandates that a core of information be readily integrated for the rapid data analysis necessary for well-designed therapeutic initiatives. The problem-based, integrated approach enables the care provider to recognize patients' complaints as readily accessible clues to solutions. Alternatively, either through printed or computer-based deductive programs, one may ignore the obvious clues and solve problems by rote, an approach which can be accomplished by health professionals other than physicians, and one that rarely leads to an understanding of disease processes. The integrated problem-based study examines the clinical presentation within a framework of structural and functional clues designed to permit the students to utilize the logical consequences of stepwise reasoning. That not all problems are readily solvable, or that there may not be an actual diagnosis, are not disconcerting issues. Myelodysplasia, for instance, is more of a convenient portmanteau term to use until the process is better understood, but it provides a biological explanation that enables one to approach case management in a rational manner. Such, indeed, is the process of medicine; and such, indeed, is typified in several of the case problems in this text.

Learning is a never-ending experience, one that is forever exciting, particularly when addressed in a scholarly and well-organized fashion. Built into the fabric of problem-oriented learning is a methodology-driven process that enables the learner to solve existing problems and to test newer approaches to seemingly insolvable problems. But unlike physics, molecular biology, or biochemistry, which may well be ends unto themselves, the practice of medicine is a totally irrelevant process when carried out without a solid core of natural and biological sciences to support decision making and new growth. Learning by evaluating clincial events with basic scientific tools appears to be an ideally suitable process, and one that profits by reinforcement. At the bedside, reinforcement is brought about by review and reanalysis, i.e., interaction. In this textbook, we provided appendices and reinforcement by adding "Tools" to the ends of certain sections.

Samuel Gross, M.D.
Stuart Roath, M.D.

Contributors

Ross A. Abrams, M.D.
Associate Professor of Oncology and
Radiologic Sciences
Johns Hopkins Oncology Center
The Johns Hopkins University School
of Medicine
Baltimore, Maryland

Daniel R. Ambruso, M.D.
Professor of Pediatrics
Associate Professor of Pathology
University of Colorado School
of Medicine
Associate Medical Director,
Bonfils Blood Center
Pediatric Hematologist,
The Children's Hospital
Denver, Colorado

Frederick R. Appelbaum, M.D.
Director, Clinical Research Division
Member, Fred Hutchinson Cancer
Research Center
Professor of Medicine, University
of Washington
Seattle, Washington

Richard P. Bakemeier, M.D.
Professor of Medicine
University of Colorado School
of Medicine
Associate Director, University of
Colorado Cancer Center
Associate Dean for Continuing
Medical Education
Denver, Colorado

Edward D. Ball, M.D.
Professor of Medicine
Chief, Division of Hematology/Bone
Marrow Transplantation
University of Pittsburgh Medical Center
Director, Bone Marrow Transplant
Program
Co-Director, Leukemia/Lymphoma
Program
University of Pittsburgh Cancer Institute
Pittsburgh, Pennsylvania

Lee-Ann Baxter-Lowe, Ph.D.
Molecular Genetics Program
Center for Cancer Treatment
and Research
Professor of Medicine
University of South Carolina
Columbia, South Carolina

Pamela S. Becker, M.D., Ph.D.
Assistant Professor of Medicine and
Cell Biology
Associate Director, Bone Marrow
Transplantation
University of Massachusetts Medical
Center
Worcester, Massachusetts

Yuval Brandstetter, M.D.
Assistant Professor
Department of Pediatrics
Division of Hematology/Oncology
University of Negev School of Medicine
Beersheva, Israel

F. C. Cabanillas, M.D.
Assistant Professor of Medicine
University of Texas College of Medicine
Houston, Texas

Nicolas Camilo, M.D.
Assistant Professor of Medicine
Wayne State University School
of Medicine
Henry Ford Hospital
Detroit, Michigan

James T. Casper, M.D.
Professor of Pediatrics
Midwest Children's Cancer Center
MACC-Fund Research Center
Milwaukee, Wisconsin

Talal Chatila, M.D.
Professor of Pediatrics
Division of Immunology/Rheumatology
Department of Pediatrics
Washington University School
of Medicine
St. Louis, Missouri

Nicholas Dainiak, M.D.
Clinical Professor of Medicine
Yale University College of Medicine
Chief, Division of Hematology
and Oncology
Bridgeport Hospital
Bridgeport, Connecticut

Albert B. Deisseroth, M.D., Ph.D.
Professor and Chief
Medical Hematology
Department of Medicine
Yale University College of Medicine
New Haven, Connecticut

Karel A. Dicke, M.D., Ph.D.
Director, Marrow Blood Transplantation
Co-Director, Arlington Cancer Center
Arlington, Texas
Clinical Professor of Medicine
University of Arkansas
Little Rock, Arkansas

John L. Francis, Ph.D., M.R.C.Path
Hemostasis and Thrombosis Research
Unit
Walt Disney Memorial Cancer Institute
at Florida Hospital
Altamonte Springs, Florida

Samuel Gross, M.D.
Professor and Chairman Emeritus
Pediatric Hematology/Oncology
University of Florida College
of Medicine
Gainesville, Florida
Distinguished Professor of Chemistry
University of Central Florida
Orlando, Florida

Michael G. Herman, Ph.D.
Assistant Director of Physics
Assistant Professor of Radiologic
Sciences
Division of Radiation Oncology
Johns Hopkins Oncology Center
The Johns Hopkins University School
of Medicine
Baltimore, Maryland

Roger H. Herzig, M.D.
Oncology Consultants, Inc.
Cincinnati, Ohio

George R. Honig, M.D., Ph.D.
Professor of Medicine
Chief, Pediatric Hematology
and Oncology
Department of Pediatrics
University of Illinois at Chicago
Chicago, Illinois

Geetha U. Joseph, M.D.
Associate Professor of Medicine
Department of Pediatrics
University of Louisville
Louisville, Kentucky

Michael J. Joyce, M.D., Ph.D.
Medical Director, Pediatric Bone
Marrow Transplant Program
Division of Hematology/Oncology
The Nemours Children's Clinic
Jacksonville, Florida

Armand Keating, M.D., F.R.C.P.C.
Director, University of Toronto
Autologous Bone Marrow Transplant
Program
The Toronto Hospital
Toronto, Ontario
Canada

Martin R. Klemperer, M.D.
Professor of Pediatrics
University of South Florida
Director, Bone Marrow Transplant Unit
All Children's Hospital
St. Petersburg, Florida

Elizabeth M. Kurczynski, M.D.
Medical Director
Department of Hematology/Oncology
Scottish Rite Children's Medical Center
Atlanta, Georgia

Joseph Laver, M.D.
Professor of Pediatrics
Pediatric Hematology/Oncology
Medical University of South Carolina
Children's Hospital
Charleston, South Carolina

Michael J.P. Lawman, Ph.D.
President and CEO
Morphogenesis, Inc.
Alachua, Florida
Director of Cell Biology Division
Walt Disney Memorial Cancer Institute
at Florida Hospital
Orlando, Florida
Clinical Professor
Department of Medicine
University of South Florida
Tampa, Florida

Naomi L.C. Luban, M.D.
Vice Chairman, Director of Transfusion
Medicine/Quality Assurance
Department of Laboratory Medicine
Professor, Pediatrics and Pathology
The George Washington University
Medical Center
Washington, D.C.

Archie MacKinney, Jr., M.D.
Alumni Professor of Medicine
University of Wisconsin Medical School
Chief of Hematology
William S. Middleton Memorial Veterans
Hospital
Madison, Wisconsin

Robert B. Marcus, Jr., M.D.
Professor
Radiation Oncology and Pediatrics
Shands Cancer Center
University of Florida
Gainesville, Florida

Judith Marsh, M.D.
Honorary Consultant Hematologist
University of London
St. George's Hospital Medical School
Department of Cellular & Molecular
Sciences
London, England

David A. Maybee, M.D.
Colonel, Medical Corps
Program Director, Pediatric
Hematology-Oncology Fellowship
Walter Reed Army Medical Center
Washington, D.C.
Associate Professor of Clinical Pediatrics
Uniformed Services University of the
Health Sciences
Bethesda, Maryland

Paulette Mehta, M.D.
Professor
Division of Pediatric
Hematology/Oncology
University of Florida College of
Medicine
Gainesville, Florida

Anthony A. Meluch, M.D.
University of Alabama at Birmingham
School of Medicine
Division of Hematology/Oncology
Birmingham, Alabama

Donald M. Miller, M.D., Ph.D.
University of Alabama at Birmingham
School of Medicine
Division of Hematology/Oncology
Birmingham, Alabama

William T. Pastuszak, M.D.
Chairman, Department of Pathology and
Laboratory Medicine
Hartford Hospital
Hartford, Connecticut

Paul A. Pitel, M.D.
Chief, Division of Hematology/Oncology
The Nemours Children's Clinic
Jacksonville, Florida

Joel M. Rappoport, M.D.
Professor of Medicine & Pediatrics
Yale University College of Medicine
New Haven, Connecticut

Yaddanapudi Ravindranath, M.D.
Co-Director, Division of
Hematology/Oncology
Children's Hospital of Michigan
Professor of Pediatrics
Wayne State University School of
Medicine
Detroit, Michigan

Peter Reuman, M.D.
Associate Professor of Medicine
Pediatric Infectious Disease Division
University of Florida
College of Medicine
Gainesville, Florida

Stuart Roath, M.D., F.R.C.Path
Professor of Pathology (Courtesy)
University of Florida College
of Medicine
Gainesville, Florida
Professor of Chemistry (Courtesy)
University of Central Florida
Orlando, Florida

Kenneth C. Robbins, Ph.D.
Professor Emeritus
Northwestern University
Division of Hematology/Oncology
Chicago, Illinois

M. A. Rodriguez, M.D.
Department of Hematology
Division of Internal Medicine
M.D. Anderson Cancer Center
Associate Professor of Medicine
University of Texas College of Medicine
Houston, Texas

Hidehiko Saito, M.D.
Chairman and Professor of Medicine
First Department of Internal Medicine
Nagoya University School of Medicine
Nagoya, Japan

Kenneth A. Schwartz, M.D.
Professor of Medicine
Division of Hematology
Michigan State University
East Lansing, Michigan

Bruce I. Sharon, M.D.
Associate Professor of Pediatrics
University of Illinois
Michael Reese Hospital
Chicago, Illinois

A. Majid Shojania, M.D.
Professor of Pediatrics
Associate Professor of Medicine and
Pathology
Faculty of Medicine
University of Manitoba
Head, Department of Laboratory
Medicine
St. Boniface General Hospital
Winnipeg, Manitoba, Canada

Peter S. Smith, M.D.
Division of Biology and Medicine
Department of Pediatrics
Brown University
Rhode Island Hospital
Providence, Rhode Island

Ricardo Uve Sorenson, M.D.
Professor and Chief
Division of Allergy, Immunology, and
Rheumatology
Department of Pediatrics
School of Medicine
Louisiana State University Medical
Center
New Orleans, Louisiana

Robert K. Stuart, M.D.
Professor of Medicine
Director, Hematology/Oncology Division
Medical University of South Carolina
Charleston, South Carolina

Leif G. Suhrland, M.D.
Professor Emeritus of Medicine
Michigan State University
East Lansing, Michigan

Junki Takamatsu, M.D.
Associate Professor of Medicine
Department of Transfusion Medicine
Nagoya University Hospital
Nagoya, Japan

David Tuck, M.D.
Associate Director
Bristol-Meyers Squibb
Wallingford, Connecticut

William H. Zinkham, M.D.
Professor of Pediatrics
The Johns Hopkins University School
of Medicine
Division of Pediatric Hematology
The Johns Hopkins Hospital
Baltimore, Maryland

Contents

INTRODUCTION

Hematopoietic Development

SAMUEL GROSS

Successful transmission of chromosomal-based genomic messages is brought about by programmed cell division and generation. This proliferative process, also known as the generative cycle of dividing tissue, is the substance of stem cell knowledge, and in a more pragmatic sense, the basis upon which chemotherapeutic principles are developed.

The generative cycle consists of five stages commencing with G_1 and cycling through stages S, G_2, M, and thence back to G_1. It also includes a resting, or G_0, stage of variable duration. G_1, G_2, and M are ongoing during mitosis. DNA synthesis occurs almost exclusively during the S phase, although markedly reduced levels of DNA synthesis may occur during the resting (G_0) phase, a likely response to DNA damage that may have arisen at that time. Both RNA and protein synthesis take place throughout the generative cycle (fig. I.1). Cell cycling times vary in accordance with the specifics of different tissues, the result, in part, of complex interactions between the various growth factors.

The four temporal components of mitosis begin with prophase, the time of the nuclear membrane dissolution; metaphase, the appearance of the spindle and the initiation of chromosomal alignment; anaphase, the completion of spindle and chromosomal alignment; and telophase, the time of completed invagination leading to division into two separate cells of equally constituted chromosomal and cytoplasmic components (fig. I.2). Although RNA and DNA synchrony during mitosis is the seemingly appropriate norm, dyssynchrony is a definitive and normal feature of certain cells and, in particular, with reference to the hematopoietic system, the multinucleated megakaryocyte. Dyserythropoietic anemia is an example of multinuclearity that is, in effect, mitosis gone amiss.

As suggested, generative times vary from one system to another, and hematopoietic stem cells are no exception. Once the ability to study hematopoietic stem cell growth in semisolid media was fully elaborated, the entire process of modeling generation times and cytokinetics, along with the ability to characterize the details of pluripotential stem cells and their self-replicating potential, as well as the replication and maturation processes of committed stem cells, became a rather standard laboratory procedure. These efforts, in turn, led to the development of a new vocabulary designed to address their dynamic nature. Included in this litany are the (elusive) pluripotential stem cell factor (SCF); the multipotential progenitor for granu-

locytes, macrophages, megakaryocytes, and erythrocytes (CFU-GEMM); the progenitor for neutrophils and monocytes (CFU-GM); for neutrophils (CFU-G); for monocytes (CFU-M); for eosinophils (CFU-Eo) and basophils (CFU-Baso); for megakaryocytes (CFU-Meg); and for the early and late erythroid progenitors, respectively (CFU-B and CFU-E), all of which are addressed in detail in the following chapters.

The cells that constitute the hematopoietic tissues begin their respective evolutionary processes as mesodermal outgrowths of nonstroma-related islands in the embryonic yolk sac. This process occurs over a period of approximately 2 weeks, following which there is a steady transition to sites in the developing spleen and liver, an event that is completed at the termination of the first trimester. By 4 months, or at the beginning of the second trimester, hematopoiesis shifts to its ultimate site in the marrow (with occasional entre into lymph nodes). These mesoblastic periods are referred to as the yolk sac, hepatic, and the myeloid periods. The term "myeloid" in this context embraces all aspects of blood cell formation and production.

Hemoglobin type changes also occur during the shift from mesoblastic via hepatic to myeloid sites. The earliest type of hemoglobin contains the ϵ- or Gower chains, which disappear and are replaced within 2 months by the development of α- and γ-chains. At parturition, α-chains are matched with 5–10% β- and 90–95% γ-chains. By the end of the first year in excess of 95% of the non-α-chain component are β-chains, with approximately 2% δ-chains (A_2 hemoglobin). Fetal hemoglobin, the mainstay during fetal life declines to 1%. Synthesis of A_2 hemoglobin begins at about the eighth month of intrauterine life, but unlike the high oxygen affinity ϵ- and γ-chains, its significance in hemoglobin ontogeny and phylogeny is unclear. As noted, the ϵ- and γ-chains enhance the neonate's ability to accept and maintain affinity for diffusible oxygen during its intrauterine (polycythemic) environment, a phenomenon that declines rapidly to the "adult" normal following delivery. The polycythemic state is an added process for enhanced oxygenation to dependent tissues. However, once parturition is attained, this state never returns as a norm.

The mechanism by which hemoglobin switching occurs is unknown, but the results are striking. For example, pAO_2 of (pH 7.4) cord blood is approximately 20 mm Hg at 50% O_2 saturation. Adult hemoglobin, at a 50% O_2 saturation and a pH of 7.4, has an oxygen tension of approxi-

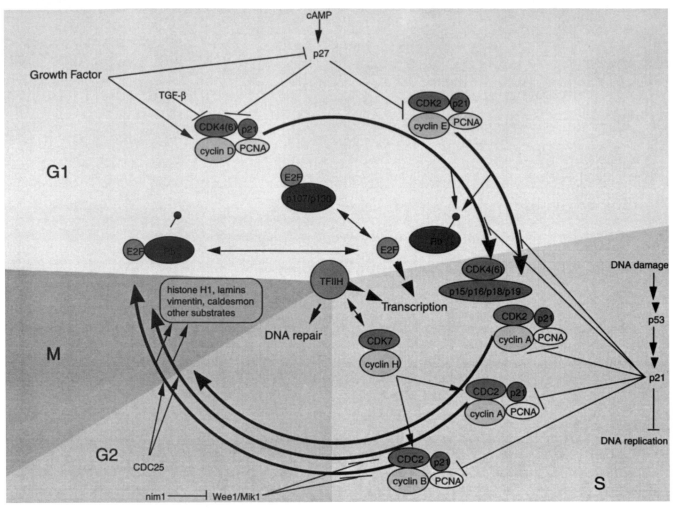

Fig I.I. The generative cycle and mechanisms of activity during the various phases.

mately 32 mm Hg. The greater oxygen affinity of fetal blood, along with the shift in the oxygen dissociation curve, is the result of impaired hemoglobin F binding with 2,3-diphosphoglyceraldehyde (DPG). Conversely, the decrease in fetal hemoglobin levels during the first year of life is associated with a corresponding increase in binding of adult hemoglobin to 2,3-DPG and an associated increase in oxygen saturation.

The red cell membrane of the neonate differs from the adult in two major respects: phospholipid distribution and antigen expression. In the neonatal red cell, sphingomyelin is increased and phosphatidyl choline levels are decreased, differences that may increase the susceptibility of these cells to increased oxidative stress. Cell sol differences between neonatal and adult red cells are related primarily to changes in the glycolytic pathway, the most important being the instability of 2,3-diphosphoglycerate. Other differences include greater instability of the redox systems and adenosine triphosphate (ATP), and decreased activity of glutathione peroxidase enzymes in the neonate, all of which, as noted, tend to increase the susceptibility of the newborn red cell to oxidative stress. In small-for-date or

premature infants, tocopherol and/or peroxidase deficiencies in the presence of increased peroxidizable fatty acid loads will lead to enhanced hemolysis.

Leukopoiesis lags behind erythropoiesis. By the end of the first trimester, granulocytes constitute 40% of the cellular elements of the bone marrow, with few, if any, found in the peripheral circulation. Granulopoiesis predominates during the first 20 weeks of extrauterine life, following which myeloid-derived cell levels decrease to approximately 40% of the total white cell count. Although granulocyte counts are highest in the neonate, sepsis, for example, usually does not result in a profound neutrophilia, because the neonate, unlike the adult, does not have sufficient marrow reserves of myeloid elements. Abnormalities in neutrophils at term include defective chemotaxis, phagocytosis, aggregation, and adherence, although not to a serious degree.

The functional abnormalities of granulocytes are reflected in monocytes as well. The reticuloendothelial system is, in essence, a monocyte-based process present in numerous sites, which, in turn, explains its recognition as the single largest system in the human body. The best ex-

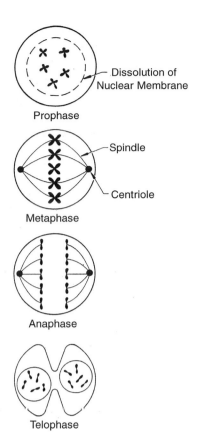

Prophase — Dissolution of Nuclear Membrane

Metaphase — Spindle — Centriole

Anaphase

Telophase

Fig. I.2. The four stages of mitosis.

ample of a reticuloendothelial organ is the spleen, with its capacity to serve both as reservoir and factory permitting the release of certain viable and entrapped hematopoietic elements while functioning as the permanent burial ground for senescent hematopoietic tissues.

Lymphopoiesis begins in the thymus and gut tissues during the latter 2 weeks of the first trimester, is present in the bone marrow at the end of the first trimester, and by 16 weeks B- and T-cell differentiation begins. Products of lymphocyte activity are initially dependent on maternal recognition. During the first 2 to 3 months of life, maturation leads to responsiveness and thence to recognition. By 3 months of life, lymphocytes respond dramatically—for example, the response of T-lymphocytes to hemagglutinin and the B-lymphocytes to pokeweed mitogen (but only in the presence of T-cells). Lymphocyte production is confined essentially to the primary lymphoid organs—that is,

the bone marrow and the thymus. Secondary lymphoid organs include the lymph nodes, which, like the spleen, consist of reticular and cellular compartments without the extensive vascularization so typical of the spleen. The lymphoid system, like the lymphocytes, per se, is not fully mature until the first few months of extrauterine life.

Although megakaryocytes are present in the yolk sac by 6 weeks of intrauterine life, it is not until midterm that platelet counts attain a level of approximately $75 \times 10^9/L$ and not until the latter part of third trimester before the levels are consonant with those at full term. At birth, the number hovers at approximately $125 \times 10^9/L$. Despite these low normal values, laboratory studies of platelet function in the immediate neonatal period tend to be somewhat abnormal, as demonstrated by defective aggregation in association with low concentrations of ADP, collagen, and thrombin. This "abnormality" rarely lasts beyond 4 to 6 weeks of age and is not associated with an abnormal bleeding time, a process that may, in fact, be more epiphenomenologic than clinically relevant. Platelets play a major interactive role with phosphatidyl inositol, arachidonic acid, activated thromboxane, calcium, and the cyclic adenosine monophosphate (AMP) catalysts as part of the events that lead to fibrinogen binding. The processes of adhesion, aggregation, and (effectively synthesized) fibrinogen binding rely on an intact vasculature endothelium capable of undergoing shape changes (e.g., contractility), as well as active protein synthesis (e.g., factor VIII subsets [vwf, plasminogen inhibitors, platelet-activating and functional products]). Defects in any of these systems lead to ineffective coagulation and clot lysis.

The coagulation proteins develop later than their cellular counterparts. Not before 30 weeks is there demonstrable evidence of significant protein coagulation factor activity. Equally germane is that vitamin K–dependent factors do not reach adult levels until parturition is completed and growth of gut bacterial flora commences. In effect, a fully developed platelet-endothelial plug depends upon adequate numbers of functional platelets interacting with appropriately activated protein clot-promoting and lysis sytems and an intact vascular component. At term the integrity of the vascular endothelium is the least mature of the clot promoting/lysing components, a feature of considerable concern for the premature neonate.

With aging, the cycle begins to fail. Hematopoiesis slows, protein synthesis lags, and the integrity of the vascular endothelium slowly deteriorates.

SECTION I

Biologic Control Mechanisms

CHAPTER 1

Biologic Control Mechanisms

STUART ROATH, JOSEPH LAVER, MICHAEL J.P. LAWMAN, SAMUEL GROSS

In 1965 Simnovitz noted that multilineage spleen colonies were capable fo self-renewal when reinserted in other spleens, therby confirming what Maximov had postulated 40 years earlier, namely, that blood cells were derived from a single class of progenitors, i.e., "the clonal origin of a single cell derivation."
—A. J. Becker, E. A. McCulloch, et al. (1967)

Introduction

Cytokines are unique proteins involved in the production and behavior of hematopoietic cells. They control stem cell replication, clonal or lineage selection, maturation rate, and growth inhibition, and are involved in interactions among a host of interleukins, interferons, and recognition and cytocidal factors. These molecules are known collectively as **biologic response modifiers.** They may initiate or contribute to pathologic states via their actions with cell surface receptors or in the intracellular environment. Since they often act in concert with other tissue products in vivo it may be difficult to predict their effects from in vitro studies, but there are now enough reports to enable us to learn more about programming of hematopoiesis by cytokines in health and disease and to some extent the therapeutic activities and potential of these moieties.

Case Report 1

A 49-year-old, nonhypertensive, white male presented with severe headaches. His family doctor noted that he had no previous history of disease, and had never smoked or been exposed to environmental or occupational hazards. Physical examination revealed normal cardiovascular and pulmonary systems. Examination of the abdomen was unrevealing—there was no adenopathy or skin lesions, but he was plethoric, a fact unnoticed by the patient, but, according to his wife, of relatively recent origin. Chest x-ray was unremarkable. Laboratory studies showed normal liver function, urea, electrolytes, and blood gases. A full blood count revealed a hemoglobin of 195 g/L, hematocrit 62%, red blood cells (RBCs) 6.8 × ^{12}/L, with normal indices. The white blood cell (WBC) count was 6.1 × 10^9/L with a normal differential and platelets of 220 × 10^9/L. A bone marrow aspiration and biopsy were remarkable only for an increase in erythroid precursors; they did not reveal other features typical of polycythemia vera.

Assessment: ***This individual had isolated erythremia, which should be distinguished from polycythemia vera. Measuring erythropoietin (Epo) levels in blood or urine is a useful means of evaluating cases of secondary polycythemia. In this individual, polycythemia was confirmed by the markedly elevated level of 720 mouse units/L (normal 5–30). Because blood gas levels were normal (there was no increase in carbon monoxide or poor oxygen saturation), less common disorders of red cell hyperproduction must be considered. The chapter on polycythemia addresses many of these diseases, as well as certain of the hemoglobinopathies characterized by abnormal oxygen dissociation curves or associated with uncommon tumors. It is also unusual to have to wait for a midlife presentation with an abnormal hemoglobin polycythemia, such as hemoglobin M and hemoglobin Heathrow. In this patient, a variety of electrophoretic studies failed to identify abnormal hemoglobins, and his oxygen dissociation curve was also normal.***

The most common tumor associated with polycythemia is renal carcinoma; it is also seen with central nervous system, ovarian, and uterine tumors, including leiomyomata.

Results of an abdominal ultrasound were inconclusive. The liver and both kidneys appeared to be of normal size, although the left one produced a doubtful small echo at the upper pole, which revealed an 8-mm diameter lesion on magnetic resonance imaging (MRI). The presumptive diagnosis was that of renal carcinoma rather than a cystic or infectious lesion. Such tumors are known to be metastatic, but repeat chest films as well as bone scans remained normal.

Management: *He received isovolemic reduction of his RBC volume to a level of 45%, at which point he underwent a left nephrectomy which revealed a 1-cm diameter clear cell carcinoma. Six months postsurgery, his hematocrit remained at 43%, and his Epo level, which had fallen to within the normal range following surgery, remained in the upper normal range.*

Discussion: This polycythemic patient had an Epo-associated kidney tumor. Erythropoietin has considerable historical interest in that it was the first biologic material to which the term **cytokine** was applied. Its action was recognized around 30 years ago by Jacobson and Goldwasser. Their experimental mice, rendered anemic by exsanguination, developed a surge in plasma activity, which increased bone marrow red cell production in nonanemic, normal animals (1). Eventually a 1 million-kd glycoprotein was identified as normally present in low amounts and increased where additional red cell production was required (2). This glycoprotein was then found to be secreted in the juxtaglomerular apparatus of the kidney in normal individuals but was understandably absent in anephric states. Cases of secondary polycythemia frequently have high levels of Epo, with the highest levels found in Epo-secreting tumors.

Epo is currently available for therapeutic use, and in anephric individuals it has been demonstrated to raise levels of hemoglobin from a base of about 60 gm/L to 100 gm/L (3). It has value in secondary chronic anemias, and has also been tried with variable results in some cases of myelodysplasia (4). However, it is not clear exactly how Epo exerts its effect on red cell production, but it likely acts on the immediate post–stem cell daughter cells, shifting them to the red cell line and also shortening the RBC period of maturation within the bone marrow itself. Epo receptors are also present on the surface of marrow erythroid precursors megakaryocytes and fetal liver cells (5). The receptor/cytokine complex appears to be internalized and degraded, but its mode of action thereafter is unclear. Epo is genetically encoded on chromosome 7 as a single copy. The gene itself may be sensitive to oxygen availability through intermediates such as heme proteins, which configurate differently depending on their oxygen content.

In polycythemia vera, plasma or urine Epo levels generally range within normal limits. The structural integrity of the Epo receptor has also been reported as normal in this disorder as has that of its messenger RNA (mRNA) (6). In effect, the role of Epo in polycythemia vera, if any, is unknown.

Biologic Features of Epo

Erythropoietin is solely responsible for the maintenance of erythrocyte mass and control of erythropoiesis. Its production is regulated by tissue hypoxia at its transcriptional level (7, 8). Both murine and human Epo have been cloned (9), and the data show it to be a single polypeptide chain of a mature protein containing 116 amino acids with a calculated molecular weight (Mr) of 18 kd. On the original precursor polypeptide there is a 27-amino acid signal peptide. Epo is also a glycoprotein containing 3 N- and 1 O-linked glycosylation sites. The difference in Mr between the recombinant (18 kd) and native forms (27–60 kd) may reflect the glycosylation rate of the two species. As with all growth factors, Epo exerts its effect via specific membrane receptors of an apparent Mr of 100 and 85 kd (10). Murine and human Epo receptors share an 82% similarity at both the amino acid and nucleic acid levels. The receptor also exhibits similarity to the β-chain of the 1L-2 receptor. There is evidence that erythroid precursors have both high- and low-affinity receptors and that the Epo receptor associates with another surface protein to create these two affinity receptors.

Case Report 2

The patient is an 18-year-old black male with end-stage renal failure of approximately 3 years' duration, following development of chronic glomerulonephritis. Initial therapy for his renal failure was peritoneal dialysis followed by a kidney transplant from his father. His posttransplant course, however, was complicated by seemingly irreversible rejection, and despite aggressive immunosuppression, his transplant had to be removed and peritoneal dialysis was resumed. He had essentially no renal function and was chronically anemic with a hematocrit in the 12–15% range. With ongoing Epo support (100 U/kg/day), his hematocrit exceeds levels of 26–28%, which is sufficient to enable him to follow his usual activities.

Discussion: Since the kidney produces >90% of Epo, the obvious candidates for this therapy are patients with end-stage renal disease (3) in whom there is a dose-dependent increase in erythropoiesis over a range of doses between 15 and 500 U/kg/day (11). Epo is also effective in the anemia of zidovudine (AZT)-treated human immunodeficiency virus (HIV) patients who have low endogenous Epo production (4) and has also been used as an effective alternative to transfusion in treating the anemia of prematurity (12, 13). In the latter instance, the hematocrit ranges between 20 and 30% and reticulocytes are below normal. In vitro studies that have identified Epo-sensitive erythroid progenitors have been borne out in clinical trials showing that Epo does, indeed, increase reticulocytes and correct the anemia (14). Epo has been successfully used in boosting the hematocrit for autologous red cell collections (15) and in certain of the anemias of chronic disease (16), including cancer (17), *wherein inadequate levels of endogenous Epo have been identified.* Conversely, those patients in whom Epo levels are normal rarely respond to added Epo; however, for reasons which are not clear, Epo has also been shown to reduce transfusion requirements in some cases of maternal deprivation syndrome (MDS) (see chap. 20), *unrelated to endogenous Epo levels.*

Case Report 3

A 56-year-old farmer presented with generalized low back pain and lethargy. This nonsmoker had an unremarkable medical history. Symptoms that had developed over a 12-month period worsened in the previous 2 months to the extent that he was unable to work. Except for low back pain and lethargy, his physical exam was unrevealing. However, his blood studies revealed a hemoglobin of 80 g/L with a normal WBC and platelet count. The peripheral blood film was characterized by RBC rouleaux formation, and his erythrocyte sedimentation rate (ESR) was 123 mm in 1 hour. Immunoglobulin assays revealed an IgG(k) paraprotein of 23 g/L with depressed normal immunoglobulin levels. X-Rays of his long bones appeared normal, but his bone marrow aspirate revealed a minor population (about 3%) of plasma cells with surface IgG(k). He had a small amount of k-light chains in his urine, and the final diagnosis was IgGK-Myeloma. Treatment with chemotherapy consisting of adriamycin, carmustine (BCNU), cyclophosphamide, and melphalan at monthly intervals was instituted. Six months later his symptoms had improved and he was back at work, free of analgesics. At that time, his paraprotein had fallen to 6 g/L, and the previously elevated β_2-microglobulin level was approaching normal limits. It was decided to discontinue therapy and observe. Three months later his symptoms reappeared, and relapse was confirmed by increases in circulating paraprotein, β_2-microglobulin levels, and >5% monoclonal plasma cells in a bone marrow aspirate. At this stage, it was decided to undertake high-dose melphalan therapy with autologous stem cell rescue.

Marrow ablation followed by autologous stem cell rescue has been shown to be an effective form of therapy for myeloma previously responsive to conventional chemotherapy (18). This form of therapy was chosen because the patient had no related donors, and it was considered important to proceed without delay in view of the rapidity of relapse. The yield of the harvested peripheral blood mononuclear cells has been found to increase following postchemotherapy stem cell rebound and to be further enhanced by the addition of granulocyte colony-stimulating factor (G-CSF). To this end, the patient received a single dose of 4 g/m² of cyclophosphamide intravenously over 4 hours, and on the following day, was begun on G-CSF in a dose of 5 µg/kg/day. By day 7 the white cell nadir was reached (0.5 × 10⁹/L). On day 9 it had risen to 2 × 10⁹/L with most of the cells being mononuclear, and at that time he underwent cytopheresis for stem cell harvesting. A total of 1 × 10⁹ mononuclear cells

slightly contaminated with neutrophils was obtained and the procedure repeated the following 2 days. A total volume of approximately 400 ml of mononuclear-rich leukocytes (equivalent to 6.4 × 10⁹/L mononuclear cells and a dose of 3.4 × 10⁹ colony-forming units/kg) was obtained. This was divided into four equal parts, frozen by a programmable freezer and stored at −178°F. The patient was next prepared for high-dose melphalan. He received 160 mg/m² intravenously, and 48 hours later his harvested mononuclear cells were reinfused. On the following day, intravenous G-CSF in a dose of 10 mg/kg/day was initiated. Treatment included antibiotics because of an unexplained fever, platelet support for levels >20 × 10⁹/L, and irradiated packed red blood cells for hematocrit levels ≥30%. On day +7 leukocytes began to reappear in the peripheral blood, and on day +12 a neutrophil count of more than 1 × 10⁹/L was achieved. G-CSF was discontinued on day +14, at which time the total WBC was 9.2 × 10⁹/L with 7.8 × 10⁹/L neutrophils. Platelet support was required for an additional 4 weeks, by which time a self-sustained level of 25 × 10⁹/L was evident. The patient was discharged from the hospital on the 14th day, and once again carefully observed as an outpatient. Three months later his clinical condition appeared to be stable, he was asymptomatic and transfusion independent with a WBC count of 6.9 × 7⁹/L and a platelet count of 52 × 10⁹/L.

Discussion: This case illustrates the effective use of **granulocyte colony-stimulating factor (G-CSF)** as a part of a therapeutic maneuver enabling otherwise lethal therapy to be given for an uncontrollable disorder. G-CSF and GM-CSF (granulocyte macrophage colony-stimulating factor), originally derived from human leukocytes or fibroblasts, are now manufactured by recombinant techniques. They have been shown to be involved in the process of proliferation and differentiation of bone marrow progenitors (19). GM-CSF is a growth factor for both macrophages and neutrophils and is presumably active slightly earlier in the differentiation pathway than G-CSF, which is restricted to the granulocyte cell line (20). Both can be given intravenously or subcutaneously depending upon circumstances. Bone pain is the major complaint registered by patients who receive G-CSF or GM-CSF, but fever, malaise, and discomfort at the injection site also occur. At higher doses (e.g., >32 µg/kg) the side effects are worsened, and a capillary leak syndrome is well known to occur with GM-CSF. (More "primitive" cytokines, e.g., Steel factor, interleukin (IL)-1, IL-6, IL-11, IL-16, have been shown in vitro to be synergistic in activities on different earlier stem cell populations (21, 22), and it is assumed that their mobilization is mediated through a variety of interacting factors such as these, all of which behave in an interlinked fashion with each other.)

Granulocyte Colony-Stimulating Factor (G-CSF)

G-CSF is known to act directly on target progenitors to induce the maturation of granulocyte colonies (23, 24). Both the human and murine homologs have been cloned (25). Two species of mRNA have been characterized and are the product of alternate use of two 5′ splice donor sites in the second intron. These two mRNAs differ in only a sequence of 9 nucleotides (3 amino acids). As with GM-CSF, G-CSF is synthesized as a 207 amino acid precursor. The mature cleavage product is 177 amino acids in length, the 3 amino acid polypeptide represents a hydrophobic signal peptide (26, 27). Native G-CSF is glycosylated, and from sequence data there appear to be potentially 3 0-glycosylation sites (residues 1, 7, and 8) (26). The G-CSF cloned product has an Mr of 18 kd but an Mr of 32 kd by gel filtration. It also appears from cloning data that there are two intrapeptide disulfide bonds, suggesting the tertiary structure for G-CSF is highly χ or α helical. Amino acid sequence homology between human and murine G-CSF is 73% in that they are highly species crossreactive. The human G-CSF receptor is an 813 amino acid glycoprotein with high homology to the IL-4 receptor. Murine G-CSF has also been cloned and is also an 812 amino acid glycoprotein with 62% sequence homology to human G-CSF (28). The number of receptor sites/cell varies from 100–700 depending on cell type and species.

Granulocyte Macrophage Colony-Stimulating Factor (GM-CSF)

Human GM-CSF stimulates the production of both granulocytes and macrophages (29). It has an Mr of between 18 and 22 kd (the recombinant form ranges from 15–19 kd). The variation in Mr (size heterogeneity) is reflective of the glycosylation of the peptide. It appears that the mature form of GM-CSF is the result of posttranslational modification on which the 144 amino acid precursor containing a 17 amino acid signal peptide is cleaved to give rise to the 127 amino acid-functional protein containing two potential N-glycosylation sites (30–32). Despite the 60% sequence homology at the amino acid level between murine and human GM-CSF, the two remain species specific. The effector function of GM-CSF is mediated through a single class GM-CSF receptor in the human (50–1000 sites/cell) and a high- and low-affinity receptor in the mouse. The GM-CSF receptor has been cloned and shown to be comprised of an α-subunit (ligand-binding chain) and a β-subunit (non-ligand-binding chain). It is interesting to note that the β-subunit is homologous to the 135-kd subunit of IL-5 receptor and IL-3 receptor.

Endotoxin stimulates GM-CSF production in monocytes. IL-1 or tumor necrosis factor (TNF) stimulates GM-CSF in endothelial, liver, lung, epidermal, and fibroblast cells, all via an RNA for GM-CSF. At present the indications for GM-CSF appear to be similar to those for G-CSF but the profile of side effects in the former is more unfavorable. However, GM-CSF may have a broader stimulating effect on other cytokines.

Macrophage Colony Stimulating-Factor (M-CSF)

M-CSF is known to stimulate the formation of macrophage colonies, activate macrophage effector function, and act as an inhibitor of bone reabsorption. Messenger RNA characterization during the cloning of M-CSF suggests the presence of two mRNA species, with a predominant transcript of 4.0 kb (kilobase), arising from alternate splicing (33, 34). The precursor polypeptide is of 61 kd Mr, comprising 554 amino acids. The mature M-CSF polypeptide of 189 amino acids is the result of cleavage to remove a 32 amino acid signal peptide and a 333 amino acid carboxyterminal peptide (33). The mature peptide is secreted as a homodimer containing both N- and O-linked sugars, and has an apparent Mr of 70–90 kd. It is interesting to note that the smaller mRNA transcript codes for a peptide that exists also as a homodimer of apparent Mr of 36–52 kd and is probably a membrane-bound form of M-CSF. A higher Mr species of M-CSF has also been described. This species of M-CSF appears to be a heterodimer of the 43-kd monomer and a 200-kd proteoglycan form of M-CSF.

Messenger RNA for M-CSF is present in endothelial cells, fibroblasts, and monocytes; G-CSF and γ-interferon induce M-CSF in monocytes; and TNF and IL-1 do likewise in endothelial cells. Endothelial cells, monocytes, and fibroblasts contain mRNA for M-CSF (35). What stimulates the production of M-CSF from fibroblasts is as yet unknown.

The receptor for M-CSF is found on all mononuclear phagocytic cells and is the well-studied cellular protooncogene c-fms, whose product is a tyrosine kinase. An evaluation of the clinical role of M-CSF, particularly any effect on stimulating phagocytic uptake of fungi is not yet available.

Case Report 4

A 23-month-old white female presented with a history of recurrent infections since 7 weeks of age. These began with otitis media and progressed to bacterial meningitis with only mononuclear cells present in the cerebrospinal fluid. She also had numerous cutaneous erythematous, burrowing lesions on her skin. Despite a WBC of 20 × 10⁹L, neutrophils were not seen. Treatment with tobramycin, ceftazidine, and amoxycillin was instituted following culture of Pseudomonas from all the infected sites. Bone marrow aspiration showed failure of granulocyte maturation at the committed cell level. WBC transfusions were given and recovery from the immediate problem ensued, primarily because of the aggressive use of antibiotics. The baby's past history had been punctuated by a series of repeated auditory and respiratory tract infections, all treated with numerous antibiotics as well as steroids. The chronicity of her disease caused her to have a mastoidectomy and a myringotomy *was also carried out. A diagnosis of **Kostmann Syndrome** (congenital agranulocytosis) was made and she was begun on rh-G-CSF with an escalating dose schedule up to 30 µg/kg/day by continuous intravenous infusion followed by 18 µg/kg/day of G-CSF subcutaneous. This therapy induced a neutrophil count of $2 \times 10^9/L$ with normal platelet and RBC counts.*

> Discussion: rh-G-CSF has been shown to be effective in the treatment of Kostmann syndrome (36). However, these patients are capable of producing G-CSF and also express the receptor for this factor; therefore the hypothesis is that the abnormality lies in the signal transduction process (37). It is suggested that G-CSF may function by the combined mass effect of adequate endogenous plus additional exogenous G-CSF (see chap. 21). G-CSF has also been effective in the treatment of cyclic neutropenia where the incidence of infections in the trough intervals has decreased (38). In a similar way it has been extensively used (as has GM-CSF) in the management of post-chemotherapy neutropenia. Quicker recovery of circulating neutrophils with shortened hospital stay and shorter intervals between treatments has been recorded in a number of trials (39). This effect has also led to amelioration of AZT toxicity in AIDS patients (40). It has been suggested that G-CSF be used with caution in myeloproliferative diseases as it may accelerate the progression of the disease; this possibility has arisen in the treatment of leukemia and MDS but has not proved to be a clinical problem (41). The question of the competence of cytokine-driven neutrophils also appears to be clinically unimportant despite data showing in vitro inadequacy (42).

Case Report 5

A 52-year-old white female presented with complaints of tiredness of several months' duration and increasing discomfort in the left hypochondrium of 4 weeks' duration. Her past medical history was unremarkable. She delivered three children in the previous 25 years without complications, and had a hysterectomy 15 years earlier. She had never had blood transfusion support before. She worked most of her life as a private secretary and was not taking medications. Physical examination showed a well-nourished, pale woman without skin lesions or evidence of subcutaneous masses. There were no palpable lymph nodes, and examination of the chest and cardiovascular system was unremarkable except for a slight tachycardia. She was normotensive. The ocular fundi showed occasional small hemorrhages with some venous dilations. On abdominal examination she had an enlarged liver, 2 cm below the costal margin, and a tender palpable spleen extending 8 cm below the left costal margin. She also had a well-healed lower abdominal hysterectomy scar.

Assessment: Clinical suspicion of anemia and an enlarged spleen in a middle-aged adult with evidence that these had not been present previously suggests an acquired hematologic or lymphoreticular disorder. Blood counts revealed the following: hemoglobin was 96 g/L, platelets $110 \times 10^9/L$, and WBC $185 \times 10^9/L$; of these $140 \times 10^9/L$ were neutrophils with an occasional myelocyte, 2 were lymphocytes, and the remainder were immature granulocytes, including a small number of blasts along with occasional nucleated RBC and megakaryocyte fragments. Urea and electrolyte levels were also within normal limits. Uric acid was in the normal range (5.5 mg/100 ml). Examination of the bone marrow showed a hypercellular marrow with loss of architecture and increase in all cell lines, especially the granulocyte compartments. Megakaryocytes were also present. Cytogenetic analysis of the bone marrow showed that all dividing cells were Philadelphia chromosome positive. Fluorescent in situ hybridization indicated the presence of the BCR/ABL oncogene complex, verifying the diagnosis of chronic myelogenous leukemia.

Management: Therapy was initiated with hydroxyurea 1 g daily and purinethol 300 mg/day. The patient progressed uneventfully, and after 6 weeks her hemoglobin had risen to 118 g/L; platelets were 180×10^9, and the WBC had fallen to $9 \times 10^9/L$. At this point, allogenic bone marrow transplantation was considered but the lack of a matched donor precluded this option and it was decided not to seek an unrelated donor. Therapy with interferon (γIFN) was instituted at a dose of 3 megaunits subcutaneously three times weekly and was incrementally increased to 6 megaunits three times a week over the next 2 months. After an additional 2 months, the WBC had fallen to $4 \times 10^9/L$. The patient did not tolerate the γIFN therapy well. She experienced lethargy, a general lack of wellbeing, occasional headaches, and low-grade fever (38°C), which necessitated antipyretics. Reexamination of the bone marrow at this time revealed some reappearance of normal architecture but still considerable activity in all hemopoietic sectors. Peripheral blood showed only normal mature leukocytes with approximately equal numbers of neutrophil and mononuclear cells. The plasma urate levels had fallen to 3 mg/dL%, and a mild aberration of liver function had disappeared. The bone marrow karyotype showed approximately 70% positive cells for the Philadelphia chromosome. The dose of γIFN was reduced to 3 megaunits three times a week, and the patient's tolerance to this medication gradually improved. The WBC remained in the $4–8 \times 10^9/L$ range. Hemoglobin remained constant between 105 and 122 g/L; platelets fell slightly to $140–180 \times 10^9/L$.

> Discussion: Although chronic myelogenous leukemia (CML) is dealt with in detail elsewhere, this case serves as a platform for discussion of the use of interferons. They have been known for many years to have antitumor activity and were originally discovered in a search for viral infection control. Presumably some of the symptoms of influenza-like disorders are in fact endogenous interferon induced. Certain tumors, espe-

cially lymphomas, are also known to provoke increased interferon levels (43). Their mass production in vitro from human leukocytes (or fibroblasts) and later by recombinant techniques made possible clinical trials where they have been shown to be valuable in treating CML, **Hairy Cell Leukemia,** myeloma, and to a lesser extent, renal cell carcinoma and melanoma (44).

Among the interferons, αIFN has been prominent in treating malignant diseases. There are two main classes of interferons, γ and α, which are used in the clinical field. An alternative to single agent therapy is the combination of interferon α and with other conventional chemotherapeutic agents or cytokines such as IL2. In vitro and in vivo studies have demonstrated synergistic and additive effects between and among interferons and different chemotherapeutic compounds (45).

Combining interferon with other cytokines has been tried, for example, in osteopetrosis; M-CSF, which is a growth factor affecting mainly the macrophage lineage, has been introduced recently in combination with interferon-γ. The rationale was that stimulation of the macrophagic lineage might induce the activity of osteoclasts that are derived from these cells (46).

Case Report 6

*The patient presented with pallor and congestion at 1 month of age. His hemoglobin was 76 g/L and platelet count was 91×10^9/L. His serum calcium was 9.1 mg/dl. An ophthalmologic evaluation demonstrated severe optic atrophy and no demonstrable vision. Abdominal ultrasound showed hepatosplenomegaly. On chest x-ray, the patient was found to have diffusely sclerotic bone. The generalized nature of the condition was confirmed by a skeletal survey, which led to the diagnosis of **Osteopetrosis.** A Port-A-Cath was placed for recurrent transfusions. By 3 months of age, the patient was being transfused every 2 weeks. His length was 53 cm (same as his birth length) and his weight was 5.8 kg. His head circumference was 42 cm. His skull had prominent scalp veins, marked frontal bossing, and a slightly open anterior fontanel. The optic disks were pale. No pupillary response was appreciated. The spleen was 7 cm below the costal margin and extended to within 2 cm of the midline. The neurologic examination, except for severely impaired vision, was normal. The patient had a normal hearing evaluation with brainstem-evoked response testing. The computed tomography (CT) of the skull showed narrowed optic canals with very dense temporal bones. The only areas of bone marrow activity noted on a technetium-labeled sulfur colloid scan were at the base of the skull and the distal ends of the long bones. Neutrophil testing showed a marked nitroblue tetrazolium reduction (NBT) (0.34 optical density units compared with 0.65 for control population). When stimulated with γIFN in vitro, the baby showed an increase in white cell NBT staining to an optical density of 0.62. The iliac crest*

biopsy showed markedly increased amounts of trabecular bone, 64.4% (normal value 21%). The urinary calcium excretion was only 0.03 mg/mg Cr.

Management: *The patient with the less aggressive form of osteopetrosis was referred for therapy with γIFN after an unsuccessful search for a marrow transplant donor. Treatment with γIFN at a dose of 1.5 μg/kg, three times a week was given for 6 months. The NBT staining in the white cells increased to 0.736 optical density units (unstimulated, in vitro). After 6 months of therapy, the trabecular bone volume in the iliac crest biopsy decreased to 26.6%. The urinary calcium excretion increased to 0.2 mg/mg Cr. The optic nerve foramina increased from 0.9 mm (narrowest point) to 3.0 mm (normal 4–6 mm). The internal auditory canals increased from 3.3 to 4.1 mm in diameter (normal 2–5 mm). The hemoglobin increased from 76 to 91 g/L. This was not a true comparison since the initial hemoglobin was obtained 3 days after a transfusion, whereas the 6 month value was obtained 5.5 months after the last transfusion. The platelet count increased from 91×10^9/L to 227×10^9/L. The patient, who had not grown from birth to 3 months of age, had an increase of 18.5 cm over the 6 months of therapy. Vision did not recover. Hearing remained normal. No other developmental anomalies were noted and the developmental assessors found the baby to have normal development for a blind child.*

Discussion: A defect in superoxide generation is present in the majority of patients with osteopetrosis (47). Osteoclasts require superoxide generation for normal bone resorption. γIFN stimulates leukocyte superoxide production in patients with osteopetrosis, and a significant rise in superoxide production was seen in our patient. In parallel to this, there was an increase in the calcium excretion and a decrease in the trabecular bone volume, suggesting an increase in osteoclastic function. This translated into an improved clinical picture with a rise in hemoglobin and platelet count, a normalization of growth, and normal neurologic development.

Osteopetrotic patients with blindness and severe anemia (<80g/L) have the worst prognosis for survival (48). Untreated, 50% die within 6 months and only 15% survive to 2 years. Thus, the almost complete reversal of the osteopetrotic state seen in this patient is remarkable. While this patient provides the most graphic response to therapy noted with this treatment, possibly because of the early initiation of treatment, similar improvement has been found in all 8 patients in a series treated and surviving for 8 months (49). In addition, no serious infections (septicemia, pneumonias, urinary tract infections, or meningitis) were seen in any patient.

γIFN has been shown to act in concert with both standard chemotherapeutic agents and M-CSF (45, 46) and to reduce the growth of progenitor cells in juvenile CML. However, clinical use in JCML has proved toxic and less successful in a small group of patients (50) than in adult CML.

Modulation of the proliferative state of cells by agents that induce differentiation are attractive alternatives or additions to established therapy. Differentiating agents have been used in hematologic and other diseases, including leukemias and MDS. The most promising results have been seen in acute promyelocytic leukemia (APML).

Case Report 7

*A 45-year-old physician presented with a 2 day history of rapidly progressive bruising over much of his body. He had been feeling tired for the previous week but otherwise enjoyed good health and had taken no medications recently. His past history was unremarkable and he had been an occasional blood donor, the last time 3 months previously. On examination, he was well nourished, in no distress but virtually covered with subcutaneous and mucous membranous ecchymoses, small and large confluent bruises of recent origin. One small retinal hemorrhage was seen and his urine contained a trace of RBCs. Gentle physical examination revealed no organomegaly or adenopathy. In a relatively well individual the differential diagnosis would initially lie between an acquired platelet or coagulation defect, but the presenting blood count showed the following: hemoglobin 115 g/L, WBC 12.3 × 10⁹/L, and platelets 60 × 10⁹/L with a peripheral blood film showing 76% promyelocytes with prominent granules and occasional faggot cells. An immediate diagnosis of **Acute Promyelocytic Leukemia (APML-M3)** was made, later confirmed cytogenetically by the presence of the characteristic 15/17 translocation. Additional laboratory testing showed a low fibrinogen at 1.5G/L and elevated fibrinogen split products.*

Management: Management represents two problems: rescue from the immediate disseminated intravascular coagulation (DIC) syndrome presumed to be occurring, and treatment of the leukemia. Most observers agree that the bleeding in APML is due to accelerated procoagulant activity rather than a pure fibrinolytic syndrome, and the increased levels of tissue factor present in APML cells may be the key to the pathology of the syndrome. Until recently strategies involving replacement therapy, the use of heparin, and fibrinolytic inhibitors such as EACA were recommended until antileukemic therapy had time to effect significant decrease in the tumor mass. APML was generally regarded as a leukemia with a bad prognosis because of deaths during induction due to bleeding (51). It had long been known that retinoic acids were capable of differentiating promyelocytic cells in culture (52), and clinical studies were carried out in China leading to the advent of therapy with retinoic acids, particularly the all trans

derivative (ATRA) (53, 54), which facilitated rapid resolution of the bleeding problem with promyelocytic differentiation. As mature myeloid cells replace the promyelocytes and cell adhesion and granule content normalize, the coagulation defect rapidly corrects (55). Alone or in combination with "standard" chemotherapy, ATRA has given remission rates of up to 95% in this disorder (56, 57). The dreaded "ATRA syndrome" which bedeviled its early use seems not to occur with added chemotherapy. Even without ATRA, outcome of this disorder had improved and it may be that bone marrow transplantation, currently regarded as the best treatment for adult acute leukemia, may not be warranted in APML (58).

The patient was begun on ATRA 60 mg daily by mouth, and carefully monitored with twice-daily blood counts, including platelets and fibrinogen levels. By the third day he had ceased to show bleeding from venipuncture sites or new bruises. Blood transfusion or platelet support was not necessary and by this time the platelet count was 70 × 10⁹/L. However the WBC had risen to 30 × 10⁹/L so cytoreductive treatment with Cytarabine and Daunorubicin begun as in described in chapter 22. The ATRA was continued for a total of 14 days, and four cycles of Cytarabin/Daunorubicin were given in all. At present the patient is in bone marrow and cytogenetic remission and a search is taking place for a possible bone marrow donor.

Retinoic Acids and Acute Promyelocytic Leukemia (APML)

APML has a typical karyotype—a 15/17 translocation (59)—resulting in a fusion gene, the RAR/PML gene. The RAR (retinoic acid α-receptor) gene found on chromosome 17 is blanked in the fusion process (60). The normal function of the gene product(s) is to work as transcription factor(s) when bound to retinoids. There are probably several closely related RARs (and RXRs whose ligands are less certain) within the cell, and they are globular proteins resembling hormone receptors such as those for thyroxine or glucocorticoids. The retinoid/receptor complexes react with specific gene sequences—retinoic acid response elements (RAREs)—whose transcription is involved in many developmental/differentiation events. Embryologic differentiation is influenced by retinoids, which are highly mutagenic, and in vitro granulocyte differentiation is promoted by them. This also takes place in cultured human lymphocyte antigen (HLA-60) cells where the RAR/PML gene is absent; it is also clear that retinoids act in APML even when the gene responsible for their binding appears to be functionally unavailable. Perhaps the gene masking is incomplete and still responsive to pharmacologic amounts of retinoids, or RAREs on distant sites may be activated. Another explanation, which also accounts for the rapid correction of the hemostatic defect, may lie in the role of

RAREs. One of these has been identified near the gene controlling thrombomodulin production at a cyclic adenosine monophosphate (cAMP) responsive area. Thrombomodulin upregulation has been noted in NB4 promyelocytic cell line cultures exposed to ATRA as has a reduction in tissue factor. cAMP amplifies both of these actions (61). Increased thrombomodulin and decreased tissue factor activity would normalize the procoagulant (and fibrinolytic) activity that is the main cause of morbidity in presenting APML.

Retinol (vitamin A) itself is a relatively feeble hemopoietic differentiating agent, but if it is terminally substituted by a carboxyl group, as in the cis or trans form, it has a markedly increased potential. Even then, retinoids alone are still poor stimulators of hemopoietic colony formation in vitro but act synergistically with G-CSF or Epo in both normal and leukemic growth studies. Differentiation occurs with decreased self-renewal capacity, which presumably accounts for the karyotypic and genetic clonal remissions seen with ATRA. In AML cultures, retinoids are also ineffective as differentiating agents and have no proven value in the treatment of AML. They are only occasionally successful in improving neutrophil counts in MDS (62). TNFα and interferons also act together with retinoids in vitro as co-differentiating agents, but they have yet to be tried clinically. Another analog of vitamin A, B-cis-retinoic acid, is known to include in vitro differentiation (52). In a recent pilot study this agent has induced durable clinical and laboratory responses in patients with JCML (63).

Other Hematologically Active Cytokines

Although **interferons (IFNs)** are mentioned in several chapters as well as earlier in this chapter, some additional information includes the following:

IFN-α-2β inhibits megakaryocyte production and has been tried in patients with essential thrombocytosis. It has a modest and nontoxic antileukemic effect in relapsed ALL in children. **IFN-α-2α** has been shown to prolong survival in many patients with chronic myelocytic leukemia. IFN-α is also effective when used as continuous therapy for hairy cell leukemia and may prolong the plateau phase of myeloma. The IFNs may inhibit hematopoiesis by (1) stimulating the inhibitory activity of tumor necrosis factor (TNF-γ) and (2) inhibiting monocyte-derived interleukin 1.

Interleukins (ILs) are best described as a diverse group of hematopoietic growth factors derived from the glycoprotein family and capable of initiating highly specified hematopoietic functions. Early on, they were categorized according to their various activities, i.e., granulocyte colony-stimulating factor (G-CSF), etc., but as additional cytokines were identified from an ever widening range of tissues, descriptive nomenclature was replaced by a numerical categorization. The following descriptions highlight their unique features.

IL-1 consists of IL-1α and IL-1β, both of which stimulate G-, GM-CSF, and IL-6 production from mesenchymal tissues such as fibroblasts and endothelial cells (L32) (64). It also induces release of TNF-γ. Both polypeptides are encoded on chromosome 2's long arm. They are synthesized as a single 31-kd precursor and the β form is found in greater amounts than the α form. IL-1 has been shown to be produced in vitro by myeloblasts, which may account for some of their growth advantage in vivo (64, 65). An antagonist for the IL-1 receptor occurs naturally and there is also a soluble incomplete form of the receptor. Both of these have been synthesized and inhibit leukemia colony formation in vitro. Clinical trials of such inhibitors are taking place. IL-1 is produced by fixed and mobile macrophages and is stimulated by TNF.

IL-2 induces cytotoxic T cell activity and proliferation of B, T, and NK lymphocytes, and TNF in monocytes.

It was one of the first ILs to be tried clinically—used as a single agent it has some effect in metastatic melanoma but is limited by its dose-related toxicity. Subsequently used with LAK cells and in combination with chemotherapy regimens and αIFN alpha, responses have been recorded in 15–50% of patients. However, usually these responses are not durable and occur at the expense of considerable toxicity. Trials in lymphoma have also suggested activity, but the value of IL-2 is not yet established. An interesting development is the use of IL-2 to initiate graft-versus-leukemia (GVL) effect in autologous bone marrow transplantation (BMT) (66). Experimental evidence suggests that it may also have a role in dealing with minimal residual disease (67). IL-2 receptors are found on lymphocytes and monocytes and their expression is modulated by TGFβ and IFNγ, for example. Its mutation has been associated with cases of X-linked immunodeficiency (68).

IL-3 is a multi-CSF capable of supporting multilineage colony formation early in their development. It is also a powerful growth factor synergizing with many of the CSFs, including stem cell factor (SCF), GM-CSF, Epo, 1L-6, and G-CSF.

Human IL-3 was identified and expressed several years after the identification of mouse IL-3. Both species have been cloned. The genes encoding the human and murine IL-3 are approximately the same length (3 kb) mRNA transcript yielding a translational product with an Mr of 15–25 kd (69). Human and murine homology at both nucleic acid and amino acid levels is 45% and 29%, respectively, which accounts for its species specificity. The IL-3 growth factor exerts its effector function through a multisubunit complex receptor (70). This includes a 70-kd β-subunit (responsible for signal transduction). It is this subunit that is shared between IL-3, IL-5, and GM-CSF receptor systems (71–73).

Because of its presumed multipotent hemopoietic-stimulating ability, IL-3 has been tried in MDS where hemopoiesis is broadly ineffective. The results of several small trials (74) show variable benefit including rises in all three blood cell lines in up to half the 32 subjects reviewed. Dysplasia persisted with side effects similar to those elicited by G-CSF.

IL-4 is an intermediate-acting, lineage nonspecific growth factor that can act alone on the proliferation and differentiation of committed and/or primitive hematopoietic progenitors. IL-4 can also act synergistically with CSF growth factors to support hematopoiesis or to inhibit CSF-induced colony formation (75). Cloning data, in particular nucleotide sequence, suggest an open reading frame coding for a 140-amino acid polypeptide, of which the first 20 amino acids from the amino terminal end act as a signal sequence. Both the human and mouse are glycosylated proteins and have a 50% amino acid sequence homology (76). However, the human and mouse 1L-4 are species specific. 1L-4 also has a high affinity receptor, approximately 140 kd in Mr, and is found on hematopoietic progenitor cells and nonhematopoietic cells (stroma, brain, spleen, melanoma, and liver) (77). IL-4 is a growth factor for most cells, including T-lymphocytes.

IL-4 as well as IL-1 has been suggested as a target for leukemia therapy and to act as in vitro modulators in CML (78). IL-4 also inhibits IL-1 activity. IL-4 may be more than one molecule, as it has effects on GM-CSF and G-CSF-modulated colony formation as well as IL-1, and may also act in concert with IL-3. Its spectrum of actions resembles those of interferons.

IL-5 is a 13-kd polypeptide of 115 amino acids. It stimulates eosinophil production and activates cytotoxic T cells (79). It may be produced by Reed Sternberg cells in Hodgkin disease and account for the eosinophilia sometimes evident there and in parasitic and possibly some allergic reactions.

IL-6 has been shown to interact with both myeloid and lymphoid progenitors and nonhematopoietic cells within the hematopoietic system (80). This cytokine has also been shown to synergize with IL-3 and M-CSF in the proliferation of hematopoietic stem cells. The sequence of mRNA for both human and murine IL-6 indicate that they code for 213 and 212 amino acid polypeptide containing a 24 and 28 amino acid signal sequence, respectively. Both species of IL-6 also contain two intra chain disulfide bonds and have both N- and O-linked glycosylation sites. Human and murine IL-6 share a 41% amino acid sequence homology (81), and human IL-6 works extremely well in the mouse systems (82). Again, the effector function of IL-6 is exerted by interacting with an IL-6 receptor. This receptor is a heterodimer of a ligand-binding chain (80 kd) and a signal transducer (non-ligand-binding chain) of 130 kd. IL-6 is produced by monocytes, T and B lymphocytes, marrow stromal cells, endothelial cells, fibroblasts, and keratinocytes among several others (83). It can be regarded as an acute phase reactant in some respects but may have a wider role (84). It stimulates megakaryopoiesis in mice. Recently it has been shown to be elevated in immunosuppressed patients.

IL-7 stimulates monocyte induced cytokines. It may also have a role in pre-B lymphocyte stimulation. It is produced by one marrow stromal fibroblast and activates the earlier pre-B lymphocytes until their gene rearrangement is complete. It improves ALL blast cell growth in vitro and

also enhances drug toxicity, acting in opposition to TGFβ in this respect.

IL-8, a member of the CXL branch of the chemokine superfamily, induces granulocyte chemotaxis and promotes leukocyte adhesion, degranulation, and the respiratory burst, and activates the 5-lipoxygenase pathway. It is secreted by endothelial cells through stimulation by IL-1 and TNF, but may have a much broader originator cell profile. Like other chemokines, it is of low molecular weight. Receptors on the polymorphonuclear leukocyte (PMN) surface show homology with those of C5a and FMLP. It is a mediator of the inflammatory response and may actually be an integral part of the inflammatory cascade.

IL-9 stimulates early red cell production. However, it also promotes AML blast cell growth in vitro and may be a critical autocrine loop factor in this disease. It is produced in Hodgkin disease, as are IL-1, IL-2, IL-4, IL-5, IL-6, and IL-9, and may account for some of the cellular aspects of its pathology and its clinical symptoms. It is both produced by and enhances production of CDX T cells.

IL-10 induces B lymphocyte and mast cell growth following its release from endotoxin-stimulated monocytes and activated T lymphocytes. It inhibits T cell proliferation. Anti IL-10 antibodies block all of the above and also inhibit monocytic and Th1 cell cytokine production, including G-CSF and GM-CSF. The CD-11b receptor for C_3bi is downgraded by IL-10 and may be a natural anti-inflammatory agent. It also has a wide (indirect?) effect on hemopoiesis, including myelopoiesis. Its signal transduction system acts through the Stat family of receptors.

Although originally discovered for its ability to stimulate the growth of a plasmacytoma cell line, **IL-11** has also been shown to be important in the proliferation of myeloid cells. The IL-11 gene was initially cloned from the cyclic DNA (cDNA) library constructed from a primate cell line and subsequently from a cDNA library from human lung fibroblasts (MRC5). The DNA for IL-11 is 597 nucleotides long, encoding 199 amino acids with an Mr of 23 kd. Adjacent to this open reading frame is a stretch of 51–60 nucleotides encoding a conventional protein leader sequence. There are no N-glycosylation sites and this polypeptide contains a high proportion of proline residues (17%) and no cysteines, features not found in any other growth factor. Primate IL-11 and human IL-11 exhibit a high degree of nucleotide sequence homology. The adipogenesis inhibitory factor (AGIF) was also recently cloned and was found to be identical to IL-11. The complete genomic sequence for IL-11 has been elucidated. The gene is 7 kb in length with 5 exons and 4 introns. Despite evidence that IL-6 and IL-11 do not compete for receptor sites on IL-6- and IL-11-sensitive cells, it has been shown that IL-11-induced bioactivity is mediated through the IL-6 signal transducer (gp 130). Receptor systems for cytokines are probably complexes of shared and unique elements combined with a signal transducer that may also be shared. The IL-11 signal transducer gp 130 is shared with

IL-6. It induces rapid transient tyrosine phosphorylation. On the 3T3-L cell line a single class of high affinity IL-11 receptor (Mr 150 kd) was found. It aids in secretion and supplements IL-3 in its ability to stimulate megakaryocyte production. IL-11 has already been tried with G-CSF in the restoration of neutrophil levels following marrow conditioning regimens (85).

IL-12 induces production of IFN and regulates T cell development. It also induces T and NK cells to produce γINF. It is produced by mononuclear antigen-presenting cells, although originally derived in the laboratory from Epstein-Barr virus (EBV)-infected B cell lines, and is also known as natural killer cell-stimulatory factor (NKCSF). It is a heterodimer with 40 and 35 kd chains. The former is encoded on chromosome 5 q31/32 in an area rich in genes for cytokines, the latter on the long arm of chromosome 3. It has been cloned and the sequences of the amino acids in the smaller monomer have areas of commonality with IL-6 and G-CSF. Its production is regulated by IFN and GM-CSF. IL-12 appears to have a central immunoregulatory role in T cell and NK cell activity and potentially might play a part with other interleukins such as IL-4 in enhancing natural or induced immune antitumor activities.

IL-13 is a T cell derived cytokine that enhances IgE, IgG, and IgM and γINF synthesis. IL-4 and IL-13 appear to share common receptors along with CD-23, MHC Class II, and CD-72 synthesis in B cells. IL-13 is interesting in that it is also part of the IL cluster on the long arm of chromosome 5, with genes for IL-3, IL-4, IL-5, IL-12, RF1, and CSF2. Its molecular weight is 12 kda and is produced by various T lymphocytes. It suppresses monocyte production of inflammatory cytokines and enhances tyrosine phosphorylation of a number of kinases critical in signal transduction.

Other Cytokines

Tumor necrosis factor (TNF) is an example of a pleiotropic gene product—one with many phenotypic effects through its actions on other genes. TNFα and its coproduct TNFβ are encoded on the chromosome 6 MHC region. TNFα may be identical with cachectin, the 17-kd protein produced by macrophages which has direct antitumor effects. However, TNFα is multifunctional and its cytocidal effects include the potentiation of oxidative stress. It may not have a role in normal hemopoiesis, but because of its synergy with IL-3 and its ability to influence other regulatory cytokines such as IL-1, MG-CSF, and GM-CSF, it may have an as yet undetermined role in hemopoietic disorders or their management. Its promise as a single agent antitumor drug has not been fulfilled.

Transforming growth factor β (TGFβ₁) has been shown to be present in eosinophils and is probably also secreted in pathologic states, such as **Hodgkin Disease**, by mononuclear cells. If it has a role in hemopoiesis it is probably as a downregulator of colony-stimulating factors.

GM-CSF-IL-3 Fusion Protein (pixy321)

In order to develop enhanced activity for some of the colony-stimulating factors, researchers have produced a fusion protein containing IL-3 and GM-CSF. This fusion protein was constructed using a plasmid containing the coding regions of GM-CSF and IL-3 connected via a sequence encoding a synthetic linker. The resulting recombinant protein (pixy321) was expressed in yeast. These workers and others have shown enhanced activity in terms of its receptor affinity, colony-forming activity, and proliferation supporting the finding that, once fused, GM-CSF and IL-3 still retain their respective native confirmation. Early clinical data have received mixed reviews primarily because of excessive toxicity (86, 87).

Stem Cell Factor (SCF)

SCF (Steel factor; C-Kit ligand, mast cell growth factor) is a multilineage growth factor exerting its effect on hematopoietic stem cells, melanocytes, mast cells, and embryonic stem cells (88, 89). SCF also exhibits a high degree of synergy with other cytokines (32–35, 88–91). Native SCF has an apparent Mr of 30 kd and is a noncovalently linked dimer under physiologic conditions. Natural SCF is highly glycosylated with N-linked and O-linked sugars. SCF exists in two forms, cell bound and/or secreted (35, 37, 91, 92). The translated, cell-bound product predicts a 25-amino acid signal sequence, a 36-amino acid intracellular domain, a 25-amino acid transmembrane domain and a 164-amino extracellular domain (91–93). The soluble form consists of the 164 extracellular domain. The production of either the soluble or membrane-bound L-form is the result of alternative splicing of the MRNA transcript. Both murine and rat SCF have a 79% sequence homology to the human at the amino acid level. Mouse and/or rat SCF have activity on human hematopoietic cells, while human SCF has no activity on either mouse or rat (92). The normal cellular receptor for SCF is the C-Kit protooncogene. The oncogene is a member of the transmembrane tyrosine kinase receptor group (94, 95). On very early progenitor cells there are approximately 100–1,000 receptors/cell.

FLt-3/FLk-2 Ligand

The ligand for the FLt-3/FLk-2 tyrosine kinase receptor was very recently cloned (40, 41, 96, 97). This growth factor has been shown to stimulate the proliferation of both murine and human hematopoietic stem cells (96). The cDNA for this growth factor encodes a type 1 transmembrane protein. The open reading frame of 696 base pairs encodes 231 amino acids. It also appears that this polypeptide has an N-terminal signal peptide of 27 amino acids, a 161-amino acid extracellular domain, a 22-amino acid transmembrane domain, and a 21-amino acid cytoplasmic domain. Furthermore, the ligand is glycosylated with two potential N-glycosylated sides. The predicted Mr of the

Table 1.1. Cytokines—Names and Sources

Name	Sources	Name	Sources	Name	Sources
Angiogenin	Fibroblasts, lymphocytes, colon epithelium	FGF-7	Stromal cells of epithelial tissue	IL-1ra	Monocytes/macrophages, endothelial cells, fibroblasts, neuronal cells, glial cells, keratinocytes, epithelial cells
EGF	Present in body fluids, low levels in tissues, EGF-like activity in platelets, secretory cells of sweat glands	G-CSF	T cells, macrophages, neutrophils, endothelial cells, fibroblasts		
		GM-CSF	Macrophages, T cells, endothelial cells, mast cells, neutrophils, eosinophils, fibroblasts	IL-2	T cells
Epo	Kidney, liver, macrophages?			IL-3	T cells, thymic epithelial cells, keratinocytes, neuronal cells, mast cells
FGF Acidic	Brain, retina, bone matrix, osteosarcomas	GROα/MGSA	Fibroblasts, chondrocytes, epithelial cells; monocytes/macrophages, neutrophils, platelets		
FGF Basic	Neural tissue, pituitary, adrenal cortex, corpus luteum, placenta			IL-4	T cells, macrophages, mast cells, basophils, B cells, bone marrow stromal cells
FGF-3	Expressed by epithelial cells of mamary tumors, expressed at various sites and times during embryonic development	HB-EGF	Macrophages	IL-5	T cells, mast cells
		HGF	Platelets, fibroblasts, macrophages, endothelial cells, smooth muscle cells	IL-6	T cells, monocytes/macrophages, fibroblasts, hepatocytes, endothelial cells, neuronal cells
FGF-4	Expressed by certain tumor cells, expressed by various tissues during embryonic development	IFNα/β	T cells, B cells, monocytes/macrophages, fibroblasts	IL-7	Bone marrow stromal cells, fetal liver cells
		IFNγ	T cells, NK cells	IL-8	Monocytes, T cells, fibroblasts, endothelial cells, keratinocytes, hepatocyes, chondrocytes, neutrophils, epithelial cells
		ICF 1 & IGF-2	Many tissues		
FGF-5	Normal fibroblasts, tumor cell lines, retinal pigment, epithelium, various tissues during embryonic development	IL-1α	Monocytes/macrophages, endothelial cells, fibroblasts, neuronal cells, glial cells, keratinocytes, epithelial cells	IL-9	T cells
				IL-10	T cells, macrophages, keratinocytes, B cells
FGF-6	Expressed during embryonic development and in adults in testis, heart, and skeletal muscle (mice): Kaposi sarcoma tissue in AIDS	IL-1β	Monocytes/macrophages, endothelial cells, fibroblasts, neuronal cells, glial cells, keratinocytes, epithelial cells		

(continued)

native protein is 23,164 daltons. It appears that the mouse and human have a high degree of sequence homology at the amino acid level. The murine FL-ligand will interact with human hematopoietic and murine stem cells. The FL-ligand and the human homolog bind to specific receptors (FLR-3/FLK-2) (98) in the mouse and STk-1 in human) (99). This receptor complex has been found in human blood and marrow and is restricted to CD-34+ cells (99).

Thrombopoietin

Megakaryopoiesis and subsequent platelet production are vital to hemostasis, wound healing, and blood coagulation. Recently the characterization of a protooncogene, c-Mpl, has led to the identification of a ligand for this protooncogene receptor (100–102). The deduced human, murine,

and canine amino acid sequences exhibited a high degree of homology (69–77% similarity) at the amino acid level. On sequence comparisons made with other growth factors it appears that thrombopoietin has 25% sequence homology to erythropoietin. The produced molecular weight of the primary translation product is 35 kd; however, the molecular weights of the purified forms of thrombopoietin (from canine aplastic plasma) are 25 and 31 kd. The total number of amino acids in the recombinant molecule equals 353 residues (100). Thrombopoietin, as stated earlier, utilizes the C-Mpl protooncogene as its receptor on thrombopoietic-sensitive cells (101, 102). Table 1.1 is a summation of the cytokine/biologic response modifier data.

It is becoming apparent that the biologic response modifiers described in this chapter are not acting in a closed hemopoietic system solely related, for instance,

Table 1.1.—*continued*

Name	Sources	Name	Sources	Name	Sources
IL-11	Stromal fibroblasts, trophoblasts	MIP-1β/ Act 2	T cells, B cells, monocytes, mast cells, fibroblasts	RANTES	T cells, platelets, renal epithelium, mesangial cells
IL-12	B cells, macrophages	NGF	Smooth muscle cells, fibroblasts, activated macrophages, epithelial cells, neurons, astrocytes, Schwann cells	SCF	Bone marrow stromal cells, endothelial cells, fibroblasts, Sertoli cells
IL-13	T cells				
IL-14	T cells			TGF-α	Macrophages, skin keratinocytes, pituitary, brain
IP-10	Monocytes, fibroblasts, endothelial cells, keratinocytes				
LIF	Bone marrow stromal cells, fibroblasts, T cells, monocytes/ macrophages, astrocytes	OSM	T cells, monocytes/ macrophages	TGF-β	Chondrocytes, osteoblasts, osteoclasts, platelets, fibroblasts, monocytes
		PD-ECGF	Platelets, Stromal cells of placenta, foreskin fibroblasts, vascular smooth muscle cells, some carcinoma cell lines		
M-CSF	T cells, neutrophils, macrophages, fibroblasts, endothelial cells			TNF-α	Neutrophils, activates lymphocytes, NK cells, LAK cells, astrocytes, endothelial cells, smooth muscle cells
LMW-BCGF	T cells				
MCP-1/ MCAF	Monocytes/macrophages, fibroblasts, B cells, endothelial cells, smooth muscle cells, glioblastoma cells	*Gliostatin*	Quiescent type 1 astrocytes	TNF-β	Lymphocytes
				VEGF	Aortic smooth muscle cells, various tumor cells, epithelial cells, macrophages
MIP-1α	T cells, B cells, monocytes, mast cells, fibroblasts	PD-DCGF	Platelets, endothelial cells, monocytes/ macrophages, smooth muscle cells, fibroblasts, cytotrophoblasts, neurons		

to growth or immune activity. In hematology there is interaction—"crosstalk"—between the coagulation, inflammatory, and myeloproliferative systems, and common cytokine receptors or messengers and transducers may be utilized. For instance, protein S, although recognized as a key natural anticoagulant, in combination with activated protein C (APC), also has a role in the inflammatory cascade through C4BP, the C4b-binding protein. Its receptors include a tyrosine kinase (tyro 3), as is common to many cytokines. However, tyro 3 is expressed in many neural tissues, and protein S itself is actually produced by some neural cell lines, also binds to monocytes and neutrophils, has a role in endothelial growth, and is found in osteoblasts, suggesting that it has a role in bone turnover. In the broadest aspect of communications and homeostasis, corticotrophins and neuroendocrine factors have leucocyte receptors, and IL-1, IL-2, and IL-6 have been postulated to act directly on the hypothalamus and pituitary (as well as have IFNa, TNFa, and PGF2a) and glial cells are being discovered to have receptors for interleukins. It is likely that interactions between cell growth, activation (e.g., through chemokines and other inflammatory mediators), endothelium, and the vascular system, and the neural and neuromuscular systems will continue to be recognized.

Conclusions

As understanding of the biologic response modifiers has been progressively refined through knowledge of their actions, chemistry, genetics, receptors, and interactions, a new degree of insight into hemopoietic cell growth and its relation to disease states has resulted. Of all the biologic response modifiers, the interferons have the longest pedigree in clinical studies. Interferons are changing our expectations and management of chronic myelogenous leukemia in particular and probably of the lymphoproliferative and immunoproliferative disorders as well. The more recent use of all trans derivative is transforming the outcome of acute promyelocytic leukemia. Erythropoietin and granulocyte colony-stimulating factor may become major supporting players in bone marrow failure and enhance other therapeutic options such as high-dose chemotherapy. Combinations of cytokines or biologic response modifiers (BMRs) with each other, with chemotherapy or immunotherapy (e.g., with primed lymphocytes), and their use in marrow and organ graft manipulation are likely to provide further advances. The use of growth factor inhibitors is an intriguing possibility in leukemia. As the use of drugs and the availability of bone marrow transplantation changed the outlook completely in hematologic malignancies in the past 30 years, so the advent of BMR usage is likely to be another major step forward.

REFERENCES

1. Jacobson LO, Goldwasser E, Curney CW, et al. Studies of Erythropoietin: the hormone regulating red blood cell production. Ann NY Acad Sci 1959;77:551.

2. Myake T, Kung CK, et al. Purification of human erythropoietin. J Biol Chem 1977;252:5558.

3. Eschbach JW, Egrie JC, Dowing MR. Corrections of the anemia of end stage renal disease with recombinant human erythropoietin. N Engl J Med 1987;316:73.

4. Baer AN, Dessypris EN, Goldwasser E, et al. Blunted erythropoietin response to anemia in rheumatoid arthritis. Br J Haematol 1987;66:559.

5. Berridge MV, Fraser JK, Carter JM, et al. Effects of recombinant human erythropoietin on megakaryocytes and on platelet production in the patient. Blood 1988;72:970.

6. Hess G, Rose P, Gamm H, et al. Molecular analysis of the erythropoietin receptor system in patients with polycythemia vera. Br J Haematol 1994;88:794.

7. Schuster SJ, Badiavas EV, Costa-Giomi P, Winmann R, Erslev AJ, Caro J. Stimulation of erythropoietin gene transcription during hypoxia and cobalt exposure. Blood 1989;73:13.

8. Goldberg MA, Dunning SP, Bunn HF. Regulation of the erythropoietin gene: evidence that the oxygen sensor is a heme protein. Science 1988;242:1412.

9. Lin FK, Suggs S, Lin CH, Browne JK, Smalling R, Egrie JC, Chen KK, Fox FM, Martin F, Stabinsky Z, et al. Cloning and expression of the human erythropoietin gene. Proc Natl Acad Sci USA 1985;82:7580.

10. Kitamura T, Tojo A, Kuwaki T, Chiba S, et al. Identification and analysis of human erythropoietin receptors on a factor-dependent cell line, TF-1. Blood 1989;73:375.

11. Bommer J, Alexiou C, Muller-Buhl U, et al. Recombinant human erythropoietin therapy in haemodialysis patients—dose determination and clinical experience. Nephrol-Dial-Transplant 1987;2:238.

12. Groopman JE. Management of hematologic complications of human immunodeficiency virus infection. Rev Infect Dis 1990;12:931.

13. Stockman JA. Erythropoietin: off again, on again. J Pediatr 1988;112:906.

14. Beck D, Masserey E, Meyes M, et al. Weekly intravenous administration of recombinant human erythropoietin in infants with anemia of prematurity. Eur J Pediatr 1991;150:767.

15. Goodnough LT, Price TH, Rudnick S, et al. Preoperative red cell production in patients undergoing aggressive autologous blood phlebotomy with and without erythropoietin therapy. Transfusion 1992;32:441.

16. Vengdemie G, Swaak AJ. The role of erythropoietin in the anemia of chronic disease in rheumatoid arthritis. Clin Rheumatol 1990;9:22.

17. Henry DH. Recombinant human erythropoietin for the treatment of anemia in patients with advanced cancer. Semin Hematol 1993;30(Suppl 6):12.

18. Barlogie B, Jagannaths Vasole D, Tricot G. Hematopoietic stem cell autograft in support of myeloablative therapy for multiple myeloma. J Hematol 1994;3:149.

19. Laver J, Moore MAS. Clinical use of recombinant human hematopoietic growth factors. J Natl Cancer Inst 1994;81:1370.

20. Souza L, Boone TC, Gabrilove J, et al. Recombinant human granulocyte colony stimulating factor: effects on normal and leukemic myeloid cells. Science 1986;232:61.

21. Moore MAS, Warren PJ. Synergy of interleukin-1 and granulocyte colony stimulating factor in vivo stimulation of stem cell recovery and hematopoietic regeneration following 5-FU treatment in mice. Proc Natl Acad Sci USA 1987;84:7131.

22. Leary AG, Ikebachi K, Hirai N, et al. Synergism between interleukin 6 and interleukin 3 in supporting proliferation of human hematopoietic cells: comparison with interleukin-1. Blood 1988;71:1754.

23. Boone TC, Gabrilove J, Souza LM, et al. Recombinant human granulocyte colony-stimulating factor: effects on normal and leukemic myeloid cells. Science 1986;232:61.

24. Metcalf D, Nicola NA. Proliferative effects of purified granulocyte colony-stimulating factor (G-CSF) on normal mouse hemopoietic cells. J Cell Physiol 1985;124:313.

25. Asano S, Nagara S, Tguchiya M, et al. Molecular cloning and expression of cDNA for human granulocyte colony-stimulating factor. Nature 1986;319:415.

26. Liu L, Platzer E, Welte K, et al. Purification and biochemical characterization of human pluripotent hematopoietic colony-stimulating factor. Proc Natl Acad Sci USA 1985;82:1526.

27. Boone TC, Lu HS, Lui PH, Souza LM. Disulfide and secondary structures of recombinant human granulocyte colony stimulating factors. Arch Biochem Biophys 1989;268:81.

28. Johnson GR, Matsumoto M, Metcalf D, Nicola NA. Purification of a factor inducing differentiation in murine myelomonocytic leukemia cells: identification as granulocyte colony stimulating factor. J Biol Chem 1983;258:9017.

29. Burgess AW, Metcalf D. The nature and action of granulocyte-macrophage colony stimulating factors. Blood 1980;56:947.

30. Gough L, Gough NM, Metcalf D. Molecular cloning of cDNA encoding a murine haematopoietic growth regulator, granulocyte-macrophage colony stimulating factor. Nature 1984;309:763.

31. Burgess AW, Metcalf D, Nicola NA. Similar molecular properties of granulocyte-macrophage-colony-stimulating factors produced by different mouse organs in vitro. J Biol Chem 1979;254:5290.

32. Temple PA, Witek JG, Wong GG. Human GM-CSF: Molecular cloning of the complementary DNA and purification of the natural and recombinant proteins. Science 1985;228:810.

33. Kawasak ES, Ladner MB, Wang AM, et al. Molecular cloning of a complementary DNA encoding human macrophage-specific colony-stimulating factor (CSF-1). Science 1985;230:291.

34. Anderson D, Cogman D, Wignall J, et al. Human macrophage colony stimulating factor (M-CSF): alternate RNA splicing generates three different proteins that are expressed on the cell surface and secreted. Behring Inst Mitt 1988;83:15.

35. Schuster SJ, Badiavas EV, Costa-Giomi P, Weinmann R, Erslev AJ, Caro J. Stimulation of erythropoietin gene tran-

scription during hypoxia and cobalt exposure. Blood 1989; 73:13.

36. Bonilla MA, Gillio AP, Driggerio M, et al. Effects of recombinant human granulocyte colony stimulating factor on the neutropenia in patients with congenital agranulocytosis. N Engl J Med 1989;320:1574.

37. Elsner J, Roester J, Emmendorfer A, et al. Abnormal regulation in the signal transduction in neutrophils from patients with severe congenital neutropenia: relation of impaired mobilization of cytosolic free calcium to altered chemotaxis, superoxide anion generation and F-actin content. Exp Hematol 1993;21:38.

38. Hammona WP, Price TH, Souza LM, et al. Treatment of cyclic neutropenia with granulocyte colony stimulating factor. N Engl J Med 1984;320:1306.

39. Gabrilove JL, Jakuboski A, Scher H, et al. Effect of granulocyte colony stimulating factor on neutropenia and associated morbidity of chemotherapy for transitional cell carcinoma of the urothelium. N Engl J Med 1988; 318:1414.

40. Mueller BU, Jacobsen F, Butler KM, et al. Combination treatment with azidothymidine and granulocyte colony stimulating factor in children with human immunodeficiency virus infection. J Pediatr 1992;121:797.

41. Estey EH. Use of colony stimulating factors in the treatment of acute myeloid leukemia. Blood 1994;83:2086.

42. Gabrilove JL, Jakubowski A. Hematopoietic growth factors: biology and clinical applications. Monogr Natl Cancer Inst 1990;10:73.

43. Hahn T, Levin S. The interleukin system in patients with malignant disease. J Interferon Res 1992;p 23.

44. Hansen RM, Borden EC. Current states of inteferons in the treatment of cancer. Oncology 1992;6:19.

45. Hoffman MA. Walder S. Mechanisms by which interferon potentiates chemotherapy. Cancer Invest 1993;11:310.

46. Rodriguiz RM, Key LL, Ries WL. Combination macrophage colony stimulating factor and interferon gamma administration ameliorates the osteopetrotic condition in microphthalmic (mi/mi) mice. Pediatr Res 1993;33:384.

47. Key LL, Ries WL, Glasscock H, et al. Osteoclastic superoxide generation: taking control of bone resorption using modulators of superoxide concentrations. Int J Tissue React 1992;14:295.

48. Shapiro F. Osteopetrosis: current clinical considerations. Clin Orthop 1993;294:52.

49. Key LL, Ries WL, Rodriguiz RM, et al. Recombinant human interferon gamma therapy for osteopetrosis. J Pediatr 1992;121:119.

50. Maybee DR, Dubowy R, Krischer J, et al. Unusual toxicity of high dose alpha interferon (aIFN) in the treatment of juvenile chronic myelocytic leukemia (JCML). ASCO Proceedings, 28th Annual Meeting, 1992;11:950a.

51. Warrel RP, Wang ZY, Degos L. Acute promyelocytic leukemia. N Engl J Med 1993;329:177.

52. Breitman TR, Collins SJ, Keene BR. Terminal differentiation of human promyelocytic leukemic cells in primary culture in response to retinoic acid. Blood 1980;57:1000.

53. Huang ME, Ye UC, Chen SR, et al. Use of all trans retinoic acid in the treatment of acute promyelocytic leuekemia. Blood 1988;72:567.

54. Castagne S, Chomienne C, Daniel MT, et al. All trans retinoic acid as a differentiating therapy for acute promyelocytic leukemia. Blood 1990;76:1704.

55. Dombret H, Scrobohaci ML, Ghorra P, et al. Coagulation disorders associated with acute promyelocytic leukemia. Leukemia 1993;7;2.

56. Avvisati G, Beccarani M, Ferrara F, et al. AIDA protocol in the treatment of newly diagnosed acute promyelocytic leukemia: a pilot study of the Italian cooperative group. Blood 1994;84(Suppl 1):1506.

57. Fenaux P, Chastang C, Chommienne C, et al. Treatment of newly diagnosed acute promyelocytic leukemia (APL) by all trans retinoic acid (ATRA) 37,38 combined with chemotherapy: the European experience. Leuk Lymphoma 1995; 16:431.

58. Tezcan H, Barnett MJ, Bredeson CN, et al. Treatment of acute promyelocytic leukemia in patients presenting at Vancouver General Hospital from 1983 to 1992. Leuk Lymphoma 1995;16:439.

59. Gillard EF, Solomon E. Acute promyelocytic leukemia and the t(15;17) translocation. Semin Cancer Biol 1993;4:359.

60. Borrow J, Goddard AD, Sheer D, et al. Molecular analysis of acute promyelocytic breakpoint cluster on chromosome 17. Science 1990;249:1577.

61. Koyama T, Hoirosawa S, Kawamata N. All trans retinoic acid upregulates thrombomodulin and downregulates tissue factor expression in acute promyelocytic leukemia cells: distinct expression of thrombomodulin and tissue factor in human leukemic cells. Blood 1994;84:3001.

62. Paquette RL, Koeffler HP. Differentiation therapy in myelodysplastic syndromes. Hemat Oncol Clin N Am 1992; 6:692.

63. Castleberry RP, Emanuel PD, Zuckerman KS, et al. A pilot study of isotretinoin in the treatment of juvenile chronic myelogenous leukemia. N Engl J Med 1994;331:1680.

64. Estrov Z, Kurzock R, Estey E, et al. Inhibition of acute myelogenous leukemia blast proliferation by IL-1 receptor antagonist and soluble IL-1 receptors. Blood 1992; 79:1938.

65. Estrov Z, Kurzock R, Wetzler ME, et al. Suppression of chronic myelogenous leukemia colony growth by IL-1 receptor antagonist and soluble IL-1 receptors: a novel application for inhibitors of IL-1 activity. Blood 1991;78:476.

66. Cahill R, Verma U, Areman C. IL-2 activated bone marrow transplantation in patients with advanced hematological malignancies. Induction of autologous GvHD. Blood 1994; 84(Suppl 1):726.

67. Yin HJ, Zhang LP. Experimental study of IL-2 and LAK cells in treatment of mouse L7911 minimal residue leukemia. Blood 1994;84(Suppl 1):588.

68. Noguchi M, Yi H, Rosenblatt HM, et al. Interleukin 2 receptor gamma chain mutation results in X-linked severe combined deficiency in humans. Cell 1993;73:147.

69. Otsuka T, Miyajima A, Brown N, et al. Isolation and characterization of an expressible cDNA encoding human IL-3 Induction of IL-3 mRna in human T-Cell clones J Immunol 1988;140:2288.

70. Nicola NA, Metcalf D. Subunit promiscuity among hemopoietic growth factor receptors. Cell 1991;67:1.

71. Sonoda Y, Yang YC, Wong GG, et al. Analysis in serum free culture of the targets of recombinant human hemopoietic growth factors; Interleukin 3 and granulocyte/macrophage colony stimulating factor are specific for early developmental stages. Proc Natl Acad Sci USA 1988;85:4360.

72. Kirshenbaum AS, Goff JP, Kessler SW, et al. Effect of IL-3 and stem cell factor on the appearance of human basophils

and mast cells from CD-34+ pluripotent progenitor cells. J Immunol 1992;148:772.

73. Donahue RE, Seehra J, Metzger M, et al. Human IL-3 and CGM- CSF act synergistically in stimulating hematopoiesis in primates. Science 1988;241:1820.

74. Ganser A, Hoelzer D. Treatment of MDS with hemopoietic growth factors. Hemat Oncol Clin N Am 1992;6:639.

75. Peschel C, Paul WE, Ohara J, et al. Effects of B-cell stimulatory factor 1/interleukin 4 on hematopoietic progenitor cells. Blood 1987;70:254.

76. Yokota T, Otsuka T, Mosmann T, et al. Isolation and characterization of a human interleukin cDNA clone, homologous to mouse B-cell stimulatory factor 1 that expresses B-cell and T-cell stimulating activities. Proc Natl Acad Sci USA 1986;83:5894.

77. Lowenthal JW, Castle BE, Christiansen J, et al. Expression of high affinity receptors for murine interleukin 4 on hemopoietic progenitor cells. J Immunol 1988; 140:456.

78. Estrov Z, Markowitz AB, Kurzrock R, et al. Suppression of chronic myelogenous leukemia colony growth by interleukin 4. Leukemia 1993;7:214.

79. Sideras P, Noma T, Honjo T. Structure and function of interleukin 4 and 5. Immunol Rev 1988;102:189.

80. Wong GG, Clark SC. Multiple actions of interleukin 6 within a cytokine network. Immunol Today 1988;9:137.

81. Van Snick J, Cayphas S, Szikora JP, et al. cDNA cloning of murine interleukin HP1: homology with human interleukin 6. Eur J Immunol 1988;18:193.

82. Wong GG, Witek-Giabnotti JS, Temple PA, et al. Stimulation of murine hemopietic colony formation by human IL-6. J Immunol 1988;140:3040.

83. Roodman GD. Interleukin 6. A potential autocrine/paracrine factor in Paget's Disease of bone. J Clin Invest 1992;89:46.

84. Hirano T. Interleukin 6 and its relation to inflammation and disease. Clin Immunopathol 1992;62:60.

85. Champlin RE, Mehra P, Kaye JA, et al. Recombinant human IL-11 following autologous BMT for breast cancer. Blood 1994:84(Suppl 1):395.

86. Curtis BM, Williams DE, Broxmeyer HE, Dunn J, Farrah T, Jeffery E, Clevenger W, DeRoos P, Martin U, Friend D, et al. Enhanced hematopoietic activity of a human granulocyte/macrophage colony-stimulating factor-interleukin 3 fusion protein. Proc Natl Acad Sci USA 1991;88:5809.

87. Williams DE, Park LS. Hematopoietic effects of a granulocyte-macrophage colony-stimulating factor/interleukin-3

fusion protein. Cancer 1991;67(Suppl):2705.

88. Witte ON. Steel locus defines new multipotent growth factor. Cell 1990;63:5.

89. Flanagan JG, Leder P. The kit ligand: a cell surface molecule altered in steel mutant fibroblasts. Cell 1990; 63:185.

90. Zsebo KM, Williams DA, Geissler EN, Broudy VC, et al. Stem cell factor is encoded at the SI locus of the mouse and is the ligand for the c-kit tyrosine kinase receptor. Cell 1990;63:213.

91. Anderson DM, Lyman SD, Baird A, et al. Molecular cloning of mast cell growth factor, a hematopoietin that is active in both membrane bound and soluble forms. Cell 1990; 63:235.

92. Martin FH, Suggs SV, Langley KE, et al. Primary structure and functional expression of rat and human stem cell factor DNAs. Cell 1990;63:203.

93. Brannan CI, Lyman SD, Williams DE, et al. Steele-Dickie mutation encodes a c-kit ligand lacking transmembrane and cytoplasmic domains. Proc Natl Acad Sci USA 1991; 88:4671.

94. Yarden Y, Kuang WJ, Rang-Feng T, et al. Human proto-oncogene c-kit: a new cell surface receptor tyrosine kinase for an unidentified ligand. EMBO J 1987;6:3341.

95. Yarden Y, Escobedo JA, Kuang WJ, et al. Structure of the receptor for platelet-derived growth factor helps define a family of closely related growth factor receptors. Nature 1986;323:226.

96. Lyman SD, James LJ, et al. Molecular cloning of a ligand for the FLt-3/FLk-2 tyrosine kinase receptor: a proliferative factor for primitive hematopoietic cells. Cell 1993; 75:1157.

97. Hannum E, Culpepper J, et al. Ligand for FLT-3/FLK-2 receptor tyrosine kinase regulates growth of hematopoietic stem cells and is encoded by variant RNAs. Nature 1994; 368:643.

98. Mathews W, Jordan CT, et al. A receptor tyrosine kinase specific to hematopoietic stem and progenitor cell-enriched populations. Cell 1991;65:1143.

99. Small D, Levenstein M, et al. STK-1, the human homolog of FLK-2/FLT-3, is selectively expressed in CD34+ human blood marrow cells and is involved in the proliferation of early progenitor/stem cells. Proc Natl Acad Sci USA 1994; 91:459.

100. Barthy TD, Bogenbarger J, et al. Identification and cloning of a megakaryocyte growth and development factor that is a ligand for the cytokine receptor c-Mpl. Cell 1994;77:1117.

EXERCISES AND TOOLS FOR BIOLOGICAL CONTROL MECHANISMS

To communicate is to participate.

1. Using the information below, develop schematic exercises in the study of control mechanisms involving the broad field of human hematopoiesis.

PLATELETS: following injury adhere to, aggregate at, and release cytokines at endothelial sites which activate complement. Released cytokines include PDGF, TGF-β, EGF, RANTES, IL-1, HGF, GRO-α, and PD-ECGF.

BASOPHILS AND MAST CELLS: the allergy cells, which activate by degranulation following release of anaphylatoxins and/or when surface IgE binds to antigens; also active against parasites. Release mast cell cytokines include GM-CSF, IL-1, 3, 4, 5, 6, 8; TNF-α; MIP-1α, MIP-1β; and from basophils, IL-4.

EOSINOPHILS: mast cell mediators with only marginal phagocytic qualities. Released cytokines include IL-1α, IL-3, 6; GM-CSF, TGF-α, TGF-β.

NEUTROPHILS: dedicated antibacterial phagocytes that migrate from the marrow following injury-initiated stimuli. Cytokines released include IL-1α, IL-1β, IL-3, 6, 8; G-, GM-, M-CSF; PAF, TNF-α, GRO-α.

MACROPHAGES: multimodal phagocytes that also present antigen. Released cytokines include IL-1, 3, 6, 8; G-, GM-, M-CSF; PDGF, HB-EGF, VGF, NGF, LIF, OSM, FGF basic, TGF-α, TGF-β; TNF-α, GRO-α, MIP-1α, and MIP-1β.

T-HELPER LYMPHOCYTES: interact with B Lymphocytes and Cytotoxic T Cells. Released cytokines from Th0, Th1, and Th2 subsets include IL-1, 2, 3, 4, 5, 6, 9, 10, 13, 14; G-, M-, GM-CSF; ILF, OSM, HMW-BCGF, RANTES, MIP-1α, MIP-1β; TNF-α, TNF-β.

CYTOTOXIC T LYMPHOCYTES: kill virus infected cells. Released cytokines include IL-2, IFN-γ; TNF-α, TNF-β.

NATURAL KILLER (NK) LYMPHOCYTES AND LEUKOCYTE ACTIVATED KILLER (LAK) LYMPHOCYTES destroy Ig coated cells; LAK cells are activated NK cells. Cytokines released include M-, GM-CSF; IL-3, IFN-γ; TNF-α, TNF-β.

B LYMPHOCYTES, once antigenically stimulated, become powerful synthesizers of Ig. Relased cytokines include IL-1, 4, 5, 6; GM-CSF, TNF-α, TNF-β; IFN-γ.

2. Review Table 1.1 and the text to develop a schema that incorporates cytokines and growth factors in hematopoietic control. Refer to fig I.1 in the Introduction to relate to events in the cell cycle.

Red Cell Disorders

CHAPTER 2

Protein Synthesis— Megaloblastic Disorders

A. MAJID SHOJANIA

Beginning in 1823 and continuing through 1872 certain morphological and clinical features of pernicious anemia were identified, but not before the passage of another 100 years (1926) did Minot and Murphy establish a linkage between nutrition, the role of the liver, and megaloblastic hematopoiesis. In 1860 the relationship between gastric secretions and pernicious anemia was first described, but there occurred a 60-year lapse before Castle, a pupil of Minot, detailed these observations.
—Editors (1996)

Patients with megaloblastic anemias often are initially seen with macrocytic anemia, but not all macrocytic anemias are megaloblastic and not all megaloblastic anemias are macrocytic. There are numerous causes for macrocytic and for megaloblastic anemias. However, familiarity with the pathophysiology of folate and cobalamin (Cbl) deficiencies, careful attention to the history and physical examination, along with a few simple laboratory tests, are usually sufficient for proper diagnosis of the cause of macrocytic or megaloblastic anemia. Only in very exceptional cases are more sophisticated techniques needed for elucidating the cause of megaloblastic anemia.

A practical and proper approach to a case of macrocytic anemia is to first determine whether or not the macrocytosis is associated with megaloblastic changes. If there are megaloblastic changes, then the anemia should be considered to be due to folate or cobalamin deficiency unless proven otherwise. If the bone marrow does not show megaloblastic changes and does not by itself provide the cause of macrocytosis, familiarity with the causes of non-megaloblastic macrocytosis should lead to the proper diagnosis. This chapter is not intended to cover every aspect of megaloblastic anemias. Rather, it will define the pathogenesis and clinical and laboratory features, concentrate on the pathophysiology of cobalamin and folate deficiencies, and describe the proper approaches to the diagnosis and management of these disorders.

Megaloblastic Anemias

Case 1

S., a 17-year-old white girl, was referred by her physician because of possible hemolytic anemia. She had been in perfect health until 6 months earlier when she began feeling tired, had a loss of energy and ambition, and progressively worsened. In the previous 4 weeks she had noted exertional shortness of breath and finally went to see her own physician who, noting her pallor and scleral icterus, examined her. Positive findings were a hemoglobin (Hb) of 78 g/L, white blood cell (WBC) count 2.3 × 10^9/L, and serum bilirubin 50 µM/L. In a previous checkup 14 months earlier, the patient's hemoglobin was 120 g/L and her WBC count was 7.2 × 10^9/L. Her diet was balanced and included an adequate supply of meat and fresh vegetables and fruits. She had lost her appetite over the past 3 months but she had forced herself to eat and maintain her regular diet. Still, she had lost 2.5 kg in the preceding 6 months. Her menstrual periods had previously been heavy, lasting about 5–6 days, but over the past 6 months had become irregular, with lighter blood flow. Her last period was 6 weeks earlier. She had experienced no paresthesia or urinary symptoms. She was born in Canada and had not visited any other country. Her mother had been getting vitamin B_{12} injections for many years.

On physical examination, she appeared pale and her sclera was slightly yellow, her tongue was smooth, and the remainder of the physical findings were not remarkable. The initial laboratory findings revealed hemoglobin of 74 g/L, WBC count 2.1 × 10^9/L, platelet count (Plt) 70 × 10^9/L, mean corpuscular volume (MCV) 96 fL, mean corpuscular hemoglobin concentration (MCHC) 32%, reticulocyte count (retic) 20 × 10^9/L, red blood cell distribution width (RDW) 22% (normal 11.5–14.5%). Examination of blood smear showed marked anisocytosis and moderate poikilocytosis, and there were many macrocytes and some microcytes and hypochromic red cells. There was increased number of hypersegmented neutrophils and platelets appeared decreased in number and some were large. Other abnormal initial laboratory findings included the following: total serum bilirubin of 54 µM/L (normal <20), uric acid 420 mM/L (normal

<360), serum lactate dehydrogenase (LDH) 1998 U/L (normal <200), serum haptoglobin 0.05 g/L (normal 0.3–1.4). Additional blood samples had been taken for serum ferritin, serum and red cell folate, and serum cobalamin, but the results were not available on the day of visit. Considering the history, the initial complete blood count (CBC), and blood smear, the diagnosis of combined megaloblastic anemia and iron deficiency was suspected, and a bone marrow examination showed the presence of advanced megaloblastic changes. The stainable iron in the bone marrow appeared adequate but less than would be expected in severe megaloblastic anemia, thus confirming the initial impression of combined megaloblastic anemia and iron deficiency.

Commentary: *This patient was diagnosed to have megaloblastic anemia. In order to understand her condition and explain her symptoms and management, we will first define the megaloblastic anemias, describe the clinicopathologic aspects of these disorders, and then return to the patient described in case 1 to see whether we can explain all of her symptoms and signs by this diagnosis before discussing her management.*

Megaloblastic Anemias are a group of disorders with distinct morphologic features, resulting from unbalanced nucleic acid synthesis when DNA synthesis and replication are impaired or slowed but RNA synthesis is completely or relatively intact. This imbalance between the synthesis of RNA and DNA results in asynchrony between maturation of cytoplasm and that of nucleus (nuclear-cytoplasmic dissociation) creates morphologic changes in hemopoietic cells (and in any other cell that has to grow and divide) that is called "megaloblastic changes."

DNA Synthesis and Biochemical Basis of Megaloblastic Changes

Human DNA consists of very long polymers of nucleotide subunits, each of which is made of a 5-carbon sugar moiety called "deoxyribose" attached to a phosphate group at 5′ carbon position and to a purine or pyrimidine base at 1′ position. A phosphodiester bond between 5′ position of one sugar and the 3′ position of adjacent sugar provide the linkages of the nucleotides. There are only four bases in DNA. Two are purines: adenosine (A) and guanosine (G), and two are pyrimidines: thymine (T) and cytosine (C). DNA is thermodynamically most stable when two strands are coiled around each other to form a double-stranded helix. The two strands are held together with hydrogen bonds between the bases of one DNA strand, with complementary bases in the other strand. Each purine or pyrimidine base is complementary base for the other nonidentical purine or pyrimidine base of DNA. The chemical composition of RNA is very much similar to that of DNA, except that the sugar is a ribose instead of deoxyribose and instead of thymine (methyl-uracil) RNA contains uracil (U). Nuclear DNA is involved in two vital processes: gene expression and replication. The first step in DNA replica-

tion is the uncoiling of double helix. Subsequently, each DNA strand acts as a template for formation of a complementary DNA strand, with the help of an enzyme, α-DNA polymerase, which uses as the substrate four deoxyribonucleoside triphosphates: dATP, dGTP, dTTP, and dCTP. Each base bonds with its complementary base pair on the DNA template, the sugar and one phosphate moiety link up to adjacent phosphate and sugar moieties to make up the backbone of the new DNA, and two of the three phosphates of triphosphate moiety are lost from each nucleotide. The deficiency of any substrate, enzymes, or cofactors needed for synthesis of purines or pyrimidines of DNA, their incorporation in DNA, or reduction of ribonucleotides may cause megaloblastic anemia.

Normally most of the cells in the body are in a resting state, and at any point in time only a very small proportion of cells are replicating and dividing. Those that are in the process of division rapidly double their DNA in order to divide to make two daughter cells with DNA content roughly similar to their own and then enter a resting phase. In megaloblastic anemias, as the result of slowed DNA synthesis, this process is slowed and, depending on the degree of DNA impairment, many of the cells spend a longer time in the process of DNA synthesis in order to divide, may not reach the point of doubling their DNA, and "die" without reproducing. Those that survive, since they are in the process of increasing their DNA, have larger nuclei, with associated changes in chromatin pattern and increased chromosome breakdown. Furthermore, their cytoplasm also tends to increase as the result of relatively unimpaired RNA and protein synthesis. Consequently, the megaloblastic cells are generally larger both as the result of increased RNA, protein (cytoplasm), and increased DNA content (1). Megaloblastic changes have been noted in any proliferating cells that have been examined, including the mucosa of the tongue, stomach, intestine, cervix, and vagina. However, the megaloblastic changes are more striking in hemopoietic cells of bone marrow and peripheral blood, partly because the bone marrow cells are rapidly replicating so that any impairment of DNA synthesis is more likely to manifest itself earlier in these cells, and partly because they are best studied due to ease of accessibility. An experienced hematologist or technologist can quickly recognize the characteristic morphologic changes in the peripheral blood or bone marrow aspirate, whereas in other cells more advanced changes are necessary before tissue preparation abnormalities are recognized by the pathologist.

Morphologic Changes in Peripheral Blood Cells

In advanced megaloblastic anemia, severe anemia is present and often leukopenia with neutropenia and thrombocytopenia. As the result of the continued RNA and protein synthesis (in the context of slowed DNA synthesis), the MCV and mean corpuscular hemoglobin (MCH) of the red cell are increased, but the MCHC remains normal. The RDW is also often increased, reflecting the increased variation in cell size due to impaired hemopoiesis (RDW is now calculated by all automated instruments performing CBC). It roughly represent the coefficient of variability of the individual red cell volume). The reticulocyte count is low due to ineffective erythropoiesis. Examination of the blood smear shows macrocytes, especially macroovalocytes, and increased number of hypersegmented neutrophils (this is defined as the presence of any neutrophil containing more than five lobes or when >5% of the neutrophils contain five lobes). Some authors have used the *average lobe index* of neutrophils (the average number of lobes of 100 consecutive neutrophils) to quantitate the segmentation of neutrophils and show its increase. However, this is time-consuming and involves much observer variation. The reported average lobe index has varied from 2.5 to 3.3, depending on the observer's definition of the lobe. The reason for the increased number of hypersegmented neutrophils is not clear. Arneth's belief that the number of neutrophil's lobes represents the age of the neutrophils, so that the hypersegmented neutrophils represent the older neutrophils, does not seem to be correct, because Fliedner et al. (2), using tritiated thymidine-labeling technique, showed that radiolabel appeared in five-lobed neutrophils of pernicious anemia at the same time that it appeared in the neutrophils with lesser lobes. Similarly, the view that the increased DNA of giant metamyelocyte is eventually packed into an increased number of mature lobes (1) is not supported by the report of normal DNA content of hypersegmented neutrophils (3), and by the fact that hypersegmented neutrophils appear in peripheral blood much earlier than giant metamyelocytes appear in the bone marrow (4) and persist in the blood for several days after the disappearance of giant metamyelocytes from the bone marrow.

The changes in platelet morphology are much more subtle and difficult to recognize under the microscope, but increased variation in platelet size (platelet distribution width [PDW]) can be detected electronically. In less severe cases, pancytopenia is not present and the patient may have only isolated cytopenia.

There is conflict of opinion about the earliest manifestation of megaloblastic anemia in peripheral blood. Herbert's widely quoted study of experimentally produced dietary folate deficiency in a man (4) showed that the earliest morphologic changes in peripheral blood were the appearance of increased hypersegmented neutrophils. Chanarin states that macrocytosis, as determined by automated electronic cell counter, is the earliest changes in the peripheral blood, and that megaloblastosis with normal MCV in the absence of conditions that may reduce the MCV (e.g., iron deficiency, thalassaemia, anemia of chronic disease) occurs only in about 1 in 200 cases of megaloblastic anemia (5). On the other hand, Carmel reported that 33% of patients with pernicious anemia had normal or low MCV (<100 fL) (6) and others have also reported a high percentage of subjects with megaloblastic changes who have normal MCV. The reasons for these discrepancies are in part due to the difference in definition of macrocytosis (different authors have considered an upper limit of normal for MCV to be 94, 95, 99, 100, 102, 103 fL) and the population studied. As more physicians routinely order serum folate and serum cobalamin determinations for patients with neuropsychiatric disorders, more cases of early megaloblastic changes with normal MCV are found. It should be stated that increased hypersegmented neutrophils are often missed on routine examination of a blood smear, unless it is specifically sought. Those who have reported its early appearance and sensitivity are those who have especially looked for it as part of their study. The use of electronic cell counters for determination of MCV by most of the laboratories has eliminated the component of observer variation and expertise, however. Thus the rise of MCV is more likely to be reported by the clinical laboratory than the increase in the number of hypersegmented neutrophils.

Megaloblastic Changes in Bone Marrow

Generally, the bone marrow in megaloblastic anemia is very cellular and the cells show the characteristic nuclear-cytoplasmic dissociation. As the cells mature and divide, this nuclear-cytoplasmic dissociation becomes more exaggerated and more easily recognizable in bone marrow smear stained with a Romanowsky stain. As the *erythroid precursors* mature and divide through the stages of pro-, basophilic, polychromatophilic, and orthochromatic erythroblasts, their cytoplasm increases and changes from deep blue in the pro- and basophilic stages to the reddish orange of completely hemoglobinized orthochromatic cell. The nucleus, on the other hand, becomes smaller, its chromatin pattern becomes coarser and clumped, and by the orthochromatic stage it is a small homogenously stained mass with no recognizable chromatin pattern. In megaloblastic anemias the promegaloblasts and basophilic megaloblasts may be increased in number. They are also a little larger, with increased amounts of cytoplasm, and their fine and uneven chromatin pattern gives a speckled pattern to the nucleus resembling "sliced salami." In the polychromatic stage, the megaloblasts are larger than their normal counterparts, and their nucleus is more open and less mature. In the orthochromatic stage when the cytoplasm is completely hemoglobinized, instead of a small, dark pyknotic nucleus, a large nucleus with a discernible chromatin pattern is seen that may be segmented or lobulated, and Howell-Jolly bodies representing nuclear fragments may be seen in the cytoplasm.

Myeloid precursors show a parallel lag in nuclear maturation, similar to that seen in erythroid precursors. The blasts may be increased in number but most easily recognizable changes are seen in metamyelocytes, bands, and segmented neutrophils. The metamyelocytes and bands are very large (giant forms) and their nuclei, instead of being kidney shaped, are very large, folded over themselves, and may give a pretzel appearance; their chromatin pattern is finer and more open than normal and may resemble those of myelocytes or promyelocytes. Occasionally the hyperactivity of very immature myeloid cells give the appearance of acute leukemia and errors in diagnosis have occurred. However, in general, the erythroid hyperactivity is more prominent and myeloid/erythroid (M/E) ratio is reduced.

Megakaryocytes are also abnormal in megaloblastic anemia, appear larger, and their nuclei tend to be hypersegmented and have finer chromatin pattern, but these changes are not as easily recognizable as those of erythroid and myeloid cells. Megakaryocyte cytoplasmic fragments may appear in bone marrow and peripheral blood in the form of giant platelets.

Lymphoid elements generally do not demonstrate recognizable morphologic changes due to the slow rate of replication, even though they do demonstrate the same biochemical defects seen in other marrow elements (7) (lymphocytes cultured in folate-free media and stimulated with phytohemagglutinin do exhibit megaloblastic changes).

The *stainable iron* is increased both in erythroid precursor and in macrophages and at times ring sideroblasts may be seen.

The patient described in case 1 demonstrates all morphologic changes of megaloblastic anemia (pancytopenia, increased number of hypersegmented neutrophils, low reticulocyte count, and megaloblastic bone marrow morphology). However, because of an associated iron deficiency, the MCV was not as high as one would expect and the bone marrow stainable iron was not increased. Other abnormal laboratory tests of this patient could all be explained by megaloblastic pattern of hemopoiesis. The indirect hyperbilirubinemia is due to ineffective erythropoiesis and shortened red cell survival. The shortened red cell survival (28–75 days) is due to a combination of intra- and extracorpuscular factors. In advanced megaloblastic anemia the combination of shortened red cell survival and ineffective erythropoiesis (low reticulocyte count) may cause a precipitous drop in hemoglobin, which may wrongly be attributed to acute hemolysis or blood loss. Other evidences of shortened red cell survival such as increased urine and stool urobilinogen, increased carbon monoxide production, and low serum haptoglobin are also seen in severe megaloblastic anemia. The high LDH is due to ineffective hemopoiesis and shortened red cell survival, while the increased uric acid is due to ineffective hemopoiesis and increased nuclear breakdown. None of these tests is needed to make the diagnosis of megaloblastic anemia, but familiarity with the tests that may be abnormal in megaloblastic anemia may prevent erroneous diagnosis or unnecessary investigations. Other abnormal tests in megaloblastic anemias

are low serum skeletal alkaline phosphatase (due to cobalamin dependency of osteoblast activity), and low blood cholinesterase. Hemoglobin A_2 and F may be increased in megaloblastic anemia, causing confusion with β-thalassaemia. Serum iron and percentage of iron saturation, as well as serum ferritin, are also high, and may mask the diagnosis of associated iron deficiency anemia. Coombs test result may be positive. Serum muramidase may be elevated due to ineffective leukopoiesis and rapid granulocyte turnover. Aminoaciduria may be present. In severe megaloblastic anemia the megaloblastic changes in intestinal mucosa may cause malabsorption of fat (steatorrhea), xylose, carotene, and cobalamin (8). The malabsorption of cobalamin in severe folate deficiency megaloblastic anemia may cause erroneous diagnosis of cobalamin deficiency megaloblastic anemia. In severe megaloblastic anemia, both platelet functions (9) and neutrophil functions (10), as well as cell-mediated immunity (11) may be impaired. Chromosomal abnormalities such as increased chromosomal breakage, elongation of chromosomes, despiralization, and centromere spreading are common in megaloblastic anemias (12).

Clinical Features of Megaloblastic Anemias

The symptoms and physical findings of the patient described in case 1, although not specific for megaloblastic anemia, are all consistent with and can be explained by megaloblastic anemia. Some of the signs and symptoms of megaloblastic anemia are related to anemia and its severity (e.g., tiredness, palpitation, exertional shortness of breath, peripheral edema, and signs of congestive heart failure). However, deficiencies of folate or cobalamin, which are the two major causes of megaloblastic anemia, may produce some symptoms specifically due to systemic effects of the deficiencies themselves, and these symptoms may be present without any significant anemia. These include slowly progressive lethargy, loss of appetite, loss of taste for food, weight loss, sore tongue, tingling or sensations of "pins and needles" in the hands and feet, numbness of the fingers and toes, mood changes and neuropsychiatric symptoms, including depression, "megaloblastic madness," and signs of subacute combined degeneration of the spinal cord. Skin pigmentation, loss of hair pigment (premature greying of hair), and alopecia may be the manifestation of such deficiencies. Infertility in both sexes and impotence in males may be seen in both folate and cobalamin deficiency (13, 14).

Causes of Megaloblastic Anemias

The numerous causes of megaloblastic anemias are listed in table 2.1. However, if those caused by cancer chemotherapeutic or immunosuppressive agents are excluded, the majority of those remaining are due either to folate or to cobalamin deficiency. Inborn errors of metabolism

Table 2.1 Causes of Megaloblastic Anemias

Folate deficiency or impaired folate metabolism (see table 2.5)

Cobalamin deficiency or impaired cobalamin metabolism (see table 2.4)

Cancer chemotherapy or use of an antimetabolite

   Purine analogs: 6-mercaptopurine, 6-thioguanine, azathioprine, acyclovir

   Pyrimidine analogs: 5-fluouracil, 5-fluorodeoxyuridne, 6-azauridine, zidovurine

   Inhibitors of ribonucleotide reduction: hydroxyurea, cytosine arabinoside

   Other chemotherapeutic agent: cyclophosphamide

Errors of metabolism other than those related to folate or cobalamin

   Orotic aciduria

   Thiamin-responsive megaloblastic anemia, DIDMOAD syndrome

   Lesh-Nyhan syndrome

   Purine nucleoside phosphorylase deficiency

   Pathogenesis unknown

Other acquired megaloblastic anemia of unexplained mechanism

   Cooper deficiency

   Arsenic intoxication

   Ascorbic acid deficiency (scurvy)

   Sarcoidosis

   Chronic analgesic ingestion (aspirin + salicylamide + caffeine)

   Refractory megaloblastic anemia, myelodysplasia

   Erythroleukemia

causing megaloblastic anemia are extremely rare. Although definitive diagnosis of folate or cobalamin deficiency requires the use of laboratory tests, taking a proper history, with particular attention to diet, bowel habits, drug intake, associated diseases, and previous gastrointestinal surgery often allows establishment of the cause of megaloblastic anemia and differentiation between folate and cobalamin deficiency. Before continuing the discussion of case 1, a discussion of these pathophysiogic characteristics of folate and cobalamin follows.

Folate Metabolism

The terms "folic acid," "folacin," "folates," and "folate compounds," which are often interchangeably used, refer to a group of compounds (vitamins) with closely similar basic structures and biologic properties. In correct terminology, "folic acid" is the name of the original synthetic form of folate that was produced commercially for the treatment and prevention of folate deficiency. Folic acid consists of a double-ringed pteridine (2-amino-4-hydroxy pteridine) moiety joined via a methylene group at the C6 position to a paraaminobenzoic acid to form pteroic acid, which in turn is joined to an L-glutamic acid to form pteroylglutamic acid or pteroylmonoglutamate (PteGlu). This compound is the oxidized stable form of folate. It is scarce in nature but has the basic structure of a parent compound

for all folates. In nature, folates occur mostly in conjugated or polyglutamate (PteGlu$_n$) form in which, instead of a single glutamic acid, multiple glutamic acids are linked by peptide bonds. Folic acid and other oxidized forms of folates are not biologically active and have to be reduced to the tetrahydrofolate (FH$_4$) form before they can participate in biologic reactions. This reduction is catalized by dihydrofolate reductase, which changes the oxidized folates first to dihydrofolate (FH$_2$) and then to FH$_4$ (15, 16). The reduced folates generally act as single carbon donors or acceptors in their biologic reactions. The significant single carbons involved are formyl ($-CH = 0$), methylene ($-CH2-$), methenyl ($-CH=$), methyl ($-CH3$), hydroxymethyl ($-CH_2OH$), and forminino ($-CH = NH$). With the exception of N^5-formyltetrahydrofolate (folinic acid, leucovorin), which is stable and is commercially available as a pharmacologic source of FH$_4$, the other reduced forms of folates are unstable and easily oxidize on exposure to air or to heat (cooking) unless they are protected by reducing agents such as ascorbic acid.

Folate Source

Folates are synthesized by higher plants and by most microorganisms. Some organisms that can not synthesize folates such as *Lactobacillus casei, Streptococcus faecalis,* or *Pediococus cerviciae* are used for microbiologic assay of folates in blood and other media. The folate-rich foods include green vegetables such as asparagus, broccoli, spinach, brussel sprouts, lettuce, green onion (top), and lima beans. Among animal products, liver and kidney are high in folates. Fruits, such as lemon, orange, peach, and banana have only moderate folate content, but, since folates are heat labile and much of folate in food is destroyed by cooking (50–96%), fresh fruits and green leafy vegetables that do not have to be cooked provide the major source of dietary folate (15). Human and unprocessed or pasteurized cow's milk have about 50–55 μg of folates (by *L. casei* assay), but goat's milk is quite low on folate (6 μg/L).

Folate Requirements

The minimal daily requirement for folate in adults is said to be about 50 μg (15). Earlier studies and reports had overestimated the daily requirement of folates. Accordingly, nutritional surveys overestimated the prevalence of dietary folate deficiency (based on dietary food folate content). Herbert has presented extensive evidence that a daily intake of 3 μg/kg of body weight of folate not only maintains the folate nutriture of adults but also provides a substantial body reserve (17). Another study (18) has shown that under normal conditions the body catabolizes only about 100 μg/day of folate, and that this rate remains relatively unchanged even in response to saturating doses of 5 mg/day of folic acid for several days, indicating that the absorption of 100 μg of folic acid meets the requirement of normal adults. The recommended dietary allowance (RDA) for folate, therefore, has been recently reduced by the Food and Nutrition Board to 200 μg and 180 μg for adult men and women (but, to 400 μg for pregnant and to 280 μg for lactating woman), 25–35 μg for infants, and 50–100 μg for children) (19).

Absorption of Folates

Folate compounds in plants and animal tissue are primarily in polyglutamate forms, whereas in human plasma they are in monoglutamate forms, mainly N^5-methyltetrahydrofolate(CH_3-FH_4). Folate polyglutamates in food have to be hydrolyzed (deconjugated) in the small bowel before absorption occurs (20). Most body tissues have the enzyme "conjugase" that is able to break down polyglutamates into monoglutamates. In the intestinal lumen, both pancreatic secretion and bile contain such conjugase. Two folate conjugases have been identified in human intestinal mucosa. One, an exopeptidase, active on the surface of jejunal brush borders, has a pH optimum of 6.5 and requires Zn^{2+} and Co^{2+}. The other, an endopeptidase, is intracellular and has pH optimum of 4.5. The luminal pH is critical for absorption. Increasing the luminal pH of the jejunum by the administration of sodium bicarbonate, antacid, or H_2 receptor antagonists reduces the absorption of folate.

The absorption of hydrolyzed polyglutamates (monoglutamates) occurs via an active carrier-mediated energy-dependent transport system in the intestinal mucosa and requires binding to brush border membrane-associated folate-binding protein, which has a high affinity for monoglutamates, and exhibit pH dependency (pH optimal of 5.0) and saturability (21).

In physiologic doses, 79–98% of monoglutamates and 25–90% of folate polyglutamates are absorbed. Folates are primarily absorbed in proximal jejunum. But unless resection or lesions of the proximal small bowel is very extensive, the remainder of the small intestine can absorb dietary folate adequately (22). Absorbed monoglutamates in physiologic doses are reduced in the enterocytes and converted mostly to CH_3-FH_4. Pharmacologic doses of folic acid can be absorbed unchanged by passive diffusion across the intestinal mucosa in a nonsaturable pH and energy-independent manner, and can produce clinical responses in the rare instances of specific congenital folate malabsorption. There is a curious absorption pattern of milk folate that is different from that of other food folates. Milk contains a high-affinity folate-binding protein (FBP) that helps to concentrate folates in milk and protects the milk folates from oxidation and proteolysis by pancreatic enzymes. In a study of suckling rats, the absorption of folate bound to FBP occurred slowly and primarily in the ileum, whereas free folate was absorbed more readily and primarily in the jejunum (23).

There is an enterohepatic cycle for the absorbed folate in which folate is excreted by the liver in the bile, primarily as N^5-methyltetrahydrofolate, and then reabsorbed by the gut mucosa (24).

Folate Transport and Cellular Uptake

FBPs are abundant in various cells and body fluids and are crucial for absorption, distribution, retention, and conservation of folates (23). The FBPs exist in two forms that have immunologic cross-reactivity, identical terminal and internal aminoacid sequences, single-chained glycoproteins, and similar molecular weight of approximately 40,000 daltons. One form is hydrophillic, soluble (S-FBP), and is present in body fluids such as plasma, milk, urine, cerebrospinal fluid (CSF), and bile. The other form is hydrophobic and present on the membrane of most of body cells (M-FBP), and is responsible for binding to folate and internalizing it (23, 25). M-FBPs (or folate receptors) are anchored in the membrane by a glycosyl-phosphatidylinositol linkage and appear to move in and out of the cell, transporting folate monoglutamates, especially CH_3-FH_4 (but also folate analogues such as methotrexate) into the cell (23, 26). Once inside the cell, the folate dissociates from the binder in the acid pH of caveolae (endosomic vesicle) and the binder returns to the cell surface (26). Plasma contains two S-FBP. One is a high-affinity binder with a very low capacity that binds PteGlu in preference to other physiologic folates and folate analogs; the other is low-affinity binder that may be albumin or another positively charged protein. Only a small portion of plasma folate is bound to S-FBP. The significance of FBP in plasma is not clear. It is possible that it has no physiologic significance and it is there as the result of random cleavage from the surface of the cells, or it might act as a minor storage protein to conserve folates or selectively clear plasma of oxidized folates (23, 25). Folate concentration in CSF is several times as high as that of plasma (27). The site of exchange is the choroid plexus, and transport occurs against a gradient. Only 5 $-CH_3$-FH_4 can pass into the CSF (27).

Once the folate monoglutamate enters the cell, it is mostly converted to polyglutamates containing three to eight or more glutamic acid residues. This process requires an ATP-dependent pteroylglutamate synthetase (16). Folate polyglutamates constitute 80% of human leukocyte and 70% of erythrocyte folate content. In human tissues folate polyglutamates are found mostly in heptaglutamate form but higher glutamates (up to decaglutamate) are also found (16). In addition to polyglutamates, a small fraction of folates in the cells is tightly associated with folate-binding proteins, three of which have been identified as enzymes involved in methyl group metabolism: mitochondrial sarcosine dehydrogenase, dimethylglycine dehydrogenase, and cytosolic glycine N-methyl transferase. Another enzyme, 10-formyltetrahydrofolate dehydrogenase, is also found to be a major cytosolic folate binder in the liver.

Folate Stores

The adult human body stores of folate are about 7.5 $\pm$ 2.5 mg (15). The liver is the major site of folate storage, with its folate content, based on several data, ranging from 0.69–17 μg/g of liver. Among 560 autopsies in Canada, the mean folate content of liver plateaued at 8.8 μg/g of liver between 11 and 20 years of age and then gradually decreased (28).

Plasma Clearance and Urinary Loss of Folate

Plasma clearance of folate is quite rapid. After an intravenous dose of folic acid (15 μg/kg), 60% of the injected dose disappears from the plasma within 3 minutes, followed by a slower rate of clearance and transport to body tissues. The daily urinary loss in normal adults is minimal (1–10 μg, with an average of 4.2 μg), and the loss does not significantly increase following an intravenous folate dose of 100 μg of folic acid.

Cobalamin Metabolism

Consideration of space does not allow coverage of the fascinating historical events leading to the isolation, characterization, and crystallization of vitamin B_{12} and treatment of pernicious anemia, a previously fatal disease. However, excellent reviews are available (14). The name "vitamin B_{12}" was selected by Rickes and colleagues at Merck Laboratories when they announced the preparation of a crystallized form of antipernicious anemia factor from the liver (14). However, the vitamin form that was originally crystallized was a cyanocobalamin, which is not a natural vitamin but a stable form of cobalamin, produced by the chance use of cyanide in the extraction process. All natural forms of vitamin B_{12} are of the cobalamin family. The cobalamin molecule consists of two major portions. One is a tetrapyrrole macrocyclic group called "corrin," which strongly resembles porphyrin, and like porphyrin, is synthesized from δ-aminolevulinic acid and porphobilinogen. At the center of corrin is a cobalt atom which is bound to the four nitrogen atoms of four pyrrole rings. Of the two remaining coordination sites of cobalt atom, one is occupied by a 5,6-dimethylbenzimidazolyl nucleotide and the other by various ligands (e.g., cyano, hydroxo, adenosyl, methyl, etc.), the identity of which determines the name of cobalamin (e.g., cyanocobalamin [CNCbl], hydroxocobalamin [OHCbl], adenosylcobalamin [AdoCbl], and methylcobalamin [MeCbl]) The first two of these compounds (CNCbl and OHCbl) are available as pharmaceutical preparations for treatment of cobalamin deficiency and can be readily converted in animal tissues to biologically active coenzymes, AdoCbl and MeCbl by a coenzyme synthetase system.

The cobalt atom in corrinoids may be in various states of oxidation, the fully reduced form Cob(I)alamin, a partially oxidized form, Cob(II)alamin, and the fully oxidized form, Cob(III)alamin. The reduction of the oxidized form is mediated by cobalamin reductases, which are present both in the cytosol and in mitochondria. The term "vitamin B_{12}" that was originally given to cyanocobalamin is often used interchangeably with cobalamins as a generic name for all cobalamins, especially in clinical medicine, but "cobalamin" is the preferred term.

Sources and Requirement of Cobalamins

Cobalamins are synthesized only by certain cobalamin-producing organisms. Plants neither synthesize nor contain cobalamin and a strict vegetarian diet is therefore devoid of cobalamin. Herbivores obtain their supply of cobalamin from the cobalamin-producing microorganisms in their gut, while carnivores, including humans, receive their supply of cobalamin by eating meat or other animal products. Beef liver is the richest dietary source of cobalamin (116 μg/100 g). Kidney has an average of 38.3 μg/100 g of cobalamin, while egg yolk and cow's milk contain 9.26 and 0.36 μg/100 g of cobalamin, respectively. Cobalamin is relatively stable with cooking. Heating in acid pH does not destroy cobalamin, but heating in alkaline pH does. The average diet supplies about 2.7–31.6 μg/day of cobalamin. Cobalamin losses from the body occurs through urine, faeces, and desquamated cells. The average daily loss of cobalamin in human is 2–6 μg. Based on the long-term biologic half-life of absorbed [^{60}Co]cobalamin in human volunteers, the turnover rate of cobalamin was estimated at 2.55 μg/day or 0.05% of body pool per day (29). A daily intake of 3.64 μg of cobalamin would be needed to keep this estimated body pool of cobalamin stable. However, this exceeds the minimum daily requirements of cobalamin. Many vegetarians with daily intakes of <1 μg of cobalamin for many years do not show any hematologic or neurologic manifestations of cobalamin deficiency (30). Furthermore, hematologic response in cobalamin deficiency megaloblastic anemia can be obtained with as little as 0.1 μg/day of parenteral cobalamin (31). The revised RDA for cobalamin of the U.S. Food and Nutrition Board, National Academy of Science, and National Research Council is 0.3 μg in infants <6 months of age, 0.5 μg for infants 6–12 months of age, 0.7 μg for children 1–3 years of age, 1.0 μg for children 4–6 years of age, 1.4 μg for children 7–10 years of age, 2 μg for persons 11–50 years of age, 2.2 μg for adults >50 years of age, and 2.6 μg for pregnant and lactating woman (19). The mean body cobalamin content of normal adult humans is 3.9–5.0 mg, and the liver is the principal site of its storage (0.6–1.5 mg, with an average of 1.0 μg/g of wet liver). This body store can supply the body's cobalamin requirement for many years. Thus, it takes an average of 5 years (range 2–10 years or more) for cobalamin deficiency megaloblastic anemia to develop following total gastrectomy (19).

Absorption of Cobalamins

Cobalamin has many unique and peculiar characteristics. The unique source of its production in nature and the very minute requirement for sustaining life have already been mentioned. As mentioned earlier, plants do not need and do not synthesise cobalamin. On the other hand, some microorganism such as *Propionibacterium shermanii* of the animal rumen or antibiotic-producing molds such as *Streptomyces griseus* and *Streptomyces aureofaciens* produce so much cobalamin that they can be used for inexpensive commercial production of cobalamins; some others cannot synthesize cobalamin but are dependent upon it (e.g., *Lactobacillus leichmannii* and *Euglena gracilis*, which are used for microbiologic assay of cobalamin) and some others neither synthesize it nor are dependent on it (e.g., *Escherichia coli*). Animals cannot synthesize cobalamin and are dependent on it, but each finds its own peculiar way of demonstrating their cobalamin deficiency (some develop megaloblastic anemia, some manifest neurologic disorder or a wasting disease, and others just die!) and each finds its own peculiar way of getting cobalamin to its needy tissues. The mechanism of cobalamin absorption is different in man, dog, rabbit, and rat (32); and in humans it somewhat resembles the game of Dungeons and Dragons: the food cobalamin must pass through "perils" at several levels and change hands several times before it finally reaches the tissues. Although scientists have provided an explanation for each step, no explanation is given for why nature has made it so complicated and why it is so different than absorption of other vitamins or nutrients.

Cobalamin is a large water-soluble vitamin that cannot readily transverse the lipid membrane of cells. Its absorption requires the presence of specific cobalamin binders, specific receptors, proper pH, digestive enzymes, and calcium ions (32). Dietary cobalamin is present largely in its coenzyme forms (methylcobalamin and adenosylcobalamin), coupled to proteins (mainly their respective intra cytosolic and intramitochondrial enzymes). In the stomach, cobalamin is released from the proteins by acid-pepsin but immediately bonds to cobalamin-binding proteins, of which two types are present in the stomach. One type consists of salivary and gastric R-proteins (R-binders) and the other is intrinsic factor (IF), a glycoprotein, which is produced and secreted by parietal cells in the fundus and cardia of the stomach. Under normal conditions, when gastric pH is low, binding of cobalamin to R-protein is greatly favored and cobalamin-R-protein complex enters the proximal intestine, where pancreatic acid protease degrades the R-protein so that the released cobalamin is then available to bind to IF. IF and cobalamin provide mutual protection for each other and the IF-cobalamin complex becomes unavailable for use by microorganisms and resistant to enzyme digestion. This allows the complex to reach the distal half of the ileum, where it binds to the specific high-affinity cobalamin receptors located on the luminal surface of ileal mucosa cells (enterocytes). This binding requires extracellular calcium ions and pH >5.4, but does not require energy. The IF-cobalamin receptor on enterocytes has been isolated and purified from several species. The receptor is highly specific for the IF-cobalamin complex and does not bind IF, cobalamin, or the cobalamin-R-protein complex. Following attachment to IF-cobalamin receptors, IF-cobalamin enters the cell via endocytosis, and there cobalamin binds to transcobalamin II (TCII)

and then enters the circulation. Absorption of cobalamin is slow. Following ingestion of radiolabeled cobalamin, radioactivity begins to appear in the plasma at 3 hours and peaks at 6–12 hours after ingestion (33). The number of ileal receptors is the limiting factor in active absorption of cobalamin. No more than 1.5–2.0 μg of cobalamin is absorbed from a single oral dose by active absorption (fig. 2.1). Further cobalamin may be actively absorbed if a second dose is given 3 hours later. About 1% of a large dose of ingested cobalamin can be absorbed by passive absorption (fig. 2.1) (34, 35), and daily doses of 1000 μg of oral vitamin B_{12} have been used successfully for the treatment and maintenance of pernicious anemia (34, 36).

Cobalamin can be absorbed rapidly and efficiently through nasal mucosa and by inhalation. It may also be absorbed through rectal mucosa, but not through colonic or buccal mucosa (35).

There is an enterohepatic cycle for cobalamin, and a large amount of cobalamin is secreted in the bile (0.5–9 μg/day). The cobalamin in the bile is bound to R-protein and $\frac{2}{3}$ to $\frac{3}{4}$ of cobalamin excreted through the bile is reabsorbed by an IF-mediated mechanism similar to that of dietary cobalamin. The existence of this enterohepatic cycle explains why cobalamin depletion occurs at much slower rates in those who do not take cobalamin in their diet such as vegans (over a 20-year period of time) (30) than in those who can not absorb cobalamin, such as those who have had total gastrectomy or ileal resection (2–10 years) (19).

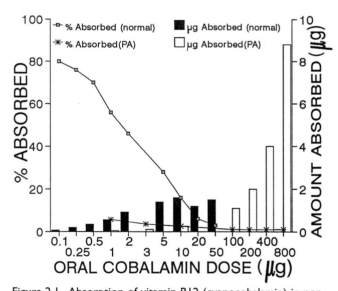

Figure 2.1. Absorption of vitamin B12 (cyanocobalamin) in normal subjects and in patients with pernicious anemia. Note that in normal subjects increasing the Cbl dose from 5–50 mg produces little change in the net amount of absorbed Cbl. This is due to limited capacity of ileal IF-Cbl receptors to absorb Cbl from a single dose. In subjects with PA receiving 100–800 mg Cbl the absorption rate is 1% (passive absorption), but the net amount absorbed increases proportional to the dose used. The slightly higher rate of absorption with lower dose of Cbl in PA is due to some residual IF in some subjects with PA (data adopted from references 34 and 35).

Cobalamin Transport

The absorbed cobalamin primarily binds to transcobalamin II (TCII), which rapidly delivers cobalamin to the tissues. TCII is a polypeptide synthesized by many tissue cells, including hepatocytes, ileal enterocytes, macrophages, fibroblasts, hematopoietic cells of the bone marrow, and endothelial cells (32, 37, 38). TCII has a high affinity for cobalamin. The TCII-cobalamin complex (1:1 molar ratio) has a plasma half-life of 6–9 minutes. The complex is delivered to cells via surface TCII receptors. The TCII-cobalamin first binds to the cell surface receptors and then enters the cell by the process of endocytosis. Subsequently, cobalamin dissociates from TCII at the low pH of lysosomes and is converted to its cobalamin coenzyme forms. The rapid plasma clearance of TCII-cobalamin keeps most of the plasma TCII unbound. In contrast, the TCI, another cobalamin binder in plasma, is found mostly bound to cobalamin due to very slow plasma clearance of TCI-cobalamin (T½ of 9–12 days) (37). TCI is an R-protein, so named because of its *rapid* electrophoretic mobility compared with that of IF. It is also called "cobalophilin," or "haptocorrin." R-Proteins are also glycoproteins, present in many cells and body fluids, including plasma, milk, and amniotic fluid. They exhibit immunologic cross-reactivity but different electrophoretic mobility, primarily due to the difference in the amount of associated sialic acid and fucose (37, 38). Contrary to IF and TCII, which have high specific binding affinity to cobalamins, TCI and other R-binders bind cobalamins, cobalamin analogs, and corrinoids with similar efficiency (39).

TCI in plasma derives primarily from granulocytes, and under normal conditions it exists mostly in bound form (TCI-cobalamin). In the fasting state, about 70% of plasma cobalamin is bound to TCI (33, 37). A third transcobalamin (TCIII) in serum is also an R-protein produced by specific granules of granulocytes and is primarily released in serum after blood is clotted. It is very similar to TCI but has less sialic acid (37).

Case 1

Historic Clues: *From the foregoing, certain important points should be considered in the patient's history, which, when present, can lead to the proper diagnosis of folate or cobalamin deficiency. The most common cause of folate deficiency is dietary deficiency. Since green leafy vegetables and fruits provide most of the dietary folate, special attention should be paid in this regard when taking a dietary history. Folate malabsorption as the cause of folate deficiency is much less common and, if it exists, it is usually part of a general food malabsorption, with the patient having symptoms of general malabsorption (e.g., chronic or recurrent diarrhea or steatorrhea). The commonest cause of cobalamin deficiency, on the other hand, is cobalamin malabsorption, which is often isolated specific cobalamin malabsorption and is not associated with evidences of general malabsorption. Considering the*

daily requirement, the body store can supply the folate requirement for only a few months (4, 40), whereas cobalamin stores can satisfy the body cobalamin requirement for several years (2–10 years for patients with cobalamin malabsorption and >20 years for patients with dietary cobalamin deficiency). Consequently, if megaloblastic anemia occurs within a few months after gastrointestinal surgery, it is probably due to folate deficiency rather than cobalamin deficiency, even if the surgery had caused cobalamin malabsorption (e.g., gastrectomy or ileal resection). Conditions that increase the requirement for folate and cobalamin (e.g., pregnancy, lactation, malignancy) or that interfere with absorption of both folate and cobalamin (e.g., tropical sprue, malabsorption syndrome, alcoholism) cause folate deficiency much earlier than the time required for cobalamin deficiency to develop, and thus patients with these conditions present with folate deficiency megaloblastic anemia.

The patient in case 1 gave no indication of dietary deficiency of folate or cobalamin, nor was she pregnant or taking any drug which could cause megaloblastic anemia. Consequently, her megaloblastic anemia should be considered to be due to either cobalamin or folate malabsorption and, since the patient had combined megaloblastic anemia and iron deficiency, we have to consider two possible diagnoses. Either this patient has cobalamin malabsorption (juvenile pernicious anemia) with associated iron deficiency related to heavy menstrual blood loss and possible decreased iron absorption due to gastric achlorhydria, or she has combined folate and iron deficiency as part of a generalized malabsorption. Considering that this patient had no symptoms of malabsorption and gave no history to indicate celiac disease or tropical sprue in the past, I favored the diagnosis of cobalamin deficiency megaloblastic anemia. After assurance that blood was taken for serum folate and serum cobalamin assays, she was given 1000 µg of intramuscular vitamin B$_{12}$ (cyanocobalamin) and asked to return for followup in 1 week. When she returned, she was feeling much better and stronger even though she still had exertional shortness of breath. Laboratory findings revealed the following: hemoglobin 78 g/L, WBC count 4.2 × 10⁹/L, and reticuloyte count 404 × 10⁹/L, indicating a good response to therapy. By then the results of original serum folate and serum cobalamin testing were also available: serum cobalamin 45 pmol/L (normal 130), serum folate 11.9 nmol/L (normal 7.6), serum ferritin 68 g/L, which, although within normal limit (20–95), was lower than the expected high level seen in severe megaloblastic anemia. These results confirmed the diagnosis of cobalamin deficiency megaloblastic anemia. The patient was started on intramuscular vitamin B$_{12}$ 1000 g once a week for 7 weeks and then 1000 µg given intramuscularly once a month. She was also given oral ferrous sulfate 300 mg three times daily for her presumed associated iron deficiency. When her hematologic parameters all returned to normal, further investigations were carried out to elucidate the cause of *her cobalamin deficiency. Not all of these investigations are necessary for most cobalamin deficiencies, but they were carried out in this case because pernicious anemia at this age is unusual, and we might have been dealing with some rare form of cobalamin deficiency. Her serum contained parietal cell antibody and blocking type of IF antibody, but her serum immunoglobulin levels were normal and tests for antinuclear antibody, immune complex, antithyroglobulin antibody, and anticardiolipin antibody were negative. Her Schilling test showed <1% excretion of radiolabeled cobalamin in 24-hour-urine (normal >7%) and a repeat Schilling test with IF was normal (11% excretion). Her total serum cobalamin-binding capacity and transcobalamin levels were normal. Gastric analysis with pentagastrin stimulation was performed, which showed gastric achlorhydria (table 2.2). No functional intrinsic factor could be identified in gastric juice.*

These results clearly establish the diagnosis of **Juvenile Pernicious Anemia,** so named because it occurs in adolescents and young adults (contrary to the more common form of pernicious anemia that occurs in middle or old age).

Pernicious Anemia (PA) is an acquired disease of unknown cause associated with the development of gastric mucosa atrophy, reduction of parietal cells, and the reduction and final absence of IF and HCl excretion, which causes cobalamin malabsorption. It generally occurs in older subjects. The mean age of 484 cases reported by Cox was 60.5 years (41). Among 2413 cases of PA, only 2.6% were <30 years of age at the time of diagnosis (35). PA is fairly common. A survey of a population of 16 million in the United Kingdom showed a prevalence of 127/100,000 population (42). A survey of Glasgow showed a frequency of 2.5% in the population >65 years of age and in northwest England a frequency of 3.7% >75 years of age (35). Although the cause of PA is not known, an inherited predisposition

Table 2.2 Gastric Analysis of Case 1 Following Pentagastrin Stimulation

Specimen (15 min)	Volume (ml)	pH	Total Acid (mM)
Basal			
1	13	7.7	0.0
2	20	7.6	0.0
3	1	8.1	0.0
4	1	8.1	0.0
Post-Pentagastrin			
1	60	7.2	0.0
2	24	7.6	0.0
3	50	7.5	0.0
4	5	8.4	0.0
5	3	8.0	0.0

Basal acid output = 0.0 mM/hr (normal 0.0–5.6); peak acid output = 0.0 mM/hr (normal 11.6–19.9.

for PA seems to exist. PA is associated more commonly with blood group A and certain HLA types. Several European surveys have indicated PA to be more common in females than males (ratio 1.4/1.0), and PA has been recognized to occur with the highest frequency among people from Scandinavia, the United Kingdom, and in other countries whose population originated from these areas (United States, Australia, New Zealand) (35). It is also common among blacks. Normal adult blacks have higher serum cobalamin and higher TCI, TCII, and TCIII than whites (unrelated to environmental factors). However, the average ages at the time of diagnosis of PA is significantly lower in blacks than in whites (43). PA is more common among the family members of PA patients than in the general population (25/1000 among the relatives of PA probands) (44), and the incidence of gastric atrophy, parietal cell antibody, and IF antibody is much higher in relatives of PA patients than in general population (45).

The primary lesion in PA is gastric atrophy. The parietal (oxyntic) cells become replaced by mucus-producing cells, and there is infiltration of the stomach wall with plasma cells and lymphocytes. The gastric antrum, however, remains relatively intact. The gastric atrophy and loss of secretory cells cause significant reduction of gastric juice at rest and following gastrin or histamine stimulation, as well as reduction of HCl production, which keeps the gastric pH <6.0 and often in alkaline range. The IF of gastric juice is often undetectable and, if present, is markedly decreased. The serum gastrin is markedly elevated in PA due to stimulation of gastrin release by food and lack of gastric acidity, which acts as a feedback inhibitor of gastrin release. Consequently, along with gastric atrophy, there is generally hyperplasia of the endocrine cells in the antral mucosa, which, in addition to gastrin, secrete more 5-hydroxytryptamine and vasoactive intestinal polypeptides. This hypertrophy may be associated with gastric carcinoid tumor, which is much more common in PA than in general population (46).

Although the cause of gastric atrophy and PA is not clear, an autoimmune disorder is favored. The high frequencies of parietal cell antibody (90%), IF antibody (54%), and cell-mediated immunity against IF (86%) in PA are in keeping with an autoimmune cause for PA. Furthermore, the lymphocytotoxins occur with high frequency in PA, and there is a significant reduction in the number of T-suppressor cells in treated PA patients with IF antibodies (47). Additionally, steroid therapy has been shown to improve cobalamin absorption, increase the number of parietal cells, and increase HCl and IF excretion in the stomach (48). The number of IgA-secreting lymphocytes in stomach mucosa is markedly increased in PA. The high association of PA with other autoimmune disorders (table 2.3) also supports an autoimmune cause of PA.

Table 2.3 Reported Association of Pernicious Anemia with Other Autoimmune or Immune-Mediated Disorders

Glandular disorders	Immunoglobulin disorders
Thyroid	Acquired hypo-γγ-globulinemia
Hypothyroidism	IgA deficiency with IgA antibody
Hyperthyroidism	Monoclonal gammopathy
Autoimmune thyroiditis	**Collagen vascullar disorders**
Parathyroid	Lupus erythematosus
Hypoparathyroidism	Rhumatoid arhritis
Hypocalcemia	Anticardiolipin antibody
Adrenal	**Autoimmune cytopenias**
Idiopathic adrenal failure	Autoimmune thrombocytopenia
(autoimmune adrenalitis)	Autoimmune hemolytic anemia
Pancreas	Autoimmune pancytopenia
Diabetes mellitus	Pure red cell hypoplasia
Ovary	**Miscellaneous disorders**
Premature ovarian failure	Celiac disease
Thymus	Allopecia
Myasthenia gravis	Vitiligo
Polyglandular deficiency syndrome	

Our case shows typical features of pernicious anemia. With demonstration of cobalamin deficiency anemia (megaloblastic cell morphology, low serum cobalamin, and normal serum folate), which is associated with an abnormal Schilling test correctable with the administration of IF and presence of IF antibody, no other diagnosis needs to be considered. However, we shall briefly mention other causes of cobalamin malabsorption that could be readily excluded in this case.

Once the diagnosis of cobalamin deficiency due to isolated cobalamin malabsorption was made, in addition to JPA due to acquired immune-mediated deficiency of IF, as discussed above, we need to consider four possible hereditary disorders that are associated with cobalamin malabsorption:

1. Congenital IF deficiency
2. Presence of abnormal IF (labile or with low-affinity binding)
3. Defective ileal IF receptors (Imerslund-Grásbeck syndrome)
4. Transcobalamin II deficiency or abnormal TCII

The presence of gastric achlorhydria and IF antibody in case 1 rules out both congenital IF deficiency and the presence of an abnormal IF, while correction of the abnormal Schilling test with IF rules out both defective ileal receptor and TCII deficiency.

Congenital IF Deficiency (32, 49, 50) is a very rare autosomal recessive disorder that generally manifests between 1 and 5 years of age, although, in few cases with partial deficiency, the megaloblastic anemia has been recognized in the second or third decade of life. In this disorder, gastric IF is absent or deficient (quantitatively or functionally), but the gastric mucosa is morphologically normal and exhibits normal secretions of HCl and pepsin. There is no evidence of the presence of IF antibody or other associated autoimmune disorders to indicate that the absence of IF is immunologically mediated. A few cases of cobalamin deficiency megaloblastic anemia have been reported in which IF is present but is labile due to increased susceptibility to proteolysis or has a reduced affinity for cobalamin or ileal IF receptors (49, 50).

Imerslund-Grásbeck Syndrome (32, 49, 50) is an autosomal recessive disorder that generally manifests between 1 and 5 years of age, but manifestation in older children and adults has also been reported. In this disease, the gastric functions and IF functions are normal, but cobalamin absorption is abnormal, either due to absence of ileal IF receptor or to a deficit after binding of IF-cobalamin to the receptors. Consequently, the abnormal Schilling test or other tests of cobalamin malabsorption do not become corrected with addition of IF. Many of these patients are also reported to have proteinuria.

Transcobalamin II Deficiency (49, 50) generally manifests itself after a few weeks of life, with failure to thrive, diarrhea, irritability, and severe megaloblastic anemia. It is a rare autosomal recessive disorder. The megaloblastic anemia in these cases is due to lack of TCII, which is required for cobalamin transport to the tissues. However, since TCII is also needed for transport of cobalamin from enterocytes into the blood, the tests of cobalamin absorption are also abnormal. Furthermore, contrary to other forms of cobalamin malabsorptions, which respond to minimal daily doses or monthly injections of vitamin B_{12}, these patients require massive doses (1000 μg) of vitamin B_{12} given parenterally once or twice a week in order to respond hematologically.

In addition to the above-mentioned hereditary TCII deficiency, which is associated with impaired cobalamin absorption and cobalamin transport, there are also very rare examples of acquired disturbance of cobalamin transport causing megaloblastic anemia. One patient had no detectable TCII but very high TCI, another had markedly elevated TCII, and a third could not maintain normal circulating level of TCII-cobalamin.

In addition to the hereditary causes mentioned above, there are numerous acquired causes of cobalamin malabsorption. These could be related to disease or lesions of the stomach in which IF production may be absent or deficient, such as in *total or subtotal gastrectomy*, corrosive destruction of gastric mucosa, or severe *simple atrophic gastritis*. In all diseases of the stomach causing cobalamin deficiency, the tests of cobalamin absorption are abnormal, but the test becomes normal if IF is provided with the radiolabeled cobalamin. The exception to this rule is the case of atrophic gastritis in which the absorption of crystalline cobalamin may be normal, but absorption of protein-bound cobalamin is decreased due to lack of HCl and pepsin required to dissociate cobalamin from proteins (51).

Abnormal events in the small bowel resulting in cobalamin malabsorption are listed in table 2.4. Many drugs interfere with cobalamin absorption. However, because of the long-lasting body cobalamin store, only the drugs that may be taken over a very long period are recognized to cause cobalamin deficiency (see table 2.4).

Dietary cobalamin deficiency occurs only in longstanding, *strict vegetarians* (*vegans*). The one exception to this is cobalamin deficiency megaloblastic anemia that occurs in the first few months of life in *infants breastfed by cobalamin-deficient mothers* (either due to a vegetarian diet or to PA) (52). These babies of cobalamin-deficient mothers are born with low cobalamin stores and are fed by cobalamin-deficient maternal milk. As a result, they have a megaloblastic anemia in early infancy that may mimic hereditary TCII deficiency or an inborn error of cobalamin metabolism, but they have normal cobalamin absorption and respond to minimal daily requirement of cobalamin even when it is given orally.

Cobalamin deficiency may occur as the result of long-term use of large doses of ascorbic acid (which destroys cobalamin [53]) or very acutely, following nitrous oxide (N_2O) inhalation either for anesthesia, accidental or intentional. N_2O rapidly inactivates cobalamin by oxidization of cobalamin and inhibition of cobalamin-dependent methionine synthase (54). Prolonged continuous exposure or repeated short exposure may cause acute megaloblastic anemia.

Table 2.4 Megaloblastic Anemias due to Deficiency or Impaired Utilization of Cobalamin

Due to decreased dietary intake (nutritional deficiency)
  Longstanding strict vegetarians
  Breastfed infants of mothers with cobalamin deficiency (vegans or those with pernicious anemia)
Due to cobalamin malabsorption
  Due to disease of stomach
    Total or subtotal gastrectomy, gastric bypass
    Atrophic gastritis
    Corrosive destruction of gastric mucosa (lye or acid ingestion)
  Due to deficiency of intrinsic factor (IF)
    Pernicious anemia (due to autoimmune destruction of IF-producing cells)
    Abnormal IF (low binding affinity, labile IF)
    Congenital IF deficiency
  Malabsorption due to abnormalities of small bowel or its content
    Chronic pancreatitis or pancreatic insufficiency, cystic fibrosis
    Gastric hypersecretion (Zollinger-Ellison syndrome)
    Bacterial overgrowth: blind loop syndrome, diverticulosis, hypo-γγ-glublinemia, impaired bowl motility (scleroderma), acquired
      immunodeficiency syndrome (AIDS)
    Diphyllobothrium latum (fish tapeworm) infestation
    Disorders of terminal ileum
      Crohn disease, tropical sprue, celiac disease, tuberculus ileitis, lymphoma, AIDS, radiation injury
      Resection of terminal ileum or jejunoileal bypass
      Hereditary cobalamin malabsorption due to defective IF receptors (Immersland-Grásbeck syndrome)
  Transcobalamin II (TCII) deficiency, abnormal TCII, acquired TCII deficiency, disturbed cobalamin binding
  Drug-induced malabsorption or destruction of cobalamin
    Slow k
    Biguanides (metformin, phenformin)
    Cholestyramin
    Colchine
    Neomycin
    PAS (paraaminosalicytic acid)
    Ethanol
    Cyproteron-acetate + ethinyl-estradiol
    H_2-receptor antagonists and antacids
Due to disorders of cobalamin transport
  Hereditary TCII deficiency
  Hereditary abnormality of TCII
  Acquired disturbances of transcobalamins
Due to destruction or inactivation of cobalamin
  Nitrous oxide (N_2O) inhalation (anesthesia, accidental, intentional)
  Ascorbic acid
Inborn errors of cobalamin metabolism (cobalamin mutants)
  Cb1C and Cb1D mutant class: defective reduction of Cob(III)alamin to Cob(III)alamin
  Cb1E and Cb1G mutant class: defect in methionine-syndthase-associated reducing system
  Cb1F mutant class: defect in transport of Cb1 from endosomes or lysosomes to cytoplasm

Finally, there are a few rare forms of inborn errors of cobalamin metabolism that are associated with megaloblastic changes (49, 50). These include *cobalamin C* and *cobalamin D* mutant classes (defective reduction of Cob(III)alamin to Cob(II)alamin), *cobalamin E* and *cobalamin G* mutant classes (defect in methionine-synthase-associated reducing system) and *cobalamin F* mutant class (defect in transport of cobalamin from endosomes or lysosomes to cytoplasm).

The Treatment of Cobalamin Deficiency

Excluding cases of dietary cobalamin deficiency which can be treated with minimal daily doses of oral cobalamin (2–5 μg), and TCII deficiency which requires very large and frequent parenteral doses of cobalamin, PA and other cases of cobalamin malabsorption that are not correctable require lifelong cobalamin therapy, either with parenteral cobalamin or massive daily oral doses of cobalamin. In PA or other cobalamin malabsorptions, a single injection of 100–1000 μg of vitamin B_{12} is sufficient to return the hematologic parameters to normal. However, more vitamin B_{12} is generally given initially to build the body store of cobalamin, at least partially, before the patient is placed on monthly cyanocobalamin or 3-monthly hydroxocobalamin injections. It takes 60×1000 μg injections of cyanocobalamin to restore body store of cobalamin to normal (29), but there is no need to restore cobalamin to normal as long as one makes sure that the patient is receiving lifelong maintenance therapy. Different authorities have chosen to give between 4 and 14 injections of 100–1000 μg of cyanocobalamin (daily, twice a week, or weekly) in order to partially restore the body store. The patient is then maintained on monthly parenteral doses of 100–1000 μg of cyanocobalamin. Monthly maintenance doses of 30–100 μg are adequate to prevent recurrence of cobalamin deficiency, and most of the larger dose of cobalamin is excreted in the urine. When vitamin B_{12} was expensive, giving smaller maintenance dose was considered economically sound, but today cyanocobalamin is very inexpensive, and since no toxicity is reported with larger doses of cyanocobalamin, most authorities recommend 1000 μg of cyanocobalamin for monthly maintenance, which results in higher retention of cobalamin than when 100 μg cobalamin is given. No patient with PA should require cobalamin injections more often than once a month (100–1000 μg) for maintenance therapy. If the patient becomes anemic or symptomatic again while taking this maintenance dose, it is not due to cobalamin deficiency, and the patient should not be given more frequent doses of cobalamin but should be fully investigated to determine the cause of the newly developed anemia (or other symptoms). Hydroxocobalamin has a higher binding affinity for TCII and other proteins. For equal parenteral doses, more hydroxocobalamin than cyanocobalamin is retained (following a 1-mg parenteral dose, only 50–80 μg of cyanocobalamin but 250–330 μg of hydroxocobalamin is retained) (29); and maintenance therapy with injections of 1000 μg of hydroxocobalamin every 3 months is feasible and is commonly used in Europe (55). However, this form of therapy has not gained much support in North America (it is not even listed in the 1992 edition of the U.S. Physicians' Desk Reference). In some patients receiving hydroxocobalamin antibody to TCII develops (55).

Maintenance therapy with oral doses of 500–1000 μg cyanocobalamin daily is also feasible (34, 36), but, again, for various reasons, has not gained much support in North America, although it is used quite frequently in Sweden (36). Oral preparations containing vitamin B_{12} and IF have also been used, but are neither as economical nor as efficacious as parenteral or oral vitamin B_{12} alone in cobalamin malabsorptions other than those due to IF deficiency. Even in PA, the development of IF antibody may cause reduced absorption of cobalamin in cobalamin-IF complex (56).

Response to Therapy and Complications

Patients with cobalamin deficiency often begin to feel better within a couple of days of cobalamin therapy, even before the level of hemoglobin shows any increase. The reticulocyte response begins in 3–4 days and peaks within 6–10 days of initiation of therapy. In uncomplicated cases, the magnitude of response is related to the severity of the anemia (the lower the hemoglobin, the greater the reticulocyte response). In severe megaloblastic anemias, the hemoglobin may continue to drop in the first week following the initiation of therapy, causing considerable anxiety for the inexperienced physician. Thrombocytopenia and neutropenia, if present initially, are corrected more rapidly than the anemia, and, in fact, thrombocytosis may follow initial therapy. A decrease in serum potassium may occur in the first few days of initiation of therapy, especially in severe megaloblastic anemia. An alarming rate of early sudden mortality from cardiovascular causes and pulmonary edema (4.3–14%) has been reported attributed to this hypopotassemia (57), although this has not been the experience of other centers (58).

Blood transfusion is rarely indicated in cobalamin deficiency. In patients with very severe anemia or with heart failure, if transfusion is needed, it should be administered very carefully and slowly in the form of packed red cells or be carried out as partial exchange transfusion, in order to prevent cardiac overload.

If, following appropriate cobalamin therapy and initial response the patient's hemoglobin fails to normalize completely, then the possibility of associated iron deficiency should be considered. Associated iron deficiency is common in patients with PA (and other causes of cobalamin deficiency). This iron deficiency may be due to decreased intake (vegetarians), decreased absorption (PA, gastrectomy), or increased loss (Crohn disease), but the megaloblastic anemia often masks its presence so that it only manifests itself when the megaloblastic anemia is corrected but the hemoglobin fails to reach the normal level.

Long-term Followup of PA

In addition to the high incidence of carcinoid tumor in PA (mentioned earlier) (46), there is a definite increase in risk of gastric carcinoma. In a followup study of PA patients at Boston City hospital, 5–8% died of gastric carcinoma (59). In another study, among 123 PA cases, 5 had malignant carcinoid tumor and 5 had adenocarcinoma of the stomach (46), and a more recent survey of 5161 cases of PA (over 34,195 person-years) showed a 3-fold increased risk of gastric carcinoma in PA patients compared with the general population. The same study also demonstrated increased risk of cancers in the buccal cavity, melanoma, multiple myeloma, and leukemia in the PA group (60).

In addition to "early" iron deficiency anemia that may be present at the time of diagnosis of PA, there is a higher incidence of later-onset iron deficiency anemia in PA, which could result from either reduced iron absorption due to gastric atrophy and lack of HCl and pepsin, or increased blood loss due to associated gastric carcinoma.

A discussion of the specific functions of cobalamins and folates follows the discussion of case 2 and causes of folate deficiency.

Case 2

Mrs. D, a 25-year-old white gravida 3 para 3 was admitted to the hospital 5 weeks postpartum because of dizziness and extreme fatigue of 3 weeks' duration. Over the past 4 years, she had given birth to 3 healthy infants. During the third pregnancy she had experienced considerable morning sickness, with nausea and vomiting up to 6 months of gestation and, although she was prescribed an iron- and folate-containing multivitamin preparation, she did not take more than a few of the tablets because she claimed the pills were making her vomit. We were told that her hemoglobin at 7 months of gestation was 120 g/L. Her diet contained adequate dairy products and meat but inadequate amount of fresh fruits and vegetables. Her delivery was uneventful and there was no excessive postpartum hemorrhage. She was breastfeeding her baby up to the time of her admission to the hospital. On the third postpartum day, when she was discharged on ferrous gluconate 300 mg three times daily, her hemoglobin was 69 g/L, WBC count was $5.0 \times 10^9/L$, and her platelet count $150 \times 10^9/L$. She took the iron tablets very irregularly, claiming that they were upsetting her stomach. She was not taking any other medication and gave no history of previous bowel problems or surgery. On the day of admission she was brought to the emergency department because of dizziness and a feeling of faintiness. Initial laboratory tests showed hemoglobin 52 g/L, WBC count $1.6 \times 10^9/L$, and platelet count $17 \times 10^9/L$, MCV 110.6 fL, MCHC 343 g/L. On physical examination, she appeared very pale, had a blood pressure of 100/60, and heart rate of 106 beats/minute. There was no evidence of bleeding, jaundice, or hepatosplenomegaly, and the neurologic examination results were normal. Examination of her peripheral blood showed many macrocytic and some hypochromic red cells. There was an increased number of hypersegmented neutrophils; platelets appeared markedly decreased and there were some large platelets. Other laboratory tests available by the time of examination included the following: reticulocyte count $26 \times 10^9/L$, serum bilirubin 16μ M/L, LDH 2830 U/L.

With pancytopenia and increased number of hyperegmented neutrophils, as well as the history and physical findings, the diagnosis of folate deficiency megaloblastic anemia, probably associated with iron-deficiency anemia was considered. A bone marrow aspiration confirmed the presence of advanced megaloblastic changes, and stainable iron was adequate but considered reduced for the severity of megaloblastic anemia. The megakaryocytes were numerically adequate. Blood was drawn for serum folate, red cell folate, serum cobalamin, and serum ferritin. Because of the marked anemia, which was making her dizzy, and marked thrombocytopenia, she was given two units of packed red cells. She was also started on oral folic acid 5 mg daily, ferrous sulfate 300 mg three times daily, and was given a single intramuscular injection of vitamin B_{12} 1000 μg (because of the very remote possibility that she may be cobalamin deficient). Six days later the hemoglobin was 92 g/L, WBC count $3.9 \times 10^9/L$, platelet count $90 \times 10^9/L$, and reticulocyte count $824 \times 10^9/L$. The admission serum folate 2.3 nM/L, red cell folate 85 nM/L, serum cobalamin 347 pM/L, serum ferritin 109 g/L.

Commentary: *At the initial visit to the emergency room, when only the results of CBC were available, megaloblastic anemia, acute leukemia, and aplastic anemia were considered in the differential diagnosis. After examination of the blood smear and finding of the increased number of hypersegmented neutrophils, in addition to macrocytosis, megaloblastic anemia became the most likely diagnosis; bone marrow examination confirmed this diagnosis and excluded other possibilities. Once the diagnosis of megaloblastic anemia was made, folate deficiency as the cause of megaloblastic anemia was strongly favored because of the patient's dietary history, recent pregnancy, and lactation, as well as her age. Subsequent results of low serum and red cell folate along with normal serum cobalamin level confirmed the diagnosis of folate deficiency and no further investigation was necessary.*

Case 2 is a young woman, with age, physical, and initial laboratory findings similar to those of case 1. The laboratory abnormalities in case 2 are more severe, but the pattern of abnormalities is the same in the 2 cases and can be explained by megaloblastic anemia and associated iron deficiency (although the serum bilirubin in case 2 is within the normal limit of <20μ M/L, it should be regarded as increased in a patient with a hemoglobin of 52 g/L). The causes of megaloblastic anemia in these 2 cases are quite different. One is due to cobalamin deficiency and the other to folate deficiency. But, in both cases, attention to the medical and dietary histories led *to the correct diagnosis even before the confirmatory laboratory tests became available.*

Causes of Folate Deficiency

Folate deficiency is one of the most common dietary deficiencies encountered in clinical practice (13, 15). Folates are labile and undergo degradation over time. Natural folate conjugases in food degrade polyglutamates to monoglotamates, and reduced monoglutamates easily oxidize with exposure to ultraviolet light or cooking, hence the reduced availability of dietary folate despite the presence of folates in most foods. The reported prevalence of folate deficiency varies, depending on the criteria used for diagnosis (folate intake below RDA, low serum folate, low red cell folate, megaloblastic changes, etc.), the population studied, and the geographic location. In recent years, with attention to prophylaxis of folate deficiency in susceptible groups, the incidence of this deficiency has been reduced, at least in the developed countries. The prevalence of folate deficiency in the United States, based on low red cell folate determined by the second National Health Examination Survey for the period 1976–1980 was 8% in adult men and 13% in premenopausal women. The prevalence among the elderly population in different parts of the word has been 8–60% and a report based on the survey of 14 reports showed 8.7% of elderly people living at home and 18% of those in institutions have low red cell folate (61). A Nutrition Canada survey from 1970–1972 defined the categories of high, moderate, and low risk for folate deficiency, based on serum folate level of <2.5 ng, 2.5–5.0 ng, and >5.0 ng/ml, respectively. In that study, 12% of subjects were at high risk, 38% at moderate risk, and 40% at low risk (62).

The *causes of folate deficiency* are listed in table 2.5 and can be categorized as follows:

Dietary Deficiency

Dietary folate deficiency is the most common cause of folate deficiency. Such deficiency can result from consuming a diet generally deficient in folate-rich foods (fresh vegetables, fruits, etc.), from a diet depleted of folate by cooking, or from special diets (e.g., goat's milk feeding of infants, *phenylketonuria* or *maple syrup urine disease diet*, some *weight-loss* diets), *anorexia nervosa*, or *bulimia nervosa*. Dietary folate deficiency is quite common among elderly or institutionalized patients in nursing home or psychiatric settings (13).

Increased Folate Requirement

Certain ages and physiologic conditions are associated with high folate requirement. Such conditions include *prematurity and infancy* (63), *adolescence* (64), *pregnancy* (13, 63), and *lactation* (63). Since folates are needed for cell production, any condition associated with increased cell production can cause folate deficiency if the increased requirement is not met. These include *hemolytic anemias, myeloproliferative disorders, leukemias, lymphomas,* other *malignancies,* and *chronic exfoliative dermatosis* (13). In the patient in case 2, Mrs. D., severe folate deficiency megaloblastic anemia developed, not only because she had a poor dietary folate intake due to nausea, vomiting, and possibly food aversions, but also because she was initially pregnant and then breastfed her baby, causing further demand on her folate stores.

Folate Deficiency in Pregnancy

Several factors contribute to the predisposition to folate deficiency in pregnancy. Excess folate is needed for donation to the rapidly growing fetus, for production of placental tissue, and for excess red cell production associated with increased blood volume in pregnancy. In addition, there is increased urinary folate excretion during pregnancy and there may be reduced dietary intake due to dietary aversion, nausea, and vomiting associated with pregnancy. Furthermore, based on massive doses of folic acid required to correct some megaloblastic anemias of pregnancy, some authors have speculated that defective folate metabolism or inadequate utilization of folates may be present at least in some pregnant women (63). The impaired folate metabolism in women taking oral contraceptives (65) also supports the possibility of defective folate metabolism due to hormonal changes in pregnancy. The incidence of folate deficiency during pregnancy varies depending on the criteria used, the diligence with which folate deficiency is sought, and the population studied. The incidence of folate deficiency based on low serum folate in different reports has been 8–100%, based on low red cell folate 5.8–40%, and based on megaloblastic changes 0–75% (63). The incidence of folate deficiency is higher in twin pregnancy than in single pregnancy and higher in multiparas than in primiparas (63). Lactation can deplete the mother of 25–51 µg/day of folate (15) and thus further aggravate or precipitate folate deficiency megaloblastic anemia.

Folate Deficiency in Prematurity and Infancy

There is an active transport of folate from mother to fetus. Serum, red cell, and liver folate content increase in the fetus with the progress of gestation. Newborns have much higher serum and red cell folate level than their mothers, but these levels fall rapidly in the first few months of life. The decrease is more rapid for serum than for red cell folate and more rapid in premature infants than in full-term infants due the greater rate of growth and lower body store of folate in the premature babies. By 6–12 weeks of age about two-thirds of small normal premature infants may show laboratory evidence of folate deficiency, as demonstrated by low serum and red cell folate, high urinary formiminoglutamic acid (FIG LU) excretion, or by megaloblastic changes (63). In full-term infants, the fall of serum and red cell folate is

Table 2.5 Megaloblastic Anemias due to Deficiency or Impaired Utilization of Folate

Dietary deficiency
  Consuming diet generally deficient in folate-rich food (fresh vegetables, fruits), or folate-depleted (by cooking and boiling)
  Special diets (goat's milk diet in infancy, phenylketonuria, maple syrup urine disease, some weight-loss diets, anorexia nervosa, bulimia nervosa
  Decreased dietary intake by elderly or institutionalized pateints in nursing home or psychiatric institute
Folate intake not meeting increased folate requirement
  Physiologic conditions
    Pregnancy and/or lactation
    Prematurity and infancy
    Adolescence
  Pathologic conditions associated with rapid cell growth and division
    Hemolytic anemias, myeloproliferative disorders, leukemias, lymphomas, or other malignancies
    Psoriasis, dermatitis herpetiform, and other chronic exfoliative dermatosis
Folate malabsorption
  With normal intestinal mucosa morphology
    Congenital folate malabsorption
    Drug-induced folate malabsorption: sulfasalazine, biguandide (metformin, phenformin), antacids (magesium or aluminum hydroxide, H_2-receptor antagonist), paraaminosalicytic acid, folate antagonists
    Diseases changing intestinal pH: chronic pancreatitis, atrophic gastritis
  With intestinal mucosa abnormalities
    Tropical or nontropical sprue (celiac disease)
    Regional enteritis (Crohn disease)
    Chronic diarrhea or recurrent gastroenteritis in infancy
    Hypothyroidism (myxedematous gut)
    Giardiasis
Defective cellular uptake or impaired folate metabolism
  Drug-induced (often with multiple effect and multiple sites)
    Folate antagonists: methotrexate, pyrimethamine, trimethoprim, triamterene, pentamidine isethionate, piritrexim
    Alcohol (ethanol)
    Anticonvulsants: diphenylhydantoin, barbiturates, primidone, valproic acid
    Antituberculus drugs: cycloserine
    Oral contraceptive
    Nitrufuratoin
    Glutethimide
  Dieatry aminoacid imbalance: glycine, serine, homocysteine, methionine, parenteral hyperalimentation in intensive care setting
  Hemodialysis
  Following bone marrow transplantation
Inborn errors of folate metabolism
  Deficiency of homocysteine: 5-methyltetrahydrofolate methyltransferase (methionine synthase)
  Deficiency of glutamate formininotransferase
  Deficiency of dihydrofolate reductase
  Familial defect in cellular folate uptake

not as rapid, but following a short period of gastroenteritis, folate deficiency anemia may easily develop even in them.

Folate Malabsorption

Folate malabsorption may be seen in the presence of normal intestinal morphology, in which case folate malabsorption is often an isolated malabsorption (e.g., congenital or drug-induced folate malabsorption), or may be seen in conditions where intestinal mucosa is abnormal in which case folate malabsorption is associated with symptoms and evidence of malabsorption of other nutrients. Some of the causes of folate malabsorption are listed in table 2.2. We shall discuss briefly only those few that are of special interest or are more common.

Congenital Folate Malabsorption is a very rare form of folate malabsorption in which there is specific folate malabsorption in the presence of normal gut mucosa morphology and in the absence of malabsorption of any other food or nutrients (66–68). Patients with this disorder generally present with folate deficiency megaloblastic anemia in the first few months of life and most have neurologic complications, including mental retardation, seizure, ataxia, extrapyramidal deficit, and peripheral neuropathy. The occurrence of at least two pairs of affected siblings and parental consanguinity in four families (66) strongly favors a hereditary disorder. Curiously, only 2 of 13 reported cases are male (67, 68). There is severe malabsorption of both mono- and polyglutamate forms of folate, as well as defective transport of folate across the blood-brain barrier. Large daily doses of folic acid (10–40 mg orally) may be needed to keep serum folate within the normal range, and even larger doses, as much as 100 mg daily, may be needed to raise the CSF folate level to normal (66). Since reduced folates are better transported through choroid plexus, the treatment with folinic acid (5-formyl-FH$_4$) is preferable in this condition. The patient in whom 40 mg of oral folic acid daily and 5 mg of intramuscular folic acid daily failed to raise CSF folate responded rapidly to 5 mg of intramuscular folinic acid daily, with his CSF folate becoming normal within 6 days. Subsequent oral folic acid (40 mg/day) and parenteral folinic acid (5 mg twice a week) reversed much of this patient's neurophysiologic abnormalities (67).

Celiac Disease (gluten-induced enteropathy or nontropical sprue) is the commonest cause of malabsorption in temperate zones and is quite often associated with folate deficiency. The disease is due to an inherited sensitivity to the glutamine-rich protein fraction (gluten, gliadin) of grains. This sensitivity causes intestinal villous atrophy associated with hypertrophy of crypts and infiltration of lamina propria with lymphocytes and plasma cells. Although the malabsorption is general, since the pathology is more prominent in the proximal small bowel where exposure to gluten occurs, cobalamin absorption is less affected. Folate deficiency is so common in this disorder that some authors have used the absence of folate deficiency as evidence against the presence of celiac disease. Anemia was present in 89% of 122 cases of celiac disease, and of the 115 who had bone marrow examinations, 45% had pure megaloblastic anemia, 52% had mixed megaloblastic and iron-deficiency anemia, and 3% had iron-deficiency anemia alone (69). The folate deficiency also occurs commonly in children with celiac disease, but the often-associated iron deficiency may mask the megaloblastic presence. The presence of splenic atrophy and hyposplenism in celiac disease may also modify the blood smear morphology through the presence of Howell-Jolly bodies and increased target cells. Folate malabsorption in celiac disease is more severe for polyglutamates than is for monoglutamates. Removal of gluten and gliadin from the diet increases the serum and red cell folate and corrects the megaloblastic anemia. However, in severe folate deficiency it is best to treat the deficiency with folic acid.

Tropical Sprue is a malabsorption syndrome of undetermined (but likely infectious) cause that is endemic to tropical regions. The disease may develop in visitors to the endemic area months or years later. The chronic diarrhea is associated with symptoms of malaise, fatigue, weight loss, and malabsorption of fat, carbohydrate, vitamins, and other nutrients. Folate deficiency due to malabsorption is quite common in this disorder, and megaloblastic anemia due to folate deficiency generally manifests itself in those who have had the disease for more than a few months. Megaloblastic anemia was re-

ported in 60–100% of cases of tropical sprue from tropical regions, in immigrants from those regions (70), and in 78% of army personnel who were stationed in Singapore and in whom tropical sprue developed (71). In addition to folate malabsorption, cobalamin malabsorption is also very common in tropical sprue (unlike celiac disease). However, because the body supply of cobalamin lasts much longer than the body supply of folate, the megaloblastic anemia in the first few months is generally due to folate deficiency, but, in chronic stage, cobalamin deficiency or combined folate and cobalamin deficiency may occur. The disease in the acute stage (<3 months' duration) often responds dramatically to folic acid therapy. More chronic forms may also respond to folic acid but the dose must be higher (5 mg daily) and taken for a longer period in order to prevent recurrence. In the chronic forms, the possibility of associated cobalamin deficiency should also be considered and cobalamin therapy be added if there is evidence of cobalamin deficiency. Neuropathy due to cobalamin deficiency following folate therapy of tropical sprue has been reported (72). The rapid and dramatic response of tropical sprue to folic acid is unexplained and is not related to correction of folate deficiency itself, because patients with severe folate deficiency from other causes do not show symptoms of tropical sprue; and response to folic acid, in the acute stage, may occur before depletion of body store of folates.

Crohn Disease often involves the ileum and is associated with cobalamin malabsorption only but sometimes may involve or extend to the proximal small bowel, causing folate malabsorption. Furthermore, sulfasalazine, which is commonly used in the treatment of Crohn disease, causes folate malabsorption and may cause folate deficiency in Crohn disease (73).

Defective Cellular Uptake or Impaired Metabolism of Folate

Numerous drugs can interfere with folate absorption, utilization, or metabolism (13, 20, 74, 75). The most-studied and understood drugs are the dihydrofolate reductase inhibitors (the so-called folate antagonists), which include: *methotrexate, pyrimethamine, trimethoprim, piritrexim, pentamidine isothionate,* and *triamterene.* These drugs bind to dihydrofolate reductase and prevent reduction and activation of folates. Methotrexate is a potent, irreversible inhibitor of dihydrofolate reductase. Once inside the cell, it is polyglutamated by the same enzyme, polyglutamate synthetase, that synthesizes folate polyglutamates, binds folate-binding proteins, and competes with folate polyglutamates. In high doses, methotrexate can cause megaloblastic changes in a matter of hours. Other dihydrofolate reductase inhibitors such as trimethoprime, pyrimethamin, piritrexim, and pentamidine have much higher affinities for bacterial or protozoal enzymes than for the mammalian enzymes. They can therefore be used for treatment of bacterial or protozoal infections with doses that would not generally cause megaloblastic changes for humans. However, prolonged use of these drugs may cause megaloblastic anemia. In addition to being inhibitors of folate reductase, the folate antagonists that have been studied (methotrexate, trimethoprim, pyrimethamine, and triamterene) also inhibit folate absorption (76).

Other drugs and nutrients that may interfere with folate metabolism include *ethanol* (77), anticonvulsant (*phenytoin, barbiturates, primidone, valproic acid*) (78), *cycloserine* (79), *oral contraceptives* ((65), *nitrofurantoin* (80), and dietary *amino acid imbalance (glycine, serine, homocysteine, methionine)* (75). Acute folate deficiency megaloblastic anemia may occur during *parenteral hyperalimentation*, as the result of decreased intake, increased requirement, amino acid imbalance, and ethanol effect (81). *Chronic hemodialysis* may cause folate deficiency as the result of removal of folate and also possibly as the result of a defect in membrane transport of folate (due to retention of anions in uremia) (82). Acute folate deficiency megaloblastic anemia may occur following *bone marrow transplantation*, due to decreased intake, decreased absorption, and increased requirement during marrow recovery.

Folate deficiency in alcoholics is quite common, especially in skid-row alcoholics who tend to buy alcohol rather than food. The cause of this folate deficiency is multifactorial. Poor dietary intake, decreased absorption, increased urinary loss, and impaired folate utilization are all contributing factors (77).

Folate deficiency in anticonvulsant users is common. It is most often reported in phenytoin users but has also been reported in primidone, phenobarbital, and valproic acid users. The postulated mechanisms of this deficiency are decreased absorption of folate, increased requirement of folate due to microsomal induction of folate-requiring enzymes, and increased catabolism of folates, as well as interference with DNA synthesis. However, evidence against all of these possibilities has been reported (83).

Oral contraceptives (OC) can interfere with folate metabolism. Compared with nonusers, OC users were shown to have lower serum and red cell folate and higher urinary FIG LU excretion. Although some reports have failed to show statistically significant differences between the serum folate of OC users and that of nonusers, the bulk of evidences supports the deleterious effect of OC on folate metabolism (65). To date, the suggested causes are reduced folate intake, increased folate requirement due to microsomal induction, decreased absorption, and inceased urinary loss (65). Megaloblastic anemia in OC users due to inhibition of folate polyglutamate absorption was described by two groups, but in two subsequent reports the absorption of folate polyglutamates in OC users was normal (65). One study suggested that abnormal folate polyglutamate absorption in OC users was due to preexisting latent folate malabsorption that had become manifest due to other effects of OC in folate metabolism (65). Several cases of megaloblastic anemia in OC users

have been described; however, the presence of associated causes for folate deficiency have not been excluded. It seems that the effect of OC on folate metabolism and folate depletion is mild, but when there are other associated problems (e.g., reduced folate intake, increased requirement, or decreased absorption), megaloblastic anemia may occur (65).

Inborn Errors of Folate Metabolism

Several cases of inborn errors of folate metabolism have been reported (66). These cases are extremely rare but have provided the "experiment of nature" that has helped our understanding of folate metabolism. They include methionine synthase (hemocysteine: 5-methyltetrahydrofolate methyltransferase) deficiency, glutamate formiminotransferase deficiency, dihydrofolate reductase deficiency, and familial defect in cellular folate uptake. These disorders often manifest themselves in small children with central nervous symptoms, neurologic abnormalities, and mental retardation. They do not all cause megaloblastic anemia, but megaloblastic anemias are reported in deficiencies of methionine synthase, glutamate formiminotransferase, and, possibly, dihydrofolate reductase.

We have discussed the megaloblastic anemias and the deficiencies of folate and cobalamin. A discussion of the metabolic functions of these two vitamins and their interaction with each other follows to review their role in the development of megaloblastic anemias and also explain the values and limitations of the laboratory tests used in investigation of folate and cobalamin deficiency.

Metabolic Functions of Folates

In mammalian cells, the folates exists almost entirely in reduced polyglutamate form, and in this form they participate in several reactions involved in the acceptance and transfer of a single carbon moiety (16). The source of single carbons are serine, methionine, formate, and histidine. The significant single carbons involved are formyl $(-CHO)$, methylene $(-CH_2-)$, methenyl $(=CH-)$, methyl $(-CH_3)$, hydroxymethyl $(-CH_2OH)$, and formimino $(-CH=NH)$. Folate coenzymes acting as single carbon donors or acceptors are involved in serine-glycine interconversion, thymidylate synthesis, histidine catabolism, purine synthesis (carbons 2 and 8 of the purine ring are contributed by 10-formyl-FH_4), methionine synthesis, methyl group oxidation to formaldehyde[16] (fig. 2.2), and possibly porphyrin synthesis (84). A description of the three reactions that are more closely involved in hematologic aspects of folate deficiency follows (in most scientific literature, as well as in this chapter, reactions involving folates are represented by monoglutamates; but, actually, the polyglutamates are the ones that are participating in the reactions, and monoglutamates, if they do participate, are less effective than the polyglutamates).

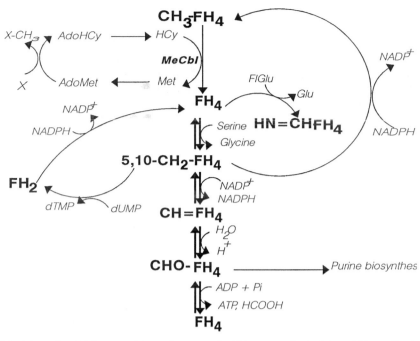

Figure 2.2. The role of folates in sigle carbon transfer. FH_4 = tetrahydrofolate, FH_2 = dihydrofolate, MeCbl = methylcobalamin, AdoHCy = adenosylhomocysteine, AdoMet = adenosylmetionine, X = methyl group acceptor, dUMP = deoxyuridine monophosphate, dTMP = deoxythymidine monophosphate.

Histidine Catabolism

In its normal catabolic pathway, histidine is transformed to urocanic acid, then to 4-imidazolene-5-propionic acid, and finally to formiminoglutamic acid (FIG LU). The later, in the presence of formiminotransferase-cyclodeaminase and FH_4, is converted to glutamic acid (fig. 2.3). This folate-dependent step provides the basis for the urinary FIG LU excretion test proposed for the diagnosis of folate deficiency. If the amount of FH_4 is reduced, FIG LU cannot be changed to glutamic acid. Thus, accumulated FIG LU enters the blood and becomes excreted in the urine. In testing urinary FIG LU excretion, a test dose of L-histidine hydrochloride (15 g for adults) is given to the patient in order to stress the metabolic pathway, and the amount of FIG LU excreted in 24-hour urine is determined by electrophoretic or enzymatic methods.

Thymidine Synthesis

The methylation of deoxyuridine-monophosphate (dUMP) to deoxythymidine-monophosphate (dTMP) requires the enzyme thymidylate synthetase (TS) and coenzyme 5,10-methylenetetrahydrofolate (5,10-CH_2-FH_4), as is shown in figure 2.4. This reaction constitutes the major pathway of dTMP production under normal condition (i.e., de novo synthetic pathway). The blockade in this reaction, which is necessary for DNA synthesis, is considered to be the basis for megaloblastic changes associated with folate deficiency. Another pathway of dTMP production—salvage pathway—involves direct utilization of thymidine with the help of thymidine kinase (TK) (fig. 2.4). The de novo and salvage pathways of dTMP production provide the basis for the deoxyuridine (dU) suppression test

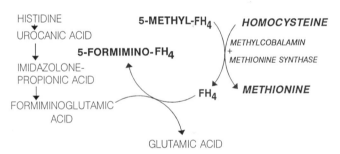

Figure 2.3. The role of folates in histidine catabolism and in methionine synthesis.

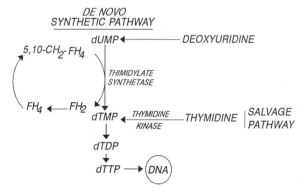

Figure 2.4. The role of folates in DNA synyhesis.

(dUST) (85), which is used in the differential diagnosis of the causes of megaloblastic anemia and will be discussed later. Although the reduced conversion of dUTMP to dTMP is generally considered to be the main cause of megaloblastic changes in folate deficiency and this defect can be demonstrated by the dU suppression test, there are some data that suggest that impaired thymidylate synthesis may not be the central defect in megaloblastic hemopoiesis. Thus, for example, it is reported that the activity of TS in bone marrow cells is reduced only in severe folate or cobalamin deficiency megaloblastic anemias, and the rate of thymidylate synthesis exceeds its rate of incorporation in DNA of both normal and megaloblastic marrow cells (86). Furthermore, the deoxyribonucleoside triphosphate content of bone marrow cells in megaloblastic anemia is much higher than that of normal or leukemic bone marrow and the excess accumulation of deoxyribonucleotide is much greater for dCTP (deoxycytidine triphosphate) than for dTTP (87).

Methionine Synthesis

In the de novo pathway of methionine synthesis, both folate and cobalamin act as coenzymes (16). In this pathway the methyl group of $N^5\text{-}CH_3\text{-}FH_4$ is transferred to Cbl to form meCbl, which in turn provides its methyl group for the methylation of homocysteine to form methionine (fig. 2.5). (In the liver, there is also a non-folate-dependent pathway of methionine synthesis in which betaine is the methyl donor and betaine homocysteine methyltransferase is the enzyme (16). This pathway, however, is not present in other tissues). The pathway of methionine synthesis is the major site of interaction of folate and cobalamin interaction and is considered to be directly or indirectly responsible for megaloblastic changes seen in cobalamin deficiency.

Metabolic Functions of Cobalamins

The coenzyme forms of cobalamin—AdoCbl and MeCbl—participate in numerous reactions in microorganisms and in animals, but most of these reactions are cobalamin dependent only in certain organisms or animals (88, 89). By analogy to folate, which participates in single-carbon unit transfer, AdoCbl participates in several reactions, which results in intramolecular transfer of hydrogen from one carbon atom to an adjacent carbon atom (89). In humans only two roles have been identified for cobalamin coenzymes: (a) the MeCbl-mediated de novo synthesis of methionine (88);

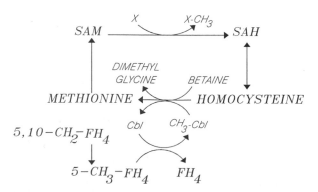

Figure 2.5. The interaction of folate and cobalamin in methionine synthesis. SAM = S-adenosylmethionine, SAH = S-adenosylhomocysteine.

(b) the AdoCbl-mediated conversion of methylmalonic acid (MMA) to succinic acid (89). The de novo synthesis of methionine, which requires both folate and Cbl has already been discussed above. A single-carbon unit from serine or formate is transferred to tetrahydrofolate polyglutamate and further reduced to methyltetrahydrofolate polyglutamate. Methionine synthase then transfers the methyl group from methyl-FH$_4$-polyglutamate to Cbl to form MeCbl, which in turn passes its methyl group to homocysteine to form methionine, which in turn is converted, in an ATP-requiring reaction, to S-adenosylmethionine.

The conversion of MMA to succinic acid requires the enzyme methylmalonyl-CoA mutase, which requires AdoCbl as a coenzyme (89). MMA is intermediary metabolite derived from the metabolism of propionic acid, leucine, isoleucine, valine, and methionine. It is normally converted to succinic acid or succinyl-CoA. In cobalamin deficiency the block in this reaction causes MMA to accumulate in blood and urine, hence the use of MMA measurement in blood or urine for the diagnosis of cobalamin deficiency (90).

Folate and Cobalamin Interaction and Pathogenesis of Megaloblastic Anemia

There is considerable interaction between folates and cobalamins. Deficiency of either vitamin causes megaloblastic anemia, which may respond at least temporarily to therapy with large doses of the other vitamin. In severe cobalamin deficiency, serum folate may be high, normal, or low, and the majority of the patients have low red cell folate and high urinary FIG LU excretions, all of which return to normal with cobalamin therapy. Similarly, in severe folate deficiency serum cobalamin level may be low, which is corrected with folate therapy.

The megaloblastic morphology in folate deficiency is attributed to impaired DNA synthesis, at least in part due to impaired (folate dependent) synthesis of deoxythymidine from methylation of deoxyuridine, as described above. The pathogenesis of the megaloblastic morphology in cobalamin deficiency, on the other hand, is not clear. Two major hypotheses have been proposed to explain the mechanism of megaloblastic anemia in cobalamin deficiency. The first hypothesis generally referred to as the "methylfolate trap hypothesis" (91), proposes that cobalamin deficiency causes the blockade of the cobalamin-dependent synthesis of methionine from homocysteine. Since, in this reaction, methyltetrahydrofolate acts as a methyl donor to become tetrahydrofolate, a block in this reaction leads to the accumulation of methyltetrahydrofolate (which is the principal folate in plasma) and prevents the recycling of folate to tetrahydrofolate and $N^{5,10}$-methylenetetrahydrofolate, which is required for thymidylate synthesis. Decreased thymidylate synthesis results in impaired DNA synthesis and megaloblastic morphology, while the trapped methyltetrahydrofolate is excreted in the urine, causing tissue depletion of folate. The other hypothesis, the so-called "formate starvation hypothesis" (92), proposes that the primary defect in cobalamin deficiency is impaired methionine synthesis. Since methionine is the major source of single carbon units, and since the substrate for folate polyglutamate is formyltetrahydrofolate, the formyl of which is derived from methionine, the decreased methionine synthesis results in reduced availability of folate coenzyme (folate polyglutamate). It is further postulated that this reduced availability of formate also leads to reduced thymidylate synthesis, because formate constitutes an important source of methylene, which is required for the methylation of deoxyuridine to deoxythymidine. Neither theory seems to provide all of the answers, and there is no reason to suppose that the two theories are mutually exclusive.

Approach to the Diagnosis of Folate and Cobalamin Deficiency

We should emphasize that the diagnosis of folate or cobalamin deficiency in the majority of cases is quite easy, provided that one takes a proper history with special attention to diet, drug intake, presence of gastrointestinal symptoms, and history of previous gastrointestinal surgery. The measurement of serum folate and serum cobalamin in the majority of the cases provides the diagnosis, as long as one is aware of limitations of these assays and the conditions under which they may produce falsely positive or negative results (the tests used in investigation of megaloblastic anemias and their limitations are discussed in the appendix). *Provided that the diagnosis of megaloblastic anemia is established,* a low serum cobalamin and normal or high serum folate establish the diagnosis of cobalamin deficiency megaloblastic anemia (fig. 2.6). If serum folate is low and serum cobalamin is normal, then the diagnosis of folate deficiency is made. It is only when both serum folate and cobalamin are low that one may have to make further efforts to determine whether the patient has a combined deficiency or if the low serum level of one vitamin is in fact due to a true deficiency of the other vitamin. In such cases, performance of tests of cobalamin absorption, after megaloblastic anemia is corrected with therapy, generally provides the answer. If the patient is not a vegetarian and tests of cobalamin absorption are normal (Schilling test and absorption of protein-bound cobalamin), one can exclude cobalamin deficiency and assume the case is one of folate deficiency. If the Schilling test or another test of cobalamin absorption is abnormal, the diagnosis of cobalamin deficiency and the need for lifelong cobalamin therapy are established. If, after correction of cobalamin deficiency, repeat serum folate becomes normal, folate deficiency is excluded, but, if it remains low, folate deficiency is confirmed. Once the diagnosis of folate deficiency is made, unless the patient is receiving drugs that can cause folate deficiency, it is assumed that the cause is dietary deficiency. However, if the patient gives an indication of good dietary folate intake or has symptoms suggestive of a mal-

absorption syndrome, then further investigation for establishing the cause of malabsorption is warranted to establish its cause. If serum folate is normal and serum cobalamin is low in the presence of megaloblastic anemia in someone >40 years of age, we can assume that the patient has PA. Tests of cobalamin absorption (with and without IF) would confirm the diagnosis of PA, but these tests are not necessary unless something in the history or presenting symptoms suggests that the patient may have a disease of the small bowel. The management of PA or cobalamin malabsorption due to asymptomatic Crohn disease or cobalamin malabsorption due to asymptomatic bowel disease is the same, so establishing the true cause of cobalamin malabsorption is only of academic interest.

There is some confusion in the interpretation of reported data with regard to folate or cobalamin deficiency. It is true that in the sequence of events in development of folate or cobalamin deficiency a decrease in the serum level of these vitamins appears before the development of anemia, so that the patient may have a true deficiency of folate or cobalamin without anemia. However, once the patient is anemic, *unless the anemia is associated with megaloblastic changes in the blood or bone marrow, the anemia should not be attributed to deficiency of one of these vitamins solely on the ground that the patient has low serum folate or low serum cobalamin.* On the other hand, patients with folate, and especially with cobalamin deficiency, may have neuropsychiatric symptoms and signs without any anemia. In these cases, if serum cobalamin is low (or MMA is high in serum or urine), the patient should be treated with high doses of cobalamin while awaiting further investigations to establish the cause of the neuropsychiatric problems or to establish the presence of cobalamin deficiency. Similarly, if neuropsychiatric symptoms are associated with low serum folate, the patient should be given folate therapy, and if serum cobalamin is borderline low the Schilling test or another test of cobalamin absorption should be performed to verify that the patient does not have a latent PA.

Other Causes of Macrocytosis

So far we have limited our discussion to megaloblastic anemias and their causes. However, since macrocytosis is the most common laboratory abnormality which brings to attention possible folate or cobalamin deficiency (CBC is routinely ordered in most patients, whereas tests of serum folate and cobalamin are not routine), we should briefly discuss other conditions that may cause macrocytosis but are not associated with megaloblastic morphology (these conditions are listed in table 2.6).

Macrocytosis, with or without anemia, is fairly common and is often due to causes other than folate or cobalamin deficiency. Some authors have described three different types of macrocytes. **Thick macrocytes** have high MCV and appear large and thick under the microscope. They oc-

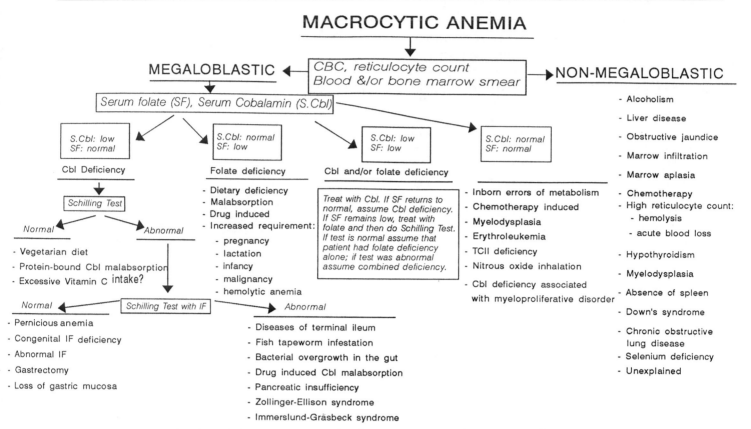

MACROCYTIC ANEMIA

CBC, reticulocyte count
Blood &/or bone marrow smear

MEGALOBLASTIC ← → NON-MEGALOBLASTIC

Serum folate (SF), Serum Cobalamin (S.Cbl)

S.Cbl: low SF: normal	S.Cbl: normal SF: low	S.Cbl: low SF: low	S.Cbl: normal SF: normal
Cbl Deficiency	Folate deficiency	Cbl and/or folate deficiency	

NON-MEGALOBLASTIC
- Alcoholism
- Liver disease
- Obstructive jaundice
- Marrow infiltration
- Marrow aplasia
- Chemotherapy
- High reticulocyte count:
    - hemolysis
    - acute blood loss
- Hypothyroidism
- Myelodysplasia
- Absence of spleen
- Down's syndrome
- Chronic obstructive lung disease
- Selenium deficiency
- Unexplained

Cbl Deficiency

Schilling Test

Normal ← → Abnormal

- Vegetarian diet
- Protein-bound Cbl malabsorption
- Excessive Vitamin C intake?

Normal ← Schilling Test with IF → Abnormal

- Pernicious anemia
- Congenital IF deficiency
- Abnormal IF
- Gastrectomy
- Loss of gastric mucosa

Folate deficiency
- Dietary deficiency
- Malabsorption
- Drug induced
- Increased requirement:
    - pregnancy
    - lactation
    - infancy
    - malignancy
    - hemolytic anemia

- Diseases of terminal ileum
- Fish tapeworm infestation
- Bacterial overgrowth in the gut
- Drug induced Cbl malabsorption
- Pancreatic insufficiency
- Zollinger-Ellison syndrome
- Immerslund-Gräsbeck syndrome

Treat with Cbl. If SF returns to normal, assume Cbl deficiency. If SF remains low, treat with folate and then do Schilling Test. If test is normal assume that patient had folate deficiency alone; if test was abnormal assume combined deficiency.

- Inborn errors of metabolism
- Chemotherapy induced
- Myelodysplasia
- Erythroleukemia
- TCII deficiency
- Nitrous oxide inhalation
- Cbl deficiency associated with myeloproliferative disorder

Figure 2.6. Simplified diagram showing classification and suggested investigation of macrocytic anemias.

cur in megaloblastic anemias and when the reticulocyte count is high. **Thin macrocytes** appear large and thin under the microscope but have normal MCV, and they are more common in liver disease, obstructive jaundice, and absence of the spleen. They result from increased red cell membrane without increase in cell volume and are attributed to changes in red cell membrane lipids. The third type of macrocyte, referred to as the **volumetric macrocyte,** has increased MCV but appears normal in size under the microscope and is seen in patients receiving chemotherapy for cancer. However, considerable overlap exists between the three types with regard to their occurrence in different conditions. Macrocytosis in the absence of significant anemia is often neglected by many physicians, and the opportunities for early diagnosis of some correctable conditions are lost. The incidence varies depending on the population studied and the criteria used for identifying macrocytosis. It was found in 3.7% of 3805 adults attending a university primary care center (MCV >98.6 fL). In this study, as well as most of the other studies in the United States and Europe, the major cause of nonmegaloblastic macrocytosis in the adult population has been *chronic alcoholism* (93).

Macrocytosis is quite common in *alcoholics.* Ethanol has several effects in hemopoietic cells. In those consuming large quantities of ethanol there may be anemia, leukopenia, thrombocytopenia, or pancytopenia. The anemia may be hyporegenerative, megaloblastic, sideroblastic, or hemolytic; and the red cells are often macrocytic with or without megaloblastic changes in the bone marrow (77, 93, 94). Ethanol is the most common cause of macrocytosis in

otherwise healthy-looking individuals who either do not admit to being alcoholic or do not think that they are more than social drinkers but do "socialize" quite often! Although folate deficiency is common in skid-row alcoholics with poor nutrition, severe alcoholics with good nutrition may have megaloblastic changes in the marrow without associated folate or cobalamin deficiency. Furthermore, ethanol intake of 40–60 g daily may cause macrocytosis without associated megaloblastic changes.

The mechanism of macrocytosis in alcoholics is not clear. Ethanol interfers with folate metabolism at the cellular level, increases folate requirement by microsomal induction, increases folate loss (in urine and in stool), and decreases folate absorption. However, macrocytosis in alcoholics persists even when they take folate supplement and continue to drink. Ethanol has toxic effects in all marrow progenitor cells, especially erythroid cells, has inhibitory effect on $Na^+–K^+$–ATPase, and causes changes in fatty acid composition, lipid content, and fluidization of the red cell membrane, all of which may contribute to macrocytosis (77, 95).

The macrocytosis of *liver disease* is due to changes in red cell membrane phospholipids as the result of deficiency of lecithin-cholesterol acyltransferase (LCAT). The deficiency of this liver enzyme in plasma causes changes in red cell membrane phospholipids (increased cholesterol and phosphatidylcholine that results in formation of thin macrocytes and target cells).

The mechanism of macrocytosis in *obstructive jaundice* is due to inhibition of LCAT enzyme activity by bile salts that are retained in plasma as the result of biliary obstruction.

Reticulocytes, especially those produced under increased erythropoietin stimulation, are larger than mature erythrocytes. When there is increased demand for erythrocyte production, erythroid precursors skip one or two mitotic division in order to enter the blood circulation earlier. This results in production of larger reticulocytes and larger mature erythrocytes. Consequently, any condition that is associated with reticulocytosis—*hemolytic anemia, following acute blood loss,* and *erythropoietin therapy*—can cause macrocytosis. The mechanism of macrocytosis in aplastic anemia or in myelophthisic conditions is not clear but may be due to increase erythropoietin stimulation. Macrocytosis in the *absence of spleen* is due to lack of "polishing effect" of the spleen, which normally removes structural imperfections from the cell membrane as well as Heinz bodies and Howell-Jolly bodies from the red cell. Most *cancer chemotherapeutic agents* cause macrocytosis by interfering with DNA synthesis and or by suppressing the erythropoiesis. The macrocytosis of *hypothyroidism* is at least in part due to increased cholesterol in red cell membranes. However, it should be noted that there is also higher association of hypothyroidism with pernicious anemia (table 2.5) and with folate deficiency (due to folate malabsorption, which itself is due to myxedematous gut). The macrocytosis of *Myelodysplasias* and *Down syndrome* are due to impaired erythropoiesis.

Table 2.6 Causes of Nonmegaloblastic Macrocytosis

Physiological cause
  Newborn
  Pregnancy
Pathological causes
  Chronic alcoholism
  Liver disease
  Obstructive jaundice
  Rapid red cell production (following acute blood loss, chronic hemolysis, erthropoietin therapy)
  Aplastic anemia or marrow suppression, chemotherapy, marrow infiltration
  Myelodysplastic syndromes ($5q^-$, sideroblastic anemia)
  Hypothyroidism
  Absence of spleen
  Down syndrome
  Chronic obstructive lung disease (COPD)
  Selenium deficiency
  Multiple sclerosis
  Hereditary hydrocytosis
  Unexplained macrocytosis of nature women (hormonal?)
Artefactual (when determined by electronic equipment)
  Presence of cold agglutinin
  Presence of very high white cell count
  Severe hyperglycemia
  Blood sample left at room temperature for several hours
  Partial blockade of instrument's aperture

Spurious macrocytosis (laboratory artifact) may be produced by electronic cell counters when there are:

1. cold agglutinin (due to clumping of red cells at room temperature);
2. very high WBC count (white cells have much higher cell volumes than red cells and they are also counted as red cells by electronic instruments);
3. partial blockade of the instrument's aperture;
4. when the blood sample is left at room temperature for several hours;
5. severe hyperglycemia (due to intracellular hyperosmolality and entry of water into red cells when blood is diluted by the electronic instruments).

The false results in the first four conditions should be picked up by a good laboratory technologist and noted on the report, but the technologist is not aware of the presence of hyperglycemia and will not comment on the false macrocytosis produced by hyperglycemia.

We should emphasize that although the conditions cited above can cause macrocytosis, one should not attribute the macrocytosis to any of these conditions without excluding cobalamin and folate deficiency by checking serum cobalamin and serum folate levels. Many of the conditions cited above may be associated with folate or cobalamin deficiency, which, if not recognized, may proceed to cause significant morbidity. Furthermore, as mentioned earlier, macrocytosis is the eariest abnormality seen in CBC of folate or cobalamin-deficient patient.

The diagnosis of megaloblastic anemia is quite easy if one pays attention to the history and to common clues available through routine laboratory tests (e.g., macrocytosis and increased number of hypersegmented neutrophils). The establishment of the cause is often easy and the management is even easier. Furthermore, the treatment is inexpensive and brings great satisfaction to the symptomatic patient and the attending physician. While hematologic abnormalities, no matter how severe, will fully resolve with treatment, the neurologic abnormalities of cobalamin deficiency may become irreversible if not treated early. Unfortunately, considerable delay in recognizing folate or cobalamin deficiency often occurs, because many physicians ignore MCV and description of blood smear unless the patient's hemoglobin is quite low or anemia is associated with leukopenia or thrombocytopenia (96, 97). Even when the possibility of folate or cobalamin deficiency is considered, there is often unnecessary delay in completing the investigation and starting therapy, causing prolonged hospitalization and possibly additional morbidity (96).

Appendix

Laboratory Investigation of Megaloblastic Anemias

Having discussed the pathophysiology of megaloblastic anemias, we can now turn to the laboratory investigation of megaloblastic anemias. Appropriate use of laboratory studies facilitates accurate diagnosis in an economical fashion. The technical aspects of the tests discussed below are beyond the scope of this chapter, but we shall discuss the basis of these tests and the proper interpretation of the test results.

Laboratory investigation of megaloblastic anemias involves three groups of tests:

Tests to Establish the Presence of Megaloblastic Anemia

These tests include examination of peripheral blood (*CBC* and *examination of blood smear*) and *bone marrow aspiration*.

Tests to Differentiate between Folate Deficiency and Cobalamin Deficiency

These tests include *serum and/or red cell folate, serum cobalamin level, urinary FIGlu excretion, urinary MMA excretion, serum MMA level, dUST*, and *therapeutic trial*.

Tests to Establish the Cause of Folate or Cobalamin Deficiency

These tests include *tests of folate or cobalamin absorption, gastric analysis, IF antibody*, and *transcobalamin levels*.

Tests to establish the presence of megaloblastic anemia, i.e., CBC, examination of peripheral blood smear, and bone marrow aspiration, have already been discussed. In megaloblastic anemia, examination of the blood smear shows the presence of macrocytosis as well as increased number of hypersegmented neutrophils. As mentioned earlier, in addition to megaloblastic anemias there are numerous conditions that cause macrocytosis of the RBCs (see table 2.6). Similarly, there are several other causes for increased number of hypersegmented neutrophils in peripheral smear: *chronic infection, myeloproliferative disorders, renal failure, severe iron deficiency anemia,* and hereditary hypersegmentation of neutrophil nuclei. However, when both macrocytosis and increased number of hypersegmented neutrophils are present, there is strong indication that megaloblastic changes are present in the bone marrow.

Tests to Diagnose Folate and Cobalamin Deficiency

Serum folate assay

Serum folate may be determined by microbiologic method using *Lactobacillus casei* or by an isotope method using competitive or noncompetitive ligand-binding principles. Low serum folate is the earliest laboratory sign of folate deficiency (4), but it often occurs without folate deficiency. In Herbert's study (4), serum folate fell below normal after 3 weeks of folate-depleted diet, whereas increased hypersegmented neutrophils occurred after 7 weeks, very mild megaloblastic changes after 10 weeks, increased urinary FIG LU excretion after 13 weeks, red cell folate below normal after 17 weeks, macroovalocytosis in peripheral blood after 18 weeks, overtly megaloblastic marrow after 19

weeks, and anemia after 20 weeks on folate-depleted diet (4). *Low serum folate does not always indicate folate deficiency.* It is common in hospitalized patients due to short-term decrease in dietary folate intake and is seen in 2–19% of patients with megaloblastic anemia due to cobalamin deficiency and in 60% of patients with viral or mycoplasma infections (98). Serum folate may also be low in iron-deficiency anemia. Similarly, acetylsalicylic acid (aspirin) ingestion may result in low serum folate level by reducing the folate-binding capacity of the serum (99). Uremia may cause falsely low serum folate results in the assays in which separation of folate from binders is not required. Familiarity with the type of assay used by the laboratory is important for the proper interpretation of the test results. Some antibiotics and antineoplastic agents, for example, may inhibit the growth of *L. casei* in the microbiologic assay, thereby again producing falsely low result (100), whereas these agents have no effect in the radioisotope assay of folates. Folate antagonists such as methotrexate, pyrimethamine, trimethoprim, etc., which may cause megaloblastic changes in the bone marrow, would result in normal serum folate by isotope assay and may produce falsely low serum folate in microbiologic assay, reflecting the greater antifolate activity of the agents on *L. casei* than on bone marrow cells. Falsely low serum folate values may be obtained in the radioisotope assay when the serum contains other radioactive materials, such as ^{99m}Tc or ^{67}Ga (5, 100). The range of normal serum folate levels reported by different laboratories also varies considerably, depending on the method of assay, and even among laboratories that are presumably using the same method of assay. Consequently, patients' serum folate results should always be compared with the normal values reported by the same laboratory that has performed the test.

Erythrocyte folate assay

Red cell folate may be measured by the same techniques with which serum folate is measured. The concentration of red cell folate normally is 20–50 times that of serum. Red cell folate is more representative of the tissue concentration of folates. In the course of the development of folate deficiency, the fall in red cell folate (below normal) occurs much later than in serum folate. The high dilution of blood required for erythrocyte folate assay generally dilutes antibiotics and antimetabolites to the point that they no longer inhibit the growth of microorganism used in the microbiologic assay. Consequently, erythrocyte folate is generally unaffected in subjects whose serum folate is falsely low due to antibiotics or antineoplastic agents (except methotrexate which also causes low red cell folate in microbiologic assay). Erythrocyte folate may remain low and informative if a folate-deficient patient has received a few doses of folic acid and the patient's serum folate has returned to normal. When folate deficiency has developed rapidly (in prematurity, pregnancy, and in total parenteral nutrition), red cell folate may remain normal despite megaloblastic morphology of the bone marrow (5, 100). Erythrocyte folate is significantly higher in iron deficiency anemia than in normal subjects.

The major disadvantage of red cell folate is that it often does not discriminate between cobalamin deficiency and folate deficiency megaloblastic anemia. In severe cobalamin deficiency anemia, more patients may have low erythrocyte folate than have low serum folate. Review of different reports has shown that 2–19% of PA patients have low serum folate but 23–62% have low erythrocyte folate. The reduced erythrocyte folate in cobalamin deficiency results from the reduced polyglutamate content of erythrocytes, which may be explained either by th "methylfolate trap" or "formate starvation" hypotheses, described above. The question of whether to order serum folate or red cell folate is often asked. Each test has its own advantages and limitations: although red cell folate is a better representative of body store of folate, once megaloblastic anemia has developed, determination of serum folate with serum cobalamin is simpler and more informative than determination of red cell folate with serum cobalamin. In a recent retrospective review of serum and red cell data, it was concluded that 95% of patients who had red cell folate determination would have had identical outcomes even if red cell folate level had not been available (101).

Serum cobalamin assay

Serum cobalamin level may be measured either by microbiologic (*Lactobacillus leichmannii* or *Euglena gracilis*) or radioisotope assay. Antibiotics and antimetabolites that give falsely low serum folate may also produce falsely low serum cobalamin in microbiologic assay (100). The use of β-lactamase to reduce interference of antibiotic has been proposed. *E. gracilis* assay is not affected by these antibiotics, but sulfonamide and chlorpromazine may produce falsely low values in the *Euglena* assay (100). The presence in serum of other radioisotope materials (^{99m}Tc or ^{67}Ga) may produce falsely low serum cobalamin in radioisotope assays. Serum cobalamin is generally low in cobalamin deficiency megaloblastic anemia but may remain normal in *TCII deficiency* or when cobalamin deficiency is associated with conditions that cause very high TCI, such as in *chronic myelocytic leukemia or some malignancies* (100). Similarly, in *hepatitis* or when there is *liver cell necrosis*, the release of cobalamin in blood circulation may raise the serum cobalamin and mask a cobalamin deficiency state. Low serum cobalamin does not necessary indicates cobalamin deficiency. There are several conditions that may be associated with low serum cobalamin but normal body stores of cobalamin. Such conditions include: *primary folate deficiency, pregnancy, iron deficiency, multiple myeloma, hereditary absence of TCI, use of oral contraceptives, hyporegenerative neutropenias* (e.g., *chemotherapy-induced granulocytopenia, aplastic anemias*, etc.), *anticonvulsants*, or *use of large doses of vitamin C* (5, 100). Unlike low serum folate, which may result from a short-term dietary deficiency or increased demand, low serum cobalamin generally implies a long-term abnormality and should be taken seriously. Since undiagnosed cobalamin deficiency may progress to cause severe morbidity and even irreversible neurologic complications, a low serum cobalamin (130 pmol/L) should be always investigated to exclude or confirm true cobalamin deficiency, which requires treatment.

Urinary FIG LU excretion test

This test, which was originally proposed for the diagnosis of folate deficiency, is now rarely used for routine investigation of megaloblastic anemias, although it may have some application in research. It may also be of use in the study of subjects receiving certain folate antagonists in whom neither microbiologic nor radioassay of serum folate provide reliable information. Urinary FIG LU is increased in folate deficiency, but may also be increased in cobalamin deficiency, in liver cirrhosis, and in certain inborn errors of metabolism.

Urinary MMA excretion

MMA is produced from the metabolism of propionic acid, valine, leucine, isoleucine, and methionine. With the exception of rare cases of hereditary inborn errors of metabolism that may cause methylmalonic aciduria, increased MMA excretion indicates deficiency of cobalamin coenzyme (AdoCbl). Urinary MMA may be measured colorimetrically, chromatographically (with paper, thin-layer, or gas) by mass spectrometry, and, more recently, by capillary gas chromatography-mass spectrometry. The test is useful for assessing the tissue level of cobalamin coenzyme, AdoCbl, when the serum cobalamin level is low, but it is not clear whether the low serum cobalamin represents true deficiency. The test is not widely available and the requirement of loading dose of valine or leucine and 24-hour urine collection diminishes its practicability.

Serum MMA and homocysteine

The recent development of the sensitive capillary gas chromatography-mass spectrometry method has allowed the measurement of serum MMA and homocysteine. Since both of these substances require cobalamin for further metabolism, their measurement allows for the assessment of cobalamin status at the cellular level. In cobalamin deficiency, both serum MMA and homocysteine are increased, whereas in folate deficiency, serum homocysteine is increased but serum MMA is normal. These tests have been reported to be abnormal in some cobalamin deficient patients with normal serum cobalamin level. In one study (102) serum MMA and/or total homocysteine were greater than 3 standard deviations above normal in 94% of cobalamin-responsive patients. Another report by the same group (90) indicated that 95% of patients who had relapsed or were suboptimally treated for cobalamin deficiency showed early elevation of serum MMA and/or total homocysteine, but only 69% showed subnormal serum cobalamin. In 419 consecutive cases of proven cobalamin deficiency, 12 patients had normal serum cobalamin but increased serum MMA and/or total homocysteine. The ratio of MMA in CSF to that in serum is reported to be higher than normal in subjects with neuropsychiatric manifestations of cobalamin deficiency

(103). The advantage of these tests is that they can be performed on the same sample as cobalamin assay in order to refine otherwise inconclusive results. The major disadvantage of these tests is that they are at present costly and complicated to perform and are only available in a very limited number of laboratories.

The deoxyuridine (dU) suppression test (dUST)

This test directly measures the incorporation of [³H]thymidine (^{3}H-TdR) in marrow culture cells in the presence of deoxyuridine and indirectly assess the adequacy or inadequacy of de novo pathway of thymidine synthesis (85). Normally, most of the thymine in DNA is derived from the de novo pathway and only a small amount is derived from direct phosphorylation of preformed thymidine (salvage pathway). In dUST, aliquots of marrow cells are cultured in the presence or absence of deoxyuridine and in the presence or in the absence of cobalamin or folate (^{3}H-TdR being supplied to all the tubes). The incorporation of ^{3}H-TdR in the cells of the tubes which have no dU represents the contribution of the salvage pathway and exhibits the highest radioactivity. The amount of radioactivity in the cells of the tubes containing dU but no cobalamin or folate represent the suppressed ^{3}H-TdR uptake due to de novo synthesis of TdR from dU. Normally, about 95% of the thymidine requirement of marrow cells is met by de novo synthesis and the ^{3}H-TdR uptake by the cells in the tube containing dU is < 5% of those in the control tube (without dU, folate, and cobalamin). In folate or cobalamin-deficient bone marrow culture, less dU is converted to TdR, so more ^{3}H-TdR is incorporated in marrow cells (>10%). In patients with cobalamin deficiency, addition of cobalamin or formyltetrahydrofolic acid, but not methyltetrahydrofolate, corrects the abnormal dUST. In patients with folate deficiency, addition of folic acid, methyl-FH$_4$, or formyl-FH$_4$ corrects the dUST, but cobalamin does not. In principle, this is a good test for differentiating between the diagnosis of folate and cobalamin deficiency and provides the answer in the same day. However, the test is not available in most hospitals. It requires fresh bone marrow aspirate (10–15 ml in standard test and 2 ml in micromethod test) and the test has to be planned in advance. In addition, the test is time consuming and expensive. The fact that it can provide rapid diagnosis of folate and cobalamin deficiency is hardly an advantage worth the cost, because there is no urgency to make the diagnosis on the same day as long as one can start treatment with cobalamin and/or folate while awaiting the result. Nonetheless, dUST is a very useful research tool in the study of the pathogenesis of, for example, drug-induced megaloblastic anemias, as well as in the elucidation of various inherited syndromes associated with cobalamin or folate deficiency or errors of folate and cobalamin metabolism. It is also useful, if available, in the study of patients with low serum folate but normal bone marrow, in the diagnosis of folate deficiency when red cell folate is normal or has become normal with transfusion, and when folate or cobalamin deficiency is suspected but blood and bone marrow morphology are normal or controversial (85).

Therapeutic trial

As stated earlier, a deficiency of either vitamin may show a hematologic response when large doses of the other vitamin is given. However, when only the minimal daily requirement of vitamin is provided, the patient will respond with reticulocytosis only if the deficiency involved that vitamin. The therapeutic trial doses for folate deficiency is 0.1 mg of folic acid daily given orally or given intramuscularly for 10 days, and for cobalamin deficiency it is 1 µg of vitamin B$_{12}$ given intramuscularly daily for 10 days. Demonstration of a significant rise in reticulocyte count in anemic patients within 10 days constitutes a satisfactory response to therapeutic trial. This method of diagnosing the vitamin deficiency was commonly employed before assays for folate and cobalamin and tests of cobalamin absorption were available.

Tests for Study of the Causes of Folate and Cobalamin Deficiency

Tests of cobalamin absorption

Cobalamin absorption may be assessed by giving a test dose of radioactive cobalamin and determining its urinary or fecal excretion, as well as its plasma level or total body retention (5, 100, 104). Tests of fecal excretion are rarely used in clinical laboratories. Hepatic uptake of radioactivity is also rarely used, but may be useful if urine collection for the Schilling test is incomplete. In such cases, counting the radioactivity over the liver after a few days can determine whether cobalamin absorption is adequate. A common method of assessing cobalamin absorption is the Schilling test, which is based on urinary excretion of radiolabeled cobalamin. In this test, the patient first receives 0.5–2 µg of radiolabeled cobalamin orally (test dose) and subsequently (1–4 hours later) receives 1 mg of vitamin B$_{12}$ intramuscularly (flushing dose). A 24-hour urine sample is then collected for measurement of radioactivity. The large, nonradioactive, flushing dose of cobalamin given parenterally is absorbed before the oral dose, and therefore saturates the cobalamin binders in the blood. Consequently, much of the absorbed radiolabeled cobalamin cannot bind the transcobalamins and so is excreted in the urine. Normally, depending on the test dose, >5–16% of radioactivity appear in the urine. If cobalamin absorption is decreased, then less than this normal amount of radioactivity will be excreted in the 24-hour urine sample. Falsely abnormal Schilling tests can occur due to *incomplete urine collection, renal failure, failure to give the flushing dose of cobalamin,* or *use of decomposed radioactive cobalamin* (5, 100, 104). Incomplete urine collection is a common source of error in the Schilling test. Unfortunately, since the pattern of absorption of cobalamin differs from that of other substances, and there is delay in absorption of cobalamin, detection and correction for incomplete collection with the use of other markers is not possible. Loss of urine in the first 3 hours may not affect the Schilling test result, but loss of urine sample between 8 and 12 hours after the test dose may significantly reduce the amount of radiolabeled cobalamin in the urine. Before performing a Schilling test, some centers collect a 24-hour urine sample as a "rehearsal" in comparison with the urine volume during the Schilling test and in order to detect radioactivity from other sources. However, this procedure causes additional hardship for the patient (especially for the outpatient). Some centers administer a second flushing dose of cobalamin after 24 hours and collect the urine for another 24 hours. This approach may eliminate the falsely abnormal Schilling test in renal impairment, and will increase the gap between normal and abnormal cobalamin excretion. Furthermore it results in the removal of a greater amount of radioactivity from the body. *Falsely normal Schilling tests may be obtained when urine is contaminated with stool or when other isotopes, such as ^{99m}Tc, are excreted in the urine following organ scanning.* Determination of *plasma radioactivity* following the administration of the test dose has been used as a test of cobalamin absorption. However, several studies have demonstrated a significant overlap in results between control subjects and PA patients (104), and it is better to use this method in conjunction with the Schilling test rather than on its own.

Irrespective of the test used for cobalamin absorption, if the result indicates cobalamin malabsorption, the test may be repeated after giving the test dose of radiolabeled cobalamin with IF. If addition of IF corrects the cobalamin malabsorption, it is assumed that cobalamin malabsorption is due to lack of IF (PA, gastrectomy, congenital absence of IF). If addition of IF does not make the correction, cobalamin malabsorption is due to an intestinal defect. When bacterial overgrowth is thought to be responsible for cobalamin malabsorption, the test of cobalamin absorption may be repeated following a course of antibiotic (tetracycline) therapy. If the test of absorption becomes normal, then it is assumed that cobalamin malabsorption was due to bacterial overgrowth.

A *double isotope technique* for assessing both free and IF-bound-cobalamin absorption is also available. In this test, ^{58}Co-labeled free cobalamin and ^{57}Co-labeled Cbl-IF are given simultaneously to the patient, and either the plasma ratio or the urinary ratio of the two isotopes is determined. In normal subjects, i.e., when IF excretion is adequate, the absorption or excretion of both free and IF-bound cobalamin is similar, so the ratio of isotopes (in urine or in plasma) is close to one. However, in PA or when IF is lacking, more of ^{57}Co than ^{58}Co is absorbed or excreted in urine. This test is simple, and in theory, has a few advantages over the standard Schilling test, since it eliminates the need for repeating the test with Cbl-IF, and the results would be reliable even if urine collection is incomplete or if there is renal failure. However, in practice, misleading results may be obtained, with an overlap between the results in normal control subjects and patients with PA. This phenomenon is attributed to exchange between free cobalamin and cobalamin bound to IF (104).

Test of Protein-Bound Cobalamin Absorption

Patients who have cobalamin deficiency but are not vegetarians are generally assumed to have cobalamin malabsorption. However, some of these patients may show a normal Schilling test. In such cases, the possibility of malabsorption of protein-bound cobalamin (food cobalamin) should be considered (51, 105, 106). The absorption of protein-bound cobalamin may be determined by use of radiolabeled cobalamin bound to chicken meat, chicken serum, egg yolk, or egg white (51, 104, 105). The transfer of protein-bound cobalamin to gastric R-binder requires acid pH and pepsinogen. Patients with simple atrophic gastritis, because of gastric hypo- or achlorhydria and deficiency of pepsinogen, cannot absorb this protein-bound cobalamin, but may still excrete enough IF to have adequate absorption of crystalline cobalamin used in the Schilling test. Nevertheless, in these patients true cobalamin deficiency may eventually develop. Since severe megaloblastic anemia from any cause may result in cobalamin malabsorption due to abnormality of the gut mucosa (megaloblastic gut), *it is best to perform the tests of cobalamin absorption after proper therapy has corrected the megaloblastic changes in the gut.* Furthermore, if a Schilling test is performed too early in the investigation of anemia, the large flushing dose of cobalamin given with the test may correct the megaloblastic changes irrespective of the deficiency, so that subsequent examination of the bone marrow may provide misleading results.

Tests of folate absorption

Tests of folate absorptions are rarely used in clinical practice because dietary deficiency constitutes the major cause. When abnormal absorption is suspected, there is often evidence of malabsorption of other nutrients, and it is inferred that folate is also not absorbed adequately. Nevertheless, numerous methods for folate absorption are available in centers interested in the study of folates. Folate absorption can be measured by administration of an oral test dose of mono- or polyglutamate folate (either cold or [^{3}H]-labeled) after tissue folate has been saturated by several days of folate administration, and then detecting a rise in serum folate or urinary excretion of folate (either *Streptococcus fecalis* or *L. casei* assay or radioactivity). Alternatively, folate absorption may be determined by measuring fecal excretion of [H_3]-labeled folate or by comparing 24-hour urinary excretion of folate after an oral test dose of folate with a 24-hour urine sample following similar dose of folate administered subcutaneously or using the double- or triple-lumen jejunal perfusion method.

Intrinsic factor and parietal cell antibodies

There are two types of IF antibody in PA, one which binds IF at its cobalamin-binding site and prevents binding of cobalamin to IF and is sometimes called "blocking" or "type I" antibody, and the other, which binds IF or IF-Cbl at the site away from its cobalamin-binding site and is called "IF binding" or "type II" antibody and may interfere with binding of IF-Cbl to intestinal receptors. Just over half of the patients with PA have blocking IF antibody, and about 35% have the binding type, but the binding type is generally seen in those who also have blocking antibody.

IF antibody may also present in gastric secretions (IgG or secretary IgA). The presence of IF antibody in cobalamin deficiency constitutes strong evidence for PA, since the presence of IF antibody other than in PA is rare. On the other hand, parietal cell antibody, which is frequently found in serum of patients with adult PA (but not in congenital absence of IF), is so commonly seen in other conditions that it has very little diagnostic value in the investigation of cobalamin deficiency.

Gastric analysis

Before the tests of cobalamin absorption and assays of serum folate and cobalamin became available, gastric analysis was frequently employed in the investigation of megaloblastic anemia, but is now seldom used in clinical practice (except in rare cases of congenital IF deficiency). In adult PA, there is a gastric achlorhydria that is permanent and remains abnormal after hematologic correction with cobalamin therapy. However, gastric achlorhydria is not unique to PA and may be seen in severe folate or iron deficiency, as well as in the elderly population. Thus, the presence of gastric achlorhydria does not constitute evidence of PA, but the absence of gastric achlorhydria excludes the diagnosis of the adult type of PA. Gastric analysis is time consuming and requires gastric intubation with considerable discomfort to the patient and should not be used except in investigation of unexplained cobalamin deficiency in childhood and adolescence. However, if one goes through the trouble of collecting gastric juice for gastric analysis, in addition to the volume and free HCl determination, IF content of gastric juice should also be determined. In PA, the IF content of gastric juice is absent or markedly decreased.

Noninvasive tests of gastric atrophy are available in some centers. *Low levels of serum pepsinogen I and low values of serum pepsinogen I/pepsinogen II ratio correlate well with the presence of gastric atrophy.*

REFERENCES

1. Herbert V. Biology of disease: megaloblastic anemias. Lab Invest 1985;52:3.
2. Fliedner TM, Cronkite EP, Killmann SÅ, Bond VP. Granulocytopoiesis: II, emergence and pattern of labelling of neutrophilic granulocytes in humans. Blood 1964; 24:683.
3. Wickermasinghe SN, Pratt JR. Myelocyte proliferation in pernicious anemia. Acta Haematol 1970;44:37.
4. Herbert V. Experimental nutritional folate deficiency in man. Trans Assoc Am Physicians 1962;75:307.
5. Chanarin I. Investigation and management of megaloblastic anemia. Clin Haematol 1976;5:747.
6. Carmel R. Pernicious anemia: the expected findings of very low serum cobalamin levels anemia and macrocytosis are often lacking. Arch Intern Med 1988;148:1712.
7. Van Der Weyden MB, Hyman RJ, Rose IS, Brumley J. Folate-deficient human lymphoblasts—changes in deoxynucleotide metabolism and thymidylate cycle activities. Eur J Haematol 1991;47:109.
8. Lindenbaum J, Pezzimenti JF, Shea N. Small intestinal function in vitamin B_{12} deficiency. Ann Intern Med 1974; 80:326.
9. Levine P. A qualitative platelet defect in severe vitamin B_{12} deficiency: response hyperresponse and thrombosis after vitamin B_{12} therapy. Ann Intern Med 1973;78:533.
10. Falcao RP. Neutrophil function in megaloblastic anemia. Braz J Med Biol Res 1988;21:939.
11. Kátká K. Immune function in pernicious anemia before and during treatment with vitamin B_{12}. Scand J Haematol 1984; 32:76.
12. Das KG, Mohanty D, Garewal G. Cytogenetics in nutritional megaloblstic anemia: prolonged persistance of chromosomal abnormalities in lymphocytes after remission. Acta Haematol (Basel) 1986;76:146.
13. Chanarin I. Folate deficiency. In: Blakely RL, Whitehead VM, ed. Folates and pterines: nutritional, pharmacological and physiological aspects. Vol. 3. New York: Wiley-Interscience, 1986.
14. Kass L. Pernicious anemia. Philadelphia: WB Saunders, 1976.
15. Rodriquez MS. A conspectus of research on folacin requirement in man. J Nutr 1978;108:1983.
16. Shane B. Folypolyglutamate synthesis and role in the regulation of one carbon metabolism. In: Auerbach GD, McCormick DB, eds. Vitam Horm 1989;45:263.
17. Herbert V. Recommended dietary intake (RDI) of folate in humans. Am J Clin Nutr 1987;45:661.
18. McNulty H, McPartlin JM, Weir DG, Scott JM. Folate catabolism in normal subjects. Hum Nutr Appl Nutr 1987; 41:338.
19. Food and Nutrition Board. Recommended dietary allowance. 10th ed. Washington, DC, 1989 (also published in Am J Diet Assoc 1989;89:1750).
20. Halstead CH. The intestinal absorption of dietary folate in health and disease. Am Col Nutr 1989;8:650.
21. Said HM, Ghishan FK, Redha R. Folate transport by human intestinal brush border membrane vesicles. Am J Physiol 1987;252:G229.
22. Said HM, Redha R, Tipton W, Nylander W. Folate transport in ileal brush border membrane vesicles following extensive resection of proximal and middle small intestine in the rat. Am J Clin Nutr 1988;47:75.
23. Henderson GB. Folate binding proteins. Annu Rev Nutr 1990;10:319.
24. Steinberg SE, Campbell CL, Hillman RS. Kinetics of normal folate enterohepatic cycle. J Clin Invest 1979;64:83.
25. Kane MA, Waxman S. Biology of disease: role of folate binding proteins in folate metabolism. Lab Invest 1989; 60:737.
26. Rothberg KG, et al. The glycophospholipid-linkled folate receptor internalized folate without entering the clathrin-coated pit endocytic pathway. J Cell Biol 1990;110:637.
27. Spector R. Cerebrospinal fluid folate and the blood brain barrier. In: Botez I, Reynold EH. Folic acid in neurology psychiatry and internal medicine. New York: Raven Press, 1979.
28. Hoppner K, Lambi B. Folate levels in human livers from autopsies in Canada. Am J Clin Nutr 1980;33:382.
29. Heinrich CH. Metabolic basis of the diagnosis and therapy of B_{12} deficiency. Semin Hematol 1964;1:199.
30. Mehta BM, Rege DV, Satoskar RS. Serum B_{12} and folic acid activity in lactovegetarian and nonvegetarian healthy adult indians. Am J Clin Nutr 1964;15:77.
31. Sulivan LW, Herbert V. Studies on minimum daily requirement of vitamin B_{12}. N Engl J Med 1965;272:340.

32. Kapadia CR, Donaldson RM. Disorders of cobalamin (vitamin B_{12}) absorption and transport. Annu Rev Med 1985; 36:93.

33. Hall CA. Transcobalamin I and II as natural transport proteins of vitamin B_{12}. J Clin Invest 1975;56:1125.

34. Berlin H, Berlin R, Brante G. Oral treatment of pernicious anemia with high doses of vitamin B_{12} without intrinsic factor. Acta Med Scand 1968;184:247.

35. Chanarin I. The megaloblastic anemias. 2d ed. Oxford: Blackwell, 1979.

36. Lederle FA. Oral cobalamin for pernicious anemia: medicine's best kept secret. JAMA 1991;265:94.

37. Jacob E, Baker SJ, Herbert V. Vitamin B_{12} binding proteins. Physiol Rev 1980;60:918.

38. Neale G. B_{12} binding proteins. Gut 1990;31:59.

39. Stupperich E, Nexø E. Effect of cobalt-N coordination on the cobamide recognition by the human vitamin B_{12} binding proteins intrinsic factor transcobalamin and haptocorin. Eur J Biochem 1991;199:299.

40. Gailani SD, Carey RW, Holland JF, O'Malley JA. Studies of folate deficiency in patients with neoplastic diseases. Cancer Res 1970;30:327.

41. Cox EV. The clinical manifestation of B_{12} deficiency in addisonian pernicious anemia. In: Heinrich HC, ed. Vitamin B_{12} and intrinsic factor. Proceedings of the Second European Symposium on Vitamin B_{12} and Intrinsic Factor. Hamburg: Enke, 1962.

42. Scott E. The prevalence of pernicious anemia in Great Britain. J Coll Gen Pract Res 1960;3:80.

43. Carmel R, Johnson CS, Weiner JM. Pernicious anemia in Latin Americans is not a disease of elderly. Arch Intern Med 1987;147:1995.

44. McIntyre PA, Hahn R, Conley CL, Glass B. Genetic factors in predisposition to pernicious anemia. Bull Johns Hopkins Hosp 1959;104:309.

45. Varis E, et al. Gastric morphology function and immunology in first-degree relatives of probands with pernicious anemia and controls. Scand J Gastroenterol 1979; 14:129.

46. Borch K. Epidemiologic clinicopathologic and economic aspects of gastroscopic screening of patients with pernicious anemia. Scand J Gastroenterol 1986;21:20.

47. Wodzinski MA, Forrest MJ, Barnett D, Lawrence ACK. Lymphocyte subpopulations in patients with hydroxycobalamin responsive anemia. J Clin Pathol 1985;38:582.

48. Ardeman S, Chanarin I. Steroids and Addisonian pernicious anemia. N Engl J Med 1965;273:1352.

49. Linnell JC, Bhatt HR. Inherited errors of cobalamin metabolism. Clin Hematol 1995;8:567.

50. Fenton WA, Rosenberg LE. Inherited disorders of cobalamin transport and metabolism. In: Scriver CR, Beaudet AL, Sly WS, Valle D. Metabolic and molecular bases of inherited diseases. 7th ed. New York: McGraw-Hill, 1995.

51. Carmel R. Malabsorption of food cobalamin. Clin Hematol 1995;8:639.

52. Doyle JJ, Langevin AM, Zipursky A. Nutritional vitamin B_{12} deficiency in infancy: three case reports and a review of the litterature. Pediatr Hematol Oncol 1989;6:161.

53. Hines JD. Ascorbic acid and vitamin B_{12} deficiency. JAMA 1975;234:24.

54. Koblin DD, et al. Effect of nitrous oxide on folate and vitamin B_{12} metabolism in patients. Anesth Analg 1990; 71:610.

55. Skouby AP. Hydroxycobalamin for initial and long-term therapy for vitamin B_{12} deficiency. Acta Med Scand 1987; 221:399.

56. Lowenstein L, Cooper BA, Brunton L, Gartha S. An immunologic basis for acquired resistance to oral administration of hog intrinsic factor and vitamin B_{12} in pernicious anemia. J Clin Invest 1961;40;1656.

57. Lawson DH, Murray RM, Parker JLW. Early mortality in the megaloblastic anemias. Q J Med 1972;41:1.

58. Carmel R. Treatment of severe pernicious anemia: no association with sudden death. Am J Clin Nutr 1988; 48:1443.

59. Zamcheck N, Grable E, Ley A, Norman L. Occurrence of gastric cancer amoung patients with pernicious anemia at the Boston City Hospital. N Engl J Med 1955;252:1103.

60. Brinton LE, et al: Cancer risk following pernicious anemia. Br J Cancer 1989;59:810.

61. Rosenberg H, et al. Folate nutrition in elderly. Am J Clin Nutr 1982;36:1060.

62. Thompson JN, Hoppner K. Folic acid deficiency in Canada. In: Botez EH, Reynolds EH, eds. Folic acid in neurology psychiatry and internal medicine. New York: Raven Press, 1979.

63. Shojania AM. Folic acid and vitamin B_{12} deficiency in pregnancy and in the neonatal period. Clin Perinatol 1984; 11:433.

64. Tsui JC, Nordstrom JW. Folate status of adolescents: effects of folic acid supplementation. J Am Diet Assoc 1990; 90:1551.

65. Shojania AM. Oral contraceptives: effects on folate and vitamin B_{12} metabolism. Canad Med Assoc J 1982; 1226:244.

66. Rosenblatt DS. Inherited disorders of folate transport and metabolism. In: Scriver CR, Beaudet AL, Sly WS, Valle D, eds. The metabolic and molecular bases of inherited diseases. 7th ed. New York: McGraw-Hill, 1995.

67. Steinschneider M, et al. Congenital folate malabsorption: reversible clinical and neurophysiological abnormalities. Neurology 1990;40:1315.

68. Urbach J, Abrahamov A, Grossowicz N. Congenital isolated folic acid malabsorption. Arch Dis Child 1987;62:78.

69. Hoffbrand AV. Anemia in adult coeliac disease. Clin Gastroenterol 1974;3:71.

70. Thomas G, Clain DJ. Endemic tropical sprue in Rodesia. Gut 1976;17:877.

71. O'Brien W. Acute military tropical sprue in South East Asia. Am J Clin Nutr 1968;221:1007.

72. River JV, Rodrique De la Obra F, Maldonado MM. Anemia due to vitamin B_{12} deficiency after treatment with folic acid in tropical sprue. Am J Clin Nutr 1964;18:110.

73. Franklin JL, Rosenberg IH. Impaired folic acid absorption in inflamatory bowel disease: effects of salacylsulfadine (Azulfidine). Gastroenterology 1973;64:517.

74. Lambie DG, Johnson RH. Drugs and folate metabolism. Drugs 1985;30:145.

75. Stebbins R, Scott J, Herbert V. Drug induced megaloblastic anemias. Semin Hematol 1973;10:2235.

76. Zimmerman J, Selhub J, Rosenberg IH. Competitive inhibition of folate absorption by dihydrofolate reductase inhibitors trimethoprim and pyrimethamine. Am J Clin Nutr 1987;46:518.

77. Hillman RS, Steinberg SE. The effects of alcohol on folate metabolism. Annu Rev Med 1982;33:345.

78. Wickramasinghe SN, Williams G, Saunders J, Durston JHJ. Megalobalstic erythropoiesis and macrocytosis in patients on anticonvulsants. Br Med J 1975;4:136.

79. Klipstein FA, Berlinger FG, Reed LJ. Folate deficiency associated with drug therapy of tuberculosis. Blood 1967;29:697.

80. Morris JS. Nitrofurantoin and peripheral neuropathy with megaloblastic anemia. J Neurol Neurosurg Psychiatr 1966;29:224.

81. Wardrop CAJ, Heatley RV, Tennant GB, Hughes LE. Acute folate deficiency in surgical patients on aminoacid/ethanol interavenous nutrition. Lancet 1975;2:640.

82. Jeanette JC, Goldman JD. Inhibition of the membrane transport of folates by anions retained in uremia. J Lab Clin Med 1975;86:834.

83. Hansen DK. Embryotoxicity of phenytoin: an update on possible mechanisms. Proc Soc Exp Biol Med 1974;361:1991.

84. Kohashi M, Clement RP, Tse J, Piper WN. Rat hepatic uroporphyringoen III co-synthase. Biochem J 1984;220:755.

85. Metz J. The deoxyuridine suppression test. CRC Crit Rev Clin Lab Sci 1984;200:205.

86. Matthews JH, Armitage J, Wickramasinghe SN. Thymidine synthesis and utilization via the de novo pathway in normal and megaloblastic human bone marrow cells. Eur J Haematol 1989;42:396.

87. Iwata N, Omine M, Yamauchi H, Tadashi M. Characteristic abnormality of deoxyribonucleoside triphosphate metabolism in megaloblastic anemia. Blood 1982;60:918.

88. Poston JM, Stadtman TC. Cobamides as cofactors. Methylcobamides and the synthesis of methionine methane and acetate. In: Babior MB, ed. Cobalamin: biochemistry and physiology. New York: Wiley Interscience, 1975.

89. Babior BM. Cobamides as cofactors: adenosylcobamide dependent reactions. In: Babior MB, ed. Cobalamin: biochemistry and physiology. New York: Wiley Interscience, 1975.

90. Lindenbaum J, Savage DG, Stabler SP, Allen RH. Diagnosis of cobalamin deficiency; II, relative sensitivities of serum cobalamin methylmalonic acid and total homocysteine concentrations. Am J Hematol 1990;34:99.

91. Shane B, Stokstad ELR. Vitamin B_{12}-Folate Interrelations. Annu Rev Nutr 1985;5:115.

92. Chanarin I, Deacon R, Lumb M, Perry J. Cobalamin and folate: recent developments. J Clin Pathol 1992;45:277.

93. Colon-Otero G, Menke D, Hook CC. A practical approach to the differential diagnosis and evaluation of the adult patient with macrocytic anemia. Med Clin North Am 1992;76:581.

94. Savage D, Lindenbaum J. Anemia in alcoholics. Medicine 1986;65:322.

95. Taraschi TF, Rubin E. Biology of disease: effects of ethanol on chemical and structural properties of biologic membrane. Lab Invest 1985;52:120.

96. Shojania AM. Physician's management of suspected vitamin B_{12} deficiency. Can Med Assoc J 1980;123:1127.

97. Carmel R, Karnaze DS. Physician response to low serum cobalamin levels. Arch Intern Med 1983;146:1161.

98. Jacobson W, Wreghitt TG, Saich T, Nagington J. Serum folate in viral and mycoplasmal infections. J Infect 1987;14:103.

99. Alter HJ, Zvaifler NJ, Rath CE. Interaction of rheumatoid arthritis, folic acid and aspirin. Blood 1971;38:405.

100. Shojania AM. Problems in the diagnosis and investigation of megaloblastic anemia. Can Med Assoc J 1980;122:999.

101. Jaffe JP, Schilling RF. Erythrocyte folate levels: a clinical study. Am J Hematol 1991;36:116.

102. Stabler SP, Allen RM, Savage DG, Lindenbaum J. Clinical spectrum and diagnosis of cobalamin deficiency. Blood 1990;76:871.

103. Stabler SP, et al. Cerebrospinal fluid methylmalonic acid levels in normal subjects and in patients with Cbl deficiency. Neurology 1991;41:10.

104. Chanarin I. Isotopes in megaloblastic anaemia. Clin Haematol 1977;6:719.

105. Carmel R, Snow RM, Karnaze DS. Atypical cobalamin deficiency is commonly demonstrable in patients without megaloblastic anemia and is often associated with protein-bound cobalamin malabsorption. J Lab Clin Med 1987; 109:454.

106. Miller A, et al. Bound vitamin B_{12} absorption in patients with low serum B_{12} levels. Am J Hematol 1992;40:163.

CHAPTER 3

Globin Synthesis— Thalassemia Syndromes

GEORGE R. HONIG, BRUCE I. SHARON

"We cannot look into the cavities and marrows of the bones unless they be first broken. I observe a threefold cavity of the bones and a threefold marrow. In the greater cavities of the larger bones, the marrow is reddish, in the lesser cavities of the smaller bones the marrow is white. In the spongy bones there is contained a marrowy liquor."
—Riolanus, *Physic and Chyrurgery* (1657)

Case 1

A 7-month-old boy was found to be anemic. The infant was born full-term following an uneventful pregnancy and delivery. He progressed well until 5 months of age, at which time he was noted to have a decreased level of activity, poor appetite, and pallor. His weight showed a decrease from the 50th to the 25th percentile for his age and his spleen was observed to be enlarged, extending 3 cm below the costal margin. The infant otherwise appeared healthy. He was receiving no medications. The child's father was of Greek heritage; his mother's parentage was French-Dutch-German. The infant's blood count showed the following: hemoglobin 65 g/L, red blood cells (RBC) 3.5×10^{12}/L, mean corpuscular volume (MCV) 61 fl, RDW 13.5%, reticulocytes 2.7%, white blood cells (WBC) 10.3×10^9/L, and platelets 214×10^9/L. A stained blood smear demonstrated hypochromia, poikilocytosis, occasional target cells, and microcytosis; nucleated red cells were also seen. The infant's serum ferritin level was 220 mg/L and his corrected erythrocyte sedimentation rate was 5 mm/hr. His hemoglobin composition included: HbA 12%, HbA_2 2.1%, and HbF 86%.

Commentary

The microcytosis and hypochromia that characterize this infant's anemia make it possible to focus immediately on the differential diagnosis of a relatively small group of hematologic entities. These include iron or copper deficiency, due either to nutritional insufficiency of these minerals or occurring as a secondary manifestation of other pathologic processes; any of the various thalassemia syndromes; or one of a distinctly uncommon group of entities, the sideroblastic anemias.

The normally very rapid growth rate of infants during the first year of life imposes a substantial nutri-

tional requirement for iron, which will result in iron-deficiency anemia if not met. As a general rule, full-term infants who have not had significant blood loss are born with sufficient iron stores to meet their needs for approximately 6 months, even if they receive little or no exogenous iron. In this patient, therefore, iron deficiency would be an unlikely cause for his microcytic anemia, unless evidence could be found indicating occult blood loss. The ample serum ferritin level provides further justification for eliminating iron deficiency from the differential diagnosis.

The clinical and hematologic features of iron-deficiency anemia can also develop in patients with nutritional iron sufficiency, although under these circumstances the anemia is not usually of a very severe degree. Conditions that give rise to this form of iron deficiency result from metabolic or other factors that interfere with iron utilization in erythropoiesis. Chronic infections and other forms of inflammatory disease are frequently accompanied by this form of anemia. Iron stores in these patients, as estimated by bone marrow-stainable iron or by the level of serum ferritin, may be normal or elevated, yet the anemia may be quite responsive to iron therapy. The normal erythrocyte sedimentation rate in the case described above militates against this type of pathophysiology. Other conditions that can produce microcytic anemia due to an inhibition of iron utilization include the effects of various drugs and chemicals (lead poisoning, isoniazid, chloramphenicol) and the presence of underlying malignancy. None of these possibilities would appear to be likely in this case.

Only trace levels of copper are needed to prevent the microcytic anemia of copper deficiency. This uncommon deficiency state is likely to be encountered only in patients receiving total parenteral nutrition with a trace mineral-deficient regimen, or in association with severe generalized malnutrition, exudative enteropathy, or in Wilson disease. None of these possibilities merits serious consideration in this patient.

Microcytic anemia is also a prominent finding in a rare and heterogeneous group of disorders that are classified as sideroblastic or iron-loading anemias. These conditions may be congenital or acquired, with the latter forms seldom occurring in children. Many of the hereditary sideroblastic anemias follow an X-linked inheritance pattern, and some forms are responsive topyridoxine. The hemoglobin composition of the blood from patients with sideroblastic anemia is characteristically normal.

The thalassemias comprise by far the most prevalent group of congenital microcytic anemias. With laboratory evidence that makes it possible largely to exclude iron deficiency in this patient (including the normal RDW value), serious consideration needs to be given to the possibility of his having some form of thalassemia. His very high percentage of fetal hemoglobin (beyond 6 months of age HbF normally represents <3% of the total) could represent either the presence of one of the syndromes of persistence of HbF synthesis, or could reflect a compensatory change in response to deficient β-chain production. None of the known forms of hereditary persistence of fetal hemoglobin synthesis produces a significant degree of anemia or microcytosis, and this finding therefore can be taken as strong evidence that the child has a form of β-thalassemia (1). Although his percentage of HbA$_2$ was within the usual range of normal, when taken as a percentage of HbA it too was elevated. As part of the further evaluation of this patient's hematologic disorder, blood counts and hemoglobin analyses of both of his parents should be included, and would be likely to provide very useful information.

Normal Human Hemoglobins and Globin Genes

Functional human hemoglobin molecules are tetramer structures comprised of pairs of protein-heme subunit dimers. Each of these dimers contains an α- or α-like globin chain and a β- or β-like chain. The α-globin genes as well as an embryonic α-like gene referred to as ζ are localized to a 40-kilobase (kb) segment of the short arm of chromosome 16 (fig. 3. 1), whereas the β-globin gene cluster is on the short arm of chromosome 11. As a consequence of their separate chromosomal origins, α- and β-globin abnormalities segregate independently and may therefore be coinherited in any possible combination.

The β-globin gene cluster extends for approximately 60 kb, encompassing the ϵ-globin, $^G\gamma$-globin, $^A\gamma$-globin, δ-globin, and β-globin genes. Interestingly, the order in which these genes are organized on the chromosome parallels their sequential expression during embryonic, fetal, and postnatal development. The ϵ-globin gene is normally expressed only during the embryonic stage of development. The γ-globin genes exist as a closely linked gene pair; the globin chains that are encoded by these genes normally differ from each other by only a single amino acid, glycine or alanine, at position 136. The γ-globin genes are the primary non-α-globins produced during fetal life; their expression normally declines beginning shortly after the time of birth to be replaced by the synthesis of β-chains. By 6 months of age the adult pattern of globin chain synthesis is reached, with γ-globin synthesis representing <3% of the total. The δ-globin gene has >90% homology with the β-globin gene, but primarily because of a dysfunctional promoter region (2) (see below), its expression is limited under normal circumstances to approximately <3% that of the β-globin gene. A pseudo-β-globin gene is normally also present, at a position between the $^A\gamma$- and the δ-globin gene. The pseudo-β-globin gene has approximately 70% homology with the normal β-globin gene, but is not expressed; it is believed to have arisen by a gene duplication event, followed by successive mutations that resulted in its inactivation (3).

In contrast to the normally present duplicated α-globin genes, only one functional β-globin gene is represented in the normal haploid genome. In the final assembly of tetrameric hemoglobin molecules, gene products from chromosome 16, i.e., α-globin chains, combine with those from chromosome 11, i.e., γ-, δ-, or β-globin chains to form, respectively, hemoglobins F, A$_2$, and A.

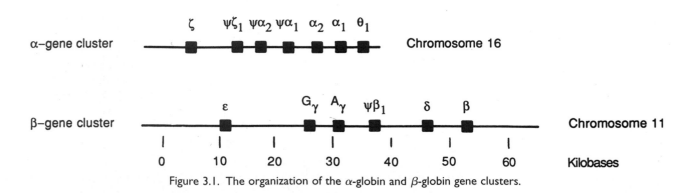

Figure 3.1. The organization of the α-globin and β-globin gene clusters.

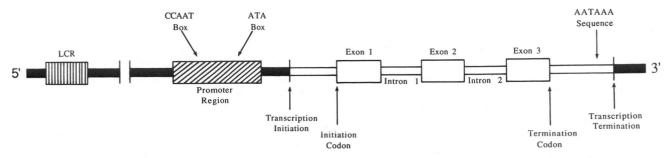

Figure 3.2. Representation of the structural organization of the genes that encode the globin chains of hemoglobin. The portion of the gene that is transcribed is represented by the unshaded segments. *LCR* represents the locus control region.

Organization and Expression of Globin Genes

The β-globin gene cluster has been studied in considerable detail, and has served as a useful model for the study of gene structure and regulation (4). A critical regulatory region, located between 5 and 20 kb 5' to the ε-globin gene (see fig. 3.2) is referred to variously as the locus control region (LCR) or locus activating region (LAR) (1). Findings from a variety of studies suggest that DNA sequences in this segment are necessary for full activation and tissue-specific expression of the globin genes. It appears that the "up" regulatory effect of the LCR is positional, i.e., it enhances transcription of the globin genes by positioning them in a favorable spatial orientation.

The promoter region of the β-globin gene is located between 20 and 110 base pairs 5' to the cap site (see below) and is required for the precise and efficient initiation of DNA transcription. This region contains specific polynucleotide sequences that also are present in numerous other gene systems, including ATAAAA, CCAAT, CACACCC, and CCTCACCC, −31, −76, −93, and −108 base pairs 5' to the cap site, respectively.

In the transcription of the globin-gene DNA to form complementary RNA copies, the segments that are transcribed include polynucleotide sequences both 5' and 3' to the portion that is translated in globin chain synthesis (see fig. 3.2). Each globin gene also contains two intervening sequences (introns) which interrupt the expressed portions (exons) that direct the amino acid sequences of the globin chains; the DNA sequences of the intron segments are transcribed into the complementary RNA product, but they subsequently are removed by an enzymatic process and the ends are rejoined in the formation of functional globin mRNA. Normal functioning of this splicing process requires the presence of specific nucleotide sequences at both the 5' ("donor") and 3' ("acceptor") ends of the introns. The donor and acceptor splice sites invariably contain GT and AG, respectively, and the adjacent 6–24 base pairs are substantially conserved as well.

The final steps in the formation of fully functional globin mRNA involve the further addition of nucleotides to both the 3' and 5' end of the RNA transcripts. A modified nucleotide structure referred to as a cap is linked to the 5' end, and appears to be important for efficient translation of the mRNA. A 50–75 base poly (A) "tail" is added at the 3' end. A hexanucleotide sequence AAUAAA) in the 3' nontranslated segment of the premRNA appears to be the necessary signal for addition of the poly (A) tail. There is evidence that this polyadenosine sequence enhances the stability of the mRNA.

Globin Chain Synthesis

The translation of the triplet nucleotide codons in the globin mRNA to form polypeptide chains takes place in the cytoplasm of the hemoglobin-synthesizing cells. Complex ribosomal structures mediate this process. An AUG codon signals the translation initiation point, and a UAA codon functions to terminate polypeptide synthesis. The final steps in the assembly of the hemoglobin molecule, including the addition of heme to the globin chains and the joining of the individual subunits, take place by processes of spontaneous association.

β-Thalassemia Mutations

Thalassemia genes have been identified with remarkably high frequency throughout much of a broad subtropical region extending from Southern Europe to Southeast Asia. The concurrence of this geographic region with the presence historically of endemic falciparum malaria has suggested that malaria may have been a potent selective force for disseminating these genes. A considerable body of epidemiologic data supports this relationship, but the biologic basis for the association between thalassemia and endemic malaria has not been satisfactorily defined. Sporadic examples of thalassemia have been found in virtually all populations in which it has been sought, and examples of apparently new thalassemia mutations have also been described.

Thus far, well more than 100 different β-thalassemia mutations have been described, and the list continues to grow (5, 6). It has become clear that a wide variety of mutations can produce essentially identical clinical syndromes, and it is seldom possible to ascertain the presence of a specific mutation from clinical findings alone. Occasionally, however, clinical heterogeneity in disease expression can be observed between individuals who apparently have identical molecular defects. In most cases, such variation in expression appears to result from differences in the genetic background upon which the primary thalassemia mutations have occurred (e.g., those which result in elevated HbF production), or from the concurrent inheritance of other globin-gene abnormalities (e.g., α-thalassemia). When thalassemia genes have been characterized among individuals from relatively isolated populations, typically one or only a small number of mutations has been found within the population.

A substantial number of β-thalassemias have been shown to result from deletion mutations that result in a loss of all or part of the β-globin gene. It is believed that these deletions may have arisen by recombination events associated with mispairing during meiosis. More extensive deletions that involve additional globin genes in the β-globin cluster are expressed as δβ- or δβ-thalassemia syndromes.

The largest group of β-thalassemia mutations exist in the form of point mutations (i.e., single-base substitutions) or as deletions or insertions of one or a small number of nucleotides (see fig. 3.3). Among the former group are the so-called nonsense mutations, which result from single-base substitutions that create synthesis termination codons in the place of codons for individual amino acids. The effect of such a mutation is an abnormally shortened and therefore nonfunctional globin chain. Because these thalassemia genes produce no functional gene product, they are characterized as β⁰-thalassemia mutations. A nonsense mutation at β-17 is the cause for one of the most common forms of β-thalassemia in Chinese individuals,

and another at β-39 accounts for >90% of β-thalassemia genes in Sardinians.

Nonfunctional globin mRNA can also be produced by frameshift mutations, which result from additions or deletions of nucleotides in exon coding regions of the genes, and which produce an alteration in the reading frame. Frameshift mutations commonly occur at sites of short direct repeats of nucleotide sequences. These types of mutations also give rise to β⁰-thalassemia.

Approximately a dozen mutations have been described that are localized to the promoter region of the β-globin gene (i.e., transcriptional mutants [5]). Most of these have been known to occur within or near to the ATA region, about 30nt upstream of the mRNA cap site, and in the CACACCC sequence, located between 105 and 90nt upstream of the gene. These mutations result in an approximately 70–80% reduction in the amount of β-chain that is synthesized, thus producing a β⁺ phenotype (see fig. 3.4). In contrast to these β-globin-promoter mutations which result in down regulation (i.e., impaired β-globin synthesis), several ᶜγ- or ᴬγ-globin gene promoter mutations have been described that cause enhanced γ-globin synthesis, producing the phenotype of hereditary persistence of fetal hemoglobin (HPFH).

Nearly half of all of the known β-thalassemia mutations produce defects in RNA splicing. Precise and efficient excision of the transcribed intervening sequences (introns) from the mRNA precursor is essential for the formation of normally functional mRNA. Specific nucleotide sequences at the exon-intron boundaries serve as identification points to direct this process. The dinucleotides GT and AG, re-

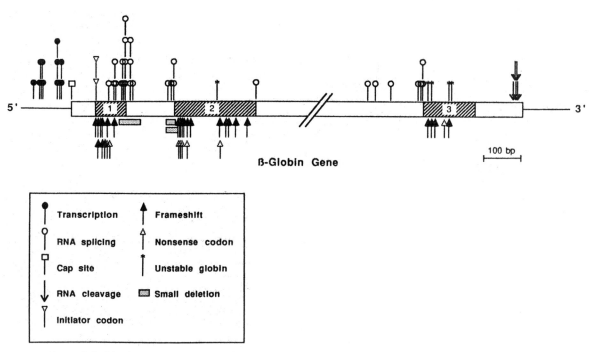

β-Globin Gene

100 bp

• Transcription	▲ Frameshift
○ RNA splicing	△ Nonsense codon
▢ Cap site	┃ Unstable globin
↓ RNA cleavage	▦ Small deletion
▽ Initiator codon	

Figure 3.3. The locations in the β-globin gene of point mutations and small deletions that have been identified in patients with β-thalassemia. (From Kazazian HH Jr. Semin Hematol 1990;27:209–228, with permission.)

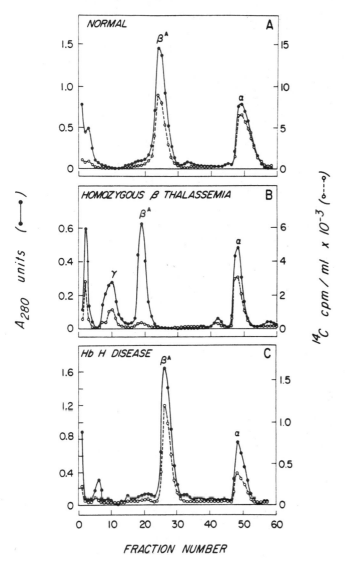

Figure 3.4. Globin synthesis patterns from erythroid cells of a normal individual and from patients with HbH disease (α-thalassemia) and homozygous β-thalassemia (Cooley anemia). The synthesis of each globin chain is proportional to the incorporation of ^{14}C-L-leucine, as represented by the *open points* and the *dashed line*. The pattern shown for the β-thalassemia patient demonstrates some synthesis of β-chains, and therefore would be characterized as β$^+$. (From Bunn HF, Forget BG. Hemoglobin: molecular, genetic, and clinical aspects. Philadelphia: WP Saunders, 1987, with permission.)

nucleotide sequences that are recognized by the splicing enzymes. As a result of these mutations, incorrectly spliced, nonfunctional globin mRNA is formed. Most of these mutations produce β$^+$-thalassemia. Point mutations involving the AAUAAA sequence at the 3' end of the globin mRNA, which appears to constitute a signal for mRNA cleavage and polyadenylation, have also been shown to produce β-thalassemia. Mutations involving this sequence cause a diminution, but not total abrogation, of normal mRNA cleavage and polyadenylation, and thus result in a β$^+$-phenotype.

A number of structurally abnormal globins have been shown to be accompanied by hematologic features of thalassemia; a variety of mechanisms account for these changes. Hemoglobin Knossos, which contains an Ala → Ser substitution at β-27, is a notable example. The DNA structure that results from this mutation also produces activation of a cryptic splice site, giving rise to a β$^+$ thalassemia-like syndrome (7). Hemoglobin Terre Haute results from a base substitution in the third exon of the β-globin gene. Its abnormal globin chain is highly unstable, undergoes very rapid catabolism within the cell, and is accompanied by an unusually severe thalassemic phenotype, even in the heterozygous state (8). Hb Tak (9) is another example of this type of abnormality (9). A mutation affecting the translation-termination codon in the gene for this hemoglobin variant results in the translation of an abnormally long globin chain containing 11 additional amino acids; the cause for its thalassemia-like expression, however, is not well understood.

Pathophysiology of β-Thalassemia

By definition, thalassemia mutations result in a quantitative decrease in the synthesis of one or more of the globin chains. In the case of β-thalassemia, the deficiency of β-chain synthesis is reflected in a decrease in the formation of HbA, and the erythrocytes are significantly underhemoglobinized. Although some degree of "compensation" can take place, with increased amounts of HbF and HbA$_2$ being synthesized, the process is always incomplete and, especially in homozygous β^0-thalassemia, anemia is characteristically severe.

A second factor that contributes to the pathophysiology of β-thalassemia derives from the imbalance between the synthesis of α- and non-α-chain synthesis in the erythroid cells of these patients (see fig. 3.4). The excess, uncombined α-chains that are formed are highly unstable and undergo a complex series of oxidative steps (see below) that ultimately contribute to a damaging of the erythrocyte membrane. These changes, in turn, produce a shortening of red cell survival. This hemolytic process adds further to severity of the patients' anemia.

Erythrocytes from individuals with thalassemia have been shown to be significantly more susceptible than normal to oxidative stress (10), because these cells contain an excess of uncombined globin chains, high concentrations of non-heme iron, and relatively low concentrations of

spectively, appear to be crucial for the recognition of the 5' ("donor") and 3' ("acceptor") splice sites of the intervening sequences. Mutations affecting these sites prevent functional mRNA formation, and produce the β^0-phenotype. Splice junction sequences immediately adjacent to these invariant dinucleotides are also substantially conserved, and mutations in these sequences typically produce β$^+$-thalassemia. Splice junction mutations, or mutations occurring well within the intervening sequences, often result in variable activation of novel (cryptic) splice sites, and may produce either β^0- or β$^+$-thalassemia. In another group of β-thalassemia mutations, single-base substitutions, either in the globin gene exons or its introns, create hemoglobin. The excess-free α-globin subunits in patients with β-thalassemia readily undergo oxidation to form methemoglobin, through a process that results in the formation of superoxide and other oxygen-free radicals. These oxygen radicals cause a variety of destructive changes, including the formation of additional methemoglobin, the production of reversible and irreversible hemichromes, membrane lipid peroxidation, and oxidative damage to both globin and cell membrane proteins (summarized in fig. 3.5). The effects on the cell membranes have been shown to produce disturbances in cation exchange that contribute importantly to the shortening of erythrocyte survival in these patients.

Hemichromes are oxidation products of globin subunits. When initially formed, hemichromes are soluble and can be fully restored to a normal functional state. Following additional successive oxidation steps, however, these proteins become irreversibly oxidized and insoluble. In the latter form they can be visualized in the red cells, after staining with a supravital redox stain as Heinz bodies. They

are eventually catabolized to separate heme and globin species, leading to deposition on the red cell membrane of excess iron, denatured globin chains, and heme. Hemichromes have a particular tendency to aggregate with membrane protein 3, and to interfere with its interaction with spectrin and ankyrin. There is also evidence that protein 4.1 is oxidatively damaged in β-thalassemia erythrocytes, and its function in mediating the binding of spectrin to actin is impaired. Hemichromes appear to increase or alter the antigenicity of the cell membrane and increase the membrane binding of autologous immunoglobulin, and this change promotes phagocytosis and early destruction of the red cells.

Erythrocyte membrane lipid peroxidation also appears to be a contributing factor to the hemolytic process in patients with β-thalassemia. Oxidative changes of the lipid components result in increased rigidity and lessened deformability of the red cells, which impedes their flow through the spleen. The oxidized membrane lipids also lead to increased antigenicity of the cell membranes,

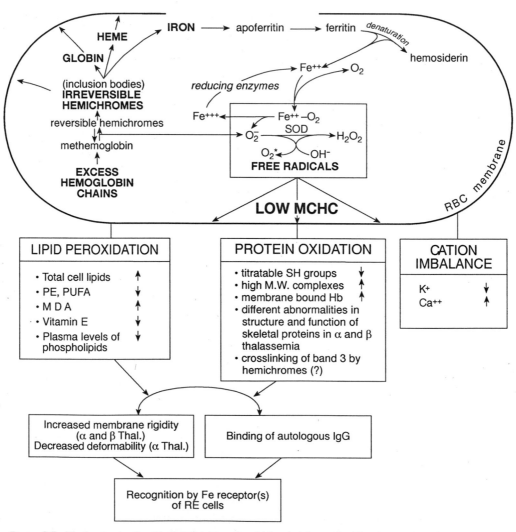

Figure 3.5. Mechanisms of oxidative damage of red blood cell membrane components in thalassemia. The injurious effects contribute to a shortening of red cell survival, adding to the severity of the anemia. (From Shinar E, Rachmilewitz EA. Semin Hematol 1990;27:70–82, with permission.)

heightened recognition of the altered red cells by macrophages, and their accelerated destruction.

The hemolytic process in patients with untreated severe β-thalassemia also includes a major intramedullary component whereby erythroid cell precursors in the bone marrow, primarily nucleated forms, are prematurely destroyed by phagocytic cells. The severe anemia in these patients, together with their ongoing generation of hemolysis products, produces an intense erythropoietin-mediated erythropoietic drive. The bone marrow becomes greatly expanded, filling all of the medullary cavities of the bones, and expanding to the point of causing characteristic bony deformities. The long bones typically develop thinned cortices that are prone to pathologic fracture. Bony deformities are particularly prominent in the face and skull, producing maxillary hypertrophy (and resultant overbite) and frontal bossing. Extramedullary sites, including the liver and spleen, may also become engorged with erythroid marrow. In some patients paravertebral masses have developed that were most easily visualized in radiographs of the chest. These could be shown to represent masses of hematopoietic tissue that expanded as nodular aggregates after breaking through the vertebral cortices.

Paradoxically, the intensely active erythropoiesis in these patients is accompanied by the release from their bone marrow of relatively small numbers of mature erythrocytes. This disparity is explained by the massive intramedullary destruction of erythroid precursors, as described above. This process of ineffective erythropoiesis is a hallmark of the severe thalassemias. A quantitative assessment of this imbalance can be obtained from ferrokinetic studies of these patients. Typically the iron clearance was found to be significantly more rapid than normal, yet with only a small fraction of the administered radioiron appearing in the patients' erythrocytes. Because of their high rate of hemolysis, jaundice is a common finding in these patients and cholelithiasis is a frequent additional complication.

Laboratory Findings in Patients with β-Thalassemia

The sine qua non of all significant forms of thalassemia is the presence of microcytosis; the accompanying anemia may vary in severity from mild to very severe, depending on the specific genetic abnormalities that are present. In mild forms of heterozygous β-thalassemia, the erythrocyte morphology may show only subtle changes from normal, with occasional target cells, basophilic stippling, and poikilocytosis, but little anisocytosis, so that the RDW typically is not increased. Patients with homozygous or severe compound eterozygous forms of β-thalassemia exhibit highly abnormal red cell changes, including degrees of hypochromia that are often striking, with other changes indicative of severe cell membrane damage; normoblastemia is also frequently present. Following splenectomy, these dysmorphic changes are often accentuated, and are accompanied by the presence of Howell-Jolly bodies.

The most meaningful assessment of the biochemical severity of α-thalassemia syndrome is the determination of the degree of imbalance between the synthesis of α-like and β-like globin chains by bone marrow cells or blood reticulocytes (see fig. 3.4). This type of assessment is not a usual part of the diagnostic evaluation of patients suspected of having thalassemia, but may be required for unusual or complex thalassemia syndromes. In general, the severity of the clinical manifestations of a thalassemic disorder will correlate well with the degree of imbalance of the complementary globin chains.

The hemoglobin composition of the blood in patients with β-thalassemia reflects the compensatory changes associated with the impairment of β-chain synthesis, as described above. Patients with homozygous β^0-thalassemia who have not been transfused will have no detectable HbA in their blood. In those with milder β-thalassemia syndromes, an elevated level of HbF with variable percentages of HbA_2 will be present. In most forms of heterozygous β-thalassemia the percentage of HbA_2 will be significantly elevated, representing the primary diagnostic finding in this condition. Variable elevations in the level of HbF can also be demonstrated in most affected individuals. The less common δβ-thalassemia syndrome characteristically produces levels of 5–20% of HbF in heterozygotes, together with normal percentages of HbA_2. The relative ease of confirmation of a diagnosis of heterozygous β-thalassemia makes it possible to identify genetic carriers of thalassemia confidently. Laboratory studies of heterozygous parents of patients with clinically significant β-thalassemia are also often very helpful in characterizing and classifying these syndromes.

A variety of relatively rapid and straightforward laboratory methods have been developed that make it possible to detect and identify most of the more frequently-occurring β-thalassemia mutations using DNA derived from a small sample of blood or amniocytes. For usual clinical diagnostic evaluation this type of determination is rarely needed. These methods do have an important diagnostic role, however, in that they make it possible to establish a diagnosis of β-thalassemia prenatally with a high level of reliability.

In the case described above, the child's hematologic picture is entirely compatible with a diagnosis of homozygous β-thalassemia, i.e. Cooley anemia. The finding of a significant percentage of HbA in his blood indicates that he has at least one β^+-thalassemia gene. Possible combinations that could give rise to this thalassemia syndrome would include: (a) homozygous β^+-thalassemia; (b) compound-heterozygous β^+/β^0- thalassemia; or (c) compound-heterozygous $\beta^+/\delta\beta$- thalassemia. As indicated earlier in this section, studies of parents or other relatives can often be very helpful for sorting out the various types of thalassemia abnormalities. Within each of the possible categories of thalassemia genes that this patient might have, any of a large number of different mutations could account for the observed abnormalities.

Clinical Management Issues for Patients with β-Thalassemia

For β-thalassemia patients with severe degrees of anemia, periodic transfusions of red cell concentrates constitute the principal element of therapy. The objectives of transfusion therapy in these patients are twofold: one goal is to correct the anemia; the other is to suppress the ineffective erythropoiesis and thereby to ameliorate the consequences of the expanded bone marrow (11). Early transfusion regimens, which corrected the patients' hemoglobin levels to a minimum of 60–80 g/L, prevented the primary effects of their anemia but were insufficient to suppress endogenous erythropoiesis and its secondary complications, including bony thinning and disfigurement, and increased gastrointestinal absorption of iron. A significant advance in the transfusion management of these patients came with the development by Wolman (12) of what has come to be known as "hypertransfusion" regimens; these were designed to maintain a hemoglobin level of at least 85–105 g/L. This approach, which usually entails transfusing packed red cells (ca. 20 ml/kg of body weight per month), has the important effect of decreasing the erythropoietic drive, and substantially diminishes or eliminates the adverse consequences of ineffective erythropoiesis, as described above.

For patients with β-thalassemia major who are clearly dependent on transfusion, the regimen of periodic transfusions should ordinarily be started as soon as the diagnosis is established. In patients who exhibit a failure of normal growth, as in the case described above, the prompt initiation of transfusion therapy would also be indicated. When uncertainty exists about whether the nadir of the patient's hemoglobin level has been reached, and if there is a question about whether the patient might have a milder thalassemia intermedia phenotype, transfusions can be delayed, with careful observation, until the situation becomes clear. Once transfusions are started, the effectiveness of the regimen can be assessed by observing the growth pattern and overall health status of the patient. Hepatitis B vaccine (Recombivax) should be given to any patient for whom repeated transfusions will be necessary.

Splenomegaly often develops in patients with thalassemia, because of expanded reticuloendothelial activity related to phagocytosis of the abnormal red cells and from the accumulation of excess iron stores; extramedullary hematopoiesis may also be a contributing factor, but is rarely important in adequately transfused patients. The age at which splenomegaly becomes prominent varies, but generally this does not become a significant problem in patients receiving hypertransfusion until they are well into their teen years. Generally accepted as being an indication for splenectomy are significant hypersplenic changes, reflected most frequently by an increasing transfusion requirement of >240 ml of packed red cells/kg/year.

With medical management, including hypertransfusion, most patients with β-thalassemia major are free of symptoms of anemia and are able to lead quite normal lives. With continuing transfusion therapy, however, chronic iron accumulation becomes a prominent secondary complication, and if not adequately managed, it is likely to contribute to a fatal outcome by early adult age. Each milliliter of red blood cells contains approximately 1 mg of elemental iron. Because there is no physiologically effective mechanism for ridding the body of excess iron, repeated red cell transfusions lead to an inexorable increase in the total body iron burden.

Untransfused patients with thalassemia major have also been shown to have excessive gastrointestinal absorption of iron, so that even without the contribution from transfusions significant iron overloading can develop in these patients. The mechanisms for this are not well understood. One intriguing hypothesis is that in such cases the erythropoietic drive is so vigorous and the requirement for iron to accommodate red cell synthesis so formidable that the erythron is functionally iron deficient, thus stimulating continued iron absorption from the gut. The excessive gastrointestinal absorption of iron appears to be proportional to the overall rate of red cell production. Patients who are appropriately transfused benefit from diminished gastrointestinal absorption of iron, but suffer from excessive iron accumulation as a result of transfusion.

The primary sites of iron toxicity are the heart, liver, and endocrine system. Cardiac sequelae are the most grave, and prior to the development of effective iron-chelation therapy this complication accounted for the majority of deaths in these patients. Iron deposition has been shown to occur in both the myocardium and the conduction system, and can give rise to both myocardial failure and lethal arrhythmias.

By the time they have reached approximately 5 years of age, intensively transfused patients with β-thalassemia could be shown from serial biopsy studies to have significant hepatic fibrosis. By their second decade of life, many of these patients exhibited findings of frank cirrhosis. Hepatic failure has led to a fatal outcome in a relatively small number of these patients.

Endocrine dysfunction in hypertransfused patients frequently becomes apparent in their preadolescent years, with delayed growth, and especially with attenuation of the adolescent growth spurt. These changes are believed to result from diminished levels of liver-derived somatomedin. Delayed puberty, which often is accompanied by a delayed bone age, has been shown to be caused by hypothalamic pituitary dysfunction. Some of these patients respond well to treatment with growth hormone. Abnormal glucose tolerance is also a frequent finding in these patients, occasionally evolving to frank diabetes mellitus. Thyroid, parathyroid, and adrenal dysfunction can sometimes be demonstrated, but usually is only subclinical.

Iron appears to mediate its toxic effects through its role in catalyzing the formation of free oxygen radicals. Normally, iron in the body is nearly completely protein bound, in which form it is incapable of generating oxygen radicals. Under conditions of transfusional overload, free iron becomes more plentiful both intracellularly and in circulating extracellular pools. Clinical assessment of the total body iron burden is usually based on the serum ferritin level, but a predictable, linear relation between serum ferritin and body iron stores exists only within a relatively limited range. The measurement of iron in liver biopsy specimens is the most accurate method for the estimation of the total body iron burden, but this method is seldom used because of its invasiveness (11).

Chelation therapy using deferoxamine (DFO) currently represents the most effective available treatment for transfusional iron overload. DFO has high affinity and specificity for iron, and it effectively chelates iron from both the intracellular and extracellular compartments. Once bound, the chelated iron complex is excreted through the kidneys and, with increasing doses, in the stool. The main pharmacologic limitations of DFO are its poor absorption from the gastrointestinal tract and its short half-life. In order for the drug to be effective, it must therefore be given parenterally and over an extended period of time.

DFO has been shown to be effective in maintaining iron balance, and capable of achieving net iron loss when given daily at doses of about 25–50 mg/kg. The drug is ordinarily administered subcutaneously over 6–12 hours, using a battery-operated portable infusion pump. Subcutaneous administration of DFO is tedious and time consuming, and its use is often accompanied by local discomfort or reaction at the site of administration. As might be anticipated, compliance is a frequent problem. For patients with severe degrees of iron overload, regimens using high-dose (>50 mg/kg/ 24 hours) DFO have recently been introduced, with promising results (13).

A number of adverse effects have been reported with use of DFO, including the development of cataracts, retinal damage, ototoxicity with tinnitus and hearing loss, and renal impairment. These untoward effects are more likely to occur with high-dose regimens, and most of these problems appear to be reversible if the medication is withheld in a timely fashion. Also, growth delay and epiphyseal changes have been observed in infants and young children who were treated with DFO. Thus, in considering when to initiate therapy with DFO, the benefit of preventing significant iron overload through early treatment must be weighed against the additional risks that may occur with treatment at a young age. There is general agreement that chelation therapy should be started when the serum ferritin level reaches ca. 1000–1500 ng/ml, which in hypertransfused children usually occurs at about 3–4 years of age.

Toxicity studies and preliminary clinical trials are currently in progress to examine the safety and efficacy of several compounds that chelate iron effectively and are well absorbed following oral administration (14). One of these agents, 1,2-dimethyl-3-hydroxypyrid-4-one (L-1) can be produced inexpensively and appears to be as effective as deferoxamine. These new agents offer the hope of being able to achieve iron balance in these patients with ease of administration and enhanced compliance, and at considerably lower cost.

Allogeneic bone marrow transplantation for patients with thalassemia major has been employed in a number of centers in recent years (15). Successful engraftment can now be achieved in well over 60% of these patients. Earlier experience suggested that only very young patients (those <5 years of age), could be candidates for bone marrow transplantation because of adverse effects of multiple transfusions. More recent reports, however, indicate that patients with β-thalassemia well into their teen years can now be transplanted with high potential for success.

In a remarkable series of experiments, human β-globin genes have been successfully introduced into the germ line of mice with β-thalassemia, resulting in a striking correction of their anemia and microcytosis (16). These results lend support to the potential for "gene therapy" for patients with severe thalassemia. Although therapeutic applications of cloned gene transfers for certain other human disorders are already being attempted, at present at least, it seems unlikely that this approach will be feasible in the near future for thalassemia patients.

Preventive Strategies for Severe β-Thalassemia

Individuals with heterozygous β-thalassemia can be readily identified by screening techniques that detect microcytosis by electronic cell counting. This approach, together with comprehensive programs of public education, has been applied extensively in a number of countries, particularly in Southern Europe. Couples at risk of having offspring with severe β-thalassemia are identified and offered the opportunity to have prenatal testing to identify affected fetuses. Many of these programs have been highly effective in reducing the numbers of births of affected infants.

Case 2

A 24-year-old school teacher of Filipino ancestry had a history of anemia extending back to her childhood. She had been treated with iron on several occasions with questionable benefit. She had not had jaundice, and she generally enjoyed good health. The patient was seen with complaints of dysuria and vomiting accompanied by pyuria, and she was given oral sulfisoxazole. On the second day of treatment, she noted mild jaundice; the following day the jaundice deepened and was accompanied by pallor with symptoms of weakness and dizziness. Her spleen was noted to be enlarged, extending 6 cm below the costal margin. Her blood count showed the following: hemoglobin 54 g/L, MCV 60 fl, and reticulocytes 10%. A stained smear of her blood (fig. 3.6) demonstrated a marked degree of red cell morphologic abnormality with severe anisopoikilocytosis. Her G-6-PD activity was 0.98 MU/mol Hb (normal equals 0.22–0.52), and her serum ferritin 1600 ng/ml. Her hemoglobin electrophoresis results, from a hemolysate that was prepared using chloroform as a destromatizing agent, demonstrated normal findings, with HbA 97.0%, HbA₂ 2.5%, and HbF 0.5%. When the electrophoresis was repeated using a hemolysate prepared only with distilled water, an anodally-migrating band was identified, representing ca. 12% of the total hemoglobin. Further analysis of this hemoglobin showed that it contained only β-globin chains. Incubation of the patients' red cells with the supravital redox stain brilliant cresyl blue produced prominent inclusions in many of the cells.

Commentary

The differential diagnosis for a patient with an acute onset of anemia following exposure to a sulfonamide, antimalarial, or other oxidant drug or chemical should appropriately focus first on the possibility of a deficiency of a red cell enzyme associated with the hexose monophosphate shunt pathway; of these, glucose-6-phosphate dehydrogenase (G-6-PD) deficiency is by far the most frequent, although as an X-linked recessive trait this condition would be unlikely to cause symptomatic disease in a female. Even without the benefit of the hemoglobin electrophoresis findings, the patient's significant microcytosis must also suggest that other diagnostic possibilities be considered. The other major category of hematologic disorders that produce oxidant drug-induced hemolysis includes a group of unstable hemoglobins that share the property of undergoing in-

tracellular precipitation under oxidative conditions. When α chain synthesis is significantly decreased in relation to β-chain synthesis, as is the case in the more severe forms of α-thalassemia (see fig. 3.4), substantial quantities of uncombined hemoglobin β-subunits may accumulate in the red cells, in the form of semistable β₄-hemoglobin tetramers that can be identified as a rapidly migrating band by hemoglobin electrophoresis.

The instability of Hbβ₄ (also referred to as HbH) is an important contributing factor to the chronic hemolysis that characteristically accompanies the symptomatic forms of α-thalassemia. A practical point in correctly identifying this condition is that the instability of HbH causes it to precipitate out of solution when it comes in contact with any of the organic solvents that are routinely used in diagnostic laboratories to remove stroma from red cell lysates. Unless proper steps are taken to modify the usual procedure when HbH is suspected, its presence will be missed, as was illustrated in case #2.

Clinical Phenotypes of α-Thalassemia

The various α-thalassemia syndromes make up a continuum of hematologic diseases that range from an abnormality so mild as to be barely recognizable, to a disease of such severity as to be virtually incompatible with extrauterine survival. Most of these syndromes fit fairly well into one of four characteristic clinical phenotypes, which correspond to an absence of function of one, two, three, or all four of the normal complement of α-globin genes.

The *silent carrier* α-thalassemia phenotype, corresponding to a loss of one functioning α-globin gene (α,α/-,α) is, as its name implies, not ordinarily accompanied by any overt clinical or hematologic abnormality. The red cell morphology of affected individuals is characteristically normal, as is their hemoglobin composition. Mild microcytosis may be present, but the MCV is almost always within the normal range. The phenotype of α-thalassemia trait ([α,α/-,-] or [-,α/-,α]) is accompanied by a hematologic picture very similar to that of β-thalassemia trait, as described in the preceding section. Mild anemia with significant microcytosis and red cell dysmorphology are the most common findings. At birth, this form of α-thalassemia is associated with substantial levels (generally ca. 4–7%) of γ₄ tetramers, sometimes referred to as hemoglobin Barts. This homotetramer, which is considerably more stable than HbH, is readily identified by routine hemoglobin electrophoresis. Within a few weeks after birth, however, the Hb Barts disappears, and apart from rare cells that may have demonstrable HbH inclusions, the hemoglobin composition of the erythrocytes from these individuals is entirely normal.

HbH disease [-,α/-,-] is a form of α-thalassemia of intermediate severity, with clinical and hematologic features generally similar to those expressed by the patient described above. A number of early reports of patients with HbH dis-

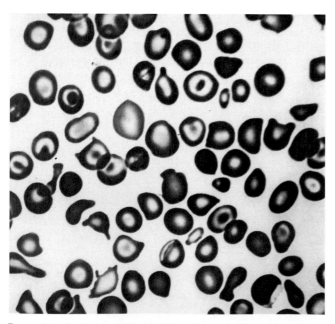

Figure 3.6. Erythrocyte morphology of patient 2.

ease, primarily originating from countries in eastern Asia, described a very serious clinical syndrome accompanied by a marked degree of anemia, hepatosplenomegaly, poor growth, and a generally debilitated condition. It later became apparent that many of these patients also suffered from chronic infections and malnutrition, which were important contributing factors to the severity of their hematologic disease. In the absence of such complicating problems, HbH disease typically presents with a moderately severe anemia, prominent microcytosis with red cell dysmorphology, and mild chronic hemolysis. Acute infections or exposure to oxidant drugs and chemicals may precipitate acute hemolytic episodes in these patients, with an abrupt fall in their hemoglobin levels such as that described in case 2. The condition is fully expressed at birth, with affected newborns having 20–30% of Hb Barts (γ_4) in their erythrocytes. During the first year of life, as HbF becomes replaced by HbA in these infants, most or all of their Hb Barts disappears to be replaced by HbH.

The clinically most severe α-thalassemia phenotype, which results from a total absence of α-globin chain synthesis [-,-/-,-], is the hydrops fetalis α-thalassemia syndrome. Inasmuch as all of the normal postnatally expressed hemoglobins (A, A_2, and F) contain α-chains, none of these hemoglobins can be produced in the red cells of fetuses with this disorder. Accordingly, a large fraction of their hemoglobin, usually more than 80%, consists of homotetramers of β and γ-chains. A notable feature of hemoglobins β_4 and γ_4 is that they have very high oxygen affinity, so much so that they release virtually no oxygen under physiologic conditions, and therefore they are unable to function as oxygen carriers in vivo. Those fetuses with this disorder who have survived in utero up to or near full term have had a substantial quantity of hemoglobin Portland ($\zeta_2\gamma_2$), a normal embryonic hemoglobin containing the α-like ζ-chain which ordinarily is not expressed beyond the first trimester of gestation. Hemoglobin Portland has been shown to have normal functional properties quite similar to those of HbA, and it appears that the presence of this hemoglobin makes it possible for at least some of these fetuses to survive the gestation period. Conversely, with α-thalassemia deletion mutations in which the ζ-globin genes are also deleted (see below), the hydrops fetalis phenotype is not observed, presumably because affected fetuses would succumb early in gestation. Most fetuses with this form of α-thalassemia, even those that had substantial amounts of Hb Portland, were stillborn, but some were born alive. They typically had severe generalized edema, massive hepatosplenomegaly, and heart failure. Only a small number of these infants survived more than a few hours, although with intensive management, including exchange transfusions, there have been a few longer-term survivors.

Pathophysiology of α-Thalassemia

Unbalanced globin chain synthesis, with a deficiency of α chains in relation to non-α-chains, is the feature common to all forms of α-thalassemia (see fig. 3.4C). The specific

mutations and gene deletions that are the underlying causes for the abnormal globin chain synthesis are discussed in the following section. As described earlier, uncombined β- and γ-globin subunits, when present in the red cells in substantial excess, are able to form semistable homotetramer hemoglobin molecules. However, when these hemoglobin species are subjected to the action of peroxide and oxygen free radicals, they undergo a series of oxidation processes, leading ultimately to the formation of irreversible hemichromes like those described above for the uncombined α-globin subunits in β-thalassemia erythrocytes (See fig. 3.5).

The β- and γ-chain hemichromes, in a similar fashion, undergo precipitation within the red cells, which causes damage to the cell membrane, with a resulting shortening of the cell's survival. This hemolytic process, added to the underhemoglobinization of the red cells that results from the deficient synthesis of normal hemoglobin, together produce the microcytic, hemolytic picture that characterizes these disorders.

The Normal Human α-Globin Gene System

The structure and organization of the genes that encode the α-globin chains are virtually identical to what was described above for the β-globin gene (see fig. 3.2), with each gene containing three exons, two intervening sequences, and a similar group of regulatory sequences. The cluster of α- and α-like globin genes have been localized to the short arm of chromosome 16. Included among the α-like globin genes are the ζ-ene, referred to in a previous section, and several nonexpressed pseudogenes termed $\psi\zeta_1$, $\psi\alpha_1$, $\psi\alpha_2$, and φ_1 (see fig. 3.1). The α_1- and α_2-globin genes have somewhat different sequences in their flanking regions, but their coding sequences are identical and their α-chain protein products are therefore indistinguishable from each other. The normal diploid complement of four α-globin genes that results from this gene representation accounts for the four major clinical forms of α-thalassemia, as described above.

The remarkable degree of similarity of the DNA sequences of the α_1- and α_2-globin genes has been explained as being the result of a process termed "concerted evolution." According to this concept, the paired α-globin genes originally arose by a process of gene duplication, and they subsequently retained virtually identical sequences, in spite of many millions of years of evolutionary history, by a process of unequal recombination that has the effect of shunting the genes from one chromosome to another. An example of this process is represented in fig. 3.7. Because of the considerable sequence homology between the α_1- and α_2-genes, it is hypothesized that mispairing between these two genes and/or their homologous flanking regions may occasionally take place during meiosis. When a crossing-over recombination event accompanies this process, the result will be a chromosome with a single α-globin locus as well as a chromosome with three loci, as illustrated in fig. 3.7. The hypothesis of concerted evolution also assumes that this process operates in reverse.

Several lines of evidence provide support for this model. Most importantly, in man as well as in a number of species of other primates, both the single locus and triplicated arrangements have been found with substantial frequency. The rightward crossover form of recombination, as shown in fig. 3.7, has been shown to occur in many different populations throughout the world, and this form of single locus α-globin gene deletion is by far the most prevalent known type of α-thalassemia gene.

Classification of the Mutations That Give Rise to α-Thalassemia

Many of the types of single base substitutions that were described above as mutation mechanisms for β-thalassemia have also been identified as the underlying cause for α-thalassemias. These various point mutations include: an alteration of an α-globin gene translation initiation codon, intron abnormalities that result in defective mRNA processing, frameshift and "nonsense" mutations, a translation termination codon abnormality, and a base substitution in the poly-A addition signal. These types of mutation mechanisms, however, account for relatively few cases of α-thalassemia, with most of the known forms resulting from mutations that involve gene deletions (18, 19).

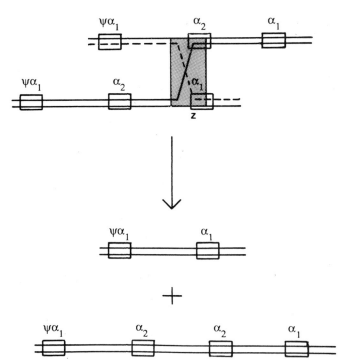

Figure 3.7. Mispairing of the α_1- and α_2-globin genes in the recombination process that is thought to be responsible for the formation of single- and triple-locus chromosomes. The *shaded area labeled ζ* is a region of considerable base-sequence homology that is believed to facilitate the mispairing.

Figure 3.8 illustrates several of the well-characterized gene deletions that produce α-thalassemias. The rightward deletions referred to earlier result in the formation of a single α-locus chromosome consisting of a fusion product of the 5′ portion of an α_1-globin gene and the 3′ portion of an α_2-gene (see figs. 3.7 and 3.8A). The leftward deletion mutation also results in a single α-locus chromosome, but in this case by a mechanism that involves deletion of the α_2-gene, leaving the α_1-gene intact (see fig. 3.8B). The various other deletion mutations illustrated in figure 3.8 result in a total or partial loss of both of the α-globin genes, and consequently chromosomes containing these abnormalities lack any α-globin gene product.

A much smaller and quite diverse group of α-thalassemia syndromes is associated with the presence of structurally abnormal hemoglobins (20). One subset of these abnormalities, of which Hb Petah Tikva and Hb Quong Sze are examples, involves the synthesis of highly unstable α-chains that undergo very rapid proteolysis within the red cells. These abnormal hemoglobins usually cannot be detected by usual laboratory procedures, and special methods are needed to demonstrate their presence. Another group of abnormal hemoglobins, of which Hb Constant Spring is the most prevalent, result from mutations in the translation termination codon of the α-globin genes. The effect of this type of abnormality is the production of longer-than-normal α-chains with additional amino acids at their carboxyl termini. Hb Constant Spring has been frequently identified in patients from Far Eastern countries who have HbH disease. HbG Philadelphia, a relatively common α-chain variant among individuals of African heritage, is often associated with α-thalassemia by yet another mechanism: the gene for this hemoglobin, and those for a number of other α-chain variants as well, have been shown to exist on single α locus chromosomes, usually in the form of a rightward deletion, as described above. Thus individuals who express HbG Philadelphia also will exhibit hematologic features of α-thalassemia.

Other α-Thalassemia Syndromes

At least 15 individuals have been described in whom the hematologic picture of HbH disease was present together with a syndrome characterized by dysmorphic changes and mental retardation (21). In one group of these patients, relatively small deletions of the short arm of chromosome 16 were identified, which included the entire a-globin gene cluster. It was hypothesized that the deleted chromosomal segment may have included one or more genes related to the mental retardation. In another subset of patients with this HbH/retardation syndrome, the a-globin gene maps were found to be entirely normal, suggesting that their underlying mutations may have affected a trans-acting factor related to the normal regulation of a-globin expression.

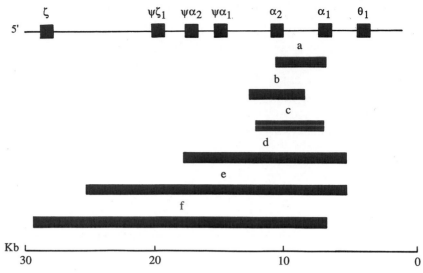

Figure 3.8. Examples of well-characterized deletions in the α-globin gene cluster that give rise to α-thalassemia. *Bar a* represents the "rightward" type of deletion and *bar b* the "leftward" type, both of which produce single-locus chromosomes. *Bars c,* *d, and e* represent deletions that encompass part or all of both of the α-globin genes while retaining the ζ-globin gene, and *bar f* depicts a more extensive deletion involving all of the functional globin genes in the α-globin gene cluster.

A hematologic picture indistinguishable from that of genetically inherited HbH disease has also been observed to occur as an acquired abnormality, in association with a variety of leukemias and myeloproliferative disorders. Studies of affected individuals with this hematologic syndrome have shown the HbH expression to be confined to a distinct red cell clone. Analyses of their α-globin genes have not demonstrated a deletion pattern in these individuals, and the underlying defect in this group of conditions has not been clearly identified.

Clinical and Management Considerations

Individuals with deletions of one or two α-globin genes require no specific form of medical management. HbH disease may produce chronic hemolytic anemia of at least moderate severity, with the full range of potential complications relatable to chronic anemia and/or hemolytic disease. Because of the risk of acute hemolytic episodes in these patients when they are exposed to oxidant drugs and chemicals, it may be desirable to provide them a list of agents to avoid, as is commonly done for individuals with G-6-PD deficiency. Hemolysis may also be accentuated in patients with HbH disease who have acute infections or during pregnancy. Splenomegaly with accompanying hypersplenism complicate this condition in some patients, necessitating a splenectomy.

When both parents carry double-deletion α-thalassemia genes, they are at risk of having affected offspring with the hydrops fetalis α-thalassemia syndrome. The fetus with this disorder can be identified in utero by reliable laboratory methods, and when recognized these pregnancies have frequently been aborted. Toxemia has been described as a common and often severe complication of such pregnancies. In the few reported examples of live-born infants with this syndrome who were successfully resuscitated and transfused, neurologic damage and other neonatal complications have apparently been quite frequent. In light of the absolute and lifelong dependence of these infants on red cell transfusions, decisions about aggressive resuscitation and transfusion at birth may require careful deliberation.

Case 3

A 4-year-old boy from a newly immigrated Vietnamese family was found to have pallor, growth retardation, a dysmorphic facial appearance with frontal bossing and maxillary prominence, and massive hepatosplenomegaly. His blood count showed the following: hemoglobin 58 g/L, MCV 54 fl, and reticulocyte count 4%. A stained blood smear showed very abnormal red cell morphology, with anisopoikilocytosis, prominent target cells, and occasional stippled cells. Electrophoresis of his hemoglobin at alkaline pH showed absent HbA, with the major hemoglobin band exhibiting mobility similar to that of HbA₂; this abnormal hemoglobin was identified by agar-gel electrophoresis as being HbE. Approximately 60% of the boy's hemoglobin consisted of HbE + HbA₂, with HbF making up the remaining 40% (see fig. 3.9). Hematologic findings from the patient's father included the following: hemoglobin 92 g/L and mean corpuscular volume 55 fl, with his hemoglobin analysis showing HbA 92%, HbA₂ 5.8%, and HbF 2.5%. The boy's mother's findings included: Hb 108 g/L and MCV 72 fl, with her hemoglobin composition consisting of HbA 55% and HbE 45%.

Commentary

HbE is a β-chain variant in which β-26 glutamate is replaced by lysine; this hemoglobin has been observed as

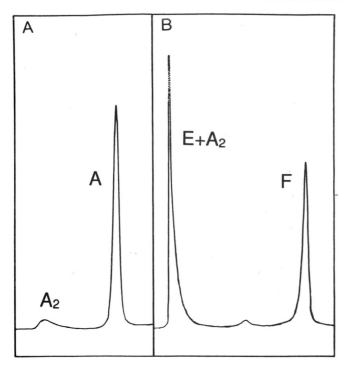

Figure 3.9. Hereditary persistence of fetal hemoglobin (HPLC) patterns from a normal individual (A), and from case 3 described in the text (B).

considered that one or both of the parents may have concomitant α-thalassemia. We could therefore conclude that the patient has HbE/β-thalassemia, and possibly some associated form of α-thalassemia.

From both the clinical and hematologic findings from this patient, it is readily apparent that this is not the usual "interacting" expression of a β-chain structural variant in combination with β-thalassemia. In the most familiar example of this type of expression, in which genes for HbS and β-thalassemia occur together, the characteristic finding is a decrease or total suppression of HbA production as a result of the β-thalassemia gene; consequently, the percentage of HbS is increased as compared with that seen in individuals with sickle-cell trait. HbF may be slightly increased in patients with HbS/β-thalassemia, but for the most part their clinical findings are generally similar to those associated with HbSS. By contrast, homozygous HbE is typically a clinically benign condition, which does not ordinarily produce anemia or other significant pathology. HbE/β-thalassemia, however, is often accompanied by a severe degree of anemia and a clinical picture very similar to that of Cooley anemia, as this case illustrates.

a rare abnormality in a number of different populations, but it has been found to occur with very high frequency (as high as q = 0.6) in parts of Southeast Asia, particularly in certain regions of Laos, Thailand, and Cambodia. This area, in which falciparum malaria formerly was endemic, also has incidence rates of both α- and β-thalassemia that are among the highest in the world (22).

In the analysis of potentially complex hemoglobinopathy/thalassemia syndromes, family studies are often invaluable. The elevated level of HbA_2 in the father in this family indicates that he has β-thalassemia trait. The mother is heterozygous for HbE. In light of their national origins the possibility also needs to be

HbE as a-Thalassemic Determinant

HbE is one of the hemoglobin structural variants that has thalassemia-like expression even in heterozygous states, i.e., it is characteristically accompanied by some degree of anemia, microcytosis, and red cell dysmorphology. A group of α-chain variants that produce the phenotype of α-thalassemia were discussed in the preceding section; a substantial number of β-chain variants are similarly associated with β-thalassemia-like hematologic findings from corresponding types of mechanisms. In the case of HbE, two different possible mechanisms may contribute to its thalassemic phenotype. For one thing, HbE has been shown to be unstable, and it readily undergoes precipita-

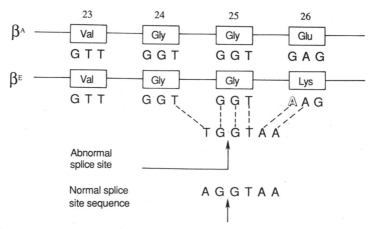

Figure 3.10. Comparison of the nucleotide base sequences of the $β^A$- and $β^E$-globin genes in the region of the bE mutation site. The newly created splice site resulting from the base substitution in the $β^E$-globin gene is compared with the 5' consensus nucleotide sequence at the normal splice site.

tion under oxidant conditions. This property may contribute to its thalassemia-like expression in a manner similar to that described earlier for abnormal hemoglobins with unstable α-chains that produce the phenotype of α-thalassemia (23).

It has also been demonstrated that β^E mRNA is substantially decreased in quantity in erythroid cells that produce this hemoglobin. The explanation for this finding came from studies of the transcription of the β^E-globin gene and the processing of its mRNA precursor. It was determined that as a result of the G → A base substitution that gave rise to the β^E mutation, a new recognition site was created for the nuclear enzymes that cleave the mRNA at intron-exon boundary sites as the normal initial step in the removal of the intron transcripts. As a result of this defect, a portion of the β^E mRNA precursor is incorrectly spliced and consequently lacks functional mRNA activity (24) (see fig. 3.10).

Clinical Implications of the HbE Syndromes

Homozygous HbE, alone or in combination with milder forms of α-thalassemia, produces a clinical picture similar to that of thalassemia trait, and no treatment is usually needed. The rare combination of HbEE with HbH disease is expressed as a severe thalassemia syndrome requiring chronic transfusion therapy.

Because of the high frequency of both HbE and β-thalassemia in Southeast Asian populations, HbE/β-thalassemia is a prevalent and significant disease. Although in the most severely affected of these patients the disorder is expressed as a transfusion-dependent, Cooley anemia-like condition, other patients with HbE/β-thalassemia have a more moderate degree of anemia and do not require transfusions. Concomitant α-thalassemia was shown to be present in a number of patients with the milder expression of HbE/β-thalassemia and has been suggested to be an ameliorating factor (25). This apparently beneficial effect of α-thalassemia could be the result of a more balanced pattern of synthesis of α- and β-chains in the erythroid cells of these patients.

REFERENCES

1. Bollekens JA, Forget BG. δβ-Thalassemia and hereditary persistence of fetal hemoglobin. Hematol Oncol Clin N Am 1991;5:399–422.
2. Humphries RK, Ley T, Turner P, et al. Differences in human alpha-, beta-, and delta-globin gene expression in monkey kidney cells. Cell 1982;30:173–183.
3. Chang L-YE, Slightom JL. Isolation and nucleotide sequence analysis of b-type globin pseudogene from human, gorilla and chimpanzee. J Mol Biol 1984;180:767–784.
4. Honig GR, Adams JG III. Human hemoglobin genetics. New York: Springer, 1986.
5. Huisman THJ. The β- and δ- thalassemia repository. Hemoglobin 1992;16:237–258.
6. Kazazian HH Jr. The thalassemia syndromes: molecular basis and prenatal diagnosis in 1990. Semin Hematol 1990;27:209–228.
7. Orkin SH, Antonarakis SE, Loukopoulos D. Abnormal processing of β^Knossos RNA. Blood 1984;64:311–313.
8. Adams JG III, Boxer LA, Baehner RL, et al. Hemoglobin Indianapolis (b 112 [G14] Arginine): an unstable β-chain variant producing the phenotype of severe β-thalassemia. J Clin Invest 1979;63:931–938.
9. Lehmann H, Casey R, Lang A, et al. Haemoglobin Tak: a β-chain elongation. Br J Haematol 1975;31(Suppl):119–131.
10. Shinar E, Rachmilewitz EA. Oxidative denaturation of red blood cells in thalassemia. Semin Hematol 1990;27:70–82.
11. Fosburg MT, Nathan DG. Treatment of Cooley's anemia. Blood 1990;76:435–444.
12. Wolman LJ. Transfusion therapy in Cooley's anemia: growth and health as related to long-range hemoglobin levels. A progress report. Ann NY Acad Sci 1964;119:736–747.
13. Cohen A, Mizanin J, Schwartz E. Rapid removal of excessive iron with daily high-dose intravenous chelation therapy. J Pediatr 1989;115:151–155.
14. Piomelli S. Oral iron chelators for the clinical management of iron overload. Ann NY Acad Sci 1990;612:311–314.
15. Lucarelli G, Galimberti M, Polchi P, et al. Bone marrow transplantation in thalassemia. Hematol Oncol Clin N Am 1991;5:549–556.
16. Costantini F, Chada K, Magram J. Correction of murine β-thalassemia by gene transfer into the germ line. Science 1986;233:1192–1194.
17. Cao A, Rosatelli MC, Leoni GB, et al. Antenatal diagnosis of beta-thalassemia in Sardinia. Ann NY Acad Sci 1990;612:215–225.
18. Higgs DR, Vickers MA, Wilkie AOM, Pretorius I-M, Jarman AP, Weatherall DJ. A review of the molecular genetics of the human α-globin gene cluster. Blood 1989;73:1081–1104.
19. Liebhaber SA. α-Thalassemia. Hemoglobin 1989;13:685–731.
20. Steinberg MH. The interactions of α-thalassemia with hemoglobinopathies. Hematol Oncol Clin N Am 1991;5:453–473.
21. Wilkie AOM, Zeitlin HC, Lindenbaum RH, Buckle VJ, Fischel-Ghodsian N, Chui DHK, Gardner-Medwin D, MacGillivray MH, Weatherall DJ, Higgs DR. Clinical features and molecular analysis of the α-thalassemia/mental retardation syndromes: II. cases without detectable abnormality of the α globin complex. Am J Hum Genet 1990;46:1127–1140.
22. Monzon CM, Fairbanks VF, Burgert EO Jr, Sutherland JE, Elliot SC. Hematologic genetic disorders among Southeast Asian refugees. Am J Hematol 1985;19:27–36.
23. Wickramasinghe SN, Hughes M, Wasi P, Fucharoen S, Modell B. Ineffective erythropoiesis in haemoglobin Eb-thalassemia: an electron microscope study. Br J Haematol 1981; 48:451–457.
24. Orkin SH, Kazazian HH Jr, Antonarakis SE, Ostrer H, Goff SC, Sexton JP. Abnormal RNA processing due to the exon mutation of β^E-globin gene. Nature 1982;300:768–769.
25. Winichagoon P, Fucharoen S, Weatherall D, Wasi P. Concomitant inheritance of α-thalassemia in β^0-thalassemia/HbE disease. Am J Hematol 1985;20:217–222.

CHAPTER 4

Hemoglobinopathies: Abnormal Structure

NICOLAS CAMILO, YADDANAPUDI RAVINDRANATH

Peculiar elongated and sickle-shaped red corpuscles. . . .
—J. B. Herrick (1910)

The sickling disorders are characterized by the presence and predominance of an abnormal hemoglobin, hemoglobin S (HbS). Hemoglobin S may be present in a heterozygous form (sickle trait), a homozygous form (hemoglobin SS disease), or in a double-heterozygous form associated with either decreased β-chain production (sickle β-thalassemia) or another abnormal hemoglobin (hemoglobin D, C hemoglobin O Arab). Historical milestones for hemoglobin S disease are presented in Table 4.1.

Case 1

D.R. is a 27-month-old black girl born 10-16-89 to a 31-year-old black female $G_3P_3A_0$, after an uncomplicated pregnancy and delivery. Hemoglobin SS disease was diagnosed in utero by amniocentesis, done because the mother had a previous child with sickle cell anemia. The mother had planned, but later changed her mind and refused, termination of pregnancy. The diagnosis was confirmed during neonatal screening by isoelectric hemoglobin focusing, which showed an FS pattern. The hemoglobin solubility was positive at this time. At age 3 months, the baby's physical examination results were negative. Laboratory evaluation showed the following: hemoglobin 93 g/L, mean cell volume (MCV) 81.1 fl, white blood cell (WBC) count $6.5 \times 10^9/L$, reticulocyte count 4.8%. Peripheral blood smear showed moderate anisocytosis but no sickled red blood cells (RBC). She was started on penicillin prophylaxis. At 6 months of age, she had an acute upper respiratory infection. Physical examination showed no acute respiratory distress, a palpable liver 2 cm below the left costal margin (LCM), and a palpable spleen tip. Complete blood count (CBC) revealed the following: hemoglobin 51 g/L, MCV 78.9 fl, reticulocyte count 13.4%, WBC $16.8 \times 10^9/L$ with differential count showing 3% myelocytes, 3% metamyelocytes, 8% bands, 7% neutrophils, 71% lymphocytes, 6% monocytes, and 38 nucleated RBC/100 WBC. Peripheral smear showed anisopoikilocytosis, polychromasia, and occasional target and sickle cells. Spontaneous recovery ensued and 1 month later CBC showed hemoglobin 81 g/L. At 12 months of age the baby had her first pain-ful episode, consisting of left leg pain. At the age of 13 months, she had her first documented episode of pneumonia. Blood counts showed hemoglobin 83 g/L, MCV 67.5 fl, red cell distribution width (RDW) 26.3%, reticulocyte count 7.2%, WBC $11.1 \times 10^9/L$, with differential count showing 1% metamyelocytes, 45% neutrophils, 22% bandforms, 25% lymphocytes, 4% monocytes, and 1% nucleated RBC. Peripheral blood smear was remarkable for moderate anisopoikilocytosis, moderate hypochromia, and some target and some sickled cells. She received intravenous cefuroxime. Blood culture was negative for pathogens. Serum iron level was 21 $\mu g/dl$ (low). The patient had an uneventful course and was sent home after 72 hours to complete 14 days of amoxicillin/clavulanate, and was placed on oral iron treatment.

At 23 months of age, she received pneumococcal and Haemophilus influenzae type B vaccines.

Diagnosis

The β^S gene is prevalent in Central Africa, the Mediterranean, the Middle East, and India (fig. 4.1). It parallels the incidence of falciparum malaria and appears to provide some protection from malaria. The current prevalence of the β^S gene in the United States, the Caribbean, and Central and South America is entirely accounted for by the movement of people of African origin following colonization of the New World. About 8% of people of African origin in the United States have the β^S gene.

The clinical course of hemoglobin SS disease is variable, with some patients being asymptomatic and others having painful episodes constantly (1). Most patients have long asymptomatic periods with occasional exacerbations or crises. The reason for this variability is not completely understood and is under intense study. Genetic factors affecting the expression of the disease include the presence of α-thalassemia, the level of fetal hemoglobin, and glucose-6-phosphate dehydrogenase (G-6-PD) deficiency. Environmental factors, such as diet, geographic location, socioeconomic conditions, and access to medical care influence certain aspects of the disease.

Table 4.1 Historical Milestones for Hemoglobin S Disease°

1910	Herrick describes the presence of elongated crescent shaped red cells in the peripheral blood smears of some black individuals with anemia.
1917	V. E. Emmel shows that virtually all red cells from an individual with sickle trait undergo sickling with prolonged anaerobic incubation.
1927	Vernon Hahn and Elizabeth Gillespie identify that hemoglobin-free red cell ghosts do not undergo sickling.
1930	Scriver and Waugh show reversible oxygen dependent sickling *in vivo*.
1940	Thomas Hale Ham and William Castle describe the relationship between sickling, increased viscosity and vasoocclusive manifestations of the disease.
1941	Irving Sherman in Wintrobe's laboratory observes that red cells from anemic patients sickled much more readily than those with sickle trait and that upon deoxygenation sickled red cells exhibit birefringence in polarized light.
1945	William Castle on a train ride from Denver to Chicago with Linus Pauling, discusses sickle cell disease and I. J. Sherman's observations and suggests that some type of molecular alignment might be occurring.
1948	Janet Watson and colleagues note that sickling did not become significant until the fetal hemoglobin in the infant is replaced by " adult" hemoglobin suggesting that an abnormal adult hemoglobin may be the culprit.
1949	L. Pauling, H. Itano, S. J. Singer, and I. C. Wells demonstrate that "sickle" hemoglobin can be separated from normal adult hemoglobin by electrophoresis of hemolysates and that individuals with trait have roughly equal amounts of normal adult and sickle hemoglobins.
1950	John Harris in Castle's laboratory concluded that sickling was due to polymerization of the abnormal hemoglobin.
1950	Perutz and Mitchison observed that crystals of deoxygenated hemoglobin S were birefringent and had decreased solubility.
1957	Vernon Ingram established that sickle hemoglobin differed from HbA by only a single amino acid substitution in the β-globin chain: β-6 glutamic acid-valine thus establishing sickle cell anemia as the first molecular disease and confirming one gene/one enzyme (polypeptide) hypothesis of Beadle and Tatum.

°Adapted from Bunn HF, Forget BG. Hemoglobin: molecular, genetic and clinical aspects. Philadelphia: WB Sanders, 1986.

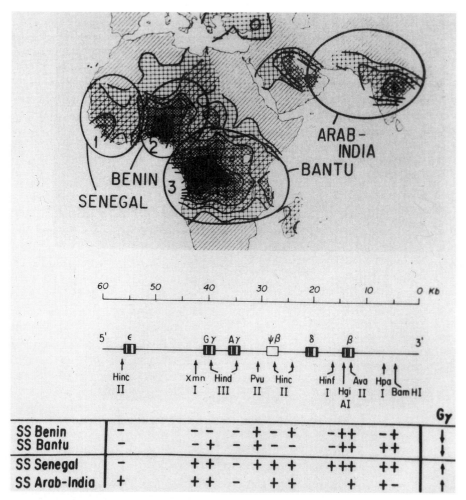

	Hinc II	Xmn I	Hind III	Pvu II	Hinc II	Hinf I / Hgi AI	Ava II	Hpa I / Bam HI	Gγ
SS Benin	−	−	−	−	+ −	+	− + +	− +	↓
SS Bantu	−	−	+	−	+ −	−	− + +	+ +	↓
SS Senegal	−	+	+	−	+ +	+	+ + +	+ +	↑
SS Arab-India	+	+	+	−	+	+	+	+ −	↑

Figure 4.1. The upper portion of the figure illustrates the origin and incidence of β^s gene and the prevalence of various β-globin haplotypes in the African continent, the Mediterranean, the Middle East, and the Indian subcontinent. The middle portion depicts the β-like gene cluster and the endonuclease definable polymorphic sites. The bottom portion shows the patterns observed in the four major β^s-linked haplotypes. The changes in the production of $^G\gamma$-chains (fetal hemoglobin) are shown in the last column to the right. (From Nagel RL, Ranney HM. [49]).

The disease severity changes with age in some patients. The pain episodes decrease in frequency and severity, but chronic organ damage ensues. After having had a mild course, bouts of multiple complications may develop in some patients in a relatively short period, with return to baseline after resolution of these (2).

The symptoms of hemoglobin SS disease are the result of intracellular polymerization of HbS, subsequent formation of erythrocytes with abnormal shape (sickle cells), and the abnormal interaction of these cells with the vascular endothelium (see below). The outcome is hemolytic anemia and vasoocclusion, with subsequent organ infarcts and damage.

Sickled erythrocytes have a decreased lifespan, 10–20 days, as compared with the normal lifespan of 120 days (3). The patient usually maintains a hemoglobin of 60 to 100 g/L by increasing erythropoiesis six- to eightfold (4). Hemolysis is predominantly extravascular, with the major sites of erythrocyte destruction being the spleen in early childhood and the liver after the spleen becomes infarcted. The compensatory mechanisms for anemia are present, including right shift in the oxygen dissociation curve and increased cardiac output.

β-Globin synthesis starts shortly before birth coincident with the rapid decline in γ-chain synthesis and is the predominant non-α-chain being produced at birth. However, at birth the γ-chain containing fetal hemoglobin still constitutes 65–90% of the hemoglobin and the β-globin containing hemoglobin does not reach adult levels of >95% until about 6 months–1 year of age. Disorders affecting the β-globin gene such as β-thalassemia major and sickle cell anemia are clinically silent at birth because of the normally low amounts of β-chains at birth. In contrast, α-thalassemias and α-globin disorders such as some of the unstable hemoglobin variants show clinical manifestations at birth.

Thus SS infants are asymptomatic at birth due to the presence of high levels of hemoglobin F (HbF). Hemolytic anemia develops concomitantly with declining levels of HbF and is evident by 4 months of age (4, 5). It results in pallor, weakness, fatigue, and jaundice. Cardiomegaly is usually present by 3 years of age (6). A left parasternal heave is common. A loud third heart sound and a left parasternal midsystolic ejection murmur are usually heard. Cardiomegaly can be demonstrated by cardiac imaging or electrocardiograph.

There is a moderate to severe normocytic normochromic hemolytic anemia (55–95 g/L), with target cells, sickled cells, Howell-Jolly bodies, polychromatophilia, reticulocytosis (5–30%), and nucleated red blood cells (NRBC) (table 4.1, fig. 4.2). The MCV is normal, unless complicated by coexistent thalassemia trait or iron deficiency, as in the case described above (table 4.1). The mean corpuscular hemoglobin concentration (MCHC) is elevated due to irreversibly sickled cells (ISC) and other dense cells. Leukocytosis ($12–15 \times 10^9$/L) due to demargination, and thrombocytosis, the result of increased platelet survival and reduced splenic reservoir, are also present. Increased reticulocytosis may be evident by 1–4 weeks of age (2). Irreversibly sickled cells appear as the hemoglobin F level declines. Erythrocyte sedimentation rate (ESR) is usually low, except during vasoocclusive episodes and infections, when it is elevated. The bone marrow is hypercellular, with erythroid hyperplasia predominating.

The **diagnosis** of hemoglobin SS disease can be made in the fetus by blood sampling and globin synthesis

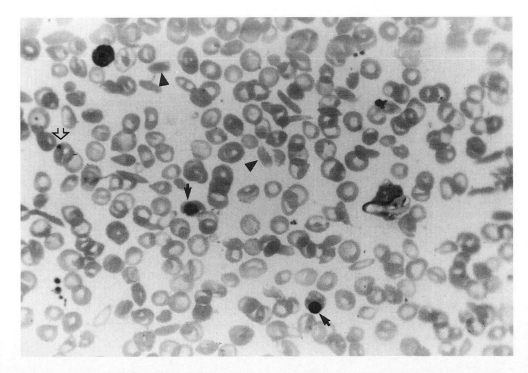

Figure 4.2. Peripheral blood smear of a child with sickle cell anemia. Straight arrows point to nucleated red blood cells. *Curved arrow* points to Howell-Jolly body.

measurement, or by amniocentesis and analysis of fetal DNA (7, 8).

In the newborn, the diagnosis can be made by citrate agar hemoglobin electrophoresis at pH 6.2. In the older child, identification of hemoglobin S can be accomplished by demonstration of sickle hemoglobin, such as in the "sickle prep" (9) and hemoglobin solubility methods (fig. 4.3A) (10). The sickle test, or sickle prep, is based on the change in morphology of the hemoglobin S–containing red cells when deoxygenated (9). One drop of 2% sodium metabisulphite is mixed with one drop of blood on a microscope slide covered with a coverslip and sealed with molten paraffin wax to exclude air and prevent drying. Sickling is demonstrated 1–24 hours later. The solubility test takes advantage of the relative insolubility of hemoglobin S in high-molarity solutions. Hemolysates with hemoglobin S become cloudy and those without it remain clear (fig. 4.3A). Solutions employed include concentrated phosphate buffers, lysing agents, and reducing agents. The definitive diagnosis is made by hemoglobin separation methods, or by DNA analysis. Hemoglobin electrophoresis is the method used most commonly. Cellulose acetate electrophoresis at alkaline pH (8.2) is the preferred test (fig. 4.3B), and citrate agar gel electrophoresis at acid pH (6.2) (fig. 4.3C)(11) is used to separate other hemoglobins, such as D and G, that comigrate with HbS on cellulose acetate. Thin-layer isoelectric focusing (12) and high-performance liquid chromatography (13) are more sensitive and have a higher resolution than conventional electrophoresis, but require greater technical skills. These methods, however, are routinely used in the mass screening of neonates for sickle cell anemia, now mandatory in many states in the United States.

Prenatal diagnosis of sickle cell anemia was initially accomplished by obtaining a sample of fetal blood from the umbilical vein or from the placenta (if situated anteriorly). The need to delay such procedures until after the 20th week of gestation posed severe time constraints on couples opting for therapeutic abortion if the fetus had SS disease. The finding of linkages between β^s gene and restriction endonuclease fragment length polymorphism (RFLP) led to its use in antenatal diagnosis at an earlier stage in gestation by analysis of genomic DNA of amniotic fluid cells (14). These techniques were further refined by the identification of restriction enzymes that specifically identify the genetic mutation (codon GAG to GTG) that results in the substitution of valine for glutamic acid in β-globin chain at position 6 (fig. 4.4). The restriction enzymes Dde I (15, 16) and Mst II (8, 16–18) both cut normal DNA at the $\beta6$ Glu site and not the β^s DNA. The development of procedures for chorionic villus sampling make possible an accurate diagnosis of

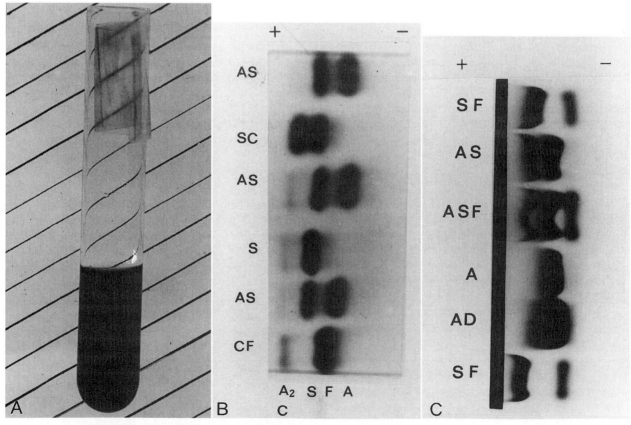

Figure 4.3**A.** Positive sickle solubility test. Note that the cloudiness caused by precipitation of hemoglobin S obscures the *lines in the background*. **B.** Cellulose acetate electrophoresis at pH 8.2. **C.** Citrate agar electrophoresis at pH 6.2.

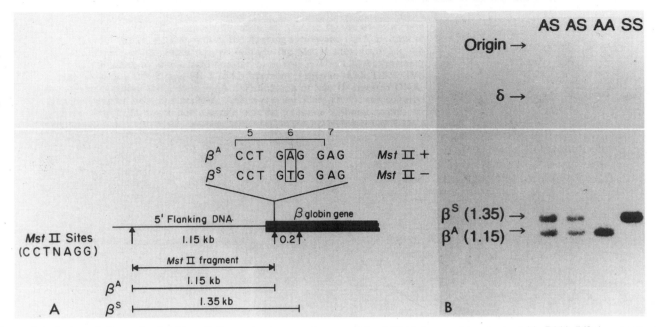

Figure 4.4. Antenatal diagnosis of sickle cell disease by the use of restriction endonuclease Mst II. **A.** Diagram of the flanking region and the 5′ portion of the β-globin structural gene. *Arrows* indicate the Mst II sites, including the one corresponding to aminoacid position 5, 6, and 7. The 1.15-kb fragment is seen in normal DNA, and the 1.35-kb fragment is seen in sickle DNA. IVS denotes intervening sequences. **B.** Autoradiograph of Mst II-digested DNA, showing samples from parents (AS, AS), a previous child (AA), and cultured ammniotic-fluid cells, which demonstrate that the fetus is a SS homozygote. (From Bunn HF, Forget BG. [57]).

sickle cell anemia and thalassemias as early as 8 weeks of gestation.

The presence of interacting α- or β-thalassemia can be suspected from peripheral blood counts (table 4.2) and identified by standard electrophoretic methods. The MCV is normal in AS and SS individuals, uncomplicated by coexistent iron-deficiency anemia or α-thalassemia trait. The MCV is reduced in the presence of thalassemia trait. The amount of HbS in AS individuals is lower when there is coexistent α-thalassemia, from the usual 40% to about 30% (2).

In the first decade of life, mortality in untreated HbSS disease can be as high as 10–15% (fig. 4.5)(2). Mortality is highest in the first 5 years (2), with the leading causes being pneumococcal septicemia and meningitis in the United States (19, 20). Other causes of death include acute splenic sequestration, acute chest syndrome, stroke, and chronic organ failure (21). Early diagnosis, comprehensive care, and prophylactic penicillin, have decreased the mortality rate to <5% (22, 23). A recent study found that, among patients >20 years of age, those with high frequency of pain episodes tended to die earlier than those with low rates (24).

Differential Diagnosis

SS disease must be distinguished from other inherited hemolytic disorders such as other hemoglobinopathies, enzymopathies, severe forms of red cell membrane disorders, and transient erythroblastopenia in the early recovery phase. The differential diagnosis of HbSS disease includes other sickle hemoglobinopathies. The disorders most likely to be confused with HbSS disease are HbSβθ-thalassemia, HbS (δβ)θθ-thalassemia, and HbS/HPFH (hereditary persistence of fetal hemoglobin). Other disorders to consider are HbSC disease, HbSβ⁺-thalassemia, HbSD disease, HbSO Arab disease, HbSE disease, and other rare variants.

Pathophysiology

Biochemistry of Sickling

Sickle cell anemia is due to the substitution of thymine for adenine in the β6 codon for glutamic acid, which results, in turn, in the substitution of valine for glutamic acid at the 6th residue in the β-globin chain. An exact explanation of how this amino acid substitution causes sickling is not yet known. The conformational changes associated with oxygenation (relaxed state, R) and deoxygenation (tense state, T) play an important part. In the deoxygenated hemoglobin molecules, the αβ-dimers move apart and rotate in relation to each other, resulting in changes in intersubunit hydrogen bonds and contact sites. The substitution of the hydrophobic valine to glutamic acid results in the formation of different (more stable) hydrophobic and electrostatic bonds in the deoxy state that favor aggregation and result in **polymerization** of hemoglobin (fig. 4.6). Electron microscopic examination shows that the hemoglobin molecules are arrayed on top of each other in a helical formation; each fiber has 14 strands (25). The process is time dependent. Initially there is the rate-limiting formation of a nucleus (15–30 HbS tetramers),

Table 4.2 Clinical and Laboratory Features of Selected Sickle Cell Syndromes°

Syndrome	Clinical Severity	Splenomegaly	Hematologic Values				Hemoglobin Electrophoresis				
			Hemoglobin (g/dl)	MCV (fl)	Retic (%)	RBC Morphology	A	A₂	F	S	C
SS	Usually marked	< 5 yr yes > 5 yr no	6–10	> 80	5–20	ISC 4+ Targets 2+ Howell-Jolly bodies	0		0–20	80–100	—
SS α-thal α,–/α,–	Variable	Variable	7–11	65–75	5–10	ISC 2+ Targets 2+			0–20	80–100	—
Sβ⁰-thal	Marked to moderate	Yes	6–10	< 80	5–20	ISC 3+ Targets 3+ Howell-Jolly bodies	0	3–6	0–20	75–100	—
Sβ⁺-thal	Asymptomatic to moderate	Yes	9–12	< 75	5–10	ISC 1+ Targets 3+	10–30	3–6	0–20	50–80	—
SC	Mild to moderate	Yes	10–15	75–95	5–10	ISC ± Targets 4+ HbC crystals	—	—	—	50	50
S HPFH	Asymptomatic	No	12–14	< 75	1–2	ISC − Targets rare	—	< 2.5	> 30	< 70	—

°Data compiled from various sources. There is considerable variability among the different syndromes and among patients. *Abbreviations:* ISC, irreversibly sickled cells; targets, target cells; HPFH, hereditary persistence of fetal hemoglobin; MCV, mean corpuscular volume.

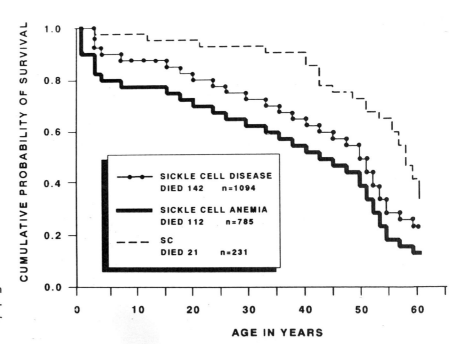

Figure 4.5 Mortality risk for patients with sickle cell disease, comparing SS and SC patients. (From Powars D, Chan LS, Schroeder WA. [41]).

followed by the formation of microtubules and fibers, and ultimately gelation (26). Thus there is a long delay before sickling occurs (27). The polymerization and sickling are reversed quite rapidly on oxygenation (in 0.5 seconds in vitro). The lag time to polymerization and the rapid reversal on oxygenation protect the patients from otherwise disastrous complications as the red cells traverse through the capillaries and venous circulation. The sol gel transition of sickle hemoglobin is also concentration, temperature, and pH dependent. Lowering concentration of S hemoglobin lengthens the time to gelation, which explains why the SS disease (as well as sickle trait) is milder when there is coexistent α-thalassemia (28, 29). The presence of other hemoglobins alters the minimum concentration of S

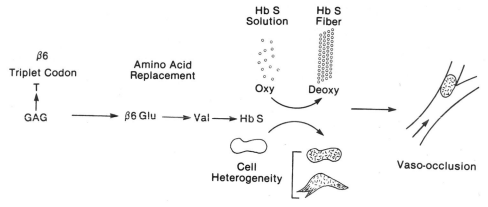

Figure 4.6 Scheme of pathogenesis of sickle cell disease. (From Bunn HF, Forget BG. [57]).

hemoglobin required for gelation (30–32). In the minimum gelation concentration (MGC) experiments it was shown that hemoglobin F retards sickling to a greater extent than does HbA or HbC (β6 Glu → Val). In contrast, HbO$_{Arab}$ (β121 Glu → Lys) and HbD$_{Los\ Angeles}$ (β121 Glu → Gln) both interact particularly strongly with HbS. These in vitro observations correlate highly with known clinical manifestation in doubly heterozygous individuals. Individuals with Sβ^+-thal, S-HPFH, and SS individuals with high F (as in some regions of Saudi Arabia and India) are almost totally asymptomatic, as are individuals with sickle trait (HbAS); SC individuals have moderate disease, while those with SO$_{Arab}$ and SD$_{Los\ Angeles}$ have symptoms comparable in severity to the homozygous state (SS).

Rheology of Sickling

The polymerization of S hemoglobin into microtubules and fibers causes great distortion of the red cell, leading to the characteristic sickling seen on wet films and peripheral blood smears. Upon reoxygenation the process is reversible and the deoxygenated sickled red cell is capable of assuming the normal discoid shape. However, after repeated cycles of sickling and desickling the cells lose this ability and are irreversibly sickled. These irreversibly sickled cells (ISCs) are dehydrated, rigid, and have little capacity for deformation (the hemoglobin-free ghosts of ISCs retain the abnormal shape), and are responsible for the increased viscosity of SS blood compared with normal. On the blood smears, the ISCs can be distinguished from the reversibly sickled cells (RSCs) by their truncated ends and a long axis that is twice the width of the cell (or greater). The RSCs, on the other hand, have the filamentous ends and are frequently curved, assuming the classic sickle configuration. The permanent distortion of the membrane in ISCs is probably due to oxidant damage to the membrane as a result of coming in contact with the polymerized hemoglobin and the resultant cross-linking of the membrane skeletal proteins.

Enumeration of ISCs from blood smears may give falsely high values. Incubation of venous blood with 100% oxygen reduces the numbers by half; further reductions can be achieved by exposure to carbon monoxide, which fixes hemoglobin in the oxy conformation. When carefully measured, the ISCs vary from 2–30%, but in a given individual with sickle cell disease the ISCs are constant in percentage. However, ISC numbers do not relate to clinical severity.

Recent studies of alterations in rheology of sickle erythrocytes, both in steady state and during painful episodes, suggest that these parameters may be useful in the laboratory confirmation of a vasoocclusive event in children with SS. It has been shown that the deformable sickle erythrocytes are more adherent to the vascular endothelium than the rigid ISCs (33). It has been observed that higher rates of painful episodes occur in patients with cells that are less dehydrated, more deformable, and have higher hemoglobin concentrations (34, 35). A negative correlation between deformability and percentage of dense cells (obtained by percoll-hypaque density gradient separation) has been noted and it has been shown that the percentage of dense cells decreases during painful episodes (36). The red cell distribution width (RDW) parallels this disappearance of dense cells during the vasoocclusive episodes (36, 37). The decrease in the ISC ric dense cell fraction presumably reflects the entrapment of the ISC at the site of vascular occlusion. This loss of ISCs is responsible for the paradoxical observation that deformability of sickle erythrocytes improves during pain episodes (Johnson RM. Unpublished observations on SS patients observed at Wayne State University Sickle Cell Center, Detroit). These observations have yet to be confirmed in children with SS disease.

Genetic Basis of Clinical Severity

The clinical severity of sickle cell anemia is highly variable. Over the years, investigators have attempted to define laboratory parameters that predict clinical severity. The task is complicated by the fact that the clinical definition of severity is difficult. The frequency of painful episodes is not the only measure of severity, for SS individuals with relatively few painful episodes may have a fatal outcome due to any of a variety of complications (overwhelming sepsis, splenic sequestration, acute chest syndrome, cerebrovascular accidents). The frequency of painful episodes may not bear any relationship to chronic debilitating sequelae (leg ulcers, chronic cardiopulmonary complications, renal disease). In earlier sections we discussed the relationship between the deformability of the red cell, the hemoglobin concentration, and the frequency of painful episodes. Another parameter that has been studied extensively in relation to severity is the level of fetal hemoglobin. The fetal hemoglobin level in SS individuals varies from 5–20%. It has been known for some time that sickle cell disease is milder in certain ethnic groups, notably in individuals from the Arabian peninsula and the Indian subcontinent (37–41). The fetal hemoglobin level in SS individuals in these two ethnic groups has been found to be relatively higher, reaching up to 15–20%. The genetic basis for this difference in the level of fetal hemoglobin is complex, but appears to be linked to DNA haplotypes, defined as patterns of DNA polymorphisms in the β-globin gene cluster (42–48).

These haplotypes are identified using various restriction endonucleases that cleave the DNA at specific sites. Using selected endonucleases, the researcher can discern specific patterns along a section of a chromosome. Using such techniques, one can identify several DNA haplotypes linked to β^S gene, of which four patterns account for the majority. These are SS Benin, SS Senegal, SS Bantu, and SS Arab-India (see fig. 4.1)(41, 49). The percentage of fetal hemoglobin varies among the different haplotypes. The highest mean hemoglobin F levels in sickle cell anemia patients have been found in those with the Arab-Indian haplotypes, followed by Senegal, Bantu, and Benin haplotypes in that order (fig. 4.7). The Senegal and the Arab-Indian haplotypes are associated with a high expression of $^G\gamma$ and maintenance of the newborn $^G\gamma{:}^A\gamma$ ratio of fetal hemoglobin

(60:40 vs the adult ratio of 40:60). The Benin, Bantu (Central African Republic), and Cameroon haplotypes are characterized by normal $^G\gamma$ levels in the adult.

An additional factor influencing fetal hemoglobin levels appears to be gender (41). The mean fetal hemoglobin level in females with SS disease has been found to be higher than in males (8.55% vs 6.09% in one study)(41). The genetic basis for this difference is under investigation.

The relationship between the inheritance of the different haplotypes and the morbidity of sickle cell disease has been reviewed (41). The frequency and intermixing of the haplotypes is highly variable in African Americans. More than half of the patients have at least one Benin haplotype, 25% have the CAR (Bantu), 12% have the Senegal, 3% have the Cameroon, and the remainder have one of several infrequently observed haplotypes (41, 50).

The patients with a Senegalese haplotype have a lower age-adjusted incidence rate in every acute clinical complication. The inheritance of a single Senegalese haplotype appears to protect against various complications (table 4.3).

The morbidity and clinical severity of SS disease is also influenced by the coinheritance of α-thalassemia, which is frequent in the populations affected by the β^S gene. The combined influence of the β^S gene haplotype and α-thalassemia on morbidity in sickle cell anemia has been examined by Poward et al. (41). A schematic representation of the relationship is presented in figure 4.8. The presence of α-thalassemia appears to have a moderating effect. This is presumably related to the decrease in MCHC, which influences the rate of polymerization of hemoglobin S, as discussed above (51).

Management

Evaluation

Evaluation starts with history and physical examination. Family history, if positive, and ethnic origin are helpful in determining the initial choice of laboratory studies. A useful battery of studies might include a direct antiglobulin test; hemoglobin electrophoresis with quantitation of hemoglobin A_2 and hemoglobin F; isopropanol precipitation test for unstable hemoglobins; red cell 2,3-diphosphoglycerase (DPG), adenosine triphosphate (ATP) and DPG/ATP ratio; and G-6-PD assay and osmotic fragility. All of these studies can be done with <5 ml of blood. It is important to recognize that there may be only one chance to obtain a pretransfusion blood sample, and anticoagulated blood should be set aside to be sent to reference laboratories if the above studies cannot be performed immediately on site.

Therapy

Transfusion Therapy

Simple transfusion is indicated to improve oxygenation in severe symptomatic anemia, such as occurs in aplastic crisis and splenic sequestration. Exchange transfusion is

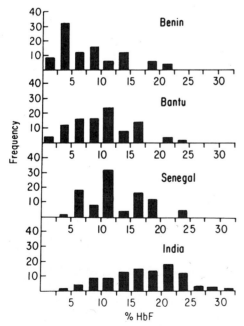

Figure 4.7. Frequency of distribution of hemoglobin F levels in homozygous carriers of the Benin, Bantu, Senegal, and Arab-Indian haplotype. (From Nagel RL, Ranney HM. [49]).

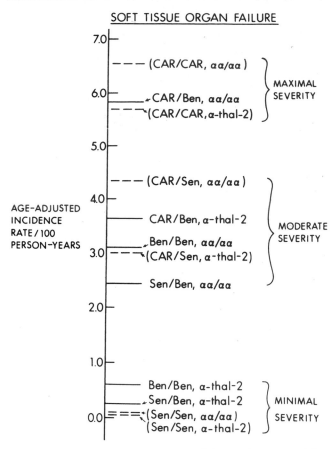

SOFT TISSUE ORGAN FAILURE

Figure 4.8. Schematic representation of the coinheritance of the β^S gene cluster haplotype and α-thalassemia-2 on the incidence of irreversible soft tissue failure in sickle cell anemia. *Solid lines* depict significant age-adjusted incidence rates. *Broken lines* are estimated rates for less common genetic combinations. (From Powars D, Chan LS, Schroeder WA. [41]).

indicated to improve microvascular perfusion by decreasing the proportion of HbS-containing erythrocytes in acute, impending, or suspected cerebrovascular accidents (CVA), acute progressive lung disease, and in priapism lasting longer than 6 hours and not responding to fluid therapy (52).

Less clear indications for exchange transfusion include prevention of recurrence of splenic sequestration, preparation for surgery under general anesthesia, intractable pain episodes, skin grafts, and chronic conditions, such as leg ulcers, and chronic organ failure. Transfusions are not indicated for chronic asymptomatic anemia, uncomplicated pain episodes, or minor infections (52). Chronic exchange transfusion regimen is indicated for a minimum of 3–5 years after CVAs. Patients on transfusion regimens for extended periods such as those with strokes are at risk for organ damage from hemochromatosis and may require iron chelation therapy. If desferrioxamine chelation is initiated, a recommended schedule is to start with a dose of 25–50 mg/kg/day administered by continuous subcutaneous infusion over 10–12 hours for 5–7 days a week. Addition of hydrocortisone 1 mg per 500 mg of desferrioxamine to the infusate reduces the local irritation.

Other complications of chronic transfusions are alloimmunization and increased risk for blood-borne infections, such as hepatitis B and C, and human immunodeficiency virus (HIV), despite donor screening. Patients on chronic transfusion regimen should undergo periodic evaluation of cardiac, liver, renal, and endocrine function, as well as screening for blood-borne infections. Semiannual studies include alanine aminotransferase (ALT), bilirubin, blood urea nitrogen (BUN), creatinine, ferritin, hepatitis A, B, and C, and HIV serology. Cardiac and ophthalmic evaluation, audiometry, and 2-hour oral glucose tolerance test are also done annually.

Several techniques of exchange transfusion are in use (52). A practical, safe, and effective method consists of the administration of 10–12 ml/kg of packed RBCs immediately following a phlebotomy of half that amount (53–55). The red cell bag is at the bedside and ready to be administered at the time of the phlebotomy. The patient's vital signs and blood pressure are monitored closely during the phlebotomy and during the administration of the packed red cells.

For acute treatment of CVAs and priapism, it is recommended that the proportion of hemoglobin S be reduced to <30%, preferably within 24 hours of diagnosis. Three partial exchange transfusions are usually required to accomplish this goal.

Other techniques include standard single or double-volume exchange transfusion, and red cell pheresis followed by packed red cell transfusion.

Chemotherapy

In the past two decades, several agents have been shown to modify the sickling process in vitro. Clinical trials with most of these agents have produced conflicting results, and controlled trials have not confirmed clinical efficacy. These chemical modifiers fall into five broad categories: (a) those that increase hemoglobin F synthesis (e.g., 5-azacytidine, hydroxyurea, erythropoietin, hydroxybutyrate); (b) noncovalent and covalent modifiers (e.g., urea, sodium cyanide, acetylic acid, pyridoxal derivatives, glutathione, cystamine); (c) membrane modifiers (zinc, procaine hydrochloride, phenothiazines, cetiedil citrate, pentoxifylline); (d) agents that improve peripheral perfusion (tolazoline, papaverine, pentoxifylline); and (e) miscellaneous compounds (acetazolamide, desamino-D-arginine vasopressin). A great impetus for the development of antisickling agents came from the initial clinical trials with oral and intravenous urea (56). However, it was quickly observed that each of these agents has its limitations, primarily due to undesirable complications that restrict clinical use. Despite these setbacks, the knowledge gained from these agents should provide the basis for future developments in this area. The mechanism by which each of these agents affect the sickling process is different (57, 58). Noncovalent modifiers such as urea interfere with polymerization by disrupting intermolecular hydrophobic bonds. The chief limitations for the use of urea are the large amount of the agent required for in vivo activity and the associated fluid load and electrolyte disturbances which might complicate the care of a sick patient. Low-dose prophylactic oral urea has shown no significant benefit. Sodium cyanate inhibits sickling by carbamylation of $\beta6$ valine and increases the oxygen affinity of hemoglobin S (59, 60). However, the irreversible binding of these covalent modifiers (such as sodium cyanate) to other proteins leads to systemic toxicity. Neurotoxicity has been frequent with sodium cyanate when it is given in clinically effective doses (61). This has led to its abandonment.

The well-known association of high fetal hemoglobin in SS patients with low clinical severity led to attempts at increasing the hemoglobin F production (62). The most extensively studied drugs are 5-azacytidine, hydroxyurea, and, more recently, butyrate. 5-Azacytidine is known to cause demethylation of genes, which results in derepression (63, 64). Although clinical trials have confirmed that hemoglobin F production indeed increases when 5-azacytidine is given, the level of increase was not sufficient to significantly alter the clinical course. The potential for mutagenesis and carcinogenesis with this chemotherapeutic agent dampens the enthusiasm for long-term use of the agent. In this regard, hydroxyurea appears to be more promising primarily because of the larger clinical experience with long-term oral treatment in patients with chronic myelogenous leukemia. Clinical trials (62, 65–69) show that a 10–15% increase in the fetal hemoglobin can be achieved with a dose of 10–30 mg/kg/day. In addition to the increase in F cells and F reticulocytes, there is also an increase in MCV and a decrease in MCHC. However, the modest increment of fetal hemoglobin may not be sufficient in patients with low baseline fetal hemoglobin levels to make significant clinical impact. There remains a potential for carcinogenesis.

The observation that infants of diabetic mothers have high fetal hemoglobin levels led to the evaluation of sodium butyrate (which is increased in these infants) as an agent to stimulate fetal hemoglobin synthesis (70). In vitro studies confirmed that butyrate indeed stimulates fetal hemoglobin synthesis (71, 72). Because of the low order of toxicity and clinical use of butyrate in other settings (e.g., in cancer patients and as a nutritional support), clinical trials were initiated in 3 patients with sickle cell anemia and 3 patients with β-thalassemia syndromes with a short course of intravenous infusion of arginine butyrate. The drug was infused continuously for either 2 or 3 weeks at doses ranging from 500–2000 mg/kg of body weight per day (73). In all 6 patients, fetal hemoglobin synthesis increased by 6–45% above pretreatment values. The proportion of F reticulocytes increased twofold and the level of globin mRNA increased twofold to sixfold. In one thalassemic patient who was treated for 7 weeks, hemoglobin increased from 4.7–10.2 gm/dl. Toxicity was minimal. These initial studies appear promising.

Membrane modifiers such as zinc inhibit sickling through membrane expansion and increase in surface area (74–76). Cetiedil citrate interferes with sickling by preventing cellular dehydration through calcium-activated potassium efflux that normally accompanies sickling (77–80). Pentoxifylline, a methylxanthine derivative, has had extensive clinical trials in adults for chronic peripheral vascular disease and dementia (74, 81–83). Pentoxifylline increases membrane fluidity, deformability, and filterability by increasing the red cell ATP content and decreasing potassium efflux. It also appears to interfere with the attachment of hemoglobin to red cell membranes. Pentoxifylline has been used successfully in a sickle cell anemia patient in the treatment of chronic leg ulcer that was unresponsive to standard therapy (84). Clinical trials suggest that there is a reduction in the duration of pain crisis in hospitalized SS patients.

Bone Marrow Transplantation

Bone marrow transplantation can be curative for sickle cell disease. Because of the risks associated with the procedure, selection of patients has been limited to those with severe disease. Ten patients 11 months to 11 years of age have undergone bone marrow transplantation for sickle cell disease (85, 86). Short-term followup of these patients has shown encouraging results. A large multicenter study is in preparation in the United States.

Gene Therapy

New techniques to attempt to insert β-globin gene in stem cells are being investigated. Several conditions must be met for successful insertion. The normal gene has to be inserted in the target cell and be expressed at a level that will correct the deficiency. In addition, the process must be safe for the patient.

Retroviral vectors are the most effective in inserting foreign genes into cells. Means of overcoming such problems as lack of transfection of enough stem cells and inhibitory effect on the retrovirus of sequences necessary for normal β-globin gene expression are being sought. Current approaches include methods to increase viral titer and methods to increase stem cell proliferation through the use of growth factors (interleukin-3, interleukin-6, interleukin-1, granulocyte-macrophage colony-stimulating factor)(87).

Health Maintenance

The approach to health maintenance at the Children's Hospital of Michigan Sickle Cell Center is outlined below. Detection is done by isoelectric focusing in neonatal blood samples. The screening is performed by the Michigan Department of Public Health Laboratory, which reports the result to the patient's pediatrician. The patient's parents and the Sickle Cell Center are notified if an abnormal hemoglobin is detected.

If one of the sickle syndromes is suspected, the parents are notified to schedule a first visit when the infant is between 6 and 8 weeks of age. At this time, complete history and physical examination are obtained. Laboratory evaluation includes complete blood count, reticulocyte count, blood group typing, as well as baseline ALT, bilirubin, blood urea nitrogen, and creatinine, ferritin, and urine analysis. Hemoglobin electrophoresis to confirm the diagnosis and hemoglobin F quantitation are done at 2–3 months of age. Genetic counseling and anticipatory guidance are given. The parents are taught to recognize such signs of illness as irritability, fever, respiratory difficulty, and the signs of splenic sequestration, and instructed to contact the physician if any of these are present. The importance of hydration is emphasized. Immunizations are initiated, and the patient is started on penicillin prophylaxis. The immunization schedule is the same as for healthy children, with the addition of 23-valent pneumococcal vaccine at 2 and 5 years of age and every 5 years thereafter. Vaccine failures have been reported, usually in children <4 years of age and usually caused by serotypes not included in the vaccine or included, but less antigenic. Penicillin is given at a dose of 125 mg orally twice daily up to 3 years of age and 250 mg twice daily thereafter. An 84% reduction in pneumococcal septicemia has been achieved with penicillin prophylaxis (22). Hepatitis B vaccine is recommended for all children with sickle cell disease and is given in three doses at the initial visit, at 1 month, and at 6 months of age.

Patients with hemoglobin SS disease are seen quarterly for routine visits. Interval history and physical examinations, complete blood count, reticulocyte count, and any other pertinent diagnostic studies are obtained. Anticipatory guidance is reinforced. Annually, the following diagnostic studies are obtained: ALT, bilirubin, blood urea nitrogen, creatinine, and urine analysis. Ultrasound of the gallbladder is done yearly until it shows positive. Lead levels are done annually until 6 years of age and more frequently in any child with pica. After 15 years of age, the patient is sent for annual ophthalmic examinations (after 10 years of age in patients with hemoglobin SC).

Case 1 (continued)

At 2 years of age, D.R. presented to the emergency room with 1 day's history of fever, rapid breathing, and pallor. On physical examination, her temperature was 40.5°C, respirations 60 breaths/minute, heart rate 200 beats/minute, blood pressure 131/62 mm Hg. The child appeared sick, lethargic but arousable, and markedly pale, had a 3/6 systolic ejection murmur at the left lower sternal border, and a palpable liver, 3 cm, and spleen, 5 cm below the costal margin. Capillary refill was 2–3 seconds. The patient was immediately given oxygen and fluid resuscitation. Blood and urine cultures, blood count, gases, blood typing, and cross-matching were obtained, and the patient was given a stat dose of cefotaxime intravenously. Hemoglobin was 27 g/L, MCV 85.6 fl, reticulocyte count 32.8%, WBC 42.5 × 10⁹/L, with differential 3% bands, 55% neutrophils, 35% lymphocytes, 7% monocytes, and 8% nucleated RBC. Platelet count was

$27 \times 10^9/L$. *Smear showed neutrophils with mild toxic granulations, RBC with moderate anisopoikilocytosis, marked polychromasia, slight target, and sickle cells. Prothrombin time (PT), partial thromboplastin time (PTT), and fibrin split products were normal. The patient was admitted to the intensive care unit. On subsequent examinations 40 minutes and 90 minutes after the first examination, the spleen was measured at 7 and 8 cm, respectively. A partial exchange transfusion was performed. The heart rate decreased to 116 beats/minute, and spleen to 6 cm 4 hours after exchange transfusion, and Hgb increased to 112 g/L. Blood, urine, and cerebrospinal culture results were negative. Subsequent course was unremarkable and the patient was discharged on the 4th day to continue penicillin prophylaxis. On followup outpatient examination 1 day after discharge, the spleen was measured at 5 cm below costal margin. A chronic transfusion regimen was recommended to prevent recurrences of sequestration episodes, but the patient's mother declined. Therefore the patient underwent surgical splenectomy 1 month later. An exchange transfusion was performed 2 days prior to the surgery to decrease hemoglobin S level and thus prevent complications of hypoxia during anesthesia and surgery.*

Acute Anemic Episodes

Diagnosis

Acute anemia is most commonly the result of splenic sequestration or erythroblastopenic episode (aplastic crisis).

Acute splenic sequestration occurs in infants and young children 5 months–2 years of age whose spleens have not yet undergone fibrosis (88, 89). The cause is unknown, but patients with low HbF levels are at greater risk (90). This is one of the most dangerous complications of hemoglobin SS disease in early life and one of the leading causes of death. Splenic sequestration is due to intrasplenic pooling of blood. There is sudden onset of weakness, pallor, dyspnea, tachypnea, tachycardia, syncope, and abdominal fullness due to massive splenomegaly. The hemoglobin drop is rapid, with marked reticulocytosis, erythroblastosis, and moderate-to-severe thrombocytopenia (88). Hypotension and shock may occur. The patient may die within hours after onset; in fact, some patients are dead on arrival at the hospital (88, 89). Recurrence rate can be as high as 47%, usually within 6 months (89), and a mortality rate as high as 14% has been reported (91). Minor episodes of splenic sequestration are frequent, presenting with moderate increases in spleen size, decrease in hemoglobin of 2–3 g/dl, and resolving spontaneously (91). These children may be at risk for more severe episodes. Sequestration may occur in the liver (sickle hepatopathy), causing liver enlargement, tenderness, hyperbilirubinemia, increased anemia, and reticulocytosis (92). Shock does not occur since the liver is not as distensible as the spleen. Sickle hepatopathy should be distinguished from acute cholecystitis.

Erythroblastopenic episodes (aplastic crises) result from the temporary suppression of erythropoiesis due to bacterial infections, such as *Salmonella* and *Streptococcus*, and viral infections, such as infectious mononucleosis (93) and especially parvovirus B19 (94). When due to parvovirus B19, acute erythroblastopenic episodes occur in an epidemic pattern (95). Parvovirus B19 is a major cause of acute erythroblastopenia in patients with chronic hemolytic anemia of any kind, in contrast to the transient erythroblastopenia of childhood, whose etiology is still unknown (96). B19 parvovirus infects hematopoietic cells, causing inhibition of colony formation of the red cell progenitors CFU-E and BFU-E in vitro (97).

During these episodes, there is weakness, listlessness, tachypnea, and tachycardia. Reticulocytes are absent, and marrow erythroblasts are markedly reduced. The anemia can become severe, resulting in congestive heart failure and even death. Erythroblastopenia usually resolves spontaneously in approximately 10 days. During recovery, there is marked reticulocytosis and erythroblastosis, with the reticulocyte count reaching 50% or more at times. The diagnosis of parvovirus B19 is made by serology (98, 99) or by demonstrating the presence of viral DNA (99).

Treatment

Evaluation of acute anemia includes taking of history and physical examination, with attention to respiratory distress, signs of circulatory failure and shock, and liver and spleen size. Complete blood count, reticulocyte count, and blood group typing are obtained. The test for parvovirus detection is sent if aplastic crisis is suspected. Septic workup and measurement of blood gases may be required if the patient looks severely ill. Admission to the hospital is usually necessary to monitor respiratory and hemodynamic status. Intensive care is the rule for acute splenic sequestration. In splenic sequestration, hemoglobin is monitored every 4 hours until stable. Hemoglobin and reticulocyte count are monitored daily in erythroblastopenic episodes.

Acute splenic sequestration is treated aggressively with oxygen and intravenous fluids, as needed, for respiratory distress and shock. Packed red cells are transfused as soon as available to raise Hb to 90–100 g/L. Antibiotics are administered empirically if the patient is febrile, very ill, or in shock, until sepsis is ruled out by negative culture results.

In patients who have had more than one episode of splenic sequestration, chronic transfusion regimens have been recommended to prevent recurrences (100). However, in a recent retrospective study, the risk of recurrence in patients in a transfusion program was similar to that in the patients who were only observed, and the recurrences occurred despite hemoglobin S levels of <30% (101).

Erythroblastopenic episodes are self-limited, however, symptomatic patients and patients with severe anemia require red cell transfusion. To avoid circulatory overload in severe anemia, the physician must give transfusions slowly, in aliquots of 3–5 ml/kg every 6–8 hours, to gain a Hb level of 50–60 g/L. Intravenous furosemide may be used in these circumstances to decrease plasma volume. A partial exchange transfusion may be required in the most severe cases.

Case 2

Case 2 is that of a 3-year-old African American boy born 6/1/88. Both parents had sickle cell trait. The diagnosis of hemoglobin SS disease was made during neonatal screening by isoelectric focusing, which showed an FS pattern. The hemoglobin solubility was positive at this time. The boy was seen for the first time in the Sickle Cell Clinic at the age of 7 months. At this time he was started on prophylactic penicillin. At 8 months of age, painful swelling developed in the fingers in the right hand. The diagnosis of dactylitis was made and he was treated with hydration and oral analgesics as an outpatient with resolution of the symptoms.

Vasoocclusive Painful Episodes

Diagnosis

The onset of vasoocclusive manifestations is variable, but 50% of patients will have symptoms by 1 year of age and most by 5–6 years of age. Vasoocclusion can lead to acute episodic events and to chronic organ damage. Acute vasoocclusive episodes and vasoocclusive-related strokes occur more often in children and young patients, while symptoms related to organ failure, in particular, cardiac and renal symptoms, are seen more often in adults. Painful episodes (pain crises) are the most common acute vasoocclusive events. The pain seems to result from inflammatory response to tissue necrosis. This has been demonstrated in the case of painful bone crises (102, 103); however, the pathophysiology of abdominal pain crises is less clear and may involve different mechanisms in different situations.

There are a number of precipitating factors, such as infections, fever, dehydration, fatigue, changes in weather, and psychological factors. Although a few patients have frequent severe pain episodes, most patients have long asymptomatic periods with few episodes of pain.

The pain is described as deep-seated, boring, and may last from minutes to days or weeks, involving single to multiple sites (2). A dull ache can persist for days after the pain crisis has resolved. A mild fever may be present. Clinical signs are often lacking, especially when the infarctions occur in deep-seated areas. The hemoglobin may fall early in the course (36). Erythrocyte deformability is further decreased (104) and density separation studies show that the dense cell fraction is also decreased during the crisis (36, 105). The red cell distribution width (RDW) has been found to be decreased during the painful crisis, possibly reflecting this trapping of ISC-rich dense cell fraction (36, 37). This finding requires confirmation.

Painful bone episodes are due to avascular necrosis of limited areas of bone marrow with inflammatory response. The marrow seems vulnerable because of its high oxygen requirement and small capillaries. Infarction of the bony cortex may occur in infants, but is uncommon after early childhood because of good collateral circulation.

The location of infarction changes with age. Infarction of metacarpals and metatarsals is most frequent in infants, whereas long bone involvement is more common in older individuals.

Painful episodes involving metacarpals and metatarsals (e.g., dactylitis, hand-foot syndrome) result from symmetrical infarction of these bones (fig. 4.9A). Often the presenting symptom of the SS disease, these episodes occur more often between the ages of 6 months and 2 years (106). There is painful swelling of the dorsa of the hands and feet, often with fever. Dactylitis is associated with low hemoglobin F levels and high reticulocyte counts (90). Radiographs show soft tissue swelling at first, and areas of osteolysis, periostitis, and bone reabsorption approximately 2 weeks later. Attacks resolve within 1 week, but recurrence is common. Occasional sequelae include premature epiphyseal fusion and bone shortening (107, 108).

Painful episodes involving long bones result from infarction in the diaphyseal-metaphyseal junction or in the intermediate segment. The bones most frequently involved are the humerus, tibia, and femur (109). The episodes begin after the third or fourth year of life. The pain is described as deep, gnawing, throbbing, and there is tenderness and sometimes swelling in the affected area (fig. 4.9B). Signs of inflammation are uncommon except when the affected area of the bone is superficial such as anterior tibia or clavicle. Mild-to-moderate fever may be present. Radiographic study results are usually negative at the onset, but may later show areas of bone infarction

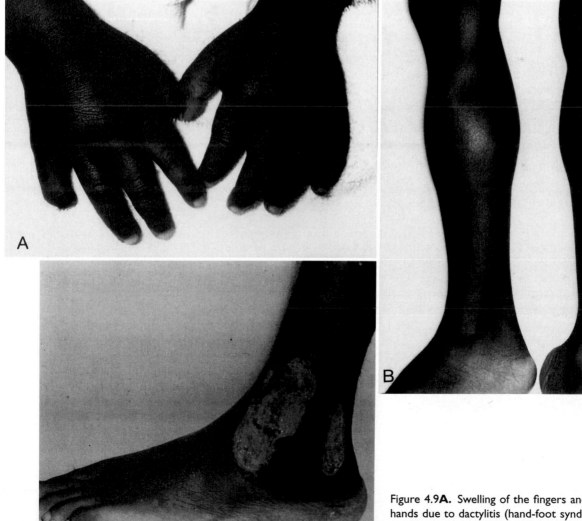

Figure 4.9A. Swelling of the fingers and dorsum of the hands due to dactylitis (hand-foot syndrome). B. Infarct of tibia causing swelling of the anterior aspect of the leg. C. Chronic leg ulcer in a patient with sickle cell anemia.

and periostitis. The attack usually resolves in 3–5 days. Distinction from osteomyelitis may be difficult when there is fever and localized pain.

Acute infarcts of other bones are seen. Skull bony infarcts with periorbital swelling with and without proptosis and/or ophthalmoplegia have been reported (110, 111). Infarcts of the mandible may occur as well (112). Rib or sternal infarcts are associated with chest pain. Some have suggested that, in many cases, rib infarcts may be the initial event in the acute chest syndrome (113). Vertebral bodies are commonly affected, causing back pain. Joint symptoms result from marrow infarction in juxta-articular areas of long bones, or from microvascular congestion or thrombosis in the synovial membrane (114). There is pain and tenderness in the affected joint, sometimes accompanied by warmth and a joint effusion, which, if aspirated, yields noninflammatory, sterile fluid (114). Some patients may have a migratory polyarthralgia (115).

Episodes of abdominal pain may occur alone or in combination with bone pain crises. The exact mechanism by which abdominal pain occurs is not known in the majority of the episodes. Mechanisms that may lead to abdominal pain in patients with hemoglobin SS disease include mesenteric arterial thrombosis (116), infarction in the vertebral marrow with either referred or root pain, and capsular stretching from infarction within abdominal structures, such as liver or spleen (117). Pneumonia, cholecystitis, pyelonephritis, and mesenteric or retroperitoneal adenopathy are other sources of abdominal pain in these patients (118).

The episodes are frequently recurrent. The pain is epigastric or central, usually mild, and may be accompanied by low-grade fever. Occasionally, the pain may be severe, localized, with tenderness, guarding, fever, and leukocytosis. The bowel sounds are usually normal, but may be decreased. These episodes may be hard to distinguish from an acute "surgical" abdomen. The crisis resolves spontaneously in a few days in most cases. Bowel perforations do not occur in abdominal pain episodes.

Management

Evaluation of pain episodes starts with taking of history and physical examination. The severity and location of pain are assessed. Fever, tachypnea, respiratory distress, localized abdominal pain, peritoneal signs, bone point tenderness, and joint swelling, although often present in sickle cell crises, mandate a careful search for other causes, especially infectious. If infection is suspected, appropriate cultures and imaging studies should be obtained and antibiotics should be started empirically. Since osteomyelitis is infrequent, the patient with bone pain and fever can be managed conservatively for 3–4 days. Thus invasive procedures such as aspiration of a bone or joint are only implemented when the clinical course is not consistent with pain crisis, since they pose a risk to these patients because of poor wound healing.

Mild-to-moderate pain can be treated on an ambulatory basis with oral hydration and oral analgesics such as acetaminophen with codeine. Oral nonsteroidal antiinflammatory drugs (NSAIDs), such as ibuprofen and naproxen may be helpful, particularly with chronic pain. Admission to the hospital is indicated if there is no response to ambulatory treatment or if there is severe pain or pain complicated by other conditions such as fever or infection. If dehydrated, the patient is hydrated orally if able to drink, or parenterally if unable. Fluid and electrolyte balance is monitored closely and care is taken not to overhydrate. Parenteral opioids are the drugs of choice for patients with severe pain. The choice of a specific agent depends on many factors, such as individual previous experience, side effects, interactions with other drugs, and patient preference. During the initial 24–48 hours, the drug is administered in a fixed schedule at an interval that does not extend beyond the duration of action. Morphine and meperidine are the drugs used most frequently; however, the use of meperidine is falling out of favor in many institutions because of its effects on the central nervous system and the risk of seizures (119). Meperidine-associated seizures tend to occur early after starting the drug (<4 days from the start of therapy), are usually generalized, and do not recur when the drug is discontinued (120, 121). Meperidine-associated seizures appear to be less common in children. The majority of meperidine-associated seizures have been reported in adults. Caution should be exercised not to oversedate. Careful monitoring of the response, by talking to the patient, family, and nurses is essential. The patient is also monitored for respiratory depression. Measures to avoid atelectasis, such as incentive spirometer and early ambulation. should be encouraged.

Hydroxyzine and promethazine may potentiate the analgesic effect of opioids. NSAIDS are used as adjuvants in some patients. Patients with very severe pain that is not responsive to the measures outlined above may require continuous infusion treatment with morphine. New modalities are under investigation for the treatment of sickle cell pain. Patient-controlled analgesia devices have been tried with promising results (122, 123). Clinical trials with Ketorolac, a new parenteral NSAID, are being conducted. This drug may prove useful as frontline therapy for moderate-to-severe pain.

Case 2 (continued)

The patient was hospitalized at age 8 months because of fever and irritability. The cultures were negative and he was discharged after 3 days of intravenous cefuroxime.

He remained well until 15 months of age when he presented to the emergency room with cough, nasal congestion, three episodes of emesis, and high fever for 1 day. Physical examination showed temperature of 39.4°C, respiratory rate 44 breaths/minute, heart rate 150 beats/minute, blood pressure 132/55 mm Hg, a grade 2–3/6 systolic ejection murmur at the left sternal border, *and a palpable spleen tip. There were no meningeal signs. Laboratory studies included the following: hemoglobin 84 g/L, MCV 77.4 fl, WBC count 33.6 × 10⁶/L,* with 1% bandforms, 54% neutrophils, 42% lymphocytes, 3% monocytes, 2% nucleated red blood cells; reticulocyte count was 14%; peripheral blood smear showed marked anisopoikilocytosis and polychromasia, moderate target cells, occasional sickle cells, and occasional Howell-Jolly bodies. A chest x-ray was negative. Blood cultures were obtained and the patient was admitted to the hospital and treated with intravenous cefuroxime. The blood cultures grew Streptococcus pneumoniae. The boy was treated for 10 days with intravenous cefuroxime and was discharged from the hospital after an uneventful course to continue prophylactic penicillin. At the age of 24 months he received the pneumococcal vaccine.*

Infectious Episodes

Diagnosis

Infections are the leading cause of death during childhood in patients with hemoglobin SS disease (19, 124). Impairment of splenic function and opsonization renders these children more susceptible to infection with *S. pneumoniae* and *Haemophilus influenzae*. Sepsis, meningitis, and pneumonia are the most common infectious syndromes.

Fulminant pneumococcal septicemia is most common in children <2 years of age (125, 126). The course may be rapid, with progression from high fever to shock and death within 12–24 hours of the onset of symptoms. Disseminated intravascular coagulation and adrenal hemorrhage may occur. Meningeal involvement may be present, despite a paucity of signs due to the rapid progression. In these cases, the cell count, glucose, and protein in the cerebrospinal fluid usually appear normal, but the bacterial cultures are positive. The incidence of osteomyelitis is increased in patients with hemoglobin SS disease. It is most common before the age of 5 years. The long bones are affected most frequently (109). Multiple lesions may occur, often bilateral and sometimes symmetrical. *Salmonella* infection accounts for >50% of cases (128, 129).

Fever, bone pain, local swelling and warmth, leukocytosis, and markedly elevated erythrocyte sedimentation rate are the usual clinical findings. Differentiating osteomyelitis from vasoocclusive episodes involving bone is often difficult (see earlier). Radiographic changes are not specific in the early stages. Bone nuclear scintigraphy may show increased uptake in osteomyelitis; however, similar findings are present in bone marrow infarction (130), thus limiting the usefulness of the test in sickle cell anemia. False negative results are common (131). Similarly, magnetic resonance imaging (MRI) studies are not always conclusive. It should be pointed out, however, that bone scans may highlight a site for needle aspiration of material for culture if the suspicion of osteomyelitis is high.

Septic arthritis may occur as a complication of osteomyelitis or of bacteremia. This condition may be difficult to differentiate from sympathetic joint effusions occurring during the course of vasoocclusive crises, since joint aspiration may yield elevated WBC count in both situations. However, it should be emphasized that septic arthritis is relatively rare. Thus, joint aspiration should be reserved for cases where the clinical course is suggestive of a septic joint.

Table 4.3 Age-Adjusted Incidence Rates Per 100 Person-Years and Relative Risks of Acute Recurrent Events in 221 SS Patients with or without a Senegal Haplotype

Clinical Event	No. of Episodes	Senegal° N = 42	Non-Senegal[†] N = 179	Relative Risk[‡]	(95% C.I.)	P-Value[§]
Hospital admission	2648	84.32	110.04	0.77	(0.69, 0.85)	<0.00001
All sickle crisis	1702	54.15	70.79	0.76	(0.67, 0.86)	<0.00003
Precipitated sickle crisis[‖]	479	12.94	20.53	0.63	(0.49, 0.81)	<0.00001
Acute chest syndrome	309	9.48	12.91	0.73	(0.54, 0.99)	0.045
Bone infarct (hand, foot, and long bones)	234	3.46	10.83	0.32	(0.20, 0.51)	<0.00001
Aplastic crisis	58	1.63	2.47	0.66	(0.33, 1.35)	NS
Meningitis/septicemia	57	2.10	2.29	0.92	(0.46, 1.82)	NS
Fracture	17	0.50	0.72	0.69	(0.20, 2.42)	NS
Priapism[¶]	15	0.33	1.30	0.25	(0.03, 1.92)	NS
Renal pap necrosis	12	0.18	0.56	0.32	(0.04, 2.44)	NS

°The patient has one or more Senegalese chromosomes.
[†]The patient has no Senegalese chromosomes.
[‡]Senegalese/non-Senegalese.
[§]Log-Rank test.
[‖]Associated with a major medical complication.
[¶]Using male patient population.
From Powars D, Chan LS, Schroeder WA. The variable expression of sickle cell disease is genetically determined. *Semin Hematol* 1990; 27:360. *Abbreviations:* NS, not statistically significant; C.I., confidence interval.

Treatment

The febrile patient with sickle cell anemia, particularly one <5 years of age, should be treated as potentially bacteremic. Evaluation should be prompt, emphasizing both the search for a source of infection and the respiratory and hemodynamic stability of the patient. Complete blood count, blood cultures, and chest radiograph are obtained, and the patient is given the first dose of intravenous antibiotic as soon as possible after the cultures are obtained. Antibiotics should cover S. pneumoniae and H. influenzae, as well as the usual microorganisms that are seen at that age. Our practice is to use cefuroxime for children <7 years of age and penicillin for older children. The patient is hospitalized and given intravenous antibiotics according to the organism isolated or until the cultures have been negative for 48–72 hours. A recent study suggests that febrile children <5 years of age with hemoglobin SS disease who are stable and do not appear toxic may be treated on an ambulatory basis using long-acting cephalosporins (132). The patient is given an initial intravenous dose of ceftriaxone or cefuroxime and is observed for several hours until initial laboratory results and chest radiograph are available. If the patient remains stable and laboratory tests (and chest radiograph and spinal fluid if indicated) do not appear significantly abnormal, an oral antibiotic such as cefaclor is prescribed and the patient is discharged home. Careful followup is essential if this approach is taken.

Osteomyelitis and septic arthritis are treated initially with intravenous antibiotics to cover salmonellae and staphylococci. Further treatment is tailored to eradicate the organism isolated. Duration of treatment for osteomyelitis is at least 4–6 weeks. Surgical drainage is carried out if indicated. Recurrences may occur months or years later (fig. 4.9C).

Case 2 (continued)

At 30 months of age, the patient presented to the emergency room with rhinorrhea, nasal congestion, cough, and fever. Laboratory investigations showed the following: hemoglobin 66 g/L, MCV 79.2 fl, WBC count 18.9 × 10⁶/L with 5% bands, 35% neutrophils, 50% lymphocytes, 10% monocytes, and 6% nucleated red blood cells; reticulocyte count 21.6%; peripheral blood smear showed moderate anisopoikilocytosis, marked polychromasia, moderate sickle and target cells, and occasional Howell-Jolly bodies. Admission chest x-ray showed bilateral infiltrates in both lung bases. Blood cultures were obtained and the patient was admitted to the hospital and treated with intravenous cefuroxime for 3 days. The patient had an unremarkable course. The blood cultures were negative and he was discharged on amoxicillin-clavulanate. However, the prescription was not obtained and 2 days later he was readmitted with fever and worsening of symptoms. Intravenous cefuroxime was resumed. Repeat blood cultures remained negative. On the second day of hospitalization, respiratory distress developed, with a respiratory rate of 60 breaths/minute, in-tercostal retractions, worsening of crackles, and poor air exchange. Arterial blood gas showed PO₂ 50 mm Hg. A double-volume exchange transfusion was performed with subsequent improvement of respiratory symptoms and decrease in respiratory rate. Postexchange Hb was 104 g/L. He continued to improve and was discharged after 7 days of antibiotic treatment.

Acute Chest Syndrome

Diagnosis

The term "acute chest syndrome" (ACS) encompasses episodes of chest pain, with or without fever, and, in the majority of cases, pulmonary infiltrate on chest radiograph. ACS is responsible for 25% of hospital admissions in patients with sickle cell anemia (21). ACS has been ascribed to pneumonia in children and to pulmonary infarction in adults (133, 134). The initiating event can be either, followed by the other as a complication. Rib infarcts can initiate ACS by causing local soft tissue reaction (113). Pleuritis with pleuritic chest pain develop, causing the patient to splint and hypoventilate, leading to atelectasis and radiographic infiltrate. Secondary infection may develop. Pleural effusion may result from pleural or pulmonary involvement. An association between severity of ACS and use of narcotic analgesics has been reported (135). It is thought that by causing respiratory depression and hypoventilation, narcotics may lead to atelectasis, hypoxia, and pulmonary intravascular sickling. Recently, it has been proposed that fat embolism occurring as a complication of vasoocclusive bone infarcts may be a common mechanism of ACS (136, 137).

When pathogens are isolated, the most common ones are *Pneumococcus, Salmonella, Klebsiella*, and *H. influenzae* (133, 138). *Mycoplasma pneumoniae, Chlamydia*, and viruses have been isolated also (139). Manifestations of ACS include cough, fever, tachypnea, dyspnea, pleuritic chest pain, and pleural rub. Rib tenderness is present when there is rib infarction (113). Mild respiratory symptoms may progress within a short time to acute deterioration. Purulent sputum and hemoptysis are uncommon (140). The syndrome may be preceded by pain elsewhere. The hemoglobin may drop, with a rise in the reticulocyte count and white blood cell count. About 50% of bacterial pneumonias can be confirmed by culture of the blood, sputum, or nasopharynx (133). Hypoxemia and respiratory failure may occur. Chest radiograph shows infiltrates or other abnormalities in >90% of cases, regardless of the cause (141). Pleural effusion may be present. Not infrequently chest x-ray is negative at presentation, but extensive consolidation and/or pleural effusion might evident 48–72 hours later. In patients with continuing chest pain and negative chest radiograph, rib infarcts must be considered. Rib infarcts can be demonstrated by radionuclide bone scan performed 48–72 hours after the onset of symptoms. ACS was the leading cause of death in patients >10 years of age in one series (2).

Some patients tend to have repeated episodes of ACS. Repeated attacks of ACS are a known risk factor for chronic lung disease (142). Reduction in peak expiratory flow rate can be demonstrated in these cases (143). Adults with hemoglobin SS disease have been shown to have reduction in total lung capacity, vital capacity, and forced vital capacity. The diffusing capacity of the alveolar membrane is also reduced, with the greatest reductions occurring in patients with a history of pulmonary complications (143).

Management

Patients with pulmonary symptoms should be examined promptly. Hospitalization for at least 24 hours for observation is advocated by some, even in patients with relatively mild symptoms. Evaluation includes the taking of history and physical examination, with attention to the presence and degree of fever, respiratory distress, and the presence of localized rib tenderness. Complete blood count, reticulocyte count, chest radiograph, and blood gas measurements should be obtained, as well as blood and sputum cultures if there is fever. Respiratory status is monitored closely to detect the early signs of respiratory distress, such as tachypnea.

Oxygen is administered if there is hypoxemia. Use of the incentive spirometer and pulmonary toilet are indicated. Hydration should be given and monitored carefully to avoid fluid overload.

Analgesics are given as necessary. Antibiotics are given if there is fever and/or respiratory distress. Initial drugs used should provide adequate coverage for *S. pneumoniae* and *H. influenzae* in children <6 years of age. Subsequent therapy is tailored according to culture results. Antibiotic cover for *Mycoplasma* with erythromycin should be considered if fever persists or if there is no clinical improvement.

Partial exchange transfusion (see section on transfusion therapy for details) is indicated to abort the vicious cycle of hypoxia and sickling when there is moderate-to-severe respiratory distress, rapid progression or failure to improve, or when there is extensive disease. Additional criteria for partial exchange transfusion include an arterial oxygen tension (PaO_2) of <70 mm Hg, and/or a 25% drop in patient's baseline PaO_2.

Following recovery from the acute event, patients should undergo baseline pulmonary function testing and arterial blood gas measurement in order to facilitate future evaluation for acute and chronic pulmonary disease.

Case 3

*N.B., now 8 years of age, was diagnosed to have sickle cell anemia at age 2 years. Her steady state laboratory values were as follows: hemoglobin 87 g/L, Hct 24.5%, MCV 78.5 fl, reticulocyte count 10.4%, hemoglobin S 91.2%, hemoglobin A₂ 3.1%, and hemoglobin F 5.7%. Both parents have sickle trait. She has had three episodes of pneumonia and several admissions for pain episodes. In January 1991, at 4 years of age, she pre-*sented to the emergency room with a 1-day history of dragging her left foot while walking. Examination showed muscle weakness with decreased deep tendon reflexes and a Babinski sign in the left lower extremity. The rest of the examination results were normal. A stroke was suspected. A computed tomographic (CT) scan of the brain showed no abnormalities. An MRI scan of the brain showed multiple areas of increased signal intensity throughout the parenchyma, suggestive of small infarcts or areas of reversible ischemia. An arteriogram showed no evidence of congenital or acquired vascular abnormalities. The child was started on a chronic transfusion program with the aim of maintaining hemoglobin S at <40%. Hepatitis B immunization was also started. Six months after starting the transfusion regimen, her serum ferritin was 1887 ng/ml (normal 10–400 mg/ml). Currently, she is being continued on the chronic transfusion program, has started to receive iron chelation therapy, and is asymptomatic at present.*

Cerebrovascular Accidents

Diagnosis

Cerebrovascular accidents (CVA) occur in all age groups, with an incidence of 6% (144). Infarction is seen primarily in children (mean age 8 years), and hemorrhage in adults (mean age 25 years) (144, 145).

Risk factors have been difficult to identify. Cerebrovascular disease is more common in patients with low hemoglobin F levels (146). There may be a familial predilection, but this is unclear at present (145).

Infarctive strokes are due to partial or complete occlusion of large vessels, most commonly the internal carotid artery and anterior and middle cerebral arteries (55, 147, 148). Collateral circulation develops after large vessel occlusion, giving a pseudomoyamoya appearance (148, 149).

Hemorrhagic strokes may result from aneurysms formed in weakened vessels or from extensive collateral vessels as a result of cerebrovascular occlusive disease.

Symptoms of either are usually sudden, and include paresis, most commonly hemiparesis, seizures, coma, and visual symptoms, such as hemianopia or blindness. Transient ischemic attacks may occur, manifested as dysarthria, dysphagia, paresthesias, paresis, or ataxia. Some patients may be seen with subtle signs. Seizures are usually generalized, but partial seizures occur. Stupor and coma indicate severe cerebrovascular disease (150).

CT scan of the brain detects small areas of infarction, cerebral edema, and other changes associated with stroke. These usually appear 2–4 days after the episode.

Stenotic lesions are demonstrated by cerebral angiography (fig. 4.10A) (147, 151). Recently, MRI, MRI angiography, and transcranial Doppler ultrasonography have been used to visualize stenotic lesions (152, 153).

Recovery from paralysis is usually slow and partial. Seizures may be recurrent (154). The prognosis depends

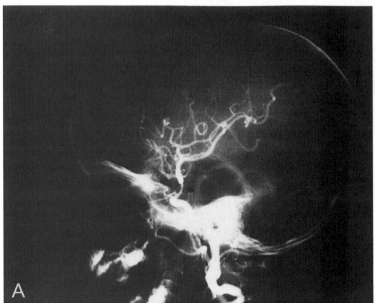
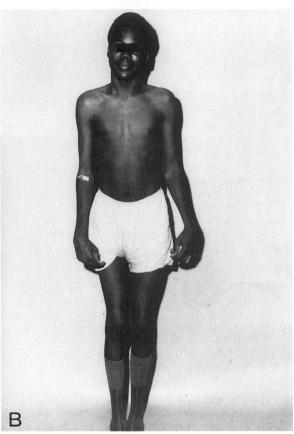

Figure 4.10**A.** Cerebral angiography showing stenosis of internal carotid artery *(arrow)* in a sickle cell anemia patient. **B.** Chronic sequelae of multiple cerebral infarcts in a patient with sickle cell anemia. Notice the mask-like fascies from bilateral facial paralysis and the contractures in the extremities.

on the cause. Mortality rate from strokes can be as high as 20% in patients who are not treated with blood transfusions (144). There is a recurrence rate of 70–90% (fig. 4.10*B*) in those who survive (144, 155), 80% of which occur within 36 months (144). Over 70% of untreated patients have permanent motor disability (fig. 4.10*B*) and a deficit in IQ (144).

Treatment

During the acute episode, rapid evaluation is essential. History is obtained, with attention to the onset and characteristics of the neurologic symptoms. Physical examination should focus on respiratory and hemodynamic status, as well as signs of increased intracranial pressure and other neurologic changes. Close monitoring for progression of symptoms is necessary. CT of the brain is done at the onset to distinguish between infarctive and hemorrhagic stroke, and to rule out other causes of neurologic symptoms. CT needs to be repeated 2–7 days later in order to demonstrate the changes in infarctive strokes. Cerebral angiography is done if no lesion is demonstrated by CT scan in the acute phase or, if hemorrhage is present, to identify surgically correctable lesions. Later, cerebral angiography may be necessary to detect areas of vessel stenosis. Cerebral angiography poses a risk to patients with sickle cell disease because of the injection of hyperosmolar contrast material. Exchange transfusion to decrease the hemoglobin S level to <30% should precede angiography. If available, newer techniques such as MRI, MRI angiography, and perhaps transcranial Doppler ultrasonography may obviate the need for contrast arteriography.

Supportive care is given as needed for maintenance of airway and ventilation. Hyperventilation should be avoided. Anticonvulsants are used if seizures are present. Drugs to decrease cerebral edema may be necessary. Rapid exchange transfusion is given as soon as blood is available to decrease the hemoglobin S level to <30%. Rapid exchange transfusion is used in both infarctive and hemorrhagic strokes. Rehabilitation is started as soon as the patient is stable and can tolerate it.

Chronic exchange transfusion is recommended to prevent recurrences. The optimal duration is not known, but since the risk of recurrence is greatest in the first 3 years after the initial event, most centers transfuse for a minimum of 3–5 years and then stop or decrease the intensity of transfusion. Some centers continue transfusion indefinitely. In such cases there is a risk for hemochromatosis; therefore chelation therapy is required eventually.

Priapism

Diagnosis

Priapism results from stasis in the vessels draining from the corpora cavernosa caused by sickling. There is evidence to suggest that priapism is not as uncommon as once thought, having a prevalence of 42–50% in one series (156). The age of onset varies from 5–40 years (156). Nocturnal erections, sexual intercourse, and masturbation may precipitate the attack.

The episodes can be prolonged and severe, lasting more than 24 hours, or short and recurrent (stuttering episodes). Short episodes may progress to major attacks. After a major attack, further episodes are unusual (156). Prolonged attacks are marked by severe penile, lower abdominal, and perineal pain. Dysuria, urinary retention, and penile and scrotal edema can occur. Symptoms are milder in the stuttering episodes. Impotence, partial or complete, has been reported following a major episode in 66% of cases (156). The prognosis is better in young children (156, 157).

Treatment

Treatment of attacks of "stuttering priapism" may prevent progression to major episodes. Minor episodes can be treated on an ambulatory basis with bedrest and oral hydration and analgesics. Stilbestrol is currently under study for prophylaxis of priapism (2). If the episode does not resolve in a few hours, the patient should be hospitalized. Adequate parenteral analgesia and sedation are used for the relief of pain. Intravenous hydration is used routinely to attempt relief of priapism. Exchange transfusion can be tried if there is no relief in 24–48 hours (157). The role of acute and chronic exchange transfusion in the treatment of priapism has not been studied in a controlled trial. Numerous other measures have been tried with little success. In severe cases regional anesthesia may be required. Surgical measures may be needed. Procedures that have been marginally successfully used include corporal aspiration and creation of shunts between the corpora cavernosa and the corpus spongiosum (158).

Chronic Syndromes

Growth and Development

Delayed physical and sexual development may be the result of multiple factors. The exact mechanism is poorly understood. Folate and zinc deficiency (159), chronic anemia, hemoglobin F level, growth hormone deficiency, and social class are among the factors thought to contribute to delayed or abnormal growth and sexual development.

Delayed sexual development is likely to be constitutional, as suggested by the relationship between weight and menarche in normal females (160). In males, there is decreased fertility with low semen volume and with low sperm number and motility (161).

Although birth weight is normal, the mean weight becomes subnormal during the first decade, which is noticeable before the first year of life (162). Patients with SS disease and $S\beta^0$-thalassemia are more affected than patients with SC disease and $S\beta^+$-thalassemia (162). The lower mean weight contributes to the typical body habitus in SS disease. Height, although delayed, approaches normal by the end of adolescence. Bone age is retarded in SS disease (163).

Musculoskeletal System

Expansion of marrow causes skeletal changes such as widening of the diploic space and thinning of the outer table in the skull, giving the radiographic appearance of "onion peel" if the trabeculae are parallel to the inner table or of "hair on end" if they are perpendicular. There is overgrowth of the anterior maxilla with dental problems and flattened vertebrae with biconcave deformity of the upper and lower surfaces (codfish vertebrae), sometimes leading to chronic back pain later in life.

Aseptic necrosis of the femoral, humeral, or fibular heads may occur as a consequence of repeated infarctions (164). Avascular necrosis of the femoral head was thought to be more common in SC disease (165); however, more recent studies fail to confirm this (166). This complication results in persistent hip pain and can lead to disability.

Cardiovascular System

Most patients with hemoglobin SS disease have cardiomegaly due to chronic anemia. Left ventricular hypertrophy is found on electrocardiography in 50% of these (167). In addition to this, a sickle cardiomyopathy has been described and is characterized by decreased left ventricular contractility and ischemic electrocardiographic changes and abnormal ejection fraction during exercise (168–170).

Immune System

The immune functions of the spleen are impaired in hemoglobin SS disease. During the first year of life a "functional asplenia" develops, with inability to clear particles from the blood; in some children this is seen as early as 3 months of age (fig. 4.11) (171). Functional asplenia may be present in spite of clinical splenomegaly. Loss of splenic function is slower in children with hemoglobin SC than in those with hemoglobin SS or hemoglobin $S\beta^0$-thalassemia (fig. 4.11) (171). In hemoglobin $S\beta^+$-thalassemia, the splenic function is nearly normal (171). Experience with patients on chronic transfusion regimens suggests that atrophic spleens may reenlarge, with restoration of splenic function (172, 173). Evidence for functional asplenia includes erythrocytes with Howell-Jolly bodies on peripheral blood smears, increased numbers of pocked red cells on phase contrast microscopy, and/or absence of uptake in spleen on radionuclide imaging (fig. 4.12) (171).

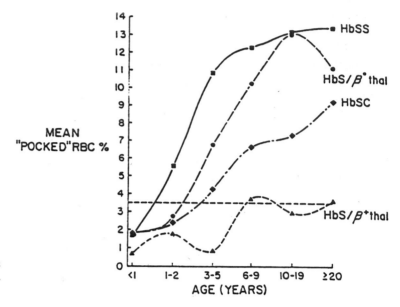

Figure 4.11. Loss of splenic function in relation to age as measured by pocked red cell count in sickle cell syndromes. (From Pearson H, et al. [171]).

ASSESSMENT OF SPLENIC FUNCTION IN HEMOGLOBIN SS DISEASE

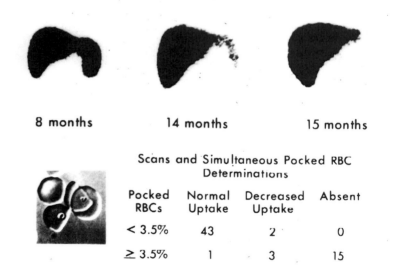

| 8 months | 14 months | 15 months |

Scans and Simultaneous Pocked RBC Determinations

Pocked RBCs	Normal Uptake	Decreased Uptake	Absent
< 3.5%	43	2	0
≥ 3.5%	1	3	15

Figure 4.12. Correlation of pocked red cell count with radionuclide imaging study of the spleen.

Renal System

Hyposthenuria, which develops early, is due to intramedullary sickling, with resultant decreased blood flow and damage of the counter current multiplier mechanism (174–177). These patients have polyuria, nocturia, enuresis, and may dehydrate easily. Hyponatremia due to excessive sodium loss in the urine can occur. Other urinary complications that can occur are papillary necrosis with hematuria and glomerulonephritis, resulting in nephrotic syndrome (178). Hematuria may be severe enough to cause iron-deficiency anemia. The left kidney appears to be more commonly involved (2). Hyposthenuria and hematuria also occur in individuals with sickle cell trait (see discussion under sickle cell trait). Coexistent α-thalassemia appears to lessen the severity of loss of urinary-concentrating ability.

Treatment of hematuria is symptomatic. ε-Aminocaproic acid (179–181) and glycopressin (182) have been used with some success in severe cases. Irrigation of renal pelvis with oxychlorosene has also been used (183). Nephrectomy has been done when the bleeding was considered life threatening (177, 184, 185).

Gastrointestinal System

A syndrome due to intrahepatic sickling has been described, with elevated liver enzymes, hyperbilirubinemia, and sometimes right upper quadrant pain (92, 186). Recurrent intrahepatic sickling can result in hepatic necrosis and cirrhosis. Gallstones are very common, ranging in incidence from 12% at 2–4 years of age to 42% at 15–18 years (187). Cholecystitis may occur as a result. Cholecystectomy is indicated after an episode of cholecystitis and for persistent *Salmonella* bacteremia if gallstones are present.

Eyes

Proliferative retinopathy, although more prevalent in hemoglobin SC disease, can also occur in SS disease. The prognosis is variable, as some lesions can progress to retinal detachment with permanent loss of vision, while others heal spontaneously by autoinfarction (188, 189). Treatment modalities used are photocoagulation and cryotherapy (189, 190).

A more benign nonproliferative retinopathy resulting from peripheral retinal hemorrhage also occurs (191).

Skin

Chronic leg ulcers (fig. 4.9), seen in adolescents and adults, result from increased venous pressure due to marrow expansion (192). The ulcers are most commonly seen in the ankles above the medial and lateral malleoli and may be bilateral (193). Minor trauma with secondary infection is a common initiating event; however, the ulcers may develop spontaneously, presumably from skin infarction. Healing is slow. Prevention of trauma is important. Treatment consists of bedrest with leg elevation, antiseptic agents, debridement when necessary, and topical antibiotics. Zinc sulphate 200 mg orally three times a day may improve healing (194). Early treatment may prevent fibrosis and relapse. Transfusion therapy and/or skin grafting should be considered for persistent cases.

Sickle Cell Trait

Sickle cell trait is the carrier (heterozygous) state for the sickle cell diseases. The affected individuals are generally asymptomatic and blood counts are normal. Red cell life span is normal. Sickle cell trait is rarely the cause of morbidity, except for a somewhat higher frequency of hematuria and pulmonary embolism (195). Loss of urine concentrating ability, well known in SS patients, is also universally present in individuals with sickle trait, and is implicated in the rare cases of sudden death resulting from massive rhabdomyolysis following severe exercise. Rarely, splenic infarction has been reported after high-altitude flying in unpressurized aircraft or after high-altitude mountain climbing, but this should not be of concern when flying in pressurized commercial airliners.

The diagnosis is made by hemoglobin electrophoresis, which shows AS pattern, indicating the presence of more hemoglobin A than hemoglobin S. This contrasts with the findings in sickle-β^+-thalassemia double heterozygotes where the amount of hemoglobin S is more than hemoglobin A.

Sickle-β-thalassemia, SC hemoglobin disease, and other double heterozygous states with hemoglobin S

Sickle cell trait is frequently coinherited with disorders of β-chain production, notably β^0- or β^+-thalassemia trait, or with other hemoglobinopathies, such as β-chain variant hemoglobins C, D or E, or α-chain variant hemoglobin G. This results in double heterozygous states for $S\beta^0/\beta^+$-thalassemia, hemoglobin SC, hemoglobin SO Arab, hemoglobin SE, hemoglobin SD, and hemoglobin SG diseases, respectively. α-Thalassemia trait can be present independently of the inheritance of the above globin chain variants. The most common of these, after SS, are Sβ-thalassemia and hemoglobin SC diseases. The distinction between these three common sickling disorders can easily be made from examination of peripheral blood smears and blood counts and confirmed by hemoglobin electrophoresis (table 4.4). Microcytosis and elevated hemoglobin A_2 differentiate Sβ-thalassemia from SS disease, whereas in SC disease the mean corpuscular volume (MCV) is normal and peripheral smears contain sickle cells only rarely but may show the characteristic hemoglobin C crystals in the RBC. Low MCV and normal level of hemoglobin A_2 in SS disease indicate the presence of coexistent α-thal trait.

Hemoglobins C, O Arab, and E comigrate with hemoglobin A_2 and hemoglobins D and G comigrate with hemoglobin S on cellulose acetate at pH 8.2, but separate from each other on acid citrate electrophoresis at pH 6.5. The clinical course and complications in Sβ^0-thal may be as severe as in SS disease and the management is similar. The manifestations are milder and less frequent in other double-heterozygous states, and many are asymptomatic until late childhood or adult life (171). Microvessel disease is more common in SC disease than in SS cases because of the increased propensity for sludging consequent to cellular dehydration associated with hemoglobin C and the resultant increased intracellular viscosity (increased

Table 4.4 Clinically Important Hemoglobin Variants*

Sickle syndromes
 Sickle cell trait
 Sickle cell disease
  SS
  SC
  $SD_{Los Angeles}$
  SO_{Arab}
  S/β-Thalassemia
Unstable hemoglobins → Congenital Heinz body anemia
 (~ 90 variants)
Hemoglobins with abnormal oxygen affinity
 High affinity → familial erythrocytosis
  (~ 40 variants)
 Low affinity → familial cyanosis (Hbs Kansas, Beth Israel, St. Mande')
M hemoglobins → familial cyanosis (6 variants)
Structural variants that result in a thalassemic phenotype
 β-Thalassemia phenotype
  Lepore hemoglobins ($\delta\beta$ fusion)
  Abnormal mRNA processing: Hbs E, Knossos
  Extreme instability: Hb Indianapolis
 α-Thalassemia phenotype
  Chain termination mutants, i.e., Hb Constant Spring
  Extreme instability: Hb Quong Sze

*From Bunn HF, Forget BG. Hemoglobin: molecular, genetic and clinical aspects. Philadelphia: WB Saunders, 1986.

MCHC). Thus, SC patients experience ophthalmic complications and avascular necrosis of femoral heads more commonly than SS patients. In contrast, large vessel complications such as CVAs are less common. In SC disease, the loss of splenic function is slower but eventually complete despite the persistence of splenomegaly into adult life. Because of the unpredictability of the degree of loss of splenic function, administration of pneumococcal vaccine is recommended just as for SS individuals.

Other Hemoglobinopathies

The most common hemoglobinopathy variants are hemoglobins S, E, C, and D$^{\text{Punjab/Los Angeles}}$ in that order, with hemoglobin S and C being African in origin, hemoglobin E arising in Southeast Asia, and hemoglobin D-Punjab via the Indian subcontinent. A recent monograph by Bunn and Forget is recommended as a quick reference guide (57) (Table 4.4). Hemoglobins C, E, and O Arab comigrate with hemoglobin A$_2$ on cellulose acetate but are present in much higher quantity (30–40%) than hemoglobin A$_2$ (normal = 1.5–3.5% and β-thal trait up to 8%) (fig. 4.3B). Hemoglobin E comigrates with hemoglobin A on acid agar, hemoglobin O Arab with hemoglobin S, while hemoglobin C is anodal to hemoglobin S. Furthermore, hemoglobin E is usually about 30% in the heterozygotes compared to the expected 40% for the β-chain variants, is unstable on isopropanol precipitation test, is highly prevalent in people of Southeast Asia and is associated with a thalassemia phenotype (microcytosis and hypochromia). Hemoglobin C originated in west Africa and O Arab in the Arabian peninsula. Hemoglobins S, D, and G$_{\text{Philadelphia}}$ comigrate on cellulose acetate at pH 8.6, but on acid agar D and G have the same mobility as hemoglobin A (fig. 4.3C), while hemoglobin S is anodal to A; hemoglobins D and G do not sickle and have the same solubility as hemoglobin A. Being an α-chain variant, hemoglobin G is lower in amount (25%) than hemoglobin D (40%) in the heterozygous state.

Unstable hemoglobins should be suspected in children with congenital nonspherocytic hemolytic anemia (CNSHA) when the hemoglobin electrophoresis shows an abnormal hemoglobin in relatively low amounts. α-Chain variants may cause jaundice in the newborn. Solubility in isopropanol or on heating is reduced. Further identification requires amino acid analysis.

When a hemoglobin variant is suspected as a cause of polycythemia, it should be recognized that some of the variants do not separate on standard cellulose acetate electrophoresis at alkaline pH but resolve from hemoglobin A on acid agar, especially those β-chain mutants that interfere with binding to 2-3,diphosphoglycerate. Isoelectric focusing may be necessary in some cases. Methemoglobinemic variants should be suspected in cases of congenital cyanosis not associated with heart disease or cor pulmonale.

Case 4

A 23-year-old African-American, self-employed male printer had completed all but 3 hours of flight time prior to initiating his solo test. He chose a warm spring day with a stable air mass to complete the remaining pre–solo flight training in the usual unpressurized aircraft. However, on this occasion he pushed the craft to its ceiling limit of around 11,000 feet. He flew at that level for approximately 15 minutes when he suddenly experienced a sharp left upper gastric pain that radiated to the midabdomen and thence to the left shoulder. The pain was followed in short order by tachycardia and diaphoresis. Because of the intense discomfort, his flight instructor took over, landed the plane, and arranged for an ambulance to meet them at the tarmac. In the ambulance, he received oxygen by nasal and intravenous fluids. His pulse rate slowly fell from 130–85 beats/minute, but the pain persisted. At the hospital his vital signs were stable and he remained afebrile. The only abnormality on his physical examination was left upper abdominal quadrant guarding without rigidity. His bowel sounds were not abnormal. An upright film of his abdomen did not demonstrate free air, and a CBC drawn prior to the radiologic study revealed a modest anemia, as follows: Hgb 110 g/L, Hct 33%, WBC count 12 × 10^9/L, a normal differential and some red cell targeting, no microcytes, and around 5–7% polychromasia. A reticulocyte count was not ordered. His platelets were adequate on smear. A sickle cell preparation with sodium metabisulfite revealed the slow appearance of sickling, and review of the smear once again failed to reveal irreversibly sickled forms. A carefully detailed history failed to identify information suggestive of sickle cell disorders in family members, and the patient denied any history of prior hematologic disorders.

It was thought that his seemingly normal existence prior to this event, along with a low-grade anemia and the slow initiation of sickling by metabisulfite deoxygenation in vitro supported the likelihood of a splenic infarct in a person with sickle trait brought about by a 15-minute flight in an atmospheric pressure 40% lower than that of sea level. A spleen scan confirmed the presence of an area of impaired uptake. He was treated supportively with intravenous fluids and analgesics; 5 days later he was discharged from the hospital with essentially unchanged blood counts. The report of the hemoglobin electrophoresis was troubling, however. It revealed a single band consistent with the sickle band of the control sample on cellulose at pH 8.6. Electrophoretic patterns of his parents and his one sibling revealed sickle and adult bands in all three individuals. By chance, metabisulfite tests were carried out concurrently and only the mother and sibling were positive. Hemoglobin electrophoreses repeated on agar gel at pH 6.8 revealed two bands on the propositus consistent with those of his family members, with following interpretation: patient—

Table 4.5 High-Affinity Hemoglobins°

Chain	(A → A)	Site	Commentary	Chain	(A → A)	Site	Commentary
α-Chain				**β-Chain—cont'd**			
α2	(Leu..Arg)	Chongqing	U	β40	(Arg..Lys)	Athens-Ga. Waco	
α6	(Asp..Ala)	Sawara			(Arg..Ser)	Austin	
	(Asp..Asn)	Dunn		β51	(Pro..Arg)	Williamette	U
	(Asp..Val)	Ferndown		β68	(Leu..His)	Brisban, Great Lakes	U
	(Asp..Tyr)	Woodville		β79	(Asp..Gly)	G-Hsi-Tsou	
	(Asp..Gly)	Swan River		β82	(Lys..Thr)	Rahere	
α14	(Trp..Arg)	Evanston			(Lys..Met)	Helsinki	
α16	(Lys..Met)	Harbin	U	β86	(Ala..Asp)	Olomouc	
α40	(Lys..Glu)	Kanya	U	β87	(Thr..O)	Tours	
	(Lys..Met)	Karagawa		β89	(Ser-Asn)	Creteil	
α44	(Pro..Leu)	Milledgeville			(Ser..Asg)	Vanderbilt	
	(Pro..Arg)	Kawachi		β90	(Gly..Asp)	Pierre Benite	
α45	(His..Arg)	Fort de France		β93	(Cys..Arg)	Okazaki	
α84	(Ser..Arg)	Etobioke		β94	(Asp..His)	Barcelona	
α85	(Asp..Asn)	G-Norfolk			(Asp..Asn)	Bunbury	
	(Asp..Tyr)	Atago		β96	(Leu..Val)	Regina	
	(Asp..Val)	Inksten		β97	(His..Gln)	Malmo	
α88	(Ala..Ser)	Loire			(His..Leu)	Wood	
	(Ala..Val)	Columbia-Missouri			(His..Pro)	Nagoya	
α90	(Lys..Met)	Handa Munatake		β99	(Asp..Asn)	Kempsey	
α92	(Arg..Gln)	J Capetown			(Asp..His)	Yakima	
	(Arg..Ser)	Chesapeake			(Asp..Ala)	Radcliffe	
α95	(Pro..Ala)	Denmark Hill			(Asp..Tyr)	Ypsilanti	
	(Pro..Ser)	Rampa			(Asp..Gly)	Hotel-Dieu	
	(Pro..Arg)	St Lukes			(Asp..Val)	Chemilly	
	(Pro..Leu)	G-Georgia			(Asp..Glu)	Cormora	
α97	(Asn..His)	Dallas		β100	(Pro..Leu)	Brigham	
α126	(Asp..His)	Sassal		β101	(Glu..Lys)	British	
	(Asp..Asn)	Tarrant			(Glu..Gly)	Columbia Alberta	
	(Asp..Val)	Fukitomi			(Glu..Asp)	Potomac	
	(Asp..Tyr)	Montefiore		β103	(Phe..Leu)	Heathrow	
α138	(Ser..Pro)	Attleboro		β105	(Leu..Phe)	South Milwaukee	
α139	(Lys..Thr)	Tokoname		β109	(Val..Met)	San Diego	
	(Lys..Glu)	Hanamaki			(Val..Leu)	Johnston	
α140	(Tyr.Arg..O)	Natal		β124	(Pro..Gln)	Ty Gard	
α141	(Arg..His)	Suresnes		β140	(Tyr.Arg..O)	Natal	
	(Arg..Cys)	Nunobiki		β141			
	(Arg..Leu)	Legnaro		β140	(Ala-Thr)	Saint Jacques	
				β142	(Ala..Asp)	Ohio	
β-Chain				β143	(His..Arg)	Abruzzo	
β2	(His..Arg)	Deer Lodge			(His..Gln)	Little Rock	
	(His..Gln)	Okayama			(His..Pro)	Syracuse	
β9	(Ser..Cys)	Porto Alegre			(His..Asp)	Rancho Mirage	
β17-18	(Lys.Val..O)	Lyon		β144	(Lys..Asn)	Andrew-Minneapolis	
β20	(Val..Mer)	Olympia			(Lys..Glu)	Mito	
β23	(Val..O)	Freiburg		β145	(Tyr..His)	Bethesda	
	(Val..Asp)	Strasbourg			(Tyr..Cys)	Rainier	
	(Val..Phe)	Palmerston North			(Tyr..Asp)	Fort Gordon	
β27	(Ala..Val)	Grange Blanche			(Tyr..Term)	Osler, Nancy McKees Rocks	
β34	(Val..Phe)	Pitie-Salpetriere		β146	(His..Asp)	Hiroshima	
β36	(Pro..Ser)	North Chicago			(His..Pro)	York	
β37	(Trp..Ser)	Hirose			(His..Leu)	Cowtown	
					(His..Gln)	Kodaira	

°U, unstable.

Table 4.6 Low-Affinity Hemoglobins°

Chain	(A → A)	Site	Commentary
α-Chain			
α94	(Asp..Asn)	Titusville	
α130	(Ala..Asp)	Yuda	
β-Chain			
β1	(Val..AcAla)	Raleigh	
β11	(Val..Phe)	Washtenaw	
β21	(Asp..Gly)	Connecticut	
β37	(Trp..Arg)	Rothschild	
β41	(Phe..Ser)	Denver	
β61	(Lys..Met)	Bologna	
β65	(Lys..Glu)	J Cairo	M
β66	(Lys..Thr)	Chico	
β73	(Asp..Tyr)	Vancouver	
	(Asp..Asn)	Korle Bu, G Accra	
	(Asp..Val)	Mobile	
	(Asp..Gly)	Tiburg	
β76	(Ala..Pro)	Calais	M
β82	(Lys..Asn)	Providence	
β83	(Gly..Asp)	Pyrgos, Mizunami	
β90	(Gly..Lys)	Agenogi	
β102	(Asn..Thr)	Kansas	C
	(Asn..Ser)	Beth Israel	C
	(Asn..Tyr)	Sante Mandé	C
β108	(Asn..Asp)	Yoshisuka	
	(Asn..Lys)	Presbyterian	
β121	(Glu..Gln)	D Los Angeles, D Punjab	

°M, methemoglobin production increased; C, cyanosis.

55% hemoglobin D, 45% hemoglobin S; father—55% hemoglobin A, 45% hemoglobin D; mother—55% hemoglobin A, 45% hemoglobin S; sibling—5% hemoglobin A, 45% hemoglobin S. The D band matched a control and was verified by fingerprinting and DNA analyses. Diagnosis: SD $\alpha^2 \beta^2$ 26 val, $\alpha^2\beta^2$ 121 glu.

For any presumptive hemoglobin S result on electrophoresis that does not bear up clinically, it is advisable to obtain a sickle cell preparation in order to determine the nature of the next test. Like homozygous CC disease, homozygous DD disease is characterized by mild hemolysis, but unlike the former, there is no associated symptomatology.

Doubly heterozygous S and C disease ($\alpha^2\beta^2$ 6 val, $\alpha^2\beta^2$ 6 lys) is a more severe hemolytic anemia than SD or SO disease and somewhat less severe than hemoglobin S β-thal. The hematocrit levels are in the upper 20s, vasoocclusive crises occur (albeit infrequently), and irreversibly sickled forms are present, as are the typical hemoglobin C intracellular crystal formations. Sickling occurs with greater frequency in SC disease than in S trait because of unbalanced chain synthesis in the direction of sickle hemoglobin, i.e., there is more S than C hemoglobin.

The reason for the crystal formation in homozygous CC disease (2 $\alpha^2\beta^2$ 2 lys) and combinations thereof is unknown, but the target formation is probably a reflection of the crystal formation. These cells tend to be drier than normal adult hemoglobin-containing cells because of water losses attendant upon excessive potassium afflux.

The severity of the anemia in hemoglobin Sβ-thal depends on the amount of the latter. Patients who are heterozygous for S and β⁰-thal have the more pronounced anemia. Patients who are doubly heterozygous for hemoglobin S and α-thal tend to be less severely anemic than the β-thal group because of an increase in cell surface volume and a lesser cation afflux, but the incidence of vasoocclusive episodes is no less frequent.

Homozygous hemoglobin O Arab (2 $\alpha^2\beta^2$ 121 lys) disease, like homozygous hemoglobin C disease, is characterized by a mild hemolytic anemia, targeting, and splenomegaly. When present with hemoglobin S, it reacts as a homozygous SS disease. Hemoglobin O migrates with hemoglobin C on cellulose acetate (pH 8.6) and is separable only on citrate agar, pH 6.0.

Hemoglobin E (2 $\alpha^2\beta^2$ 26 lys), unlike all of the aforementioned and which appears to have arisen predominately from the subequatorial belt in Africa, is the most common hemoglobinopathy in the Indian subcontinent and the second most common hemoglobinopathy worldwide. It is the only microcytic, hypochromic hemoglobinopathy with target formation, and with its modest splenomegaly and low-grade anemia, is often confused with thalassemia minor. Its close relation with thalassemia in that part of the world gives rise to many instances of hemoglobin E β-thal, which is clinically indistinguishable from homozygous β-thal (196–204).

Hereditary persistence of fetal hemoglobin (HPFH) is not a hemoglobinopathy in the amino acid substitution sense but rather a chain deletion disorder in the thalassemia sense. In this situation, the deletions involve both α- and β-chains without untoward results. Splenomegaly and modest anemia are the typical clinical features. There are three variants of this disorder, based on their "origins" or locale: black, Greek, and Kenyan. In the black variant, the disease, as noted, is mild and in the doubly heterozygous state modifies other hemoglobinopathies because of the presence of hemoglobin F in every cell. In this group, both γ^G and γ^A (3:2) are present.

In the Greek variant only γ^A is present, and as in the black variant, produces essentially no clinical problems. In the Kenyan variant, only γ^G is present and is the result of a γ/β crossover. It, too, is clinically silent. A fourth type, not truly a variant, per se, is the heterocellular form of HPFH, so-called because of its heterogeneous cellular distribution (205–209).

Along with the above, there are various low- and high-affinity oxygen, as well as stable and unstable, hemoglobinopathies (as enumerated in tables 4.4–4.7),

Table 4.7 Unstable Hemoglobins°

Chain	(A → A)	Site	Commentary
α-Chain			
α6	Asp..O	Boyle Heights	H
α24	Tyr..His	Luxembourg	
α26	Ala..Glu	Shenyang	
α27	Glu..Lys	Shuangfeng	
α31	Arg..Ser	Prato	
α43	Phe..Val	Torino	L
	Phe..Leu	Hirosaki	
α47	Asp..Gly	Kokura, Umi Belinson	H
	Asp..His	Hasharon, Sealy L-Ferrara	
	Asp..Asn	Arya	
	Asp..Ala	Cordele	
α50	His..Arg	Aichi	
α53	Ala..Asp	J-Rovigo	
α59	Gly..Val	Tetton	
α62	Val..Met	Evans	
α63	Ala..Asp	Pontoise	
α80	Leu..Arg	Ann Arbor	
α86	Leu..Arg	Moabit	L
α87	His..Arg	Iwata	
α91	Leu..Pro	Port Philip	
α103	His..Arg	Contaldo	
α109	Leu..Arg	Suan-Dok	
α110	Ala..Asp	Petah Tikva	
α112	His..Asp	Hopkins II	H
α130	Ala..Pro	Sun Prairie	
α131	Ser..Pro	Questembert	
α136	Leu..Pro	Bibba	
	Leu..Art	Toyama	
β-Chain			
β6	Glu..O	Leiden	
β7	Blu..Gly	G-San Jose	
β11	Val..Asp	Windsor	H
β14	Leu..Arg	Sogn	
	Leu..Pro	Saki	
β15	Trp..Arg	Belfast	L
	Trp..Gly	Radwick	
β22	Glu..Lys	E-Saskatoon	
β23	Val..Gly	Miyashiro	H
β24	Gly..Arg	Riverdale-Bronx	H
	Gly..Val	Savannah	H
	Gly..Asp	Moscva	
β26	Glu..Lys	E	
	Glu..Val	Mondor	
β27	Ala..Asp	Volga, Drenthe	
β28	Leu..Gln	St. Louis	H
	Leu..Arg	Chesterfield	
	Leu..Gro	Genova, Hyogo	H
β29	Gly..Asp	Lufkin	
β30	Arg..Ser	Tacoma	
β31	Leu..Pro	Yokohama	
β32	Leu..Pro	Perth, Lincoln	
	Leu..Arg	Kobe	
	Leu..Val	Castilla Muscat	
β33	Val..O	Korea	
β35	Tyr..Phe	Philly	H

Chain	(A → A)	Site	Commentary
β-Chain			
β36	Pro..Thr	Linkoping	
β38	Thr..Pro	Hazebrouck	
β39	Gln..Glu	Vassa	
β41	Phe..O	Bruxelles	
β42	Phe..Ser	Hammersmith	L
	Phe..Leu	Chiba	L
	Phe..Val	Louisville, Bucuresti	L
		Sendagi, Warsaw	L
β43	(Phe-Glu-Ser)..O or (Glu-Ser-Phe)..O	Niteroi	L
β45	Phe..Ser	Cheverly	L
β48	Leu..Arg	Okaloosa	L
β49	Phe..Val	Las Palmas	
β54	Sen..Pro	Jacksonville	H
β55	Met..Lys	Mtera	
β56	(Gly-Asn-Pro-Lys)..O	Tochigi	
β57	Asn..Lys	G-Ferrara	
β60	Val..Ala	Collingwood	
	Val..Glu	Cagliari	
β62	Ala..Pro	Duarte	H
β63	His..Pro	Bicerte	M
	His..Arg	Zurich	
β64	Gly..Asp	J-Calabria, J Bari	H
β66	Lys-Glu	I-Tolouse	M
β67	Val..Asp	Bristol	L
	Val..Ala	Sydney	
β68	Leu..Pro	Mizuho	
β70	Ala..Asp	Seattle	
β71	Phe..Ser	Christchurch	
β74	Gly..Val	Bushwick	
	Gly..Arg	Aalborg	
	Gly..Asp	Shepherds Bush	H
β74-75	(Gly-Leu)..O	St. Antoine	
β75	Leu..Pro	Atlanta	
	Leu..Arg	Pasadena	H
β81	Leu..Arg	Baylor	H
β83	Gly..Cys	Ta-Li	
β85	Phe..Ser	Buenos Aires Bryn Mawr	H
β87	Thr..O	Tours	
β88	Leu..Arg	Boros	
	Leu..Pro	Santa Ana	
β91	Leu..Pro	Sabrine	
	Leu..Arg	Carribean	L
β91	(Leu-His-Cys-Asp-Lys)..O	Gun Hill	
β92	His..Gln	St. Etienne Istanbul	H
	His..Asp	J-Altgeld Gardens	
	His..Pro	Newcastle	H
	His..Arg	Moshaisk	
	His..Asn..Asp	Redondo,	

Table 4.7 Unstable Hemoglobins°—cont'd

Chain	(A → A)	Site	Commentary	Chain	(A → A)	Site	Commentary
β-Chain				**β-Chain—cont'd**			
β97	His..Pro	Nagoya		β128	Ala..Asp	J-Guantanamo	
β98	Val..Met	Koln,	H	β129	Ala..Pro	Crete	
		San Franciso,			Ala..Val	LaDesirade	L
		Ube		β130	Tyr..Asp	Wien	
	Val..Gly	Nottingham	H	β131	Gln..Lys	Shelby	
	Val..Ala	Djelfa	L		Gln..Pro	Shanghai	
β101	Glu..Gln	Rush			Gln..Arg	Sarrebourg	
β106	Leu..Pro	Southampton,	H	β134	Val..Glu	North Shore	
		Casper		β135	Ala..Pro	Altdorf	
	Leu..Gln	Tubingen	H		Ala..Glu	Beckman	
	Leu..Arg	Terre Haute		β136	Gly..Asp	Hope	
β107	Gly..Arg	Burke	L	β138	Ala..Pro	Brackton	
β111	Val..Phe	Peterborough	L	β139	Asn..Asp	Geelong	
	Val..Ala	Stanmore	L	β140	Ala..Asp	Himeji	L
β112	Cys..Arg	Indianapolis		β141	Leu..Arg	Olmsted	
β113	Val..Glu	New York,	L		Leu..O	Coventry	
		Kaohsiung		β142	Ala..Pro	Toyoake	
β115	Ala..Pro	Madrid					
β117	His..Pro	Saitama		**δ-Chain**			
β119	Gly..Asp	Fannin-Lubbock		δ98	Val..Met	A₂ Wrens	
	Gly..Val	Bougardirey-		δ121	Glu..Val	A₂ Menzanares	
		Mali					
β124	Pro..Arg	Khartoum		**ᴳγ-Chain**			
β126	Val..Glu	Hofu		γ130	Trp..Gly	F-Poole	
	Val..Gly	Dhonburi,					
		Neapolis		**ᴬγᵀ-Chain**			
β127	Gln..Lys	Brest		ᴬγᵀ25	Gly..Arg	F-Xin Jiang	

°H, high affinity; M, medium affinity; L, low affinity.

Table 4.8 Methemoglobinopathies°

Chain	(A → A)	Site	Commentary
α-Chain			
α58	(His..Tyr)	Boston	C−
α87	(His..Tyr)	Iwate	C−
β-Chain			
β67	(Val..Glu)	Milwaukee	C−
β63	(His..Tyr)	Saskatoon	C+
β92	(His..Tyr)	Hyde Park	C−

°C+, rapid conversion to methemoglobin; C−, slow conversion to methemoglobin.

which include 144 α-chain, 277 β-chain, 25 δ-chain, and 44 γ-chain abnormalities, of which S, C, D, E, and 0 Arab, in addition to the thalassemias, are of major clinical relevance (210, 211).

REFERENCES

1. Serjeant GR, Richards R, Barbor PRH, Milner PF. Relatively benign sickle-cell anaemia in 60 patients aged over 30 in the West Indies. Br Med J 1968;3:86.
2. Serjeant GR. Sickle cell disease, New York: Oxford, 1985.
3. Erlandson ME, Schulman L, Smith CH. Studies on congenital hemolytic syndromes: III, rates of destruction and production of erythrocytes in sickle cell anemia. Pediatrics 1960;25:629.
4. Serjeant, GR, et al. The development of haematological changes in homozygous sickle cell disease: a cohort study from birth to 6 years. Br J Haematol 1981;48:533.
5. Hayes RJ, et al. The haematology of steady state homozygous sickle cell disease: I, frequency distribution, longitudinal observations, effects of age and sex. Br J Haematol 1985;59:369.
6. Stevens MCG, Crooks GW, Serjeant GR. The development of cardiomegaly in homozygous sickle cell disease. West Indian Med J 1985;34:253.
7. Alter B. Prenatal diagnosis of hemoglobinopathies and other hematologic diseases. J Pediatr 1979;95:501.
8. Orkin SH, Litle, PFR, Kazazian HH, Boehm CD. Improved detection of the sickle mutation by DNA analysis. N Engl J Med 1982;307:32.
9. Daland GA, Castle WB. A simple and rapid method for demonstrating sickling of the red blood cells; the use of reducing agents. J Lab Clin Med 1949;33:1082.
10. Itano HA. Solubilities of naturally occurring mixtures of human hemoglobin. Arch Biochem Biophys 1953;47:148.
11. Robinson AR, et al. A new technique for differentiation of hemoglobin. J Lab Clin Med 1957;50:745.
12. Galacteros F, et al. Cord blood screening for hemoglobin abnormalities by thin layer isoelectric focusing. Blood 1980;56:1068.
13. Wilson JB, Headlee ME, Huisman THJ. A new high performance liquid chromatographic procedure for the separa-

tion and quantities of various hemoglobin variants in adult and newborn babies. J Lab Clin Med 1983;102:174.

14. Kan YW, Dozy AM. Antenatal diagnosis of sickle cell anaemia by DNA analysis of amniotic fluid cells. Lancet 1978;2:910.

15. Geever RF, et al. Direct identification of sickle cell anemia by blot hybridization. Proc Natl Acad Sci USA 1981;78:5081.

16. Chang JC, Kan YW. Antenatal diagnosis of sickle cell anaemia by direct analysis of the sickle mutation. Lancet 1981;2:1127.

17. Wilson, JT, Milner PF, Summer ME. Use of restriction endonucleases for mapping the allele for β^S globin. Proc Natl Acad Sci USA 1982;79:3628.

18. Chang JC, Kan YW. A sensitive new prenatal test for sickle cell anemia. N Engl J Med 207:30, 1982.

19. Powars, DR. The natural history of sickle cell disease—the first ten years. Semin Hematol 1975;12:267.

20. Robinson MG, Watson RJ. Pneumococcal meningitis in sickle cell anemia. N Engl Med 1966;274:1006.

21. Thomas AN, Pattison C, Serjeant GR. Causes of death in sickle-cell disease in Jamaica. Br Med J 1982;285:633.

22. Gaston MH, Verter JI. Prophylaxis with oral penicillin in children with sickle cell anemia: a randomized trial. N Engl J Med 1986;314:1593.

23. Vichinsky E, et al. Newborn screening for sickle cell disease: effect on mortality. Pediatrics 1988;81:749.

24. Platt OS, et al. Newborn screening for sickle cell disease: rates and risk factors. N Engl J Med 1991;325:11.

25. Hofrichter J, Hendricker D, Eaton WA. Structure of hemoglobin S fibers: optical determination of the molecular orientation in sickled erythrocytes, Proc Natl Acad Sci USA 1973;70:3604.

26. Hofrichter J, Ross PD, Eaton WA. Kinetics and mechanism of deoxyhemoglobin S gelation: a new approach to understanding a sickle cell disease. Proc Natl Acad Sci USA 1974;71:4864.

27. Eaton WA, Hofrichter J, Ross PD. Delay time of gelation: a possible determinant of clinical severity in sickle cell disease. Blood 1976;47:621.

28. Noguchi CT, et al. α-Thalassemia changes erythrocyte heterogeneity in sickle cell disease. J Clin Invest 1985;75:1632.

29. Embury SN, Clark MR, Monroy G, Mohandas N. Concurrent sickle cell anemia and α-Thalassemia: effect on pathological properties of sickle erythrocytes. J Clin Invest 1984;73:116.

30. Bookchin RM, Nagel RL, Ranney HM. Structure and properties of hemoglobin C-Harlem, a human hemoglobin variant with amino acid substitutions in 2 residues of the β-polypeptide chain. J Biol Chem 1967;242:248.

31. Bookchin RM, Nagel RL, Ranney HM. The effect of $\beta^{73 \, Asn}$ on the interactions of sickling hemoglobins. Biochim Biophys Acta 1970;221:373.

32. Nagel RL, et al. β-Chain contact sites in the haemoglobin S polymer. Nature 1980;283:832.

33. Mohandas N, Evans E. Sickle cell adherence to vascular endothelium. J Clin Invest 1985;76:282.

34. Ballas S, et al. Rheologic predictors of the severity of the painful sickle cell episodes. Blood 1988;72:1216.

35. Lande WM, et al. The incidence of painful episodes in homozygous sickle cell disease: correlation with red cell deformability. Blood 1988;72:2056.

36. Fabry ME, Bemjamin L, Lawrence C, Nagel RL. An objective sign in painful crisis in sickle cell anemia: the concomitant reduction of high density red cells. Blood 1984;64:559.

37. Batabyal JN, Wilson JMG. Sickle cell anemia in Assam. J Indian Med Assoc 1958;30:8.

38. Brittenham G, et al. Sickle cell anemia and trait in southern India: further studies. Am J Hematol 1979;6:107.

39. Lehman H, Cutbush M. Sickle cell-train in Southern India. Br Med J 1952;1:389.

40. Perrine RP, et al. Benign sickle cell anaemia. Lancet 1972;1:1163.

41. Powars D, Chan LS, Schroeder WA. The variable expression of sickle cell disease is genetically determined. Semin Hematol 1990;27:360.

42. Kan YW, Dozy AM. Polymorphism of DNA sequence adjacent to the human beta-globin structural gene: relationship to sickle mutation. Proc Natl Acad Sci USA 1978;75:5631.

43. Kan YW, Dozy AM. Evolution of the hemoglobin S and C genes in world populations. Science, 1980;209:388.

44. Antonarakis SE, et al. Nonrandom association of polymorphic restriction sites in the beta globin gene cluster. Proc Natl Acad Sci USA 1982;79:137.

45. Antonarakis SE, Kazazian HH Jr, Orkin SH. DNA polymorphism and molecular pathology of the human globin gene clusters. Hum Genet 1985;69:1.

46. Nagel RL. The origin of the hemoglobin S gene: clinical, genetic and anthropological consequences. J Biol Med 1984;2:53.

47. Nagel RL, et al. Hematologically and genetically distinct forms of sickle cell anemia in Africa. N Engl J Med 1985;312:880.

48. Nagel RL, et al. The hematological characteristics of sickle cell anemia bearing the Bantu haplotype: the relationship between $^G\gamma$ and Hb F levels. Blood 1987;69:1026.

49. Nagel RL, Ranney HM. Genetic epidemiology of structural mutations of the β-globin gene. Semin Hematol 1990;27:342.

50. Schroeder WA, et al. β Cluster haplotypes, α gene status, and hematological data from SS, SC, and S-β thalassemic patients in Southern California. Hemoglobin 1989;13:325.

51. Embury SH, et al. Concurrent sickle cell anemia and α-thalassemia: effect on severity of anemia. N Engl J Med 1982;306:270.

52. Charache S, Lubin B, Reid CD, eds. Management and therapy of sickle cell disease. NIH Pub No. 91 2117, 1991.

53. Anderson R, Cassell M, Mullinax GL, Chaplin H. Effect of normal cells on viscosity of sickle-cell blood: *in vitro* studies and report of six years' experience with a prophylactic program of "partial exchange transfusion." Arch Intern Med 1963;111:286.

54. Lusher JM, Haghighat H, Khalifa S. A prophylactic transfusion program for children with sickle cell anemia complicated by CNS infarction. Am J Hematol 1976;1:265.

55. Sranaik SA, et al. Periodic transfusions for sickle cell anemia and CNS infarction. Am J Dis Child 1979;133:1254.

56. Nalbandian RM, et al. Sickle cell crisis terminated by intravenous urea in sugar solutions—a preliminary report. Am J Med Sci 1971;261:309.

57. Bunn HF, Forget BG. Hemoglobin: molecular, genetic and clinical aspects. Philadelpha: WB Saunders, 1986.

58. Cooperative Urea Trials Group: Clinical trails of therapy for sickle cell vaso-occlusive crises. JAMA 1974;228:1120.

59. Cerami A, Manning JM. Potassium cyanate as an inhibitor of the sickling of erythrocytes *in vitro*. Proc Nat Acad Sci USA 1971;68:1180.

60. Ueno H, Bai Y, Manning JM. Covalent chemical modifiers of sickle cell hemoglobin. Ann NY Acad Sci 1989; 565:239.

61. Peterson CM, et al. Sodium cyanate induced polyneuropathy in patients with sickle-cell disease. Ann Intern Med 1974;81:152.

62. Charache S. Hydroxyurea as treatment for sickle cell anemia. Hematol Oncol Clin N Am 1991;5:571.

63. Ley TJ, et al. 5-Azacytidine selectively increases γ-globin synthesis in a patient with β^+ thalassemia. N Engl J Med 1982;307:1469.

64. Ley TJ, et al. 5-Azacytidine increases γ-globin synthesis and reduces the proportion of dense cells in patients with sickle cell anemia. Blood 1983;62:370.

65. Charache S, Dover GJ, Moyer MA, Moore JW. hydroxyurea-induced augmentation of fetal hemoglobin production in patients with sickle cell anemia. Blood 1987;69:109.

66. Rodgers GP, et al. Hematologic responses of patients with sickle cell disease to treatment with hydroxyurea. N Engl J. Med 1990;322:1037.

67. Platt OS, et al. Hydroxyurea enhances fetal hemoglobin production in sickle cell anemia. J Clin Invest 1984; 74:652.

68. Dover GJ, et al. Hydroxyurea induction of hemoglobin F production in sickle cell disease; relationship between cytotoxicity and F cell production. Blood 1986;67:735.

69. Veith R, Galanello R, Papayannopoulou T, Stamatoyannopoulos G. Stimulation of F-cell production in patients with sickle-cell anemia treated with cytarabine or hydroxyurea. N Engl J Med 1985;313:1571.

70. Perrine SP, Greene MF, Faller DV. Delay in featal hemoglobin switching in infants of diabetic mothers. N Engl J Med 1985;313:1571.

71. Perrine SP, et al. Sodium butyrate infusions in the ovine fetus delay the biologic clock for fetal globin gene switching. Proc Natl Acad Sci USA 1988;85:8540.

72. Perrine SP, et al. Sodium butyrate enhances fetal globin gene expression in patients with hemoglobin SS and β thalassemia Blood 1979;74:454.

73. Perrine SP, et al. A short-term trial of butyrate to stimulate fetal globin-gene expression in the beta globin disorders. N Engl J Med 1993;328:81.

74. Benjamin LJ. Membrane modifiers in sickle cell disease. Ann NY Acad Sci 1989;565:247.

75. Brewer GJ, Oelschlegel FJ Jr. Antisickling effects of zinc. Biochem Biophys Res Commun 1974;58:854.

76. Brewer GJ, Brewer LF, Prasad AS. Suppression of irreversibly sickled erythrocytes by zinc therapy in sickle cell anemia. J Lab Clin Med 1977;90:549.

77. Benjamin LJ, et al. A collaborative double-blind randomized study of cetiedil citrate in sickle cell crisis. Blood 1986;67:1442.

78. Benjamin LJ, Kokkini G, Peterson CM. Cetiedil: Its potential usefulness in sickle cell disease. Blood 1980;55:265.

79. Orringer EP, et al. A single-dose pharmacokinetic study of the antisickling agent cetiedil. Clin Pharmacol Ther 1986; 39:276.

80. Stuart J, Stone PCW, Bilto YY, Keidan AJ. Oxpentifylline and cetiedil citrate improve deformability of dehydrated sickle cells. J Clin Pathol 1987;40:1182.

81. Teuscher T, Weil Von Der Ahe C, Bailod P, Holzer B. Double-blind randomised clinical trial of pentoxiphyllin: I, vasoocclusive sickle cell crisis. Trop Geogr Med 1989; 41:320.

82. Billett HH, et al. Pentoxifylline (Trental) has no significant effect on laboratory parameters in sickle cell disease. Nouv Rev Fr Hematol 1989;31:403.

83. Poflee VW, Gupta OP, Jain AP, Jajoo UN. Haemorheological treatment of painful sickle cell crises: use of pentoxifylline. J Assoc Physicians India 1991;39:608.

84. Frost ML, Treadwell P. Treatment of sickle cell leg ulcers with pentoxifylline. Int J Dermatol 1990;29:375.

85. Vermeylen C, Fernandez Robles E, Ninane J, Cornu G. Bone marrow transplantation in five children with sickle cell anaemia. Lancet 1988;1:1427.

86. Ferster A, et al. Bone marrow transplantation for severe sickle cell anaemia. Br J Haematol 1992;80:102.

87. Hesdorffer C, Markowitz D, Ward M, Bank A. Somatic gene therapy. Hematol Oncol Clin N Am 1991; 5:423.

88. Seeler RA, Shwiaki MZ. Acute splenic sequestration crises (ASSC) in young children with sickle cell anemia. Clin Pediatr 1972;11:701.

89. Emond AM, et al. Acute splenic sequestration in homozygous sickle cell disease; natural history and management. J Pediatr 1985;197:201.

90. Stevens MCG, Padwick M, Serjeant GR. Observations in the natural history of dactylitis in homozygous sickle cell disease. Clin Pediatr 1981;20:311.

91. Topley JM, Rogers DW, Stevens MCG, Serjeant GR. Acute splenic sequestration and hypersplenism in the first five years in homozygous sickle cell diseaes. Arch Dis Child 1981;56:765.

92. Buchanan GR, Glader BE. Benign course of extreme hyperbilirubinemia in sickle cell anemia: Analysis of six cases. J Pediatr 1977;91:21.

93. Megas H, Papadaki E, Constantinides B. Salmonella septicemia and aplastic crisis and aplastic crises in a patient with sickle-cell anemia. Acta Pediatr 1969;50:517.

94. Pattison JR, et al. Parvovirus infections and hypoplastic crises in sickle-cell anaemia. Lancet 1981;1:664.

95. Serjeant GR, et al. Outbreak of aplastic crises in sickle cell anaemia associated with parvovirus-like agent. Lancet 1981; 2:595.

96. Bhambhani K, et al. Transient erythroblastopenia of childhood not associated with human parvovirus infection. Lancet 1986;1:509.

97. Mortimer PP, et al. A human parvovirus-like virus inhibits hematopoietic colony formation *in vitro*. Nature 1983; 302:426.

98. Cohen BJ, Mortimer PP, Pereira MS. Diagnostic assays with monoclonal antibodies for the human serum parvovirus-like virus. J Hyg 1983;91:113.

99. Anderson MJ, Jones SE, Minson AC. Diagnosis of human parvovirus invection by dot-blot hybridization using cloned viral DNA. J Med Cirol 1985;15:163.

100. Rao S, Gooden S. Splenic sequestration in sickle cell disease: role of tranfusion therapy. Am J Pediatr Hematol Oncol 1985;7:298.

101. Kinney TR, Ware RE, Schultz WH, Filston HC. Long-term management of splenic sequestration in children with sickle cell disease. J Pediatr 1990;117:194.

102. Charache S, Page DL. Infarction of bone marrow in the sickle cell disorders. Ann Intern Med 1967;67:1195.

103. Alavi A, Bone JP, Kuhl DE, Creech RH. Scan detection of bone marrow infarcts in sickle cell disorders. J Nucl Med 1974;15:1003.

104. Kenny MW, Mcakin M, Worthington DJ, Stuart J. Erythrocyte deformability in sickle-cell crisis. Br J Haematol 1981;49:103.

105. Warth JA, Rucknagel DL. Density ultracentrifugation of sickle cells during and after pain crisis: increased dense echinocytes during crisis. Blood 1984;64:507.

106. Watson RJ, Burko H, Megas H, Robinson M. The hand-foot syndrome in sickle cell disease in young children. Pediatrics 1963;31:975.

107. Bohrer SP. Bone ischemia and infarction in sickle cell disease. St. Louis: Warren H. Green, 1981.

108. Serjeant GR, Ashcroft MT. Shortening of the digits in sickle cell anaemia—a sequela of the hand-foot syndrome. Trop Georgr Med 1971;34:341.

109. Keeley K, Buchanan GR. Acute infarction of long bones in children with sickle cell anemia. J Pediatr 1982;191:170.

110. Blank JP, Gill FM. Orbital infarction in sickle cell disease. Pediatrics 1981;67:879.

111. Al-Rashid RA. Orbital apex syndrome secondary to sickle cell anemia. J Pediatr 1979;95:426.

112. Hammersley N. Mandibular infarction occurring during a sickle cell crisis. Br J Oral Maxillofac Surg 1984;22:103.

113. Rucknagel DL, Kalinyak KA, Gelfand MJ. Rib infarcts and acute chest syndrome in sickle cell diseases. Lancet 1991;337:831.

114. Schumacher HR, Andrews R, McLaughlin G. Arthropathy in sickle-cell disease. Ann Intern Med 1973;78:203.

115. Hanissian AS, Silverman A. Arthritis of sickle cell anemia. South Med J 1974;67:28.

116. Kimmelstiel P. Vascular occlusion and ishemic infarction in sickle cell disease. Am J Med Sci 1948;216:11.

117. Diggs LW. Anatomic lesions in sickle cell disease. In: Abramson H, Bertles JF, Wethers DL, eds. Sickle cell disease: diagnosis, management, education and research. St. Louis: CV Mosby, 1973.

118. Crastnopol P, Stewart CF. Acute abdominal manifestations in sickle cell disease. Arch Surg 1949;59:993.

119. Payne R. Pain management in sickle cell disease: rationale and techniques. Ann NY Acad Sci 1989;565:189.

120. Tang R, Shimomura SK, Rotblatt M. Meperidine-induced seizures in sickle cell patients. Hosp Formul 1980;76:764.

121. Nadvi S, Sranaik S, Ravindranath Y. Prevalence of seizures in sickle cell disease; it is associated with vaso-occlusive pain or merperidine. Blood 1994;84 (Suppl):556.

122. Schechter NL, Berrien FB, Katz SM. The use of patient-controlled analgesia in adolescents with sickle cell pain crisis. A preliminary report. J Pain Sympt Manag 1988;3:109.

123. Gonzalez ER, et al. Intermittent injection vs patient-controlled analgesia for sickle cell crisis pain: comparison in patients in the emergency department. Arch Intern Med 1991;151:1373.

124. Seeler RA. Deaths in children with sickle cell anemia. A clinical analysis of fatal instances in Chicao. Clin Pediatr 1972;11:634.

125. Overturf GD, Powars D, Baraff LJ. Bacterial meningitis and septicemia in sickle cell disease. Am J Dis Child 1977;131:784.

126. Lobel JS, Bove KE. Clinicopathologic characteristics of septicemia in sickle cell disease. Am J Dis Child 1977;131:784.

127. Kabins SA, Lerner C. Fulminant pneumococcemia and sickle cell anemia. JAMA 1970;211:467.

128. Barrett-Connor E. Bacterial infection and sickle cell anemia: an analysis of 25 infections in 166 patients and a review of the literature. Medicine 1971;50:97.

129. Robinson MG. Clinical aspects of sickle cell disease. In: Levere RD, ed. Sickle cell anemia and other hemoglobinopathies. New York: Academic Press, 1975.

130. Amundsen TR, Siegel MJ, Siegel BA. Osteomyelitis and infarction in sickle cell hemoglobinopathies: differentiation by combined technetium and gallium scintigraphy. Radiology 1984;153:807.

131. Rao S, Strashun A, Miller S. Bone scintigraphy in patients with sickle cell disease and osteomyelitis. Ann NY Acad Sci 1989;565:452.

132. Rogers ZR, Morrison RA, Vedro DA, Buchanan GR. Outpatient management of febrile illness in infants and young children with sickle cell cell anemia. J Pediatr 1990;117:736.

133. Barrett-Connor E. Acute pulmonary disease and sickle cell anemia. Ann Rev Resp Dis 1971;104:159.

134. Charache S, Scott JC, Charache P. "Acute chest syndrome" in adults with sickle cell anemia. Arch Intern Med 1979;139:67.

135. Palmer J, Broderick KA, Naiman JL. Acute lung syndrome during painful sickle cell crisis-relation to site of pain and narcotic requirement. Blood 1983;62:59.

136. Styles L, et al. The predictive value of secretory phospholipase A^2 in acute chest syndrome. Pediatr Res 1995;37:166.

137. Lane PA, O'Connell JL, Hassell KL, Weil JV. Free fatty acids increase permeability of cultured pulmonary artery endothelium: implications for pathogenesis of acute chest syndrome in sickle cell disease. Pediatr Res 1995;37:161A.

138. Barrett-Connor E. Pneumonia and pulmonary infarction in sickle cell anemia. JAMA 1973;224:997.

139. Miller ST, et al. Role of Chlamydia pneumoniae in acute chest syndrome of sickle disease. J Pediatr 1991;118:30.

140. Bromberg PA. Pulmonary aspects of sickle cell disease. Arch Intern Med 1974;133:652.

141. Davies SC, et al. Acute chest syndrome in sickle cell disease. Lancet 1984;1:36.

142. Poward D, et al. Sickle cell chronic lung disease: prior morbidity and the risk of pulmonary failure. Medicine 1988;67:66.

143. Bowen EF, Crowston JG, De Ceulaer K, Serjeant GR. Peak expiratory flow rate and the acute chest syndrome in homozygous sickle cell disease. Arch Dis Child 1991;66:330.

144. Poward D, et al. The natural history of stroke in sickle cell disease. Am J Med 1978;65:461.

145. Sarnaik SA, Lusher JM. Neurological complications of sickle cell anemia. Am J Pediatr Hematol Oncol 1982;4:386.

146. Powars DR, et al. Lack of influence of fetal hemoglobin levels or erythrocyte indices on the severity of sickle cell anemia. J Clin Invest 1980;65:732.

147. Stockman JA, Nigro MA, Mishkin MM, Oski FA. Occlusion of large cerebral vessels in sickle-cell anemia. N Engl J Med 1972;287:846.

148. Seeler RA, Royal JE, Powe L, Goldbarg HR. Moyamoya in children with sickle cell anemia and cerebrovascular occlusion. J Pediatr 1978;93:808.

149. Garza-Mercado R. Pseudomoyamoya in sickle cell anemia. Surg Neurol 1982;18:425.

150. Portnoy BA, Herion JC. Neurological manifestations in sickle cell disease. Ann Intern Med 1972;76:643.

151. Gerald B, Seves JI, Langston JW. Cerebral infarction secondary to sickle cell disease: arteriographic findings. AJR 1980;134:1209.

152. Wiznitzer M, et al. Diagnosis of cerebrovascular disease in sickle cell anemia by magnetic resonance angiogaphy. J Pediatr 1990;117:551.

153. Adams, R et al. The use of transcranial ultrasonogaphy to predict stroke in sickle cell disease. N Engl J Med 1992; 326:605.

154. Greer M, Schotland D. Abnormal hemoglobin as a cause of neurologic disease. Neurology 1962;12:114.

155. Russell MO, et al. Effect of transfusion therapy on arteriographic abnormalities and on recurrence of stroke in sickle cell disease. Blood 1984;63:162.

156. Emond AM, Homan R, Hayes RJ, Serjeant GR. Priapism and impotence in homozygous sickle cell disease. Arch Intern Med 1980;140:1434.

157. Seeler RA. Intensive transfusion therapy for priapism in boys with sickle cell anemia. J Urol 1973;110:360.

158. Noe HN, Williams J, Jerkins GR. Surgical management of priapism in children with sickle cell anemia. J Urol 1981;126:770.

159. Prasad AS, Cossasck ZT. Zinc supplementation and growth in sickle cell disease. Ann Intern Med 1984;100:367.

160. Alleyne SI, D'Hreus Rauseo R, Serjeant GR. Sexual development and fertility of Jamaican female patients with homozygous sickle cell disease. Arch Intern Med 1981; 141:1295.

161. Osegbe DN, Akinyanju O, Amaku EO. Fertility in males with sickle cell disease. Lancet 1981;2:275.

162. Platt OS, Rosenstock W, Espeland MA. Impact of sickle hemoglobinopathies on growth and development. N Engl J Med 1984;311:7.

163. Whitten CF. Growth status of children with sickle cell anemia. Am J Dis Child 1961;102:101.

164. Diggs LW. Bone and joint lesions in sickle-cell disease. Clin Orthop 1967;51:119.

165. Hill MC, et al. Abnormal epiphyses in sickling disorders. AJR 1975;124:34.

166. Sebes JI, Kraus AP. Avascular necrosis of the hip in the sickle cell hemoglobinopathies. J Canad Assoc Radiol 1983; 34:136.

167. Lindsay J Jr., Meshel JC, Ptterson RH. The cardiovascular manifestations of sickle cell disease. Arch Intern Med 1974; 133:643.

168. Rees AH, et al. Left ventricular performance in children with homozygous sickle cell anaemia. Br Heart J 1978; 40:690.

169. Alpert BS, et al. Hemodynamic and ECG response to exercise in children with sickle cell anemia. Am J Dis Child 1981;135:362.

170. Covitz W, et al. Exercise-induced cardiac dysfunction in sickle cell anemia: a radionuclide study. Am J Cardiol 1983; 51:570.

171. Pearson H, et al. Developmental pattern of splenic dysfunction in sickle cell disorders. Pediatrics 1985;76:392.

172. Buchanan GR, et al. Splenic phagocytic function in children with sickle cell anemia receiving long-term hypertransfusion therapy. J Pediatr 1989;115:568.

173. Ozkaynak MF, Ortega JA. Reversibility of anatomical and functional asplenia by chronic transfusion in a child with sickle cell anemia. Am J Pediatr Hematol Oncol 1989; 11:445.

174. Schlitt LE, Keital HG. Renal manifestations of sickle cell disease: a review. Am J Med Sci 1960;239:773.

175. Hatch FE, Culbertson JW, Diggs LW. Nature of the renal concentrating defect in sickle cell disease. J Clin Invest 1967;46:336.

176. Statius Van Eps LW, Pinedo-Veels C, DeVries GH, De Konig J. Nature of concentrating defect in sickle cell nephropathy: microradioangiographic studies. Lancet 1970; 1:450.

177. Buckalew VM, Someren A. Renal manifestations of sickle cell disease. Arch Intern Med 1974;133:660.

178. Bernstein J, Whiten CF. A histologic appraisal of the kidney in sickle cell anemia. Arch Pathol 1960;70:407.

179. Bilinski RT, Kandel GL, Rabiner SF. Epison aminocaproic acid therapy of hematuria due to heterozygous sickle cell diseases. J Urol 1969;102:93.

180. Black WD, Hatch FE, Acchiardo S. Aminocaprioc acid in prolonged hematuria of patients with siclemia. Arch Intern Med 1976;136:678.

181. McInnes BK. The management of hematuria associated with sickle hemoglobinopathies. J Urol 1980;124:171.

182. John EG, et al. Effectiveness of triglycyl vasopressin in persistent hematuria associated with sickle cell hemoglobin. Arch Intern Med 1980;140:1539.

183. Goodman MS, Jacobs JA. Sickle cell hematuria controlled by intrarenal oxychlorosene irrigation. J Urol 1983;130:326.

184. Lucas WM, Bullock W. Hematuria in sickle cell disease. J Urol 1960;83:733.

185. Lief PD, Sullivan A, Goldberg M. Physiological contributions of thin and thick loops of Henle to the renal concentrating mechanism (abstract). J Clin Invest 1969;48:52.

186. Sheehy TW. Dickle hepatopathy. Soc Med J 1977;70:533.

187. Sarnaik S, et al. Incidence of cholelithiasis in sickle cell anemia using the ultrasonic gray-scale technique. J Pediatr 1980;96:1005.

188. Condon PI, Serjeant GR. Behavior of untreated proliferative sickle retinopathy. Br J Ophthalmol 1980;64:404.

189. Condon PI, Serjeant GR. Photocoagulation in proliferative sickle retinopathy: results of a 5 year study. Br J Ophthalmol 1980;64:832.

190. Goldbaum MH, Fletcher RC, Jampol LM, Goldberg MF. Cryotherapy of proliferatiave sickle retinopathy: II, triple freeze-thaw cycle. Br J Ophthalmol 1979;63:97.

191. Condon PI, Serjeant GR. Ocular findings in homozygous sickle cell anemia in Jamaica. Am J Ophthalmol 1972; 73:533.

192. Thrall JH, Rucknagel DL. Increased bone marrow blood flow in sickle cell anemia demonstrated by thalium-210 and Tc 99m human albumin micropheres. Radiology 1978; 127:817.

193. Serjeant GR. Leg ulceration in sickle cell anemia. Arch Intern Med 1974;133:690.

194. Serjeant GR, Galloway RE, Gueri MC. Oral zinc sulphate in sickle-cell ulcers. Lancet 1970;2:891.

195. Heller P, Best WR, Nelson RB, Becktel J. Clinical manifestations of sickle-cell trait and glucose-6-phosphate dehydrogenase deficiency in hospitalized black patients. N Engl J Med 1970;300:1001.

196. Ballas SK, et al. The xerocytosis of HbSC disease. Blood 1987;69:124.

197. Chernoff A. The hemoglobin D syndromes. Blood 1958; 12:116.

198. Efremov SD, et al. Homozygous O-Arab in a Gypsy family in Yugoslavia. Hemoglobin 1977;1:389.

199. Fairbanks VF, et al. Homozygous hemoglobin E mimics β-thalassemia minor without anemia or hemolysis: hematologic, functional, and biosynthetic studies of first North American cases. Am J Hematol 1980;8:109.

200. Ibrahim SA, Mustafa D. Sickle-cell haemoglobin O disease in a Sudanese family. Br Med J 1967;3:715.

201. Biggs LW, et al. Intraerythrocytic crystals in a white patient with hemoglobin C in the absence of other types of hemoglobin. Blood 1954;9:1172.

202. Bunn HF, et al. Molecular and cellular pathogenesis of hemoglobin SC disease. Proc Nat Acad Sci USA 1982; 79:7527.

203. McCurdy PR. Hemoglobin S-G (S-D) syndrome. Am J Med 1974;57:665.

204. Benz EJ, et al. Molecular analysis of the β-Thalassemia phenotype associated with inheritance of hemoglobin E ($\alpha_2\beta_2^{26}$ Glu→Lys). J Clin Invest 1981;68:118.

205. Charache S, Conley CL. Heriditary persistence of fetal hemoglobin. Ann NY Acad Sci 1969;165:37.

206. Huisman THJ, et al. Heriditary persistence of fetal hemoglobin. N Eng J Med 1971;285:711.

207. Sofronidou K, et al. Globin chain synthesis in the Greek Type ($^a\gamma$) of hereditary persistence of fetal haemoglobin. Br J Haematol 1975;29:137.

208. Wood WG, et al. $^G\gamma\delta\beta$ Thalassemia and $^G\gamma$HPFH (Hb Kenya type): comparison of 2 new cases. J Med Genet 1977;14:237.

209. Weatherall DG, et al. Fetal haemoglobin. Clin Haematol 1974;3:467.

210. Perrine RP, et al. Natural history of sickle cell anemia in Saudi Arabs. Ann Intern Med 1978;88:1. Br J Haematol 1978;40:415.

211. Schneider RG, et al. Abnormal hemoglobins in a quarter million people. Blood 1976;48:629.

CHAPTER 5

Heme Synthesis Degradation and Porphyrin Disorders

SAMUEL GROSS

. . . because this disease caused them to have red teeth and to be disfigured, hirsute and nocturnal, persons with erythropoietic porphyria may have been responsible for the werewolf legend.
—L. Illis (1964)

Introduction

Heme, or ferrous (Fe^{++}) protoporphyrin IX, is an iron-complexed tetrapyrrole, derived from the decarboxylation of ketoglutarate to form succinyl CoA. Although porphyrin synthesis takes place in both liver and erythrocytes, heme (as in ferrous protoporphyrin IX, and unlike the ferric protoporphyrin of peroxidase or the ferric or ferrous protoporphyrin of cytochrome c) is synthesized solely in developing erythrocytes. The first and final phases of the heme biosynthetic pathway, i.e., the condensation of glycine and succinyl CoA to form 5-aminolevulinic acid, and the conversion of protoporphyrinogen III to protoporphyrin IX, respectively, take place in the mitochondria. The intermediate metabolites porphobilinogen, hydroxymethylbilane, uroporphyrinogen III, and coproporphyrinogen III, are synthesized in the cell sol. A number of potentially severe disorders, principally affecting the liver and/or the red blood cells, occur along this pathway, the result of either inborn or exogenously induced metabolic defects; and their infrequent occurrence is all the more remarkable when one considers the number of enzyme systems involved in the overall process.

Case 1

A 14-month-old boy was brought to the local pediatrician for a routine examination that yielded normal results in all respects. Because the child lived in an old, low-rent building, he was tested for lead levels, and a hematocrit was also obtained. The sample was collected on a piece of filter paper and sent to the board of health for analysis. One week later the report returned with the following information: erythrocyte protoporphyrin (EP): 120 μg/dl (normal <70 μg/dl; blood lead level: 28 μg/dl (normal <1 μg/dl). One commonly assesses lead and red cell protoporphyrin levels on the same sample because of the known exponential increase in EP

with increasing lead levels (1). Synthesis of red cell δ-aminolevulinic acid (ALA) dehydratase is inhibited by lead (2), and with ever-increasing amounts of lead there is a corresponding decline in the enzyme, which in turn accounts for the exponential increases in serum and urine ALA. The sulfhydryl groups of ferrochetalase, the final enzyme in the heme synthesis pathway, ferrochetalase sulfhydryl groups (3) are also inactivated by lead, as a consequence. This impedes the enzyme's ability to incorporate iron into protoporphyrin. The net effect is a rise in "free" protoporphyrin (4).

A confirmatory venous blood sample, including complete blood count and iron studies, was then obtained, along with further history regarding diet in which the possibility of lead ingestion/exposure was emphasized. This, in turn, was followed by abdominal and long bone x-rays in search of lead-containing paint chip densities in the abdomen and "growth arrest" (lead) lines in the long bones, respectively, which were not forthcoming (5, 6). The history did not show lead ingestion. The only untoward elicited event was an excessive intake of cow's milk, almost to the exclusion of many solid foods.

The blood test results returned with the following information: hemoglobin 105 g/L, hematocrit 33.5%, red blood cells (RBCs) 4.5 × 10⁹/L (mean corpuscular volume [MCV] 68 fL, mean corpuscular hemoglobin [MCH] 22 pg, and mean corpuscular hemoglobin concentration [MCHC] 30%). He had a white blood cell (WBC) count of 6.1 × 10⁹/L, a normal age-related differential, and a blood film that was minimally microcytic, hypochromic, and poikilocytotic. There was no basophilic stippling. Platelet count was 230 × 10⁹/L, and the reticulocyte count was 1.5%. His bound serum iron level was 70 μg/dl, total iron-binding capacity was 450 μg/dl, with a serum ferritin level of 6 ng/L. A repeat blood lead level carried out on venous blood was 4 μg/dl.

Table 5.1. CDC Classification of Childhood Lead Poisoning; 1992[a]

Proposed Risk Classification for Asymptomatic Children

Blood Lead Level μg/dl	Recommended Action
0–9	No immediate concern
10–14	Community/environmental survey
15–19	Retest, educational intervention
20–24	Medical attention, monitor periodically, house visit
25–54	Remove Pb source, medical attention, CaNaEDTA test
55–69	Remove Pb source, treat with CaNaEDTA, return to "clean" home
≥70	Emergency hospitalization, treat with BAL and CaNaEDTA; return to "clean" home

[a]Abbreviations: BAL, British Anti-Lewisite; CaNaEDTA, calcium sodium ethylene diamine tetraacetate.

Table 5.2. Common High-Risk Lead Sites for Children in North America

Paint lead	In old houses
Air lead	Greater in urban areas
Dust lead	Greater in urban areas (greatest in old houses)
Food lead	Greater in canned food

Note that all sources are additive.

Table 5.1 lists the Centers for Disease Control (CDC) Classification of Lead Poisoning. So-called "normal" blood lead levels refer to levels obtained in inhabitants of pristine areas of the world, such as the Himalayas, the Andes, the Amazon basin, and the like, where normal values range from <1 to a high of 4 μg/dl (5).

The boy's pediatrician concluded that the child did not have lead poisoning but was rather in the early anemic stages of nutritional iron deficiency. He prescribed a 3-month course of oral iron and offered instructions on proper nutrition. Recovery was uneventful, and at the end of the proscribed course of therapy, the child's hemoglobin and MCV had risen to 117 g/L and 80 fL, respectively.

Case 2

A 12-month-old boy child living in a home with flaking lead-based paint had blood lead level testing performed in a mobile city unit designed specifically for house-to-house screening surveys in high-risk, lead-prevalent areas.

Table 5.2 identifies common high-risk lead sites for children in North America.

The serum lead level was 48 μg/dl and the screening EP level was 112 μg/dl (repeat determination, 125 μg/dl), data consistent with lead poisoning. Additional blood tests revealed the following: hemoglobin 112 g/dl, MCV 78 fL, no red cell stippling. WBC was normal with normal differential, and platelet numbers,

and reticulocyte count. The boy's bound serum iron was 92 μg/dl, total iron binding capacity was 347 μg/dl, serum ferritin was 238 ng/L. A repeat blood lead level was 55 μg/dl.

Physical and psychologic evaluations of the child were within normal limits. X-rays of the long bones revealed growth arrest lines, but there was no radiologic evidence of opaque material in the abdominal films. Inspection of the dwelling revealed numerous flakes of lead-based paint.

The blood lead level fell to 6 μg/dl following a 5-day inpatient course of edetic acid (EDTA) chelation therapy (6, 7), after which the child was discharged to a temporary shelter pending repair of his home. Repeat blood lead and EP levels 2 weeks later were 38 μg/dl and 147 μg/dl, respectively (7). Oral chelation therapy with dimethyl succinic acid (DMSA) was administered for an additional 3 weeks after the family returned to a lead-free home. Repeat blood lead and EP levels were 25 μg/dl and 168 μg/dl, respectively. At 3 and then 4 months later, both blood lead and EP levels declined to 15 μg/dl and 28 μg/dl, and then to 7 μg/dl and 18 μg/dl, respectively.

Tables 5.3 and 5.4 enumerate the methods for treating asymptomatic and symptomatic lead poisoning in children.

For this child, therapy was tailored to treat asymptomatic lead poisoning with parenteral EDTA followed by DMSA, an oral, water-soluble preparation derived from British anti-lewisite (BAL). Because DMSA has a powerful affinity for lead, its use is restricted and can be administered only when the contaminating source has been removed, which was the situation in this case.

Heme Synthesis

Heme synthesis is initiated by amino levulinic acid synthetase (synthase)-induced condensation of glycine and succinyl CoA. This irreversible change forms δ-aminolevulinic acid (ALA), which, in turn, is followed by the catalytic condensation of two molecules of ALA in the presence of ALA dehydrase to yield a monopyrole, porphobilinogen (PBG), and two molecules of water (8–11).

ALA synthase activity occurs in the cytosolic polyribosomes and it is the precursor of the functional enzyme found in the mitochondria. Two forms have been identified, one encoded on chromosome X (erythroid ALA), the other nonerythroid form on chromosome 3 (12–14). ALA dehydrase, whose codon is found on chromosome 9, requires both sulfhydryl groups and zinc to maintain activity (15).

PBG, the substance upon which many of the tetrapyrroles, including heme, chlorophyll, cobalamin, and the like are built, is a relatively unstable molecule, which, when exposed to light, changes from a colorless to a dark red compound (16). Four molecules of PBG are deaminated by hydroxymethylbilane synthase (formerly PBG deaminase or uroporphyrinogen 1 synthase), to form hydroxymethylbilane (HMB) (17), which, in the presence of uroporphyrinogen III cosynthetase, loses water and forms

Table 5.3. Treatment of Asymptomatic Lead Poisoning in Children[a]

Blood lead	Treatment	Details
>70 μg/dl	BAL and CaNaEDTA	Start BAL 50 mg/m² i.m. every 4 hr (300 mg/m²/d). At 4 hr add CaNaEDTA 1000 mg/m²/d. Treatment with CaNaEDTA for 5 d. BAL may be discontinued after 3 days if blood Pb <50 mg/dl. Repeat cycle if Pb levels rebound.
56–69 μg/dl	CaNaEDTA	CaNaEDTA 1000 mg/m²/d 5 d, continuous infusion. If lead exposure controlled, give CaNaEDTA as a single outpatient i.m. dose. Repeat outpatient i.m. dose. Repeat cycle if Pb levels rebound.
25–55 μg/dl		Perform CaNaEDTA provocation test to assess lead exertion ratio: μg of Pb excreted/mg of CaNaEDTA given.
Ratio: >0.70	CaNaEDTA or DMSA	CaNaEDTA 1000 mg/m²/d 5 d, continuous infusion or divided doses (with a heparin lock). If lead is controlled, CaNaEDTA may be given as a single outpatient i.m. dose. Alternatively, treat with oral DMSA. Repeat cycle if Pb levels rebound.
0.60–0.69	CaNaEDTA or DMSA	3 d with CaNaEDTA i.m. as above.
Age <3 yr		Alternatively, treat with oral DMSA.
	No treatment	Repeat blood Pb and EP every 2 wk.
Age >3 yr		Repeat CaNaEDTA provocation test if Pb rises.
	No treatment	
>0.60		Repeat blood Pb and EP every mo.
		Repeat CaNaEDTA provocation test if Pb rises.

[a]Based on pretreatment lead levels. Abbreviations: BAL, British Anti-Lewisite; CaNaEDTA, calcium sodium ethylene diamine tetraacetate; DMSA, dimethyl succinic acid; EP, erythrocyte protoporphyrinogen; Pb, lead.

Table 5.4. Treatment of Symptomatic Lead Poisoning

Treatment	Details
Control convulsions	Assisted respiration requipment at bedside. Valium 0.15 mg/kg slowly. Repeat 0.10 mg/kg as needed. Spinal puncture (to rule out meningitis, <1 ml of fluid).
Maintain diuresis	i.v. ¼ mg Saline, 5% dextrose for urine flow 350–500 ml/m²/d.
BAL and CaNaEDTA	Start with BAL 75 mg/m² i.m. every 4 hr (450 mg/m²/d). After 4 hr CaNaEDTA 1000 mg/m²/d continuous infusion. Discontinue BAL after 3 d if blood Pb <50 μg/dl. Repeat cycles if Pb rebounds.

uroporphyrinogen III (18). There are two HMB synthase isoenzymes encoded on chromosome 11(q23) (19).

Uroporphyrinogen lll is the first macrocyclic tetrapyrrole precursor (20), the acetic acid side chains of which, once decarboxylated by uroporphyrinogen III decarboxylase, form the reduced tetrapyrrole, coprophorphyrinogen III (21). The decarboxylations occur as four sequential events, presumptively by four isomers of the enzyme, which in vitro can be carried out by a single enzyme (22). All of the aforementioned reactions occur in the cell sol.

Once synthesized, coproporphyrinogen III is transported to the mitochondria, at which site its propionic acid side chains are sequentially decarboxylated by coproporphyrinogen oxidase to form vinyl groups (23). The resultant protoporphyrinogen IX is oxidized by protoporphyrinogen IX oxidase to form protoporphyrin lX (24). This is the single example in heme biosynthesis of an oxidized porphyrin functioning as a substrate. The final step in heme synthesis requires ferrochetalase (heme synthase) to enzymatically link ferrous iron and protoporphyrin in the formation of iron protoporphyrin IX (heme) (3).

Untoward biomedical events with clinical sequelae may occur at any step along the heme biosynthetic pathway, commencing with pyridoxal phosphate, the cofactor for the catalytic condensation of succinyl CoA and glycine (25). In pyridoxine-deficient animals, their defective heme synthesis is corrected by the administration of pyridoxal phosphate (26).

ALA synthetase plays an important interacting role with heme. In cell-free systems, heme directly inhibits the activity of the preformed enzyme. Within the cell, heme regulates its synthesis: low cellular concentrations of heme induce additional synthesis of ALA synthetase; and, conversely, when the cellular concentration of heme is high, the enzyme synthesis is decreased. Products or processes that interfere with heme synthesis can increase ALA synthetase production. Included in these events are clinical exacerbations of acute intermittent porphyria and related disorders (to be discussed). Figure 5.1 outlines the steps in heme biosynthesis.

Defects in Porphyrin Metabolism Due to Lead Toxicity

Lead inhibits most of the heme biosynthesis steps. Its most marked effect is on **ALA dehydratase,** followed in de-

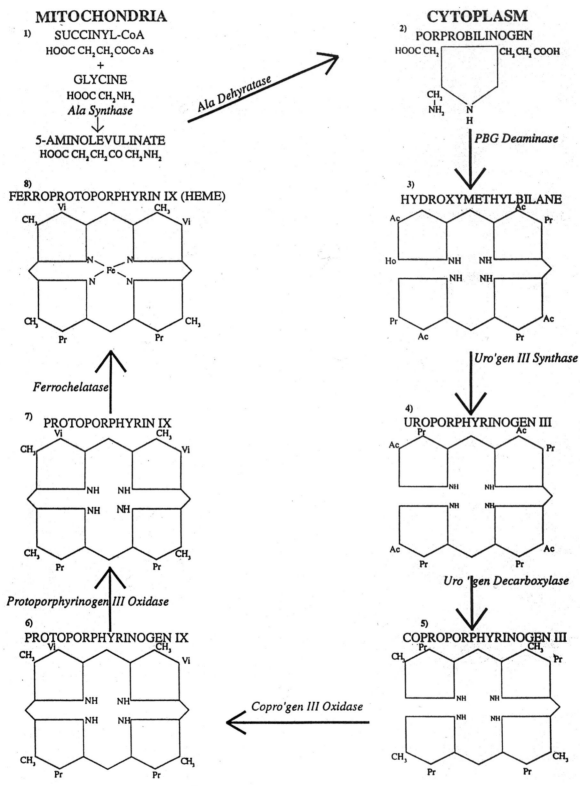

Figure 5.1. Heme biosynthetic pathway.

creasing order of sensitivity, by ferrochetalase, coproporphyrinogen oxidase, and hydroxymethylbilane synthetase (PBG deaminase). It also impairs delivery of iron to ferrochelatase (27), which, in turn, results in the accumulation of a *zinc* rather than an *iron* metalloporphyrin (28). This substitution accounts for the rare occurrence of ringed sideroblasts in lead toxicity, since there is little hemosiderin deposited.

Lead poisoning effects ALA metabolism. Both serum and urinary ALA dehydratase activity decrease along with urinary ALA excretion, a process that distinguishes lead-induced changes from those seen in **Acute Intermittent Porphyria,** wherein PBG is excreted at levels far greater than ALA. Increased urinary and zinc coproporphyrin levels are also increased in lead poisoning.

The red cell basophilia seen in lead poisoning is the result of lead-induced impairment of **pyrimidine 5'-nucleotidase synthesis** (29). Ordinarily, in normal reticulocytes pyrimidine 5'-nucleotidase degrades residual ribosomal RNA, which in effect clears out unwanted pyrimidine breakdown products via enzymatic dephosphorylation (30). Failure to do so, as in **Congenital Pyrimidine 5'-Nucleotidase Deficiency** (31), results in a buildup of ribosomal RNA aggregates, which are manifest cytologically as punctate RBC basophilia in association with an intravascular hemolytic anemia. An essentially similar but *acquired* disorder occurs in lead poisoning.

Pentose phosphate shunt activity is impaired in lead poisoning. Lead directly inhibits **glucose-6-phosphate-dehydrogenase (G-6-PD)** synthesis, which is further altered by lead-induced pyrimidine nucleotide accumulation.

Prolonged lead exposure also impairs **globin synthesis** (32).

"Lead colic," i.e., pain and ileus, often in association with palsy, occurs as a consequence of lead-induced toxic impairment of neuroregulation (33).

The anemia of lead poisoning is probably multivariant. It is in part hemolytic (34), is often associated with iron deficiency (which may be the major factor), and may directly affect red cell production, which early on is manifest by a hypercellular marrow. Later, this is manifest by marrow hypocellularity, an appearance that is reminiscent of the progression from early to advanced iron deficiency (35–37).

Defects in Porphyrin Metabolism due to Inborn Errors

Not only is heme biosynthesis prey to intoxicants such as lead, it is also vulnerable to genetic (and occasionally acquired) defects along each step of the pathway, which, in turn, lead to errors in pyrrole metabolism that range from mild to severe and complex. The following is a case in point.

Case 3

An 8-year-old boy of Irish, Scotch, and Slovenian descent was admitted to the hospital by referral with a diagnosis of congenital nonspherocytic hemolytic anemia. He was the 3rd of 5 healthy siblings and the offspring of 2 healthy parents. There were no unusual illnesses in any of the known relatives. At 7 months of age he was examined because of pallor noted 1 month after a full-term, uneventful birth. His physical examination was characterized by pallor, frontal bossing, and hepatosplenomegaly, and his laboratory data were as follows: hemoglobin 55 g/L, RBC count 2×10^{12}/L, WBC count 11.4×10^9/L, platelet count 100×10^9/L, with numerous nucleated RBCs in the blood film, and 6% reticulocytes. The red cell morphology was described as hypochromic, microcytic, anisocytotic, poikilocytotic, and occasionally spherocytic.

Numerous tests in search of antibodies were negative. He received iron therapy (without benefit) along with transfusions and shortly thereafter it became apparent that he was transfusion dependent. By 6 months of age he was beginning to blister in the sunlight. His first dentition was brownish in color and thought to be due to the oral iron that he had earlier received. A splenectomy performed at 9 months of age failed to relieve his symptoms. Over time his platelet counts showed a steady, insidious decline. His mother also reported that commencing with birth his diapers stained pink; and his physician, after noting that his urine tested negative for heme, suggested that the color was due to urates. His vesicular eruption increased in number and size and progressed to serosanguinous bullae. Hypertrichosis and the brown staining of his teeth steadily worsened. His need for transfusions did not abate, and his platelets continued their downward spiral.

At the time of his first hospital session in the most recent setting, his examination and blood tests were essentially unchanged. A bone marrow biopsy revealed massive increases in hemosiderin, marked fluorescence in most of the developing red cell precursors, and megaloblastic maturation. He had a fully saturated iron-binding protein, along with a serum folate level of 2.5 µg/L and (elevated) urinary coproporphyrin and uroporphyrin levels of 700 and 7500 µg/24 hours, respectively. Under appropriately regulated ultraviolet (UV) light, approximately one half of both immature and mature red cells fluoresced, and the same "burned out" appearance was seen by electron microscopy.

*History and physical examination, along with laboratory studies, confirmed the diagnosis of **Congenital Erythropoietic Porphyria** complicated by a superimposed folate deficiency. The latter process was readily corrected with oral folic acid supplementation, which effected a rise in platelets and a decrease in transfusion requirements. The boy died 10 years later as a consequence of transfusion-induced iron overload.*

Comment: *Congenital erythropoietic porphyria (CEP) is inherited as an autosomal recessive trait characterized biochemically by excessive production of uroporphyrinogen I because of defective synthesis of uroporphyrinogen III cosynthase (38).*

Singular among the initial findings in this disease were the pink-stained diapers.

Beets, heme, PBG, urates, and certain antimetabolites (daunomycin and related compounds) lend a pink-to-red coloration to the urine, but only PBG becomes pink on standing.

Skin photosensitivity first appeared in the third month and over time progressed to fluorescing fluid-containing vesicles and disfiguring, poorly healing and often necrotic bullae.

Excessive hair growth leading to hypertrichosis follows upon the skin disfigurement (39), and the brownish dental discoloration, which appeared with the first eruptions, is the result of porphyrin deposition in the dentin (40).

Like virtually all similarly afflicted patients, this child had a hemolytic anemia in association with ineffective erythropoiesis and a steadily enlarging spleen. The late-occurring folate deficiency developed in response to intake insufficient to meet the demands of accelerated red cell production. The morphologic aspects of the anemia included alterations in size and shape, basophilic stippling, and normoblastemia in excess of reticulocytosis, findings consistent with disordered maturation. Electron microscopy and fluorescent excitation studies of both developing and mature red cells supported the presence of bilineage red cell production, as shown by both fluorescing and nonfluorescing cells.

The clinical expression of disordered accumulation and excretion of biologically excessive and useless material has puzzled investigators for years, both because of its obvious heterogeneity and its rarity. The nature of the biosynthetic defect is well established, i.e., an abnormality resulting from accumulation of uroporphyrin I and not (as was formerly held) underproduction of uroporphyrinogen III. This feature, however, is but one part of what is likely to be a syndrome. It has been proposed that the full clinical expression of this disease is the inheritance of two recessive traits, namely, a defect in uroporphyrinogen III cosynthase and **Congenital Type I Dyserythropoiesis.** Although this may explain why some cases of erythropoietic porphyria have minimal or late onset anemia and others are rampant, it is more likely a single disease with a phenotypic heterogeneity (39–42).

Measures designed to treat the deleterious effects of this disorder, or syndrome, include avoidance of UV exposure, splenectomy, hypertransfusion, and oral porphyrin absorption agents. Splenectomy may reduce the severity of the hemolysis and thus the frequency of transfusions, but it is not curative. Hypertransfusion therapy with aggressive, ongoing iron chelation appears to have value, but whether these approaches, with or without the addition of porphyrin-absorbing agents such as charcoal or hematin or the addition of hydroxyurea have any long-term efficacy in the severe cases, awaits further studies. The one form of therapy with reasonable expectation of success in the severe cases is allogeneic bone marrow transplantation (43–47).

Including congenital erythropoietic porphyria, as in the above case, there are seven well-defined disorders of porphyrin metabolism that occur along the heme biosynthetic pathway. These disorders are usually classified by clinical expression as well as the underlying biochemical abnormality.

Disorders of porphyrin-induced cutaneous photosensitivity include **Congenital Erythropoietic Porphyria, Porphyria Cutanea Tarda,** and **Protoporphyria.**

Disorders of porphyrin-induced neurologic disturbance include **Acute Intermittent Porphyria** and **Homozygous ALA Dehydratase Deficiency.**

Disorders of porphyrin-induced cutaneous and neurologic defects include **Variegate Porphyria** and **Hereditary Coproporphyria.**

Deficiency of ALA dehydratase, the enzyme responsible for the conversion of δ-ALA to hydroxymethylbilane, is an example of a porphyrin-induced neurologic disorder: **ALA Dehydratase Porphyria (ADP)** (48). Probably a mutation at the ALA dehydrase gene site is the underlying cause (49). This, the rarest of all of the porphyrias, is inherited as an autosomal dominant (50). The principal biochemical derangement occurs in the liver and results in markedly elevated urinary excretion of ALA and coproporphyrin. Symptoms, which are essentially neurovisceral, range from mild to severe. Many of the symptoms of ADP are similar to those of severe lead poisoning, and to a lesser extent, tyrosinemia (51), from which both are readily distinguished by addressing the nature of the intoxicants and/or the secretory products.

In the hydroxymethylbilane-uroporphyrinogen pathway two porphyrias occur. Deficiency of uroporphyrinogen III cosynthetase results in congenital erythropoietic porphyria, as illustrated in the case described above. The other disorder in this pathway, **Acute Intermittent Porphyria (AIP),** is an autosomal dominantly inherited abnormality causing partial HMB synthase (PBG deaminase) deficiency (52). In fact, there are at least four different variants or genetic mutations leading to this deficiency which lead, in turn, to four different expressions, all characterized by episodes of mental, neurologic, and abdominal impairment (53, 54). This mutant-induced partial synthesis of HMB synthase results in excessive quantities of hepatic-derived ALA and PBG, both of which are excreted in the urine (55). They are also present in lesser quantities in the urine of carriers. Urinary PBG is readily detected because of its deep red color on exposure to light and air. This disorder is particularly prevalent amongst peoples of northern Scandinavia and the British Isles (56). Unlike all other porphyrias, the full-blown defect tends to occur in older patients and only rarely before the early to midthirties (56). Most individuals with this disorder do not manifest symptoms, and those who do may experience them as infrequently as yearly or less. However, when full-blown, the symptoms are striking and often begin with severe abdominal pain, which then progresses to debilitating neuropathies and mental aberrations (57–61). A variety of steroids and related pharmacologic substances have been implicated in precipitating these attacks via mechanisms that are as yet unclear (56). Treatment with analgesics and antianxiety drugs (62) is essentially supportive. For uncontrollable cases, hematin, which blocks the activity of ALA synthetase, has been shown to have variable success (63), but it is best reserved for severe, unrelenting events because it tends to (mildly) suppress platelet production and impair synthesis of protein clotting factors. Certain of the H_2 antagonists, which function by inhibition of cytochrome metabolism with resultant increases in heme and corresponding decreases in ALA synthase, may prove to be helpful in dealing with exacerbations. Barbiturates must *never* be used for the control of seizures, because of the symptom-initiating effects (64). Endogenous estrogen production can also be controlled by the use of oral contraceptives, which on occasion may actually precipitate attacks (60). Studies of experimental porphyria indicate that diets rich in carbohydrates may also prevent and sometimes control the severity of attacks.

Defects in conversion of uroporphyrinogen III to coproporphyrinogen III brought about by uroporphyrinogen decarboxylase deficiency result in one of the porphyria cutanea tarda (PCT) triads (65). Of all of the pyrrole metabolic disorders, the porphyria cutanea tarda triad is the most common. The underlying defect, which is inherited as an autosomal dominant, is the impaired synthesis of hepatic uroporphyrinogen decarboxylase. The defect involves mainly hepatic tissue, and, to a lesser degree, red cells (66). Familial porphyria cutanea tarda is characterized almost exclusively by skin photosensitivity (67). **Hepatoerythropoietic Porphyria,** the most severe form of the triad, is inherited in the homozygous state (68). Sporadic porphyria cutanea tarda, with the decarboxylase abnormality restricted to the liver, is clinically less severe than hepatoerythropoietic porphyria (65). Its inheritance pattern (if, indeed, it is inherited) is unclear, and so too is the mechanism by which exogenous material seemingly initiates its sporadic eruption (69).

With the exception of its mild hematologic defect, all other aspects of this disease strongly resemble congenital erythropoietic porphyria, namely, photosensitivity, poor skin healing, vesicles, hyperpigmentation, hypertrichosis, and occasionally hepatosplenomegaly. The scleroderma that is common in this group of disorders is the result of uroporphyrin-induced stimulation of collagen synthesis (70). It is also likely that the deposition of porphyrin in the skin enhances generation of superoxides and other free-oxygen radicals, which, in turn, adversely effect the integrity of the skin. Aggressive avoidance of alcohol and/or estrogens will minimize the manifestations of this disease (71). Chloroquine therapy, which induces formation of a readily excretable, water-soluble chloroquine-uroporphyrin complex, has gained some success (72), but phlebotomy continues to be the treatment of choice because it removes large quantities of iron, another disease-enhancing oxidant (73). Not only is iron deleterious (as an oxidant), it also inhibits uroporphyrinogen decarboxylase activity, which is further reason to avoid its use in patients with both congenital and acquired disease. Low-dose chloroquine infusion is recommended for patients in whom phlebotomy, for whatever reason, is ineffective.

The model example of **acquired porphyria cutanea tarda** is the wheat fungicide (hexachlorobenzine) exposure in Turkey, which intoxicated large numbers of citizens. In these individuals the disorder was characterized by skin pigmentation, hepatomegaly and photosensitivity (74, 75).

Deficiency of coproporphyrinogen oxidase, the enzyme responsible for conversion of coproporphyrinogen III to protoporphyrinogen IX, results in the autosomal dominant inheritance of **Hereditary Coproporphyria (HCP)** (76). This disorder is characterized by large quantities of coproporphyrin lll excreted in the feces and urine (77). Well over half the patients are asymptomatic and are, therefore, considered latent (76). Clinical manifestations are similar, albeit milder than those of ALA dehydratase deficiency porphyria, and include abdominal pain, neuropathies, psychiatric disturbances, and in somewhat fewer patients, photosensitivity-induced skin lesions (77, 78). Treatment, like that with all other porphyrias, includes avoidance of precipitating drugs (barbiturates, lead, steroidal contraceptive agents, diaminodiphenylsulfone) and the possible use of a high-carbohydrate diet along with supportive measures for acute attacks.

Variegate (or Mixed) Porphyria (VP) is the result of impeded conversion of protoporphyrinogen IX to protoporphyrin IX because of defective or deficient protoporphyrinogen oxidase synthesis (79). This disorder is inherited as an autosomal dominant with both neurologic and cutaneous manifestations. Onset is early in childhood, and it is particularly prominent in South Africa, the result of a small inbred group of early Dutch settlers (80). During acute episodes, both ALA and PBG are secreted in large amounts, whereas their excretion during latency remains normal. Clinical findings include the broad range of moderate-to-severe neurovisceral complaints with striking cutaneous findings (81). Therapy consists of both preventative and symptomatic supportive measures as with other similar disorders. It is important to distinguish this disorder from AIP. In the latter disorder, urinary excretion of ALA and PBG is present after the acute episode. This is not the case in variegate porphyria.

Protoporphyria, or **Erythropoietic Protoporphyria (EEP)** is the result of a defect in heme synthase (ferrochelatase), the enzyme responsible for the conversion of protoporphyrin IX to heme. It is inherited as an autosomal dominant (82). Protoporphyria is characterized by distinct cutaneous manifestations. It occurs more commonly than congenital erythropoietic porphyria and does not manifest itself until late childhood or early adolescence (83). The cutaneous manifestations do not resemble those of erythropoietic porphyria or porphyria cutanea tarda. In response to sunlight, patients with this disorder develop paresthesias, which precede the development of edema and erythema (84). The signs and symptoms involve only those areas exposed to sunlight, and any individual so afflicted will experience light-induced skin damage secondary to protoporphyrin deposition (85). It is commonly held that this disease, like porphyria cutanea tarda, is worsened by oxygen-dependent free radicals (86). A few patients with this disorder develop anemia and/or cholelithiasis (87). Liver damage following upon protoporphyrin deposition in hepatobiliary tracts and resultant "store formation" may be large enough to cause biliary obstructive disease (88). However, overall the disease is mild. Cholestyramine binds to protoporphyrin, increases its fecal elimination, and, in addition, effects losses in erythrocyte and plasma protoporphyrin concentrations, which further lessens the extent of protoporphyrin-induced liver disease (89). β-Carotene, in doses as high as 150 mg/day, along with sunscreen agents, have produced modest-to-good results in acute cases (90, 91). Figure 5.2 is a recapitulation of porphyrin biosynthesis and defects related to inborn errors.

The study of *endogenous* metabolic errors that occur along the heme synthetic pathway are as intellectually ap-

pealing as they are societally important. However, the societal issues relative to these disorders pale in comparison to the *exogenous*-induced problems brought about by lead intoxication. Lead poisoning continues to be the single most important pediatric environmental health problem in the United States. It is as prevalent as it is insidious. It is no less distressing when benefit ratios, often

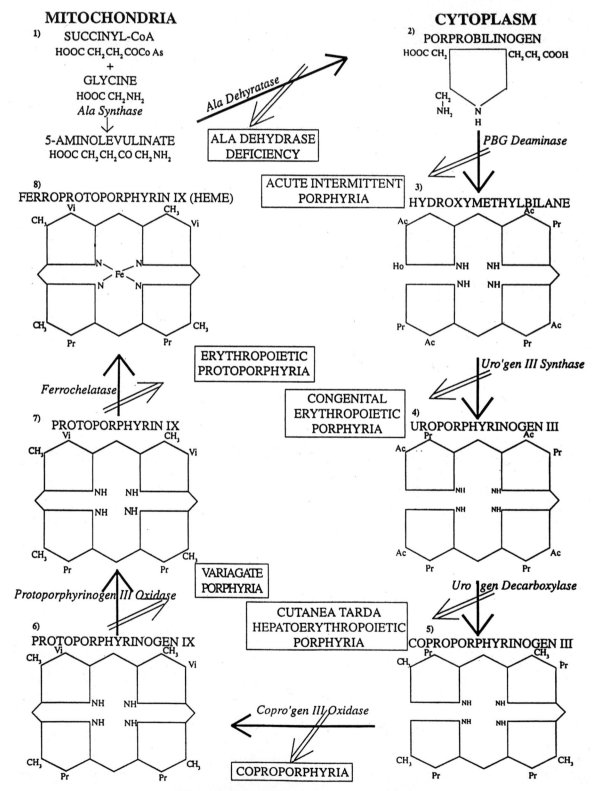

Figure 5.2. Inborn errors in porphyrin metabolism.

used to enforce lead-control regulations, are not as easily applied to old household paint as they are to lead in gasoline or lead in drinking water.

The most damaging effects of lead poisoning are behavioral difficulties and impaired cognitive function, problems that are not limited to disadvantaged populations. The effects are so dramatic that any threshold effect, presumed to be >10 $\mu g/dl$, is not apparent all the way down to 1 $\mu g/dl$ in studies of IQ in children.

The cost needed to address the hazards of leaded paint pollution must be measured in terms of the vast quantity of dollars used to develop programs for individuals whose cognitive functions mandate extensive medical care, along with other sources of additional education.

The inherent abnormalities of porphyrin metabolism are identifiable, usually predictable, and often preventable and/or treatable, but the frequency and the cost involved in all of these procedures is a pittance compared with the enormous burden of exogenously impaired porphyrin metabolism brought about by chronically low-level exposure to lead (92–96).

Heme Degradation: Bilirubin Metabolism

Once the process of heme synthesis is completed, the mature, enucleated red cell begins its extramedullary voyage on a programmed path to senescence. The process is on occasion discontinuous, but the net effect is the same—cell death. With the exception of overt blood loss, >90% of heme degradation occurs within macrophages. The final product, the opposite end of the porphyrin synthetic process, is bilirubin. A summation of factors that participate in the red cell aging process is listed in table 5.5.

The initial enzymatic processes involved in heme degradation are carried out by an integrated multienzyme system that includes heme oxygenase, P-450 reductase, and biliverdin reductase, a reaction mixture that requires NADPH and O_2. The multiple, and as yet incompletely understood, steps in the degradation of heme (initially as

Table 5.5. Changes in the Erythrocyte Associated with Aging

Decrease in glycolytic rate and in enzyme activity
Decrease in pentose shunt activity
Decrease in cellular components, including glutathione, K, Ca, Na, thiols, and ubiquitin
Decrease in membrane constituents including lipids, glycoproteins, and sialyl residues
Increase in lipid peroxidation
    Increase in membrane polymers, copolymers, membrane-bound hemichromes, spectrin hemoglobin aggregates, galactosyl residues, and protein kinase-C
Decrease in purine and pyrimidine enzymes
Increase in methemoglobin, hemoglobin A_2, oxygen affinity, red blood cell density, osmotic and mechanical fragility, and viscosity
Decreased red blood cell deformability

hemin) through hydroxy-, oxy-, and verdoheme to biliverdin and thence to bilirubin occurs within the macrophage before entering the plasma en route for processing in the hepatocyte. Heme is further degraded in the liver by specific transferases, i.e., Y-ligands or proteins, and, following a series of controlled plasma reflexes, it is then excreted into the gut. Excretion follows conjugation in the hepatocyte to a (water-soluble) glucuronide before entry into the gall bladder.

Case 4

An otherwise normal-appearing full-term infant, the first offspring of an apparently healthy 25-year-old mother, was noted to be icteric 24 hours after an uneventful birth and delivery. The icterus appeared initially on the brow and then spread diffusely thereafter. The mother received prenatal medications and had no untoward symptomatology throughout the entire pregnancy. At the delivery site it was noted that the mother was type O, Rh+, the baby was type B, Rh+, and the father was type B, Rh+. The infant had an Apgar score of 9 at the time of delivery, and he was breastfeeding well 24 hours later. His physical examination was entirely within normal limits, and he was in the 60–70th percentile for weight and length. He had a normal complete blood count (CBC), including a hemoglobin of 165 g/L and a total bilirubin level of 8.5 mg/dl with a direct reacting level of 2.5 mg/dl and a negative Coombs test. Blood film revealed 30–40% spherocytes. Because of the uncertainty regarding the elevation in direct-reacting bilirubin, a variety of studies was ordered, including a search for potential infectious agents as well as abnormal metabolites. The most likely cause seemed to be an ABO incompatibility despite the negative Coombs test. Twenty-four hours later, on day +3, the bilirubin had risen to a level of 11 mg/dl with a direct component of 3.5 mg/dl. His toxoplasma, rubella, cyomegalovirus, and herpes simplex virus (TORCH) titers, including serologic tests for syphilis, were negative. His hematocrit had fallen slightly, and there were numerous spherocytes on the peripheral smear. A repeat Coombs test, reviewed by microscopic analysis, proved to be positive. The physician explained that the child probably had a mild ABO incompatibility but could neither rule out the possibility of congenital spherocytosis nor could he readily explain the elevated direct bilirubin level. She thought that it might be due to inspissated bile secondary to mild dehydration and ordered supplemental sugar water feedings. At that point the mother recalled having severe gall bladder disease with gallstones when she was in her early teens and that she was told that she had an unusual familial type of blood disease with "round red cells." She then showed the physician an abdominal scar that essentially covered the undersurface of the rib cage and which represented surgery that included simultaneous removal of her gall bladder and her spleen. The mother further noted that she received penicillin for approximately 3 years following her surgery and then voluntarily stopped it. A review of the maternal blood smear showed that she had nu-

merous spheroidal red blood cells. Her record also indicated that an osmotic fragility test performed prior to surgery showed increased lysis of red cells in hypotonic saline characteristic of spherocytosis. The baby's course was uneventful; the bilirubin never rose above 12 mg/dl, always with an elevated direct-reacting component. On day +4 the baby was discharged to home, and over the next month his bilirubin level declined to 4.0 mg/dl with a direct level of 1.5 mg.dll. At 2 months of age the Coombs test was no longer positive. The spherocytes persisted and no other abnormalities except for the typical decline in hemoglobin during the first 6 months of life, were identified. The mother was advised not to breastfeed the child because of concern over the rare instance of breast milk inhibition of glucurnyl transferase further enhancing a preexisting ecteric state. The child thrived on cow's milk, and ate a balanced diet. By 1 year of age he was noted to be chronically anemic with a hemoglobin value approximately 1 standard deviation below the age-related mean.

Increased osmotic lysis in hypotonic saline confirmed the presence of spherocytes and supported the diagnosis of **Hereditary Spherocytosis.**

The persistence of an elevated direct-reacting bilirubin continued to be puzzling. It was recommended that if he were to become symptomatic by age 3 or 4 years, a splenectomy be carried out. Preparations were made to immunize the child at approximately 2 years of age with pneumococcal, hemophilus, and meningococcal vaccines in anticipation of such an event. Despite the fact that the child was chronically anemic, the mother refused permission to carry out a splenectomy except as an emergency, because she recalled her own extended illness at the time of her surgery. Thus, at the completion of his immunization schedule, the mother no longer brought the child to the physician.

At 10 years of age, the boy's physician received a frantic call from the family indicating that the child was listless and appeared to be very pale and yellow. On examination, pertinent findings included pallor, marked icterus, and a palpable spleen tip. An automated hematology profile included a hemoglobin of 70 g/L, WBC count of 8.0×10^9/L, platelet count of 120×10^9, RBC count of 2.7×10^{12}/L, packed cell volume of 21%, and reticulocyte count of 0.3%. His total bilirubin was 7.0 mg/dl direct and 16.5 mg/dl total. Liver enzymes were

Table 5.6. Defects in Bilirubin Metabolism

Conjugated Disorders	
Inherited	
Dubin-Johnson (A)	Accumulation of pigment in hepatocytes
	Nonvisualized gall bladder
	Mild disorder
Rotor syndrome (B)	Defect in transport system
	Both A & B have increased urinary coproporphyrin I
	Total bilirubin range 2–10 mg/dl, occasionally higher
	Mild disorder
α^1-Antitrypsin deficiency	Hepatocytes are PAS positive
	Homozygous form leads to cirrhosis
	Potentially fatal disorder, treated with liver transplant
Galactosemia/tyrosinemia	Both are mild, easily diagnosed in newborn
	Treated by dietary controls
Congenital	
Obliterative cholangiopathy (biliary artresia)	Liver transplant is ultimate therapy when all else fails
Choledochal cyst	Surgical excision is the treatment of choice
Intrahepatic chlestasis (Byler disease)	Often progresses to cirrhosis
Acquired	
Chemical	Antimetabolites, hyperalimentation, toxins, industrial
Infection	Bacterial, protozoal, viral, fungal
Unconjugated disorders	
Inherited	
Crigler-Najjar disease	Total (Ho) to partial (He) absence of glucoronyl transferase
Homozygous (Ho)/Heterozygous (He)	(Ho) leads to bilirubin encephalopathy; (He) mild
Gilbert disease	Apparent in early teen years, mild disease, etiology unknown
Acquired	
Neonatal noninherited disorders	
Breast milk jaundice	Mild, disappears following interruption in breastfeeding
Transient familial jaundice	High levels of unconjugated bilirubin, treated by exchange transfusion
Drug-induced hyperbilirubinemia Vitamin K	Competition for binding sites
Hormonal disorders	
Thyroid deficiency	Delayed glucuronide synthesis
Infants of mothers w/diabetes mellitus	
Hemolytic disease of newborn	High bilirubin levels following excessive hemolysis and failure at conjugation

marginally elevated. The initial impression was an aplastic crisis in a person spherocytosis-induced hemolysis, the former probably secondary to a viral infection. Flat film of the abdomen revealed a half-dozen opacities in a visualized gall bladder. The boy's parents reluctantly agreed to both cholecystectomy and splenectomy. An endoscopic attempt to empty the gallbladder of stones failed, and a two-stage procedure was carried out. A liver biopsy carried out at the time of cholecystectomy revealed hepatocytes free of bile retention. Review of urinary excretory elements identified low excretory levels of urinary coproporphyrin.

In effect, the patient had 3 disorders: viral-induced pancytopenia, hereditary splenocytosis, and, as a cause of the direct biliruninemia, **Rotor Syndrome,** *which is readily distinguishable from* **Dubin-Johnson Syndrome,** *which, unlike rotor syndrome, does not show gallbladder visualization and has abnormal pigment storage in the hepatocytes.*

Comment: *Just as there are a number of inherited and acquired red cell compartment defects that result both in a shortened life span and heightened bilirubin production, so, too, are there inborn and acquired defects in bilirubin metabolism that result in a spectrum of mild-to-serious diseases. Table 5.6 is a compendium of disorders in conjugated and unconjugated bilirubin metabolism.*

The final stage of bilirubin metabolism occurs within the gut. Hydrolysis of bilirubin diglucuronide occurs in the terminal ileum. Of note is the fact that at times of gut stasis bilirubin readily loses its conjugate, which, in turn, leads to reabsorption into the vascular space and, if persistent, a further worsening of a preexisting hyperbilirubinic state.

Urobilinogen formed by the bacteria-derived deconjugating enzymes is oxidized to its final fecal-containing product, urobilin. Most of the urobilinogen enters this process directly, with about 20% coming into the system indirectly following reabsorption from the enterohepatic circulation. A small amount of this cycled urobilogen winds up in urine following glomerular filtration. Other urobilin intermediates, namely, mesobilinogen and stercobilinogen, also contribute to the ultimate urobilin pool, but the explanation for these alternative pathways is as yet unclear (97–111).

Conclusion

In summary, hemoglobin degradation proceeds along two major routes. Intravascular hemolysis occurs in the liver, wherein hemoglobin in its oxidated form is totally bound to haptoglobin and deposited as a methemoglobin-haptoglobin complex before further degradation occurs. In the same setting, heme is released from methemalbumin and methemopexin complexes, respectively, once the haptoglobin-binding complex is fully saturated. Extravas-

cular hemolysis occurs in the spleen, in which setting there are no intermediates, i.e., hemoglobin is directly degraded to heme and globin. At both sites, iron, once released from heme, is recycled via the storage pool, the porphyrin ring is further degraded to bilirubin, the globin chains are degraded to amino acids, and the cycle begins again.

REFERENCES

1. Lamola AA, Piomelli S, et al. Erythropoietic protoporphyria and Pb intoxication: the molecular basis for difference in cutaneous photosensitivity; II, different binding of erythrocyte protoporphyrin to hemoglobin. J Clin Invest 1975;56:1528.
2. Moore MR, Meredith PA. The association of δ-aminolaevulinic acid with the neurological and behavioural effects of lead exposure. In: Hemphill DD, ed. Trace metals in environmental health. Columbia: University of Missouri Press, 1976:363–371.
3. Porra RA, Jones OTG. Studies on ferrochetalase; II, an investigation of the role of ferrochelatase in the biosynthesis of various heme prosthetic groups. Biochem J 1963;87:186.
4. Needleman H, Schell A, et al. Long-term effects of childhood exposure to lead at low dose. N Engl J Med 1990; 322:83.
5. Lin-Fu JS. Vulnerability of children to lead exposure and toxicity. N Engl J Med 1973;289:1229.
6. Chisolm JJ Jr. The use of chelating agents in the treatment of acute and chronic lead intoxication in childhood. J Pediatr 1968;73:1.
7. Piomelli S, Rosen JF, et al. Management of childhood lead poisoning. J Pediatr 1984;105:523.
8. McKay R, Druyan, et al. Intramitochondrial localization of δ-aminolevulinic synthetase and ferrochelatase in rat liver. Biochem J 1969;114:445.
9. Jordan PM, Seehra JS. Mechanism of action of δ-aminolevulinic acid dehydratase stepwise order of addition of the two molecules of δ-aminolevulinic acid in the enzyme synthesis of porphobilinogen. J Chem Soc Chem Commun 1980;4:240.
10. Tsukamoto I, Yoshinga T, Sano S. The role of zinc with special reference to the essential thiol groups in δ-aminolevulinic acid dehydratase of bovine liver. Biochim Biophys Acta 1979;570:167.
11. Wetmur JG, Bishop DF, et al. Molecular cloning of a cDNA for human δ-aminolevulinate dehydratase. Gene 1986; 43:123,
12. Yamamoto M, Fujita H, et al. An immunochemical study of δ-aminolevulinate synthase and δ-aminolevulinate dehydratase in liver and erythroid cells of rat. Arch Biochem Biophys 1986;245:76.
13. Sassa S, Granick S, Bickers DR, Levere RD, Kappas A. Studies on the inheritance of human erythrocyte δ-aminolevulinate dehydratase and uroporphyrinogen synthetase. Enzyme 1973;16:326.
14. Srivastava G, Borthwick IA, Brooker JD, et al. Purification of rat liver mitochondrial δ-aminolevulinate synthase. Biochem Biophys Res Commun 1982;109:305.
15. Potluri VR, Astrin KH, et al. Human 5-aminolevulinate dehydratase: chromosomal localization to 9q34 by in situ hybridization. Hum Genet 1987;76:236.
16. Battersby AR, Fookes CJR, Matcham GWJ, et al. Biosynthesis of the pigments of life: formation of the macrocycle. Nature 1980;285:17.

17. Raich N, Romer PH, et al. Molecular cloning and complete sequence of human erythrocyte porphobilinogen deaminase. Nucleic Acids Res 1986;14:5955.

18. Bogorad L. The enzymatic synthesis of porphyrins from porphobilinogen; II, uroporphyrin III. J Biol Chem 1958; 233:510.

19. Grandchamp B, de Verneuil H, et al. Tissue-specific expression of porphobilinogen deaminase: two isozymes from a single gene. Eur J Biochem 1987;162:105.

20. Frydman RB, Feinstein G. Studies on porphobilinogen deaminase and uroporphyrinogen III cosynthetase from human erythrocytes. Biophys Acta 1974;350:358.

21. Straka JG, Kushner JP. Purification and characterization of bovine hepatic uroporphyrinogen decarboxylase. Biochemistry 1983;22:4664.

22. Jackson AH, et al. Macrocytic intermediates in the biosynthesis of porphyrins. Philos Trans R Soc Lond (Biol) 1976; 273:191.

23. Grandchamp B, et al. The mitochondrial localization of coproporphyrinogen III oxidase. Biochem J 1978;176:97.

24. Jackson AH, et al. Mesoporphyrinogen IV: a substrate for coproporphyrinogen oxidase. J Chem Soc Chem Commun 1976;1:322.

25. Labbe RF, Nielsen L. Clinical-biochemical interpretations of erythrocyte protoporphyrin: ferrochetalase-pyridoxal phosphate studies. In: Doss, M, ed. Porphyrins in human disease. Basel: Karger, 1976.

26. Cartwright GE, et al. Hematologic response of pyridoxine deficient swine to pyridoxine. Proc Soc Exp Biol Med 1963; 114:7.

27. Labbe RF, Rettmer RL. Zinc protoporphyrin: a product of iron-deficient erythropoiesis. Semin Hematol 1989; 26:40.

28. Labbe RF, Rettmer RL, Shah AG, Turnlund JR. Zinc protoporphyrin: past present and future. Ann NY Acad Sci 1987;514:7.

29. Lachant NA, Tomoda A, Tanaka Kr. Inhibition of the pentose phosphate shunt by lead: a potential mechanism for hemolysis in lead poisoning. Blood 1984;63:518.

30. Piddington SK, White JM. The effect of lead on total globin and α- and β-chain synthesis; in vitro and in vivo. Br J Haematol 1974;27:415.

31. Paglia DE, Valentine WN. Hereditary and acquired defects in the pyrimidine nucleotidase of human erythrocytes. Curr Top Hematol 1980;3:75.

32. Ali MAM, Quinlan A. Effect of lead on globin synthesis in vitro. Am J Clin Pathol 1977;67:77.

33. Dagg JH, Goldberg A, Lochhead A, Smith JA. The relationship of lead poisoning to acute intermittent porphyria. Q J Med 1965;34:163.

34. Berk P, et al. Hematologic and biochemical studies in a case of lead poisoning. Am J Med 1970;

35. Clark M, Royal J, Seeler R. Interaction of iron deficiency and lead and the hematologic findings in children with severe lead poisoning. Pediatrics 1988;81:247.

36. Cullen MR, Robins JM, Eskenazi B. Adult inorganic lead intoxication: presentation of 31 new cases and a review of recent advances in the literature. Medicine 1983; 62:221.

37. Schwartz J, et al. Lead-induced anemia: dose-response relationships and evidence for a threshold. Am J Public Health 1990; 80:165.

38. Nordmann Y, Deybach JC: Congenital erythropoietic porphyria. Semin Liver Dis 1982;2:154.

39. Gross S, et al. Hematologic studies on erythropoietic porphyria: a new case with severe hemolysis, chronic thrombocytopenia and folic acid deficiency. Blood 1964; 23:762.

40. Weston MC, et al. Congenital erythropoietic uroporphyria (Gunther's disease) presenting in a middle-aged man. Int J Biochem 1978;9:921.

41. Kushner JP, et al. Congenital erythropoietic porphyria, diminished activity of uroporphyrinogen decarboxylase and dyserythropoiesis. Blood 1982;59:725.

42. Weiming X, Warner CA, Desnick RJ. Congenital erythropoeitic porphyria: identification and expression of 10 mutations in the uroporphyrinogen III synthase gene. J Clin Invest 1995;95:905.

43. Piomelli S, Poh-Fitzpatrick KM, Seaman L, et al. Complete suppression of the symptoms of congenital erythropoietic porphyria by long-term treatment with high-level transfusions. N Engl J Med 1986;314:1029.

44. Haining RG, et al. Congenital erythropoietic porphyria: the effects of induced polycythemia. Blood 1970;36:297.

45. Rank JM et al. Hematin therapy in late onset congenital erythropoietic porphyria. Br J Haematol 1990;75:617.

46. Piomelli S, et al. Current strategies in the management of Cooley's anemia. Ann NY Acad Sci 1985;256:267.

47. Pimstone NR, et al. Therapeutic efficacy of chronic charcoal therapy in congenital erythropoietic porphyria. N Engl J Med 1987;316:390.

48. Bird TD, et al. Inherited deficiency of delta-aminolevulinic acid dehydratase. Am J Hum Genet 1979;31:662.

49. Brandt A, Doss M. Hereditary porphobilinogen synthase deficiency in humans associated with acute hepatic porphyria. Hum Genet 1981;58:194.

50. Doss M, et al. New type of acute porphyria with porphobilinogen synthase (δ-aminolevulinic acid dehydratase) defect in the homozygous state. Clin Biochem 1982; 15:52.

51. Sassa S, Kappas A. Hereditary tyrosinemia and the heme biosynthetic pathway: profound inhibition of δ-aminolevulinic and dehydratase activity by succinylacetone. J Clin Invest 1983;71:625.

52. Strand L, et al. Heme biosynthesis in intermittent acute porphyria: decreased hepatic conversion of porphobilinogen to porphyrins and increased delta-aminolevulinic acid synthetase activity. Proc Natl Acad Sci USA 1970; 67:1315.

53. Desnick RJ, et al. Acute intermittent porphyria: Characterization of a novel mutation in the structural gene for porphobilinogen deaminase. J Clin Invest 1985;76:865.

54. Stein JA, Tschudy DP. Acute intermittent porphyria. Medicine 1970;49:1.

55. Kaelbing R, et al. Urinary porphobilinogen: Results of screening 2500 psychiatric patients. Arch Gen Psychiatry 1961;5:494.

56. Kappas A, et al. The porphyrias. In: Stanbury JB, et al, ed. The metabolic basis of inherited disease, 5th ed. New York: McGraw-Hill, 1983.

57. Bonkowsky HL, Schady W. Neurologic manifestations of acute porphyria. Semin Liver Dis 1982;2:108.

58. Beattie Ad, Goldberg A. Acute intermittent porphyria: natural history and prognosis. In: Doss, M, ed. Porphyrins in human diseases. Basel: Karger, 1976.

59. Sorensen AW, With TK: Persistent pareses after porphyric attacks. Acta Med Scand 1971;190:219.

60. Stein JA, et al. Abnormal iron and water metabolism in acute intermittent porphyria with new morphologic findings. Am J Med 1972;41:2530.

61. Carney MWP. Hepatic porphyria with mental symptoms. Lancet 1972;2:100.

62. Monaco RN, et al. Intermittent acute porphyria treated with chlorpromazine. N Engl J Med 1957;256:309.

63. Pierach CA. Hematin therapy for the porphyric attack. Semin Liver Dis 1982;2:125.

64. Larson AW, et al. Post traumatic epilepsy and acute intermittent porphyria: effects of phenytoin, carbamazepine and clonazepam. Neurology 1978;28:824.

65. Elder GH, et al. Immunoreactive uroporphyrinogen decarboxylase in sporadic porphyria cutanea tarda. N Engl J Med 1978;299:274.

66. Felsher BF, et al. Decreased hepatic uroporphyrinogen decarboxylase activity in porphyria cutanea tarda. N Engl J Med 1982;306:766.

67. Grossman ME, Poh-Fitzpatrick MB. Porphyria cutanea tarda: clinical features and laboratory findings in 40 patients. Am J Med 1979;67:277.

68. Fujita H, et al. Immunochemical study of uroporphyrinogen decarboxylase in a patient with mild hepatoerythropoietic porphyria. J Clin Invest 1987;79:1533.

69. Elder GH, et al. Immunoreactive uroporphyrinogen decarboxylase in the liver in porphyria cutanea tarda. Lancet 1986;2:229.

70. Grossman ME, Poh-Fitzpatrick MB. Porphyria cutanea tarda: diagnosis and management. Med Clin North Am. 1980;64:807.

71. Lundvall O. Phlebotomy treatment of porphyria cutanea tarda. Acta Derm Venereol (Stockh) 1982;100:107.

72. Kordac V. Frequency of occurrence of hepatocellular carcinoma in patients with porphyria cutanea tarda in long-term follow up. Neoplasma 1972;19:135.

73. DiPadova C, et al. Effects of phlebotomy on urinary porphyrin pattern and liver histology in patients with porphyria cutanea tarda. Am J Med Sci 1983;285:2.

74. Cam C, Nogogosyan G. Acquired toxic porphyria cutanea tarda due to hexachlorobenzene. JAMA 1963;183:88.

75. Cetingil AI, Ozen AM. Toxic porphyria. Blood 1960;15:1002.

76. Andres J, et al. Hereditary coproporphyria: incidence in a large English family. J Med Genet 1984;21:341.

77. Brodie MJ, et al. Hereditary coproporphyria. Demonstration of the abnormalities in haem biosynthesis in peripheral blood. Q J Med 1977;182:229.

78. Ditrapani G, et al. Peripheral nerve findings in hereditary coproporphyria. Acta Neuropathol (Berl) 1984;63:96.

79. Deybachj JF, et al. The inherited enzymatic defect in porphyria variegata. Hum Genet 1981;58:425.

80. Eales L, et al. The clinical and biochemical features of variegate porphyria: an analysis of 300 cases studied at Groote Schuur Hospital, Captetown. Int J Biochem 1980;12:837.

81. Mustajoki P. Variegate porphyria Ann Intern Med 1978;89:238.

82. Reed WB, et al. Erythropoietic protoporphyria: a clinical and genetic study. JAMA 1970;214:1060.

83. Prentice RTW. Goldberg A. Photosensitivity: familial incidence, clinical features and incidence of erythropoietic protoporphyria. Br J Dermatol 1969;81:414.

84. DeLeo VA, et al. Erythropoietic protoporphyria: ten years' experience. Am J Med 1976;60:8.

85. Magnus IA, et al. Erythropoietic protoporphyria: A new porphyria syndrome with solar urticaria due to protoporphyrinemia. Lancet 1961;2:448.

86. Lim HW, et al. Activation of the complement system in patients with porphyrias after irradiation in vivo. J Clin Invest 1984;11:1103.

87. Cripps DJ, Scheuer PJ. Hepatobiliary changes in erythropoietic protoporphyria. Arch Pathol Lab Med 1965;80:500.

88. Bloomer JR. Protoporphyria. Semin Liver Dis 1982;2:143.

89. Strathers GM. Porphyrin-binding effect of cholestyramine: results of in vitro and in vivo studies. Lancet 1966;2:780.

90. Mathews-Roth MM, et al. Beta-carotene therapy for erythropoietic protoporphyria and other photosensitivity diseases. Arch Dermatol 1977;113:1229.

91. Mathews-Roth MM. Anemia in erythropoietic protoporphyria. JAMA 1974;230:824.

92. Bellinger D, Leviton A, Waternaux C, Needleman H, Rabinowitz M. Low level lead exposure, social class, and infant development. Neurotoxicol Teratol 1989;10:473.

93. The nature and extent of lead poisoning of children in the United States: a report to Congress. Washington, DC: Agency for Toxic Substances and Disease Registry, 1988. DHHS Publication 99-2966.

94. Schwartz J. Societal benefits of reducing lead exposure. Environ Res 1994;66:105.

95. Sciarillo W, Alexander G, Farrell KP. Lead exposure and child behavior. Am J Pub Health 1992;82:1356.

96. Schwartz J. Low-level lead exposure and children's IQ: a meta-analysis and search for a threshold. Environ Res 1994:65:42.

97. Berk PD, Wolkoff AW, et al. Inborn errors of bilirubin metabolism. Med Clin North Am 1975;59:803.

98. Gilbert A, Lereboullet P. La cholemie simple familale. Semaine medicale 19091;21:241.

99. Sieg A, Stiehl A, et al. Gilbert's syndrome: diagnosis by typical serum bilirubin patters. Clin Chem Acta 1986;154:41.

100. Crigler JR Jr, Najjar VA. Congenital familial nonhemolytic jaundice with kernicterus. Pediatrics 1952;10:169.

101. Odell GB, Cukier JO, Gourley GR. The presence of a microsomal UDP-glucuronyl transferase for bilirubin in homozygous jaundiced Gunn rats and in the Crigler-Najjar syndrome. Hepatology 1981;1:307.

102. Hunter JO, Thompson PH, et al. Inheritance of type 2 Crigler-Najjar hyperbilirubinemia. Gut 1973;14:46.

103. Newman AJ, Gross S. Hyperbilirubinemia in breast-fed infants. Pediatrics 1963;32:995.

104. Dubin IN, Johnson FB. Chronic idiopathic jaundice with unidentified pigment in liver cells: a new clinico-

pathologic entity with a report of 12 cases. Medicine 1954;
33:155.

105. Rotor AB, Manah AN, Florentin A. Familial nonhemolytic
jaundice with direct van dan Bergh reaction. Acta Med Phil
1948;5:37.

106. Koskelo P, Toivonen I, Aldercreutz H. Urinary coropor-
phyrin isomer distribution in Cubin-Johnson syndrome.
Clin Chem 1967;13:1006.

107. Shimizu Y, Naruto H, et al. Urinary coproporphyrin isomers
in Rotor's syndrome: a study of eight families. Hepatology
1981;1:173.

108. Sharp HL. The current status of alpha-I-antitrypsin, a protease inhibitor, in gastrointestinal disease. Gastroenterology
1976;70:611.

109. Fitzgerald JF. Cholestatic disorders of infancy. Pediatr Clin
North Am 1988;35:357.

110. Nahmias AJ, Walls KW, et al. The TORCH complex-
perinatal infections associated with toxoplasma, rubella,
cytomegalo- and herpes simplex viruses. Pediatr Res 1971;
5:405.

111. Gautier M, Eliot N. Extrahepatic biliary atresia. Arch
Pathol Lab Med 1981;105:397.

CHAPTER 6

Disorders of Iron Metabolism

SAMUEL GROSS

The anemia with the longest list of mythical, romantic, societal and dietary notions is the one resulting from iron lack. In Greek mythology a potion of iron rust and wine cured Iphicles of impotence. Chlorosis, "the green sickness" or "De Morbo Virgineo," was, in part, an iron deficiency state brought about by poor diet, societal prejudice against meat eating, and restrictive attire (corsets) that led to impaired appetite and reflux (bloody) esophagitis. Iron salts were recommended as the treatment of choice for chlorosis as early as 1730. One hundred years later ferrous sulfate improved the hypochromic anemia of iron deficiency. Yet, the stereotype of the female as a pale, weak and hysterical individual dressed in an hour glass corset tragically persisted well into the 19th century. Only when these stereotypes and prejudices abated did the corset, along with at least one cause of iron deficiency, disappear.
—Editors

In the porphyrin chapter (chap. 5), the emphasis lay on the mechanism by which a pair of simple precursors condense and ultimately form a highly specialized pyrrole capable of accepting valent iron in order to form heme. This process, as noted, unfolds along a pathway highly susceptible to inherited or exogenously induced defects.

In this chapter, discussion focuses on disorders related to iron, as: (a) the centerpiece of red cell and myoglobulin oxygen carriage, (b) the key to effective electron transfer in a number of enzymatic reactions, (c) an element highly vulnerable to vagaries in transportation, and (d) an element capable of initiating oxidative damage.

Introduction

During the latter half of the third trimester of pregnancy, iron diffuses from the mother across the placenta along a steadily increasing gradient. At full-term the infant is endowed with approximately 220–250 mg of total body iron, three-fourths of which is present in hemoglobin, the remainder in myoglobin, enzymes, transport systems, and newly emerging storage depots (1). With growth and development, effective realignment into red cells and the other compartments occurs in a manner designed to maintain efficient utilization. Once birth is completed and oral nutrition commences, iron enters the body for the first time via the alimentary tract, where both its absorption and its distribution are regulated. Iron deficiency, or lack, however, does occur and is brought about by failure (a) to address inadequacies of prematurity (2), (b) to supply the amounts needed to support growth during the first year

of life (3), (c) by losses due to bleeding (4–7), or (d) by the rare example of grossly abnormal diets.

Once body growth and marrow demands attain maturity (a steady state of iron flux), iron partition is maintained in a fairly uniform pattern. Table 6.1 identifies the iron distribution pattern in normal adults compared with premature, full-term and 1-year-old infants.

Storage of iron is carried out primarily in macrophages of the liver and marrow (8). Once it leaves its storage site, iron serves an integral role in the red cell for 120 days in the adult; 90 days in the premature neonate. At the time of red cell degradation and senescence, hemoglobin is oxidized to methemoglobin, and iron is oxidatively split from heme and incorporated into ferritin. Its release from ferritin for subsequent transportation occurs in the cell sol in a complex and as yet poorly understood process.

Iron is transported via transferrin (9), an 86-kd β_2-globulin, which, during normal daily flux, is on the average, one-third iron saturated. With decreases in iron levels, as in nutritional (10) (non–protein losing) iron deficiency or chronic blood loss, the unbound portion of transferrin rises in a seemingly teleologic manner, increasing in response to iron receptor increases brought about by lack of iron. With protein-losing disorders, both saturated and unsaturated losses occur (11) as, for example, in protein-losing enteropathies (12) and cystic fibrosis (13). In protein-calorie malnutrition (14), there is insufficient transferrin synthesized to transport iron. The net effect of all of the above is an iron-deficiency state.

Ease of iron absorption depends, in part, on the iron source. Ferrous (Fe^{++}), or heme, iron is rapidly absorbed.

Nonheme, or ferric, iron (Fe^{+++}) requires "corrective" oxidation, which is facilitated by gastric juice, in order to be readily absorbed. The largest and most readily available sources of heme iron are derived from animal products. Neither fowl nor fish are good sources of heme iron. Unlike ascorbate-rich foodstuffs, which enhance iron absorption (15–17), diets rich in calcium and/or phosphorous, both of which form insoluble iron complexes, and tea (tannic acid), which alters its valence, impede iron absorption.

Once absorption is completed, transportation begins and is indirectly influenced by hemoglobin production, by uncoupling and coupling of iron by ferritin, and by the number of external transferrin receptors (18).

Nutritional inadequacy, the result of (a) start-up insufficiency, (b) unaddressed lack of iron due to prematurity, (c) iron-poor cow's milk feeding of premature infants, (d) unsupplemented cow's milk or unsupplemented breast milk feeding in full-term infants, or, less commonly, (e) cow's milk–induced gastrointestinal (GI) blood loss, are among the likely causes of iron deficiency in the growing neonate (19–23). Almost all adult iron deficiencies are related to blood loss. Unless proper nutritional intake is compromised by excessive alcohol intake, iron-poor diets in adults may take years to become manifest. In the non-menstruating adult whose iron losses do not exceed 0.5–1.0 mg/day (in stool, sweat, nail growth), it is calculated that failure to ingest iron would take well over 3 years to decrease the 3–4 g of body iron to a clinically deficient entity.

Blood loss–induced iron deficiency may be the result of (a) intrauterine blood losses (infant to maternal, infant to infant), (b) external losses (at birth) following abruptio placenta, placenta previa, or early cord clamping, (c) severe inflammatory disease, (d) excessive acute menstrual and GI losses, (e) chronic bleeding syndromes, (f) vascular diseases, (g) intravascular hemolysis that exceeds haptoglobin binding, and (h) factitious losses (2, 4, 24–26).

Hypochromic, Microcytic Anemia of Iron Lack

Iron-deficiency anemia is a universal problem involving individuals of all ages and both sexes. It is the most common nutritional deficiency of the hematopoietic system and, in fact, may be the most common disorder seen by primary care physicians. Wherever seen, in developed or developing countries, the approach to its investigation and subsequent therapy depends upon a comprehensive understanding of the biology of heme synthesis. In the final analysis the presumption of iron deficiency as the cause of a hypochromic, microcytic anemia mandates evidence of proof, and once proven, treatment must be appropriate and include corrective replenishment of body stores. Table 6.2 is a summation of the laboratory correlates in iron deficiency.

Case 1

A 46-year-old athletic Greek-American woman sought help from her physician because of a 6-week history of generalized fatigue and irritability. Her systems review disclaimed dizziness, headache, or palpitations, and she had normal dietary and excretory habits. The only other positive finding was the occasional appearance of dark-colored urine in the morning, which she attributed to irregular menses. Her physical examination was marked by minimal pallor and a palpable spleen tip. Her nails were flat but not brittle, there was no atrophy or redness of her lingual papillae, she was not dysphagic or unable to swallow solids, and she had no symptoms of gastritis. Her menstrual periods lasted 6 days but were occasionally irregular and heavy in flow. Except for a rare analgesic, she took medicine infrequently and never took iron. Her dietary history was above suspicion. She enjoyed eating, consumed all forms of heme-containing foodstuffs and was neither anorectic nor bulimic. She

Table 6.1. Iron Partition (%)

	Adult	Premature	Term	One Year
Hemoglobin	66.0	77.0	77.0	81.0
Myoglobin	3.0	2.0	3.0	3.0
Enzyme Iron	0.1	0.1	0.1	0.1
Storage Iron	30.0	20.0	19.0	15.0
Transport Iron°	0.9	0.9	0.9	0.9

°Includes iron in the process of being incorporated into any of the above.

Table 6.2. Laboratory Correlates of Iron Deficiency

	Hemoglobin Concentration g/dL	Serum Ferritin ng/I	Transferrin Saturation %	Erythrocyte Protoporphyrin ug/g Hgb	Cell Volume (MCV) fl
Normal values	>11	7–70	>20	<3	>70
Fe stores depleted	—	<7	<20	—	—
Erythropoiesis impaired	—	<7	<10	>3	—
Erythropoiesis decreased	—	<7	<5	>4	<70
Anemia, subclinical	<11 >8	<7	<5	>5	<65
Anemia, clinical	<8	<7	<5	>8	<60
Anemia, severe°	<4	<7	<5	>10	<60

°Congestive heart failure.

was para 2+0, and she and her husband, who was also of Greek descent, had 2 healthy children, 15 and 18 years of age.

A complete blood count (CBC) revealed the following: hemoglobin 80 g/L, erythrocytes 4.25×10^{12}/L, hematocrit 29%; mean corpuscular volume (MCV) 68 fl, mean corpuscular hemoglobin concentration (MCHC) 27.6 g/dl, mean corpuscular hemoglobin (MCH) 19 pg, reticulocytes 0.2%, white blood cell (WBC) count 7.6×10^9/L, and platelets 375×10^9/L. A blood film was predominantly hypochromic with microcytosis and poikilocytosis; WBC and platelet features were unremarkable. Urine was trace positive for heme and protein. Stools were negative for heme, and a serum ferritin level was 1 mg/L (normal 7–70 mg/L).

The initial impression of the (hypochromic, microcytic, hypoferremic) anemia was iron deficiency, presumably due to excessive menstrual loss. Treatment consisted of 3 months of orally administered ferrous sulphate in a dose of 250 mg (three-fifths of which is elemental iron) three times daily. One week later, the dose was reduced to 200 mg three times daily because of abdominal discomfort. Fourteen days into her therapy, the patient's reticulocyte count was 2.1%, and repeat tests 1 month into therapy demonstrated a suboptimal response, i.e., hemoglobin 93 g/L with 2.0% reticulocytes, MCV of 70 fl, and serum ferritin of 3 mg/L. Serum folate and vitamin B_{12} levels were 9.5 ng/L and 350 ng/L, respectively, both well within the normal range. Hemoglobin A_2 accounted for 2.2% and hemoglobin F 1.2% (both within normal range) of her total hemoglobin. Repeat examination results (pelvis and rectum included) were again normal. On the basis of calculated iron needs, the presumption being that either she was not absorbing the medication or was, in fact, noncompliant, the patient was treated with intravenously administered iron in quantities sufficient to correct the anemia and repair the stores. Given her weight of 44 kg, her calculated blood volume would be 3.5 liters. Normal blood has 500 mg/L of Fe, virtually all from hemoglobin that contains 3.5 mg/g of Fe. Thus her ideal blood iron content would be 1.75 g if she had a normal hemoglobin such as 130 g/L. Her hemoglobin was only 93 g/L, however; therefore her total blood iron content was approximately 1 g ($93 \times 3.5 \times 35$), giving a deficit of 750 mg. It can be assumed that the body iron store of about 250 mg would also be exhausted, as would be any circulating iron, for a total deficit of about 1 g. In order to provide the needed 1 g of iron to repair the iron loss, she received a 5-hour infusion at 150 ml/hr of 1000 mg of elemental iron dispersed in 600 ml of 0.5% NaCl containing 5% dextrose. The infusion, included a 3-month schedule of oral iron in the previous oral dose schedule, at the end of which time her blood counts had essentially normalized to hemoglobin 135 g/L, MCV 85 fl, ferritin 10 µg/L.

Five months later she returned to her physician with recurrence of previous symptoms. She was again found to have a microcytic anemia: hemoglobin 98 g/L, MCV 71 fl, and ferritin 3 µg/L. However, her white cell and platelet counts were lower than heretofore: 3.1×10^9/L and 135×10^9/L, respectively, and on repeat history, the patient admitted to having short-term, repeat bouts of nagging low back pain, which she attributed to jogging. She also noted that her urine samples were more frequently dark colored, which when tested were positive for free hemoglobin. A red blood cell (RBC) acid hemolysis test (acidified normal serum plus suspect RBCs) was positive, and further verified by a positive (low ionic strength gradient) sucrose test. Spun sediments of urine demonstrated hemosiderin in cellular elements. It thus appeared that the iron deficiency was the result of both heavy menstrual flow and, more important, urinary iron losses secondary to intravascular hemolysis, which, in concert with the foregoing laboratory data, firmly established the diagnosis of **Paroxysmal Nocturnal Hemoglobinuria (PNH)** (26). Of note regarding the severity of the PNH were the ongoing iron losses in the presence of adequate amounts of therapeutic iron. Further studies of her red cells revealed both deficient decay accelerating factor (DAF) and membrane inhibitor of reactive lysis (MIRL), respectively (26). Deficiency of DAF and MIRL renders the red cells more sensitive to the lysing effects of complement, further confirmation of a clinical PNH class II diagnosis.

Several months later, because of the continual decrease in WBC and platelet numbers, a marrow aspirate revealed a slightly hypocellular organ with no increase in myeloblasts and a normal karyotype. A repeat sample 6 months later revealed blatant acute myelocytic leukemia.

In summary, the foregoing individual experienced iron losses secondary to heavy and uncompensated menstrual flow, to which were added urinary losses secondary to complement-induced intravascular hemolysis.

Causal Relationships

Diet

There was no evidence to support a lack of dietary iron to account for this patient's anemia. She ate a mixed diet replete with heme-containing iron, which sets her apart from individuals who are economically deprived or who otherwise choose non–meat-containing meals. In the latter two groups, with diets lacking in heme (which also aids in non–heme iron absorption) (27), iron deficiency prevails. However, initiation of aggressive fortification measures employing readily absorbable iron has successfully reduced the degree and incidence of iron deficiency in those individuals whose diets do not contain sufficient quantities of heme iron (28).

Growth and sex also affect iron requirements. The rapidly growing newborn, particularly the premature newborn, has much higher iron needs on a per kilogram basis during the first 12–18 months of extrauterine life than do individuals at any other age (3). In populations that consume balanced diets, including heme iron, the average daily iron requirement is approximately 10 mg/day—slightly less for men, as little as 5 mg/day, and slightly more for women, as much as 20 mg/day (29).

Uptake

Individuals (a) who lose portions of their gut, including the duodenum (where most iron absorption occurs) following surgery; (b) who have gastric bypass procedures; (c) whose stomachs become dysfunctional following vagotomy or gastrostomy; or (d) who ingest excessive quantities of antacids or H_2 blockers, experience varying degrees of impaired, predominantly nonheme, iron absorption. Individuals with severe and prolonged intestinal disease, including any of the so-called celiac syndromes, often experience a mixed anemia, characterized by iron, folate, and vitamin B_{12} deficiency. The clinical appearance is predominantly hypochromic and microcytic (30–35). Of note is the fact that a mixed macrocytic/hypochromic anemia will have a peripheral blood appearance more like the latter, and only by marrow analysis will it be easy to appreciate the megaloblastic maturation. Pica, particularly if the ingested material is starch-like, or clay, may also interfere with absorption. Ice, a relatively common but unnatural material for ingestion, seemingly does not impair iron absorption; and, indeed, pica is probably as much a response to iron deficiency as it is a cultural process (36–39).

There was nothing in this person's history to suggest any of the above as etiologic.

Blood loss that is the result of (a) adventitious losses, a pathologic state of self-induced blood loss, or blood loss from (b) GI and urinary tract parasitic infestation (*Schistosoma, Necator, Ancylostoma, Trichuris* (40–42); (c) anatomic defects, e.g., hiatal hernias, GI ulcers, diverticula, telangiectasia, and/or hemorrhoids; (d) inflammatory diseases; (e) malignancies; (f) drug-induced mucosal toxicity (salicylate inhibition of prostaglandin function); and (f) unregulated frequent blood donations may result in iron deficiency (4, 24–26). *None of the above applied to the patient in question.*

Iron deficiency secondary to pulmonary alveolar hemorrhage is a rare disorder of young people, is usually allergic in origin (43), and like the iron losses following long-term renal dialysis (44), will produce an iron-deficient state.

None of the above applied to this patient.

The fact that her jogging was limited to daily mile runs lessened the likelihood that she had the triad of (long-distance) runner's anemia: hemolysis, hematuria, and GI bleeding (45). During one of the later examinations, she admitted that she was no longer running with ease.

Hypochromia and Microcytic Indices

Patients with either β- or α-thalassemia minor (46), because of disordered or minimally ineffective heme synthetic pathways, tend to be moderately anemic with indices, particularly MCV and MCH, which mimic those of

Table 6.3. Age-Related Red Cell Indices

	MCV (fl)	MCH(pg)	MCHC(g/dL)
Term	105–110	32–36	30–32
6 months	89–93	28–32	31–35
2 years	76–80	25–29	31–35
10 years	84–88	27–31	32–36
15 years°	88–92	28–32	32–36
>20 years°	88–92	28–32	32–36

Calculations:

1. Mean corpuscular volume (MCV)

$$= \frac{\text{Packed cell volume (L/L)} \times 1000 \text{ (Hct)}}{\text{Red cell count } (\times 10^{12}/\text{L})}$$

$$= - \times 10^{15}/\text{L (femtoliters)}$$

2. Mean corpuscular hemoglobin content (MCH)

$$= \frac{\text{Hemoglobin (g/L)}}{\text{Red cell count } (\times 10^{12}/\text{L})}$$

$$= - \times 10^{12}\text{g (picograms)}$$

3. Mean corpuscular hemoglobin concentration (MCHC)

$$= \frac{\text{Hemoglobin (g/dL)}}{\text{HCt (L/L)}}$$

$$= \text{g/dL}$$

4. Red cell distribution width
   Automated determination (%)

°Females: 0.5 S.D. below males commencing with catamenia.

mild iron deficiency. The MCHC decreases late in iron deficiency. The newest addition in red cell indices is the automated measurement of RBCs sizes (RDW), an index that is increased in iron deficiency states but is often incapable of distinguishing such events from the anemia of chronic disease (ACD) or thalassemia trait. It remains to be seen whether this additional index may have value in screening for iron deficiency (47, 48). However, elevations in serum ferritin, iron saturation, and hemoglobin A_2 clearly distinguish between thalassemia and iron deficiency. In this patient, irrespective of her Mediterranean origins, thalassemia was not a factor. Her modest increase in hemoglobin F was probably related to her PNH, as it is with any number of dysplastic syndromes.

Table 6.3 is a summation of age-related RBC indices.

Signs and Symptoms of Iron Deficiency

Fatigue is specific only in association with other symptoms. Hemoglobin levels <40 g/L have been reported in the absence of the usually identified symptoms of *dyspnea, irritability, headache, lethargy, poor attention span, and palpitations.* Slow-onset anemia may evoke no symptoms at all until the hemoglobin level is so low that it causes cardiac failure. As a general guideline only, symptoms begin to occur at hemoglobin levels <80 g/L. It is important to point out in this context that placebos have been shown to abolish symptoms of fatigue in patients with storage iron deficiency only (49). *This patient's fatigue, in all likelihood, was the result of rapid changes in hemoglobin levels.*

Neurologic and musculoskeletal systems are impaired in iron deficiency. Muscular performance is disturbed, and serum lactate levels usually increase *(they were not measured in this patient)* (50, 51). Intracranial pressure may increase, and there are often behavioral disturbances.

Developmental defects, koilonychia, glossitis, papillary atrophy of the tongue, stomatitis, pharyngeal webs, splenic enlargement, hair-on-end osseous changes, gastritis, impaired phagocytosis, and immune function—all of varying degree—have been described in iron deficiency (52–66). *Except for the palpable spleen, none of the above were identified in this patient.*

Laboratory Correlates

In iron deficiency the absolute granulocyte count is generally normal or slightly elevated, platelet levels are often elevated, and the red cells are essentially reduced to empty rings, and when exposed to graded solutions of sodium chloride, resist hypotonic lysis. The granulocytosis and thrombocytosis are attributable to increased marrow activity. Only when the iron deficiency leads to further nutritional impairment does one see the onset of granulocytopenia and thrombocytopenia, often the result of a superimposed nutritional folate deficiency (67).

In this case, the low white blood cell and platelet counts were a manifestation of an early leukemic conversion process, not a mark of severe iron deficiency.

Hypochromic, Microcytic Disease and Heme Biology

Red cell indices echo the morphologic changes, which range from normochromic/normocytic cells to hypochromic/microcytic/anisocytotic and poikilocytotic cells in accordance with disease duration and severity. Thus, both MCV and MCH, which reflect the numbers of red cells in a specified volume and the level of hemoglobin, respectively, tend to fall well in advance of the MCHC, which is a reflection of the ratio of hemoglobin concentration to packed cell volume. The percentage of increase in red cell distribution width (RDW) is yet another measurement of the early morphologic detection of iron-deficiency anemia (68) (table 6.3).

RDW is paralleled by the rise in level of free erythrocyte protoporphyrin (FEP). The rise in FEP is the result of insufficient elemental iron to bind to already formed protoporphyrin in the heme synthesis pathway (69).

The iron-binding β_2-globulin, transferrin, is markedly increased in iron deficiency (normal 170–450 μg %) in concert with low levels of bound iron (normal 60–150 μg %). The increase in the iron-binding protein is mirrored by an increase in red cell transferrin receptors (70). Normally, the portion of protein-bound iron is approximately 33% of the total binding protein. A bound iron of <15% is strong evidence of iron deficiency. As stated previously, patients with protein-losing enteropathy, as in sprue or similar gut disturbances, have depleted protein levels. This leads to low bound iron and a low iron-binding protein (and transferrin receptors), i.e., the one exception to the typical low bound

iron and elevated iron-binding protein of iron deficiency. Decreased levels of transferrin receptors in the anemia of chronic disease also distinguish it from the increased numbers in iron deficiency (71). This sensitive immunologic assay, however, is not capable of identifying early (latent) iron deficiency.

Serum ferritin levels (normal 25–100 μg/L) measure iron storage and are, accordingly, early indicators of iron deficiency (72). They are best assessed in conjunction with other parameters because of possible coexisting alterations wherein ferritin behaves like a phase reactant as, for example, the elevated levels noted in malignant and inflammatory diseases. In the elderly, ferritin levels may be normal in the presence of iron-deficient erythropoiesis, which also lends difficulty in interpretation (73). A virtually unimpeachable approach to the analysis of iron levels is evaluation of bone marrow for hemosiderin-laden macrophages, the absence of which is the sine qua non of iron deficiency (74). Table 6.4 is a summation of clinical and hematologic sequences in iron deficiency.

Nonheme iron enzymes are the first systems to be depleted in iron deficiency. In addition to myoglobin, iron is a major constitutive component of a number of enzyme systems, including catalase, peroxidase, metalloflavoproteins, certain of the oxidases, the succinic dehydrogenases, aconitase, and many of the cytochromes. Deficiency of muscle oxidases accounts for impaired muscle performance. Decreased levels of monoamine oxidase account at least in part for the increased levels of circulating catecholamines, which in turn probably leads to behavioral problems and impaired mentation. Decreases in yet other of the oxidases account for impairment in both immune and gut-secretory function, the latter of which may explain at least some of the cases of GI bleeding seen late in iron deficiency and not otherwise accounted for by an intrinsic gut defect (75–83).

Case 2

Parents from a nearby farming community brought their 12-month-old infant to the regional hospital emergency ward because of severe lethargy and a progressively "waxy" skin appearance. Both parents were in their

Table 6.4. Clinical and Hematologic Sequences in Iron Deficiency

I. Loss of iron stores–no evidence of anemia
    Normal hematological values and indices
    Low normal ferritin and transferrin saturation

II. Early anemia
    Low MCV and MCH and low normal MCHC
    Elevated ferritin and low transferrin saturation
    Elevated iron-binding capacity (transferrin)

III. Decreased enzyme production and clinically
    blatant anemia
    Abnormally low indices, ferritin and markedly elevated
    transferrin
    Irritability, pallor, weakness, poor mental performance

early 20s, raised on farms, and pursued farming as their vocation. They were unrelated, and this child was the first offspring of their first pregnancy. Both parents were vegans. As an infant, the mother had repeated episodes of diarrhea attributed to an "allergy," and for which, among a variety of other measures, she received boiled milk because of her mother's alleged inability to provide sufficient quantities of breast milk. This presumed "milk allergy" disappeared after the first year of life, and she tolerated unmodified cow's milk thereafter. In fact her consumption increased markedly during pregnancy. Prenatal care was minimal. She went to a local health clinic in the early part of her second trimester, had blood tests, type and results unknown (other than the fact that she was told that all was well), was given some "pregnancy tablets" and told to return in 2 months for another examination and more tablets. She did not keep her next appointment and returned to the clinic only when labor began. When the tablets ran out, she did not take further medicine and maintained that her health during the remainder of her pregnancy was excellent. Labor and delivery were uneventful and atraumatic. She gave birth to a normal full-term male weighing 6.6 pounds (3 kg) and measuring 20 inches in length (50.8 cm). According to the mother, all measurements, including head circumference, were in the 50th percentile. Both mother's and infant's blood types were the same.

The baby cried spontaneously, apparently had a normal Apgar score, no evidence of early jaundice, and remained in the birthing clinic for 24 hours. Mother and baby then returned to the farm with directions concerning total care, including the umbilical stump, along with nutritional advice and scheduled immunization plans. The child was breastfed and, as directed, returned to the clinic at 6 weeks for the first course of immunization. Three months later, at followup for additional immunization, the baby weighed 16.5 pounds. No further testing was done, and the family departed with advice regarding intake of solid foodstuff. The family never returned to the clinic. The events that unfolded thereafter were as follows: the volume of the mother's breastmilk began to diminish fairly rapidly; within 4 weeks breastfeedings were discontinued, replaced by intake of boiled whole cow's milk and followed with the introduction of an admixture of rice and boiled milk. Shortly after this change, and over the ensuing 3–4 weeks, there was a change in stool volume and characteristics. They became larger, mushy, more frequent, i.e., after each feeding, and brown-green in color compared with the smaller, yellow-colored, semi-formed, seedy stools associated with breastmilk feedings. The mother introduced the use of boiled cow's milk rather than formula because of her concern that her child might be experiencing the same problems that she presumably had as an infant. Ironically, however, because of the persistence of signs and symptoms (of allergy?) much like those the mother experienced during her infancy, she elected instead to use boiled goat's milk on the advice of family and friends. Initially, the baby appeared to thrive on this regimen along with gradual introduction of cere-

als admixed with goat's milk, fruit sauces, and occasional pureed yellow vegetables. No explanation was forthcoming for the failure to maintain updated immunizations. The expected developmental landmarks over the ensuing interval through 9 months of age were intact according to the parents, but shortly thereafter the child became increasingly more irritable and was appeased only by increasing the frequency of milk feedings to the virtual exclusion of all solids. The mother also evinced concern over the fact that her child was slow in clearing a "cold" acquired 1 month earlier. By 12 months of age, lethargy predominated, although the child still experienced intervals of irritability, along with discontinuous efforts to roll over, crawl, or reach up. It was the extreme lethargy that precipitated the visit to the emergency ward at the regional hospital.

On examination, the child was afebrile, markedly pale without obvious icterus or other skin changes, and had a sinus tachycardia with hyperdynamic heart sounds, a grade III/IV holosystolic murmur, and rapid respirations without rhonchi or rales. Except for irritability alternating with lethargy, the remainder of the neurologic examination results were normal. There was minimal mucous crusting of the nares, but otherwise both upper and lower airways were clear. The liver and spleen were modestly increased in size. There was no edema or obvious muscle wasting, and the external genitalia appeared to be normal. The baby weighed 20 pounds, which placed him in the 20th percentile for weight, and he was also in the 35th percentile for length and head circumference, all of which were lower than that obtained at the 3 month examination.

Laboratory data revealed a hemoglobin of 26 g/L, hematocrit of 11%, and red cell count of 3.1×10^{12}/L (MCV 33.5 fl, MCH 12 pg, MCHC 23.6%; RDW was not available). The platelet and reticulocyte counts were 75×10^9/L and 1.1%, respectively. Total WBC count was low normal. Serum ferritin was <1 µg/L.

The peripheral blood film revealed severe hypochromia, marked anisocytosis, target formation, poikilocytosis, and decreased numbers of large and small platelets. Urinalysis results were normal and stools were weakly positive for heme.

It was the impression of the attending physician that the patient had a severe, nutritional iron deficiency with pending cardiac decompensation (tachycardia, hepatosplenomegaly). The low platelet count along with the bizarre RBC and platelet morphology were thought to be due to the severely prolonged iron-deficiency process, but the possibility of multiple deficiencies, although discussed, was not addressed. It was thought that the baby needed additional hemoglobin with minimal blood volume and he was, accordingly, transfused slowly with 5 ml/kg (46 ml, 9 g hemoglobin) of packed red cells, with an accompanying removal of 50 ml of the patient's blood. He also received daily oral, dropper-administered ferrous sulfate in an elemental iron dose of 5 mg/kg in combination with liquid vitamin C. Within 48 hours, he became more alert and within 10 days his irritability dis-

appeared, at which time his reticulocyte count rose to 7%, but he continued to resist the introduction of solids. By 14 days, it was thought that he was progressing well enough to leave for home, and his parents were given detailed instructions regarding iron-dosing sequences, the role of iron-fortified formula, and a solid (vegan) foodstuff regimen along with a followup appointment to the clinic. On the day of discharge the infant's reticulocyte count had fallen to 3% and his hemoglobin remained at 45 g/L. One week later, on schedule, he returned to clinic. At that time, his hemoglobin and hematocrit were unchanged, and his smear showed an admixture of the original bizarre morphology along with both spheroidal and oval-shaped red cells (presumably the transfused population). Platelets appeared reduced in number, and there were occasional hypersegmented granulocytes.

Because of the seemingly slow repair of the anemic process, alongside persistent thrombopenia and the new appearance of misshapen granulocyte nuclei, a marrow aspirate, performed in search of other concomitant diseases revealed megaloblastic maturation and markedly diminished hemosiderin. His serum folate was <1 ng/ml (0.5 nmol/L) in the presence of a low normal vitamin B_{12} level (310 ng/L [180 pmol/L]). The diagnosis was adjusted to include nutritional folate deficiency in association with nutritional iron deficiency.

In this particular case the cause of the iron deficiency was directly attributable to the use initially of cow's milk, which has approximately 1.0 mg/L of iron of poor bioavailability (likely the result of impaired absorption due to the elevated calcium and phosphorus levels in cow's milk protein [84]).

Breast milk has the same iron content but one-half to two-thirds the amount of protein, calcium, and phosphorous of cow's milk and, on a milligram-to-milligram basis, greater iron bioavailability. Breastfed full-term infants maintain their hemoglobin levels longer than their cow's milk-fed counterparts before embarking on diets rich in iron (85).

Inadequate content of milk iron is further worsened by boiling, which reduces whatever iron is available by about 50%. Lack of any significant quantity of iron-containing solid foodstuffs adds to the dilemma. Scalding or boiling also destroys folate, but in this instance the folate deficit was brought about by the use of goat's milk, which has somewhat (<6 µg/L of folate), adequate content for adult requirements but not at all sufficient for the rapidly growing infant, whose requirements approximate 50 µg/day (86–92).

Without proper supplement, the diet of strict vegetarians is poor in vitamin B_{12}. Because of the markedly reduced amounts of the vitamin in breastmilk, breastfed infants of vegans are at serious risk for rapid development of B_{12} deficiency (93). On the other hand, because dietary folate sources are usually high in these individuals, folate deficiency is rarely a factor in the development of megaloblastic erythropoiesis.

Commentary: *The mother of this child was not a strict vegan. She ate dairy products and, in fact, once the*

diagnosis of folate deficiency was established in her offspring, maternal serum folate and vitamin B_{12} levels were tested and found to be normal. However, her serum bound iron level was slightly decreased in association with a moderately elevated iron-binding protein, and she, too, was instructed on the amount and duration of iron administration for herself.

Iron Metabolism and Growth and Development

As noted, the full-term newborn has an overall total body iron endowment of approximately 250 mg, slightly >30% of which crosses the placenta in the final 2 months of pregnancy. Even in the iron-deficient mother, iron is phagocytized in favor of the neonate. Following birth and over the ensuing 12 months, total body iron increases by 75% in order to account for the spectacular growth in total body hemoglobin and need for iron in other systems. It is not surprising that premature infants are at high risk for the development of severe iron-deficiency anemia, with the severity proportional to the degree of prematurity. For this reason, parenteral iron may be administered to severely premature infants (who also can suffer considerable procedural blood loss) in sufficient quantity to make up for the estimated full-term deficit. These infants are then maintained on at least 5 mg/kg of elemental iron as ferrous sulfate for the first 6 months of life in order to address their generally rapid growth.

At full-term birth, 70% of the total body iron is present as hemoglobin iron, 24% as storage, and 6% as muscle and enzyme iron, with <1% as transport iron. Because daily iron losses are minimal, i.e., <0.3 mg/day in the growing full-term neonate, iron reserves are sufficient to serve iron requirements without iron supplementation for the first 4–5 months, at which time stores generally fall to approximately 10% of the total body iron and remain in that range for the first year. Nonstorage iron level increases, assuming there is sufficient iron from solid foods to accommodate the increase in total body hemoglobin, myoglobin, and enzyme iron.

At the time of red cell death, iron released from the catabolism of heme (the ultimate bilirubin source) (94) is phagocytized by macrophages, with some of the iron immediately finding its way into the heme synthetic pathway; the remainder enters the storage pool. In patients with chronic inflammatory disorders and those with malignancies as well, the storage route apparently is the overriding site (95). Failure to release iron from storage sites accounts for the hypoferremia of chronic disease, but it doesn't explain the low transferrin levels, nor is there an explanation for the phenomenon of slow release, per se. One possible explanation for the decrease in transferrin is the competitive role played by lactoferrin in patients with chronic infection (96). Iron-free lactoferrin, released by neutrophils during infection, has a greater affinity for iron than does transferrin, but it does not transport it to the developing erythron. Rather it is taken up by macrophage receptors and stored as ferritin in the liver and spleen (97). Another possible explanation for this situation is the chronic disease-induced increase in apoferritin synthesis, which, in turn, binds iron to the exclusion of transferrin. Although tempting, this explanation is yet to be confirmed, as is the suggestion that low levels of circulating iron and high levels of macrophage iron impede aggressive bacterial growth and impair toxin release (98–101).

Included among the rare and unusual causes of iron deficiency are idiopathic pulmonary hemosiderosis (43), expressed as interstitial red cell losses leading to iron entrapment in pulmonary macrophages, hypoferremia, hypertransferrinemia, and, ultimately, anemia. Additional examples in this category include cow's milk-induced red cell and secretory IgA stool losses (102), the Goodpasture syndrome variant (pulmonary hemosiderosis with glomerulonephritis) (103), and autoantibody to transferrin receptors (104).

Case 3

A 64-year-old white male bus driver complained to his physician of increasing fatigue and mild exertional dyspnea. Physical examination revealed an obese individual with slight pallor and fingernails that had been heavily trimmed because of easy breakage. The patient's oropharynx was clean, moist, and free of webbing. There were no signs of cardiac or pulmonary decompensation, and examination of the abdomen did not reveal organomegaly or masses. Rectal examination left a trace of fresh blood on the glove, and proctoscopy reveled internal hemorrhoids. Occult blood examination of the stool was not carried out. On further questioning, the patient stated that he never observed his stools and had no symptoms related to piles. He denied large bowel–associated symptoms or weight loss, took no medications, and enjoyed a diet rich in meat products. He drank alcohol moderately and had recently given up smoking. His hemoglobin was 85 g/L with an MCV of 65 fl, WBC count of 8.5×10^9/L, and platelets 430×10^9/L. The blood film showed microcytosis and hypochromia. His erythrocyte sedimentation rate (ESR) was 44 mm in the first hour. Liver and renal function test results were normal. Immunoglobulins showed a slight polyclonal increase in γ-globulins. Serum bound iron was 5 μg/dl and total iron-binding capacity (TIBC) was 66 μg/dl. Ferritin estimation or further hematologic tests were not done.

A diagnosis of iron deficiency due to blood loss from hemorrhoids was made and treatment with 300 mg of oral iron sulphate three times daily was instituted. His piles were ligated uneventfully at a local day surgical unit.

Iron deficiency in adults should always be analyzed critically before iron treatment is instituted. First, it must be established that it is truly iron deficiency and not the anemia of chronic disease or a late-diagnosis thalassemia. In iron deficiency unencumbered by other diseases, the bound serum iron level is low. Unless the accompanying TIBC is correspondingly high, a serum ferritin level estimation will distinguish between these disorders, with low

levels in iron deficiency and normal to slightly elevated levels in the anemia of chronic infection. With the microcytosis of thalassemia or the refractory anemias, both serum iron and ferritin levels are elevated. When the test results are unclear, a bone marrow examination for iron should not be deferred.

Neither ferritin nor marrow analyses were done on this patient.

Iron deficiency, as noted, is an indicator of an underlying disturbance. In premenopausal women, if menorrhagia is felt to be severe enough to cause iron deficiency, then gynecologic opinion must be obtained. In postmenopausal women and in all males, not only must the iron deficiency be confirmed (or an alternative category of anemia be applied), the etiology of the deficiency must also be identified. Blood loss from the GI tract is insufficient as a diagnosis in itself. Both site and underlying cause must be sought. Stool occult blood testing is reliable, when positive, if strict attention is paid to dietary and tooth cleaning practices in order to lessen the incidence of false positive tests. In effect, if the GI tract has no overt pathology in the presence of stools that show occult blood, the search for an etiologic process must continue and malignancy must be highly suspect.

In this case, the low TIBC suggested that the diagnosis either was incorrect or incomplete.

After 3 months of well-tolerated oral iron therapy, a repeat hemoglobin was 105 g/L, with an MCV of 75 fl and an RDW within normal limits. The reticulocyte count was 0.8% and the ESR was 56 mm/hour. At this point, the patient was referred for hematologic evaluation. The serum iron and TIBC were essentially unchanged from the previous level, but a serum ferritin of 60 μg/L was recorded. Bone marrow iron staining showed abundant iron macrophage stores.

Examination of both the lower and upper GI tract by endoscopy and contrast study did not show a lesion to account for blood loss, chronic inflammatory disease, or neoplastic disease. The search continued. An abdominal CT scan revealed a 3-cm diameter mass at the upper pole of the left kidney. This was confirmed at exploration, and a renal carcinoma was removed. Within 2 months and without further treatment, the anemia resolved. It did not reappear over the ensuing 3 years, at which time the patient was evaluated for seizures shown to be the result of a solitary cerebral metastasis.

Commentary: *This case illustrates the necessity to ensure that all of the iron-related assays concur diagnostically and that they be used to confirm or deny a suspected process. A common disorder such as hemorrhoids should not make one overlook inconsistent laboratory findings that require further consideration and investigation. A carefully obtained history and a thorough examination should readily direct the examiner to the appropriate diagnostic test(s). This case also underscores the failure to explain aberrant laboratory findings (the low serum iron and low TIBC) in the presence of an apparently straightforward diagnosis. Hemorrhoids are not uncommon in obese, middle-aged individuals with sedentary occupations, and they are also increased in incidence in lower GI tract tumors. The low TIBC should have raised suspicion of a more complex disorder before the poor response to iron led to reconsideration. Table 6.5 is a summary assessment of iron deficiency.*

Treatment of Iron Deficiency

Oral Iron

The principles of iron replacement therapy have not changed from the time of definition by Blaud in 1832 (105).

The easiest, safest, and cheapest way to treat iron deficiency is the use of orally administered and readily absorbable ferrous iron salts (Fe^{++}). With ferric iron intake, reduction to the ferrous state must be carried out in order to facilitate absorption. The most reliable iron preparations are ferrous sulphate, ferrous gluconate, and ferrous fumarate, and the therapeutic aim is the provision of 3–5 mg/day of elemental iron for children and adults. Although iron absorption is optimal on an empty stomach, gastric irritation can be a problem, and, thus, iron in either liquid or tablet form is best administered with meals or preferably with vitamin C no more frequently than every 6–8 hours. Iron should not be administered with milk because of its binding with phosphorous as an insoluble complex. Liquid preparations are preferable in children or in adults who have difficulty in swallowing.

Iron-induced side effects include abdominal distension and either constipation or diarrhea, both of which can be managed by reducing the dose to twice or even once daily. Ferrous sulfate causes severe discoloration of encased dentition in developing infants. This is readily overcome by the use of concentrated preparations in dropper form, which do not tend to linger in the oropharynx.

The only indication for iron therapy is proven iron deficiency. Apart from the risk of iron overload, when inappropriately administered to children, such practice delays the correct diagnosis of the cause of anemia. When correctly applied, iron replacement therapy coupled with appropriate response monitoring complements investigation. The pattern and speed of response provides useful additional clinical information.

Unless the patient is bleeding dramatically, the response to oral iron supplements, as measured by improvement in hemoglobin and mean cell volume, is readily predictable. Failure to respond questions the diagnosis, the validity of the patient's history or compliance, or the extent of the disease if the diagnosis is correct. Coupled with the measured hematologic improvements, there is usually marked early symptomatic improvement. Once a normal hemoglobin level has been achieved, therapy should be continued for at least 3 additional months in order to replenish iron stores.

Iron supplementation, properly administered, produces a 1% increase in the hemoglobin concentration each day. Concomitant with an increase in hemoglobin is the rise in MCV. Reticulocyte response to iron therapy is rapid and peaks in 10–12 days, with symptomatic responses apparent within a few days. In irritable, iron-deficient infants, a favorable response may occur in 2–3 days. Failure to respond to iron administration is most often the result of an incorrect diagnosis (table 6.6).

Parenteral Iron

Iron may also be administered parenterally. It is highly effective, but the overall rate of response is hardly more than that obtained with oral iron therapy. It is more expensive and carries associated risks, including anaphylaxis and hypotension. Following carefully calculated doses based on patient's ideal body weight and hemoglobin deficit, together with an allowance for body iron stores, intravenous preparation of iron dextran diluted in 5% dextrose solution can be slowly infused. The slow infusion rate lessens the potential for a hypotensive episode secondary to rapid infusion–induced ferritin mobilization. Nonetheless, all

Table 6.5. Assessment of Iron Deficiency

Clinical	
Historical Assessment	Pregnancy and delivery history; degree of prematurity (if present); nutritional and menstrual history; history of blood donations, drug use, chronic illness, bowel disease, cancer or bleeding diatheses.
Physical Assessment	Check for esophageal web, glossitis, koilonychia, pallor, decreased attention span, irritability, poor work performance.
Laboratory	
Blood Values	Reduced Hgb, Hct, RBC count, indices (MCV first to decline, then followed by MCH and finally MCHC, increased RDW0; platelet count elevated early.
Serum Bound Iron (BI) and TIBC	Bound iron <50 µg% and <15% of total iron binding protein (TIBC). Not a good indicator of latent iron deficiency. TIBC low in protein losing disorders.
Transferrin Receptor	Temporal sequence similar to BI/TIBC.
Serum Ferritin	When <10 µg/dL, good indication of latent iron deficiency (depleted iron stores). Not helpful in situation of combined iron deficiency and inflammatory disease.
RBC Protoporphyrin (EP)	Follows ferritin and BI/TIBC as indicator of iron deficiency.
Marrow Hemosiderin	Absent in all stages of Iron Deficiency. Elevated in the sideroblastic anemias.

Table 6.6. Common Reasons for Nonresponse to Iron Therapy

Incorrect diagnosis of iron deficiency anemia
Complicating illness or illnesses
Noncompliance
Inadequate preparation
Continued iron losses in excess of replacement therapy
Malabsorption syndromes

Table 6.7. Use of Parenteral Iron

Demonstrated intolerance to oral iron
Proven patient noncompliance
Clinical needs to replenish stores rapidly
  Complicated pregnancy
  Before initiating major surgery

patients so treated must be supervised in facilities with readily available resuscitation procedures. Table 6.7 summarizes parenteral iron usage.

Red Cell Transfusion

Red cell transfusion has no place in the routine management of iron deficiency. Apart from being wasteful and exposing patients to unnecessary transfusion risks, this approach fails to address the fundamental clinical problem, i.e., lack of iron. Patients with severe iron-deficiency anemia are often well adapted to their anemia, and rapid normalization of the hemoglobin via transfusion may pose undue strains on the cardiovascular system. In any patient who appears to be in borderline cardiac failure, judicious use of concentrated red cells in a dose of 5 ml/kg can be of value in tiding a patient over the most severe symptoms pending an iron response to appropriate therapy.

Hypochromic Anemia with Iron Excess

Sideroblastic anemias occur either as inherited or acquired hypochromic (and microcytic) disorders. The red cells in these individuals are typically laden with nonutilizable iron localized to the mitochondria of the developing erythroblast. Following nuclear ejection, the iron is deposited as a perinuclear ring, the so-called "ringed sideroblast," of the marrow, or circulating "siderocyte." This heterogeneous group of disorders arises as a result of either defective porphyrin synthesis, defective iron insertion into protoporphyrin, or both; and because of ineffective production, red cells frequently undergo early death, usually within the intramedullary space. The net serologic effect is an elevated bound serum iron and reduced iron-binding protein. Because these disorders typically fail to produce adequate numbers of mature, long-lived red blood cells, the resultant anemia paradoxically effects an increase in iron absorption, which further complicates the preexisting iron overload (106–109).

Of the inborn defects, **X-linked inheritance** is the commonest abnormality, followed in turn by autosomal dominant, autosomal recessive, and the rare pansystemic presentation (110–113). In approximately one-third of these patients, the administration of pyridoxine evokes a favorable, albeit a variable and only partial response, for which maintenance therapy is a proven necessity. These patients are not pyridoxine deficient but rather physiologically nonresponsive (114).

Acquired Sideroblastic Disorders include the idiopathic variety, which evolves as an insidious process in middle-aged individuals. The net effect is an anemia of sufficient severity to require red cell support. In this group, the increase in marrow turnover enhances dietary iron absorption, which in combination with multiple red cell transfusions, leads to progressive iron overload (115).

Reversible Acquired Sideroblastic Disorders include (a) alcoholism, a complex process that encompasses multiple nutritional deficiencies, (b) antituberculosis therapy, (c) hypothermia, (d) lead poisoning, and (e) (in animals) copper deficiency. Both excess lead and alcohol interact unfavorably along the heme synthetic pathway. However, lead intoxication, unlike chronic alcoholism, does not produce ringed sideroblasts, probably because the anemia of lead intoxication impairs multiple heme synthetic sites, which in turn results in an absolute cellular iron deficiency rather than the typical sideroblastic process, such as the hypochromic anemia with excess (nonutilizable) iron of chronic alcoholism. Although pyridoxine improves the defect, it functions best in concert with cessation of alcohol consumption and initiation of a proper diet (116–123). Isoniazid (INH) and similarly structured preparations used in the treatment of tuberculosis, block vitamin B_6 synthesis, which in turn adversely effects its role in pyridoxine metabolism. Hypothermia effects a total impairment of heme synthesis as well as iron incorporation into hemoglobin, which in turn is readily corrected by normalizing body temperature (124).

Table 6.8 includes both a classification and the nature of the physiologic changes that occur in disorders of iron excess.

Iron Chelation

In patients with deliberately imposed iron overload, as in transfusion-requirement disorders, daily iron chelation with subcutaneous desferrioxamine (DFO) should be carried out. DFO has a 10-fold increase over transferrin in affinity for iron. It is typically infused subcutaneously in a dose of 50 mg/kg/day (not to exceed 3 g/day) over 12 hours, usually during the overnight sleep period. Chelation therapy is not without risk. Ascorbate in combination with chelation therapy, designed to enhance chelation efficacy, may give rise to increased iron deposition when used in excess. When used sensibly and under appropriate supervision, iron chelation is a singularly successful procedure. Attention must be paid to the fact

Table 6.8. Red Blood Cell and Serology in Disorders of Iron Excess

	Iron Absorption	Transferrin	Transferrin Saturation	Storage Iron	Erythropoiesis
Transfusion overload	N	⇑	⇑	⇑	⇓
Hereditary hemochromatosis	⇑	⇑	⇑	⇑	N
Ineffective erythropoiesis	⇑	⇓	⇑	⇑	⇑°
Congenital or acquired hemolytic disorder	⇑	⇓	⇑	⇑	⇑

°Increase in intramarrow death; N = normal.

that DFO, when used in excess, may induce ocular toxicity, and the catheter itself may be the source of serious and sometimes fatal infections. Efforts to develop suitable oral chelation are as yet unavailable for widespread clinical use (125–130).

REFERENCES

1. Josephs HW. The iron of the newborn baby. Acta Paediatr 1959;4:03.
2. Woodruff CW, et al. Multiple causes of iron deficiency in infants. JAMA 1958;167:715.
3. Schulman I. Iron requirements in infancy. JAMA 1961;175:118.
4. Beveridge BR, et al. Hypochromic anemia. Q J Med 1965;34:135.
5. Witts LF. Hypochromic anemia. Philadelphia: FA Davis, 1969.
6. Silverstein FE, Feld AD, Gilbert DA. Upper gastrointestinal tract bleeding. Arch Intern Med 1981;141:322.
7. Palmer ED. Upper gastrointestinal bleeding. Springfield, IL: Charles C Thomas, 1970:6, 101.
8. Bothwell TH, Charlton RW, et al. Iron metabolism in man. Oxford: Blackwell, 1979:576.
9. Alsen P, Listowsky I. Iron transport and storage proteins. Ann Rev Biochem 1980;49:357.
10. Dallman PR. Iron deficiency in the weanling: a nutritional problem on the way to resolution. Acta Paediatr Scand 1986;323:59.
11. Lundström U, Perkkiö M, et al. Iron deficiency anemia with hypoproteinemia. 1983;58:438.
12. Apt L, Pollycove M, et al. Idiopathic pulmonary hemosiderosis: a study of the anemia and iron distribution using radioiron and radiochromium. J Clin Invest 1957;36:1150.
13. Vichinsky EP, Pennatha-Das R, et al. Inadequate erythroid response to hypoxia in cystic fibrosis. J Pediatr 1984;105:15.
14. Olson RE. Protein-calorie malnutrition. New York: Academic Press, 1975.
15. Hallberg L. Bioavailability of dietary iron in man. Ann Rev Nutr 1981;1:123.
16. Charlton RW, Bothwell TH. Iron absorption. Ann Rev Med 1983;34:55.
17. Jacobs P, Bothwell T, et al. Role of hypochloric acid in iron absorption. J Appl Physiol 1964;19:187.
18. Casey JL, DiJeso B, et al. The promoter region of the human transferrin receptor gene. NY Acad Sci Am 1988;526:54.
19. Saarinen UM, Simes MA, et al. Iron absorption in infants: high bioavailability of breast milk iron as indicated by the extrinsic tag method of iron absorption and by the concentration of serum ferritin. J Pediatr 1977;91:36.
20. Rios E, Hunter RE, et al. The absorption of iron as supplements in infant cereal and infant formulas. Pediatrics 1975;55:686.
21. Stekel A, Olivares M, et al. Absorption of fortification iron from milk formulas in infants. Am J Clin Nutr 1986;43:917.
22. Tunnessen WW, Oski FA. Consequences of starting whole cow milk at 6 months of age. J Pediatr 1987;111:813.
23. Walter T, Hertrampf E, et al. Effect of different milk diets on gastrointestinal blood loss in infancy. In: Hercberg S, ed. Recent knowledge on iron and folate deficiencies in the world. Paris: INSERM, 1989.
24. Hallberg L, et al. Menstrual blood loss and iron deficiency. Acta Med Scand 1966;180:639. Acta Obstet Gynecol Scand 1966;45:320. Scand J Clin Lab Invest 1964;16:244. Scand J Haematol 1979;22:17.
25. Hartmann RC, et al. Paroxysmal nocturnal hemoglobinuria: clinical and laboratory studies relating to iron metabolism and therapy with androgen and iron. Medicine 1966;45:331.
26. Barosi G, et al. Abnormal splenic uptake of red cells in long-lasting iron deficiency anemia due to self-induced bleeding (factitious anemia). Blut 1978;35:75.
27. Cook JD, Reusser ME. Food iron absorption in human subjects; III, comparison of the effects of animal proteins on nonheme iron absorption. Am J Clin Nutr 1976;29:859.
28. Committee on Dietary Allowances-Food and Nutrition Board: Recommended dietary allowances. Washington, DC: National Academy of Sciences, 1980.
29. Committee on Iron Deficiency, AMA Council on Foods and Nutrition: Iron deficiency in the United States. JAMA 1968;203:497.
30. Simon SR, Zemel R, Betancourt S, Zidar BL. Hematologic complications following gastric bypass operation. Blood 1987;70:50.
31. Adams JF. The clinical and metabolic consequences of total gastrectomy. Scand J Gastroenterol 1968;3:145.
32. Hallberg L, Rossander-Hulthen L, Gramatkovski E. Iron fortification of flour with a complex ferric orthophosphate. Am J Clin Nutr 1989;50:129.
33. Magnusson BEO: Iron absorption after antrectomy with gastroduodenostomy. Scand J Haematol 1976;26(suppl):1.
34. Kilpatrick ZM, Katz J. Occult celiac disease as a cause of iron-deficiency anemia. JAMA 1969;208:999.
35. Skikne BS, Lynch SR, Cook JD. Role of gastric acid in food iron absorption. Gastroenterology 1981;81:1068.
36. Coltman CA Jr. Pagophagia and iron lack. JAMA 1969;207:513.
37. Callinan V, O'Hare JA. Cardboard chewing: cause and effect of iron-deficiency anemia (letter). Am J Med 1988;85:449.
38. Crosby WH. Pica. JAMA 1976;235:2765. Arch Intern Med 1971;127:960.

39. McDonald R, Marshall R. The value of iron therapy in pica. Pediatrics 1964;34:558.

40. Fleming AF. Iron deficiency in the tropics. Clin Haematol 1982;11:365.

41. Giles HM, et al. Hookworm infection and anaemia. Q J Med 1964;33:1.

42. Roche M, Layrisse M. The nature and causes of hookworm anemia. Am J Trop Med Hung 1966;15:1031.

43. Kuhn MJ. Idiopathic pulmonary hemosiderosis: the importance of a chest radiograph in children with unexplained anemia. Mt. Sinai J Med (NY) 1985;52:358.

44. Parker PA, Izard MW, Maher JF. Therapy of iron deficiency anemia in patients on maintenance dialysis. Nephron 1979; 23:181.

45. Dufaux B, et al. Serum ferritin, transferrin, haptoglobin and iron in middle and long-distance runners, elite rowers and professional racing cyclists. Int J Sports Med 1981;2:42.

46. Pearson HA, et al. Screening for thalassemia trait by electronic measurement of mean corpuscular volume. N Engl J Med 1973;288:351.

47. Marsh WL, Bishop JW, Carcy TP. Evaluation of red cell volume distribution width (RDW). Haematol Pathol 1987; 1:117.

48. Houwen B. The use of inferrant strategies in the differential diagnosis of microcytic anaemia. Blood Cells 1989; 15:509.

49. Elwood PC, et al. Symptoms and circulating hemoglobin level. J Chronic Dis 1969;21:615.

50. Dallman PR. Manifestations of iron deficiency. Semin Hematol 1982;19:19.

51. Schoene RB, et al. Iron repletion decreases maximal exercise lactate concentrations in female athletes with minimal iron deficiency anemia. J Lab Clin Med 1983;102:306.

52. Lozoff B, et al. Developmental deficits in iron-deficient infants: Effects of age and severity of iron lack. J Pediatr 1982; 101:948.

53. Capriles LF. Intracranial hypertension and iron deficiency anemia. Arch Neurol 1963;9:147.

54. Hogan GR, Jones B. The relationship of koilonychia and iron deficiency in infants. J Pediatr 1970;77:1054.

55. Baird IM, et al. The tongue and oesophagus in iron deficiency anaemia and the effect of iron therapy. J Clin Pathol 1961;14:603.

56. Ekberg O, Malmquist J, Lindgren S. Pharyngo-oesophageal webs in dysphageal patients. A radiologic and clinical investigation in 1134 patients. ROFO 1986;145:75.

57. Khosla SN. Cricoid webs-incidence and follow-up study in Indian patients. Postgrad Med J 1984;60:346.

58. Hutton CF. Plummer-Vinson syndrome. Br J Radiol 1956; 29:81.

59. Anderson NP. Syndrome of spoon nails, anemia, cheilitis and dysphagia. Arch Dermatol 1938;37:816.

60. Aksoy M, et al. Radiographic bone changes in chronic iron deficiency anemia. Blood 1966;27:677.

61. Davidson WMB, Markson JL. The gastric mucosa in iron deficiency anemia. Lancet 1955;2:639.

62. Dallman PR. Iron deficiency and the immune response. Am J Clin Nutr 1987;46:329.

63. Piedras J, Alcocer-Varela J, Lopez-Karpovitch X, Cardenas MR. Decreased interleukin-2 production by peripheral blood cells of iron-deficient children. Blood 1987; 70:103.

64. Kuvibidila S, et al. Influence of iron deficiency anemia on selected thymus function in mice: thymulin biological activity, T-cell subsets, and thymocyte proliferation. Am J Clin Nutr 1990;51:228.

65. Murakawa H, Bland CE, Willis ST, Dallman PR. Iron deficiency and neutrophil function: different rates of correction of the depression in oxidative burst and myeloperoxidase activity after iron treatment. Blood 1987;69:1464.

66. Chandra RK. Reduced bacteriocidal capacity of polymorphs in iron deficiency. Arch Dis Child 1973;48:864.

67. Matoth Y, Zamir R, et al. Studies of folic acid in infancy; II, folic and folinic acid blood levels in infants with diarrhea, malnutrition and infection. Pediatrics 33: 1964; 33:694.

68. Marsh WL, Bishop JW, Carcy TP. Evaluation of red cell volume distribution width (RDE). Haematol Pathol 1987; 1:117.

69. Koller JE, et al. The diagnosis of iron deficiency by erythrocytic protoporphyrin and serum ferritin analyses. Acta Paediatr Scand 1978;67:361.

70. Flowers CH, Skikne BS, Covell AM, Cook JD. The clinical measurement of serum transferrin receptor. J Lab Clin Med 1989;114:368.

71. Ferguson BJ, Skikne BS, Simpson KM, Baynes RD, Cook JD. Serum transferrin receptor distinguishes the anaemia of chronic disease from iron deficiency anaemia. J Lab Clin Med 1992;119:385.

72. Lipschitz DA, Cook JD, Finch CA. A clinical evaluation of serum ferritin as an index of iron stores. N Engl J Med 1974;290:1213.

73. Holyoake TL, Stott DJ, McKay PJ, Hendry A, MacDonald JB, Lucie NP. Use of plasma ferritin concentration to diagnose iron deficiency in elderly patients. J Clin Pathol 1993;46:857.

74. Gale E, et al. The quantitative estimation of total iron stores in human bone marrow. J Clin Invest 1963;42:1076.

75. Hagler L, et al. Influence of dietary iron deficiency on hemoglobin, myoglobin, their respective reductases, and skeletal muscle mitochondrial respiration. Am J Clin Nutr 1981;34:2169.

76. Dallman PR, et al. Myoglobin and cytochrome response during repair of iron deficiency. J Clin Invest 1965; 44:1631.

77. Celsing F, Ekblom B, et al. Effects of chronic iron deficiency anaemia on myoglobin content, enzyme activity, and capillary density in the human skeletal muscle. Acta Med Scand 1988;223:451.

78. Jain SK, Yip R, et al. Evidence of peroxidative damage to the erythrocyte membrane in iron deficiency. Am J Clin Nutr 1983;37:26.

79. Dillmann E, Johnson DG, Martin J, Mackler B, Finch DA. Catecholamine elevation in iron deficiency. Am J Physiol 1979;237:R297.

80. Beutler E. Iron enzymes in iron deficiency. J Lab Clin Med 1959;52:694.

81. Gardner GW, Edgerton VR, et al. Physical work capacity and metabolic stress in subjects with iron deficiency. Am J Clin Nutr 1977;30:910.

82. Weinberg J, Levine S, et al. Long-term consequences of early iron deficiency in the rat. Pharmacol Biochem Behav 1979;11:631.

83. Simes AL, et al. Decreased monoamine oxidase activity in liver of iron deficient rats. Can J Biochem Cell Biol 1969; 47:999.

84. Saarinen UM, Simes MA, et al. Iron absorption in infants: high bioavailability of breast milk iron as indicated by the

extrinsic tag method of iron absorption and by correlation of serum ferritin. J Pediatr 1977;91:136.

85. Saairen UM. Need for iron supplementation in infants on prolonged breastfeeding. J Pediatr 1978;93:177.

86. Layrisse M, Martinez-Torres C. Food absorption: iron supplementation of food. In: Brown EB, Moore CV, eds. Progress in hematology VII. New York: Grune & Stratton, 1971:137.

87. Sullivan LW, et al. Studies of the daily requirement for folic acid in infants and the etiology of folate deficiency in goat's milk megaloblastic anemia. Am J Clin Nutr 1966; 18:311.

88. Davis LJ. Macrocytic anaemia in children. Arch Dis Child 1944;19:147.

89. Emerson PN, Wilkinson JH. Lactate dehydrogenase in the diagnosis and assessment of response to treatment of megaloblastic anemia. Br J Haematol 1966;12:678.

90. Elliott BA, Fleming AF. Source of elevated serum enzyme activities in patients with megaloblastic erythropoiesis secondary to folic acid deficiency. Br Med J 1965;1:626.

91. Ellegaard J, Esmann V. Folate deficiency in malnutrition, malabsorption, and during phenytoin treatment diagnosed by determination of serine synthesis in lymphocytes. Eur J Clin Invest 1972;2:315.

92. Mahmood T, et al. Macrocytic anemia, thrombocytosis and nonlobulated megakaryocytes. The 5q-syndrome, a distinct entity. Am J Med 1979;66:946.

93. Higginbottom MC, et al. A syndrome of methylmalonic aciduria, homocystinuria, megaloblastic anemia and neurologic abnormalities in a vitamin B-12 deficient breast-fed infant of a strict vegetarian. N Engl J Med 1984;310:789.

94. London IM, et al. On the origin of bile pigment in normal man. J Biol Chem 1950;184:351.

95. Fillet G, Dook JD, Finch CA. Storage iron kinetics; VII, a biologic model for reticuloendothelial iron transport. J Clin invest 1974;53:1527.

96. Karle H. The pathogenesis of the anaemia of chronic disorders and the role of fever in erythrokinetics. Scand J Haematol 1974;13:81.

97. Lynch SR, et al. Iron and the reticuloendothelial system. In: Jacobs A, Worwood M, eds. New York: Academic Press, 1974.

98. Lash JA, et al. Plasma lactoferrin reflects granulocyte activation in vivo. Blood 1983;61:885.

99. Birgens HS, et al. Lactoferrin-mediated transfer of iron to intracellular ferritin in human monocytes. Eur J Haematol 1988;141:52.

100. Bodel P. Studies on the mechanisms of endogenous pyrogen production; III, human blood monocytes. J Exp Med 1974;140:954.

101. Cortell S, Conrad ME. Effect of endotoxin on iron absorption. Am J Physiol 1967;213:43.

102. Perkkio M, et al. sIgA and IgM containing cells in the intestinal mucosa of iron-deficient rats. Am J Clin Nutr 1987; 46:341.

103. Rees AJ. Pulmonary injury caused by antibasement membrane antibodies. Semin Resp Med 1984;5:264.

104. Larrick JW, Human ES. Acquired iron-deficiency anemia caused by an antibody against the transferrin receptor. N Engl J Med 1984;311:214.

105. Blaud P. Sur les maladies chlorotiques, et sur une mode de traitement specifique dans ces affections. Rev Med Franc Strange 1832;45:341.

106. Bottomley SS. Sideroblastic anaemia. Clin Haematol 1982; 11:389.

107. Cooley TB. A severe type of hereditary anemia with elliptocytosis: interesting sequence of splenectomy. Am J Med Sci 1945;209:561.

108. Pasanen AVO, Salmi M, Vuopio P, Tenhunen R. Heme biosynthesis in sideroblastic anemia. Int J Biochem 1980; 12:969.

109. Soslan G, Brodsky I. Hereditary sideroblastic anemia with associated platelet abnormalities. Am J Hematol 1989; 32:298.

110. Brien WF, Mant JM, Etches WS. Variant congenital dyserythropoietic anaemia with ringed sideroblasts. Clin Lab Haematol 1985;7:231.

111. Amos RJ, Miller ALC, Amses JAL. Autosomal inheritance of sideroblastic anaemia. Clin Lab Haematol 1988;10:347.

112. Hamel BCJ, Schretlen EDAM. Sideroblastic anaemia: a review of seven paediatric cases. Eur J Pediatr 1982; 138:130.

113. Pearson HA, et al. A new syndrome of refractory sideroblastic anemia with vacuolization of marrow precursors and exocrine pancreatic dysfunctional J Pediatr 1979;95:976.

114. Harris JW, Horrigan DL. Pyridoxine-responsive anemia. Analysis of 62 cases. Adv Intern Med 1964;12:103.

115. Cazzola M, et al. Natural history of idiopathic refractory sideroblastic anemia. Blood 1988;71:305.

116. Hines JD. Reversible megaloblastic and sideroblastic marrow abnormalities in alcoholic patients. Br J Haematol 1969;16:87.

117. Savage D, Lindenbaum J. Anemia in alcoholics. Medicine 1986;65:322.

118. Eichner ER, Hillman RS. The evolution of anemia in alcoholic patients. Am J Med 1971;50:218.

119. Bottomley SS. Sideroblastic anaemia. In: Jacobs A, Worwood, eds. Iron in biochemistry and medicine, II. London: Academic Press, 1980.

120. Dunlap WM, James GW, Hume DM. Anemia and neutropenia caused by copper deficiency. Ann Intern Med 1974;80:470.

121. Moore MR, Meredith PA, Goldberg A. Lead and heme biosynthesis. In: Singhal RL, Thomas JA, eds. Lead toxicity. Baltimore: Urban & Schwarzenberg, 1980.

122. Labbe RF. Lead poisoning mechanisms. Clin Chem 1990; 36:1870.

123. Haden HT. Pyridoxine-responsive sideroblastic anemia due to anti-tuberculosis drugs. Arch Intern Med 1967; 120:602.

124. O'Brien H, Amens JAL, Molin DL. Recurrent thrombocytopenia, erythroid hypoplasia and sideroblastic anemia associated with hypothermia. Br J Haematol 1982;51:451.

125 Hoffbrand AV, Gorman A, et al. Improvement in iron status and liver function in patients with transfusional overload with long-term subcutaneous desferrioxamine. Lancet 1979;1:947.

126. Peppard M, Callendar ST, et al. Ferrioxamine excretion in iron-overloaded man. Blood 1982;60:288.

127. Nathan DG, Oral iron chelators. Semin Hematol 1990; 27:83.

128. Daly AL, Velazquez LA, et al. Mucormycosis: association with deferroxamine therapy. Am J Med 1989;87:468.

129. O'Brien RT. Ascorbic acid enhancement of desferrioxamine induced urinary excretion in thalassemia major. Am NY Acad Sci 1974;232:221.

130. McLaran CJ, Bett JHN, et al. Congestive cardiomyopathy and hemochromatosis; rapid progression possibly accelerated by excessive ingestion of ascorbic acid. Aust NZ J Med 1982;12:187.

CHAPTER 7

Red Cell Membrane Defects

PAMELA S. BECKER

The resistance (fragility) of erythrocytes to various fluids was first studied by Malassez in 1873, and the mechanism of the destruction of the red blood-cell has been more or less imperfectly understood since the time of Hamburger's investigations on the osmosis of body fluids.
—Pearce (1918)

Introduction

The red blood cell membrane provides the cell with the durability it requires to endure its numerous turbulent circulations through the heart and the tortuous, inhospitable climate of the spleen. In addition, it provides the flexibility to negotiate narrow capillary channels less than half its diameter and minute slits between the splenic cords and sinuses. A number of defects intrinsic to the membrane proteins can lead to hereditary hemolytic anemias. These include hereditary spherocytosis, hereditary elliptocytosis, hereditary pyropoikilocytosis, and hereditary stomatocytosis, as well as other rare conditions.

Case 1

An 18-year-old male presented with complaint of a recent flu-like syndrome consisting of fever, vomiting, malaise, abdominal pain, headache, and arthralagias. On physical examination, he was and his spleen tip was 2 cm below the costal margin, without lymphadenopathy or abdominal tenderness. A complete blood count (CBC) demonstrated a white blood cell (WBC) count of 3.2 × 10⁹/L, (53% neutrophils, 30% lymphoctyes, 15% monocytes, 2% eosinophils) hematocrit 24%, reticulocyte count 0.1%, platelet count 110 × 10⁹/L. Prothrombin and partial thromboplastin times were normal. The mean corpuscular volume (MCV) was 84 fL; mean corpuscular hemoglobin concentration (MCHC) 36%. The total bilirubin was 3.2 mg/dl, direct 0.6 mg/dl, the alanine transaminase (ALT) was 28 U/L, the aspartate transaminase (AST) 60 U/L, the alkaline phosphatase 104 U/L, and the lactic dehydrogenase (LDH) 340 U/L. An ultrasound revealed calcified gallstones.

Comment: *The patient appeared to have a viral syndrome, with suppression of blood counts. Important clues to the underlying diagnosis included the splenomegaly and presence of gallstones in a young individual. There was pancytopenia with an inappropriately low reticulocyte count. The MCHC was slightly increased.*

The elevated LDH and indirect bilirubin suggested a hemolytic process.

> *Peripheral blood smear:* spherocytes, occasional microsphorocytes (fig. 7.1)
> *Bone marrow biopsy:* cellular marrow with decreased to absent erythroid precursors

Comment

Spherocytes are small, spheroidal cells which lack the central pallor seen in biconcave discs. The MCHC is increased, presumably due to cellular dehydration. The presence of up to 10% spherocytes on the peripheral blood smear can be normal or artifactual. Spherocytes can be seen in autoimmune hemolytic anemia or in hereditary spherocytosis. Both of these conditions are associated with reticulocytosis and increased erythroid activity on bone marrow examination. The most important differentiating laboratory study is the Coombs test, which will demonstrate the presence of antibody directed against red cell antigens in autoimmune hemolytic anemia.

After 10 days from the onset of the initial symptoms, the reticulocyte count began to rise, and peaked at 30% at 10 days after presentation. The hematocrit eventually reached 35%, and stabilized with 5% reticulocytes. The WBC eventually reached 7.0 × 10⁹/L at 14 days after the onset of symptoms.

> *Special tests:*
> Glucose 6-phosphate dehydrogenase (G-6-PD): 10 (normal range 4.6–13.5 U/g of hemoglobin)
> Coombs test: negative direct and indirect
> IgM for parovirus B-19: positive
> Osmotic fragility, both incubated and unincubated: increased
> Serum haptoglobin: 0 mg/dl

Evaluation of the patient's family members demonstrated the presence of mild anemia and mild reticulocytosis in both his father and sister. The mother and another

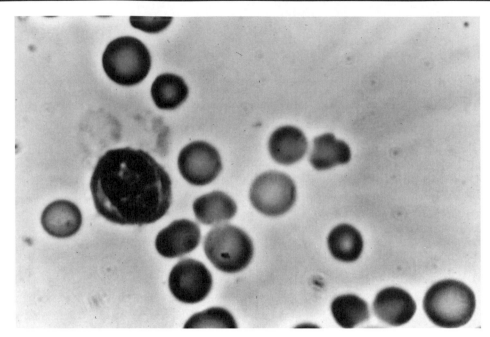

Figure 7.1. Peripheral blood smear from patient described in case 1. There are numerous spherocytes present.

sister were unaffected. Red cells from the affected individuals demonstrated increased osmotic fragility.

*Diagnosis: **Aplastic crisis induced by parvovirus B-19 infection in a young man with occult hereditary spherocytosis.***

Comment

Parvovirus is the etiologic agent for the childhood illness known as fifth disease (erythema infectiosum). The bone marrow can be a target for parvovirus infection, and in individuals with chronic hemolytic anemia this results in anemia and reticulocytopenia (1–3). Erythroid production is suppressed, leading to a rapid drop in hematocrit. Parvovirus can also suppress proliferation of all bone marrow progenitor cells, resulting in leukopenia and mild thrombocytopenia. Viral-associated hemophagocytosis has also been implicated as a cause of the neutropenia and thrombocytopenia, since the myeloid and megakaryocyte cell lineages are not directly infected by the virus. A profound anemia can become manifest in patients with hemolytic anemias who are dependent on accelerated red blood cell (RBC) production to maintain an adequate hematocrit.

The Coombs's test was negative, ruling out the possibility of the other major cause of spherocytic hemolytic anemia, autoimmune hemolytic anemia. Other causes of hemolytic anemia include deficiencies of red cell glycolytic enzymes, but the cells are generally not spheroidal.

The serum haptoglobin was 0 g/L, indicating that hemolysis had been ongoing. Haptoglobin is cleared when it binds the free hemoglobin released by lysis of red cells.

The **Osmotic Fragility** is a reflection of the sensitivity of the erythrocyte to lysis in low ionic strength. It reflects the surface-to-volume ratio. The less surface area, the

more spheroidal the cell shape, and it takes less influx of volume to lyse the cell. There can also be increased osmotic fragility in immune hemolytic anemia or bacterial sepsis. Incubation of the blood at 37°C for 24 hours (the "incubated" osmotic fragility test) can improve the sensitivity because of metabolic depletion, which makes the cells more susceptible to osmotic lysis. This sensitivity to metabolic depletion is also reflected in the **Autohemolysis Test,** which demonstrates increased numbers of lysed hereditary spherocytes as compared with normal red cells, with only partial protection by the addition of glucose.

Therapy

Maintenance of adequate folic acid stores may be critical to keep up with the increased erythropoiesis required to compensate for the hemolytic anemia. Intravenous immune globulin may have some efficacy in parvovirus infection. Packed red cell transfusions may be administered for a profound drop in hematocrit and absent reticulocytes, or may be occasionally chronically required in the more severe form of the disorder.

Clinical Features

Hereditary spherocytosis is most often mild and clinically insignificant, but in its severe form it can be associated with pallor, jaundice, and splenomegaly. It can present at any age, but most usually, manifests in childhood. Occasionally, there is a more severe neonatal presentation with high serum bilirubin when exchange transfusion is sometimes needed because of the risk of kernicterus. The condition then gradually improves, although a few transfusions may be needed. In about 20–30% of pa-

Chapter 7 / Red Cell Membrane Defects

tients, there is a very mild course and the hemolysis is well compensated for by amplified red cell production. These patients are largely asymptomatic. About two-thirds of patients have a mild-to-moderate anemia, with palpable splenomegaly. Their course is complicated by events such as hemolytic, aplastic, or megaloblastic crises, and gallbladder disease. The **Hemolytic Crises** can occur in the setting of acute infection, the **Aplastic Crises** in the setting of viral infection (e.g., parvovirus B-19), and **Megaloblastic Crises** in the setting of folate deficiency, such as in pregnancy. Pigment gallstones are formed due to the chronically elevated levels of bilirubin resulting from the hemolytic anemia, and can be detected as early as adolescence. A small percentage of patients have a severe, transfusion-dependent course with chronic jaundice. Except for these extremely severe cases, there is generally an excellent response to splenectomy. After splenectomy, the most highly conditioned microspherocytes disappear and the anemia, reticulocytosis, and jaundice resolve.

Pathophysiology

There are several types of inherited hemolytic anemia due to defects in the protein components of the RBC membrane. These include hereditary spherocytosis (HS), hereditary elliptocytosis (HE), hereditary pyropoikilocytosis (HPP), and hereditary stomatocytosis.

Hereditary spherocytosis is a clinically and genetically heterogeneous disorder of the RBC characterized by increased osmotic fragility and spheroidal shape. There is a classical, autosomal dominant type and a more severe, recessively inherited form. The biochemical defects in these disorders have been related to abnormalities in the RBC membrane proteins, although in many cases of HS, the specific molecular defects have not yet been identified.

The erythrocyte membrane consists of lipid bilayer traversed by integral membrane proteins and bordered by peripheral membrane proteins. The lipid bilayer consists of the phospholipids, phosphatidylcholine (PC), phosphatidylethanolamine (PE), sphingomyelin (SM), phosphatidylserine (PS), and cholesterol, with a few other minor components (4). Each layer is arranged such that the polar head groups are aligned at one surface and the hydrophobic fatty acid side chains are buried internally. The glycolipids that carry the major red cell antigens (e.g., A, B) are located in the external half of the bilayer. There is an asymmetric distribution of the phospholipids, such that PC and SM are concentrated in the outer half, and PE and PS are located in the inner half (5).

The integral membrane proteins are composed of an outer, glycosylated portion, a transmembrane hydrophobic sequence, and internal cytoplasmic domain. The peripheral membrane proteins associate with the internal or external face, largely through interactions with the transmembrane proteins. A number of the red cell membrane proteins were named for their position of relative migration on SDS-polyacrylmide gels (6). These include α- and β-spectrin (bands 1 and 2, respectively), ankyrin (band 2.1), the anion transport channel (band 3), proteins 4.1, 4.2, dematin (band 4.9), actin (band 5), glyceraldehyde-3-phosphate dehydrogenase (band 6), and bands 7 and 8 (fig. 7.2). Table 7.1 lists the red cell membrane proteins and indicates features such as size, oligomeric state, chromosome location of the gene encoding the protein, and disease states resulting from abnormalities in these proteins.

Transmembrane Glycoproteins and Associated Proteins

There are two major types of erythrocyte transmembrane glycoproteins, the glycophorins (reviewed in references 7 and 8) and band 3 (reviewed in reference 9). There are four types of glycophorins: A, B, C, and D (also known as glycoproteins α, δ, β, and γ). Glycophorin A is the major sialoglycoprotein in the red cell. The extracellular region is quite polar, with abundant carbohydrate, and bears the M and N blood group antigens, lectin-binding sites for phytohemagglutinin and wheat germ agglutinin, and viral receptors. Glycophorin A is believed to exist as a dimer in the membrane. It is a specific marker for erythroid cells. Glycophorin B shares its first 26 amino acid residues with glycophorin A, but lacks an oligosaccharide chain at position 21, and is believed to have arisen from the latter pro-

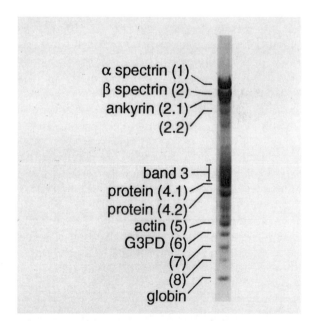

Figure 7.2. Eryathrocyte membrane protein: SDS polyacrylamide gel electrophoresis. The red cell membrane proteins are designated numerically by their relative migration on SDS polyacrylamide gels. Bands 1 and 2 are the spectrin α- and β-chains, respectively. Band 2.1 is ankyrin. Band 3 is the anion transport channel. Band 4.9 is dematin. Band 5 is erythrocyte actin. Band 6 is glyceraldehyde-3-phosphate dehydrogenase (G-6-PD). Band 7 includes stomatin (band 7.2). Band 8 contains residual hemoglobin.

Table 7.1. Erythrocyte Membrane Proteins

SDS Gel Band	Protein	Mol Wt (Gel) (x10³)	Mol Wt (Calc) (x10³)	Oligomeric State	Chromosome Location	Associated Diseases
1	α-Spectrin	240	281	Heterotetramer	1q22-q25	HE, HPP, HS
2	β-Spectrin	220	246	Heterotetramer	14q23-q24.2	HE, HPP, HS
2.1	Ankyrin	210	206	Monomer	8p11.2	HS
2.9	α-Adducin	103	81	Tetramer	4p16.3	
	β-Adducin	97	80			
3	AE1	90−100	102	Dimer or tetramer	17q12-q21	HS, SAO, HAc
4.1	Protein 4.1	80+78	66	Monomer	1p33-p34.2	HE
4.2	Pallidin	72	77	?Dimer or trimer	15q15-q21	HS
4.9	Dematin	48+52	43+46	Trimer		
	p55	55	53	?Dimer	Xq28	
5	β-Actin	43	42	Oligomer (−14)	7pter-q22	
	Tropomodulin	43	41	Monomer	9q22	
6	G3PD	35	36	Tetramer	12p13	
7	Stomatin	31	32			?HS
	Tropomyosin	27+29	28	Heterodimer	1q31	
8	Protein 8	23				
PAS-1	Glycophorin A	36	14	Dimer	4q31	Non
PAS-2	Glycophorin C	32	14		2q14-q21	HE
PAS-3	Glycophorin B	20	8	?Dimer	4q31	Non

tein by gene duplication. It carries the S, s, and U antigens and has N blood group activity. Glycophorin C is distinct from glycophorins A and B, but glycophorin D may arise from the same gene product as C by alternative RNA splicing or differential processing.

There are numerous anomalies of the glycophorins, including the En(a-) phenotype, in which glycophorin A is absent or exists as a fusion of the amino terminal end of glycophorin A with the carboxy terminal end of glycophorin B (Finnish and English types, respectively), the S-s red cells which lack glycophorin B, and Gerbich negative (Ge−) red cells, which lack glycophorin C. The glycophorin A and B variant erythrocytes, including those that totally lack these proteins, have no detectable change in red cell physiology. In contrast, the Leach phenotype of Ge− red cells, which totally lacks glycophorin C, is associated with elliptocytes but minimal hemolysis. Another type of Ge − is associated with a hybrid glycophorin C-D gene product and no elliptocytes. Glycophorin C deficiency can also arise in patients with protein 4.1 deficiency. In fact, the amount of GP-C appears to be directly related to the amount of protein 4.1 (10): with total absence of protein 4.1, there is 9% of the usual quantity of glycophorin C; when half of the protein 4.1 is present, there is 44% of the normal quantity of glycophorin C. Thus, protein 4.1 must serve an anchoring role in the attachment of glycophorin C.

Band 3 (anion exchange protein 1) is the 102 kd glycoprotein that serves as the major anion transport channel (9). In the membrane, its million copies per cell exist as dimers or tetramers. Its N-terminal end is cytoplasmic and contains a binding site for several cytoplasmic proteins, including the glycolytic enzymes, glyceraldehyde-3-phosphate dehydrogenase (11, 12), aldolase (13), and phosphoglycerate kinase (14), hemoglobin (15),

and proteins 2.1 (ankyrin) (16–18), 4.1 (19), and 4.2. The C-terminal region is glycosylated and possesses the function of chloride-bicarbonate exchange. The nucleotide sequence predicts multiple transmembrane helices which contribute to formation of the anion transport channel.

Pallidin (protein 4.2) is a 77,000-kd peripheral membrane protein present in about 500,000 copies per cell (reviewed in reference 20). Pallidin binds to band 3 (21) and probably to ankyrin (21), and it is deficient in some patients with spherocytosis. There is a recessive murine mutant designated **pallid** which is characterized by hypopigmentation, prolonged bleeding time, and defective lysosomes (22).

The Erythrocyte Membrane Skeleton

There is an elaborate network of proteins (23, 24) underlying the surface of the lipid bilayer which provides structural support known as the "membrane skeleton." The major components are spectrin, actin protofilaments, proteins 4.1 and 4.9, myosin, tropomyosin, and adducin. Negative-staining electron microscopy has revealed the fine details of the lattice. There are junctional complexes composed of protein 4.1 and F-actin protofilaments joined in a hexagonal pattern (25) by spectrin tetramers or oligomers. Spectrin dimers self-associate at one end to form tetramers and higher oligomers (26, 27), and at the opposite end, bind to F-actin protofilaments under the enhancing influence of protein 4.1 (see diagram in fig. 7.3) (28, 29). Moreover, the abnormalities encountered by similar electron microscopy studies of defective red cell membranes are striking (30). Spectrin comprises nearly 70% of the membrane skeleton protein content by weight. It is a heterodimer of the long intertwined α- and β-chains, bands 1 and 2, respectively, on SDS gels. Their sizes are formidable, the

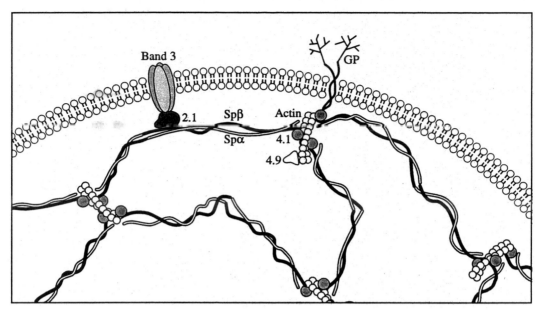

Figure 7.3. The erythrocyte membrane skeleton. Spectrin heterodimers of the α- and β-chains interact at one end to form tetramers and higher oligomers. At the opposite end, they bind to short filaments of F-actin and protein 4.1. The membrane skeleton is anchored to the lipid bilayer through the binding of β-spectrin to ankyrin and of ankyrin to band 3.

α-chain is 267 kd and the β-chain is 246 kd (molecular weights predicted by nucleotide sequence) (31, 32). They are arranged in antiparallel alignment with respect to their N and C termini. The original structural model for spectrin was a linear arrangement of globular domains separated by protease-sensitive regions (33, 34). These were designated α1 through α5, and β1 through β4. The current model depicts both chains as consisting of multiple 106 amino acid repeating segments of triple α-helices (35). There are 21 on the α-chain and 17 on the β-chain. In addition, there are regions of nonrepetitive sequence that appear to have specialized functions.

Spectrin is a member of a gene superfamily including such proteins as fodrin (nonerythroid spectrin), α-actinin, and dystrophin. All such proteins share the homologous repeating subunits and have similar N-terminal β- and C-terminal α-chains (36). The former region contains the actin-binding domains of the proteins and the latter, two EF hand structures with calcium-binding function in all of the proteins except erythroid spectrin.

Anchoring Proteins: Proteins 2.1 (Ankyrin) and 4.1

Ankyrin contains the high-affinity binding site that mediates attachment of spectrin to the lipid bilayer via band 3 (16, 37, 38). It is a pyramidal molecule (39) of 206 kd and has three domains. The 89 kd N-terminal region consists of twenty-two 33 amino acid repeats and contains the binding site for band 3 (40). The repeats are similar to those found in proteins that control the cell cycle. The central 62-kd domain contains the spectrin-binding site (40). The 55-kd C-terminal domain contains regulatory sequence that modulates the binding of ankyrin to spectrin and band 3 (40). Alternative splicing of these sequences produces isoforms of different size and function. Protein 2.2 arises by alternative splicing, lacks a negative regulatory region (41), and therefore binds more tightly to spectrin and band 3.

Protein 4.1 is a globular 80-kd phosphoprotein. It migrates as a doublet on discontinuous SDS-polyacrylamide gels due to deamidation of asparagine 502, which occurs gradually with red cell aging (42), and results in progressively increased 4.1a, present in older cells (43). A central 10-kd chymotryptic peptide retains the capacity to enhance spectrin-actin binding (44) and bind to myosin (45), and an N-terminal 30-kd peptide binds to glycophorin and calmodulin. In nonerythroid cells, an elongated 135-kd isoform is present. There are about ten nucleotide sequence motifs that are alternatively spliced in or out to produce a number of isoforms. Motif I encodes a 21-amino acid segment that contains the binding site for spectrin and actin (46). Its expression is linked to terminal erythroid maturation (47). The splicing in of motif IV in conjunction with the splicing out of motif V is required to produce the elongated form. The functions of the other motifs are presently unknown. Protein 4.1 also binds to glycophorins A (48) and C (49), and band 3 (50), but the predominant linkage to the transmembrane glycoproteins is via glycophorin C (51).

Actin and Its Associated Proteins

Red cell actin is the β form of actin (52), identical to that expressed in skeletal muscle (53). However, it does not exist as the long filaments present in muscle; rather, it exists as protofilaments (54), of 12–16 monomers, arranged in double-helical fashion (54). These short filaments are stabilized by their interactions with spectrin, protein 4.1, and tropomyosin, and by capping of the slow growing or "pointed" end of actin by tropomodulin (55).

Compounds that inhibit actin polymerization increase membrane flexibility, while compounds that promote its polymerization rigidify the membrane (53), indicating that the state of actin polymerization can regulate membrane flexibility. Spectrin tetramers bind to the side of actin filaments, via the N-terminal region of β-spectrin (56, 57); because they are bivalent, they cross-link actin filaments, and this interaction is greatly amplified by protein 4.1 (28, 29).

Dematin (protein 4.9). This 48- and 52-kd pair of proteins form a core skeletal component along with spectrin, actin, and protein 4.1 (23). The protein must also attach to a lipid or integral membrane protein, since it remains associated with the membrane when the other skeletal proteins are extracted; however, this attachment site has not been identified. The native protein is a trimer and is phosphorylated by a cAMP-dependent kinase and protein kinase C (58–60). It binds to actin and bundles actin filaments into cables (61). This action is abolished by phosphorylation at the cAMP-dependent site (62).

Adducin. This protein is a heterodimer containing α- (81 kd) and β- (80 kd) subunits (63). Adducin is believed to play a role in the early assembly of the spectrin-actin network. The protein binds to actin and, like protein 4.1, increases the binding of spectrin to actin (63). The adducin-spectrin-actin complex promotes binding of a second spectrin, a reaction that is blocked by calmodulin (63). The protein is phosphorylated by protein kinase C and protein kinase A, but the function of the phosphorylation is unknown.

Tropomyosin. Erythrocyte tropomyosin is a heterodimer of 27,000- and 29,000-dalton subunits that run on SDS gels in the region of band 7 (64). The red cell analog is similar to other nonmuscle tropomyosins by many criteria (64). There is one copy for each 6 to 8 actin monomers, which is just enough to cover all of the red cell actin protofilaments. The length of tropomyosin and the length of the protofilaments also correspond. This suggests a model in which each protofilament bears two tropomyosins, one in each of the two filament grooves. The possible functions include stabilization of the short actin filament and conferring specificity to the site of spectrin interactions along the actin protofilaments.

Tropomodulin. Tropomodulin is a 43 kd protein which binds to tropomyosin in a 2:1 molar ratio with a K_d of 5×10^{-7} M (55, 65). In erythrocytes, there are 30,000 copies per cell, suggesting that one associates with each actin filament. Tropomodulin appears to associate with the pointed end of the filament and block growth at that end (66). Tropomyosin amplifies this effect. Tropomodulin remains attached to the membrane when spectrin, actin, and tropomyosin are removed, but the membrane-binding site has not yet been identified.

The Role of the Spleen

Although the molecular lesions responsible for HS are intrinsic to the RBC, the pathophysiology of the hemolysis is related to the presence of the spleen. In most patients with typical autosomal dominant HS, removal of the spleen will result in resolution of the hemolysis. Even in patients with severe hemolytic anemias, splenectomy generally affords some improvement. The theories that have been proposed to explain the deleterious environment of the spleen are focused on a few concepts: the inability of nondeformable spherocytes to traverse the splenic fenestrations, the acidic environment during detention in the spleen, and the direct effect of macrophages in the process of "splenic conditioning."

Molecular Defects in Hereditary Spherocytosis

Defects in ankyrin, spectrin, band 3, and pallidin have been found in hereditary spherocytosis. Erythrocyte membranes from the majority of HS patients are deficient in spectrin, including both the dominant and recessive (67) forms of the disease, and the degree of spectrin deficiency correlates closely with the severity of the disease (68). Recently, it has been found that the degree of spectrin deficiency closely correlates with the degree of ankyrin deficiency in the most common type of autosomal dominant HS (69). Specific molecular defects have recently been identified in ankyrin. Deficiency of band 3 accounts for a smaller proportion of patients, and deficiency of protein 4.2 is associated with a recessively inherited spherocytic hemolytic anemia associated with the presence of elliptocytes as well. The molecular defects in HS are summarized in table 7.2.

Mouse Mutants

There are naturally occurring murine mutants with an autosomal recessive condition similar to this human disorder, and the molecular defects identified in these mutants have significant relevance to the human conditions. There are six types of such mutants in the common house mouse, *Mus musculus*: sph/sph (spherocytosis), sph^{ha}/sph^{ha} (hemolytic anemia), sph^{2J}/sph^{2J}, sph^{2BC}/sph^{2BC}, ja/ja (jaundice), and nb/nb (normoblastosis) (70, 71). Anemia is observed only in the homozygous state, and these mutants represent mutations at three alleles: sph, ja, and nb. The clinical features include spherocytosis, reticulocytosis of 60–90%, jaundice, marked hepatosplenomegaly, and reduced RBC life span to <1 day (normally 48 days). The sph mutants have defects in α-spectrin (for example, absent α-spectrin mRNA in the sph/sph mutant) (71). The ja/ja mutant has a termination codon position 1160 in β-spectrin (72) and the nb/nb mouse has a defect in ankyrin that gives rise to a truncated 150-kd (instead of 210 kd) protein (73). The ja/ja phenotype could be transferred to the hypoplastic W/W^v mouse by bone marrow transplantation (70), but as of yet, successful transplantation of normal bone marrow into these mice has not been achieved. Similarly, the nb mouse totally lacks the full-length ankyrin, the protein which attaches spectrin to the transmembrane protein band 3, and is consequently deficient in spectrin by about 50% (71). Unlike the human

Table 7.2. Molecular Defects in HS

Type	Clinical Condition	Protein Abnormality	Molecular Defect
SPECTRIN			
Autosomal recessive spherocytosis	Severe HS in homozygote	Spectrin severe deficiency	Linkage to a spectrin polymorphism
Spectrin Kissimmee	Moderate severity	Defective protein 4.1 binding function	β Spectrin Trip202→Arg
ANKYRIN			
Ankyrin deficiency	Mild to moderate in heterozygote	Concomitant spectrin/ ankyrin deficiency (60–90%)	Multiple defects: point mutations in 5′ untransslated region and codon 463, extra base in codon 572, 4 bp deletion in codons 797-798, premature terminations, ankyrin gene deletion, translocation at site of ankyrin gene
Ankyrin Prague		Truncated ankyrin	Unknown
BAND 3			
Band 3 deficiency	Mild HS	Bank 3 deficiency (65–85%)	
Band 3 Prague			Duplication of 10 bases after codon 818
Band 3 Montefiore	Spherocytic hemolytic anemia	Band 3 mutation leading to protein 4.2 deficiency	Glu 40→Lys
Band 3 Tuscaloosa	Hemolytic anemia	Band 3 mutation leading to protein 4.2 deficiency	Pro 327→Arg
PALLIDIN (PROTEIN 4.2)			
Pallidin deficiency	Severe Hemolytic anemia in homozygotes (spherocytes, elliptocytes, or ovalostomatocytes)	Pallidin deficiency primary or secondary to band 3 mutation (see above)	See variants below
Pallidin Nippon			Ala 142→Thr
Pallidin Lisboa			Codon 88 or 89-1 bp deletion
Pallidin Tozeur			Arg 310→Gln

conditions thus far associated with defective ankyrin, the nb defect is associated with deficient ankyrin in the Purkinje and granule cells of the cerebellum, and therefore results in a psychomotor disorder at the age of 6 months (74). The defect in ankyrin is in the *Ank-1* gene, which is also highly expressed in those tissues. There is an Ank-1 related protein (165 kd) expressed in fetal reticulocytes which can compensate for the lack of ankyrin during fetal life such that the mice do not become anemic until the 1st day of life (75, 76).

Combined Spectrin/Ankyrin Deficiency

Deficiency of the erythrocyte membrane skeleton protein, spectrin, has been demonstrated in patients with recessive HS (67) and a majority of patients with autosomal dominant HS (77), and the degree of deficiency appears to correlate with clinical severity (68). The degree of spectrin deficiency is directly related to the degree of hemolysis, degree of anemia, transfusion requirement, and response to splenectomy. Moreover, in one child with hydrops fetalis due to severe HS, there was a virtual absence of α-spectrin syn-

thesis (78). The precise mechanism that causes the spectrin deficiency is thought to be related in some cases to a defect in ankyrin. As already noted, there is a direct relationship between the degree of the deficiency of the two proteins, and concomitant spectrin and ankyrin deficiency has been identified in 19 of 20 kindreds with HS (69).

The initial clue in pinpointing the molecular origin of the defect resulting in spectrin deficiency was derived from the description by two groups of families with translocations involving chromosome 8 and concomitant HS (79, 80), suggesting that this chromosome was in some way related to HS. A heterozygous deletion of the short arm of chromosome 8, 8p11.1-8p21.2, was then found to be associated with HS and neurologic symptoms in one individual (81), and this patient and another unrelated patient with a similar clinical condition were found to completely lack the gene encoding ankyrin (82), located on chromosome 8. In one large kindred with HS and no chromosome deletion, linkage of HS was demonstrated to the ankyrin gene (83). Another kindred with dominant HS was found to have a truncated ankyrin protein (ankyrin Prague) (84). Eight mutations in ankyrin have recently been identified in patients with dominant and recessive HS (85). These include those designated ankyrin Stuttgart, ankyrin Einbeck, ankyrin Marburg, ankyrin Bovenden, ankyrin Walsrode, and ankyrin Dusseldorf. The mutations found include those leading to frameshift or termination, as well as heterozygous mutations in the 5′ untranslated region found in the recessive condition (85).

Protein 4.2 (Pallidin) Deficiency Arising from Defects in 4.2 and Band 3

Abnormalities of protein 4.2 and band 3 have also been related to HS. Several patients of Japanese descent, one Portuguese patient, and one Tunisian patient have been described with an apparently recessive disease characterized by moderately severe anemia and complete or nearly complete absence (~99%) of pallidin. In the first Japanese patients, the red cells contained only a trace quantity of a 74/72 kd pallidin doublet instead of the usual abundant 72 kd species, because of an Ala142 to Thr mutation (86) that affects the processing of pallidin mRNA. Other Japanese patients have had the same mutation, designated pallidin^{Nippon} (87). The Portuguese variant (pallidin^{Lisboa}) is caused by a single-base deletion in codon 88 or 89 (88). No detectable pallidin is synthesized. The Tunisian variant (pallidin^{Tozeur}) is caused by a substitution of Gln for Arg at position 310 (88) and is stable enough to accumulate to low levels in the red cell. Finally, red cell pallidin deficiency has also been associated with mutations in the cytoplasmic domain of band 3 in 2 patients. One of the mutations lies near the N-terminus of the cytoplasmic domain, Glu^{40} to Lys, designated band 3^{Montefiore}; the other is near the C-terminal end of the domain, Pro^{327} to Arg, designated band 3^{Tuscaloosa} (89), and is associated with a spherocytic hemolytic anemia. Presumably, these amino acids form part of the pallidin-binding site.

Band 3 Deficiency

Deficiency of band 3 has also been demonstrated in hereditary spherocytosis (90–92). As many as 10–15% of dominant HS patients may have a primary deficiency of band 3. Their red cells contain 25–40% less band 3 than normal. In many cases, a small proportion of "mushroom-shaped" cells is present in addition to the usual spherocytes. The band 3 molecule is progressively lost as the cells circulate, particularly the "mobile" fraction. This fraction represents band 3 that is not bound to the skeleton, which suggests the primary defect may affect self-association of band 3 rather than its interactions with various skeletal proteins. In one family, a 10 bp segment of the band 3 gene is duplicated near the C-terminal end of the protein, leading to a shift in the reading frame and an altered C-terminus after amino acid 821 (band 3 Prague) (90). This mutation affects the last transmembrane helix, probably alters insertion of band 3 into the membrane, and abolishes the transport channel function.

β-Spectrin Defect Associated with Defective Protein 4.1 Binding

Three kindreds have been previously described in whom the spectrin is defective in its ability to bind protein 4.1 (93, 94). These kindreds have autosomal dominant HS, and likely represent only a small subset of patients with HS. For one of the kindreds, early studies had demonstrated that approximately 40% of the spectrin was unable to bind protein 4.1 (94), and that there was abnormal chymotryptic digestion of the isolated β-spectrin in individuals form this kindred (95). A point mutation has now been identified in β-spectrin at position 202, TGG to CGG (Trp to Arg), in the three affected members of one of these kindreds (spectrin Kissimmee) (96) in the region of protein 4.1 binding (97).

Deficiency of Stomatin (Protein 7.2) in Hereditary Stomatocytosis

Hereditary stomatocytosis, also known as hydrocytosis, is similar to spherocytosis in that there is a more severe decrease in the surface area-to-volume ratio, resulting in a shape change to the stomatocyte (reviewed in reference 98). These cells are spheroidal, and slit-like regions of pallor can be observed on peripheral blood smears. There is failure of the Na$^+$, K$^+$ pump, leading to accumulation of Na$^+$, then gain of water, and, consequently, cell swelling. One of four red cell membrane proteins in the region of protein 7, protein 7.2b or stomatin, is absent from these patients (99, 100), as well as a patient with another disorder, cryohydrocytosis (101), in which the red cells swell in the cold. This protein has now been cloned and sequenced (102), and its function is currently under study.

Case 2 (Adapted from Reference 103)

A newborn infant boy born at 38 weeks' gestation was noted to be jaundiced with hepatomegaly at 6 hours of life. He had hemoglobinuria and hyperbilirubinemia (240 mmol/L). The hemoglobin was 83 g/L, hematocrit 23%, and reticulocyte count 17% (uncorrected). The peripheral blood smear exhibited anisocytosis, poikilocytosis, and nucleated red cells.

Comment

This child presented with neonatal hemolytic jaundice. The differential diagnosis includes infection, immune hemolytic anemia (including hemolytic disease due to Rh, ABO, or minor group maternal-fetal incompatibility), hemoglobinopathy, hemolytic anemia due to deficiencies of glycolytic enzymes, or hereditary hemolytic anemias due to membrane defects. These can be distinguished by red cell morphology, Coombs's test, hemoglobin electrophoresis, and red cell enzyme assays. Infections such as viral respiratory infections, infectious mononucleosis, cytomegalovirus, and *Mycoplasma pneumoniae* can be associated with autoimmune hemolytic anemia.

The patient was afebrile without signs of respiratory infection. Serologic tests for rubella, herpes, toxoplasmosis, and Epstein-Barr virus were negative. Both the mother and child were blood type O, Rh positive. The Coombs's test was negative. The bone marrow showed erythroid hyperplasia with iron overload. The bilirubin was >550 mmol/L.

Comment

The treatment for hyperbilirubinemia in the newborn is exchange transfusion when it exceeds or is projected to exceed critical levels.

Exchange transfusions were administered at 16 and 26 hours of life. The infant also required transfusions on days 6, 14, and 26. The hemolytic anemia persisted through early childhood, such that he remains dependent on red cell transfusions at his current age of 3 years. Hemoglobin electrophoresis demonstrated the presence of sickle cell trait. Assays of the red cell enzymes glucose-6-phosphate dehydrogenase (G-6-PD) and pyruvate kinase were normal. Subsequent studies on the patient were complicated by the presence of a high proportion of transfused red cells; therefore, the patient's family was examined. There was no known family history of hemolytic anemia, although a brother was stillborn at 36 weeks' gestation. Examination of parents' peripheral blood smears demonstrated that both exhibited anisocytosis, and 2–3% elliptical cells were observed in the father. Both parents and two sisters demonstrated decreased red cell deformability; all had normal red cell thermal sensitivity.

Subsequent reevaluation of the peripheral smear in the patient demonstrated microcytosis (mean corpuscular volume [MCV] 75), microspherocytes, ovalocytes, and microovalocytes.

Comment

The greatest clue to the origin of the severe hemolytic anemia in the newborn or young child was the presence of poikilocytes, and later, ovalocytes, on the peripheral blood smear, as well as the small number of elliptical cells seen on the father's blood smear, suggesting a defect in the erythrocyte membrane skeleton. Study of this family in a research laboratory (103) demonstrated a defect in spectrin self-association in both parents, a characteristic feature of hereditary elliptocytosis or hereditary pyropoikilocytosis. In addition, the ektacytometry measurements obtained in the family members were consistent with hereditary elliptocytosis. The interpretation of the analysis was that the parents and two siblings had heterozygous hereditary elliptocytosis, and the proband, homozygous HE. The severe phenotype could arise from homozygous expression of the same HE defect or compound heterozygosity for two different HE defects. Alternatively, if the low expression allele (LELY) for α-spectrin was inherited in trans to the allele bearing the HE defect, the relative amount of the abnormal α-chain would be exaggerated and give the phenotype of a more severe disorder.

Hereditary Elliptocytosis (HE): Clinical Features

There are multiple clinical syndromes of HE, including common HE (HPP in homozygogous or compound heterozygous form), spherocytic HE, and ovalocytosis. The hallmark feature of HE is the elliptical, cigar-shaped erythrocyte. The course in the overwhelming majority of patients is quite benign. In some patients, there is a more severe hemolytic anemia in neonatal life that generally resolves and the usual mild anemia ensues. HPP can be viewed as a more severe form of HE, with red cells that exhibit increased thermal sensitivity and a peripheral blood smear remarkable for microcytosis and poikilocytosis.

Common HE

Common HE, the most frequent type, is the mild autosomal dominant condition. The most mild form is the silent carrier state, usually identified because a relative presents with a more severe condition. The red cell morphology is normal, and the patients are not anemic, although in vitro research analysis can demonstrate a defect in the erythrocyte membrane skeleton (104, 105). Mild HE describes the usual form where patients exhibit no anemia, but have a well-compensated mild hemolytic anemia and prominent elliptocytosis on the peripheral blood smear. Occasionally, more severe hemolysis may occur, especially in a setting of splenomegaly due to other causes (106), infection (107, 108), or, occasionally, pregnancy (107). HE with infantile poikilocytosis is the variant characterized by excessively severe hemolysis (hyperbilirubinemia, poikilocytosis) in the newborn period, followed by a gradual transition to more classical HE over 6–24 months (109–112).

Spherocytic HE

Spherocytic HE is a condition that features the presence of both spherocytosis and elliptocytosis (113, 114). There is mild-to-moderate hemolysis, with increased osmotic fragility, as in HS. Splenic sequestration may occur, and splenectomy results in resolution of the hemolysis, as in cases of classical, autosomal dominant HS.

Southeast Asian Ovalocytosis

Southeast Asian ovalocytosisis a variant form found among inhabitants of Melanesia and Indonesia (115–117). It is characterized by stomatocytic elliptocytes, and its prevalence has been attributed to the relative resistance of the cells to infection by malarial organisms in vitro (118–121),

Table 7.3. Molecular Defects in HE

Type	Clinical Condition	Protein Abnormality	Molecular Defect
α SPECTRIN			
Spectrin α$^{I/78}$	Silent carrier to moderate HE in heterozygote	78 kd peptide on domain map	Arg 41→Trp
Spectrin Tunis (α$^{I/78}$)	Silent carrier to moderate HE in heterozygote	78 kd peptide on domain map	Arg 45→Ser
Spectrin α$^{I/74}$	Silent carrier to moderate HE in heterozygote/ severe HE to HPP in homozygote	74 kd peptide domain map	Arg28 Four point mutations
Spectrin Genova	Same as above	74 kd peptide on domain map	Arg 34→Trp
Spectrin Culoz	Same as above	74 kd peptide on domain map	Gly 46→Val
Spectrin Lyon	Same as above	74 kd peptide doman map	Lys 48→Arg
Spectrin α$^{I/165 \text{ or } 68}$	Silent carrier to mild HE in homozygote	65 kd peptide on domain map	Leu 49→Phe
Spectrin Ponte de Sor	Silent carrier in heterozygote moderate He in homozygote	65 kd peptide on domain map	Gly151→Asp
Spectrin α$^{I/61}$	Silent carrier in heterozygote/HPP in homozygote	61 kd peptide on domain map	?
Spectrin α$^{I/46}$	Mild HE in heterozygote/ HPP in homozygote	46 kd peptide on domain map	Deletion amino acids 178-226
Spectrin α$^{I/502}$	Mild HE in heterozygote/ HPP in hemozygote	50 kd peptide on domain map	Leu 207→Pro Leu 260→Pro Ser 261→Pro
Spectrin α$^{I/506}$	Mild HE in heterozygote	50 kd peptide on domain map	His 469→Arg Gun 471→Pro
Spectrin Alexandria	Mild to moderate HE in heterozygote	50 kd peptide on domain map	Deletion His 469
Spectrin α$^{I/43}$	Mild HE in heterozygote	43 kd peptide on domain map	?
Spectrin Sfax	Mild HE in heterozygote	36 and 33 kd peptides	Deletion amino acids 363-371
β SPECTRIN			
Associated with α$^{I/74}$ peptide	Silent carrier to moderate HE in heterozygote/severe HPP to hydrops fetalis in homozygote	β spectrin mutation leads to production of 74 kd alpha spectrin peptide on domain map	Ala 2053→Pro or other variants below

although this protection may be incomplete in vivo (122). The red cell morphology is remarkable for rounded elliptocytes, often with one or two transverse bars (123, 124). The rigidity of the elliptocytes is attributed to increased oligomerization of a mutant band 3 molecule, leading to increased association with the membrane skeleton (125). This latter mutant band 3 is described in a later section.

Pathophysiology

The defects in hereditary elliptocytosis and hereditary pyropoikilocytosis have been linked to defects in α- and β-spectrin, protein 4.1, and band 3. The membrane skeletons exhibit increased mechanical fragility under shear stress that can be demonstrated by ektacytometry. The spectrin defects lead to functional impairment in the ability of spectrin to self-associate, and include abnor-

malities in both the α- and β-chains. Several of the variants are named on the basis of the city of origin of the propositus, analogous to the hemoglobin variants. The molecular defects in HE are summarized in table 7.3.

Molecular Defects in Hereditary Elliptocytosis (Also Hereditary Pyropoikilocytosis [HPP] and Southeast Asian Ovalocytosis [SAO])
α-Spectrin defects

All the α-spectrin mutations in HE result in defective spectrin self-association, except for spectrin Jendouba (126). The consequence is mechanical instability of the red cell membrane and disordered structure of the membrane skeleton, as assessed by EM. HPP may arise by one of three mechanisms: homozygous HE mutations, compound heterozygosity for two different HE muta-

Table 7.3. Molecular Defects in HE, continued

Type	Clinical Condition	Protein Abnormality	Molecular Defect
β SPECTRIN, continued			
Spectrin Cagliari	Silent carrier to moderate HE in heterozygote/ severe HPP to hydrops fotalis in homozygote	β spectrin mutation leads to production of 74 kd alpha spectrin peptide on domain map	Ala 2018→Gly
Spectrin Providence	Silent carrier to moderate HE in heterozygote/ severe HPP to hydrops fetalis in homozygote	β spectrin mutation leads to production of 74 kd alpha spectrin peptide on domain map	Ser 2019→Pro
Spectrin β$^{220/218}$ (Rouen)	Moderate HE in heterozygote	Truncated β spectrin 218 kd	G→T in donor splice situ, exon skipping
Spectrin β$^{220/216}$ (Nice)	Moderate HE in heterozygote	Truncate β spectrin 216kd	AG dpulication at codon 2045/2046
Spectrin β$^{220/216}$ (Tandil)	Hemolytic HE	Truncate β spectrin 216 kd	Deletion 7bp at codon 2041
Spectrin β$^{220/216}$ (Tokyo)	Mild hemolytic HE	Truncate β spectrin 216 kd	Deletion C in condon 2059
Spectrin β$^{220/214}$ (Gottingen)	Moderate HE	Truncate β spectrin 214 kd	T→A in donor splice site, exon skipping
Spectrin β$^{220/214}$ (LePuy)	Moderate HE		A→G in donor splice site, exon skipping
PROTEIN 4.1			
Protein 4.1 deficiency	Mild HE in heterozygote/ severe hemolytic HE in homozygote	Heterozygote 50% protein 4.1 Homozygote 0% protein 4.1	In one kindred deletion of 318bp including erythroid translation initiation site
Protein 4.1 Madrid	Silent carrier in heterozygote/ severe HE in homozygote	Heterozygote 50% protein 4.1 Homozygote 0% protein 4.1	ATG→AGG at initiation codon
Protein 4.1$^{68/65}$	Mild HE in heterozygote	Truncated peptides 65 and 68 kd	Deletion amino acids 407-486
Protein 4.1^{95}	Mild HE	Elongated 95 kd peptide	Duplication amino acids 407-529
GLYCOPHORIN C			
Glycophorin C deficiency	Silent carrier in heterozygote/ mild HE in homozygote	Heterozygote: 50% glyco- phorin C homozygote: 0% glycophorin C	Deletion of exons 3 & 4 or deletion of 2bp in codons 44-45 and frameshift
BAND 3			
Southeast Asian ovalocytosis	Stomatocytic elliptocytosis in heterozygote	Abnormal anion transport, band 3 oligomerization	Deletion amino acids 400-408 alters signal sequence in first transmembrane helix, linked to silent Band 3 Memphis polymorphism (Lys 56→Glu)

tions, or an HE mutation with a defect in α-spectrin synthesis in the other allele (LELY allele). A "low expression" (LELY = Low Expression LYon) α-spectrin allele arises from skipping of exon 46 and occurs in association with a polymorphism of the $\alpha^{V/41}$ tryptic peptide (exon 40 mutation) (127, 128). The LELY allele can affect the relative expression of the normal to HE alleles and, thus, the clinical severity. If an HE mutation is on a chromosome bearing the α^{LELY} mutation, a mild defect can be converted into a silent one or a severe one into a mild one. In contrast, a defective HE allele inherited trans (on the opposite chromosome) to the low expression allele results in a more severe clinical condition.

During limited tryptic digestion of normal spectrin (86), the 80-kd αI domain, undergoes a second cleavage at Lys 45 or Lys 48 to produce the 74-kd domain. When abnormally high levels of the 74-kd peptide are produced compared with the 80-kd peptide, the $\alpha^{I/74}$ defect is identified. Similarly, when peptides of other molecular weight are produced instead of the 80-kd peptide, the disorders are designated by the size of those peptides. Identification of these peptide abnormalities led to the localization of the defect necessary to define the DNA mutations.

In order to identify the mutation responsible at the nucleotide sequence level, reverse transcription (RT) and polymerase chain reaction (PCR) are performed, utilizing specific primers flanking the region suspected to contain the mutation. Reticulocyte mRNA is isolated from the peripheral blood. The cDNA product is subcloned and subjected to nucleic acid sequencing. Several subclones must be obtained and sequenced in the heterozygous patients, because, on average, only half of the subclones will have the mutant allele. Many variations of this technique have been used to identify the mutations described in the following sections. In addition, other techniques, such as allele-specific oligonucleotide hybridization and heteroduplex mapping have also been used.

The majority of the spectrin mutations are characterized by a decrease or absence of the normal αI 80-kd domain, and appearance of smaller proteolytic fragments, including a new 78-kd peptide ($\alpha^{I/78}$) (129), a new 74-kd peptide ($\alpha^{I/74}$) (103, 105, 130, 131), a new 65-kd (or 68-kd) peptide ($\alpha^{I/65}$) or ($\alpha^{I/68}$) (132–135), a new 61-kd peptide ($\alpha^{I/61}$) (136), two new 46- and 17-kd (or, in other reports, 50- and 21-kd) peptides ($\alpha^{I/46}$ or $\alpha^{I/50a}$) (105, 137, 138), another 50-kd peptide with a more basic isoelectric point ($\alpha^{I/50b}$) (138), a defect with two new 42 and 43-kd peptides ($\alpha^{I/42–43}$) (139), or a new peptide of 36 kd ($\alpha^{I/36}$).

The precise mutations responsible for hereditary elliptocytosis have been identified for most of the α-chain variants. Figure 7.4 indicates the positions of many of these mutations. Of interest, a large number of the mutations occur in the helix 3 segments. The $\alpha^{I/78}$ defect can arise due to changes in codons 41 or 45, CGG to TGG (Arg to Trp) (spectrin Tunis) (140) or AGG to AGT (Arg to Ser) (141), respectively. The $\alpha^{I/74}$ defect can arise from four mutations in codon 28 (142–144) or from changes in codons 46 (GGT to GTT, Gly→Val:spectrin Culoz) (145), 48 (144), or 49 (CTT to TTT, Leu→Phe:spectrin Lyon) (145) (all helix 3 mutations). Codon 28 must therefore be a "hot spot" for mutations. Interestingly, the mutations arising in codon 45 or 48 result in severe HPP, whereas those arising in codons 41, 46, or 49 produce a milder HE phenotype. The $\alpha^{I/65}$ defect is a mild condition arising from the duplication of ^{154}Leu or in spectrin Ponte de Sor, ^{151}Gly→Asp^{138} (146). The mutation responsible for the $\alpha^{I/61}$ defect has not yet been defined. The $\alpha^{I/50a}$ defect results in the substitution of proline, an amino acid known to restrict mobility at three different positions: ^{207}Leu→Pro, ^{260}Leu→Pro, or ^{261}Ser→Pro^{138} (147, 148). The $\alpha^{I/50b}$ defect arises by three different mechanisms: ^{469}His→Pro, ^{471}Glu→Pro, or dele-

tion of ^{469}His (spectrin Alexandria) (138, 148, 149). The $\alpha^{I/36}$ defect (spectrin Sfax) results from deletion of codons 363–371, helix 3 of repeat 4, due to activation of a cryptic splice site (150).

There are two variants of the αII domain associated with asymptomatic HE in the heterozygous state: $\alpha^{II/31}$ defect (spectrin Jendouba)^{126} and $\alpha^{II/21}$ defect (spectrin Oran) (151). Spectrin Oran arises from a deletion of amino acids 822 to 862, due to a mutation A→G in the acceptor splice site for exon 18, resulting in skipping of exon 18.

One final α-spectrin abnormality in HE is a truncated chain (234 kd). Although spectrin containing this mutant chain is defective in self-association, studies thus far suggest that the primary defect may lie at the opposite end of the molecule, in the αIV domain (152).

Several clinical syndromes are associated with these α-chain defects. There appears to be an inverse relationship between the distance of the mutation from the self-association site and the clinical severity: the closer to the self-association site, the greater the functional defect, and the more severe the clinical illness (153). For example, the $\alpha^{I/74}$ defect produces severe disease with a greater proportion of spectrin dimers. The homozygous state results in life-threatening hemolytic anemia. In contrast, homozygous $\alpha^{I/65}$ spectrin is associated with only mild hemolysis and a more minor defect in spectrin self-association. The $\alpha^{I/46}$ mutation appears to be of intermediate severity.

In addition, patients with HPP have also been found to be deficient in spectrin (~30% less than the normal quantity) (154), which may be due to one of two mechanisms: reduced synthesis of α spectrin or increased degradation of mutant spectrin prior to assembly on the membrane. The latter hypothesis is supported by one study (155).

β-Spectrin defects

The β-spectrin abnormalities include truncations, which delete various amounts of the C-terminus, as well as missense mutations. Both groups of mutations alter spectrin

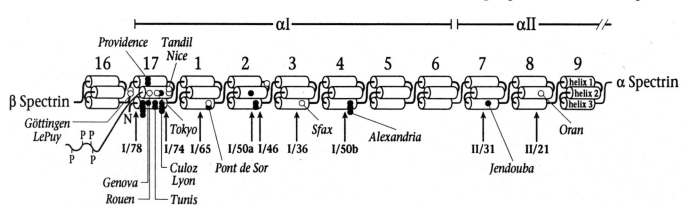

Figure 7.4. Location of mutations leading to hereditary elliptocytosis and hereditary pyropoikilocytosis. The circles represent the locations of mutations in C-terminal β-spectrin and N-terminal α-spectrin at the contact site between the two chains. (Adapted from Gallagher PG, Tse WT, Forget BG. Semin Perinatol 1992;14:351; figure 115-20 from The metabolic and molecular basis of inherited disease, 7th ed, 1995).

self-association. For example, for one of the β-spectrin truncated variants, $β^{220/216}$, in which ~4 kd is lost from the C-terminus, low-temperature spectrin extracts contain increased spectrin dimer ~50% of the dimer-tetramer pool, compared with normal value of 5–10%) and nearly all of the deleted $β^{216}$-spectrin is found in the dimer fraction (156, 157), indicating that $β^{216}$ is responsible for the functional defect. Seven different defects causing truncated β-spectrin chains have thus been identified on a molecular level: spectrin Rouen (158), spectrin Nice (159), spectrin Tandil (160), and spectrin Tokyo (161), due to frameshift mutations; spectrin LePuy (162) or spectrin Gottingen (163), due to exon skipping; and finally, spectrin Yamagata (a 210-kd variant for which the mechanism is as yet undefined) (164). The mutations are localized within helix 2 of repeat segment β17 (see fig. 7.4), and can lead to the $α^{I/74}$ abnormality on limited tryptic domain maps. Moreover, point mutations in this same region of β17 at codon 2053 (Ala to Pro), at codon 2019 (Ser→Pro) (spectrin Providence) (165) or at codon 2018 (Ala→Gly) (spectrin Cagliari) (166) can lead to the $α^{I/74}$ abnormality on domain maps and severe HPP in the homozygous state, or in the case of spectrin Providence, to lethal hydrops fetalis (165).

> Clinically, the patients with the β-spectrin truncations have mild-to-moderate hemolysis with prominent elliptocytosis and some fragmented red cells. Thermal stability is unusual; the red cells become echinocytic at 47°C (normal = 49°C), but do not fragment.

Protein 4.1 Deficiency

In several kindreds with HE, protein 4.1 was found to be either partially deficient or completely absent (167, 168). These variants appear to be more common in patients of French and North African descent. Protein 4.1 is decreased about 50% in heterozygotes and is absent in homozygotes. Clinically, the heterozygotes have mild HE with little or no hemolysis. In contrast, homozygotes have a severe transfusion-dependent hemolytic anemia with marked osmotic fragility, normal thermal stability, bizarre red cell morphology, and a very good response to splenectomy. The homozygous 4.1-deficient membranes are very fragile, but stability can be restored by reconstitution with purified protein 4.1 or even a recombinant peptide containing the region critical for spectrin-actin binding.

Molecular genetic studies in one Algerian kindred show that the disease is caused by a 318nt deletion that eliminates the initiation codon that gives rise to the 80-kd erythroid isoform of protein 4.1 (169, 170). A second family has an altered downstream initiation codon (ATG to AGG, 4.1^{Madrid}), which presumably blocks expression of the erythroid protein 4.1 isoform (171).

In addition to deficiency in protein 4.1, some of these patients are also missing (partially) other proteins, such as protein 4.9 or glycophorin C (172). Patients with complete protein 4.1 deficiency have only 9% of the normal amount of glycophorin C. This lends strong support to the theory that protein 4.1 binds to glycophorin C in the membrane.

Structural and Functional Defects of Protein 4.1

Three structural anomalies of protein 4.1 have been described. One of these occurred in two generations of a French family with mild HE and moderate chronic hemolysis (173). The disorder is characterized by prominent elliptocytosis with mechanically fragile membranes. Osmotic and thermal stability and spectrin self-association are normal. SDS gels show a 50% reduction in protein 4.1 and two faint new bands, 65 and 68 kd, that are immunologically related to 4.1. Functionally, the patient's 4.1 bind to a crude mixture of normal spectrin and actin only 40% as well as normal. A similar variant has been observed in the dog (76/78 kd) (174). Molecular studies demonstrated that protein $4.1^{68/65}$ was due to a deletion of 80 amino acids, Lys^{407}-Gly^{486}, which includes the entire spectrin-actin binding domain, Lys^{407}-Glu^{427}, whereas the canine protein $4.1^{78/76}$ results from a deletion of precisely the 21-amino acid peptide that arises by alternative splicing of a 63nt exon critical for spectrin-actin binding. The second defect has been identified in a single kindred with mild HE. The patients are heterozygous for an elongated (95-kd) variant of protein 4.1, designated protein 4.1^{95} (175), that comigrates with protein 3 and is detected with immunoblots. This anomaly results from the internal duplication of a 369nt segment consisting of three exons that encodes for Lys^{407}-Gln^{529} (176), thus producing two spectrin-actin-binding domains. Fortunately, this latter insertion does not markedly alter spectrin-actin binding, which probably accounts for its relatively mild clinical phenotype.

The third variant, designated $4.1^{Presles}$ is a shortened protein 4.1 that migrates as a doublet with an apparent molecular weight of 73 and 74 kd (177). This is caused by skipping of one exon that encodes 34 amino acids near the beginning of the C-terminal 22/24-kd domain (178). The clinical condition is apparent only in the homozygous state.

Deficiency of Glycophorin C

Deficiency of this minor sialoglycoprotein occurs in homozygous protein 4.1 deficiency, as described above, and in patients with the rare Leach phenotype of Gerbich-negative (Ge−) red cells. The Gerbich antigen system is carried on glycophorins C and D. Patients with the Leach subtype of Ge− lack both glycophorin C and D (179). These patients, but not other patients with Ge− red cells (who lack the antigen but not glycophorins C and D), have mild elliptocytosis with increased fragility. Their red cells contain only 30% of the normal amount of protein 4.1 (172), which may account for the elliptocytic phenotype. This information strongly suggests that glycophorin C is an important binding site for protein 4.1 in normal red cells.

In contrast, patients lacking glycophorin A, B, or both A and B are entirely asymptomatic and have normal red cell morphology.

Defects of Band 3

Band 3 Memphis. The band 3 Memphis polymorphism results from the point mutation Lys^{56} to Glu (180, 181). This changes the electrophoretic mobility such that the variant band 3 migrates more slowly and the N-terminal chymotryptic fragment has a molecular weight of 63 instead of 60 kd (182). Six to seven percent of the normal population is heterozygous for this variant, but the polymorphism is entirely silent, even in the homozygous state, unless accompanied by the deletion of amino acid residues 400–408, the lesion identified in patients with Southeast Asian ovalocytosis.

Southeast Asian Ovalocytosis (SAO). The prevalence of this condition has been attributed to the resistance of the ovalocytes to invasion by *Plasmodium falciparum* (120). The affected individuals are heterozygous for a band 3 variant designated band 3 SAO which has an electrophoretic migration identical to band 3 Memphis. Molecular genetic analysis has revealed two abnormalities in the SAO allele: (a) the band 3 Memphis polymorphism, $Lys^{56} \rightarrow Glu$, and (b) the deletion of amino acid residues 400–408 at the junction between the cytoplasmic and membrane domains (117, 183, 184). This deletion removes part of the first transmembrane α-helix, which is thought to serve as an internal signal sequence and probably disrupts the structure of the membrane region. As a consequence, band 3 SAO lacks anion transport activity. This may explain why homozygous band 3 SAO is not observed (presumably lethal).

As noted earlier, SAO red cells are extraordinarily rigid, the most rigid red cells known. This impedes entry of malarial parasites, which may account for the high frequency of the mutations in the indigenous populations of Southeast Asia. Moriyama and colleagues (185) have observed that band 3 is nonspecifically trapped in isolated skeletons from SAO red cells, while Liu and colleagues have described increased oligomerization of band 3 SAO associated with the membrane skeleton which they propose as the mechanism for the increased rigidity (186). Remarkably, the rigid SAO red cells negotiate the circulation normally and do not lead to impaired tissue perfusion or hemolysis.

Hereditary acanthocytosis. One band 3 variant associated with acanthocytosis has been described with increased anion transport activity, decreased ankyrin binding sites, and slightly slowed mobility on SDS gels (187). Peptide mapping suggested that there was an alteration in the membrane domain. The effect on ankyrin binding might reflect changes in band 3 oligomerization or indicate previously unrecognized interactions between the C-terminal end of the protein, which lies inside the membrane, and the ankyrin-binding site on the N-terminal, cytoplasmic domain. The mutation has been identified as Pro868→Leu (188).

Summary

HS and HE are thus very heterogeneous disorders associated with a large number of molecular defects. In many kindreds, the actual mutations have been identified. However, despite our knowledge of the defective structure and function of the specific membrane proteins, we still do not understand how those abnormalities lead to a spheroidal or an elliptical shape.

Regarding the shape of elliptocytes, it has been noted that *nucleated* elliptocyte precursors are round, and the cells only elongate or fragment gradually as they circulate. This process resembles the progressive development of spherocytosis in hereditary spherocytes, and is consistent with the concept that the change in shape is secondary to the intrinsic structural instability of the skeleton. Mild skeletal defects lead to elliptocytosis by increasing membrane plasticity. As noted earlier, normal red cells rapidly regain their shape if they are transiently deformed, but they remain misshapen if the distortion is maintained for long periods of time (minutes to hours). Presumably, protein skeletal interactions realign in response to stress. In a cell with weakened skeletal interactions, like the hereditary elliptocyte, this process would be accelerated. In vivo red cells are deformed into a stable elliptical or torpedo shape in very small capillaries and are sometimes detained for short periods of time. It is easy to imagine how this distortion, repeated thousands of times per day, could cause red cells to gradually elongate and assume their characteristic shape in typical mild HE. This hypothesis remains to be proved.

Red cells with more severe skeletal defects would also tend to elongate, but if skeletal instability were sufficiently compromised, they would be unable to withstand the shear stresses experienced in the normal circulation, and fragmentation would predominate. This process would explain the nearly identical morphology observed in homozygous HE and hereditary pyropoikilocytosis (HPP), and in neonates with mild HE and poikilocytosis.

In spite of the uncertainties about the molecular mechanisms involved in the different subtypes of HE, the available information suggests that red cell death in the various hemolytic forms follows a similar pathway. In all cases hemolysis is markedly ameliorated by splenectomy, and where examined, splenic pathology shows cordal congestion essentially identical to that observed in HS.

In contrast, in HS, there is progressive membrane loss related to defective attachment of the membrane skeleton to the lipid bilayer. The progressive loss of membrane leads to a decreased surface area-to-volume ratio, and hence a more spheroidal cell than the biconcave disc. The spheroidal cells have decreased deformability and become entrapped in the spleen. Retention in the harsh environment of the spleen leads to progressive membrane damage and eventual hemolysis.

As summarized in this chapter, numerous types of molecular defects have been identified in these conditions that contribute to the pathophysiology of the hereditary hemolytic anemias.

REFERENCES

1. Saarinen UM, Chorba TL, Tattersall R, Young NS, Anderson LJ, Palmer E, Cocela PF. Human parovirus B-19 induced epidemic acute red cell aplasia in patients with hereditary hemolytic anemia. Blood 1986;67:1411.

2. Lefrere JJ, Courouce MA, Girot R, Bertrand Y, Soulier JP. Six cases of hereditary spherocytosis revealed by human parovirus infection. Br J Haematol 1986;62:653.

3. Schwartz RS, Chiu DT, Lubin B. Plasma membrane phospholipid organization in human erythrocytes. Curr Top Hematol 1985;5:63.

4. Verkleij AJ, Zwaal RFA, Roelofsen B, Confurius P, Kastelijn D, van Deenen LLM. The asymmetric distribution of phospholipids in the human red cell memabrane: a combined study using phospholipase and frees-etch electron microscopy. Biochim Biophys Acta 1973;323:178.

5. Steck TL. The organization of proteins in the human red cell membrane. J Cell Biol 1974;62:1.

6. Fukuda M. Molecular genetics of the glycophorin A gene cluster. Semin Hematol 1993;30:138.

7. Cartron JP, Le Van Kim C, Colin Y. Glycophorin C and related glycophorins: structure, function, and regulation. Semin Hematol 1993;30:152.

8. Tanner MJA. Molecular and cellular biology of the erythrocyte anion exchanger (AE1). Semin Hematol 1993; 30:34.

9. Reid MD, Takakuwa Y, Conboy J, Tchernia G, Mohandas N. Glycophorin C content of human erythrocyte membranes is regulated by protein 4.1. Blood 1990;75:2229.

10. Kliman HJ, Steck TL. Association of glyceraldehyde-3-phosphate dehydrogenase with the human red cell membrane: a kinetic analysis. J Biol Chem 1980;255:6314.

11. Tsai I-H, Prasanna-Murthy SN, Steck TL. Effect of red cell membrane binding on the catalytic activity of glyceraldehyde-3-phosphate dehydrogenase with the human red cell membrane. J Biol Chem 1982;259:1438.

12. Jenkins JD, Madden DP, Steck TL. Association of phosphofructionkinase and aldolase with the membrane of the intact erythrocyte. J Biol Chem 1984;259:9374.

13. De BK, Kirtley ME. Interaction of phosphosphoglycerate kinase with human erythrocyte membranes. J Biol Chem 1977;252:6715.

14. Walder JA, Chatterjee R, Steck TL, Low PS, Musso GF, Kaiser ET, Rogers PH, Arnone A. The interaction of hemoglobin with the cytoplasmic domain of band 3 of the human erythrocyte membrane. J Biol Chem 1984;259:10238.

15. Bennett V, Stenbuck PJ. The membrane attachment protein for spectrin is associated with band 3 in human erythrocyte membranes. Nature 1979;280:468.

16. Bennett V, Stenbuck PJ. Association between ankyrin and the cytoplasmic domain of band 3 isolated from the human erythrocyte membrane. J Biol Chem 1980;255:6424.

17. Hargreaves WR, Giedd KN, Verkleij A, Branton D. Reassociation of ankyrin with band 3 in erythrocyte membranes and in lipid vesicles. J Biol Chem 1980;255:11965.

18. Lombardo CR, Willardson BM, Low PS. Localization of the protein 4.1-binding site on the cytoplasmic domain of erythrocyte membrane band 3. J Biol Chem 1992; 267:9540.

19. Johnsson R. Red cell membrane proteins and lipids in spherocytosis. Scand J Haematol 1978;20:341.

20. Korsgren C, Cohen CM. Associations of human erythrocyte protein 4.2: binding to ankyrin and to the cytoplasmic domain of band 3. J Biol Chem 1988;263:10212.

21. White RA, Peters LL, Adkinson LR, Korsgren C, Cohen CM, Lux SE. The murine pallid mutation is a platelet storage pool disease associated with the protein 4.2 (pallidin) gene. Nature 1992;2:80.

22. Sheetz MP. Integral membrane protein interaction with Triton cytoskeletons of erythrocytes. Biochim Biophys Acta 1979;557:122.

23. Yu J, Fischman DA, Steck TL. Selective solubilization of proteins and phospholipids of red blood cell membranes by nonionic detergents. J Supramol Struct 1973; 1:233.

24. Liu S, Derick LH, Palek J. Visualization of the hexagonal lattice in the erythrocyte membrane skeleton. J Cell Biol 1987;104:527.

25. Ungewickell E, Gratzer W. Self-association of human spectrin: a thermodynamic and kinetic study. Eur J Biochem 1978;88:379.

26. Liu SC, Windisch P, Kim P, Palek J. Oligomeric states of spectrin in normal erythrocyte membranes. Cell 1984; 37:587.

27. Cohen CM, Foley SF. The role of band 4.1 in the association of actin with erythrocyte membranes. Biochim Biophys Acta 1982;688:691.

28. Ohanian V, Wolfe LC, John KM, Pinder JC, Lux SE, Gratzer WB. Analysis of the ternary interaction of the red cell membrane skeletal proteins spectrin, actin and protein 4.1. Biochemistry 1984;23:4416.

29. Liu SC, Derick LH, Agre P, et al. Alteration of the erythrocyte skeletal ultrastructure in hereditary spherocytosis, hereditary elliptocytosis and pyropoikilocytosis. Blood 1990;76:198.

30. Sahr KE, Laurila P, Kotula L, Scarpa AL, Coupal E, Leto TL, Linnenbach AJ, Winkelmann JC, Speicher DW, Marchesi VT, Curtis PL, Forget BG. The complete cDNA and polypeptide sequences of the cDNA for human erythroid alpha spectrin. J Biol Chem 1990; 265:4434.

31. Winkelmann JC, Chang JG, Tse WT, Marchesi VT, Forget BG. Full length sequence of the cDNA for human erythroid beta-spectrin. J Biol Chem 1990; 265:11827.

32. Speicher DW, Morrow JS, Knowles WJ, Marchesi VT. Identification of proteolytically resistant domains of human erythrocyte spectrin. Proc Natl Acad Sci USA 1980; 77:5673.

33. Speicher D, Morrow JS, Knowles WJ, Marchesi VT. A structural model of juman erythrocyte spectrin: alignment of chemical and functional domains. J Biol Chem 1982; 257:9093.

34. Speicher DW, Marchesi VT. Erythrocyte spectrin is comprised of many homologous triple helical segments. Nature 1984;311:177.

35. Speicher DW. The present status of erythrocyte spectrin structure: the 106-residue repetitive structure is a basic feature of an entire class of proteins. J Cell Biochem 1986; 30:245.

36. Luna EJ, Kidd GH, Branton D. Identification by peptide analysis of the spectrin-binding protein in human erythrocytes. J Biol Chem 1979;254:2526.

37. Yu J, Goodman SR. Syndeins: the spectrin-binding protein(s) of the human erythrocyte membrane. Proc Natl Acad Sci USA 1979;76:2340.

38. Tyler JM, Reinhardt BN, Branton D. Associations of erythrocyte membrane proteins: binding of purified bands 2.1 and 4.1 to spectrin. J Biol Chem 1980;255:7034.

39. Lux SE, John KM, Bennett V. Analysis of cDNA for human erythrocyte ankyrin indicates a repeated structure with homology to tissue-differentiation and cell-cycle control proteins. Nature 1990;344:36.

40. Davis LH, Davis JQ, Bennett V. Ankyrin regulation: an alternatively spliced segment of the regulatory domain functions as an intramolecular modulator. J Biol Chem 1992; 267:18966.

41. Inaba M, Gupta KC, Kuwabara M, Takahaski T, Benz EJ, Maede Y. Deamidation of human erythrocyte protein 4.1: possible role in aging. Blood 1992;79:3355.

42. Mueller TJ, Jackson CW, Dockler ME, Morrison M. Membrane skeletal alterations during in vivo mouse red cell aging. Increase in the band 4.1a:4.1b ratio. J Clin Invest 1987;79:492.

43. Correas I, Leto TL, Speicher DW, Marchesi VT. Identification of the functional site of erythrocyte protein 4.1 involved in spectrin-actin associations. J Biol Chem 1986; 261:3310.

44. Pasternack GR, Racusen RH. Erythrocyte protein 4.1 binds and regulates myosin. Proc Natl Acad Sci USA 1989; 86:9712.

45. Horne WC, Huang S, Becker PS, Tang TK, Benz Jr. Tissue-specific alternative splicing of protein 4.1 inserts an exon necessary for formation of the ternary complex with erythrocyte spectrin and actin. Blood 1993; in press.

46. Chasis JA, Coulombel L, Conboy J, McGee S, Andrews K, Kan YW, Mohandas N. Differentiation-associated switches in protein 4.1 expression: synthesis of multiple structural isoforms during normal human erythropoiesis. J Clin Invest 1993;91:329.

47. Anderson RA, Lovrien RE. Glycophorin is linked to band 4.1 protein to the human erythrocyte membrane skeleton. Nature 1984;307:655.

48. Mueller TJ, Manson M. Glycoconnectin (PAS2), a membrane attachment site for the human erythrocyte cytoskeleton. In: Krockeberg W, Eaton J, Greuner G, eds. Erythrocyte membranes: 2. Clinical and experimental advances. New York: Alan R. Liss, 1981:95.

49. Pasternack GR, Anderson RA, Leto TR, Marchesi VT. Interactions between protein 4.1 and band 3: an alternative binding site for an element of the membrane skeleton. J Biol Chem 1985;260:3676.

50. Pinder JC, Chung A, Reid ME, Gratzer WB. Membrane attachment sites for the membrane cytoskeletal protein 4.1 of the red blood cell. Blood 1993;82:3482.

51. Pinder JC, Gratzer WB. Structural and dynamic states of actin in the erythrocyte. J Cell Biol 1983;96:768.

52. Nakaskima K, Beutler E. Comparison of structure and function of human erythrocyte and human muscle actin. Proc Natl Acad Sci USA 1979;76:935.

53. Byers T, Branton D. Visualization of the proteins associations in the erythrocyte membrane skeleton. Proc Natl Acad Sci USA 1985;82:6153.

54. Fowler VM. Tropomodulin: a cytoskeletal protein that binds to the end of erythrocyte tropomyosin and inhibits tropomyosin binding to actin. J Cell Biol 1990;111:471.

55. Karinch AM, Zimmer WE, Goodman SR. The identification and sequence of the actin-binding domain of human red blood cell β-spectrin. J Biol Chem 1980; 265:11833.

56. Bresnick AR, Janmey PA, Condeelis J. Evidence that a 27-residue sequence is the actin-binding site of ABP-120. J Biol Chem 1991;266:12989.

57. Siegel DL, Branton D. Partial purification and characterization of an actin-binding protein, band 4.9, from human erythrocytes. J Cell Biol 1985;100:775.

58. Husain-Chishti A, Levin A, Branton D. Abolition of actin-bundling by phosphorylation of erythrocyte protein 4.9. Nature 1988;334:718.

59. Gardner K, Bennett V. Modulation of spectrin-actin assembly by erythrocyte adducin. Nature 1987;328:359.

60. Fowler VM, Bennett V. Tropomyosin: a new component of the erythrocyte membrane skeleton. In: Kruckeberg WC, Eaton JW, eds. Erythrocyte membrane 3: Recent clinical and experimental advances. New York: Alan R. Liss, 1984:57.

61. Fowler VM. Identification and purification of a novel Mr 43,000 tropomyosin-binding protein from human erythrocyte membranes. J Biol Chem 1987;262:12792.

62. Fowler VM, Sussmann MA, Miller PG, Flucher BE, Daniels MP. Tropomodulin is associated with the free (pointed) ends of the thin filaments in rat skeletal muscle. J Cell Biol 1993;120:411.

63. Agre P, Orringer EP, Bennett V.: Deficient red-cell spectrin in severe, recessively inherited spherocytosis. N Engl J Med 1982;306:1155.

64. Agre P, Asimos A, Casella JF, McMillan D. Inheritance pattern and clinical response to splenectomy as a reflection of erythrocyte spectrin deficiency in hereditary spherocytosis. N Engl J Med 1986;315:1579.

65. Savvides P, Shalev O, John KM, Lux SE. Combined spectrin and ankyrin deficiency is common in dominant hereditary spherocytosis. Blood 1993;82:2953.

66. Bernstein SE. Inherited hemolytic disease in mice: a review and update. Lab Anim Sci 1980;30:197.

67. Bodine DM, Birkenmeier CS, Barker JE. Spectrin-deficient inherited hemolytic anemias in the mouse: characterization by spectrin synthesis and mRNA activity in reticulocytes. Cell 1984;37:721.

68. Bloom ML, Barker JE. A C to T transition in the beta spectrin gene found in the jaundiced mouse DNA. Blood 1993; 82:308a.

69. White RA, Birkenmeier CS, Lux SE, Barker JE. Ankyrin and the hemolytic anemia mutation, nb, map to mouse chromosome 8: presence of the nb allele is associated with a truncated erythrocyte ankyrin. Proc Natl Acad Sci USA 1990;87:3117.

70. Peters LL, Birkenmeier CS, Bronson RT, White RA, Lux SE, Otto E, Bennett V, Barker JE. Purkinje cell degeneration associated with erythroid ankyrin deficiency in nb/nb mice. J Cell Biol 1991;114:1233.

71. Peters LL, Birkenmeier CS, Barker JE. Fetal compensation of the hemolytic anemia in mice homozygous for the normoblastosis, nb, mutation. Blood 1992;80:2122.

72. Peters LL, Turtzo C, Birkenmeier CS, Barker JE. Distinct fetal Ank-1 and Ank-2 related proteins and mRNAs in normal and nb/nb mice. Blood 1993; 81:2144.

73. Agre P, Casella JF, Zinkham WH, McMillan C, Bennett V. Partial deficiency of erythrocyte synthesis in burst-forming units-erythroid in lethal hereditary spherocytosis. Nature 1985;314:380.

74. Whitfield CF, Follweiler JB, Lopresti-Morrow L, Miller BA. Deficiency of α-spectrin synthesis in burst-forming units-erythroid in lethal hereditary spherocytosis. Blood 1991; 78:3043.

75. Kimberling WJ, Taylor PA, Chapman RG, Lubs HA. Linkage and gene localization of hereditary spherocytosis (HS). Blood 1978;52:859.

76. Bass EB, Smith SW, Stevenson RE, Rosse WF. Further evidence for location of the spherocytosis gene on chromosome 8. Ann Intern Med 1983;99:192.

77. Chilcote RR, LeBeau MM, Dampler C, Pergament E, Verlinsky Y, Mohandas N, Frischer H, Rowley JD. Association of red cell spherocytosis with deletion of the short arm of chromosome 8. Blood 1987;69:156.

78. Lux SE, Tse WT, Menninger JC, John KM, Harris P, Shalev O, Chilcote RR, Marchesi SL, Watkins PC, Bennett V, McIntosh S, Collins FS, Francke U, Ward DC, Forget BG. Hereditary spherocytosis associated with deletion of the human erythrocyte ankyrin gene on chromosome 8. Nature 1990;345:736.

79. Costa FF, Agre P, Watkins SM, Winkelmann JC, Tang TK, John KM, Lux SE, Forget BG. Linkage of dominant hereditary spherocytosis to the gene for the erythrocyte membrane-skeleton protein ankyrin. N Engl J Med 1990; 323:1046.

80. Jarolim P, Brabec V, Lambert S, Liu SC, Zhou Z, Palek J. Ankyrin Prague: a dominantly inherited mutation of the regulatory domain of ankyrin associated with hereditary spherocytosis. Blood 1990;76(Suppl 1):37a.

81. Eber SW, Lux ML, Gonzalez JM, Scarpa A, Tse WT, Gallagher PG, Pekrun A, Forget BG, Lux SE. Discovery of 8 ankyrin mutations in hereditary spherocytosis (HS) indicates that ankyrin defects are a major cause of dominant and recessive HS. Blood 1993(Suppl) in press.

82. Elgsaeter A. A classical light scattering study. Biochim Biophys Acta 1978;536:235.

83. Bouhassira EE, Schwartz RS, Yawata Y, Ata K, Kanzaki A, Qui JJ-H, Nagel RL, Rybicki AC. An alanine-to-threonine substitution in protein 4.2 cDNA is associated with a Japanese form of hereditary hemolytic anemia (protein 4.2^{NIPPON}). Blood 1992;79:1846.

84. Shotton DM, Burke BE, Branton D. The molecular structure of human erythrocyte spectrin: biophysical and electron microscopic studies. J Mol Biol 1979;131:303.

85. Jarolim P, Palek J, Rubin HL, Prchal JT, Korsgren C, Cohen CM. Band 3 Tuscaloosa: Pro^{327}Arg^{327} substitution in the cytoplasmic domain of erythrocyte band 3 protein associated with spherocytic hemolytic anemia and partial deficiency of protein 4.2. Blood 1992;80:523.

86. Jarolim P, Rubin HL, Brabec V, et al. Band 3 Prague: a duplication of 10 bases in the erythroid band 3 gene in a kindred with hereditary spherocytosis with band 3 deficiency. Blood 1992;80(Suppl 1):277a.

87. Miraglia del Giudice E, Perrotta S, Pinto L, Cappellini MD, Fiorelli G, Cutillo S, Iolascon A. Hereditary spherocytosis characterized by increased spectrin/band 3 ratio. Br J Haematol 1992;80:133 (letter).

88. Lux S, Bedrosian C, Shalev O, Morris M, Chasis J, Davies K, Savvides P, Telen M. Deficiency of band 3 in dominant

89. Goodman SR, Shiffer KA, Casoria LA, Eyster ME. Identification of the molecular defect in the erythrocyte membrane skeleton of some kindreds with hereditary spherocytosis. Blood 1982;60:772.

90. Wolfe LC, John KM, Falcone JC, Byrne AM, Lux SE. A genetic defect in the binding protein 4.1 to spectrin in a kindred with hereditary spherocytosis. N Engl J Med 1982; 307:1367.

91. Becker PS, Morrow JS, Lux SE. Abnormal oxidant sensitivity and beta-chain structure of spectrin in hereditary spherocytosis associated with defective spectrin-protein 4.1 binding. J Clin Invest 1987;80:557.

92. Becker PS, Tse WT, Lux SE, Forget BG. β-Spectrin Kissimmee: a spectrin variant associated with autosomal dominant hereditary spherocytosis and defective binding to protein 4.1. J Clin Invest 1993;92:612.

93. Becker PS, Schwartz MA, Morrow JS, Lux SE. Radiolabel-transfer cross-linking demonstrates that the protein 4.1 binds to the N-terminal region of beta spectrin and to actin in binary interactions. Eur J Biochem 1990;193:827.

94. Lande WM, Mentzer WC. Haemolytic anaemia associated with increased cation permeability. Clin Haematol 1985; 14:89.

95. Morle L, Pothier B, et al. Reduction of membrane band 7 and actovatopm pf vp;i,e sto,i;ated (K$^+$, Cl$^-$)-contrasport in a case of congenital stomatocytosis. Br J Haematol 1989;71:141.

96. Eber SW, Lande WM, et al. Hereditary stomatocytosis: consistent association with an integral membrane protein. Br J Haematol 1989;72:452.

97. Lande WM, Thiemann PV, et al. Missing band 7 membrane protein in two patients with high Na, low K erythrocytes. J Clin Invest 1982;70:1273.

98. Hiebl-Dirschmied C, Entler B, et al. Cloning and nucleotide sequence of cDNA encoding human erythrocyte band 7 integral membrane protein. Biochim Biophys Acta 1991;1090:123.

99. Dhermy D, Lecomte MC, Garbarz M, Feo C, Gauter H, Bournier O, Galand C, Herrera A, Gretillat F, Boivin P. Molecular defect of spectrin in the family of a child with congenital hemolytic poikilocytic anemia. Pediatr Res 1984;18:1005.

100. Lawler J, Liu SC, Palek J, Prchal J. Molecular defect of spectrin in hereditary pyropoikilocytosis: alterations in the trypsin-resistant domain involved in spectrin self-association. J Clin Invest 1982;70:1019.

101. Lawler J, Liu SC, Palek J, Prchal J. Molecular defect of spectrin in a subgroup of patients with hereditary elliptocytosis: alteration in the alpha subunit involved in spectrin self association. J Clin Invest 1984;73:1688.

102. Ozer L, Mills GC. Elliptocytosis with haemolytic anaemia. Br J Haematol 1964;10:468.

103. Jensson O, Jonasson TH, Olafsson O. Hereditary elliptocytosis in Iceland. Br J Haematol 1967;13:844.

104. Nkrumah FK. Hereditary elliptocytosis associated with severe haemolytic anaemia and malaria. Afr J Med Sci 1972; 3:131.

105. Josephs HW, Avery ME. Hereditary elliptocytosis associated with increased hemolysis. Pediatrics 1965;16:741.

106. Austin RF, Desforges FJ. Hereditary elliptocytosis: an unusual presentation of hemolysis in the newborn associated

with transient morphologic abnormalities. Pediatrics 1969; 44:196.

107. Carpentieri U, Gustavson LP, Haggard ME. Pyknocytosis in a neonate: an unusual presentation of hereditary elliptocytosis. Clin Pediatr 1977;16:76.

108. Zarkowsky HS, Mohandas N, Speaker CB, Shohet SB. A congenital haemolytic anaemia with thermal sensitivity of the erythrocyte membrane. Br J Haematol 1975; 29:537.

109. Cutting HO, McHugh, Conrad FG, Marlow AA. Autosomal dominant hemolytic anemia characterized by ovalocytosis: a family study of seven involved members. Am J Med 1965; 39:21.

110. Greenberg LH, Tanaka KR. Hereditary elliptocytosis with hemolytic anemia—a family study of five affected members. Calif Med 1969;110:389.

111. Amato D, Booth PB. Hereditary ovalocytosis in Melanesians. Papua New Guinea Med J 1977;20:26.

112. Fix AG, Baer AS, Lie-Injo LE. The mode of inheritance of ovalocytosis/elliptocytosis in Malaysian Orang Asli families. Hum Genet 1982;61:250.

113. Liu S, Zhai S, Palek J, Golan DE, Amato D, Hassan K, Nurse G, Babona D, Coetzer T, Jarolim P, Zaik M, Borwein S. Molecular defect of the band 3 protein in Southeast Asian ovalocytosis. N Engl J Med 1990;323:1530.

114. Kidson C, Lamont G, Saul A, Nurse G. Ovalocytic erythrocytes from Melanesians are resistant to invasion by malaria parasites in culture. Proc Natl Acad Sci USA 1981;78:5829.

115. Hadley T, Saul A, Lamont G, Hudson DE, Miller LH, Kidson C. Resistance of Melanesian elliptocytes (ovalocytes) to invasion by *Plasmodium knowlesi* and *Plasmodium falciparum* malaria parasites in vitro. J Clin Invest 1983;71:780.

116. Mohandas N, Lie-Injo LE, Friedman M, Mak JW. Rigid membranes of Malayan ovalocytes: a likely genetic barrier against malaria. Blood 1984;63:1385.

117. Saul A, Lamont G, Sawyer WH, Kidson C. Decreased membrane deformability in Melanesian ovalocytes from Papua New Guinea. J Cell Biol 1984;98:1348.

118. Serjeantson S, Bryson K, Amato D, Babona D. Malaria and hereditary ovalocytosis. Hum Gent 1977;37:161.

119. Harrison KL, Collins KA, McKenna HW. Hereditary elliptical stomatocytosis; a case report. Pathology 1976;8:307.

120. Booth PB, Sevjeantson S, Woodfield DG, Amato D. Selective depression of blood group antigens associated with hereditary ovalocytosis among Melanesians. Vox Sang 1977;32:99.

121. Liu SC, Nichols PE, Yi SJ, Derick LH, Chiou SS, Amato D, Palek J. Southeast Asian ovalocytosis. Blood 1993;82.

122. Alloisio N, Wilmotte R, Morle L, Baklouti F, Marechal J, Ducluzeau M, Denoroy L, Feo C, Forget BG, Kastally R, Delaunay J. Spectrin Jendouba: an $\alpha^{II/31}$ spectrin variant that is associated with elliptocytosis and carries a mutation distant from the dimer self-association site. Blood 1992; 80:809.

123. Alloisio N, Morle L, Marechal J, Roux A-F, Ducluzeau MT, Guetarni D, Pothier B, Baklouti F, Ghanem A, Kastally R, Delaunay J. Sp$\alpha^{v/41}$: a common spectrin polymorphism at the α^{IV}–α^{V} domain junction: relevance to the expression level of hereditary elliptocytosis due to α-spectrin variants located in *trans*. J Clin Invest 1991;87:2169.

124. Wilmotte R, Marechal J, Morle L, Baklouti F, Philippe N, Kastally R, Kotula L, Delaunay J, Alloisio N. Low expression allele α^{LELY} of red cell spectrin is associated with mutations

in exon 40 ($\alpha^{V/41}$ polymorphism) and intron 45 and with partial skipping of exon 46. J Clin Invest 1993; 91:2091.

125. Morle L, Alloisio N, Ducluzeau MT, Pothier B, Blibech R, Kastally R, Delaunay J. Spectrin Tunis ($\alpha^{1/78}$): a new I variant that causes asymptomatic hereditary elliptocytosis in the heterozygous state. Blood 1988;71:508.

126. Palek J, Liu SC, Liu PY, Prchal J, Castleberry RP. Altered assembly of spectrin in red cell membranes in hereditary pyropoikilocytosis. Blood 1981;57:130.

127. Lecomte MC, Dhermy D, Garbarz M, Gautero H, Bournier O, Galand C, Boivin P. Hereditary elliptocytosis with spectrin molecular defect in a white patient. Acta Haematol (Basel) 1984;71:235.

128. Garbarz M, Lecomte MC, Dhermy D, Feo C, Chaveroche I, Gautero H, Bournier O, Picat C, Goepp A, Boivin P. Double inheritance of an alpha I/65 spectrin variant in a child with homozygous elliptocytosis. Blood 1986;67:1661.

129. Lecomte MC, Dhermy D, Solis C, Ester A, Feo C, Gauters H, Bournier O, Boivin P. A new abnormal variant of spectrin black patients with hereditary elliptocytosis. Blood 1985;65:1208.

130. Alloisio N, Guetorni D, Morle L, Pothier B, Duchizeau MT, Soun A, Colonna P, Clerc M, Philippe N, Delaunay J. Sp alpha I/65 hereditary elliptocytosis in North Africa. Am J Hematol 1986;23:113.

131. Lawler J, Coetzer TL, Palek J, Jacob HS, Luban N. Sp $\alpha^{1/65:}$ a new variant of the alpha subunit of spectrin in hereditary elliptocytosis. Blood 1985;66:706.

132. Alloisio N, Morle L, Bachir D, Guetarni D, Colonna P, Delaunay J. Red cell membrane sialoglycoprotein beta in hemozygous and heterozygous 4.1(-) hereditary elliptocytosis. Biochim Biophys Acta 1985;816:57.

133. Lecomte MC, Dhermy D, Garbarz M, Feo C, Gautero H, Bournier O, Picat C, Chareroche I, Ester A, Galard C. Pathologic and non-pathologic variants of the spectrin molecule in two black families with hereditary elliptocytosis. Hum Genet 1985;71:351.

134. Marchesi SL, Letsinger JT, Speicher DW, Marchesi VT, Agre P, Hyun B, Gulati G. Mutant forms of spectrin alpha-subunits in hereditary elliptocytosis. J Clin Invest 1987; 80:191.

135. Lambert S, Zail S. A new variant of the α-subunit of spectrin in hereditary elliptocytosis. Blood 1987;69:473.

136. Morle L, Morle F, Roux AF, Godet J, Forget BG, Denoroy L, Garbarz M, Dhermy M, Kastally R, Delaunay J. Spectrin Tunis (Sp $\alpha^{1/78}$), an elliptocytogenic variant, is due to the CGG→TGG codon change (Arg→Trp) at position 35 of the αI domain. Blood 1989;74:828.

137. Lecomte MC, Garbarz M, Grandchamp B, Feo C, Gautero H, Devaux I, Bournier O, Galand C, d'Auriol L, Galibert F, Sahr KE, Forget BG, Boivin P, Dhermy DL. Sp $\alpha^{1/78:}$ a mutation of the αI spectrin domain in a white kindred with HE and HPP phenotypes. Blood 1989;74:1126.

138. Garbarz M, Lecomte MC, Feo C, Devanx I, Picat C, Lefebvre C, Galibert F, Gautero H, Bournier O, Galand C, Forget BG, Boivin P, Dhermy D. Hereditary pyropoikilocytosis and elliptocytosis in a white French family with the spectrin $\alpha^{1/74}$ variant related to a CGT to CAT codon change (Arg to His) at position 22 of the spectrin αI domain. Blood 1990;75:1691.

139. Coetzer T, Sahr K, Prchal J, Blacklock H, Peterson L, Koler R, Doyle J, Manaster J, Forget BG, Palek J. Four different mutations in codon 28 of α-spectrin are associated

with structurally and functionally abnormal spectrin α$^{I/74}$ in hereditary elliptocytosis. J Clin Invest 1991;88:743.

140. Floyd PB, Gallagher PG, Valentino LA, Davis M, Marchesi SL, Forget BG. Heterogeneity of the molecular basis of hereditary pyropoikilocytosis and hereditary elliptocytosis associated with increased levels of the spectrin α$^{I/74}$-kilodalton tryptic peptide. Blood 1991;78:1364.

141. Morle L, Roux AF, Alloisio N, Pothier B, Starck J, Denoroy L, Morle F, Rudigoz RC, Forget BG, Delaunay J, Godet J. Two ellipocytogenic α$^{I/74}$ variants of the spectrin αI domain spectrin Culoz (GGT→GTT; αI 40 GLY→Val) and Spectrin Lyon (CTT→TTT; αI 43 Leu→Phe). J Clin Invest 1990;86:548.

142. Roux AF, Morle F, Guetarni D, Colonna P, Sahr K, Forget BG, Delaunay J, Godet J. Molecular basis of Sp α$^{I/65}$ hereditary elliptocytosis in North Africa: insertion of a TTG triplet between codons 147 and 149 in the α-spectrin gene from five unrelated families. Blood 1989;73:2196.

143. Gallagher PG, Tse WT, Coetzer T, Lecomte MC, Gabarz M, Zarkowsky HS, Baruchel A, Ballas SK, Dhermy D, Palek J, Forget BG. A common type of the spectrin α-I 46-50a-kD peptide abnormality in hereditary elliptocytosis and hereditary pyropoikilocytosis is associated with a mutation distant from the proteolytic cleavage site—evidence for the functional importance of the triple helical model of spectrin. J Clin Invest 1992;89:892.

144. Sahr K, Tobe T, Scarpa A, Laughinghouse K, Marchesi SL, Agre P, Linnenbach AJ, Marchesi VT, Forget BG. Sequence and exon-intron organization of the DNA encoding the αI domain of human spectrin: application to the study of mutations causing hereditary elliptocytosis. J Clin Invest 1989; 84:1243.

145. Gallagher PG, Roberts WE, Benoit L, Speicher DW, Marchesi SL, Forget BG. Poikilocytic hereditary elliptocytosis associated with spectrin Alexandria: an α$^{I/50b}$ variant that is caused by a single amino acid deletion. Blood 1993;82.

146. Baklouti F, Marechal J, Wilmotte R, Alloisio N, Morle L, Ducluzeau MT, Denoroy L, Mrad A, Ben Aribia MH, Kastally R, Delaunay J. Elliptocytogenic α$^{I/36}$ spectrin Sfax lacks nine amino in helix 3 of repet 4: evidence for the activation of a cryptic 5′-splice site in exon 8 of spectrin α-gene. Blood 1992;79:2464.

147. Alloisio N, Morle L, Pothier B, et al. Spectrin Oran (α$^{II/21}$), a new spectrin variant concerning the αII domain and causing severe elliptocytosis in the homozygous state. Blood 1988;71:1039.

148. Lane PA, Shew RL, Iarocci TA, Mohandas N, Hays T, Mentzer WC. Unique alpha-spectrin mutant in a kindred with common hereditary elliptocytosis. J Clin Invest 1987; 79:989.

149. Coetzer T, Palek J, Lawler J, Liu S-, Jarolim P, Lahav M, Prchal JT, Wang W, Alter BP, Schewitz G, Mankad V, Gallanello R, Cao A. Structural and functional heterogeneity of α spectrin mutations involving the spectrin heterodimer self-association site: relationships to hematologic expression of homozygous hereditary elliptocytosis and hereditary pyropoikilocytosis. Blood 1990;75:2235.

150. Coetzer TL, Palek J. Partial spectrin deficiency in hereditary pyropoikilocytosis. Blood 1986;67:919.

151. Hanspal M, Hanspal J, Sahr KE, Fibach E, Nachman J, Palek J. Molecular basis of spectrin deficiency in hereditary pyropoikilocytosis. Blood 1993;82:1652.

152. Dhermy D, Lecomte MC, Garbarz M, Bournier O, Galand C, Gauters H, Feo C, Allisio N, Delaunay D, Boivin P. Spectrin beta-chain variant associated with hereditary spherocytosis. J Clin Invest 1982;70:707.

153. Eber SW, Morris SA, Schroter W, Gratzer WB. Interactions of spectrin in hereditary elliptocytes containing truncated spectrin β-chains. J Clin Invest 1988;81:523.

154. Garbarz M, Tse WT, Gallagher PG, Picat C, Lecomte MC, Gallbert F, Dhermy D, Forget B. Spectrin Rouen (β$^{218/220}$), a novel shortened β-chain variant in a kindred with hereditary elliptocytosis. J Clin Invest 1991;88:76.

155. Tse WT, Gallagher PG, Pothier B, Costa FF, Scarpa A, Delaunay J, Forget BG. An insertional frameshift mutation of the β-spectrin gene associated with elliptocytosis in spectrin Nice (β$^{220/216}$). Blood 1991;78:517.

156. Garbarz M, Boulanger L, Pedroni S, Lecomte MC, Gautero H, Galand C, Boivin P, Feldman L. Spectrin β^{Tandil}, a novel shortened β-chain variant associated with hereditary elliptocytosis is due to a deletional frameshift mutation in the β-spectrin gene. Blood 1992;80:1066.

157. Kanzaki A, Rabodonorina M, Yawata Y, Wilmotte R, Wada H, Ata K, Yamada O, Akatsuka J, Iyori H, Horiguchi M, Nakamura H, Mishima T, Morle L, Delaunay J. A deletional frameshift mutation of the β-spectrin gene associated with elliptocytosis in spectrin Tokyo (β$^{220/216}$). Blood 1992; 80:2115.

158. Gallagher PG, Tse WT, Costa F, Scarpa A, Boivin P, Delaunay J, Forget BG. A splice site mutation of the β-spectrin causing exon skipping in hereditary elliptocytosis. J Biol Chem 1991;266:15154.

159. Yoon SH, Yu H, Eber S, Prchal JT. Molecular defect of truncated β-spectrin associated with hereditary elliptocytosis. J Biol Chem 1991;266:8490.

160. Takanashi K, Sugawar T, Sakurai K, et al. A trait of hereditary elliptocytosis with truncated β-spectrin (spectrin Yamagata β$^{220/210}$). Jpn J Clin Hematol 1991;32:1365a.

161. Gallagher PG, Tse WT, Mohandas N, et al. Spectrin Providence: a defect of erythrocyte beta spectrin (β$^{2109 Ser-Pro}$) for which homozygosity is associated with fatal hydrops fetalis. Blood 1992;80(Suppl 1):145a.

162. Sahr KE, Coetzer TL, Moy LS, et al. An Ala to Gly substitution in β-spectrin associated with spectrin α$^{I/74}$ in hereditary elliptocytosis (HE) and hereditary pyropoikilcytosis (HPP). Blood 1992;80(Suppl 1):276a.

163. Knowles WJ, Morrow JS, Speicher DW, Zarkowshy AS, Mohandas N, Mentzer WC, Shohet SB, Marchesi VT. Molecular and functional changes in spectrin from patients with hereditary pyropoikilocytosis. J Clin Invest 1983;71:1867.

164. Mueller TY, William J, Wang W, Morrison M. Cycloskeletal alterations in hereditary elliptocytosis. Blood 1981;58:47a.

165. Conboy J, Mohandas N, Tchernia G, Kan YW. Molecular basis of hereditary spherocytosis due to protein 4.1 deficiency. N Engl J Med 1986;315:680.

166. Conboy JG, Chasis JA, Winardi R, Tchernia G, Kan YW, Mohandas N. An isoform-specific mutation in the protein 4.1 gene results in hereditary elliptocytosis and complete deficiency of protein 4.1 in erythrocytes but not nonerythroid cells. J Clin Invest 1993;91:77.

167. Dalla Venezia N, Gilsanz F, Alloisio N, Ducluzeau M, Benz Jr, Delaunay J. Homozygous 4.1(−) hereditary elliptocytosis associated with a point mutation in the downstream initiation codon of protein 4.1 gene. J Clin Invest 1992; 90:1713.

168. Reid M, Takakuwa Y, Conboy JG, Tchernia G, Mohandas N. Glycophorin C content of human erythrocyte membrane is regulated by protein 4.1. Blood 1990;75:2229.

169. Garbarz M, Dhermy D, Lecomte MC, Feo C, Shaveroche I, Galand C, Bournier O, Bertrand O, Boivin P. A variant of erythrocyte membrane skeletal protein band 4.1 associated with hereditary elliptocytosis. Blood 1984;64:1006.

170. Conboy JG, Shitamoto R, Parra M, Winardi R, Kabra A, Smith J, Mohandas N. Hereditary elliptocytosis due to both qualitative and quantitative defects in membrane skeletal protein 4.1. Blood 1991;78:2438.

171. Marchesi SL, Conboy J, Agre P, Letsinger JT, Marchesi VT, Speicher DW, Mohandas N. Molecular analysis of insertion/deletion mutations in protein 4.1 in elliptocytosis I: biochemical identification of rearrangements in the spectrin/actin binding domain and functional characterization. J Clin Invest 1990;86:516.

172. Conboy J, Marchesi S, Kim R, Agre P, Kan YW, Mohandas N. Molecular analysis of insertion/deletion mutations in protein 4.1 in elliptocytosis: II, determination of molecular genetic origins of rearrangements. J Clin Invest 1990;86:524.

173. Morle L, Garbarz M, Alloisio N, et al. The characterization of protein 4.1 Presles, a shortened variant of RBC membrane protein 4.1. Blood 1985;65:1511.

174. Feddal S, Hayette S, Baklaouti F, Rimokh R, Wilmotte R, Mayaud JP, Marechal J, Benz Jr, Girot R, Delaunay J, Morle L. Prevalent skipping of an individual exon accounts for shortened protein 4.1 Presles. Blood 1992;80:2925.

175. Anstee DJ, Ridgewell K, Tanner MJ, Daniels GL, Parsons SF. Individuals lacking the Gerbich blood-group antigens have alterations in the human erythrocyte membrane sialoglycoproteins beta and gamma. Biochem J 1984;221:97.

176. Jarolim P, Rubin HL, Zhai S, et al. Band 3 Memphis: a widespread polymorphism with abnormal electrophoretic mobility of erythrocyte band 3 protein caused by the substitution AAG→GAG (Lys→Glu) in codon 56. Blood 1992;80:1592.

177. Yannoukakos D, Vasseur C, Driancourt C, et al. Human erythrocyte band 3 polymorphism (band 3 Memphis): characterization of the structural modification (Lys56→Glu) by protein chemistry methods. Blood 1991;78:1117.

178. Mueller TJ, Morrison M. Detection of a variant of protein 3, the major transmembrane protein on the human erythrocyte. J Biol Chem 1977;252:6573.

179. Jarolim P, Palek J, Amato D, et al. Deletion in erythrocyte band 3 gene in malaria-resistant Southeast Asian ovalocytosis. Proc Natl Acad Sci USA 1991;88:11022.

180. Mohandas N, Winardi R, Knowles D, Leung A, Parra M, George E, Conboy J, Chasis J. Molecular basis for membrane rigidity of hereditary ovalocytosis—a novel mechanism involving the cytoplasmic domain of band 3. J Clin Invest 1992;89:686.

181. Moriyama R, Ideguchi H, Lombardo CR, Van Dort HM, Low PS. Structural and functional characterization of band 3 from Southeast Asian ovalocytes. J Biol Chem 1992;267:25792.

182. Liu SC, Nichols PE, Yi SJ, Derick LH, Chiou SS, Amato D, Palek J. Molecular basis of membrane rigidity in Southeast Asian ovalocytosis: oligomerization of the mutant band 3 protein and its increased association with the membrane skeleton. Blood 1993;82(Suppl 1):308a.

183. Kay MMB, Gieljan JC, Bosman GJCG, Lawrence C. Functional topography of band 3: specific structural alteration linked to functional aberrations in human erythrocytes. Proc Natl Acad Sci USA 1988;85:492.

184. Bruce LJ, Kay MM, Lawrence C, Tanner MJ. Band 3 HT, a human red-cell variant associated with acanthocytosis and increased anion transport, carries the mutation Pro868→Leu in the membrane domain of band 3. Biochem J 1993; 293:317

CHAPTER 8

Enzyme Defects

WILLIAM H. ZINKHAM

The indiscriminate selection of a battery of hematologically oriented tests, such as obtaining a Coombs' test and levels of serum iron, vitamin B_{12} and folic acid, in every anemic patient, is wasteful, unwise and unnecessary.

—Maxwell Wintrobe (1930)

Over the years the red cell has been the focus of a variety of research pursuits designed to further our understanding of factors that are essential for its function and survival. Foremost in these pursuits was the demonstration in the middle of this century that genetically determined abnormalities of erythrocyte enzymes were associated with a variety of clinically important hematologic disorders, ranging from the selective hemolytic action of drugs to the etiology of previously unidentified congenital hemolytic disorders. Although the red cell at one time was thought of as the "impoverished nomad that starts with little and ends with less" (1), a more recent characterization appropriately calls the red cell "a tiny dynamo" (2). As in other cells, enzymes are essential for energizing the dynamo.

From a conceptual viewpoint, three levels of organization constitute the architectural composition of the red cell: hemoglobin, enzymes, and the membrane. Defects, either acquired or inherited, may effect abnormalities at any one of these sites and thereby result in premature cell death and/or cellular dysfunction. Collectively these abnormalities are referred to as hemoglobinopathies, enzymopathies, and membranopathies, respectively.

The objectives of this chapter are to review two of the most common enzymopathies affecting the red cell, one a deficiency of glucose-6-phosphate dehydrogenase (G-6-PD) and the other pyruvate kinase (PK). A case presentation will precede each review, followed by a discussion of possible pathophysiologic mechanisms, clinical recognition and management of the disorders, genetic determinants and patterns of inheritance, and, finally, how knowledge accrued from these observations may elucidate factors that lead to the death of the normal red cell.

Glucose-6-Phosphate Dehydrogenase

Case 1 (3, 4)

B.H., a black infant boy, was transferred to the pediatric service when 12 hours old because of jaundice that appeared at 7 hours of age. The infant was the product of a full-term pregnancy and a spontaneous delivery and weighed 2600 g at birth. Lethargy and jaundice were observed at 7 hours of age. The liver and spleen were palpated 2–3 cm below the costal margins. There were no other physical abnormalities.

Peripheral blood findings included a venous hematocrit of 43%. The leukocyte count was $31.4 \times 10^9/L$. There were 83% polymorphonuclear neutrophils, 11% immature neutrophils, 6% lymphocytes, and 37 nucleated erythrocytes per 100 leukocytes. A Wright stained smear of the peripheral blood revealed striking abnormalities of red cell morphology including marked anisocytosis, fragmented cells, and polychromatophilia (fig. 8. 1). A few mononuclear erythrophages were present. The reticulocyte count was 18.5%. Heinz bodies were present in approximately 20% of the red cells.

The urine was dark yellow and tested negative for albumin and sugar. The urinary sediment exhibited a rare hyaline cast. Concentrations of blood urea nitrogen (BUN), calcium, and phosphorus were 40, 8.6, and 4.0 mg/dl, respectively. The total serum protein was 5 g/dl with an albumin level of 3.4 g/dl. A blood culture was sterile and results of the serologic test for syphilis were negative.

The patient's blood group was O Rh negative and the mother's, O Rh negative. Direct Coombs' test results were negative, and incubation of mother's serum with the patient's red cells revealed no incompatibility, either by the albumin and indirect Coombs' techniques.

At 12 hours of age the serum bilirubin was 6.4 mg/dl and rose to a peak of 21.6 mg/dl (2.4 mg/dl direct). During this time the hematocrit decreased to 28.5%. Accordingly, an exchange transfusion using 500 ml of O Rh negative blood was accomplished. Afterward the bilirubin level became normal and the infant was discharged on the 18th day of life weighing 2420 g.

At 5 months of age the patient weighed 5390 g and physical examination results were normal. His hematocrit was 34% and red cell morphology was normal.

Mother: B.H.'s mother was a 19-year-old black who on the second postpartum day was noted to have a hemolytic anemia. This pregnancy was the mother's second; her first resulted in the delivery of a normal black girl. The family history was negative for any type of blood disorder.

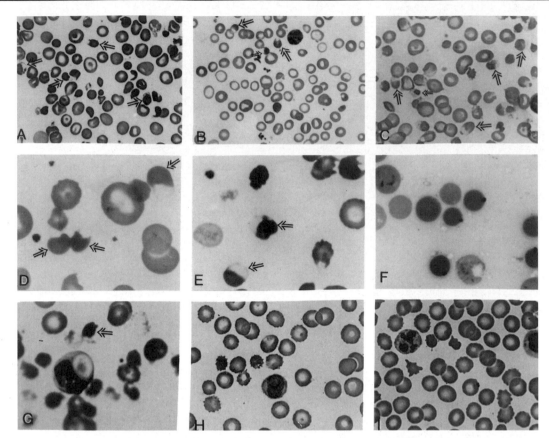

Figure 8.1. Wright-stained smears of the peripheral blood. *Arrows* point to cells exhibiting oxidant damage: "eccentrocytes," "drug reacting" cells, and "bite" or "pincer" cells. **A.** Two-day-old black infant boy with G-6-PD deficiency exposed to naphthalene in utero (×750). **B.** The same infant's mother, who also had G-6-PD deficiency and was exposed to naphthalene during pregnancy. Smear obtained on the second postpartum day (×750). **C.** A 5-year-old black boy with with G-6-PD deficiency in whom a hemolytic anemia developed soon after the boy ingested naphthalene mothballs (×750). **D.** A higher magnification of the smear shown in **C** (×1350). **E.** A 35-year-old white woman with Hb Zurich in whom a hemolytic anemia developed after she received phenazopyridine (Pyridium) (×1200). **F.** A Heinz body preparation of the same patient utilizing rhodanile blue, a neutral supravital dye. Heinz bodies appear as small, round dark inclusions at the edges of four red cells. Rhodanile blue also stains the reticulum of the reticulocytes, two of which are present (×1200). **G.** A 10-day-old black G-6-PD-deficient full-term infant who received 10 mg of menadione sodium bisulfite (Hykinone) at 8½ days of age. The leukocyte containing a red cell is an erythrophage (×1000). **H.** A 6-year-old white boy with pyruvate kinase deficiency. Splenectomy was performed at 3 years of age (×750). **I.** An 8-year-old white girl with pyruvate kinase deficiency. Splenectomy was performed at 3 years of age (×750).

Her current pregnancy was complicated by the development of preeclampsia, for which she received phenobarbital and magnesium sulfate during the last trimester. Throughout the pregnancy she had a fondness for naphthalene moth balls which she intermittently smelled, chewed, or sucked on, especially during the last trimester. Documentation of this perversion for naphthalene was provided by the patient's husband, who reported a housewide distribution of moth balls. Also he noted that the patient frequently slept at night with mothballs clutched in her hands.

On the second postpartum day the patient exhibited moderate pallor, but the remainder of the physical examination results were normal. At that time the blood count revealed a hemoglobin of 5.9 g/dl and a hematocrit of 23.3%. The reticulocyte count was 16.4%. The leukocyte count was 13,250 10⁹/L with a differential count of 3.0% juvenile neutrophils, 80% polymorphonuclear neutrophils, 1.0% eosinophils, 12.0% lymphocytes, 1.0% atypical lymphocytes, and 3.0% monocytes. Abnormalities of red cell morphology included polychromasia and moderately fine basophilic stippling (fig. 8.1). A rare red cell contained a Heinz body. A bone marrow aspirate revealed erythroid hyperplasia and an increase in the number of phagocytic macrophages, many of which contained hemosiderin. The total bilirubin was 1.8 mg/dl (0.3 direct). Values for BUN and total albumin and protein were normal.

Results of qualitative tests for naphthalene and naphthalene metabolites in the mother's and infant's urines approximately 60 hours after delivery were negative. The weight of the placenta was 600 g and a small area of the placental surface appeared to be infarcted.

Two weeks after delivery the mother's hematocrit was 31.6% and her reticulocyte count 0.6%. Physical examination revealed no abnormalities.

Pathogenetic Mechanisms

One of the most constant biologic values in man is the hematocrit, a determination that reflects the constancy of the red cell mass. Such a finely tuned homeostatic phenomenon is regulated by a variety of physiologic factors, both humoral and cellular. Reduced to simple terms, however, the constancy of the hematocrit represents a carefully controlled balance between red cell formation and red cell destruction. Stated another way, the number of red cells entering the circulation equals the number exiting. Based on this concept, a variety of diagnostic schemes for demonstrating the cause of anemia have been formulated (5–7). Pertinent to this review are the observations noted concerning our 2 patients. Both exhibited a significant degree of anemia accompanied by a marked elevation of the reticulocyte count, and, in the infant, hyperbilirubinemia as well. Hence, it appeared that the anemia was secondary to some type of hemolytic process. If so, then several questions have to be answered. What is the relationship between the exposure to naphthalene and the occurrence of hemolysis? Would a hemolytic process develop in anyone ingesting naphthalene or is the phenomenon unique to someone with an inherited abnormality of the red cell, be it at the membrane, enzyme, or hemoglobin level, thus reflecting an interplay between extra- and intra-corpuscular events?

Biochemical Studies on Infant and Maternal Red Cells: *The absence of complications usually associated with neonatal anemia, e.g., isoimmunization, infection, or bleeding, together with the occurrence of a similar hemolytic disorder in the mother, led to the supposition that naphthalene, a potent oxidant, might have been the factor causing hemolysis (8, 9). Accordingly, in vitro studies were designed to evaluate the effects of several oxidants on the sulfhydryl content of the patient's red cells. Two groups of agents were tested: one, acetylphenylhydrazine (APH), a compound first shown by Beutler et al. (10) to oxidize intraerythrocytic-reduced glutathione (GSH), the GSH stability test, and the other, naphthalene metabolites, α- and β-naphthol and α- and β-naphthoquinone. Results of glutathione studies are shown in table 8.1.*

At the time of the first observations, maternal and infant reticulocyte counts were 16.4 and 18.5, respectively. Hence the GSH values reflect the presence of a large population of young red cells. The exchange transfusion in the infant was accomplished with donor red cells in which the GSH stability test had demonstrated a normal postincubation value of 76 mg/dl of red blood cells (RBCs). Approximately 5 months after delivery GSH values before and after incubation with APH were markedly reduced, an abnormality that had previously been demonstrated in African-American subjects predisposed to the development of a hemolytic anemia after ingesting therapeutic doses of the antimalarial drug, primaquine (10). In these primaquine-sensitive subjects, the abnormality of GSH metabolism was proven to be secondary to a deficiency of G-6-PD (11). Assays for red cell G-6-PD activities performed several years later in our 2 patients revealed abnormally low values, indicating that the infant is a hemizygote, and the mother, a homozygote, their most probable genotypes being Gd^{A-} and $Gd^{A-}Gd^{A-}$, respectively (12).

G-6-PD Deficiency and Mechanisms of Hemolysis: *The mother and infant in the above-described case report eventually recovered from their episodes of hemolysis. Although the deficiency of G-6-PD is an inherited and lifetime abnormality of their red cells, neither should experience subsequent bouts of hemolysis unless exposed to other oxidants such as naphthalene. Thus, two factors must be operative to explain the development of hemolysis, one the underlying enzymopathy and the other, an environmental factor, naphthalene.*

Table 8.1 Glutathione Studies on the Infant's and Mother's Red Cells

Date of Determination	Age of Infant (hr)	Reduced GSH (mg/100 ml RBC)				Comment
		Whole Blood		After Incubation APH		
		Infant	Mother	Infant°	Mother°	
1/17	18	67	67	18	23	
1/17	30	74		27		
1/18	49	87		39		Exchange transfusion done at age 36 hr
1/23		67	67	29	22	
2/1		94		25		
2/8		75	75	35	10	
2/23			74		13	
3/15		61	70	25	6	
4/18		59		15		
6/7		43	43	9	8	
8/16			43		6	

°In older infants and adults, values for GSH after incubation of blood with APH are always >40 mg/100 ml of RBCs (125). *Abbreviations:* APH, acetylphenylhydrazine; GSH, glutathione.

The normal red cell during its finite life span of 120 days in adults and 60 days in newborns is constantly exposed to oxidizing events. Evidence for this phenomenon derives from observations that Heinz bodies, the products of aging processes, are continually being formed in the red cells of normal subjects, but only become visible in individuals with congenital or acquired forms of splenic agenesis (13). In the G-6-PD-deficient subject, as well as in some patients with unstable hemoglobinopathies, the aging process accelerates, especially in the presence of environmental oxidants.

The series of morphologic and metabolic events accompanying the exposure of G-6-PD deficient cells to drug or chemical is complex but appears to be secondary to at least two factors. One is the oxidative potential of the offending agent—in our two patients, naphthalene. Naphthoquinones, the metabolites of naphthalene, are potent oxidizing agents with oxidation potentials of −0.47 volts and −0.55 volts for naphthoquinones, respectively (14). Their oxidative capacity can be demonstrated in vitro by noting the formation of methemoglobin (MHb) in whole blood to which these agents have been added (15). Most likely MHb formation results from a two-electron reduction of molecular oxygen bound to the heme iron. One electron is donated by the ferrous iron, producing MetHb, and the other from the naphthoquinones, producing superoxide, drug-free radicals, and hydrogen peroxide. Removal of these species is mediated by GSH peroxidase, with GSH as an essential cofactor. Activation of the hexose-monophosphate shunt pathway (HMP) ensues secondary to the requirement of reduced nicotinamide adenine dinucleotide phosphate (NADPH), a cofactor for the enzyme glutathione reductase, the function of which is to reduce the oxidized GSH generated by the GSH peroxidase reaction. A metabolic scheme for this sequence of events is displayed in fig. 8.2. A deficiency of G-6-PD, the enzyme initiating the HMP, is one of only two enzymes capable of generating NADPH in the red cell, the other being the third enzyme in the HMP, 6-phosphogluconic dehydrogenase. Hence, a deficiency of G-6-PD impairs the ability of red cells to withstand oxidant stresses.

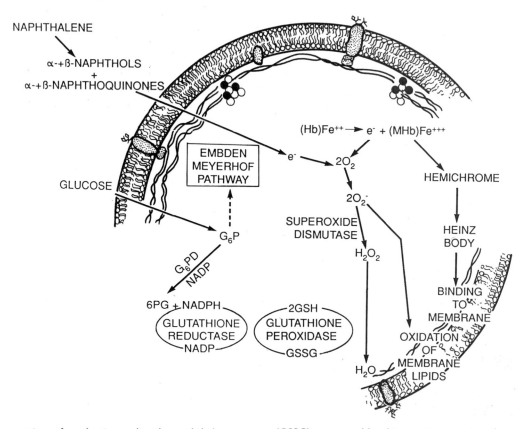

Figure 8.2. An overview of mechanisms whereby naphthalene mediates oxidative injury to red cells. Naphthalene, a water-insoluble chemical, is metabolized to water-soluble α- and β-naphthols and α- and β-naphthoquinones. These metabolites traverse the red cell membrane. One electron ($\bar{e}$) from ferrous iron, and another from the naphthalene metabolites result in the formation of superoxide (O_2^-), which in turn is converted to H_2O_2 by super oxide dismutase. Catabolism of is H_2O_2 regulated by glutathione peroxidase, an enzyme for which reduced glutathione (GSH) is an essential cofactor. Oxidized glutathione (GSSG) generated by this reaction requires the enzyme glutathione reductase and nicotinamide adenine dinucleotide phosphate (NADPH). The most important mechanism for generating NADPH in the red cell is by the first enzyme regulating the hexose monophosphate shunt pathway, G-6-PD.

Oxidative injury to the red cell is mediated by at least two other mechanisms. One is the formation of methemoglobin (MHbFe^{+++}), hemichromes, and Heinz bodies, which in turn bind to the membrane. The other is oxidation of membrane lipids by superoxide. Details of these reactions are noted in the text.

The end result of these metabolic sequences is the development of dense red cells with a low mean corpuscular volume (MCV) and a high mean corpuscular hemoglobin concentration (MCHC), cells that can be separated by centrifugation and recovered in the bottom layer of the centrifuge tube or by density gradient techniques (16). In addition to being dense and dehydrated, these cells are rigid, as reflected by their decreased filterability through microfilters (16).

What is the relationship then between oxidation of GSH and the eventual demise of the cell? A variety of hypotheses have been proposed, and recently some investigators have even questioned the role of GSH and have indicated that NADPH, and not GSH, is essential for protecting normal and G-6-PD-deficient erythrocytes from oxidant stress (17).

Additional studies have shown that the oxidative pathway for hemoglobin involves the formation of MetHb, which then degrades to a group of compounds called reversible and irreversible hemichromes (18). Presumably these compounds then form Heinz bodies, which, in turn, bind to and alter both the stability and function of membrane constituents (19–21). Hemoglobin (Hb) and MHb stabilize the membrane, whereas the hemichromes and possibly hemin from the hemichromes, are destabilizing factors (22).

As knowledge of red cell membrane proteins increases, more information should develop regarding the final events in the demise of normal and G-6-PD-deficient red cells. In 1975 Kay demonstrated the binding of autologous serum antibodies to normal high-density red cells, presumably those cells that are the oldest (23, 24). Recently Sorette et al. have shown that at least two of the antibodies are antiband 3 and anti-Gal-α-(1-3)-Gal, a galactose compound (25). They even suggest that other antibodies are present, since these antibodies constitute only 35% of the total.

Other studies demonstrating the possible mechanisms whereby Heinz bodies are related to red cell death include the demonstration that band 3, a membrane protein that regulates anion transport, aggregates in areas in which Heinz bodies have formed (26, 27). It is in these regions of the cell membrane that autologous band 3 antibody binds and in turn leads to phagocytosis by macrophages and/or cell lysis, depending on the extent of oxidative injury.

During the past several years a number of reports have focused on the important role of oxidative damage to membrane lipids as an accompaniment of cell death (28). Here again, the initiating event is exposure to environmental factors, leading to the generation of reactive oxygen molecules.

Pending the development of future knowledge, our current concept of cellular events preceding the death of G-6-PD-deficient and possibly normal red cells involves the following sequence of events: oxidant exposure, formation of peroxides, oxidation of GSH and NADPH, conversion of Hb to MetHb, formation of hemichromes and Heinz bodies that bind to and destabilize cell membrane components, and, finally, the attachment of autologous membrane antibodies or cell lysis. It is important to note, however, that several of the events preceding cell destruction have been questioned, including the binding of antibodies to senescent antigens (29).

Pertinent to this sequence of events is the knowledge that the clinical expression of the selective hemolytic action of drugs is extraordinarily similar for two different inherited red cell defects, G-6-PD deficiency, and the unstable hemoglobins. Subjects with Hb Zurich (His E7(63)$\beta \rightarrow$ Arg) are asymptomatic until exposed to what appears to be the same group of agents that hemolyze G-6-PD-deficient red cells. Especially impressive are the similarities of the morphologic changes that characterize the two disorders (fig. 8.1). In the G-6-PD-deficient subject the generation of peroxides is secondary to an enzymopathy, whereas in the Hb Zurich subjects, a structural abnormality of hemoglobin leads to the development of superoxide and drug-free radicals. Although the site of oxidant injury differs, the terminal events appear to be quite similar.

Another area to explore is the enhanced susceptibility of red cells from premature and full-term newborns to oxidant injury (30, 31). Early observations suggested that this phenomenon may be secondary to an increased instability of GSH when red cells of normal newborns are exposed to APH in vitro (32, 33). Values for G-6-PD activity were approximately two- to three-fold higher than those observed in red cells from adults (32). Glucose consumption by newborn red cells was approximately twice that of the adult, eventually leading to depletion of glucose during the 2-hour duration of the GSH stability test. Although this finding is based on in vitro events, it is possible that severe degrees of hypoglycemia in vivo may decrease the antioxidant potential of newborn red cells.

Other explanations for the increased reactivity of newborn cells to oxidant stress are the following: (a) decreased activities of catalase, GSH peroxidase, and NADH-dependent MHb reductase, (b) the increased propensity of fetal hemoglobin (HbF) to undergo oxidation, and (c) possibly a deficiency of vitamin E (30, 34). Recently Linderkamp et al. (35) have shown that unchallenged newborn red cells are less deformable than adult red cells because of their large size, an inherent property that compromises the life span of the red cell under normal conditions, and possibly more so when the red cell is exposed to oxidants.

Detection of G-6-PD-Related Hemolysis

Since millions of people have G-6-PD-deficient red cells, the demonstration of the defect in anemic subjects, especially those of certain ethnic groups, does not establish an etiologic relationship. For example, in the infant and mother with hemolytic disorder we described, how could we be certain that hemolysis was secondary to a deficiency of G-6-PD? Furthermore, the selective hemolytic effects of drugs or infections observed in G-6-PD-deficient subjects may be secondary to other pathophysiologic mechanisms, such as an unstable hemoglobin or a drug-induced Coombs' positive hemolytic process. Guidelines for definitive diagnosis are outlined in table 8.2.

The first and most important approach is to elicit a detailed reporting of exposure to any type of agent prior to the illness, including over-the-counter remedies which are often not considered to be drugs but contain chemicals such as phenacetin. In addition, possible routes of exposure should be explored: inhalation, percutaneous absorption, or ingestion. Finally, have similar episodes been experienced by the patient or members of his or her family in the past.

The clinical expression of the disorder involves different degrees of pallor, possibly scleral icterus, and a history of dark urine, sometimes referred to as "Coca-Cola colored." Splenomegaly may be present.

The hematologic findings vary according to the severity of the hemolytic anemia. With mild degrees, red cell morphologic changes and the degree of reticulocytosis are minimal, and only a 10–20 g/L decrease in hemoglobin values ensues. Changes observed with primaquine and those observed with naphthalene and fava beans are more dramatic, including the presence of Heinz bodies, the hallmark of oxidative injury to the red cell, and the appearance of "bite cells" or "drug reacting cells" in the peripheral blood (fig. 8.1). A search for Heinz bodies should be initiated immediately after the patient is first seen. Such cells rapidly disappear from the circulation, especially if the drug exposure predates the hospital admission by several days and a large population of reticulocytes with elevated G-6-PD activities has emerged. In this situation it may be difficult to distinguish Heinz bodies from the precipitates within the reticulocytes that appear during exposure to supravital stains (fig. 8.1).

The final step in defining the G-6-PD-deficient type of hemolysis is a demonstration of the enzyme abnormality in the red cells. A variety of quantitative and qualitative

Table 8.2 Identification of Patient with Hemolytic Anemia Secondary to G-6-PD Deficiency*

- **History of exposure to hemolytic agent**
  Infection, drug, chemical, fava bean
- **Characteristics of anemia**
  Slight to marked. Mild to marked reticulocytosis.
  Hemoglobinemia and hemoglobinuria with severe hemolysis
- **Red cell morphology**
  Polychromatophilia. "Drug reacting" cell changes ("bite cells," "degmacytes," "eccentrocytes")
  Heinz bodies
- **Enzyme defect**
  Qualitative or quantitative methods—Both may give high values if large population of young cells is present
  Family studies important

*Patients with congenital forms of nonspherocytic hemolytic anemia due to deficiency of G-6-PD have a chronic hemolytic process which may or may not exacerbate following ingestion of or exposure to hemolytic agents.

methods are available (36). The most extensively utilized screening tests are a dye-decolorization technique, and a fluorescent spot test (37, 38). Each method has its advantages, the major ones being reliability, cost of the chemicals, and simplicity of performance. Pitfalls are also evident. Missiou-Tsagaraki recently noted that the fluorescent spot test as performed on newborn capillary bloods collected on a special type of paper has to be performed within 2 weeks after collection, and the specimens have to be protected from high temperatures and humidity (39). A more important shortcoming of qualitative technology is its frequent failure to identify the heterozygous female. For this and other reasons quantitative methodologies are necessary.

One of the first quantitative methods for identifying more precisely the heterozygous female was a modification of the method of Glock and McLean (40, 41). The third enzyme in the HMP is 6-phosphogluconic dehydrogenase, another red cell enzyme that, like G-6-PD, generates NADPH. In order to rule out the contribution of this enzyme to the formation of NADPH in the reaction mixture, a three-cuvette system is utilized. The first is a blank. The second contains 6-phosphogluconic acid, and the third, both G-6-P and 6-PG as substrates. G-6-PD activity is calculated by subtracting the activity measured in the second from that exhibited by the third cuvette. Invariably this value is 5–10% less than when G-6-PD activity is measured with only G-6-P as substrate. Utilization of this technique has led to the demonstration of a trimodal distribution of the enzyme defect in a female G-6-PD-deficient population.

Another pitfall in quantitating G-6-PD activity is failure to remove platelets and white cells from red cells prior to preparation of the hemolysate. For this reason washing with normal saline and removing the buffy coat which contains these elements is important. Unfortunately, aspirating the buffy coat may also remove the reticulocyte layer, that portion of the sample which usually exhibits the highest enzyme activity.

Whatever method is chosen for definition of the G-6-PD abnormality, it is important to realize that reticulocytes and young red cells in G-6-PD-deficient subjects have only moderately decreased to even increased levels of G-6-PD activity, depending on the ethnic origin of the patient (42). By the time the patient presents with anemia, a major portion of the older, enzyme-deficient population of red cells will have been destroyed, so that data derived from quantification of enzyme activity in the remainder of the cells could be misleading. Several approaches have been developed and utilized to circumvent this problem. One is a centrifugation technique, in which, as a result of increased density, the older cells are present in the bottom layer of the spun preparation. After separation and lysis, enzyme determinations are performed on this population (43).

Often overlooked is the informative data that can be generated by measuring enzyme levels in other members of the family.

Figure 8.3 displays the course of enzyme activities in a 2-year-old black female who had ingested mothballs (44). At the time of these observations our hypothesis was that naphthalene-induced hemolysis occurred only in G-6-PD-deficient subjects. In this patient, enzyme values were markedly elevated (300 and 500 U/dl of RBCs prior to transfusion). The following day enzyme assays of the girl's parents' red cells revealed markedly reduced activities, suggesting that the patient had to have G-6-PD-deficient cells. Subsequent assays on the patient's red cells after the recovery phase proved this to be so.

Hemolytic Factors and G-6-PD Deficiency

The discovery of the G-6-PD-deficient red cell by the Chicago group represented the high point of a number of investigations to elucidate the mechanism of the selective hemolytic action of the antimalarial drug primaquine (45, 46). Although primaquine was the first agent identified as causing a hemolytic anemia in G-6-PD-deficient adult black males, it soon became apparent that many other drugs had a similar potential (47–49).

As noted in the case histories of our mother and infant with hemolytic anemia, the mother was directly exposed to naphthalene by sucking and ingesting mothballs. By doing so, she exposed her fetus in utero to the same toxic agent by the transplacental passage of naphthalene metabolites. As demonstrated in other subjects with naphthalene-associated hemolysis, the genetically determined deficiency of red cell G-6-PD predisposed the mother and her infant to the hemolytic effects of the agent (3, 4).

The list of drugs, chemicals, and other factors hemolyzing G-6-PD-deficient red cells has changed considerably over the years, with some of the previously suspected agents omitted, and a few of the more recently compounded drugs being added (table 8.3). Unfortunately, methodologies for demonstrating the hemolytic potential of any given drug are limited. Furthermore, on the basis of clinical observations it is difficult to differentiate the impact of the patient's illness (e.g., typhoid fever or hepatitis) on red cell survival from that of the drug. A detailed discussion of this problem is presented by Beutler in a recent review (50). Two agents formerly thought to cause hemolysis, acetylsalicylic acid and acetaminophen, now appear to

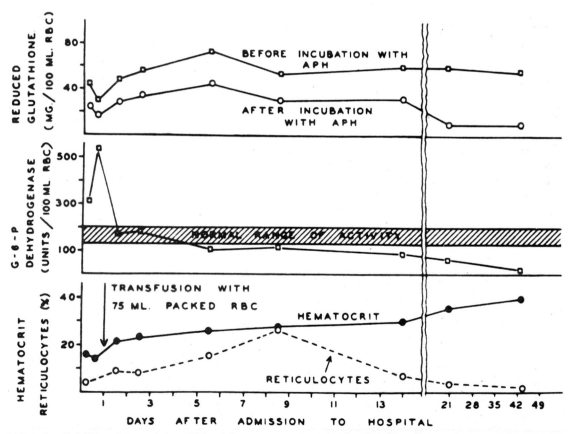

Figure 8.3. Values for G-6-PD activity and the GSH stability test in blood obtained from a 2-year-old black girl who ingested several mothballs approximately 3 days prior to admission. In blood from G-6-PD-normal white and black adults, the range of G-6-PD activity is 150–216 IU/dl of RBCs as quantified by a modification of the Glock and McLean technique (40). Note that the value for G-6-PD activity at the time of admission was 300 u/dl of RBCs, and 12 hours later, 545 u/dl of RBCs. Family studies revealed that both the father and mother were enzyme deficient, thereby suggesting that the patient had to be a homozygote ($Gd^{A-}Gd^{A-}$). Subsequent enzyme determinations proved this presumption to be true. From Zinkham (44).

Table 8.3 Factors Hemolyzing G-6-PD-Deficient Red Cells

Drugs
  Antimalarials—Primaquine, pamaquine
  Sulfonamides—Sulfanilamide, sulfacetamide, sulfamethoxa-
      zole (a major component of Bactrim), sul-
      fapyridine
  Sulfones—Thiazolesulfone, dapsone
  Nitrofurans—Nitrofurantoin
  Antipyretic—Acetanilid
  Analgesic—Phenazopyridine (Pyridium)
  Other drugs—Nalidixic acid, niridazole, vitamin K (water sol-
      uble analogs—not vitamin K$_1$)
Chemicals
  Naphthalene, phenylhydrazine, toluidine blue, methylene
  blue
Vegetables
  Bean—*Vicia faba*
  Herb—? Senna, henna
Infections
  Bacterial
  Catalase positive—*Salmonella*, coagulase +
      Staphylococci, *Escherichia coli*,
      K. pneumonia
      Chromabacterium violaceum
  Viral
      Hepatitis (usually A and possibly other types)

be innocuous. Current pediatric practice dictates that acetylsalicylic acid no longer be used for its antipyretic effect because of its etiologic role in Reye syndrome. Hence the opportunity to detect hemolysis due to this agent in the pediatric age group is quite remote. On the other hand, acetaminophen is widely used in infants and children, so it is reassuring to know that it lacks hemolytic capability.

The degree of hemolysis produced by each of the drugs or other agents varies widely. Naphthalene and fava beans promote a catastrophic hemolytic anemia, eventuating in death in some patients unless they are transfused. For this reason, these agents deserve special attention.

Naphthalene and Related Compounds

In spite of earlier reports describing the hemolytic potential of naphthalene, many physicians believed it was a harmless compound because of its water insolubility. An important contribution by Zeulzer and Apt in 1947 described a fulminating hemolytic anemia in 4 black children who accidentally swallowed naphthalene mothballs (51). Furthermore, these authors were able to reproduce the phenomenon in dogs by the oral administration of either naphthalene or naphthalene mothballs. Following this report, physicians in this and other countries recounted similar experiences in children exposed to naphthalene (3, 4, 52–57).

The characteristic features of a naphthalene-induced hemolytic anemia are the following: Heinz bodies (denatured hemoglobin) appear in the circulating red cells, followed by a marked decrease in hemoglobin values asso-

ciated with hemoglobinemia and hemoglobinuria, and death in some patients unless they are transfused. In addition to the appearance of Heinz bodies, there are remarkable changes in red cell morphology, both in dogs given naphthalene and in humans with accidental exposure (4, 51, 57). Many of the cells exhibit a densely packed portion of hemoglobin on one side of the cell and what appears to be a pale portion of cell membrane on the opposite side (fig. 8.1). Other cells appear to have lost a portion of their membrane and/or hemoglobin. A variety of names have been applied to these bizarrely shaped red cells: eccentrocytes (16), bite cells (58), pincer cells (59), and drug-reacting cells (60).

Hemolytic anemia only develops in a small percentage of children exposed to naphthalene. Several explanations have been proposed. The amount of chemical swallowed, absorbed through the skin, or inhaled may have been insufficient to cause hemolysis. Even so, reports in the literature indicate that percutaneous absorption or inhalation of the naphthalene vapors are injurious (52, 55, 61–63, 64). Another observation of interest was a study by Smille, who noted that parasiticidal doses of β-naphthol, a metabolite of naphthalene, administered to 79 Brazilian blacks induced a severe hemolytic anemia in only 4 (65). Smille suggested that certain predisposing factors were essential for the occurrence of hemolysis. Also it had been observed that the majority of other cases in the literature occurred in black individuals, implying that the unique susceptibility to hemolysis may be a characteristic of certain ethnic groups. Early studies in this and other countries demonstrated that the predisposing factor in most, but not all, patients was a deficiency of red cell G-6-PD (3, 4, 44, 57, 64, 66–68). Exceptions were noted in a series of Greek newborns in whom severe hemolysis was associated with normal G-6-PD activities (63). The primary source of exposure was a blanket stored in naphthalene mothballs, and most of the patients were infants whose ages ranged from 3–42 days, the average age being 10 days. Twelve of the infants received an exchange transfusion, eight developed kernicterus, and two died. This experience also suggests that naphthalene vapors are an important cause of neonatal jaundice in infants with the Mediterranean type of G-6-PD deficiency, an observation that may contribute to the higher incidence of neonatal icterus in this group.

Details of how naphthalene causes lysis of red cells are not yet available. A previous study indicates that naphthalene metabolites rather than naphthalene are the injurious agents. Rieders and Brieger identified four metabolites of naphthalene in the urine of their patient with naphthalene poisoning: α- and β-naphthol and α- and β-naphthoquinone (14). Addition of these compounds to blood in vitro caused hemolysis, whereas naphthalene had no effect. The oxidant potential of these chemicals was demonstrated later by measuring the conversion of reduced to oxidized glutathione in G-6-PD normal and G-6-PD^{A-} blood (4, 57). As little as 0.025 mg/10 ml of α-naphthoquinone caused an abnormal decrease of reduced glutathione in G-6-PD-deficient blood in vitro but had no effect on normal blood (fig. 8.4).

Gasser described a group of premature infants in whom a spontaneous Heinz body hemolytic anemia developed (69, 70). The detailed reporting of these cases provided a clue concerning the nature of the problem. Microphotographs of the peripheral blood smears exhibited red cell morphologic changes that are seen in patients with naphthalene-induced hemolysis (fig. 8.5). Graphs of the clinical and laboratory findings revealed that each of the premature infants received Synkavite, a tetrasodium diphosphate salt of menadione, 5–10 mg/day for a period of 1–2 weeks.

This observation by Gasser and another by Varadi and Hurworth (71), together with reports of a relationship between large doses of vitamin K and the occurrence of kernicterus in premature infants (72), suggested that the water-soluble analogs routinely used to prevent hemorrhagic disease in the newborn might have been a factor contributing to the development of hyperbilirubinemia, especially in those ethnic groups with a high incidence of G-6-PD deficiency. Further confirmation of this hypothesis was the striking structural similarity between the synthetic vitamin K compounds and the naphthalene metabolites (fig. 8.6). For these reasons, our group designed a study to determine the effect of various vitamin K preparations on the blood and bilirubin levels of full-term G-6-PD-normal and G-6-PD-deficient black infants. Thirty infants were divided into three groups of 10

each, one group given no vitamin K, another group a water-soluble analog of vitamin K_3, and the third group, vitamin K_1 (73). The only difference noted was a lowering of bilirubin values in those infants receiving vitamin K_1, suggesting that it may favorably affect bilirubin metabolism in these infants. This observation, together with the finding that vitamin K_1 does not oxidize glutathione in vitro, suggested that vitamin K_1 is the agent of choice for the treatment of vitamin K deficient states. As a prophylactic dose to prevent hemorrhagic disease of the newborn, 1.0 mg can be given.

Fava Beans

For centuries the harmful effects of fava beans (*Vicia faba*) in certain individuals had been realized, probably dating from early Greek and Roman times as reflected by the often-quoted observations attributed to Pythagoras and Hippocrates, "avoid fava beans." The major features of the disorder are an acute, severe, intravascular hemolytic episode associated with Heinz bodies and drug-reacting cells, occurring most often in persons from the Mediterranean littoral, Israel, and the Far East, and according to most reports more commonly affecting males (74–78). Another characteristic is the occurrence of several cases in the same family (79). Such a racial, sexual, and familial distribution suggests that red cells from these patients may have a defect similar to that observed

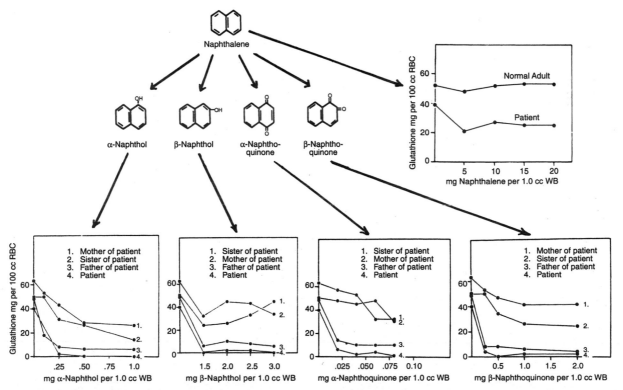

Figure 8.4. The metabolites of naphthalene and their effect on the GSH content of whole blood obtained from a black G-6-PD-deficient male with a history of a naphthalene-induced hemolytic anemia. The patient's father was enzyme deficient (Gd^A−) and his mother and sister were heterozygotes (Gd^A d^A−). From Zinkham and Childs (4).

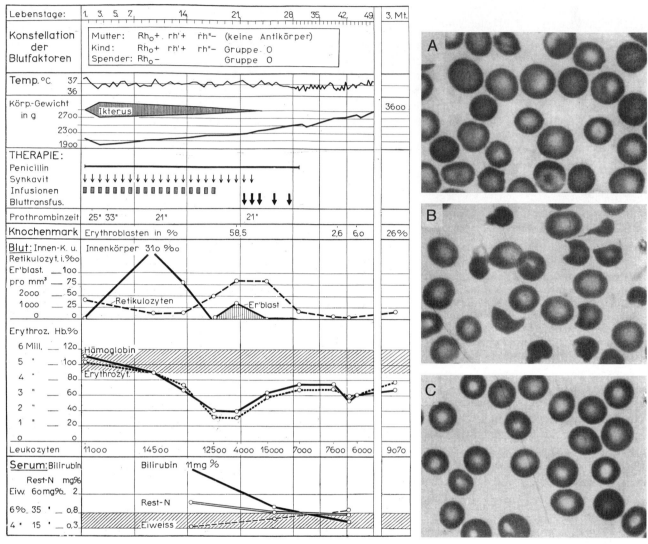

Lebenstage:	1. 3. 5. 7.	14	21	28	35	42	49	3. Mt.
Konstellation der Blutfaktoren	Mutter: Rho+. rh'+ rh"- (keine Antikörper) Kind: Rho+ rh'+ rh"- Gruppe. O Spender: Rho- Gruppe O							

Temp. °C 37 / 36

Körp.-Gewicht in g 2700 / 2300 / 1900 — Ikterus — 3600

THERAPIE:
Penicillin
Synkavit
Infusionen
Bluttransfus.

| Prothrombinzeit | 25" 33" | 21" | 21" | | | | | |
| Knochenmark | Erythroblasten in % | 58,5 | | 2,6 | 6,0 | | | 26% |

Blut: Innen-K. u. Retikulozyt. i.‰ Innenkörper 310 ‰
Er'blast. ___100
pro mm³ ___ 75
2000 ___ 50
1000 ___ 25
0 ___ 0
Retikulozyten   Er'blast

Erythroz. Hb.%
6 Mill. ___ 120 Hämoglobin
5 " ___ 100 Erythrozyt.
4 " ___ 80
3 " ___ 60
2 " ___ 40
1 " ___ 20
0 ___ 0

| Leukozyten | 11000 | 14500 | 12500 | 4000 | 15000 | 7000 | 7600 | 6000 | 9070 |

Serum: Bilirubin   Bilirubin 11mg %
Rest-N mg%
Eiw 60mg% 2
6% 35 ' ___ 0,8   Rest-N
4 ' 15 ' ___ 0,3   Eiweiss

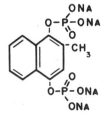

A

B

C

Figure 8.5. Graph displaying the clinical and laboratory findings in a premature infant with "spontaneous Heinz body anemia." Note that the infant received "Synkavit" (menadione diphosphate), 5–10 mg daily from the 1st–23d day of life. Heinz bodies, "Innenkörper," peaked at day 10 and disappeared at day 16. A sequence of Giemsa-stained smears of peripheral blood obtained from this infant are shown: (d) day 1, (e) day 12, and (f) day 30 of life. From Gasser (70).

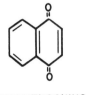

1,4 - NAPHTHOQUINONE

2 - METHYL -
1,4 -NAPHTHOQUINONE
(MENADIONE)

MENADIONE
SODIUM BISULFITE
(HYKINONE)

MENADIONE
DIPHOSPHATE
(SYNKAVITE)

Figure 8.6. Structural similarities between α-naphthoquinone, one of the four major metabolites of naphthalene, and menadione and its water-soluble analogs.

in patients with drug-induced hemolytic anemias. A large number of studies, especially in Italy, Greece, and Israel, as well as a few in the United States, have unequivocally shown that favism occurs only in subjects with G-6-PD-deficient red cells (80–83). However, favism does not develop in all G-6-PD-deficient subjects after ingesting the beans (75, 79). Also, the occurrence of hemolysis is sporadic, even in those individuals with one episode of favism. Some patients have ingested beans before and after a hemolytic episode without demonstrable hemolysis developing. For these reasons, other etiologic factors have been considered, but none have been proven.

The nature of the hemolytic agent in the bean remains unknown. Most of the hemolytic episodes occur after ingestion of fresh beans during the harvest season or after eating uncooked dry beans (78, 83, 84). There is disagreement concerning the hemolytic potential of the plant pollen (75). In this regard, earlier papers reported a decrease in reduced glutathione levels when G-6-PD-deficient red cells were incubated with extracts of the bean, pistils, or pollen (85, 86). Other workers have indicated that divicine and isouramil are the active compounds in the beans (87, 88). Clearly, there appears to be some type of hemolytic agent in the bean. If so, then variations in the concentration of the hemolytic agent or its metabolism may underlie the variable expression of favism. A report suggesting a familial predisposition to favism is already available (79). Further studies are necessary to identify the nature of these inheritable factors.

Drugs and Infections

A current listing of commonly used drugs that can induce hemolysis in G-6-PD-deficient subjects is given in table 8.3. The entry or exit of agents over the years has depended on a variety of selection processes, many by the historical recording of hemolysis in the G-6-PD subject receiving the offending agent. Obviously, more than one report is necessary to incriminate the hemolytic potential of an agent based on this type of selection process, and even then other mechanisms may be the cause of hemolysis. Another method involves the administration of Cr^{51}-labeled G-6-PD-deficient cells into a normal subject, who is then given the suspect agent (45). As noted previously, in vitro techniques are not definitive. For example, the parent compound may be without effect when added to blood in vitro, as is true for naphthalene (4). Furthermore, knowledge of the naphthalene metabolites directed attention to the water-soluble analogs of vitamin K as possible hemolytic agents because of their structural similarities.

Several large studies have reported the frequency of drug related hemolytic episodes in G-6-PD-deficient subjects. In a group of 129 patients with hemolytic events in Israel, Herman and Ben-Meir (89) stated that 14 were secondary to fava bean exposure, 10 to drugs administered to

patients with a variety of illnesses, and 1 was undetermined. Of interest was the occurrence of a hemolytic anemia in only 3 of 6 patients who received nitrofurantoin, a well-known hemolytic agent, not only in G-6-PD subjects of Mediterranean origin, but also in G-6-PD^A-subjects (90).

In another large survey, Burka et al. retrospectively analyzed the circumstances of 139 episodes of hemolysis in 63 enzyme-deficient subjects (91). Seventy three appeared to be secondary to some underlying illness, e.g., bacterial or viral infections and diabetic ketoacidosis, and 46 were attributed to drugs. In this latter group, possible offending agents were aspirin in 7, chloramphenicol in 3, streptomycin in 1, and phenytoin in 1. More recent surveys have shown that each of these agents administered in therapeutic doses does not cause hemolysis, leaving 34 attributable to some drug, the most frequent offender being a sulfonamide.

A more recent study by Shannon and Buchanan indicates the minor role of drugs as hemolytic agents in hospitalized black G-6-PD-deficient children with a hemolytic anemia (68). Of the 14 hemolytic episodes, 11 appeared to be secondary to some bacterial or viral infection and 3 to naphthalene. None could be attributed to a drug. Excluded from consideration were aspirin and acetaminophen that had been administered to many of the patients prior to hospitalization.

In summary, certain drugs or chemicals should be avoided in G-6-PD-deficient subjects. Past and current reports, however, indicate that infections, rather than drugs, are more common precipitating events.

Neonatal Jaundice and G-6-PD Deficiency

The development of a mild degree of jaundice occurs in almost every neonate, more so in premature than full-term infants. For this reason it is frequently referred to as physiologic jaundice. Sometimes the dividing line between normal and abnormal bilirubin values is difficult to establish. In general, if values for unconjugated bilirubin exceed 12 mg/dl, then certain investigative techniques should be instituted. The two most common causes associated with anemia and hyperbilirubinemia are isoimmunization (AB-O or Rh incompatibilities), and infection. Neither of these were demonstrated in the infant described in the above case report at a time when the bilirubin level peaked at 21.6 mg/dl. Consequently, other etiologic factors were explored.

G-6-PD Deficiency and Neonatal Hyperbilirubinemia

At least three explanations have been proposed to explain the occurrence of this phenomenon: (a) the common enzyme variant in different world population groups is responsible, (b) an uncommon G-6-PD mutant associated with a moderate-to-severe lifelong hemolytic anemia is the cause, and (c) some extracorpuscular factor injures the G-6-PD-deficient red cell. The majority of the reports on G-6-PD deficiency and neonatal hyperbilirubinemia focus on the first possibility, namely, that the enzyme deficiency per se is the sole etiologic agent.

Valaes et al. in Greece (92–95), Weatherall (96) and Smith and Vella in Malaya (97), Segni in Italy (98), and Panizon and Meo in Sardinia (99) were among the first to report on the development of extreme hyperbilirubinemia and even kernicterus and death in infants with G-6-PD-deficient red cells. It was impossible to calculate the frequency of the phenomenon on the basis of these early reports, because the sample size was too small and the extent of the enzyme abnormality in the general population was unknown. Furthermore, in those infants in whom hematologic data were available, there was evidence of a hemolytic process. For example, in the report of Valaes et al. (92), case 1 was anemic, with a hemoglobin of 12.1 g/dl, and this infant's red cell morphologic changes, as exhibited in fig. 8.1, are indicative of those observed in subjects with a chemical or drug-induced hemolytic disorder. In case 3, there was a history of exposure to naphthalene mothballs approximately 7 days after the appearance of jaundice at 36 hours of age. The three subjects of Weatherall's report (96) were anemic, with hemoglobin values of 6.0, 7.2, and 9.6 g/dl, respectively. However, studies of 9 additional Malayan families revealed "one or more infants" with jaundice from the third day to the second week of life. None of these infants were anemic and none exhibited a deficiency of red cell G-6-PD.

Anemia or alterations in red cell morphology did not develop in all Greek infants with G-6-PD deficiency-related hyperbilirubinemia (93, 95). Also, a thorough search for environmental factors such as drugs, chemicals, fava beans, or infections as predisposing factors for the development of hyperbilirubinemia was unrevealing. Hence, it appeared that the enzyme deficiency was solely responsible for the hyperbilirubinemia, and in some the eventual development of kernicterus and death.

Subsequent reports from Greece (100, 101), together with those from other parts of the world, including Israel (102–105), India (106, 107), Thailand (108, 109), Ghana (110), Nigeria (111), South Africa (112), Turkey (113), Sardinia (114), China (115), and Singapore (116) have indicated that G-6-PD-deficient infants in these countries are susceptible to the development of protracted hyperbilirubinemia and in most without any other demonstrable etiology. The incidence of the phenomenon is extremely varied, even within the same country (101). Finally, data from two other countries, Sweden (117) and Hungary (118), demonstrated no relationship between neonatal hyperbilirubinemia and G-6-PD deficiency. In these countries G-6-PD deficiency is a rare event.

The importance of sample size in investigating the relationship between neonatal hyperbilirubinemia and G-6-PD deficiency is illustrated by the report of Szeinberg et al. (105). Three groups of infants were studied. Group 1 involved 203 infants born to Kurdish and Iranian Jews, ethnic groups in which the incidence of G-6-PD deficiency in adult males is 58.2% and 15.1%, respectively. No cases of

neonatal hyperbilirubinemia attributable to G-6-PD deficiency were identified, although the expected number of deficient males was 122 and of heterozygous females 42. In another village of 61 Kurdish and 59 Iranian neonates, none exhibited severe jaundice or kernicterus. Groups 2 and 3 comprised observations on 12,389 infants born at the Kaplan Hospital and another 32,000 infants born at four government hospitals. From this extensive survey, the authors identified 8 Iraqi Jewish infants whose hyperbilirubinemia could not be attributed to factors other than G-6-PD deficiency. One required an exchange transfusion on the sixth day of life, in another the bilirubin level was 17.5 mg/dl, and in the remaining 6, <15 mg/dl. The authors conclude that "the present investigation does not suggest that G-6-PD deficiency constitutes a major etiological factor in the causation of severe neonatal jaundice in Israel."

In contrast to the many reports from other countries, remarkably few papers from North America address the issue of G-6-PD-deficient-related hyperbilirubinemia in the newborn (73, 119–121). A project by our group was designed to answer two questions: (a) is the full-term black newborn with G-6-PD deficiency predisposed to the development of hyperbilirubinemia? and (b) what is the effect of various vitamin K compounds on the peripheral blood and serum bilirubin values of these infants (73)? Thirty full-term enzyme-deficient infants were divided into three groups of 10 each, with one group receiving no vitamin K, another group receiving water-soluble analogs of vitamin K, and a third group, vitamin K_1. Ten enzyme-normal infants served as control subjects for each group. None of the infants exhibited bilirubin levels >14.5 mg/dl. However, the G-6-PD-deficient infants not receiving vitamin K had significantly higher bilirubin values than the other infants at the fifth and eighth days of life. Reticulocyte counts were slightly elevated in all of the G-6-PD-deficient infants. None of the enzyme-deficient group could be differentiated from the enzyme-normal group on the basis of hematocrit values, the occurrence of Heinz bodies, or red cell morphology. Since this initial study, approximately 30,000 full-term black infants have been delivered at our hospital. The incidence of G-6-PD deficiency in the African-American population of Baltimore, Maryland, is as follows: hemizygote males (Gd^{A-}) 14.2%, homozygote females ($Gd^{A-}Gd^{A-}$) 2%, and female heterozygotes ($Gd^{A-}Gd^{A}$) 24% (122). Based on these data, approximately 2000 infant boys and 300 infant girls born at our hospital, together with another small percentage of the female heterozygotes should be predisposed to the phenomenon of G-6-PD-deficient-related hyperbilirubinemia. Although bilirubin data are not available on each infant, there is no instance in which an exchange transfusion was performed in a G-6-PD-deficient infant with unexplained hyperbilirubinemia. Unfortunately, no data are available on the rate of utilization of phototherapy in our full-term nurseries. Possibly, phototherapy is responsible for the absence of exchange transfusions.

Another study in this country by Wolff et al. suggested that the incidence of jaundice was the same in G-6-PD-deficient infants as in those with enzyme normal red cells (120). Specifically, of 119 randomly selected black full-term infant boys, 8 exhibited a deficiency of G-6-PD. Only 1 of the 8 had a maximum bilirubin level >10 mg/dl. In an earlier portion of this study, 18 of 844 black and white infants weighing more than 1900 g exhibited a deficiency of red cell G-6-PD. Of the 18, 2 babies were Puerto Rican and 16 were black. Only one of the infants was icteric, with a maximal bilirubin value of 15.1 mg/100 ml. Other reports from the United States implicate a combination of events preceding the development of hyperbilirubinemia, including acidosis, hypoxia, and prematurity (121, 123).

In contrast to full-term African-American G-6-PD-deficient newborns, premature African-American infants with enzyme deficiency are prone to the development of hyperbilirubinemia (123). During a 4 month period of observation, 10 of 87 black male infants were found to be G-6-PD deficient, 5 of the 10 eventually requiring an exchange transfusion. Of the 77 enzyme-normal infants, only 8 needed an exchange transfusion.

In summary, a survey of the world literature indicates that G-6-PD deficiency per se can be associated with severe degrees of hyperbilirubinemia. The frequency of the event is quite variable, being most common in certain ethnic groups (Iraqi Jews, Italians and Greeks living in or from the Mediterranean littoral, and Chinese) and a rarity in full-term African-American infants, but present to a moderate degree in premature African-American infants. Since pathologic bilirubin levels do not develop in all G-6-PD-deficient infants, even in those countries with a high incidence of G-6-PD-related hyperbilirubinemia, other factors must be operative. Factors to consider include quantitative and/or qualitative differences in the mutant forms of the enzyme, epistatic factors that affect the activity of the Gd locus, and inherited or ontogenetic events that modify the metabolism of bilirubin. Previous and current reports have suggested but not proven that the life span of the neonatal G-6-PD-deficient red cell is reduced as it is in certain G-6-PD-deficient adults, thereby increasing the amount of bilirubin to be metabolized (124–126). Another possibility is the immaturity of the bilirubin glucuronidation pathway in some infants, which in turn leads to elevated plasma bilirubin values, especially in those infants in whom the rate of heme catabolism is increased as a result of decreased red cell survival.

Another explanation for the inter- and intra-ethnic variability of the phenomenon is the possibility that the enzyme deficiency is expressed to different degrees in hepatocytes, thereby impairing the hepatic metabolism of bilirubin. A recent report addresses this possibility by investigating the ability of enzyme-normal and enzyme-deficient newborns to glucuronidate salicylates (127).

A final consideration is the suggestion that the list of environmental agents capable of causing hemolysis and hyperbilirubinemia in the G-6-PD-deficient neonate is incomplete. Clinical reports to date of environmental agents associated with neonatal hyperbilirubinemia include naphthalene, breast milk of mothers who have ingested fava beans, menthol-containing dusting powders, and possibly herbal medicines (124, 234). A recent search for another hemolytic agent was prompted by the observation that in the Middle East, some babies with unexplained neonatal hyperbilirubinemia exhibited staining of the skin following the topical application of henna (F. A. Oski, personal observation). Henna is a dye, the source of which is the shrub *Lawsonia alba*. The plant is grown extensively in North Africa, the Middle East, and India, and large amounts are imported into the United States. When the dried leaves are soaked in water and applied to the skin, hair, or nails, an auburn-to-red color develops—hence its worldwide use as a cosmetic agent.

An important chemical ingredient of henna is lawsone (2-hydroxy-1,4-naphthoquinone), composing about 1% by weight of the crushed leaves. The structure and redox potential of lawsone is similar to that of one of the naphthalene metabolites to 1,4-naphthoquinone, an already recognized potent oxidant of G-6-PD-deficient red cells (fig. 8.7). The addition of lawsone to G-6-PD A whole blood in vitro in concentrations ranging from 1.4 to 8.6 × 1^{-3} caused a four- to eight-fold increase in methemoglobin formation and a simultaneous decrease in GSH levels to values <40 mg/ml of red cells (235). These observations indicate that lawsone is an agent capable of causing oxidative hemolysis and in concentrations similar to those observed for α-naphthoquinone. In regions of the world where there is a high incidence of G-6-PD deficiency and unexplained hyperbilirubinemia, oxidative hemolysis secondary to the cutaneous application of henna could be the initiating event.

Genetics of G-6-PD Deficiency

Knowledge that the abnormality was limited to certain individuals and to certain ethnic groups suggested a genetic basis for the disorder. Indeed, studies performed on a

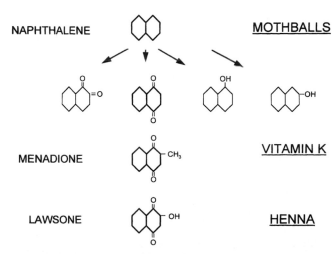

Figure 8.7. Structural similarities between α-naphthoquinone, one of the four major metabolites of naphthalene, menadione, and lawsone, a chemical derived from henna *(Lawsonia alba)*.

large number of families in which a G-6-PD subject had been identified demonstrated that the defect was transmitted by a sex-linked gene of intermediate dominance (128). To date, it is one of the most common genetic disorders in man, involving millions of people of many different ethnic groups (129).

Enzyme Polymorphisms

A large number of polymorphisms have been identified, approximately 400 to date (36). Many are silent mutations; others are associated with drug-induced hemolysis or neonatal jaundice, as noted in previous sections; and another polymorphism is associated with the occurrence of a congenital nonspherocytic hemolytic anemia. This last group is especially informative since it exhibits so well the essential role of G-6-PD in regulating the life span of the red cell. A marked deficiency of G-6-PD in spite of the presence of a large number of reticulocytes is associated with a severe hemolytic anemia, which in some patients has led to a splenectomy.

Further characterization of the mutant enzymes based on levels of enzyme activity indicated five different classes: class I variants occur in subjects with nonspherocytic hemolytic anemia; class II variants exhibit <10% of normal activity; class III, 10–60% of normal activity; class IV variants represent those with a normal range of enzyme activity; and class V, above normal activities (130). Within each group there are variations in the electrophoretic mobilities of the enzyme, together with differences in pH optima, thermolability, and kinetic properties. The magnitude of the enzyme polymorphisms is almost equal to that of the hemoglobinopathies and may even surpass those as the techniques of molecular genetics are utilized for characterization of the G-6-PD mutants.

Elucidation of the amino acid sequences in the hemoglobin variants was expedited by the fact that grams of protein could be isolated and purified quite easily. In contrast, G-6-PD constitutes far less than 1% of the total red cell protein, thereby making it extremely difficult to obtain sufficient amounts of protein for molecular characterization. Yoshida was the first to accomplish this feat by identifying the amino acid differences between G-6-PD-B and G-6-PD-A (131).

It has now became possible to identify the molecular structure of the mutant enzymes with some precision. Once the G-6-PD gene was cloned and its complementary DNA sequenced, several interesting findings emerged. As noted by Beutler, mutations in patients with congenital nonspherocytic hemolytic anemia cluster near the carboxyl end of the enzyme, whereas the more silent mutations cluster near the amino end (50). Application of this technique to many of the mutants previously identified on the basis of their kinetic and electrophoretic properties has revealed that some have similar sequence analyses (50). Thus, the discriminatory power of molecular genetics exceeds that of the biochemical approach.

Population Screening

Several bulletins published by the World Health Organization, together with reports from countries in which there is a high incidence of G-6-PD deficiency, have recommended screening for the abnormality in newborns (129). Their concern is the occurrence of neonatal jaundice days after discharge of the infant from the nursery. A recent study determined the prevalence of G-6-PD deficiency in 1,286,000 Greek newborns (39). In another report, 6,366 African-American infants were screened (132), and in yet another, 700 Chinese newborns (133). Support for a screening program is provided by Meloni et al., who have focused on creating approaches for detecting the early development of neonatal hyperbilirubinemia, together with its prevention in G-6-PD-deficient newborns (134).

Should screening programs to define the G-6-PD-deficient newborn be continued? The enormous number of G-6-PD-deficient infants raises questions about the feasibility of conducting a successful screening program, one in which the parents of the G-6-PD-deficient infants are counseled and appropriate followup is instituted to insure that the counseling program has been effective. For example, in how many of screened G-6-PD-deficient newborns does anemia later develop after exposure to some hemolytic agent? Another deficiency of a screening program, especially in those countries with a high incidence of G-6-PD deficiency, is the inability to identify the heterozygous female with some of the qualitative methodologies usually employed in these screening programs.

In North America, clinical problems secondary to G-6-PD deficiency in full-term infants are extremely rare. Rather than developing screening programs, the emphasis has been placed on identifying the causes of neonatal hyperbilirubinemia.

Once a patient with a drug- or chemical- induced hemolytic episode is identified, the family is counseled regarding other hemolytic agents and should be given a laminated card listing those agents. G-6-PD testing should be also offered to other family members.

Another possible role of counseling may be in those families in which a child with G-6-PD-deficient type of nonspherocytic hemolytic anemia requires frequent transfusions, even after splenectomy. Should in utero diagnosis be offered to these families? Probably so since severe anemia in utero may lead to hydrops fetalis as well as severe postnatal anemia. Cases of this type have not been described previously. However, a severe deficiency of G-6-PD or some other enzyme should be considered as a cause of nonisoimmune hydrops fetalis secondary to anemia.

Lyon Hypothesis

In 1961 Lyon (135) and Russell (136) proposed that only one X chromosome in each somatic cell of the female was active. The identification of the G-6-PD abnormality and the demonstration of its electrophoretic forms led to a testing of the hypothesis in humans. Davidson et al., utilizing skin biopsies, were able to identify the electrophoretic characteristics of cells cloned from a single cell (137). In heterozygous black females ($Gd^A Gd^{A-}$), both fast and slow bands were present in sonicates of skin cells. In skin cells cloned from a single skin cell, only one electrophoretic band appeared, either fast or slow, never a mixture of the two as observed in uncloned skin cultures. These findings confirmed the Lyon hypothesis.

An earlier paper by Beutler et al. also provided evidence for inactivation of one of the two female X chromosomes by studying the rate of oxidation of GSH in mixtures of normal and G-6-PD-deficient red cells (138). The slope of the curves in red cells from heterozygous females compared with artificial mixtures of G-6-PD-normal and G-6-PD-deficient cells were quite similar. Later studies utilizing a methemoglobin elution assay confirmed this observation by showing two types of elution patterns in red cells from heterozygous females (139).

Tissue Distribution

The anatomic distribution of many monogenic disorders is quite variable. Clinical observations, together with enzyme analysis of individual tissues, is necessary to determine the extent of the defect and its impact on tissue function. In the mother and infant of the case reported above with a naphthalene-induced hemolytic anemia, the red cell appeared to be the major target of the naphthalene. Even so, the possibility existed that other systems may have been injured. For example, naphthalene has been administered experimentally to rabbits in order to study those factors leading to the development of cataracts (140).

Leukocytes

The most extensively studied cell, other than the red cell in G-6-PD-deficient subjects, is the leukocyte. Several factors account for this interest: the accessibility of the white cells, although they are difficult to obtain in pure form; reports that there is a high incidence of infections in G-6-PD-deficient subjects; and similarities in the clinical presentation of subjects with chronic granulomatous disease (CGD) and G-6-PD variants associated with infections.

One of the first reports on G-6-PD activities in leukocytes from African Americans indicated that they were no different than those observed in G-6-PD-normal subjects (141). A later study from Israel demonstrated a significant reduction of G-6-PD activities in both white cells and platelets (142). Values for 6-phosphogluconic dehydrogenase activities were normal. Presumably the subjects in this study were Sephardic Jews, an ethnic group in which the enzyme defect is quantitatively and qualitatively different than the one occurring in blacks.

The physicochemical properties of the enzyme in leukocytes from two normal, one primaquine-sensitive (probably Gd^{A-}), one Mediterranean deficient, and one black with

a congenital nonspherocytic hemolytic anemia were similar to those of red cells obtained form the same subjects (143). Both the leukocytes and the platelets exhibited a moderate-to-marked reduction of enzyme activity.

A large number of studies have been designed to determine whether the G-6-PD deficiency of leukocytes in certain ethnic groups may be associated with an increased susceptibility to infections. In Saudi Arabia, G-6-PD-deficient children experienced a greater number of infections than did control subjects who were enzyme normal (144). Another report from the same country suggested that G-6-PD-deficient newborns were especially susceptible to the development of late sepsis and infections by catalase-positive organisms (145). Studies in Thailand (146), Ghana (147), and India (148) noted a higher frequency of typhoid fever, pneumococcal infections, leprosy, and tuberculosis in G-6-PD-deficient males and heterozygous females. Hospitalized G-6-PD-deficient patients in Iran also had a higher incidence of infections (149). Opposing views have been offered by workers in Sardinia (150) and Nigeria (151), countries in which G-6-PD-deficient children do not exhibit an increased incidence of infections.

Although the number of patients is small, several reports have shown a definite relationship between a severe deficiency of leukocyte G-6-PD and an increased incidence of infections (152–156). With one exception, all of the patients have been white, with a severe reduction of both red cell and leukocyte G-6-PD. In contrast to patients with chronic granulomatous disease (CGD), most of these patients experience infections later in life. However, infections in both conditions are usually due to catalase-positive rather than catalase-negative organisms. Leukocytes from subjects with a severe deficiency of G-6-PD, like those from subjects with CGD, lack a respiratory burst with failure to stimulate HMP activity, failure to reduce nitro-blue tetrazolium to formazan, and nongeneratation of hydrogen peroxide. The last characteristic explains the propensity of these subjects to have infections with catalase-positive organisms.

Liver

Oluboyede et al. observed a statistically significant difference between G-6-PD activities in livers from G-6-PD-normal and G-6-PD-deficient Nigerians, 25 males and 6 females, in whom liver biopsies were performed as part of a diagnostic evaluation (157). Using postmortem tissues, Chan et al. demonstrated a deficiency of liver G-6-PD activity in 6 G-6-PD-deficient subjects compared to 7 subjects with normal activity (158). In 2 African Americans, Marks et al. observed slightly reduced activities in two liver biopsies (141).

Factaors contributing to the severity of viral-induced hepatitis are unknown. Some reports suggest that the course of hepatitis in these patients is longer and is associated with higher bilirubin levels (159–163). Possibly, this phenomenon is secondary to the hemolytic anemia that occurs in G-6-PD-deficient patients with viral-induced hepatitis, an occurrence which in some patients is associated with renal failure (164, 165).

Another reason for the elevated bilirubin levels in G-6-PD-deficient subjects with hepatitis, as well as G-6-PD-deficient neonates with hyperbilirubinemia, is the observation that bilirubin uptake by the liver is mediated by ligandin, a cytosol protein with glutathione *S-transferase activity (158)*. Since reduced glutathione may be required for this reaction, a deficiency of G-6-PD in hepatocytes may impede the transfer of bilirubin from the serum to the hepatocytes.

Lens

Interest in G-6-PD activity of the lens was prompted by the knowledge that there are many structural and metabolic similarities between the erythron mass and the lens: both contain nonnucleated cells that are unable to synthesize protein; both exhibit a high concentration of reduced glutathione, the reduction of which is dependent on the HMP; and, finally, naphthalene, a potent hemolytic agent, also induces the formation of cataracts (140). Furthermore, L-buthionine sulfoximine, a specific inhibitor of γ-glutamyl-cysteinylglycine, induces a severe deficiency of GSH and the appearance of cataracts in male suckling mice by 9–10 days of age (166).

In one study, activities of G-6-PD and 6-PGD were determined in erythrocytes and lens from African-Americans and white individuals with senile cataracts (167). Two G-6-PD-deficient black males manifested a significantly reduced value for G-6-PD in their lens. 6-PGD activity was normal. G-6-PD activity in lenses from 35 black males at autopsy was reduced in 5, as was red cell activity. This study unequivocally showed that the G-6-PD defect exhibited by the red cell was also present in the lens of the eye. It did not indicate, but suggested, that there may be an association between the development of senile or chemically induced cataracts and the G-6-PD deficiency state. For this reason, every child who has a naphthalene-induced hemolytic anemia is followed-up for the development of cataracts.

Subsequent reports have provided evidence that other variant forms of G-6-PD deficiency may be operative in the development of cataracts. One Puerto Rican patient had a severe hemolytic anemia, cataracts, and some type of neurologic disorder (168). Two boys from a Danish family had severe nonspherocytic hemolytic anemia due to deficiency of G-6-PD. At 2 years of age, one of them exhibited cerebral palsy and lamellar cataracts (169).

Other Cells

A variety of other cell types have been investigated for G-6-PD activity. Deficiencies have been defined in platelets (170, 171), saliva (172), muscle (173), kidney (158), and sperm (174). As yet no one has demonstrated a relationship between these abnormalities and disease.

Management of G-6-PD Deficiency

The question most often asked is what type of blood should be transfused into G-6-PD-deficient subjects with drug-induced hemolysis. Survival times of G-6-PD-deficient red cells are decreased in normal volunteers following the administration of a variety of hemolytic agents (45). For this reason it is rational to use nondeficient blood in any G-6-PD-deficient subject with severe anemia secondary to drug exposure. If G-6-PD-deficient cells were transfused, their fate would be the same as the patient's red cells, providing that the hemolytic agent was still present.

Another clinical situation in which it would be advisable to use nondeficient blood is in G-6-PD-deficient newborns requiring exchange transfusions because of hyperbilirubinemia. Two objectives would be accomplished, supplanting the enzyme-deficient population of red cells with normal red cells and removal of bilirubin.

Careful monitoring of bilirubin levels in newborns of ethnic groups predisposed to the development of hyperbilirubinemia could result in the early application of phototherapy, thereby preventing the need for an exchange transfusion. Phototherapy in those infants is effective (175, 176), and contrary to some reports (177) does not appear to elevate bilirubin levels or cause anemia. Another approach in these infants has been the administration of barbiturates to enhance bilirubin glucuronidation by the liver (178).

Because of its antioxidant effects, vitamin E, with or without selenium, has been administered to G-6-PD-deficient subjects, including those with nonspherocytic hemolytic anemia. Corash et al. stated that vitamin E administered to 23 G-6-PD Mediterranean subjects prolonged the survival of their red cells (179). Red cell survival also lengthened in a patient with a severe form of G-6-PD deficiency and another patient with glutathione synthetase deficiency (180). Vitamin E, with or without selenium, reduced the rate of hemolysis in 36 G-6-PD-deficient Egyptian boys (181). Other workers, however, have indicated that vitamin E is without effect in G-6-PD-deficient subjects (182, 183). Hence the efficacy of vitamin E in those subjects with severe deficiencies of G-6-PD remains controversial. To pursue this question further, two groups have shown that the addition of vitamin E to G-6-PD-deficient blood in vitro did not alter the rate of GSH oxidation after the addition of APH (3, 183).

Pyruvate Kinase

For many years the term "congenital nonspherocytic hemolytic anemia" was used to designate a group of hemolytic disorders that escaped definition on the basis of characteristic morphologic changes (184). Hence the diagnosis was made only after conditions such as thalassemia, hereditary spherocytosis, hereditary elliptocytosis, and certain hemoglobinopathies had been excluded. A review of case reports revealed features that were common to all of them: alterations in osmotic fragilities, reduced survival of red cells in the patient as well as normal recipients, clustering in families, and variable therapeutic effectiveness of splenectomy. Unshared characteristics included heavy stippling of the red cells, and in some, an accelerated rate of autohemolysis.

The first elucidation of a metabolic, and possibly biochemical, abnormality in nonspherocytic red cells was by Selwyn and Dacie (185). On the basis of in vitro observations on glucose consumption, they were able to distinguish two varieties. Later, Newton and Bass defined an abnormality of glutathione metabolism secondary to a marked deficiency of G-6-PD in red cells from 3 Italian children with nonspherocytic hemolytic anemia, the first demonstration of an enzymopathy as a cause of a congenital hemolytic disorder (186).

Since then, many other enzyme defects have been associated with the occurrence of a variety of chronic and inherited forms of hemolytic anemia. Some of the defective enzymes regulate the flow of glucose through the Embden-Meyerhof pathway of glycolysis, while the hemolytic effects of the others are mediated via the HMP and its related enzymes. This section will focus on the most common enzymopathy of the Embden-Meyerhof pathway, a deficiency of pyruvate kinase. Less common enzyme defects affecting both pathways will be mentioned. A recent and detailed review of the subject has been presented by Valentine et al. (187), a pioneering group in the discovery of enzymopathies involving the Embden-Meyerhof pathway.

In 1959 red cells from a group of 6 patients with congenital nonspherocytic hemolytic anemia were examined for an abnormality of glutathione metabolism (40). Three white males exhibited a marked deficiency of G-6-PD; in 1, GSH values before and after incubation of whole blood with APH were decreased, together with a marked increase in G-6-PD activity; and in 2, GSH and G-6-PD values were normal. The case history of 1 of these last 2 patients, together with more recently developed enzyme data, follows.

Case 2

The patient, a 12-year-old African-American girl, was transferred to this hospital at 10 days of age because of anemia and jaundice. Her birth weight was 2500 g. Jaundice appeared at 5 days, the spleen was palpable 4 cm below the costal margin, and the girl's hemoglobin value was 50 g/L. The patient received a transfusion of 18 ml of whole blood, and because of persistent and deepening jaundice was transferred to our hospital.

The patient was pale, listless, and intensely jaundiced. Both the liver and spleen were palpable 3–4 cm

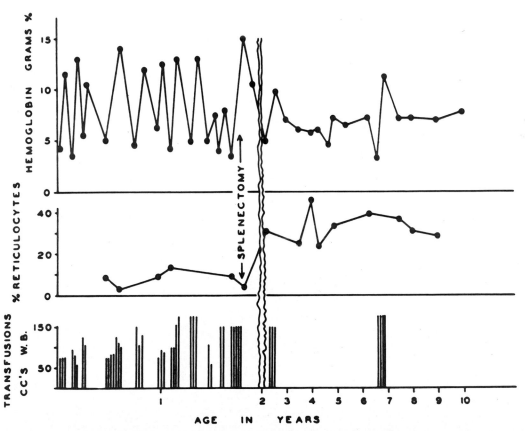

Figure 8.8. Course of hemoglobin and reticulocyte values pre- and postsplenectomy in a black girl with pyruvate kinase deficiency. Splenectomy was performed at $1^{10}/_{12}$ years of age. Note the marked rise in the percentage of reticulocytes after splenectomy. From Zinkham et al. (40).

below the costal margins. Her hemoglobin value was 42 g/L, with a reticulocyte count of 14.0%; the total nucleated count was 11 × 10⁹/L; the differential count showed 50% polymorphonuclear neutrophils, 42% lymphocytes, 7% monocytes, and 8 nucleated erythrocytes per 100 leukocytes. Cultures of the blood and urine were sterile. The total bilirubin was 16.8 mg/dl (direct, 1.2 mg %). The Coombs test, the serologic test for syphilis, and tests for circulating antibodies in the mother's serum, were negative. Later studies for an abnormal hemoglobin, utilizing a variety of techniques, were unrevealing. Nonincubated and incubated osmotic fragility test results and mechanical fragility test results were normal.

As shown in figure 8.7, the patient required transfusions every 4–6 weeks during the first 2½ years of life. After splenectomy at 1½ years of age, the reticulocyte count rose from 10% to a range of 30–40%. Only several transfusions have been given, usually during periods of severe anemia accompanying infections. At 20 years of age leg ulcers developed on the patient, and a cholecystectomy was performed at 25 years of age.

Assays for pyruvate kinase activities in the red cells of the patient and her parents revealed a marked reduction of activity in the patient, and a moderate reduction in both parents.

Pyruvate Kinase (PK) Deficiency and Hemolysis

Several features of this patient's hemolytic disorder merit special consideration. How does the PK deficiency shorten the survival time of the red cells? What is the etiologic role of the spleen and how does splenectomy result in a three- to fourfold increase in the reticulocyte count, accompanied by a significant decrease in transfusion requirements? Answers to these questions require a review of the Embden-Meyerhof pathway and its metabolic role in regulating red cell survival and function (fig. 8.9).

Glucose, the primary energy source for the red cell, freely traverses the red cell membrane, an equilibrium is established, and the amounts of intracellular and extracellular glucose are approximately equal. The cell membrane is impermeable to the phosphorylated derivatives of glucose. Intracellular glucose is phosphorylated by the enzyme hexokinase (HK), a reaction that requires ATP. Glucose-6-phosphate (G-6-P), the product of this reaction,

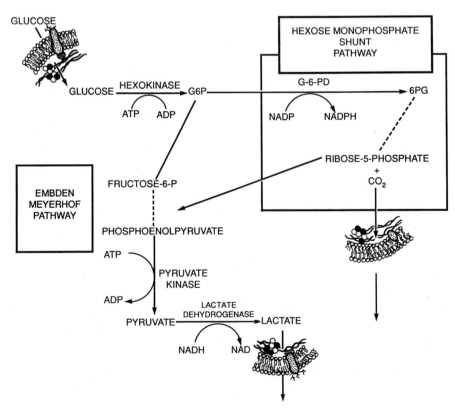

Figure 8.9. An abbreviated sketch of the two major enzyme-catalyzed pathways in the mature red cell, one, the Embden-Meyerhof pathway, and the other, the hexose monophosphate shunt pathway. Under normal conditions, >90% of glucose entering the cell is metabolized via the Embden-Meyerhof pathway. For each mole of glucose entering this pathway, 2 moles of adenosine triphosphate (ATP) are generated, this net gain of ATP resulting from the conversion of phosphoenolpyruvate

to pyruvate, a reaction that is catalyzed by the enzyme pyruvate kinase. A deficiency of pyruvate kinase results in a deficiency of ATP, a high-energy compound that is essential for maintaining the water and electrolyte composition of the red cell. A deficiency of hexokinase, the enzyme that phosphorylates glucose, as well as other enzymes of the Embden-Meyerhof pathway, may have a similar effect for ATP generation.

may then proceed into one of two metabolic pathways—the Embden-Meyerhof or the hexose monophosphate shunt. Under physiologic conditions, the major portion of the G-6-P is converted through a series of enzymatic reactions to lactate, 2 moles of lactate being generated for each mole of glucose catabolized. The mature red cell, lacking mitochondria, is unable to transform pyruvate to high-energy phosphates via the Krebs cycle. Hence, the Embden-Meyerhof pathway remains the major source of ATP, a net gain of 2 moles of ATP being generated for each mole of glucose entering the cycle.

A deficiency of PK affects red cell metabolism in a variety of ways. An important byproduct of the PK-catalyzed conversion of phosphoenolpyruvate to pyruvate is ATP. Thus, deficiency of any enzyme preceding this step will result in limited availability of ATP, and secondary to these changes, loss of water and potassium, decreased plasticity of the membrane, and early sequestering of cells in the reticuloendothelial system (188).

Reticulocytes, unlike mature cells, still retain some mitochondrial activity, together with the ability to synthesize proteins. PK-deficient reticulocytes utilize more oxygen than do normal reticulocytes, suggesting that mitochondrial oxidative activities are increased (189). Another study has demonstrated that more ATP is generated by oxidative phosphorylation in the mitochondria than by the Embden-Meyerhof pathway of the PK-deficient reticulocyte (188). These observations suggest that the PK-deficient reticulocyte should be a better survivor than the PK-deficient nonreticulated cell. Possibly, this is one of the reasons for the increased number of reticulocytes appearing in the blood of the PK-deficient patient following splenectomy (190).

On the other hand, why should the reticulocyte count be lower presplenectomy than postsplenectomy? Several papers have addressed this question, utilizing autologous red cell survival and sequestration studies in PK-deficient patients, as well as heterologous survival of PK cells in normal and splenectomized subjects. On the basis of these observations, the very immature PK cells appear to contain a population of cells that are predisposed to early removal by the liver (191). These cells might be severely deficient in PK activity, especially susceptible to the anoxic and acidic environment of the spleen, and then removed by the liver. If this is true, then what determines which cells will escape the splenic macrophages to be ingested by the Kupffer cells of the liver? Here again, the severity of the PK deficiency may be a decisive factor. A corollary phenomenon is the fate of antibody-sensitized or chemically damaged red cells (192). Those cells with the least amount of antibody or chemical damage are sequestered in the spleen. Cells exposed to larger amounts of antibody or chemical are removed by all portions of the reticuloendothelial system, including spleen, liver, and bone marrow, with some of the cells being lyzed in the circulation. Could the different degrees of severity of the PK abnormality be related to the proportions of the PK red cell isozymes, R_1 and R_2. As noted later, the catalytic characteristics of the mu-

tant R_1 form may contribute to the early demise of the PK-deficient reticulocyte (193).

Another consequence of the PK deficiency state is the accumulation of 2,3-diphosphoglycerate (2,3-DPG). In some patients this compound attains levels that in turn suppress HMP activity in oxidant-stressed red cells (194). Possibly this phenomenon accounts for the exacerbation of hemolysis that sometimes occurs during infections.

A favorable effect of the increased levels of 2,3-DPG in PK-deficient cells is a marked shift to the right of the oxygen dissociation curve (195, 196). For this reason, exercise tolerance is remarkably well preserved even in the presence of severe anemia (fig. 8.9). In contrast, enzyme deficiencies preceding the 2,3-DPG-generating portion of the Embden-Meyerhof pathway (e.g., hexokinase) result in decreased levels of 2,3-DPG, a leftward shift of the oxygen dissociation curve, and reduced exercise tolerance (195, 196).

Clinical and Hematologic Findings

The range of clinical presentation of PK deficiency is quite broad. One of our patients died in utero as a result of severe hydrops fetalis. In this same family, the fetus of

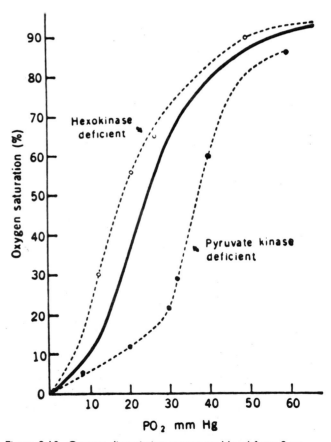

Figure 8.10. Oxygen dissociation curves on blood from 2 patients with a congenital nonspherocytic hemolytic anemia, one due to deficiency of hexokinase, and the other to pyruvate kinase. Deviations of the curves from normal are secondary to differences in the intraerythrocytic levels of 2,3-diphosphoglycerate, being depressed in hexokinase-deficient red cells and elevated in pyruvate kinase-deficient cells. From Delivoria-Papadopoulous et al. (195).

a subsequent pregnancy was transfused in utero when sonograms revealed splenomegaly and amniocentesis demonstrated the presence of heme pigments. Characteristics of the disorder in the neonatal period are the early appearance of jaundice, hepatosplenomegaly, and anemia with reticulocytosis. Anemia continues, and in some, as in the patient presented, frequent transfusions are necessary. Exacerbations of anemia may be a consequence of two phenomena, both probably due to an intercurrent infection: one, an aplastic crisis, and the other, a hyperhemolytic event (187). An aplastic crisis secondary to human serum parvovirus has been demonstrated in one patient (197). Later in life, in some patients gallstones develop and in some leg ulcers (198). Other complications include frontal bossing secondary to bone marrow hyperplasia (199), spinal compression due to extramedullary hemopoiesis (200), and iron overload (201, 202).

Hematologic findings vary according to the severity of the disease. Hemoglobin values may be extremely low in some patients and normal in those with a compensated hemolytic disorder (187). Most patients experience a marked increase in reticulocyte counts after splenectomy (189). Another feature of the postsplenectomy state is the appearance of spiculated cells in the peripheral blood (203) (fig. 8.1). The MCHC of these cells is quite high, secondary to a loss of water. For this reason they are sometimes referred to as "desiccytes" (204).

The hemoglobin pattern of the PK deficient cell is normal. Normal amounts of HbF and HbA$_2$ are present (187). Heinz body formation in vitro is increased, an abnormality that may reflect the inhibitory effect of 2,3-DPG on HMP activity (194).

Pattern of Inheritance

Multiple reports have shown that the PK defect is inherited as an autosomal recessive trait (187). Of special interest has been the finding that most patients are compound heterozygotes, having inherited one mutant form of the enzyme from one parent, and a different mutant form from the other. A major exception are those families in which consanguineous matings have occurred, in which case each parent has the same mutant enzyme and the patient is a homozygote.

The incidence of the heterozygous state varies from 1–3%, with the mutation appearing in many different ethnic groups (187). Enzyme polymorphism is extremely common and it is predicted that the number of mutations will exceed those defined for G-6-PD.

In most mammals four isozymes of PK have been identified: L, R, M$_1$, and M$_2$ (205). Each is a homotetramer with different enzymatic properties. Ontogenetic and tissue-specific patterns occur (206). M$_2$ is the only isozymic form in early fetal tissues (205). In adults, L$_1$ is the major isozyme of the liver, and M$_1$, the major molecular species in muscle. The R type is present in red cells. By electrophoretic analysis two R forms have been

demonstrated: R$_2$, the major isozyme in mature red cells, and R$_1$, the predominant form in immature cells. The isozymic form in the PK-deficient reticulocyte is a mutated form of R$_1$, the catalytic properties of which favor removal of immature red cells. For a more extensive review of these PK subsets and their pathophysiologic significance the reader is referred to Valentine et al. (187). Pertinent to this discussion is the demonstration that those PK variants associated with anemia exhibit very low enzymatic activity, are very thermolabile, and have decreased affinity for phosphoenolpyruvate. Recent isolation and sequencing of complementary DNA for the L-type isozyme has led to the characterization of the amino acid substitution and the structural conformation of two of the variants (207, 208).

Definition and Treatment

An assay for red cell PK activity should be performed in any patient with an undiagnosed congenital and nonspherocytic form of hemolytic anemia. Several methods are available. Quantification of the enzyme in hemolysates prepared from leukocyte-poor red cells is accomplished by measuring the rate of oxidation of reduced nicotinamide dinucleotide in the presence of phosphoenolpyruvate, adenosine diphosphate, and purified lactate dehydrogenase (209). By this method, three phenotypes can usually be defined: normal, heterozygous, and homozygous states, although a few exceptions have been noted (199, 210). Several screening methods are available, but none have been used extensively (211).

Management of the patient with a PK-deficient type of hemolytic anemia involves several therapeutic approaches. The first and most important is the question of splenectomy. Should it be done and, if so, when. Patients with a mild or compensated form of hemolytic anemia will not require a splenectomy, but those with more severe anemia will. In doing so, it is important to caution the parents and the patient that splenectomy will alleviate but not cure the anemia. In general, however, the procedure reduces the frequency of transfusions.

Genetic counseling should be offered to those families in which a fetus in utero or a newborn has been severely affected, as evidenced by the development of nonisoimmune hydrops fetalis or early neonatal jaundice. Prenatal diagnosis is possible, and in the fetus with life-threatening anemia, in utero transfusions may be lifesaving.

Other Enzymopathies

The number of congenital nonspherocytic hemolytic disorders due to an enzyme abnormality is quite large. It is beyond the scope of this chapter to discuss each one in detail. For this reason, those enzymopathies identified to date, together with pertinent genetic and phenotypic data, are presented in table 8.4. For more extensive information the reader is referred to other recent reviews (187, 210).

Table 8.4 Enzymopathies Associated with Congenital Nonspherocytic Hemolytic Anemia (CNSHA)

Enzyme Deficiency	No. of Cases	Genetic Transmission	Phenotype Clinical	Phenotype Laboratory	References
Embden-Meyerhof pathway					
Hexokinase (HK)	20	AR° ?AD[†] in 2	Neonatal jaundice, CNSHA—mild to marked	Red cell morphology normal except for macrocytosis and polychromatophilia	187, 210
Glucosephosphate Isomerase (GPI)	40	AR	Hydrops fetalis, neonatal jaundice, CNSHA—marked	Macrocytosis, marked reticulocytosis, few spiculated cells post-splenectomy	187, 210
Phosphofructokinase (PFK)	21	AR	Myopathy—muscle cramps in some, mild-to-moderate CNSHA	Decreased PFK in muscle	187, 210
Aldolase (ALD)	3	AR	Mental retardation and malformations (1 patient), mild-to-marked CNSHA	Normal red cell morphology, poly-chromatophilia	187, 210
Triosephosphate isomerase (TPI)	16	AR	Progressive neurologic dysfunction starting at 6–7 mo, Infections, cardiac arrhythmia, and sudden death, "cat cry" (2 patients) moderate-to-severe CNSHA	Macrocytosis, Poly-chromatophlia, marked reticulo-cytosis	187, 210
Glyceraldohyde-3-phosphate dehydro-genase (G-3-PD)	3	Probably AR	Mild CNSHA—exacerbation with drug and infection	Mild reticulocytosis	210
Phosphoglycerate kinase (PGK)	14 Males 5 Females	Sex linked	Mild-to-marked CNSHA, neurologic abnormali-ties, rhabdomyolysis (1 patient) Myoglobin-uria (1 patient)	Mild-to-marked anemia	187, 210
2,3-Diphospho-glycerate mutase (2,3-DPG)	5	AR	Mild CNSHA to polycythemia	2,3-DPG, affinity of Hb for O_2	187, 210
Enolase	1	?	No anemia, nitrofuran-toin induced hemolysis	RBC morphology abnor-mal only during drug induced hemolysis	210
Lactate dehydro-genase (LDH)	1	AR	No anemia	Deficiency of LDH B, the heart isozyme	187, 210
Hexose monophosphate shunt and related enzymes					
6 Phosphogluconate de-hydrogenase (6-PGD)	16 Heterozygotes 3 Homozygotes	AD	None in heterozygote, CNSHA in homozygotes	Anemia	213–17
Glutathione peroxidase	3 Homozygote Many heterozygote	AR	CNSHA, drug induced most normal		218–23
Glutathione reductase	3	AR	Favism (1 patient), cataracts (2 patients)	Hemolysis during episode of favism, abnormal GSH sta-bility test	224, 225
γ-Glutamylcysteine synthetase	2	AR	CNSHA, spinocerebellar ataxia	Low GSH in RBCs, Amino aciduria	226
Glutathione synthetase	7	AR	Hemolytic anemia	Markedly decreased RBC GSH,	227–229
	7	AR	Hemolytic anemia + neu-rologic deficit	5-oxoproline in plasma and urine of patients with neuro-logic defect	230–233

°Autosomal recessive.

[†]Autosomal dominant.

In general the number of patients with any one of these enzymopathies is quite small. With one exception, most are inherited as autosomal recessive traits, and in a few, extra-erythrocytic manifestations of the defect are present. The muscular and central nervous systems are those most commonly affected. Any patient with a hemolytic disorder in combination with some type of neurologic or muscular abnormality should be investigated for an underlying enzymopathy.

A final question concerns the incidence of enzymopathies as a cause of congenital hemolytic disorders without demonstrable etiology. Hirono et al. (212) reviewed their findings on the frequency of enzyme abnormalities in 722 blood samples obtained from subjects with an unknown type of hemolytic disorder. All of the known types of membrane and hemoglobin abnormalities had been excluded. Activities of 26 enzymes were measured, including members of both the Embden-Meyerhof and hexose monophosphate shunt pathways. Hemolysis was secondary to an enzymopathy in 81 patients, an abnormality of PK in 55, G-6-PD in 15, primidine 5'-nucleotidase in 5, glucose phosphate isomerase in 3, adenylate kinase in 2, phosphoglycerate kinase in 1, and glutathione synthetase in 1. Approximately 75% of the group demonstrated no evidence of an enzymopathy in the panel of 26 enzymes surveyed. Thus the majority of hereditary nonspherocytic hemolytic anemias remains unexplained. Could these disorders be secondary to a membranopathy, an enzymopathy yet to be discovered, or some other etiology? The answers to these questions are for the future, as are areas of red cell biology still to be explored.

REFERENCES

1. Valentine WN. Introduction: hereditary enzymatic deficiencies of erythrocytes. In: Valentine WN, ed. Seminars in hematology. New York: HM Stratton, 1971;8:307–310.
2. Beutler E. The red cell: a tiny dynamo. In: Wintrobe MM, ed. Blood, pure, and eloquent. New York: McGraw-Hill, 1980:141–164.
3. Zinkham WH, Childs B. Effect of vitamin K and naphthalene metabolites on glutathione metabolism of erythrocytes from normal newborns and patients with naphthalene hemolytic anemia. J Dis Child 1957;94:420–422.
4. Zinkham WH, Childs B. A defect of glutathione metabolism in erythrocytes from patients with a naphthalene-induced hemolytic anemia. Pediatrics 1958;22:461–471.
5. Oski FA. The Erythrocyte and its disorders. In: Nathan DG, Oski FA, eds. Hematology of infancy and childhood. Philadelphia: WB Saunders, 1993:18–43.
6. Adamson JW. The erythron. In: Lichtman MA, ed. Hematology and oncology. New York: Grune & Stratton 1980: 7–22.
7. Harris JW, Kellermeyer RW. Classification of the anemias. In: The red cell. Cambridge: Harvard University Press 1970:272–278.
8. La Mer VK, Baker LE. Effect of substitution on free energy of oxidation-reduction reactions: 1, benzoquinone derivatives. J Am Chem Soc 1922;44:1954–1964.
9. Berenblum I, Schoenthal R. Metabolism of chrysene in rat. Biochem J 1945;39:abstract 44.
10. Beutler E, Dern RJ, Flanagan CL, Alving AS. The hemolytic effect of primaquine: VII, biochemical studies of drug-sensitive erythrocytes. J Lab Clin Med 1955;45: 286–295.
11. Carson PE, Flanagan CL, Ickes CE, Alving AS. Enzymatic deficiency in primaquine-sensitive erythrocytes. Science 1956;124:484–486.
12. Betke K, Beutler E, Brewer GJ, Kirkman HN, Luzzatto L, Motulsky AG, Ramot B. Siniscalco M. Standardisation of procedures for the study of glucose-6-phosphate dehydrogenase: report of a WHO scientific group. WHO Tech Rep Ser 366, 1967;1–53.
13. Gasser C, Willi H. Spontane Innenküorper-bildung bei Milzagenesie. Helv Paediatr Acta 1952;4:369–382.
14. Rieders F, Brieger H. Acute hemolytic anemia due to ingestion of naphthalene mothballs: II, hemolytic action of naphthalene and its oxidation products. Pediatrics 1951;7: 725–728.
15. Harley JD, Robin H. Adaptive mechanisms in erythrocytes exposed to naphthoquinones. Aust J Exp Biol Med Sci 1963;41:281–292.
16. Ham TH, Grauel JA, Dunn RF, Murphy JR, White JG, Kellermeyer RW. Physical properties of red cells as related to effects in vivo: IV, oxidant drugs producing abnormal intracellular concentration of hemoglobin (eccentrocytes) with a rigid-red-cell hemolytic syndrome. J Lab Clin Med 1973;82:898–910.
17. Scott MD, Zuo L, Lubin BH, Chiu DT-Y. NADPH, not glutathione, status modulates oxidant sensitivity in normal and glucose-6-phosphate dehydrogenase-deficient erythrocytes. Blood 1991;77:2059–2063.
18. Rachmilewitz EA, Peisach J, Blumbert WE. Studies on the stability of oxyhemoglobin A and its constituent chains and their derivatives. J Biol Chem 1971;246:3356–3366.
19. Jandl H, Engle LK, Allen DW. Oxidative hemolysis and precipitation of hemoglobin: I, Heinz body anemias as an acceleration of red cell aging. J Clin Invest 1960;39: 1818–1836.
20. Jacob HS, Brain MC, Dacie JV. Altered sulfhydryl reactivity of hemoglobins and red cell membranes in congenital Heinz body hemolytic anemia. J Clin Invest 1968;47: 2664–2677.
21. Lubin A, Desforges JF. Effect of Heinz bodies on red cell deformability. Blood 1972;39:358–365.
22. Jarobin P, Lin S-C, Palak J. Effect of hemoglobin oxidation products on the stability of red cell membrane skeletons and the associations of skeletal proteins: correlation with a release of hemin. Blood 1990;76:2125–2131.
23. Kay MMB. Mechanism of removal of senescent cells by human macrophages in situ. Proc Natl Acad Sci USA 1975; 72:3521–3525.
24. Kay MMB, Goodman SR, Sorensen K, Whitfield CF, Wong P, Zaki L, Rudloff V. Senescent cell antigen is immunologically related to band 3. Proc Natl Acad Sci USA 1983;80: 1631–1635.
25. Sorette MP, Galili U, Clark MR. Comparison of serum anti-band 3 and anti-Gal antibody binding to density separated human red blood cells. Blood 1991;77:628–636.
26. Low PS, Waugh SM, Zinke K, Drenckhahn D. The role of hemoglobin denaturation and band 3 clustering in red blood cell aging. Science 1985;227:531–533.

27. Schluter K, Drenckhahn D. Co-clustering of denatured hemoglobin with band 3: its role in binding of autoantibodies against band 3 to abnormal and aged erythrocytes. Proc Natl Acad Sci USA 1986;83:6137–6141.

28. Chiu D, Kuypers F, Lubin B. Lipid peroxidation in human red cells. Semin Hematol 1989;26:257–276.

29. Johnson GJ, Allen DW, Flynn TP. Oxidant-induced membrane damage in G-6-PD deficient red cells. In: Yoshida A, Beutler E, eds. Glucose-6-phosphate dehydrogenase. Orlando, FL: Academic Press, 1986:153–177.

30. Jain SK. The neonatal erythrocytes and its oxidative susceptibility. Semin Hematol 1989;26:286–300.

31. Shahal Y, Bauminger ER, Zmora E, Katz M, Mazor D, Horn S, Meyerstein N. Oxidative stress in newborn erythrocytes. Pediatr Res 1991;29:119–122.

32. Zinkham WH. An in-vitro abnormality of glutathione metabolism in erythrocytes from normal newborns: mechanism and clinical significance. Pediatrics 1959;23:18–32.

33. Szeinberg A, Ramot B, Sheba C, Adam A, Halbrecht I, Rikover M, Wishnievsky S, Raban E. Glutathione metabolism in cord and newborn infant blood. J Clin Invest 1958;37:1436–1441.

34. Oski FA. The erythrocyte and its disorders. In: Nathan DG, Oski FA, eds. Hematology of infancy and childhood. Philadelphia: WB Saunders, 1987:21–23.

35. Linderkamp O, Nash GB, Wu PYK, Meiselman HJ. Deformability and intrinsic material properties of neonatal red blood cells. Blood 1986;67:1244–1250.

36. Luzzato L, Mehta A. Glucose-6-phosphate dehydrogenase deficiency. In: Scriver R, Beaudet AL, Sly WS, Valle D, eds. The metabolic basis of inherited disease. New York: McGraw-Hill, 1989:2237–2265.

37. Motulsky AG, Campbell-Kraut JM. Population genetics of glucose-6-phosphate dehydrogenase deficiency of the red cell. In: Blumberg BS, ed. Proceedings of the Conference on Genetic Polymorphisms and Geographic Variations in Disease. New York: Grune & Stratton, 1961:159–180.

38. Beutler E. Specific modification of the fluorescent screening method for glucose-6-phosphate dehydrogenase deficiency. Blood 1968;32:816–818.

39. Missiou-Tsagaraki S. Screening for glucose-6-phosphate dehydrogenase deficiency as a preventive measure: prevalence among 1,286,000 Greek newborn infants. J Pediatr 1991;119:293–299.

40. Zinkham WH, Lenhard RE Jr. Metabolic abnormalities of erythrocytes from patients with congenital nonspherocytic hemolytic anemia. J Pediatr 1959;55:319–336.

41. Glock GE, McLean P. Further studies on the properties and assay of glucose-6-phosphate dehydrogenase and 6-phosphogluconate dehydrogenase of rat liver. Biochem J 1953;55:400–408.

42. Piomelli S, Corash LM, Davenport DD, Miraglia J, Amorosi EL. In vivo lability of glucose-6-phosphate dehydrogenase in Gd^{A-} and Gd^{Mediterranean} deficiency. J Clin Invest 1968; 47:940–948.

43. Herz F, Kaplan E, Scheye ES. Diagnosis of erythrocyte glucose-6-phosphate dehydrogenase deficiency in the Negro male despite hemolytic crisis. Blood 1970;35:90–93.

44. Zinkham WH. Metabolism of glucose by erythrocytes from patients with congenital hemolytic disorders. J Pediatr 1962;60:614–622.

45. Beutler E. The hemolytic effect of primaquine and related compounds: a review. Blood 1959;14:1103–1139.

46. Tarlow AR, Brewer GJ, Carson PE, Alving AS. Primaquine sensitivity. Arch Intern Med 1962;109:209–234.

47. Gordon-Smith EC. Drug-induced oxidative hemolysis. Clin Haematol 1980;9:557–562.

48. Wintrobe MM, Lee GR, Boggs DR, Bitbell, Foerster J, Athens JW, Lukens JN, eds. Clinical hematology, 8th ed. Philadelphia: Lea & Febiger, 1981:786–802.

49. Beutler E. Hemolytic anemia in disorders of red cell metabolism. New York: Plenum, 1978:75–96.

50. Beutler E. Glucose-6-phosphate dehydrogenase deficiency. N Engl J Med 1991;324:169–174.

51. Zuelzer WW, Apt L. Acute hemolytic anemia due to naphthalene poisoning: a clinical and experimental study. JAMA 1949;141:185–190.

52. Schafer WB. Acute hemolytic anemia related to naphthalene: report of a case in a newborn infant. Pediatrics 1951; 7:172–174.

53. Mackell JV, Bauer EL. Acute hemolytic anemia due to ingestion of naphthalene moth balls: I, clinical aspects. Pediatrics 1951;7:722–725.

54. Chusid E, Fried CT. Acute hemolytic anemia due to naphthalene ingestion. AMA J Dis Child 1955;89:612–614.

55. Cock TC. Acute hemolytic anemia in the neonatal period. AMA J Dis Child 1957;94:77–79.

56. MacGregor RR. Naphthalene poisoning from ingestion of moth balls. Canad Med Assoc J 1954;70:313–314.

57. Sansone G. L'Anemia emolitica acuta da ingestione accidentale di naftalina nel bambino contributo clinico e cosiderazioni patogenetiche. Hematol Latina 1958;1:45–60.

58. Greenberg MS. Heinz body hemolytic anemia. "Bite cells"—a clue to diagnosis. Arch Intern Med 1976;136: 153–155.

59. Sullivan DW, Glader BE. Erythrocyte enzyme disorders in children. Pediatr Clin North Am 1980;27:449–462.

60. Zinkham WH. G-6-PD deficiency. In: Hartmann PM, ed. Guide to hematologic disorders. New York: Grune & Stratton, 1980:101–105.

61. Hanssler H. Lebensbedrohliche Naphtholinvergiftung bei Einem Süangling durch Vaporin-Düampfe. Dtsch Med Wochenschr 1964;89:1794–1797.

62. Irle U. Akute hüamolytische Anüamie durch Naphthalin-Inhalation bei Zwei Frühgeborenen und Eine Neugeboren. 1964;89:1798–1800.

63. Valaes T, Doxiadis SA, Fessas P. Acute hemolysis due to naphthalene inhalation. J Pediatr 1963;63:904–915.

64. Piomelli S. G6PD-related neonatal jaundice. In: Yoshida A, Beutler E, eds. Glucose-6-phosphate dehydrogenase. Orlando, FL: Academic Press, 1986:101.

65. Smillie WG. β-Naphthol poisoning in the treatment of hookworm. JAMA 1920;74:1503–1506.

66. Zinkham WH, Childs B. Effect of naphthalene derivatives on glutathione metabolism of erythrocytes from patients with naphthalene hemolytic anemia. J Clin Invest 1957; 36:938.

67. Athreya BH, Swain AK, Dickstein B. Acute hemolytic anemia due to the ingestion of naphthalene. Indian J Child Health 1961;10:305–308.

68. Shannon K, Buchanan GR. Severe hemolytic anemia in black children with glucose-6-phosphate dehydrogenase deficiency. Pediatrics 1982;70:364–369.

69. Gasser C. Die hüamolytische Früohgeburtenanüamie mit spontanei Innenküorperbildung: Ein neues Syndrom, Beobachtet an 14 Füallen. Helv Paediatr Acta 1953;8:491–529.

70. Gasser C. Hüamolytische Früohgeburten-Anüamie mit Spontan-Innenküorperbildung. In: Die hamolytischen Syndrome im Kindesalter. Stuttgart: Georg Thieme, 1951: 177–183.

71. Varadi S, Hurworth E. Heinz-body anaemia in the newborn. Br Med J 1957;1:315–318.

72. Laurance B. Danger of vitamin K analogues to newborns. Lancet 1955;1:319.

73. Zinkham WH. Peripheral blood and bilirubin values in normal full-term primaquine-sensitive Negro infants: effect of vitamin K. Pediatrics 1963;31:983–995.

74. Kattamis CA, Kyriazakou M, Chaidas S. Favism: clinical and biochemical data. J Med Genet 1969;6:34–41.

75. Kattamis CA. Favism: epidemiological and clinical aspects. In: Yoshida A, Beutler E, eds. Glucose-6-phosphate dehydrogenase. Orlando, FL: Academic Press, 1986: 25–43.

76. Szeinberg A, Sheba C, Hirshorn N, Bodonyi E. Studies on erythrocytes in cases with past history of favism and drug-induced acute hemolytic anemia. Blood 1957;12: 603–613.

77. Vella F. Favism in Asia. Med J Austr 1959;2:196–197.

78. Chang H-H. Favism: clinical analysis of 228 cases. Chin J Pediatr 1959;10:63–69.

79. Stamatayannopoulos G, Fraser GR, Motulsky AG, Fessas Ph, Akrivakis A, Papayannopoulou T. On the familial predisposition to favism. Am J Hum Genet 1966;18:253–263.

80. Sansone G, Segui G. Nuvoi Aspetti dell'Alterato Biochimismo Degli Eritrociti di Favici: Assenza Pressach Completa Della Glucoso-6-P Deidrogenasi. Boll Soc Ital Biol Sper 1958;34:327–329.

81. Zannos-Mariolea L, Kattamis C. Glucose-6-phosphate dehydrogenase in Greece. Blood 1961;18:34–47.

82. Szeinberg A, Asher Y, Sheba C. Studies on glutathione stability in erythrocytes of cases with past history of favism or sulfa-drug-induced hemolysis. Blood 1958;13:348–358.

83. Zinkham WH, Lenhard RE, Childs B. A deficiency of glucose-6-phosphate dehydrogenase activity in erythrocytes from patients with favism. Bull Johns Hopkins Hosp 1958; 102:169–175.

84. Marcolonzo F. Favismo Ittero-Emoglobinurico. Minerva Med 1953;44:1963–1968.

85. Walker DG, Bowman JE. In vitro effect of Vicia faba extracts upon reduced glutathione of erythrocytes. Proc Soc Exp Biol Med 1960;103:476–477.

86. Bowman JE, Walker DG. Action of Vicia faba on erythrocytes: possible relationship to favism. Nature 1961;189: 555–556.

87. Arese P, Mannuzzu L, Turrini F, Galiano S, Gaetani GF. etiological aspects of favism. In: Yoshida A, Beutler E, eds. Glucose-6-phosphate dehydrogenase. Orlando, FL: Academic Press, 1986:45–75.

88. De Flora A, Benatti V, Guida L, Zocchi E. Divicine and G6PD-deficient erythrocytes: an integrated model of cytotoxicity in favism. In: Yoshida A, Beutler E, eds. Glucose-6-phosphate dehydrogenase. Orlando, FL: Academic Press, 1986:77–93.

89. Herman J, Ben-Meir S. Overt hemolysis in patients with glucose-6-phosphate dehydrogenase deficiency: a survey in general practice. Israel J Med Sci 1975;11:340–346.

90. Kimbro EL, Sachs MV, Torbert JV. Mechanism of the hemolytic anemia induced by nitrofurantoin (Furadantin^R). Bull Johns Hopkins Hosp 1957;101:245–257.

91. Burka ER, Weaver Z III, Marks PA. Clinical spectrum of hemoltyic anemia associated with glucose-6-phosphate dehydrogenase deficiency. Ann Intern Med 1966;64:817–825.

92. Valaes T, Fessas PH, Doxiadis SA. Kernicterus in full-term infants without isoimmunization (4 cases). Proc Roy Soc Med 1961;54:331–333.

93. Valaes T. Red-cell enzymes and severe neonatal jaundice. Cerebral Palsy Bull 1961;3:431–434.

94. Doxiadis SA, Fessas PH, Valaes T. Erythrocyte enzyme deficiency in unexplained kernicterus. Lancet 1960;2:44–46.

95. Doxiadis SA, Fessas PH, Valaes T, Mastrokalos N. Glucose-6-phosphate dehydrogenase deficiency; a new aetiological factor of severe neonatal jaundice. Lancet 1961;1:297–298.

96. Weatherall DH. Enzyme deficiency in haemolytic disease of the newborn. Lancet 1960;2:835–837.

97. Smith GD, Vella F. Erythrocyte enzyme deficiency in unexplained kernicterus. Lancet 1960:1133–1134.

98. Segni G. Su Due Casi di Ittero Nucleare in Neonati Con Difeto Enzimatico Eritrocitario. Minerva Pediatr 1959;11:1420–1425.

99. Panizon F, Meo R. Problem Profilattici e Terapeutici di un Porticolare Ittero Grave Neonatale Individualto in Sardegua. Acta Paediatr Lat 1959;12:404–408.

100. Malaka-Zafiriu K, Tsiures I, Danielides B, Cassimios C. Salicylamide glucuronide formation in newborns with severe jaundice of unknown etiology and due to glucose-6-phosphate deficiency in Greece. Helv Paediatr Acta 1973;28: 323–329.

101. Valaes T, Karaklis A, Stravrakakis D, Bavela-Stravrakakis B, Perakis A, Doxiadis SA. Incidence and mechanism of neonatal jaundice related to glucose-6-phosphate dehydrogenase deficiency. Pediatr Res 1969;3:448–458.

102. Freier S, Mayer K, Levene K, Abrahamov A. Neonatal jaundice associated with familial G-6-PD deficiency in Israel. Arch Dis Child 1965;40:280–285.

103. Milbauer B, Peled N, Soirsky S. Neonatal hyperbilirubinemia and glucose-6-phosphate dehydrogenase deficiency. Israel J Med Sci 1973;9:11–16.

104. Ashkenazi F, Mimouni F, Merlob P, Reisner SH. Neonatal bilirubin levels and glucose-6-phosphate dehydrogenase deficiency in preterm and low-birth-weight infants in Israel. Israel J Med Sci 1983;19:1056–1061.

105. Szeinberg A, Oliver M, Schmidt R, Adam A, Sheba C. Glucose-6-phosphate dehydrogenase deficiency and haemolytic disease of the newborn in Israel. Arch Dis Child 1963; 38:23–28.

106. Baxi AJ, Undevia JV, Bhatia HM. Role of glucose-6-phosphate dehydrogenase deficiency in acute hemolytic crisis and neonatal jaundice. Indian J Med Sci 1964;18: 574–583.

107. Majid JD, Hasan MI. Neonatal jaundice due to glucose-6-phosphate dehydrogenase deficiency. J Indian Med Assoc 1965;44:143–148.

108. Flatz G, Springam S, Komkris V. Neonatal jaundice in glucose-6-phosphate dehydrogenase deficiency. Lancet 1963; 1:1382–1383.

109. Phornphutkul C, Whitaker JA, Worathumrong N. Severe hyperbilirubinemia in Thai newborns in association with erythrocyte G6PD deficiency. Clin Pediatr 1969;8: 275–278.

110. Nkrumoh FK. A severe neonatal jaundice—analysis of possible associated factors in infants from Accra. Ghana Med J 1973;1:160–167.

111. Bienzle U, Effioing C, Luzzato L. Erythrocyte glucose-6-phosphate dehydrogenase deficiency (G6PD type A⁻) and neonatal jaundice. Acta Paediatr Scand 1976;65:701–703.

112. Levin SE, Charlton RW, Freiman I. Glucose-6-phosphate dehydrogenase deficiency and neonatal jaundice in South African Bantu infants. J Pediatr 1964;65:757–764.

113. Say B, Ozand P, Berkel I, Cevik N. Erythrocyte glucose-6-phosphate dehydrogenase deficiency in Turkey. Acta Paediatr Scan 1965;54:319–324.

114. Sanna G, Fran F, De Virgiliis S, Piu P, Bertolino F, Cao A. Glucose-6-phosphate dehydrogenase red cell phenotype in Gd Mediterranean heterozygous females and hemizygous males at birth. Pediatr Res 1981;15:1443–1446.

115. Lu T-C, Wei H, Quentin Blackwell R. Increased incidence of severe hyperbilirubinemia among newborn Chinese infants with G-6-PD deficiency. Pediatrics 1968;37:994–999.

116. Brown WR, Wong HB. Hyperbilirubinemia and kernicterus in glucose-6-phosphate dehydrogenase-deficient infants in Singapore. Pediatrics 1968;41:1055–1062.

117. Englesou G, Kjellman B. Red cell glucose-6-phosphate dehydrogenase and glutathione stability in neonatal hyperbilirubinemia. Acta Paediatr 1963;52:82–86.

118. Sulyok E, Cholnoky P. The role of erythrocyte glucose-6-phosphate dehydrogenase deficiency in icterus gravis neonatorum. Acta Paediatr Acad Scient Hung 1967;8:323–326.

119. O'Flynn MED, Hsia DY-Y. Serum bilirubin levels and glucose-6-phosphate dehydrogenase deficiency in newborn American negroes. J Pediatr 1963;63:160–161.

120. Wolff JA, Bertram HG, Paya K. Neonatal serum bilirubin and glucose-6-phosphate dehydrogenase–relationship of various perinatal factors to hyperbilirubinemia. Am J Dis Child 1967;113:251–254.

121. Lopez R, Cooperman JM. Glucose-6-phosphate deficiency and hyperbilirubinemia in the newborn. Am J Dis Child 1971;122:66–70.

122. Childs B, Zinkham WH. The Genetics of primaquine sensitivity of the erythrocytes. In: Wolstenhohme GEW, O'Connor CM, eds. Biochemistry of human genetics. Ciba Foundation Symposium. Boston: Little, Brown, 1959:76–89.

123. Eshaghpour E, Oski FA, Williams M. Relationship of erythrocyte glucose-6-phosphate dehydrogenase deficiency to hyperbilirubinemia in Negro premature infants. J Pediatr 1967;70:595–601.

124. Piomelli S. G6PD-related neonatal jaundice. In: Yoshida A, Beutler E, eds. Glucose-6-phosphate dehydrogenase. Orlando, FL: Academic Press, 1986:95–108.

125. Piomelli S, Spada U, Bernini L, Siniscalco M, Adinolfi M, Mollison DL, Latte B. Survival of ⁵¹Cr-labelled red cells in subjects with thalassemia trait or G6PD deficiency or both abnormalities. Br J Hematol 1964;10:171–180.

126. Kellermeyer RW, Tarlow AR, Schrier SL, Carson PE, Alving AS. The hemolytic effect of primaquine: XIII, gradient susceptibility to hemolysis of primaquine-sensitive erythrocytes. J Lab Clin Med 1961;58; 225–233.

127. Cassimos C, Malaka-Zafiriu K, Tsiures T, Danielides B. Variations in salicylamide glucuronide formation in normal and in G-6-PD deficient children. J Pediatr 1974;84:110–111.

128. Childs B, Zinkham WH, Browne EA, Kimbro EL, Torbert JV. A genetic study of a defect in glutathione metabolism of the erythrocyte. Bull Johns Hopkins Hosp 1958;102:21–37.

129. Glucose-6-phosphate dehydrogenase deficiency: report of a WHO Working Group. WHO Reprint No. 5020, 1989:601–611.

130. Standardization of procedures for the study of glucose-6-phosphate dehydrogenase. Report of a WHO Scientific Group. WHO Tech Rep Ser, No. 366, 1967:2–53.

131. Yoshida A. A single amino acid substitution (asparagine to aspartic) between normal (B+) and the common Negro variant (A+) of human glucose-6-phosphate dehydrogenase. Proc Natl Acad Sci USA 1967;57:835–840.

132. Calvert AF, Trimble GE. Glucose-6-phosphate dehydrogenase in an Afro-American population. Human Hered 1980;30:271–277.

133. Fung RH, Keung YK, Chung GSH. Screening of pyruvate kinase deficiency and G6PD deficiency in Chinese newborns in Hong Kong. Arch Dis Child 1969;44:373–376.

134. Meloni T, Costa S, Cutillo S. Three years experience in preventing severe hyperbilirubinemia in newborn infants with erythrocyte G-6-PD deficiency. Bio Neonate 1976;28:370–374.

135. Lyon MF. Gene action in the X-chromosome of the mouse (Mus musculus L.). Nature 1961;190:372–373.

136. Russell LB. Mammalian X-chromosome action: inactivation limited in spread and in region of origin. Science 1963;140:976–978.

137. Davidson RG, Nitowsky HM, Childs B. Demonstration of two populations of cells in the human female heterozygous for glucose-6-phosphate dehydrogenase variants. Proc Natl Acad Sci USA 1963;50:481–485.

138. Beutler E, Yeh M, Fairbanks VF. The normal human female as a mosaic of X-chromosome activity: studies using the gene for G-6-PD deficiency as a marker. Proc Natl Acad Sci USA 1962;48:9–16.

139. Gall JC Jr, Brewer GJ, Dern RJ. Studies of glucose-6-phosphate dehydrogenase activity of individual erythrocytes: the methemoglobin elution test for detection of females heterozygous for G6PD deficiency. Am J Hum Genet 1965;17:359–368.

140. Gifford H. Determination of the oxidation-reduction mechanism in the lens of rabbits with naphthalene cataract. Arch Ophthalmol 1932;7:763–765.

141. Marks PA, Gross RT, Hurwitz RE. Gene action in erythrocyte deficiency of glucose-6-phosphate dehydrogenase: tissue enzyme-levels. Nature 1959;183:1266–1267.

142. Ramot B, Fisher S, Szeinberg A, Adam A, Sheba C, Gafni D. A study of subjects with erythrocyte glucose-6-phosphate dehydrogenase deficiency: II, investigation of leukocyte enzymes. J Clin Invest 1959;38:2234–2237.

143. Justice P, Shih L-Y, Gordon J, Grossman A, Hsia DY-Y. Characterization of leukocyte glucose-6-phosphate dehydrogenase in normal and mutant human subjects. J Lab Clin Med 1966;68:552–559.

144. Mallauh AA, Abu-Osba YK. Bacterial infections in children with glucose-6-phosphate dehydrogenase deficiency. J Pediatr 1987;11:850–854.

145. Abu-Osba YK, Mallouh AA, Hann RW. Incidence and cause of sepsis in glucose-6-phosphate dehydrogenase deficient newborn infants. J Pediatr 1989;114:748–752.

146. Lampe RM, Kirdpon S, Mansuwan P, Benenson MW. Glucose-6-phosphate dehydrogenase deficiency in Thai children with typhoid fever. J Pediatr 1975;87:576–578.

147. Owusu SK, Foli AK, Konotey-Ahulu FID, Janosi M. Frequency of glucose-6-phosphate dehydrogenase deficiency in typhoid fever in Ghana. Lancet 1972;1:320–321.

148. Khev M, Grover S. Glucose-6-phosphate dehydrogenase deficiency in leprosy. Lancet 1969;1:1318–1319.

149. Clark M, Root RK. Glucose-6-phosphate dehydrogenase deficiency and infection: a study of hospitalized patients in Iran. Yale J Biol Med 1979;52: 169–179.

150. Meloni T, Forteleoni G, Ena F, Meloni GF. Glucose-6-phosphate dehydrogenase deficiency and bacterial infections in Sardinia. J Pediatr 1991;118: 909–911.

151. Dawodu AH, Owa JA, Familusi JB. A prospective study of the role of bacterial infections and G6PD deficiency in severe neonatal jaundice in Nigeria. Trop Geogr Med 1984; 36:127–132.

152. Cooper MR, DeChatelet LR, McCall CE, La Via MF, Spurr CL, Baehner RL. Complete deficiency of leukocyte glucose-6-phosphate dehydrogenase with defective bactericidal activity. J Clin Invest 1972;51:769–778.

153. Baehner RL, Johnston RB Jr, Nathan DG. Comparative study of the metabolic and bactericidal characteristics of severely glucose-6-phosphate dehydrogenase deficient polymorphonuclear leukocytes and leukocytes from children with chronic granulomatous disease. J Reticuloendothel Soc 1972;12:150–169.

154. Gray GR, Stamatoyannopoulos G, Naiman SC, Kliman MR, Klebanoff SJ, Austin T, Yoshida A, Robinson GCF. Neutrophil dysfunction, chronic granulomatous disease, and non-spherocytic haemolytic anaemia caused by complete deficiency of glucose-6-phosphate dehydrogenase. Lancet 1973;2:530–538.

155. Vives Corrous JL, Feliu E, Pujades MA, Cardellach F, Rozman C, Carreras A, Jon JM, Vallespi Zuazu FJ. Severe glucose-6-phosphate dehydrogenase (G6PD) deficiency associated with chronic hemolytic anemia, granulocyte dysfunction, and increased susceptibility to infections: description of a new molecular variant (G6PD Barcelona). Blood 1982;59:428–434.

156. Mamlok RJ, Mamlok V, Mills GC, Daeschner CW III, Schmalstieg FC, Anderson DC. Glucose-6-phosphate dehydrogenase deficiency, neutrophil dysfunction, and chromobacterium violaceum sepsis. J Pediatr 1987;111: 852–854.

157. Oluboyede OA, Esau GJF, Francis TI, Luzatto L. Genetically determined deficiency of glucose-6-phosphate dehydrogenase (type A⁻) is expressed in the liver. J Lab Clin Med 1979;93:783–789.

158. Chan TK, Todd D, Wong CC. Tissue enzyme levels in erythrocyte glucose-6-phosphate dehydrogenase deficiency. J Lab Clin Med 1965;66:937–942.

159. Morrow RH Jr., Smetana HF, Sai FT, Edgcomb JH. Unusual features of viral hepatitis in Accra, Ghana. Ann Intern Med 1968;68:1250–1264.

160. Kattamis CA, Tjortjatou F. The Hemolytic process of viral hepatitis in children with normal or deficient glucose-6-phosphate dehydrogenase activity. J Pediatr 1970;77: 422–430.

161. Berry E, Melmed RN. Infectious hepatitis and glucose-6-phosphate dehydrogenase deficiency. Israel J Med Sci 1977;13:600–603.

162. Choremis C, Kattamis Ch A, Kyriazakou M, Gavriilidou E. Viral hepatitis in G-6-PD deficiency. Lancet 1966;1: 269–270.

163. Salen G, Goldstein F, Haurani F, Wirts CW. Acute hemolytic anemia complicating viral hepatitis in patients with glucose-6-phosphate dehydrogenase deficiency. Ann Intern Med 1966;65:1210–1220.

164. Phillips SM, Silvers NP. Glucose-6-phosphate dehydrogenase deficiency, infectious hepatitis, acute hemolysis, and renal failure. Ann Intern Med 1969;70:99–104.

165. Grollman AP, Odell GB. Removal of bilirubin by albumin binding during intermittent peritoneal dialysis. N Engl J Med 1962;267:279–282.

166. Calvin HI, Medvedovsky C, Wargul BV. Near-total glutathione depletion and age-specific cataracts induced by buthionine sulfoximine in mice. Science 1986;233:553–555.

167. Zinkham WH. A deficiency of glucose-6-phosphate dehydrogenase activity in lens from individuals with primaquine-sensitive erthrocytes. Bull Johns Hopkins Hosp 1961;109:206–216.

168. Westring DW, Pisciotta A. Anemia, cataracts, and seizures in patient with glucose-6-phosphate dehydrogenase deficiency. Arch Intern Med 1966;118:385–390.

169. Cohn J, Carter N, Warburg M. Glucose-6-phosphate dehydrogenase deficiency in a native Danish family: a new variant. Scand J Haematol 1979;23:403–406.

170. Ramot B, Szeinberg A, Adam A, Sheba C, Gafni D. A study of subjects with erythrocyte glucose-6-phosphate dehydrogenase deficiency: investigation of platelet enzymes. J Clin Invest 1959;38:1659–1661.

171. Wurzel H, McCreary T, Baker L, Gumerman L. Glucose-6-phosphate dehydrogenase in platelets. Blood 1961;17: 314–318.

172. Ramot B, Sheba C, Adam A, Ashkenazi I. Erythrocyte glucose-6-phosphate dehydrogenase-deficient subjects: enzyme-level in saliva. Nature 1960;185:931.

173. Bresolin N, Bet L, Moggio M, Meola G, Comi G, Gilardi A, Scarlato G. Muscle G6PD deficiency. Lancet 1987;1: 212–213.

174. Sarkar S, Nelson AJ, Jones OW. Glucose-6-phosphate dehydrogenase (G6PD) activity of human sperm. J Med Genet 1977;14:250–255.

175. Meloni T, Costa S, Dare A, Outillo S. Phototherapy for neonatal hyperbilirubinemia in mature newborn infants with erythrocyte G-6-PD deficiency. J Pediatr 1974;85: 560–562.

176. Tan KL. Phototherapy for neonatal jaundice in erythrocyte glucose-6-phosphate dehydrogenase deficient infants. Pediatrics (Neonate Suppl) 1977;59:1023–1026.

177. Kopelman AE, Ey JL, Lee H. Phototherapy in newborn infants with glucose-6-phosphate dehydrogenase deficiency. J Pediatr 1978;93:497–499.

178. Meloni T, Costa S, Cutillo S. Three years experience in preventing severe hyperbilirubinemia in newborn infants with erythrocyte G-6-PD deficiency. Biol Neonate 1976;28: 370–374.

179. Corash L, Spielberg SP, Bartsocas C, Boxer L, Steinherz R, Sheetz M, Egan M, Schlessleman J, Schulman JD. Reduced chronic hemolysis during high-dose vitamin E administration in Mediterranean-type glucose-6-phosphate dehydrogenase deficiency. New Engl J Med 1980;303: 416–420.

180. Spielberg SP, Boxer LA, Corash LM, Schulman JD. Improved erythrocyte survival with high dose vitamin E in chronic hemolyzing G6PD and glutathione synthetase deficiency. Ann Intern Med 1979;90:53–54.

181. Hafez M, Ancar E-S, Zedan M, Hammad H, Sorour AH, El-Desouky El-SA, Ganul N. Improved erythrocyte survival with combined vitamin E and selenium therapy in children with glucose-6-phosphate dehydrogenase deficiency and mild chronic hemolysis. J Pediatr 1986;108:558–561.

182. Johnson GJ, Vatassery GR, Finkel B, Allen DW. High-dose vitamin E does not decrease the rate of chronic hemolysis in G-6-PD deficiency. N Engl J Med 1983;303:432–436.

183. Newman GJ, Newman TB, Bowie LJ, Mendelsohm J. An examination of the role of vitamin E in G-6-PD deficiency. Clin Biochem 1979;12:149–151.

184. Dacie JV, Mollison PL, Richardson N, Selwyn JG, Shapiro L. Atypical congenital hemolytic anemia. J Med 1953;22:79–98.

185. Selwyn JG, Dacie JV. Autohemolysis and other changes resulting from the incubation in vitro of red cells from patients with congenital hemolytic anemia. Blood 1954;9:414–438.

186. Newton WA, Bass JC. Glutathione-sensitive chronic non-spherocytic hemolytic anemia. AMA J Dis Child 1958;96:501–502.

187. Valentine WN, Tanaka KR, Paglia DE. Pyruvate kinase and other enzyme deficiency disorders of the erythrocyte. In: Scriver CR, Beaudet AL, Sly WS, Valle D, eds. The metabolic basis of inherited disease. New York: McGraw-Hill, 1989:2341–2365.

188. Keitt AS. Pyruvate kinase deficiency and related disorders of red cell glycolysis. Am J Med 1966;41:762–785.

189. Mentzer WC Jr, Baehner RL, Schmidt-Schonbein H, Robinson SH, Nathan DG. Selective reticulocyte destruction in erythrocyte pyruvate kinase deficiency. J Clin Invest 1971;50:688–699.

190. Leblond PF, Lyonnais J, Delage JM. Erythrocyte populations in pyruvate kinase deficiency following splenectomy: I, cell morphology. Br J Haematol 1978;39:55–61.

191. Nathan DG, Oski FA, Miller DR, Gardner FH. Life-span and organ sequestration of the red cells in pyruvate kinase deficiency. New Engl J Med 1968;278:73–81.

192. Wagner HN Jr, Razzak MA, Gaetner RA, Caine WP Jr, Feagin OT. AMA Arch Intern Med 1962;110:90–97.

193. Kahn A, Marie J, Garreau H, Sprengers ED. The genetic system of the L-type pyruvate kinase forms in man: subunit structure, interrelation and kinetic characteristics of the pyruvate kinase enzymes from erythrocytes and the liver. Biochim Biophys Acta 1978;523:59–74.

194. Tomoda A, Lachant NA, Noble NA, Tanaka KR. Inhibition of the pentose phosphate shunt by 2,3-diphosphoglycerate in erythrocyte pyruvate kinase deficiency. Br J Haematol 1983;54:475–484.

195. Delivoria-Papadopoulos M, Oski FA, Gottlieb AJ. Oxygen-hemoglobin dissociation curves: effect of inherited enzyme defects of the red cell. Science 1969;165:601–602.

196. Oski FA, Marshall BE, Cohen PJ, Sugerman HJ, Miller JD. Exercise with anemia: The role of the left-shifted or right-shifted oxygen-hemoglobin equilibrium curve. Ann Intern Med 1971;74:44–46.

197. Duncan JR, Potter CG, Cappellini MD, Kurtz JB, Anderson MJ, Weatherall DJ. Aplastic crisis due to parvovirus infection in pyruvate kinase deficiency. Lancet 1983;2:14–16.

198. Vives-Carrons JL, Marie J, Pujades MA, Kahn A. Hereditary erythrocyte pyruvate-kinase (PK) deficiency and chronic hemolytic anemia: clinical, genetic, and molecular studies in six new Spanish patients. Hum Genet 1980;53:401–408.

199. Tanaka KR, Paglia DE. Pyruvate kinase deficiency. Semin Hematol 1971;8:367–396.

200. Rutgers MJ, Van Der Lugt PJ, Van Turnhout JM. Spinal cord compression by extramedullary hemopoietic tissue in pyruvate kinase-deficiency-caused hemolytic anemia. Neurology 1979;29:510–513.

201. Salem HH, Van Der Weyden MB, Firkin BJ. Iron overload in congenital erythrocyte pyruvate kinase deficiency. Med J Aust 1980;1:531–532.

202. Rowbotham B, Roeser HP. Iron overload associated with congenital pyruvate kinase deficiency and high-dose ascorbic acid ingestion. Aust N Z J Med 1984;14:667–669.

203. Oski FA, Nathan DG, Sidel VW, Diamond LK. Extreme hemolysis and red-cell destruction in erythrocyte pyruvate kinase deficiency: I, morphology, erythrokinetics, and family enzyme studies. New Engl J Med 1964;270:1023–1030.

204. Nathan DG, Shohet SB. Erythrocyte ion transport defects and hemolytic anemia: "hydrocytosis" and "desiccytosis." Semin Hematol 1970;7:381–408.

205. Imamura K, Tanaka T. Multimolecular forms of pyruvate kinase from rat and other mammalian tissues. J Biochem 1972;71:1043–1051.

206. Imamura K, Tanaka T. Pyruvate kinase isozymes from rat. In: Colowick SP, Kaplan NO, Wood WA, eds. Methods in enzymology: vol 90, Carbohydrate metabolism, part E. New York: Academic Press, 1982:150.

207. Kenzaburo T, Hisaichi F, Shigekazu N, Miwa S. Human liver type pyruvate kinase: complete amino acid sequence and the expression in mammalian cells. Proc Natl Acad Sci USA 1988;85:1792–1795.

208. Neubauer M, Lakomeh HW, Parke M, Hofferbert S, Schrüoter W. Point mutations in the L-type pyruvate kinase gene of two children with hemolytic anemia caused by pyruvate kinase deficiency. Blood 1991;77:1871–1875.

209. Tanaka KR. Pyruvate Kinase. In: Yunis JJ, ed. Biochemical methods in red cell genetics. New York: Academic Press, 1969:167.

210. Mentzer WC Jr. Pyruvate kinase deficiency and disorder of glycolysis. In: Nathan DG, Oski FA, eds. Hematology of infancy and childhood. Philadelphia: WB Saunders, 1987:561–569.

211. Beutler E. A Series of new screening procedures for pyruvate kinase deficiency and glutathione reductase deficiency. Blood 1966;28:553–562.

212. Hirono A, Forman L, Beutler E. Enzymatic diagnosis in non-spherocytic hemolytic anemia. Medicine 1988;67:110–117.

213. Brewer GJ, Dern RJ. A new inherited enzymatic deficiency of human erythrocytes: 6-phosphogluconate dehydrogenase deficiency. Am J Hum Genet 1964;16:472–476.

214. Dern RJ, Brewer GJ, Tashian RE, Shows TB. Hereditary variation of erythrocytic 6-phosphogluconate dehydrogenase. J Lab Clin Med 1966;67:255–264.

215. Lansecker C, Heidt P, Fisher D, Hartleyb H, Lohr GW. Anemie hemolytique constitutionnelle avec deficit en 6-phosphogluconate dehydrogenase. Arch Fr Pediatr 1965;22:789–797.

216. Parr CW, Fitch LI. Hereditary partial deficiency of human erythrocyte phosphogluconate dehydrogenase. Biochem J 1964;93:28–30.

217. Scialom C, Najean Y, Bernard J. Anüemie hüemolytique congnitale non-sphrocytaire avec deficit incomplet en 6-phosphogluconate dehydrogenase. Nouv Rev Fr Hematol 1966;69:452–457.

218. Necheles TF, Steinberg MH, Cameron D. Erythrocyte glutathione peroxidase deficiency. Br J Haematol 1970;19: 605–612.

219. Necheles TF, Maldonado N, Barquet-Chediak A, Allen DM. Homozygous erythrocyte glutathione peroxidase deficiency: clinical and biochemical studies. Blood 1969;33: 164–169.

220. Boivin P, Galand C, Hakim J, Blery M. Deficit en glutathion-peroxydase erythrocytaire et anüemie hemolytique medicamenteuse. Presse Med 1970;78:171–174.

221. Steinberg MH, Necheles TF. Erythrocyte glutathione peroxidase deficiency. Am J Med 1971;50:542–546.

222. Steinberg MH, Brauer MJ, Necheles TF. Acute hemolytic anemia associated with erythrocyte glutathione-peroxidase deficiency. Arch Intern Med 1970;125:302–303.

223. Beutler E, Matsumato F. Ethnic variation in red cell glutathione peroxidase activity. Blood 1975;46:103–110.

224. Loos H, Roos D, Weening R, Houwerzl J. Familial deficiency of glutathione reductase in human blood cells. Blood 1976;48:53–62.

225. Beutler E. Effect of flavin compounds on glutathione reductase activity: in vivo and in vitro studies. J Clin Invest 1969;48:1957–1966.

226. Konrad PN, Richards F II, Valentine WN, Paglia DE. Gamma glutamyl-cysteine synthetase deficiency. New Engl J Med 1972;286:557–561.

227. Oort M, Loos JA, Prins HK. Hereditary absence of reduced glutathione in the erythrocytes—new clinical and biochemical entity? Vox Sang 1961;6:370–373.

228. Boivin P, Galand C, Andre R, Debray J. Anüemies hemolytiques congnitales avec deficit isol en glutathion reduit par deficit en gluthion synthtase. Nouv Rev Fr Hematol 1966; 6:859–865.

229. Mohler DN, Majerus PW, Minnick V, Hess CE, Garrick MD. Glutathione synthetase deficiency as a cause of hereditary hemolytic disease. New Engl J Med 1970:283: 1253–1257.

230. Larsson A, Zetterstrüom R, Hagenfeldt L, Anderson R, Dreborg S, Hüormel H. Pyroglutamic aciduria (5-oxoprolinuria)—an inborn error in glutathione metabolism. Pediatr Res 1974;8:852–856.

231. Spielberg SP, Kramer LI, Goodman SI, Butler J, Tietze F, Quinn P, Schulman JD. 5-Oxoprolinuria: biochemical observations and case report. J Pediatr 1977;91:237–241.

232. Wellner VP, Sekura R, Meister A, Larsson A. Glutathione synthetase deficiency: an inborn error of metabolism involving the gamma-glutamyl cycle in patients with 5-oxoprolinuria (pyroglutamic aciduria). Proc Natl Acad Sci USA 1974;71:2505–2509.

233. Jellum E, Kluge T, Bresen HC, Stokke O, Eldjarn L. Pyroglutamic aciduria—a new inborn error of metabolism. Scand J Clin Lab Invest 1970;26:327–335.

234. Owa JA. Relationship between exposure to icterogenic agents, glucose-6-phosphate dehydrogenase deficiency and neonatal jaundice in Nigeria. Acta Paediatr Scand 1989; 78:848–852.

235. Zinkham WH, Oski FA. Henna: a potential cause of oxidative hemolysis. Pediatr Res 1995;35:993A.

CHAPTER 9

The Anemias of Chronic Diseases

DANIEL R. AMBRUSO

Nurse, it was I who discovered that leeches have red blood.
—Baron Cuvier (1769–1832), French zoologist, on his deathbed when the nurse came to apply leeches.
—Enright, *The Oxford Book of Death* (1850)

Introduction and Definition

The anemia of chronic diseases is a heterogeneous group of underproduction anemias associated with a variety of diseases and syndromes. Although diverse in nature, these clinical disorders share common pathophysiologic mechanisms affecting anemia. The recognition of the hematologic effects of chronic diseases began in the nineteenth century with association of chronic infections such as tuberculosis with anemia and its related symptoms (1). As the laboratory procedures for defining anemia came into more general use, other types of infections (osteomyelitis, subacute bacterial endocarditis, etc.) and infections agents (syphilis, typhoid, etc.) became associated with anemia and referred to as the anemia of chronic infection (2). Since the early part of the twentieth century noninfectious diseases such as rheumatoid arthritis, ulcerative colitis, and others have become better defined, with anemia recognized as a prominent feature of these conditions (3). Anemias associated with these disease states have all been classified under the term "anemia of chronic diseases." Recently, anemia of acute infection has been described; it has features in common with the anemia of chronic infections (4).

It was apparent from early studies that the severity of anemia was proportionate to the severity of the infection and its symptoms. In addition, the effects of the pathologic process on production and survival of red cells take place over a long period of time, requiring 4–8 weeks for the full extent of anemia to be reached (5). Advances in medical care over the last half-century have altered the clinical spectrum of anemias associated with chronic diseases. With the development of potent antibiotics and aggressive management schemes, chronic infections such as chronic osteomyelitis, subacute bacterial endocarditis, pulmonary abscess, and empyema have been considerably decreased. Because treatment for inflammatory diseases is not as effective as treatment for infectious diseases, anemia of chronic disease has become more commonly associated with noninfectious or chronic inflammatory diseases and other collagen vascular disorders (3). Anemia of this type may also be seen in Hodgkin disease, lymphomas, and syndromes with carcinoma (6, 7).

Anemias associated with chronic diseases share a number of clinical laboratory features. The anemia is usually mild to moderate (hemoglobin concentration of 7–11 g/dl). That it may be classified as an anemia of underproduction is confirmed by a low reticulocyte count for the hemoglobin concentration and red cell count. In addition, serum iron is decreased concomitantly with normal or decreased serum iron-binding capacity. However, tissue iron stores defined by serum ferritin or iron stain of marrow or other tissue are normal. Although the term "anemia of chronic disease" does not summarize precisely the major pathophysiologic features, it is simpler than others that have been proposed and is more appropriate for the inclusion of the wide variety of disorders associated with this type of anemia.

Case 1

A.J.H., a 14-year-old white adolescent, was admitted to the hospital with a history of weight loss, and intermittent episodes of fever, diarrhea, and vomiting over the prior 2–3 months. The illness began approximately 5–6 months before admission when the patient had intermittent, vague cramping and abdominal pain. These episodes occurred several times a week and lasted only an hour or so.

Two and a half months before admission, the adolescent had his first episode of fever with abdominal pain and diarrhea while visiting with his father. This resolved in several days. On his return home, he chills, fever (up to 102°F), nausea, vomiting, and diarrhea again developed. These symptoms continued over the next 10 weeks. The vomitus was yellow, mixed material including recent undigested food and occurred without relation to time of day, eating, type of food, activity, or sleep. Fever usually occurred in the late afternoon and was associated with decreased appetite, fatigue, and malaise. Sometimes fever responded to Tylenol. Over time, a consistent pat-

tern developed; chills began at 2–3 P.M. each day followed by fever by 5 P.M. A.J.H.'s stools were light brown, watery, and occurred 2–4 times a day. His symptoms became continuous and he was so ill that for 3 months prior to the hospital admission, he had not attended a full week of school. The family history was positive for colitis and irritable bowel syndrome in several family members on the paternal side.

On physical examination, the patient's vital signs were as follows: temperature 37.6°C, pulse rate 80 beats/min, respiratory rate 20 breaths/min, blood pressure 110/80 mm Hg, and weight 92 pounds. A.J.H. appeared to be an alert, active but histrionic male. His skin was normal except for a pruritic patch on the right scapula. He had several 2-cm diameter anterior cervical nodes bilaterally and a submandibular node (1 × 2 cm) which was tender. His chest and heart appeared normal when examined. Abdominal examination revealed no splenomegaly and a liver that was palpable at the right costal margin without enlargement or tenderness. The rectal examination

results were normal, as were the genital, skeletal, and neurologic exam results. A summary of diagnostic studies is included in table 9.1.

Comment: *This adolescent male presented with generalized symptoms and signs of a protracted illness of 3–4 months' duration. The significance of this illness to the general health of this individual was illustrated by the 30-pound weight loss and extensive absence from school during this time period. The differential diagnosis included infection (bacterial, fungal, or parasitic enteritis, tuberculosis, histoplasmosis, autoimmune disease syndrome [AIDS]), malignancy (lymphoma), and inflammatory bowel disease (Crohn disease, regional enteritis). The heme-positive stools, radiologic findings of the upper gastrointestinal (GI) series, and biopsy of the small bowel confirmed the diagnosis of ulcerative jejunitis (table 9.1). Subsequently, the patient was demonstrated to have a protein-losing enteropathy. This inflammatory bowel disease responded very rapidly over the next few months to steroids, with*

Table 9-1. Diagnostic Procedures and Tests for the Clinical Case

Test	Patient	Nor	Test	Patient	Nor
1. *Hematology/ Coagulation*			Serum iron binding capacity	196 μg/dl	250
Hemoglobin concentration	11 gm/dl	14-	Serum ferritin	65 ng/ml	15-
Hematocrit	34%	42-	3. *Serology/ Immunology/ Infectious Disease*		
MCV	69 fl	80-			
MCH	22.9 pg	28-			
MCHC	32.6 gm/dl	33-	Skin Tests:		
White Blood Count	9.8 × 10³/μl	4.8	Histoplasmosis	Negative	
Differential	31% seg		Tuberculosis	Negative	
	28% band		Heterophile antibody	Negative	
	19% lumph		Serum immunoglobulins:		
	17% mono-		IgG	1230 mg/dl	
	5% eos		IgA	152 mg/dl	
Platelet Count	573 × 10³/μl	150	IgM	64 mg/dl	
ESR	36 mm/hr	<8	HIV serology	Negative	
PTT	30 sec	37-	ANA	Negative	
PT	11 sec	11-	Rheumatoid factor	Negative	
Fibrinogen	540 mg/dl	200	VDRL	Negative	
Fibrin Split Products	<10 μg/ml	<10	Stool cultures for bacteria and exam for ova and parasites	Negative	
VIII Activity	2.32 u/ml	0.8			
*Results for adult values shown			4. *Radiology*		
2. *Chemistry* (Results for sodium chloride, potassium, bicarbonate were all normal)			Chest X-ray	Normal cardiac silhouette, lungs fields clear, no bony abnormalities	
			Upper GI series, small bowel follow-through and barium enema	Mucosal folds throughout small bowel were thickened. There is a nodular appearance to the loops, especially in the jejunum. The colon is normal.	
Total protein	5.4 g/dl	4.6			
Albumin	2.1 g/dl	3.2			
BUN	13 mg/dl	10-	Abdominal CT scan	Normal study.	
Creatinine	0.7 mg/dl	0.6	Gallium scan	No focal areas of uptake or other abnormalities	
ALT	24 IU/L	7-4			
Bilirubin (total)	0.8 mg/dl	0.1	5. *Other*		
Serum iron	26 μg/dl	59-	Biopsy of jejunal mucoa	Results consistent with nonspecific, intense jejunitis.	

weight gain, loss of symptoms, and reversal of gastrointestinal dysfunction.

Of interest was the patient's hematologic status. The hemoglobin concentration was low for age and was accompanied by a low mean corpuscular volume (MCV), diminished mean corpuscular hemoglobin (MCH), and a low normal mean corpuscular hemoglobin concentration (MCHC). The white blood cell (WBC) count was normal but the differential exhibited a shift to the left with increased numbers of band forms, suggesting infection or inflammatory disease state. The platelet count was also increased, consistent with this diagnosis. Examination of the peripheral blood smear demonstrated microcytic red cell morphology, toxic granulations in the neutrophils, and normal lymphocyte, monocyte, and platelet morphology. The erythrocyte sedimentation rate (ESR) was increased and clotting studies were consistent with inflammation or infection with a normal prothrombin time (PT), short partial thromboplastin time (PTT), elevated fibrinogen, and increased factor VIII activity.

In summary, the patient had a mild but definite microcytic anemia. With the primary diagnosis of inflammatory bowel disease, the most likely diagnosis was anemia of chronic inflammation. However, with heme-positive stools, the concomitant or separate existence of an iron deficiency state needed further evaluation. The family history was not consistent with a thalassemia.

Results of the red cell count and red cell indices may be helpful in differentiating the latter two disorders. In thalassemia, the MCV is usually well below the normal range, but there is also an erythrocytosis. In contrast, the red cell count is usually decreased but the MCV may be normal to decreased in iron deficiency. The MCHC is usually normal in thalassemia and iron deficiency with the hypochromic appearance reflecting small red cell size, decreased hemoglobin content, and high surface-to-volume ratio. Anemia of chronic diseases shares similar characteristics such as iron deficiency with a normal-to-decreased MCV and deficient red cell numbers.

Several discriminant indices may be helpful in eliminating the possibility of thalassemia. The most easily used is the Mentzer index, which is the MCV/red cell count (8). If this index is <13 then the diagnosis is more likely thalassemia, while if it is >13 iron deficiency probably exists. For A.J.H., the value is 14.5, suggesting that his disorder was not thalassemia. Although these types of indices are helpful in a relative sense, they will not be helpful in 10–15% of cases. This may be related to fact that mixed conditions may occur. Iron deficiency can be found concurrently with other conditions that cause anemias. In certain disease states, loss of iron, especially from the gastrointestinal tact, may be excessive. Mixed anemias can occur for other reasons, particularly when nutrition is poor and diminished intake of calories, protein, vitamins, or other constituents may adversely affect hemoglobin production. The primary considerations in evaluating this patient's anemia are differentiating iron deficiency from anemia of chronic diseases.

Studies of iron transport/iron storage are helpful in differentiating iron-deficiency anemia from the anemia of chronic disease. With iron deficiency, there is progressive loss of iron stores. Iron is stored within the ferritin molecule, a glycoprotein shell that contains iron phosphate salts. After depletion of ferritin stores, the serum iron decreases and in compensation total iron-binding capacity (TIBC) increases. In contrast, in anemia of chronic diseases, iron stores are not diminished and serum ferritin levels do not drop below normal values. While serum iron levels are decreased, TIBC is normal to decreased. In A.J.H., ferritin levels were normal, serum iron diminished, and TIBC low, all signs that are consistent with anemia of chronic disease. The diagnosis was further confirmed by his response to treatment. On prednisone alone, within 6 months his anemia completely resolved and all laboratory values returned to normal.

Etiology and Pathogenesis

A number of factors mediate the anemia of chronic diseases. The most prominent is abnormal iron metabolism characterized by shunting of iron to the reticuloendothelial system and withholding of iron in mononuclear phagocytes so that it is not available for erythropoiesis (9). Other important factors include inhibition of erythroid progenitors and erythropoietin (Epo) production (9). In addition, a mild decrease in red cell life span is a factor. These processes may be part of a generalized response to infection or inflammation, resulting in a number of other hematologic changes, besides anemia.

Distribution, Biochemistry, and Physiology of Iron

A detailed description of iron and iron metabolism is not appropriate to this chapter. However, several features of iron are critical to its role in the pathophysiology of the anemia of chronic diseases. Iron exists in two redox states and at physiologic pH is predominantly found in the ferric form unless biochemical pathways, such as those found in red cells, are present to keep it in the ferrous state (10). In addition, iron salts do not exist in a free state in living tissues and fluids but are bound to proteins. Most (70%) of the body's iron is found in hemoglobin. In normal individuals, as much as 25% is found in storage in the form of ferritin or hemosiderin. In steady state the predominant form is ferritin, a glycoprotein that encases ferric phosphate salts that are soluble within the cell (11, 12). Finally, a small amount of total body iron (1%) is associated with carrier/transport proteins. In health and disease, the iron carrier in the body making up the vast majority of iron-binding capacity is transferrin.

Unlike most important divalent actions, iron levels are controlled by modulating absorption; there is no other physiologic mechanism except sloughing of epithelial cells by which the body controls iron stores in the body. To a large extent, absorption is determined by the amount of iron stores in the body reflected in the ferritin stores of epithelial cells lining the gut (13). The rate of erythropoietic activity and normal body growth are also factors that enhance the absorption of iron from the gut. A number of other dietary factors are crucial to absorption, including enteral iron-carrying proteins, pH, presence of reducing substances, and presence of food as well as other local factors.

Iron Cycle

Iron recovered from turnover of senescent red blood cells or kept in the ferrous state in epithelial cells of the small bowel is taken up by transferrin. Transferrin is a plasma protein of molecular weight 84 kd, each molecule of which binds two atoms of iron (14). The affinity for iron is very high and binding of iron very specific. The direction of iron in the cycle is provided by transferrin receptors found in highest concentration in maturing erythroid cells. Once bound to transferrin receptors, iron-saturated transferrin is taken up by the erythroid precursors in an energy-requiring process (15). The iron is then stored in these cells in the form of ferritin until it can be utilized in hemoglobin synthesis.

Abnormalities in Iron Metabolism in Anemia of Chronic Diseases

Low serum iron and normal-to-decreased levels of transferrin in the presence of normal tissue stores of iron suggest that alterations in iron metabolism play a major role in the anemia of chronic disease or infection. In studies of animal models of inflammation as well as investigation of humans with infection, cancer, or inflammatory diseases, poor reutilization of iron from radio-labeled senescent red blood cells or hemoglobin solutions has been documented (16, 17). Since iron from senescent cells and hemoglobin solution is cleared by macrophages of the reticuloendothelial system and hepatic parenchymal cells, respectively, and uptake of iron and ferritin stores is normal, the data suggests an inability to mobilize sequestered iron stores. Iron absorption from the gut is moderately impaired (18). As with macrophages and liver parenchymal cells, the defect in iron is not in uptake and storage of iron but in mobilization from intracellular stores. Thus, in all three types of cells critically involved in iron metabolism defective mobilization of stored iron is a common theme.

The exact biochemical abnormality for this poor mobilization of iron is not known. One possibility lies in production of ferritin. Apoferritin is an acute phase reactant whose synthesis is stimulated by IL-1, a cytokine elevated in inflammation and infection (19–21). However, iron bound to ferritin is in chemical equilibrium with other intra- and extracellular pools of iron. Thus, decreased mobilization from this storage form seems an unlikely cause. Hemosiderin is another storage form of iron in macrophages and parenchymal cells. Unlike ferritin, the iron in hemosiderin is not soluble or as chemically or biologically available. It would seem possible that transfer of iron into a less accessible storage form of iron such as hemosiderin in response to inflammation or infection induces a state of tighter binding of iron stores within the reticuloendothelial system restricting the transfer of iron to or within the marrow.

Poor mobilization of iron cannot explain all of the abnormalities in iron metabolism seen in patients with chronic diseases. Hypoferremia is a common finding in these patients and is also an early event in acute infections, surgery, and pyrogen-induced fever (1). Although transferrin is the major iron carrier in serum in a normal steady state, a second iron-carrying protein, lactoferrin, may compete with transferrin for serum-bound iron. Lactoferrin, a protein of approximately 94 kd, is found in all exocrine secretions as well as polymorphonuclear leukocytes (22). Like transferrin, it has two iron-binding sites, but its avidity for iron remains high even at low pH (22). It is released from neutrophils during phagocytosis and found in high concentrations at sites of infection or inflammation. Lactoferrin plays a role in myelopoiesis and neutrophil function (23, 24). Its release and its increased serum levels during inflammatory disease states have been well documented (25, 26).

Macrophages and monocytes express specific receptors for lactoferrin (27). Studies on cultured macrophages demonstrate binding of lactoferrin to these cells, internalization of the lactoferrin to these cells, internalization of the lactoferrin-bound iron and transfer over 24 hours into ferritin stores (28). Since proliferating erythroid precursors in the marrow do not contain receptors for lactoferrin, it has been hypothesized that lactoferrin secreted from neutrophils under an infectious or inflammatory stimulus acts as a shunt to transport iron directly into the reticuloendothelial system where it is inserted into a less readily mobilizable form (29). A tentative scheme summarizing the known abnormalities is presented in figure 9.1.

Teleologically, withholding iron during an infectious or inflammatory disease state may be advantageous in minimizing an essential growth factor from microbes. In addition, withholding a catalyst responsible for toxic oxygen metabolites may be a means to ameliorate oxygen-mediated damage to tissues related to the inflammatory response. However, as this process becomes more chronic, iron is also withheld from developing erythroid cells, ultimately resulting in a condition deleterious to the body, anemia.

One additional feature of anemia of chronic disease may explain some of its manifestations. Often transferrin levels in the serum are reduced in this condition (30). Both decreased production and increased uptake of transferrin by macrophages have been identified as possible causes. This change, taken together with a low serum iron level, results in a diminished saturation of transferrin. The level of

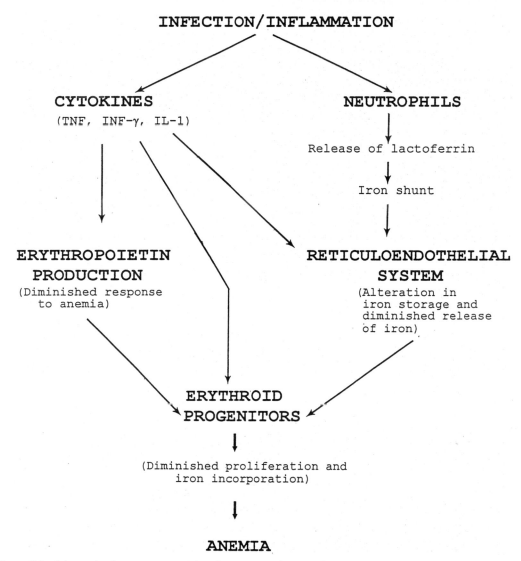

INFECTION/INFLAMMATION

CYTOKINES
(TNF, INF-γ, IL-1)

NEUTROPHILS

Release of lactoferrin

Iron shunt

ERYTHROPOIETIN PRODUCTION
(Diminished response to anemia)

RETICULOENDOTHELIAL SYSTEM
(Alteration in iron storage and diminished release of iron)

ERYTHROID PROGENITORS

(Diminished proliferation and iron incorporation)

ANEMIA

Figure 9.1. Schematic diagram summarizing the major pathogenic features of the anemia of chronic disease.

transferrin saturation in the anemia of chronic disease, however, is not as low as that found in iron deficiency. This may explain why the degree of anemia, microcytosis, and hypochromia are not as severe in most cases of anemia of chronic disease compared with iron deficiency anemia. While the precise cause of the abnormalities in iron metabolism in the anemia of chronic disease is not understood, recent studies suggest a role for cytokines such as interferon γ (INF-γ), tumor necrosis factor (TNF), and IL-1.

Other Abnormalities Contributing to Anemia

Although abnormalities with iron metabolism play the most significant role in the pathogenesis of the anemia of chronic diseases, other factors contribute to this state. Red cell life span is mildly to moderately diminished (31). The exact mechanism is not clear, but enhanced activity of the reticuloendothelial system in infectious, malignant, or inflamma-

tory states has been suggested (32). The decreased survival, however, could also be explained by minor structural changes in the red cells related to underlying conditions.

The anemia of chronic disease is more severe than would be expected for the moderate decrease in red cell survival, however. Decreased marrow production is a hallmark of the anemia of chronic diseases. Several possibilities exist for this problem with production. Early studies implicated diminished Epo response to the anemia in patients with rheumatoid arthritis, chronic infections, and malignancy (33). In other studies, however, the decrease was not as consistent (34). With the recent development of radioimmunoassays for Epo, levels of this cytokine in patients with anemia of chronic disease appear no different than levels documented in anemic patients without chronic diseases (35). Investigation of animal models and in vitro studies of progenitor cells have documented diminished numbers of erythroid progenitor cells in the presence of adequate erythropoietin levels (9). Cell-cell interactions with mononuclear phagocytes or malignant cells do not completely explain these findings (9). However, a number of inhibitors of erythropoiesis such as prostaglandins, acidic isoferritins, and the cytokines, INF-γ, TNF, IL-1, are released during inflammation and may play a role in the impaired erythropoiesis in the anemia of chronic disease (9). These compounds, however, are not specific for erythroid precursors, and their exact role in the isolated cytopenia associated with chronic disease has not been clearly defined.

Insight into the relative importance of various mechanisms in the anemia of chronic disease may be provided by use of recombinant erythropoietin in various diseases associated with this type of anemia. In a small series of patients with rheumatoid arthritis administration of Epo and iron resulted in normalization of the hematocrit, whereas iron alone had no effect (36). This might suggest that the abnormalities in iron metabolism are not the predominant factors in pathogenesis of anemia of chronic disease. Further studies, however, are necessary to reach a conclusion on this issue.

Related Disorders

Chronic disorders which are associated with the anemia described above can have a number of complications which themselves cause anemia. The diagnosis of the anemia of chronic disease or infection rests not only on the existence of clinical and laboratory characteristics noted above, but also the exclusion of other causes for anemia that may be present. These conditions may not necessarily be separate but, in fact, may add to or obscure the anemia of chronic diseases.

Most commonly in these disorders, iron loss or poor absorption may contribute to the anemia. The distinctions between iron deficiency and anemia of chronic diseases were described earlier. In complex cases, it may not be possible to reliably distinguish between these conditions, so it may be reasonable, under certain conditions, to embark on a therapeutic trial of iron. With severe inflammation or infection, however, this maneuver may only replete iron stores and not affect the anemia until the sequestration of iron and poor reutilization are resolved.

Endocrine diseases result in definite but mild hematologic abnormalities, including effects on red blood cells. Because of their extensive effects on metabolism as well as the fact that they may alter erythropoietin production directly, many hormones have dramatic effects on erythropoiesis and the metabolism of red cells. Thyroid disorders have been studied in the most detail. Hyperthyroidism may be associated with anemia that is usually characterized as normochromic and normocytic. Occasionally, the anemia may be macrocytic. In adults, hyperthyroidism is associated with a higher incidence of iron deficiency and pernicious anemia, confounding the effects of the endocrinopathy. In uncomplicated hyperthyroidism, anemia is rare and red cell indices are normal. In adrenal deficiency, mild-to-moderate anemia may occur associated with decreased metabolism. Decreased plasma volume that accompanies adrenal deficiency mitigates the effects of diminished red

cell mass. The different response rates of these two factors to treatment accounts for a paradoxical fall in hemoglobin concentration early after treatment of Addison disease and as well as an increase later in the treatment course. Mild erythrocytosis may occur with Cushing disease. Hematologic abnormalities are rare in gonadal dysfunction. In diseases of the pituitary, red cell abnormalities occur as a consequence of the altered production of trophic hormones and of specific endocrine dysfunction.

Other conditions associated with chronic anemia include drug-induced effects of marrow suppression or hemolysis, severe renal impairment, hemodilution, or replacement of bone marrow by malignant process. The anemia of chronic renal dysfunction is not directly associated with low serum iron or ferritin but rather failure of erythropoietin production. Viral infections may be associated with anemia by causing diminished production, increased destruction of red cells, or both. Diminished red cell production, due to direct viral replication erythroid precursors in the bone marrow, has been well documented in infection with human parvovirus B_{19} (37). Anemia has also been associated with thymic tumors, the exact etiology of which is unknown. Drug-related causes should always be considered as possibilities within this setting. Exclusion of these clinical conditions as well as documentation of appropriate clinical laboratory studies confirms the anemia of chronic diseases.

Management

The first step in management of anemia of chronic disease rests on the diagnosis of the infection, inflammatory disease, or malignancy, definition of the specific laboratory parameters that are abnormal, and elimination of other causes. The anemia and related symptoms may be so mild that no further intervention for the anemia is necessary. In all cases, successful treatment of the underlying disease will improve the hematologic status of the patient. As mentioned before, if the possibility of concurrent iron deficiency cannot be eliminated, a trial of iron may be attempted but failure to improve anemia may not disprove the sufficiency of iron stores. Transfusions should be considered only in life-threatening anemia, which occurs rarely in these patients. The administration of recombinent erythropoietin may be helpful to these patients if the underlying disease cannot be ameliorated by standard therapy.

Summary

In summary, anemia of chronic disease refers to anemia associated with a heterogeneous group of disorders, usually of infectious or inflammatory character. The mild-to-moderate anemia is related primarily to underproduction, resulting from abnormalities in iron metabolism. Decreased survival of red cells, diminished production of erythropoietin, and inhibition of red cell progenitors are other factors producing anemia. Definition and successful treatment of the underlying disease is the hallmark of managing the anemia. Use of iron or Epo therapy may be helpful in selected patients.

REFERENCES

1. Cartwright GE, Wintrobe MM. The anemia of infection: XVII, a review. In: Dock W, Snapper J, eds. Advances in internal medicine. Chicago: Year Book, 1952.
2. Cartwright GE. The anemia of chronic disorders. Semin Hematol 1966;3:351.
3. Wallner SF. The anemia of chronic disorders: clinical and pathologic features. In: Dunn C.D.R., ed. Current Concepts in Erythropoiesis. New York: John Wiley, 1983.
4. Abshire TC, Reeves J. The anemia of acute inflammation in children. J Pediatr 1983;103:868.
5. Lee GR. The anemia of chronic disease. Semin Hematol 1983;20:61.
6. Hyman GA. Anemia in malignant neoplastic disease. J Chron Dis 1963;16:645.
7. Friedell GH. Anemia in cancer. Lancet 1965;1:356.
8. Mentzer WC Jr. Differentiation of iron deficiency from thalassemia trait. Lancet 1973;1:882.
9. Means RT, Krantz SB. Progress in understanding the pathogenesis of the anemia of chronic disease. Blood 1992; 80:1639.
10. Spira TG. Chemistry and biochemistry of iron. In: Brown EB, Aisen P, Fielding J, Crichton RR, eds. Proteins of iron metabolism. New York: Grune & Stratton, 1977.
11. Hershko C. Storage iron regulation. Prog Hematol 1977; 10:105.
12. Deiss A. Iron metabolism in reticuloendothelial cells. Semin Hematol 1983;20:81.
13. Peters TJ, et al. Mechanisms and regulation of iron absorption. Ann NY Acad Sci 1988;526:141.
14. Aisen P, Listowski I. Iron transport and storage proteins. Ann Rev Biochem 1980;49:357.
15. Finch CA, Huebers H. Perspectives in iron metabolism. N Engl J Med 1982;306:1520.
16. Freireich EM, Miller A, Emerson CP, Ross JF. The effect of inflammation on the utilization of erythrocyte and transferrin-bound radio-iron for red cell production. Blood 1957;12:972.
17. Haurani FI, Burke W, Martinez EJ. Defective utilization of iron in the anemia of inflammation. J Lab Clin Med 1965; 65:650.
18. Haurani FI, Green D, Young K. Iron absorption in hypoferremia. Am J Med Sci 1965;249:537.
19. Koniju AM, Hershko C. Ferritin synthesis in inflammation. I. Pathogenesis of impaired iron release. Br J Haematol 1977; 37:7.
20. Platanias LC, et al. Interleukin-1: biology, pathophysiology and clinical prospects. Am J Med 1990;89:621.
21. Rogers J, et al. A motif within the 5 non-coding regions of acute phase mRNAs mediates translation by IL-1 and may contribute to the anemia of chronic disease. Blood 1991; 78:367a.
22. Malmquist J, Hansen NE, Karle H. Lactoferrin in haematology. Scand J Haematol 1978;21:5.
23. Peterson V, et al. Inhibition of colony-stimulating factor (CSF) production by postburn serum: negative feedback inhibition mediated by lactoferrin. J Trauma 1988;28:533–540.
24. Malech HL, Gallin JI. Current concepts: immunology. Neutrophils in human disease. N Engl J Med 1987;317:687.
25. Malmquist J, Thorell JI, Wollheim FA. Lactoferrin and lysozyme in arthritic exudates. Acta Med Scand 1977; 202:313.
26. Zebrak J, et al. Proteins in bronchial secretion of children with chroniqweruopc pulmonary diseases: II, relation to bronchoscopic and bronchographic examination. Scand J Resp Dis 1979;60:69.
27. Van Snick JL, Masson PL. The binding of human lactoferrin to mouse peritoneal cells. J Exp Med 1976;144:1568.
28. Van Snick JL, Markowetz B, Masson PL. The ingestion and digestion of human lactoferrin by mouse peritoneal macrophages and the transfer of its iron into ferritin. J Exp Med 1977;146:817.
29. Van Snick JL, Masson PL, Heremans JF. The involvement of lactoferrin in the hyposideremia of acute inflammation. J Exp Med 1974;140:1068.
30. Huebers HA, Finch CA. Transferrin: physiologic behavior and clinical implications. Blood 1984;64:763.
31. Dinant HJ, deMaat CEM. Erythropoiesis and mean red cell life span in normal subjects and in patients with anemia of active rheumatoid arthritis. Br J Haematol 1978;39:437.
32. Jandl JH, Jacob HS, Daland GA. Hypersplenism due to infection: study of five cases manifesting hemolytic anemia. N Engl J Med 1961;264:1063.
33. Wallner SF, et al. Levels of erythropoietin in patients with anemias of chronic diseases and liver failure. Am J Haematol 1977;3:37.
34. Douglas SW, Adamson JW. The anemia of chronic disorders: studies of marrow regulation and iron metabolism. Blood 1975;45:55.
35. Birgegard G, Hallgren R, Caro J. Serum erythropoietin in rheumatoid arthritis and other inflammatory arthritides: relationship to anemia and the effect of anti-inflammatory treatment. Br J Haematol 1987;65:479.
36. Pincus T, et al. Multicenter study of recombinant human erythropoietin in correction of anemia in rheumatoid arthritis. Am J Med 1990;89:161.
37. Potter CG, et al. Variation in erythroid and myeloid precursors in bone marrow and peripheral blood of volunteers infected with human parvovirus. J Clin Invest 1987;79:1486.

CHAPTER 10

Aplastic Anemias— Pancytopenias

JUDITH MARSH, ARMAND KEATING

The concept, along with the calculations, for Red Cell Indices, was introduced in 1929 by Maxwell Wintrobe, and a scientific rationale for the study of hematology was underway.

Introduction

Aplastic anemia refers to the marked diminution to total extinction of formed hematopoietic elements in the peripheral circulation. In order to address a rational approach to therapy, it is generally accepted that severe aplastic anemia is characterized by the following criteria: a reticulocyte count <1.0%, a platelet count <20 × 10⁹/L, and a granulocyte count of <0.5 × 10⁹/L in association with a biopsy-proven hypocellular marrow. The following case studies are designed to highlight measures taken to investigate aplasia, its etiologic events, and related treatment patterns.

Case 1

An 8-year-old boy was initially seen with a 4-week history of intermittent epistaxis and easy bruising after playing sports. His past medical history revealed normal gestation and delivery and normal developmental milestones. He had had no serious illnesses and had never required hospitalization. A family history revealed no bleeding disorders, and he had two siblings (age 2 and 4 years, respectively) who were both healthy. He had received no medications prior to this episode and there had been no obvious exposure to toxins or chemicals. Clinical examination revealed a well-nourished child at the 50th percentile for height and weight with no obvious skeletal anomalies. The skin appeared normal apart from scattered ecchymoses. There was no lymphadenopathy or hepatosplenomegaly, and the rest of the physical examination was normal. X-ray of the forearms was normal. Complete blood count (CBC) showed a hemoglobin of 100 g/L, white blood cell (WBC) count of 2.5 × 10⁹/L, neutrophils 1.0 × 10⁹/L, lymphocytes 1.1 × 10⁹/L, monocytes 0.4 × 10⁹/L, and platelets 50 × 10⁹/L. See table 10.1 for normal ranges of blood parameters.

Approach to Diagnosis of Pancytopenia: *This patient presented with a peripheral blood pancytopenia, that is, a combined deficiency of blood cells with anemia, leucopenia (associated with neutropenia), and thrombocytopenia. As with isolated deficiencies of blood cells,*

this may be due to impaired production or increased peripheral destruction of mature blood cells.

Table 10.2 illustrates the causes of pancytopenia subdivided into these two main categories. Further investigations need to be performed to determine which of the disorders listed in table 10.2 is the likely cause of the pancytopenia in this patient. A check list of investigations is shown in table 10.3. Microscopy of the peripheral blood film with examination of red cell indices is perhaps the first basic investigation to be done. Circulating blasts in leukemia, or plasma cells in myeloma, may be present, although in the case of leukemia, particularly childhood acute lymphoblastic leukemia (ALL), it may be difficult to differentiate small blasts from normal lymphocytes on routine blood smear without performing immunophenotyping of the cells. The presence of rouleaux, with a background blue staining (due to the presence of paraprotein, and usually visible to the naked eye) and a markedly elevated erythrocyte sedimentation rate (ESR) are typical hematologic findings in myeloma. A normocytic, or sometimes macrocytic normochromic, anemia is also associated with myeloma, and leucopenia and thrombocytopenia may be present in advanced disease. As with myeloma, myelofibrosis is a disease of the elderly, occurs less commonly in middle age, and is rare in young adults. Peripheral blood counts show anemia, and the white cell and platelet count initially may be normal or increased but usually are reduced later. The blood film typically shows a leukoerythroblastic anemia, tear drop poikilocytes, and often platelet anisocytosis with large, bizarre forms. Pancytopenia may occur in advanced megaloblastic anemia due to vitamin B₁₂ or folate deficiency, and the presence of oval macrocytes, tear drop poikilocytes, and hypersegmented neutrophils in the blood film with an elevated mean red cell volume (MCV) are characteristic findings. Dysplastic neutrophils (agranular, hypogranular, and pseudo-Pelger forms) are features of the myelodysplastic syndrome (MDS), where there is a qualitative defect resulting in ineffective hemopoiesis affecting any or

Table 10.1. Normal Values for Hematological Investigations Used in Case Presentations

Peripheral Blood Count	Adults			Children 10–12 yrs
	Males	Females	Both	
Hemoglobin (g/L)	130–180	115–165		115–145
Mean red cell volume (FL)			85–87	77–91
Reticulocytes ($\times 10^9$/L)			25–85	
or (%)			0.2–2.0	
Platelets ($\times 10^9$/L)			150–400	
White cell count ($\times 10^9$/L)			4–11	4.5–13.5
Neutrophils ($\times 10^9$/L)			2.0–7.5	
Lymphocytes ($\times 10^9$/L)			1.5–4.0	
Monocytes ($\times 10^9$/L)			0.2–0.8	
NAP score			35–100	
Hemoglobin F (%)			0.5–0.8	
Fibrinogen (mg/dL)			200–400	
Bone marrow:				
% blasts			0.1–3.5	
% lymphocytes			5–20	
Ferrokinetics				
Fe^{59} clearance $t_{1/2}$ (min)			60–140	
Iron utilization (%) at 10 d			70–80	

all of the three blood cell lines to result usually in pancytopenia. Often the pancytopenia is associated with a mild macrocytosis. An elevated serum lactate dehydrogenase (LDH) in MDS (and sometimes also in aplastic anemia [AA]) reflects the intramedullary destruction of cytoplasm associated with the dyserythropoiesis. With AA, there is commonly some degree of macrocytosis (usually mild) at initial presentation. The reticulocyte count is important for differentiating between impaired production of, as in AA, and increased destruction of, red cells, as, for example, in hypersplenism and paroxysmal nocturnal hemoglobinemia (PNH). The neutrophil alkaline phosphatase (NAP) score is classically low with PNH and often elevated with AA. A positive Ham-Dacie test, deficient expression of phosphatidyl inositol glycan (PIG)-anchored proteins on blood cells, with detectable urine hemosiderinemia confirms the diagnosis of PNH, which is an acquired clonal disorder that may arise from AA or progress to AA later in its course. A serum screen for autoantibodies, particularly antinuclear antibodies (ANA), is important to exclude disorders such as systemic lupus erythematosus (SLE), which can present with anemia, leucopenia or thrombocytopenia, or pancytopenia.

Although these hematologic abnormalities are usually immune-mediated, rarely a picture of true bone marrow failure may develop with SLE.

Bone marrow examination is central to the further diagnosis of pancytopenia. The degree of marrow cellularity will differentiate between impaired production of blood cells and increased peripheral destruction. At this juncture, one must emphasize the importance of performing not only a marrow aspirate but also a bone marrow (trephine) biopsy. The biopsy gives a more accurate

Table 10.2. Causes of Pancytopenia

	Marrow Cellularity
1. Mainly due to failure of production of blood cells:	
a. Bone marrow infiltration:	
Aleukemic leukemia	↑ or (↓)
Hairy cell leukemia	↑ or (↓)
Metastatic carcinoma	↑ or (↓)
Lymphoma	↑ or (↓)
Myeloma	↑ or (↓)
Myelofibrosis	↑ or (↓)
Gaucher's disease	↑ or (↓)
Niemann-Pick	↑ or (↓)
b. Vitamin B_{12} or folate deficiency	↑ or (↓)
c. Aplastic anemia	↓ or (↓)
2. Ineffective hemopoiesis:[a]	
Myelodysplastic syndrome	↑, → or (↓)
3. Mainly due to increased destruction of blood cells:	
a. Hypersplenism[b]	↑
b. Autoimmune disorders:	
Systemic lupus erythematosus	↑ (rarely ↓)
c. Overwhelming infections	↑ or (↓)
d. Paroxysmal nocturnal hemoglobinuria	↑

[a]A degree of ineffective hemopoiesis is common in megaloblastic anemia and aplastic anemia.
[b]Hypersplenism contributes to pancytopenia in lymphoma, leukemia, metabolic disorders.

Table 10.3. Further Investigation of Pancytopenia

1. Microscopic examination of peripheral blood film
2. Red cell indices, particularly mean red cell volume (MCV)
3. Reticulocyte count and erythrocyte sedimentation rate (ESR)
4. Biochemical profile, to include serum calcium, liver function tests, and lactate dehydrogenase
5. Bone marrow aspirate and trephine biopsy with cytogenetic analysis and cell marker studies
6. Serum B_{12} and red cell folate levels
7. Neutrophil alkaline phosphatase (NAP) score
8. Ham-Dacie test
9. Urine hemosiderin
10. Autoantibodies, particularly antinuclear antibodies
11. If available, ferrokinetic studies

representation of true cellularity, the marrow architecture is preserved, a biopsy is much more likely to detect abnormal marrow infiltration than an aspirate, and, finally, marrow reticulin can only be assessed on a biopsy as an indicator of marrow fibrosis. It is sometimes not possible to aspirate marrow fragments (a "dry tap"). This may indicate increased marrow fibrosis, marked marrow infiltration, or a technical failure. A severely hypocellular marrow as in AA is not a cause of a dry tap. In fact, if it is not possible to aspirate marrow fragments in a patient labeled as having AA, the diagnosis should be questioned. A dry tap is always an indication for a trephine biopsy. Increased marrow fibrosis is characteristic of idiopathic myelofibrosis but may also sometimes occur secondary to acute leukemia, particularly acute myeloid leukemia (AML) FAB type M7 (megakaryoblastic type), chronic myeloid leukemia, lymphoma, carcinoma, or tuberculosis.

A hypocellular bone marrow without increased reticulin or abnormal infiltration in the presence of pancytopenia is diagnostic of AA. There is an increase in fat cells. Macrophages, plasma cells, lymphocytes, and mast cells often appear prominent among the few residual hemopoietic cells. Because the disease is often patchy, a marrow aspirate may hit on a cellular area and so give a false impression of cellularity, whereas the marrow biopsy will usually reveal the true cellular pattern, provided that a sufficiently long core is obtained. Repeat samples, preferably from different sites, may help clarify the situation.

In leukemia, lymphoma, carcinoma, myeloma, and Gaucher disease, it is more common to find a hypercellular marrow, although hypocellularity may occur. ALL in children (and more rarely, AML) can present with pancytopenia and a hypocellular marrow (1, 2). In this situation, the marrow aspirate may only show the hypocellularity and miss the blasts, which the trephine will usually demonstrate. Examination of a peripheral blood buffy coat preparation is often a useful means of detecting circulating lymphoblasts. In vitamin B$_{12}$ or folate deficiency the marrow is usually hyper- or normocellular, but occasionally erythroid hypoplasia may occur. The marrow is megaloblastic and giant metamyelocytes are present.

MDS is also associated with a hyper- or normocellular marrow in most cases, but approximately 10–15% of cases have a hypocellular bone marrow (3). The dysplastic features of MDS are present in all three cell lines (4). Dyserythropoietic changes include nonhemoglobinized areas in the cytoplasm of late and intermediate normoblasts, bilobed or multilobed nuclei of erythroblasts, nuclear budding, cytoplasmic bridging, and ringed sideroblasts. Dysgranulopoietic features have been described earlier (see above). Dysmegakaryopoiesis can manifest as large mononuclear megakaryocytes, micromegakaryocytes (small mononuclear forms), or megakaryocytes with multiple discrete nuclei. However, difficulty can sometimes arise when the clinician tries to differentiate between hypocellular MDS and AA, because in the latter there is frequently dyserythropoiesis and there may be too few or no megakaryocytes and/or granulocytic precursors to look for dysplastic changes properly. In such cases, ferrokinetic studies are particularly helpful (5). A prolonged Fe^{59} t$\frac{1}{2}$ clearance time and reduced or absent uptake of isotope by the marrow with increased delayed uptake and accumulation in the liver are typical findings in AA. In MDS there is active uptake and retention of iron by the marrow, indicating ineffective erythropoiesis. Iron utilization (an expression of the incorporation into red cells) is reduced to about 30–50% compared with the usual 10–15% in AA. Whole body marrow scanning using Fe^{52} (or Fe^{59} or indium) can provide a useful assessment of the distribution and degree of marrow activity, demonstrating the patchy nature of erythropoiesis when it occurs (6).

Results of Investigations in Case 1: *The patient's MCV was elevated at 100 fL and his reticulocyte count was <1%. The blood film confirmed a moderate thrombocytopenia and there was anisopoikilocytosis, but no dysplastic neutrophils or blasts were seen. Serum electrolytes, urea, creatinine, liver function tests, vitamin B$_{12}$, and folate levels were all normal. A bone marrow aspirate was mildly hypocellular with reduction in all three cell lines. No dysplastic features or excess of blasts were present. Marrow biopsy confirmed moderate hypocellularity, no abnormal infiltration, and normal reticulin. Chromosome analysis of bone marrow cells revealed a normal karyotype, and culture of peripheral blood lymphocytes showed no increase in spontaneous or diepoxybutane (DEB)-stressed chromatid breakages. Viral serum screen was negative for hepatitis C, A, and B, cytomegalovirus, Epstein-Barr virus, and parvovirus B19. Ham-Dacie test was negative and hemosiderinuria was not detected. The patient was monitored over the next 3 weeks, when fever, sore throat, headache, and spontaneous bleeding developed. Clinical examination was unchanged apart from pallor, petechiae on the lower limbs, and bilateral flame-shaped fundal hemorrhages but no papilloedema. Hemoglobin had fallen to 70 g/L, reticulocytes were <0.1%, WBC 0.6 × 10^9/L, neutrophils 0.15 × 10^9/L, and platelets 10 × 10^9/L. A repeat marrow aspirate and biopsy were now severely hypocellular with <10% hemopoietic cells and no excess of blasts. The boy was treated with red cell and platelet transfusions and broad spectrum intravenous antibiotics. Earlier human lymphocyte antigen (HLA) typing of the patient and his siblings had shown that his youngest sibling was HLA identical.*

Conclusion: *This patient presented at a young age with aplastic anemia that progressed rapidly to severe aplasia. This necessitated early specific treatment, the nature of which is disclosed later. Further assessment of his aplasia in terms of whether it may have been con-*

genital or acquired, the disease severity, and its possible pathogenesis also will be discussed later in detail.

Case 2

A 48-year-old secretary had bilateral wrist pain for which a nonsteroidal antiinflammatory agent was prescribed. Two months later she complained of lethargy and scattered bruises. Past medical history was unremarkable and she had taken no other medication recently or been exposed to chemicals. She had no siblings. Clinical examination revealed pallor and scattered ecchymoses but the patient otherwise appeared normal. Complete blood count (CBC) showed hemoglobin 84 g/L, MCV 104 fL, reticulocytes 0.6%, WBC 2.0×10^9/L, neutrophils 1.1×10^9/L, lymphocytes 0.4×10^9/L, and platelets 30×10^9/L. Blood film showed anisopoikilocytosis. Serum vitamin B_{12} and folate levels were normal. A bone marrow aspirate was normocellular with dyserythropoiesis. Myelopoiesis and megakaryocytopoiesis were not dysplastic. Iron stain revealed normal stores and occasional ringed sideroblast (<5%). Bone marrow biopsy was moderately hypocellular (30%) with reduced activity in all three cell lines, and no increase in reticulin or blasts. Marrow cytogenetics were normal and the Ham-Dacie test was negative. Hemoglobin F was 2.0%. Ferrokinetics demonstrated a plasma Fe^{59} clearance $t^{1}/_2$ of 180 minutes and a reduced iron utilization of 15% on day 14. Whole body Fe^{52} scanning showed slow accumulation in the liver and reduced, patchy skeletal erythropoiesis.

A diagnosis of nonsevere AA was made. The patient later required intermittent red cell and platelet transfusions and was treated with antilymphocyte globulin (ALG) and androgens. Three months after treatment she was transfusion-independent and her blood count continued gradually to improve to the extent that at 12 months, her hemoglobin was 118 g/L, MCV 98 fL, reticulocytes 1.5%, WBC 4.8×10^9/L, neutrophils 1.8×10^9/L, and platelets 112×10^9/L. She remained clinically well and hematologically stable over the following 6 years, maintaining a near-normal blood count with persistent macrocytosis and negative Ham-Dacie test on yearly followup. However, a routine bone mar-

row at this time was moderately hypocellular and revealed hypogranular neutrophils and dysplastic megakaryocytes with no increase in blasts. Iron stain showed 30% ringed sideroblasts, and chromosome analysis revealed trisomy 6 in 10 of 20 metaphases examined. She was treated with low-dose cytosine arabinoside, but over the next 12 months there was a progressive decrease in her hemoglobin and platelets with the appearance of blasts in the peripheral blood and marrow characteristic of AML. She was treated with intensive chemotherapy, but her marrow failed to regenerate after one course and she died from septicemia.

Conclusion: In the patient in case 2 bone marrow failure developed at a later age than in the patient in case 1 and appeared to progress through a myelodysplastic phase despite showing a response to ALG, and eventually frank AML developed. This raises the question of the true nature of the patient's original disease—in particular, whether she had a preleukemic disorder at the outset. Nevertheless, at presentation she fulfilled all the diagnostic criteria for AA.

Analysis

Normal Hemopoiesis

Because AA represents the failure of normal hemopoiesis in vivo, it is relevant to review briefly the normal organization of the hemopoietic system in order to ascertain later where potential defects may occur.

The Hemopoietic System

Hemopoiesis begins in the yolk sac. Mesoderm cells located in the visceral mesoderm of the wall of the yolk sac differentiate into blood cells and blood vessels. As the embryo develops, the liver takes over as the major site of hemopoiesis, and later hemopoietic cells migrate to the bones where hemopoiesis persists throughout life. The hemopoietic cells develop in intimate association with the stromal cell microenvironment of the marrow, cells of which are also derived from the mesoderm germ layer.

The mature blood cells are ultimately derived from the hemopoietic stem cells. Stem cells can proliferate to pro-

Multipotent Cells			Progenitor Cells	Mature Cells
			Megakaryocyte-CFC	Megakaryocytes and platelets
			GM-CFC	Neutrophils
				Macrophages
Pluripotent	CFU-S	Mix-CFC	Eos-CFC	Eosinophils
Stem Cells	HPP-CFC		Bas-CFC	Basophils and mast cells
			BFU-E CFU-E	Erythrocytes
			Pre-B cells	B-lymphocytes
			Pre-T cells	T-lymphocytes

Figure 10.1 Normal stem cell development. Legend: *CFU-S,* murine spleen colony forming cells; *HPP-CFC,* high proliferative potential colony forming cell; *CFU-Mix,* multipotent CFC; *GM-CFC,* granulocyte/macrophage CFC; *Eos-CFC,* eosinophil CFC; *Bas-CFC,* basophil/mast cell CFC; *BFU-E,* primitive erythroid colonies; *CFU-E,* late erythroid colonies.

duce more stem cells (self-renewal), and also differentiate into progenitor cells committed to many separate lineages that give rise to all the mature functional end cells (7): hence, the stem cell is pluripotent (see fig. 10.1). Pluripotent stem cells account for only a very small percentage of marrow cells. The mature blood cells are postmitotic, with a relatively short lifespan, and about 3.7×10^{11} are lost each day (8). Steady-state hemopoiesis is maintained by cellular amplification alongside a progressively restricted developmental potential in the hemopoietic hierarchy, with enormous reserve for increased production of mature end cells in times of stress. Exhaustion of this reserve capacity, such as occurs in severe bone marrow failure, implies a very major marrow insult, perhaps acting at a very early stage of hemopoiesis. Following damage to the hemopoietic system, whether following bone marrow transplantation, severe damage by irradiation or chemotherapy, or some unidentified insult, initial recovery (and survival) is due to rapid proliferation and development of the more mature progenitor cells, whereas long-term recovery of hemopoiesis depends on the more primitive stem cells (9). The regulation of this hemopoietic hierarchy is dependent on growth-promoting agents (hemopoietic growth factors), negative regulatory factors, and the stromal cell microenvironment.

Hemopoietic Growth Factors and Negative Regulators

An increasing number of cytokines that stimulate the growth and development of blood-forming cells have recently been identified and cloned. These include so-called "lineage specific" factors such as macrophage colony-stimulating factor (M-CSF) (10), granulocyte-CSF (G-CSF) (11) and erythropoietin (Epo), and early acting cytokines, namely stem cell factor (SCF) (12), interleukin-3 (IL-3) (13), granulocyte-macrophage CSF (GM-CSF) (14), IL-1 (15), and IL-6 (16). These factors show extensive overlap of their biologic activities and marked synergisms, for example, stem cell factor (SCF 17) and IL-1 (15) have little and no colony-stimulating activity on their own but in combination with other cytokines exhibit profound effects on hemopoiesis. Some cytokines (for example IL-4, 5, and 6) influence the development of T- and B-lymphocytes as well as myeloid cells (see chapter 1 for details).

The recent identification of SCF may be of particular importance in the pathogenesis of congenital (and possibly acquired) forms of bone marrow failure in man. The c-kit protooncogene, allelic to the W locus in mice (18, 19), encodes a tyrosine kinase receptor, and SCF (encoded by the SL locus) is a ligand for the c-kit receptor (12). These observations explain the hemopoietic defects in two genetically anemic strains of mice: the stromal cell defect of the Sl/Sl^d strain results in defective production of SCF and the stem cell defect in the W/W^v strain is due to an absence or defective production of the SCF receptor. SCF is an earlier acting cytokine than IL-3 or GM-CSF with greater proliferative potential for Epo-dependent immature progenitor cells (CFU-Mix, and BFU-E) (20).

Important negative regulators of hemopoiesis include stem cell inhibitor/macrophage inflammatory protein 1α (M1P-1α) (21), which selectively inhibits proliferation of very immature progenitors. The presence of detectable levels of M1P-1α in bone marrow under steady-state conditions may explain the fact that only a small proportion of stem cells are proliferating at any one time. The inhibitory effect of transforming growth factor β (TGFβ) is less specific than M1P-1α, appears to be quicker acting (over hours rather than days), is differentiation linked, and is dependent on the presence of the cytokines (22). Negative regulators along with the growth-promoting factors all contribute to the maintenance of normal hemopoietic homeostasis.

The Stromal Cell Microenvironment

Studies using the Dexter long-term bone marrow culture (LTBMC) system have shown that hemopoiesis depends on intimate cell-cell interactions between hemopoietic cells and stromal cells (23, 24) (see fig. 10.2). The latter are composed of fibroblasts, macrophages, fat cells, and endothelial cells. Within the stromal (adherent) layer, once formed, early hemopoietic foci develop, and as these progenitor cells differentiate they are shed into the supernatant (nonadherent layer) (see fig. 10.2) of the culture. They can be counted and assessed in clonogenic culture. Each week the cultures are fed by replacing half the medium with fresh medium. Furthermore, long-term hemopoiesis is maintained in this system in the absence of added growth factors. These observations suggest that locally acting (rather than free) cytokines secreted by stromal cells provide the stimuli for hemopoietic cell growth. These cytokines are sequestered in the extracellular matrix (ECM) of the microenviron-

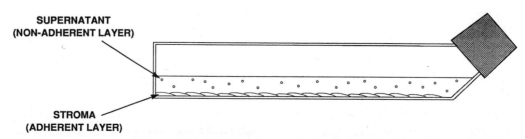

Figure 10.2 Long-term bone marrow culture (Dexter).

ment. An important component of the ECM includes the proteoglycans. Both GM-CSF and IL-3 bind to the heparin sulphate glycosaminoglycan side chain of proteoglycans, which presents the growth factor locally to the target hemopoietic cells (25, 26). In addition, adhesion molecules appear to enable hemopoietic cells to attach to specific regions of the microenvironment prior to responding to the locally presented growth factors (27).

The increasingly favored concept of stromal cell-mediated hemopoiesis suggests that the decision for stem cells to undergo self-renewal or differentiation is a reflection of the stromal cells, ECM, hemopoietic growth factors, and negative regulators that are present around them (28). Within this complex but highly organized structure of the hemopoietic system, there are clearly many possible defects that could theoretically produce hemopoietic failure. The evidence for the various proposed pathogenetic mechanisms in AA will be discussed later.

AA—The Failure of Normal Hemopoiesis

Types of AA

A brief classification of the types of AA will illustrate the marked heterogeneity of the disorder with respect to its etiology, disease severity, and possibly pathogenesis (see fig. 10.3).

Congenital AA

Although congenital AA is much less common than acquired AA, it is vital not to overlook this diagnosis so that early genetic counseling can be performed and treatment can be modified—for example, a reduction in pretransplant conditioning that is necessary in *Fanconi anemia (FA)* on account of the increased sensitivity to chemotherapy and radiation. FA is the commonest form of congenital AA. Frequent clinical abnormalities include short stature, skeletal abnormalities (particularly of thumbs, hands, wrists, and forearms), skin pigmentation, and renal and genital anomalies (29) (see table 10.4), underlining the importance of careful clinical examination of any child or

Congenital
Acquired
  • inevitable (postchemotherapy or irradiation)
  • transient (e.g., infectious mononucleosis, systemic lupus erythematosis)
  • idosyncratic-idiopathic
    • drugs
    • chemicals
    • viruses
    • paroxysmal nocturnal hemoglobinuria
    • systemic lupus erythematosis
      • pregnancy

Figure 10.3 Types of aplastic anemia.

Table 10.4. Somatic Abnormalities in Fanconi Anemia

	Approximate Incidence (%)
Skin pigmentation	75
Generalized hyperpigmentation	
Café au lait spots	
Depigmented patches	
Skeletal abnormalities	60
Thumbs	
Hands/wrists	
Forearms	
Low birth weight	55–60
Growth retardation	
Microcephaly	50
Micro-ophthalmia	
Microstomia	
Renal abnormalities	30
Horseshoe kidney	
Pelvic kidney	
Strabismus	25
Genital abnormalities	20
Cryptorchism	
Hypoplasia	
Mental retardation	20

From Gordon-Smith EC, Rutherford TM (1989) (29) with permission.

young adult initially seen clinically with AA. The underlying defect in FA is one of faulty DNA repair, which probably accounts for the high incidence of malignancy. It is uncertain whether the high incidence of hepatocellular carcinoma is due to prolonged androgen therapy. In probably at least 10%, acute leukemia develops, usually myeloid, although acute monocytic, myelomonocytic, megakaryoblastic (30), and very rarely lymphoblastic leukemia (31) have been reported. The increased risk of leukemia supports an underlying stem cell defect in the pathogenesis of FA, and the frequent finding of somatic abnormalities suggests that the defect occurs at a very primitive stage of embryogenesis prior to the hemopoietic stem cell. Not all cases of FA show the typical clinical features of the disorder (32). Approximately 30% of patients appear normal, and since the diagnosis in these patients is often overlooked they are usually diagnosed later in life with pancytopenia, for example. Nevertheless, all patients with FA demonstrate increased chromatid breakage following culture of peripheral blood lymphocytes (or skin fibroblasts or chorionic vili) with the DNA cross-linking agent diepoxybutane (DEB) (33). This test is specific for FA and is also used for prenatal diagnosis.

Dyskeratosis congenita (DC) more commonly presents at a later age than FA, although there is great overlap between the two (34, 35). In most cases inheritance of DC is X-linked recessive in contrast to autosomal recessive in FA, although some cases of autosomal inheritance (recessive and dominant) have been described in DC (36). The classical clinical signs in DC consist of leukoplakia, reticular pigmentation, and nail dystrophy. AA develops in 50% of such patients. Leukemia had not previously been documented in DC, but 2 cases have recently been reported (37). Malignant mucosal tumors, especially squamous cell carcinoma, occur more frequently than expected in DC (39). Recent in vitro studies using long-term bone marrow cultures suggest that the hemopoietic defect in DC is of stem cell origin, with normal stromal function (38). Some of the forms of congenital AA resemble phenotypically and hematologically the *Sl/Sl*^d and *W/W*^v mice (see above). These mice have abnormalities in coat color, macrocytic anemia, abnormalities of granulopoiesis and megakaryocytopoiesis, and are sterile. The evidence in favor of an underlying stem cell defect in congenital AA suggests that as for the *W/W*^v mouse, administration of SCF in vivo would not be expected to cure the hemopoietic defect in DC and FA. The recently described syndrome of late onset bone marrow failure with radioulnar fusion in 2 families sharing autosomal dominant inheritance highlights the need for careful clinical examination even in adults, with radiologic investigation advised in suspected cases (40). These patients were unable to supinate their forearms because of the skeletal abnormality. Such a diagnosis, if due to a primary stem cell defect, would suggest that only bone marrow transplant (BMT) would be curative. ALG was ineffective in both of the cases. The autosomal dominant defect in these 2 families also illustrates that as in FA, potential family donors who may or may not be hematologically normal must be screened beforehand to exclude a similar disorder.

There also exist rare cases of *congenital cytopenias,* which may later progress to generalized bone marrow failure. These can affect the megakaryocytic lineage (amegakaryocytic thrombocytopenia) or granulocytic lineage as in Shwachman-Diamond syndrome (41). The latter may less commonly present with AA. Kostmann syndrome is an autosomal recessive congenital neutropenia, but no cases of AA have risen from this disorder or from Diamond-Blackfan anemia, characterized hematologically by red cell aplasia.

Acquired AA

Etiology. Most cases of AA that are reported are idiosyncratic, have a prolonged course, and develop unpredictably in a small proportion of individuals after exposure to an identifiable (or unidentifiable) agent. Inevitable AA describes those patients developing the disorder predictably after chemotherapy or irradiation who are dose dependent and recover after 2–4 weeks unless supralethal treatment has been given. Systemic lupus erythematosus or an episode of infectious mononucleosis may be complicated by transient AA that may be immune mediated or result from direct infection of hemopoietic cells. However, prolonged aplasia may rarely occur in both these situations (42).

Most cases (75–80%) of idiosyncratic AA are idiopathic—that is, no obvious cause can be identified. Although many drugs have been implicated in the etiology of AA, there is strong evidence for only a small number of drugs causing the disorder (42).

A careful study in 1986 by the International Agranulocytosis and Aplastic Anemia Group (43) showed that the best-documented cases of drug-induced AA were due to chloramphenicol, phenylbutazone (and to a lesser extent, indomethacin), and gold. Other examples cited were usually based on a small number of reported cases. Prolonged AA has been reported after exposure to aniline dyes, organic solvents, and benzene. A myelodysplastic syndrome rather than true AA is seen after benzene exposure in most cases, and transient cytopenias, nonclonal changes, or clonal cytogenetic changes may also occur (44).

Since bone marrow failure develops in only a small minority of individuals exposed to these drugs, these individuals may have an underlying (? genetic) susceptibility to bone marrow damage that later manifests as AA when exposed to the particular agent. The same reasoning could be applied to virally induced AA, where viruses, particularly non-A, non-B hepatitis, but also hepatitis A, hepatitis B, and Epstein-Barr virus, have been implicated in some cases. The more recently identified hepatitis C virus responsible for most cases of non-A, non-B hepatitis was shown not to occur commonly in AA in one study (45). The time incidence of posthepatitic AA is difficult to determine because of incomplete serologic investigation in early cases and relatively few reported cases. Although the B19 parvovirus is the cause of aplastic crises seen in congenital hemolytic anemias such as sickle cell disease, pyruvate kinase deficiency, and hereditary spherocytosis, and persistent infection can lead to chronic bone marrow failure in patients with congenital or acquired immunodeficiency (48), no etiologic link has been shown with classical AA.

As discussed earlier, PNH is an acquired clonal disorder closely associated with AA (47). In a small proportion of patients with PNH, AML later developed. Some patients with MDS share the laboratory features of PNH (48). The association between AA and pregnancy is difficult to prove because of the development of a rare disorder in the presence of a common occurrence such as pregnancy. Nevertheless, there are well-documented reports of spontaneous resolution of the aplasia after delivery or abortion, and recurrence of aplasia with subsequent pregnancies or worsening of preexisting AA during pregnancy (49–51).

Laboratory Features of AA and Assessment of Disease Severity

AA is defined on the basis of the hematologic abnormalities usually seen in the peripheral blood and bone marrow. It is associated with pancytopenia and a hypocellular bone marrow. The degree of pancytopenia varies depending on the severity and stage of the disease. Often one (or two) cell line(s) are affected to a greater degree than the other(s). A normal white cell count and neutrophil count may occasionally be seen in the early stages, although thrombocytopenia is almost always present. The leucopenia is usually associated with a lymphopenia and monocytopenia. The anemia occurs with a reticulocytopenia, often a mild macrocytosis, an elevated hemoglobin F level and frequent dyserythropoietic features in the bone marrow. An elevated NAP score is often seen in association with coarse "toxic" granulation of neutrophils on examination of the blood film. The degree of marrow hypocellularity seen will depend partly on disease severity. In general, however, the peripheral blood count provides the best assessment of disease severity (52). The criteria for severe and very severe AA are shown in table 10.5; the remaining patients who do not fulfil these criteria have nonsevere AA. These criteria have prognostic value and are also important for determining the specific treatment for a particular patient.

Incidence of Acquired AA

The incidence of AA varies considerably worldwide. A large, thorough prospective study recently estimated an incidence of 2 cases per million population per year in seven regions of Europe and Israel (53). Similar figures have recently been reported from France (54) (1.4 per million) and the United Kingdom (55) (2.3 per million). This is in contrast to earlier studies in Europe that have reported an incidence varying between 5 and 25 per million (56–58) when less rigid diagnostic criteria were used. Apart from being retrospective, these studies performed in the 1960s and early 1970s probably included cases of MDS, particularly in older patients, and often bone marrow biopsy was not performed. In the Far East, China, and Japan, the incidence of AA is higher than in Europe, and this may be due to more frequent hepatitis and greater exposure to insecticides and other chemicals. An incidence of 7.2 per million in Bangkok was recently reported among young adults (15–24 years of age). The large study from Europe (and Israel) showed that equal numbers of males and females were affected, with two peaks in age incidence for males (ages 15–25 years and >60 years) and one peak for females (>60 years), although the disease shows a male preponderance in the European studies as well as that from Bangkok. The high incidence and a male-to-female ratio of 1.9 in Bangkok may suggest a specific environmental etiologic factor(s) in this region of Asia.

Table 10.5. International Aplastic Anemia Study Group Criteria

Criteria for severe aplastic anemia (141)
1. Bone marrow hypocellularity
   <25% of normal or 25–50% of normal and
   <30% residual hemopoietic cells
   and
2. Peripheral blood criteria
   Neutrophils   <0.5 × 10⁹/L
   Platelets   <20 × 10⁹/L   } 2 of 3
   Reticulocytes <1% corrected for hematocrit
Criteria for very severe aplastic anemia
Patients fulfill Camitta's criteria for severe aplastic anemia and have neutrophils <0.2 × 10⁹/L (104)

Pathogenesis

New insight into the pathogenesis of AA has been gained from (a) ongoing clinical studies, and (b) the application of preexisting in vitro techniques in addition to the availability of new laboratory methodology. Previously, many different and poorly understood pathogenetic mechanisms had been proposed to explain the bone marrow failure of AA. A better understanding of the pathogenesis is now providing more of a rationale for the different therapeutic options currently available, and this will be discussed later with particular reference to the two case presentations.

Clinical Observation

The following description summarizes the contribution of clinical observations to the understanding of the pathogenesis of AA. Between 30 and 50% of syngeneic transplants for AA are successful if a simple marrow infusion is given without any pretransplant immunosuppression (60, 61), implying that some cases of AA are due to a primary deficiency of stem cells. Further evidence supporting this theory is provided by the recognized association of AA with clonal disorders such as PNH, MDS, and AML. Approximately 25% of patients with PNH later have generalized marrow failure, and 5–10% of patients with AA later acquire a PNH clone (62). Appelbaum reported that 4% of patients with otherwise typical AA have an acquired clonal cytogenetic abnormality (63). With long-term followup of patients treated with ALG since the late 1970s, it has become apparent that the risk of MDS or AML is much higher than previously believed. One study from Europe reported that in 10% of patients treated with ALG and surviving 2 or more years AML developed (64), and a separate European study demonstrated a 57% cumulative risk of MDS, AML, or PNH developing in patients 8 years after ALG treatment (65). Similar findings, although perhaps less common, have also been seen in patients treated with androgens or symptomatic care alone (66). It is significant, however, that following allogeneic BMT for severe AA, providing irradiation is not used in the conditioning regimen, there is no known increased risk of acute leukemia developing, and PNH has not been reported in this situation (67, 68), suggesting that BMT possibly cures the disease whereas ALG or androgens do not, and that residual disease at the stem cell level may therefore predispose patients to later clonal disorders.

The theory of immune-mediated suppression of hemopoiesis in AA was based on the following clinical findings. First, complete autologous hemopoietic reconstitution occurs in a small proportion of patients following allogeneic BMT for AA. Second, it was argued that because 50–70% of syngeneic transplants were unsuccessful unless immunosuppressive preconditioning was given, immunologic factors were responsible for the aplasia (62). However, the possibility that these immunologic processes may be secondary to an underlying intrinsic stem cell defect cannot be excluded. Third, response to ALG was used as supportive evidence for an immune-mediated disease in responding patients, based on its lymphocytotoxic effect acting against a population of activated T-suppressor cells. There is now also evidence for an immunostimulating effect of ALG through its mitogenic effect on lymphocytes resulting in release of hemopoietic growth factors (69, 70). ALG may in addition directly stimulate hemopoietic progenitors. An increase in circulating T-suppressor cells seen in some AA patients (71, 72) has not been confirmed by all groups of workers (73, 74) and may be related to multiple blood transfusions in these patients. Likewise, reports of an increase in γ-interferon and/or interleukin 2 levels are not reproducible universally. Transfusion-induced sensitivity resulting in inhibition of marrow progenitors, rather than primary cellular or humoral inhibition, may have been responsible for the findings in many earlier studies that were not controlled to exclude this possibility. Significantly, Kaminiski and colleagues have recently shown that alloreactive CD8+ cytotoxic T-lymphocytes are generated by blood transfusions, in contrast to low numbers found in untransfused patients (75). Furthermore, correlation between these in vitro studies and clinical and hematologic response to ALG is poor.

Recurrent graft failure after syngeneic BMT for AA despite not only high-dose cyclophosphamide but also irradiation (76–78), particularly in the absence of a detectable serum or humoral inhibitor against donor marrow, may suggest a defect in the stromal cell microenvironment. Alternatively, recurrence of graft failure may be due to reemergence of an abnormal population of T-cells responsible for the original disease (76). Goss has reported natural killer (NK) cell-mediated inhibition of donor marrow in one such case (79).

Cell Culture and Molecular Studies

Initial studies assessing the in vitro hemopoietic potential of bone marrow cells from AA patients involved the use of clonogenic cultures. Marrow mononuclear cells are cultured in semisolid medium with the addition of various hemopoietic growth factors, and the ability of the cells to then give rise to individual colonies derived from all lineages (see fig. 10.1) can be assessed after 11–14 days. Studies in AA at diagnosis have consistently demonstrated either a lack or a marked reduction of all types of marrow hemopoietic progenitor cells (80, 81). However, progenitor cell assays do not take account of overall marrow cellularity; only the concentration and not the absolute number of colonies are assessed. The long-term bone marrow culture (LTBMC) system (see above and fig. 10.2) provides a more physiologic assessment of hemopoiesis since the long-term generation (over several months) of hemopoietic progenitors is dependent on the intimate interaction of stem cells with the stromal cell microenvironment. LTBMC studies in AA have shown normal stromal formation in most cases but severely defective hemopoiesis as evidenced by an absence or marked reduction in the generation of hemopoietic progenitors (82–84). This defect was of "stem cell" origin in all cases examined in two studies (84, 85). AA marrow cells inoculated onto irradiated normal LTBMC stromas did not generate progenitor cells. In contrast, stromal function in AA, as assessed by the ability of irradiated AA LTBMC stromas to support the generation of progenitor cells from normal marrow, was normal in 18 of 19 cases reported from two studies of patients with longstanding AA who had "recovered" after ALG treatment and in untreated patients. A third study reported defective stromal function in 3 of 9 patients with acute severe AA (86).

In order to examine further the nature of this "stem cell" defect, purified populations of hemopoietic progenitor cells expressing the CD34 antigen have been isolated from AA patients (87). The CD34 antigen is expressed on all colony-forming cells (CFC), precursors of CFC, pre-T cells, and pre-B cells. It is not present on more mature cells. The proportion of normal bone marrow mononuclear cells that expresses this antigen ranges from 1–4% (88). This population of cells probably does contain the pluripotent stem cell, since infusion of CD34+ cells into lethally irradiated baboons results in long-term lymphohemopoietic reconstitution (89). A recent study of patients with end-stage breast carcinoma or neuroblastoma with short followup has shown that autologous CD34+ marrow cells are capable of successful engraftment (90). Analysis of marrow CD34+ cells in a small series of patients with treated nonsevere AA showed a reduction in the percentage of CD34+ cells compared with normal control subjects, and the CD34+ cells demonstrated reduced clonogenic potential in short-term culture (87). Morphologically within the CD34+ cell fraction from normal bone marrow, a small proportion appear to resemble small blasts of lymphocyte size. Andrews has shown by fluorescence-activated cell sorting (FACS) analysis that these cells represent the precursors of CFC with marrow-repopulating ability, express the phenotype CD33-/CD34+, and account for approximately 1% of the CD34+ population (91). Morphologic examination of AA CD34+ cells revealed that small blasts were either absent or severely reduced. When these AA CD34+ cells were inoculated onto normal LTBMC stromas, generation of hemopoietic progenitors was severely deficient (87). Gibson and colleagues (unpublished observation) have recently isolated CD34+/CD33− marrow cells from patients with AA and demonstrated a reduced percentage compared with normal controls. Thus the hemopoietic defect in AA appears to be due to a deficiency of cells with marrow-repopulating ability. If these highly purified CD34+/CD33− cells fail to generate colonies in progenitor assays and are unable to repopulate irradiated marrow stromas, one may infer that the hemopoietic defect in most patients with AA is due to an intrinsic stem cell defect.

The levels of circulating hemopoietic growth factors in AA patients, for example, G-CSF, GM-CSF, Meg-CSF, and erythropoietin are generally greatly elevated (recently reviewed by Young [92]). The only reported deficiency is of IL-1. Nakao (93) showed that production of IL-1 by monocytes in patients with severe AA was defective. More recently, this has been reported to correlate with response to ALG (94). However, it is uncertain whether IL-1 deficiency represents a secondary response to an underlying stem cell defect rather than a primary event, particularly since a recent study reported no response hematologically to administration of recombinant human IL-1 given to 4 patients with refractory severe AA despite demonstrating a reduction in the lymphocytes in these patients (95).

Further examination of the stem cell compartment is possible by X-chromosome inactivation analysis in female individuals. This is a useful tool to determine whether hemopoiesis is monoclonal or polyclonal. The principles of this methodology are based on the Lyon hypothesis, as detailed in table 10.6. Previously, glucose-6-phosphate dehydrogenase (G-6-PD) enzyme variant heterozygosity was used, but this approach is limited by the very low incidence of heterozygotes in the white population. In 1 patient with nonsevere AA who was heterozygous for G-6-PD, the red cells, neutrophils, platelets, CFU-GM, most BFU-E, and T-cells expressed only one G-6-PD enzyme type, inferring that these cells were derived from a single clone. This patient had a normal marrow karyotype and no morphologic evidence of MDS or acute leukemia (96). More recently, DNA probes for two polymorphic genes (hypoxanthine phosphatidyl ribosyl transferase [HPRT] and phosphoglycerate kinase [PGK]) on the X-chromosome have become available to assess clonality in a much larger proportion of females (97). The principles are the same as for G-6-PD enzyme variant analysis, and a description (see table 10.6), with predicted patterns on Southern analysis for the PGK probe, is shown in fig. 10.4. A third X-linked DNA probe, M27β (98), detects multiallelic variation on the X-chromosome and heterozygosity rates are even higher than for the HPRT and PGK probes combined (see fig. 10.5). Using the DNA probes, one group has recently reported that 10 of 16 patients with AA showed apparent monoclonal patterns of hemopoiesis on analysis of peripheral blood mononuclear

Table 10.6. Principles of Clonality Analysis Based on X-Chromosome Inactivation

1. Only one X-chromosome is active in each female cell, the other is inactive (Lyon hypothesis).
2. X-inactivation is random, occurring early in embryonic life, and results in normal females being mosaic for heterozygous loci. In contrast, in a *monoclonal* tumor the same X-chromosome will be active in all cells.
3. On a molecular level, changes in the activation state of the X-chromosome are accompanied by changes in the methylation of cytosine residues of the DNA: inactive loci are hypermethylated. The active and inactive loci can be distinguished by cleavage with methylation sensitive restriction endonucleases, for example, HpaII or HhaI, which cut only at nonmethylated recognition sites.
4. The maternal and paternal copies of an X-chromosome gene can be distinguished by using restriction fragment length polymorphisms (RFLP), e.g., of the human hypoxanthine phosphoribosyl transferase (HPRT) and phosphoglycerate kinase (PGK) genes.

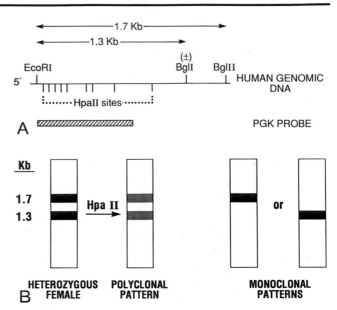

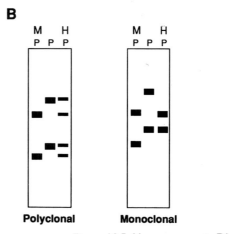

Figure 10.4 Assessment of clonality using the x-linked DNA probe PGK. **A,** 5' end of restriction map of PGK gene; **B,** predicted patterns of clonality seen on Southern analysis.

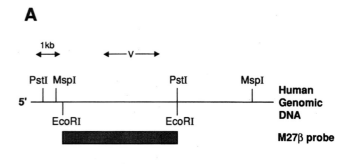

Figure 10.5 Human genomic DNA.

cells (MNC) (99–101). However, appropriate controls to exclude extreme lyonization (which can mimic a monoclonal pattern, and may occur in up to 23% of normal females) were not performed, so interpretation of these results remains uncertain (102). In contrast, a second study reported polyclonal hemopoiesis in 5 of 6 AA patients (103), a not dissimilar finding to results from a combined study from two centers reporting only 2 of 21 AA patients with monoclonal hemopoiesis, after excluding patients with extreme lyonization or those in whom control DNA was not analyzed (Janssen et al., unpublished results). Furthermore, Mehta demonstrated the absence of T-cell receptor β- and γ-gene rearrangements in all of 21 patients with AA (104). The finding of a monoclonal pattern (not due to extreme lyonization) in the presence of a normal marrow karyotype and in the absence of morphologic evidence of MDS or acute leukemia in a patient may reflect stem cell depletion or reconstitution by a resistant defective stem cell clone that survived the initial marrow insult that produced earlier bone marrow failure. An isolated monoclonal pattern in such a case of typical AA may not represent a premalignant state, whereas the finding of a clonal cytogenetic abnormality probably does indicate preleukemia.

Conclusions

Results from ongoing clinical studies and in vitro and molecular investigation indicate that an intrinsic stem cell defect or deficiency may be the major pathogenetic mechanism responsible for the bone marrow failure of acquired AA. The initial trigger(s) precipitating stem cell damage may be one or several factors. There may be an underlying genetic event at the stem cell level which predisposes to a later insult such as a virus or drug that manifests as marrow failure with cytopenias. Another view proposed by Young (94) is that there are two distinct forms of acquired AA, one which is virally induced and results in immune-mediated suppression of hemopoiesis but is not associated with later malignancy, and the other form of AA due to an intrinsic stem cell defect as in congenital aplasia which carries a risk of evolution to MDS and/or leukemia.

The Nature of the Bone Marrow Failure in Patients 1 and 2

Patient 1 was initially seen clinically with nonsevere AA, as he did not fulfill the criteria for severe AA (see table 10.5). Over a short period of time his aplasia worsened, progressing to very severe AA. It is important to identify this particularly severe subgroup of patients since a neutrophil count of $<0.2 \times 10^9/L$ is associated with a very low chance of responding to ALG, especially in young children. This observation suggests that in some children AA may be more likely to arise from an intrinsic stem cell defect (it may be unreasonable to expect ALG to correct such a defect). There was nothing clinically to suggest that the AA of patient 1 was congenital since he was of normal height and had no somatic abnormalities. A diagnosis of Fanconi anemia was excluded by the absence of increased chromatid breakages on culturing his peripheral blood lymphocytes with DEB. His acquired AA was idiopathic—i.e., no obvious cause could be identified. There was no evidence of hepatitis, exposure to drugs or chemicals associated with AA, and no evidence of PNH, as discussed earlier.

Patient 2 was initially seen with mild pancytopenia and macrocytosis. Although the marrow aspirate was normocellular, a bone marrow biopsy was moderately hypocellular, illustrating the importance of routine trephine biopsy as well as marrow aspirate in all cases of AA. At this stage, the patient had no evidence of MDS. Dyserythropoiesis alone is insufficient to make a diagnosis of MDS, and it is also frequently seen in AA. Marrow cytogenetic analysis results were normal, and about 50% of primary MDSs and most AAs have a normal karyotype. Ferrokinetic studies were more in keeping with aplasia (see above). A diagnosis of nonsevere AA in this patient was most likely, probably secondary to ingestion of a nonsteroidal antiinflammatory drug. However, it was important to exclude a possible diagnosis of SLE in this patient in view of her initial joint pains and the rare but well-documented association of SLE with AA (103, 104). Vitamin B_{12} and folate deficiency were excluded by normal serum levels and the absence of megaloblastic features in the marrow. There was no evidence of PNH. A good hematologic response was seen after ALG therapy, although the blood count did not completely normalize, a frequent finding after ALG treatment. The late development at 6 years of dysplastic features in the granulocytic series and megakaryocytes, the clonal cytogenetic abnormality in the absence of overt leukemia, and the presence of increased ringed sideroblasts (>15%) without an increase in peripheral blood or marrow blasts was consistent with MDS subtype refractory anemia with ringed sideroblasts (2). The fact that her marrow was hypocellular could either reflect previous marrow aplasia or hypocellular MDS. It is impossible to know whether the dysplastic and subsequent leukemic transformation in this patient was part of the natural history of her disease or whether it was secondary to her treatment. Similar evolution has also been seen in AA following androgen therapy. It is possible that hypocellular MDS represents an intermediate stage in the progression of AA through classical MDS and leukemia. Did this patient have a clonal disorder at diagnosis? There was no morphologic evidence of MDS or leukemia, marrow cytogenetics were normal, and the Ham-Dacie test was negative. Perhaps an abnormal clone was present but at such a low level as not to be detected by conventional laboratory techniques. Sequential analysis of clonality using X-linked DNA probes may in the future help to shed further light on the pattern of hemopoiesis in such a patient. The clinical importance of these findings is demonstrated by the management problems that such a case raises.

Rationale for Different Therapeutic Modalities

Because AA shows marked heterogeneity in all aspects of disease discussed thus far, several different therapeutic options are available. Criteria exist to help in the choice of treatment for a particular patient based on clinical factors (see below).

Supportive Care

Prior to the instigation of specific treatment of the disease, the immediate management involves supporting the patient with red cell and platelet transfusions, antibiotics, and antifungal agents, depending on the disease severity and clinical condition. For patient 2, with nonsevere AA at diagnosis, immediate supportive treatment was not required, whereas patient 1 represented a medical emergency when his disease progressed rapidly to very severe AA, necessitating urgent intensive supportive care.

In AA a balance should be achieved between preventing life-threatening hemorrhage and avoiding unnecessary transfusions in order to minimize the alloimmunization that results in resistance to random donor platelet transfusions and an increased incidence of graft rejection after allogeneic BMT.

The quality of supportive care has improved substantially with the routine use of leucocyte-depleted blood products, the availability of cytomegalovirus (CMV)-seronegative blood products, increased availability of platelet transfusions, including HLA matched paltelets and new antibiotics.

Bone Marrow Transplantation

A patient with AA is eligible for allogeneic BMT if he or she has (a) severe AA, (b) an HLA-identical sibling donor and, (c) is <45 years of age. A recent study from Europe suggested that patients >20 years old with neutrophils $0.2–0.5 \times 10^9/L$ did better with ALG (105), but this data was analyzed with insufficiently long followup to detect later clonal disorders. Therefore, if the aim is to try to cure the disease, BMT is preferable in this group. Current regimens employ high-dose cyclophosphamide only as the immunosuppressive preconditioning, with cyclosporin (to reduce graft-vs-host disease [GVHD] and to prevent graft failure) on its own or with methotrexate. Recent data from the International Bone Marrow Transplantation Registry reports no advantage in survival with the additional use of irradiation to reduce graft failure (106, 107). Indeed, with allogeneic BMT for AA the use of irradiation should be avoided due to the increased risk of GVHD (acute and chronic), sterility, impaired growth, and second malignancies. A recent study describes a cumulative incidence of 25% of second malignancies at 8 years post-BMT for severe AA using total lymphoid irradiation (108). In contrast, Witherspoon has reported a cumulative incidence of only 1.4% at 10 years in AA patients transplanted with cyclophosphamide alone as conditioning (67). Long-term actuarial survival following BMT is 60–75% for multiply transfused patients (109–111), 80% for "untransfused" patients (112), and at least 90% for children (113).

Unfortunately, only about 30% of patients in Western Europe and North America with severe AA have an HLA-identical sibling donor. For those who are young with very severe AA, without such a donor, an alternative donor should be sought since these patients respond very poorly

to ALG (114, 115). One to two percent will have an HLA phenotypically identical family member, and results for BMT using these donors are comparable to those using HLA genotypically identical donors. For BMT from mismatched family donors, results are unacceptably poor if more than a one antigen mismatch is used (116, 117). Results of BMT in children using either a one-antigen mismatch family donor or an HLA-"matched" unrelated donor have improved (118) with the use of more intensive pretransplant conditioning to reduce graft failure, increased anti-GVHD prophylaxis, better selection of recipients (only young patients with very severe disease, who are not infected at time of transplant), and new, more rapid HLA-typing techniques that allow BMT to be performed as early as possible (119–122).

ALG. The use of ALG in severe AA with or without high-dose methyl prednisolone, androgens, or cyclosporin results in variable response and survival rates of 30–70% (123–127). For those with nonsevere disease, about 80% will respond (126), although not all studies have shown improved response in nonsevere AA compared with severe AA. Children, especially if <6 years of age, respond poorly even if they have nonsevere AA (115, 128). The use of ALG is associated with relapse in 25–30% of patients (129, 130) and an incidence of clonal disorders occurring late (maximum >8 years) after therapy (65). Recent in vitro data using LTBMC indicate that all patients who have been treated with ALG have residual stem cell defects despite hematologic recovery, indicating that they are not cured of their disease. The rationale for using ALG in the treatment of AA was based on its supposed immunosuppressive action directed against circulating cytotoxic T-suppressor lymphocytes. As discussed earlier (see Pathogenesis), an immunostimulating role may also be relevant, resulting in increased release of hemopoietic growth factors.

Hemopoietic Growth Factors

The recent use of growth factors such as GM-CSF as single agents in AA has resulted in only transient increases in neutrophils, monocytes, eosinophils, and sometimes lymphocytes (131–135). No consistent effect has been seen on platelets or reticulocytes. G-CSF results in a greater increase in neutrophils and only a modest increase in monocytes. It is also less toxic that GM-CSF or IL-3 (136–137). The effect of IL-3 on blood counts in AA is similar to that of GM-CSF but with even smaller increments in the neutrophil count (139). As single agents, G-CSF or GM-CSF have potential in the treatment of serious infective episodes, or when used in combination with ALG to shorten the period of neutropenia associated with ALG therapy. The use of combinations of hemopoietic growth factors given simultaneously or concomitantly has not been fully assessed, but should perhaps be approached with great caution. Because AA is associated with a reduction in numbers of primitive hemopoietic cells (see section on The Hemopoietic System), there is the theoretical potential for stem cell exhaustion if a combination is used that preferentially stimulates stem cell differentiation rather than stem cell renewal.

Treatment of Patients 1 and 2

Patient 1 received the treatment of choice for his very severe AA, namely allogeneic BMT. Had he not had an HLA-compatible sibling, an alternative would have been a course of ALG and consideration of later transplant from either an unrelated donor. In this case it would have been reasonable to have given a course of ALG while such a donor was being sought. If one could not be found, the patient would need intensive supportive therapy while waiting for a response to ALG. However, it is unlikely that he would have been cured of his disease in view of the possible long-term complication of such treatment, as discussed above. In this context it is important to note that this risk of later clonal disease has not been reported after allogeneic BMT for AA, implying that BMT does result in true cure of a disease that probably is most often due to an intrinsic stem cell defect.

Since patient 2 was 48 years old, had nonsevere AA, and did not have an HLA-compatible sibling donor, she did not fulfill the criteria for treatment with BMT. The mild aplasia with an intermittent transfusion requirement responded predictably to ALG. Unfortunately, later MDS and subsequent AML developed. The poor response to low-dose cytosine arabinoside and later intensive chemotherapy without hematologic regeneration may have reflected a background of marrow aplasia with reduced stem cell reserve, as well as a qualitative defect due to abnormal dysplastic stem cells. Had she been younger and had an HLA-compatible sibling donor, it would have been reasonable to have contemplated allogenic BMT when MDS developed prior to AML. It has been shown that results of BMT for MDS are superior if performed in the early stage of the disease before a large tumor load develops (140). If patient 2 had a clonal preleukemic disorder at presentation it is likely that only BMT would have cured her aplasia and eradicated her abnormal clone (141).

Transient Erythroblastopenia of Childhood (TEC)

Two nonpancytopenic disorders that merit attention include pure red cell aplasia and transient erythroblastopenia of childhood. There are many cases of pure red cell aplasia, but in contrast to adults, the causes in children are more restricted, and two examples are unique to children—namely transient erythroblastopenia of childhood (TEC) and Diamond-Blackfan Anemia (DBA). TEC is a common cause of red cell aplasia that is probably viral induced, and spontaneous recovery is the rule.

TEC is an acquired disorder characterized by a normocytic, normochromic anaemia with reticulocytopenia, bone marrow erythroid hypoplasia or erythroid aplasia, and spontaneous recovery. Typically, the child is initially seen clinically with anemia, usually after 1 year of age, having been previously healthy. There is frequently a history of preceding viral infection, for example, parvovirus, which is thought to result in transient immune-mediated suppression of erythropoiesis. A serum inhibitor of erythroid bone marrow colonies can be demonstrated in more that half the cases, or less commonly a cellular inhibitor. Sometimes TEC is associated with neutropenia, and bone marrow examination may show either granulocytic hypoplasia or maturation arrest. Erythroid marrow colony numbers may be reduced or normal. It has been suggested that the neutropenia may also be immune mediated. Spontaneous recovery usually occurs within 4–8 weeks and later recurrence is very rare. TEC may present simultaneously among siblings, and clusters of cases have been reported at particular times of the year, lending more support to a viral etiology (142).

It is important to distinguish acquired TEC from the congenital form of pure red cell aplasia, Diamond-Blackfan anemia (DBA). DBA is sometimes inherited, but occurs sporadically in most cases. Unlike TEC, most cases of DBA present with anemia within the first year of life. Congenital anomalies may occur in DBA but only 30% of affected children, so that the absence of anomalies does not exclude a diagnosis of DBA. Unlike TEC, DBA is a chronic disorder that usually requires lifelong blood transfusion support, and is associated with an increased risk of acute leukemia. There is no association of TEC with leukemia. At diagnosis, red cell parameters are frequently "fetal-like," with macrocytosis, increased % hemoglobin F and i antigen expression on red cells in patients with DBA. In contrast, in TEC the red cells have normal "adult/child" values while the patient is reticulocytopenic (143).

TEC is a common cause of red cell aplasia in children. It is a transient, self-limiting condition and the prognosis is excellent. It has no long-term sequelae, no specific treatment is needed, and blood transfusion is only given if clinically indicated. It is vital to differentiate TEC from the rare but more serious, chronic form of red cell aplasia in childhood, DBA, where treatment with regular red cell transfusions and corticosteroids are necessary. An early diagnosis of TEC will avoid the inappropriate exposure to corticosteroids.

REFERENCES

1. Melhorn DK, Gross S, Nowmann MS. Acute childhood leukemia presenting as aplastic anemia: the response to corticosteroids. J Pediatr 1970;77:647.
2. Breatnach F, Chessells JM, Greaves MF. The aplastic presentation of childhood leukemia—a feature of common ALL. Br J Hematol 1981;49:387.
3. Fohlmeister J, Fischer R, Modder B, Rister M, Schaefer HE. Aplastic anemia and the hypocellular myelodysplastic syndrome: histomorphological, diagnostic and prognostic features. J Clin Pathol 1985;38:1218.
4. Bennett JM, Catovsky D, Daniel MT, Frandrin G, Galton DAG, Gralnick HR, Sultan C. Proposals for the classifica-

tion of the myelodysplastic syndromes. Br J Haematol 1982; 51:189–199.

5. Dacie JV, Lewis SM. Erythrokinetics. In: Dacie JV, Lewis SM, eds. London: Churchill Livingstone, 1984:288–312.

6. Hotta T, Murate T, Inoue C, Kagami T, Tsushita K, Wang JY, Saito H. Patchy hemopoiesis in long-term remission of idiopathic aplastic anemia. Eur J Hematol 1990;45:73.

7. Metcalf D. Hemopoietic colonies. Berlin: Springer, 1977.

8. Cronkite EP, Feinendegen, LE. Notions about human stem cells. Blood Cells 1976;2:263.

9. Jones RJ, Celano P, Sherkis SJ, Semerbrenner LL. Two phases of engraftment established by serial bone marrow transplantation in mice. Blood 1989;73:397.

10. Metcalf D. The hemopoietic colony stimulating factors. Amsterdam: Elsevier, 1984.

11. Nicola NA. Granulocyte colony-stimulating factor. In: Dexter TM, Garland JM, Testa NG, eds. Colony stimulating factors: molecular and cellular biology. New York: Marcel Decker, 1990:77–109.

12. Witte ON. Steel locus defines new multipotent growth factor (published erratum appears in Cell 1990;30;63, following 1112). Cell 1990;63:5.

13. Moore MAS. Interleukin 3: an overview. In: Schrader JW, ed. Interleukin 3: the panspecific hemopoietin; vol 15, lymphokines. New York: Academic Press, 1988: 219–280.

14. Metcalf D. The granulocyte macrophage colony stimulating factors. Science 1985;229:16.

15. Heyworth CM, Ponting IL, Dexter TM. The response of hemopoietic cells to growth factors: developmental implications of synergistic interactions. J Cell Science 1988: 91:239.

16. Ikebuchi K, Wang GG, Clark SC, Ihle JN, Hirai Y, Ogawa M. Interleukin-6 enhancement of interleukin-3 dependent proliferation of multipotential progenitors. Proc Natl Acad Sci USA 1987;84:9035.

17. McNiece IK, Langley KE, Zsebo KM. Recombinant human stem cell factor synergizes with GM-CSF, G-CSF, IL-3 and Epo to stimulate human progenitor cells of the myeloid and erythroid lineages. Exp Hematol 1991;19:226.

18. Chabot B, Stephenson DA, Chapman VM, Besmer P, Bernstein A. The proto-oncogene c-kit encoding a transmembrane tyrosine kinase receptor maps to the mouse W locus. Nature 1988;335:88.

19. Geissler EN, Ryan MA, Housman DE. The dominant white- spotting (w) locus of the mouse encodes the c-kit proto-oncogene. Cell 1988;55:185.

20. Broxmeyer HE, Cooper S, Lu L, et al. Effect of murine mast cell growth factor (c-kit proto-oncogene ligand) on colony formation by human marrow hematopoietic progenitor cells. Blood 1991;77:2142.

21. Graham GJ, Wright EG, Hewick R, et al. Identification and characterization of an inhibitor of hemopoietic stem cell proliferation. Nature 1990;344:442.

22. Hooper CW. The role of transforming growth factor-beta in hemopoiesis: a review. Leukemia Res 1991;15:179.

23. Dexter TM, Allen TD, Lajtha LG. Conditions controlling the proliferation of hemopoietic stem cells in vitro. J Cell Physiol 1977;91:335.

24. Dexter TM, Coutinho LH, Spooncer E, et al. Stromal cells in hemopoiesis. In: Dexter TM, Allen TD, eds. Molecular control of hemopoiesis. Ciba Foundation Symposium 148. Chichester: Wiley, 1990:76–95.

25. Gordon MY, Riley GP, Watt SM, Greaves MF. Compartmentalization of a hematopoietic growth factor (GM-CSF) by glycosaminoglycans in the bone marrow microenvironment. Nature 1987;326:403.

26. Roberts R, Gallagher JT, Spooncer E, Allen TD, Bloomfield F, Dexter TM. Heparan sulphate bound growth factors: a mechanism for stromal cell mediated hemopoiesis. Nature 1988;332:376.

27. Tavassoli M, Hardy CL. Molecular basis of homing of intravenously transplanted stem cells to the marrow. Blood 1990;76:1059.

28. Dexter TM. Stem cells in normal growth and disease. Br Med J 1987;295:1192.

29. Gordon-Smith EC, Rutherford TR. Fanconi anemia—constitutional, familial aplastic anemia. In: Gordon-Smith EC, ed. Aplastic anemia, clinical hematology-international practice and research. Vol 2. East Sussex: Bailliere Tindall, 1989:139–152.

30. Dharmasena F, Catchpole M, Erber W, Mason D, Gordon-Smith EC. Megakaryoblastic leukemia and myelofibrosis complicating Fanconi anemia. Scand J Haematol 1986; 36:309.

31. Smith S, Marx MP, Jordaan CJ, van Niekerk CM. Clinical aspects of a cluster of 42 patients in South Africa with Fanconi anemia. In: Auerbach AD, ed. Fanconi anemia, clinical, cytogenetic and experimental aspects. Berlin: Springer, 1989:34–46.

32. Auerbach AD, Rogatko A, Schroeder-Kurth TM. International Fanconi anemia registry: relation of clinical symptoms to diepoxybutane sensitivity. Blood 1989;73:391.

33. Auerbach AD, Adler B, Chaganti RS. Prenatal and postnatal diagnosis and carrier detection of Fanconi anemia by a cytogenetic method. Pediatrics 1981;67:128.

34. Sirinavin C, Trowbridge AA. Dyskeratosis congenita: clinical features and genetic aspects. J Med Genet 1975; 12:339.

35. Womer R, Clark JE, Wood P, Sabio H, Kelly TE. Dyskeratosis congenita: two examples of this multisystem disorder. Pediatrics 1983;71:603–609.

36. Pai GS, Morgan S, Whetsell C. Etiologic heterogeneity in dyskeratosis congenita. Am J Med Genet 1989;32:63.

37. Marsh JCW, Geary CG. Is aplastic anemia a preleukemic disorder? Br J Hematol 1991;77:447.

38. Marsh JCW, Will AJ, Hows JM, et al. "Stem cell" origin of the hematopoietic defect in dyskeratosis congenita. Blood 1992;79:3138–3144.

39. Feinberg AP, Coffey DS. Organ site specificity for cancer in chromosomal instability disorders. Cancer Res 1982; 42:3252.

40. Dokal I, Ganly P, Riebero I, Marsh J, Steed A, Kendra J, Drysdale C, Hows J. Late onset bone marrow failure associated with proximal fusion of radius and ulna: a new syndrome. Br J Hematol 1989;71:277.

41. Evans DIK. Congenital defects of the marrow stem cell. In: Gordon-Smith EC, ed. Aplastic anemia; vol. 2, clinical hematology—international practice and research. East Sussex:Bailliere-Tindall, 1989:163–190.

42. Gordon-Smith EC. Aplastic anemia. Med Int 1983;26: 1195.

43. International Agranulocytosis and Aplastic Anemia Study. Risks of agranulocytosis and aplastic anemia: a first report of their relation to drug use with special reference to analgesics. JAMA 1986;256:1749.

44. Jacobs A. Benzene and leukemia. Br J Haematol 1989; 72:119.

45. Pol S, Driss F, Devergie A, Brechot C, Berthelot P, Gluckman E. Is hepatitis c virus involved in hepatitis-associated aplastic anemia? Ann Int Med 1990;113:435.

46. Kurtzman G, Young N. Viruses and bone marrow failure. In: Gordon-Smith EC, ed. Aplastic anemia; Vol. 2, clinical hematology—international practice and research. East Sussex: Bailliere-Tindall, 1989:51–67.

47. Rotoli B, Luzzatto L. Paroxysmal nocturnal hemoglobinuria. In: Gordon-Smith EC, ed. Aplastic anemia; Vol. 2, clinical hematology—international practice and research. East Sussex: Bailliere-Tindall, 1989:113–138.

48. Ricard MF, Sigaux F, Imbert M, Sultan C. Complementary investigations in myelodysplastic syndromes. In: Schmalzl F, Hellriegel KP, eds. Preleukemia. Berlin: Springer, 1979: 56–66.

49. Fleming AF. Hypoplastic anemia in pregnancy. Br Med J 1973;3:166.

50. Krispel JW, Lynch VA, Viele BD. Aplastic anemia in pregnancy: a case report, review of the literature and a re-evaluation of management. Obstet Gynecol Surv 1976;31:523.

51. Aitchison RG, Marsh JC, Hows JM, Russell NH, Gordon-Smith EC. Pregnancy associated aplastic anemia: a report of five cases and review of current management. Br J Haematol 1989;73:541.

52. Lewis SM. Course and prognosis in aplastic anemia. Br Med J 1965;1:1027.

53. International Agranulocytosis and Aplastic Anemia Study. Incidence of aplastic anemia: the relevance of diagnostic criteria. Blood 1987;70:1718.

54. Mary JY, Baumelou E, Guiguet M. The French Cooperative Group for Epidemiological Study of Aplastic Anemia. Epidemiology of aplastic anemia in France: a prospective multicentre study. Blood 1990;75:1646.

55. Cartwright RA, McKinney PA, Williams L, Miller JG, Evans DIK, Bentley DP, Bhavnani M. Aplastic anaemia incidence in parts of the United Kingdom in 1985. Leuk Res 1988;12:459.

56. Wallerstein RO, Condit PK, Kasper CK, Brown JW, Morrison FR. Statewide study of chloramphenicol therapy and fatal aplastic anemia. JAMA 1969;208:2045.

57. Bottiger LE. Epidemiology and etiology of aplastic anemia. In: Heimpel H, Gordon-Smith EC, Heit W, Kubanek B, eds. Aplastic anemia—pathophysiology and approaches to therapy. Berlin: Springer, 1979:27.

58. Szlo M, Sensenbrenner L, Markowitz J, Weida S, Warm S, Lineth M. Incidence of aplastic anemia in metropolitan Baltimore: a population-based study. Blood 1985;65:115.

59. Issaragrisil S, Sriratanasataram C, Piankijagum A, et al. Incidence of aplastic anemia in Bangkok. Blood 1991;77: 2166.

60. Champlin RE, Feig SA, Sparkes RS, Gale RP. Bone marrow transplantation from identical twins in the treatment of aplastic anemia: implication for the pathogenesis of the disease. Br J Haematol 1984;56:455.

61. Champlin RE, Horowitz MM, van Bekkum DW, Camitta BM, Elfenbein GE, Gale RP, Gluckman E, Good RA, Rim AA, Rozman C, Speck B, Bortin MM. Graft failure following bone marrow transplantation for severe aplastic anemia: risk factors and treatment results. Blood 1989; 73:606.

62. Camitta BM, Storb R, Thomas ED. Aplastic anemia (first of two parts), pathogenesis, diagnosis, treatment and prognosis N Engl J Med 1982;306:645.

63. Appelbaum FR, Barrall J, Storb R, Ramberg R, Doney K, Sale GE, Thomas ED. Clonal cytogenetic abnormalities in patients with otherwise typical aplastic anemia. Exp Hematol 1987;15:1134.

64. dePlanque MM, Klein-Nelemans JC, van Krieken HJ. Evolution of acquired severe aplastic anemia to myelodysplasia and subsequent leukemia in adults. Br J Haematol 1989;73:121.

65. Tichelli A, Gratwohl A, Wursh A, Nisser C, Speck B. Late hematological complications in severe aplastic anemia. Br J Haematol 1988;69:413.

66. Najean Y, Haguenauer O, for the Cooperative Group for the Study of Aplastic and Refractory Anemia. Long-term (5 to 20 years) evolution of non-grafted aplastic anemias. Blood 1990;76:2222.

67. Witherspoon RP, Storb R, Pepe M, Longton G, Sullivan KM. Cumulative incidence of secondary solid malignant tumors in aplastic anemia patients given marrow grafts after conditioning with chemotherapy alone. Blood 1992; 79:289.

68. Speck B. Allogeneic bone marrow transplantation for severe aplastic anemia. Semin Haematol 1991;28:319.

69. Tong J, Bacigalupo A, Piaggio G, Figari O, Sogno G, Marmont A. In vitro response of T cells from aplastic anemia patients to antilymphocyte globulin and phytohemagglutinin: colony stimulating activity and lymphokine production. Exp Haematol 1991;19:312.

70. Nimer SD, Golde DW, Kwan K, Lee K, Clark S, Champlin R. In vitro production of granulocyte-macrophage colony stimulating factor in aplastic anemia: possible mechanism of action of antilymphocyte globulin. Blood 1991;78:163.

71. Gascon P, Zoumbos NC, Scala G. Lymphokine abnormalities in aplastic anemia: implications for the mechanism of action of anti-thymocyte globulin. Blood 1985; 65:407.

72. Zoumbos NC, Gascon BP, Djeu JY, Trost SR, Young NS. Circulating activated suppressor T lymphocytes in aplastic anemia. N Engl J Med 1985;312:257.

73. Torok-Storb B, Sieff C, Storb R, Adamson J, Thomas ED. In vitro tests for distinguishing possible immune-mediated aplastic anemia from transfusion-induced sensitization. Blood 1980;55:211.

74. Hanada T, Yamamaru H, Ehara T, Iwasaki N, Shin R, Nakahara S, Takita H. No evidence for gamma-interferon mediated hematopoietic inhibition by T cells in the course of immunosuppressive therapy. Br J Haematol 1987;67:123.

75. Kaminsky ER, Hows JM, Goldman JM, Batchelor JR. Pre-transfused patients with severe aplastic anemia exhibit high numbers of cytotoxic T lymphocyte precursors probably directed at non-HLA antigens. Br J Haematol 1990;76:401.

76. Appelbaum FR, Cleever M, Fefer A, Storb R, Thomas ED. Recurrence of aplastic anemia following cyclophosphamide and syngeneic bone marrow transplantation: evidence for two mechanisms of graft failure. Blood 1985;65:553.

77. Marsh JCW, Harhalakis N, Dowding C, Laffan M, Gordon-Smith EC, Hows JM. Recurrent graft failure following syngeneic bone marrow transplantation for aplastic anemia. Bone Marrow Transplant 1989;4:581.

78. Matsue K, Niki T, Shiobara S, et al. Transient engraftment of syngeneic bone marrow after conditioning with high dose cyclophosphamide and total abdominal irradiation in a patient with aplastic anemia. Am J Hematol 1990; 33:56.

79. Goss GD, Wittner MA, Bezwoda WR, Herman J, Rabson A, Seymour L, Derman DP, Mendelow B. Effect of natural killer cells on syngeneic bone marrow: in vitro and in vivo studies demonstrating graft failure due to NK cells in an identical twin treated by bone marrow transplantation. Blood 1985;66:1043–1046.

80. Kern P, Heimpel H, Heit W, Kubanek B. Granulocytic progenitor cells in aplastic anemia. Br J Haematol 1977;35:613.

81. Hara H, Kai S, Fushimi M, et al. Pluripotent hemopoietic precursors in vitro (CFU-Mix) in aplastic anemia. Exp Hematol 1980;8:1165.

82. Juneja HS, Lee S, Gardner FH. Human long-term bone marrow cultures in aplastic anemia. Int J Cell Clon 1989; 7:129.

83. Gibson FM, Gordon-Smith EC. Long-term culture of aplastic anemia bone marrow. Br J Haematol 1990;75:421.

84. Marsh JCW, Chang J, Testa NG, Hows JM, Dexter TM. The hematopoietic defect in aplastic anemia assessed by long-term marrow culture. Blood 1990;76:1748.

85. Gibson FM, Scopes J, Laurie A, Gordon-Smith EC. Contribution of the marrow stroma to the pathogenesis of aplastic anemia. Exp Haematol 1990;18:303a.

86. Hotta T, Kato T, Maeda H, Yamao H, Yamada H, Saito M. Functional changes in marrow stromal cells in aplastic anemia. Acta Haematol 1985;74:65.

87. Marsh JCW, Chang J, Testa NG, Hows JM, Dexter TM. In vitro assessment of marrow "stem cell" and stromal cell function in aplastic anemia. Br J Haematol 1991;78:258.

88. Civin CI, Trishmann TM, Fackler, et al. Report on the CD34 cluster workshop. In: Knapp W, Dorker B, Gilks WR, Rieber EP, Schmidt RE, Stein H, van dem Borne AEG, eds. Leukocyte typing; IV, white cell differentiation antigens. Oxford: University Press, 1989:818.

89. Berenson RJ, Andrews RG, Bensinger WI, Kalamasz D, Krilter G, Buckner CD, Bernstein ID. Antigen CD34+ marrow cells engraft lethally irradiated baboons. J Clin Invest 1988;81:951.

90. Berenson RJ, Bensinger WI, Hill RS, et al. Engraftment after infusion of CD34+ marrow cells in patients with breast cancer or neuroblastoma. Blood 1991;77:1717.

91. Andrews RG, Singer JW, Bernstein ID. Precursors of colony-forming cells in humans can be distinguished from colony forming cells by expression of the CD33 and CD34 antigens and light scatter properties. J Exp Med 1989; 169:1721.

92. Young NS. The pathogenesis and pathophysiology of aplastic anemia. In: Hoffman R, Benz EJ, Shaltil SJ, Furie B, Cohen HJ, eds. Haematology, basic principles and practice. New York: Churchill Livingstone, 1991:122–159.

93. Nakao S, Matshushima K, Young N. Decreased interleukin-1 production in aplastic anemia. Br J Haematol 1989; 71:431.

94. Childs B, Chasseing NA, Tomelden C, O'Reilly RJ, Castro-Malaspina H. Hypoproduction of interleukin-1β (IL-1β) by activated monocytes is specific for severe aplastic anemia. Exp Hematol 1991;19:260a.

95. Walsh CE, Liu JM, Stacie M, Anderson Rossio JL, Nienhuis AW, Young NS. A trial of recombinant human interleukin-1 in patients with severe refractory aplastic anemia. Br J Haematol 1992;80:106.

96. Abkovitz JL, Fialkow PJ, Niebrugge DJ, Raskind WH, Adamson JW. Pancytopenia as a clonal disorder of a multipotent hematopoietic stem cell. J Clin Invest 1984; 73:258.

97. Vogelstein B, Fearon ER, Hamilton SR, Preisinger AC, Willard HF, Michelson AM, Riggs AD, Orkin SM. Clonal analysis using recombinant DNA probes from the X-chromosome. Cancer Res 1987;47:4806.

98. Abrahamson G, Fraser NJ, Boyd Y, Craig I, Wainscoat JS. A highly informative X-chromosome probe M27ß can be used for determination of tumour clonality. Br J Haematol 1990;74:371.

99. van Kamp H, Landegent JE, Jansen RPM, Willemze R, Fibbe WE. Clonal hematopoiesis in patients with acquired aplastic anemia. Blood 1991;78:3209.

100. Gale RE, Wheadon H, Linch DC. X-Chromosome inactivation patterns using HPRT and PGK polymorphisms in hematologically normal and post-chemotherapy females. Br J Haematol 1991;79:193.

101. Josten KM, Tooze JA, Borthwick-Clarke C, Gordon-Smith EC, Rutherford TR. Acquired aplastic anemia and paroxysmal nocturnal hemoglobinemia: studies on clonality. Blood 1991;78:3162.

102. Mehta AB, Chiu E, Harhalakis N, Economou K, Foroni L, Luzzatto L, Gordon-Smith EC. A T cell lymphoma of suppressor phenotype arising in a patient with severe aplastic anemia. Br J Hematol 1989;72:287.

103. Fitchen JN, Cline MM, Saxon A, Golde DW. Serum inhibitors of hematopoiesis in a patient with aplastic anemia and systemic lupus erythematosis. Am J Med 1979;66:537.

104. Roffe C, Cahill MR, Samanta A, Bricknell S, Durrant S. Aplastic anemia in systemic lupus erythematosis: a cellular immune mechanism? Br J Rheumatol 1991;30:301.

105. Bacigalupo A, Hows J, Gluckman E, et al. Bone marrow transplantation (BMT) versus immunosuppression for the treatment of severe aplastic anemia (SAA): a report of the EBMT SAA Working Party. Br J Haematol 1988;70:177.

106. Hows JM, Bacigalupo A, Gluckman E, on behalf of the EMBTG Severe Aplastic Anemia Working Party. Impact of conditioning protocols on improved outcome of BMT for severe aplastic anemia. Bone Marrow Transplantation 1990; 5(suppl 2):52a.

107. Gluckman E, Horowitz MM, Champlin RE, et al. Bone marrow transplantation for severe aplastic anemia: influence of conditioning and graft versus host disease prophylaxis regimens on outcome. Blood 1992;79:269.

108. Socie G, Henry-Amar M, Cosset JM, Devergie A, Girusky T, Gluckman E. Increased incidence of solid malignant tumors after bone marrow transplantation for severe aplastic anemia. Blood 1991;78:277.

109. Storb R, Doney KC, Thomas ED, et al. Marrow transplantation with or without donor buffy coat cells for 65 transfused aplastic patients. Blood 1982;59:236.

110. Ramsay NK, Trewan K, Nesbith ME, et al. Total lymphoid irradiation as preparation for bone marrow transplantation for severe aplastic anemia. Blood 1980;55:344.

111. Hows JM, Marsh JC, Yin JL, et al. Bone marrow transplantation for severe aplastic anemia using cyclosporin: long-term follow-up. Bone Marrow Transplant 1989;4:11.

112. Anasetti C, Doney KC, Storb R, et al. Marrow transplantation for severe aplastic anemia: long-term outcome in fifty untransfused patients. Ann Intern Med 1986;104:461.

113. Storb R, Sanders JE, Pepe M, et al. Graft versus host disease prophylaxis with methotrexate/cyclosporin in children with severe aplastic anemia treated with cyclophosphamide and HLA-identical marrow grafts. Blood 1991; 78:1144.

114. Hows JM. The use of unrelated marrow donors for transplantation. Br J Haematol 1990;76:1.
115. Locasciulli A, Porta F, Vossen JM, Bacigalupo A. Treatment of acquired severe aplastic anemia (SAA) in children: an analysis of the EBMT-SAA Working Party. Bone Marrow Transplant 1989;4(suppl 2):90a.
116. Hows JM, Yin JL, Marsh J, et al. Histocompatible unrelated volunteer donors compared with HLA nonidentical family donors in marrow transplantation for aplastic anemia and leukemia. Blood 1986;68:1322.
117. Beatty PE, DiBartolomeo P, Storb R, et al. Treatment of aplastic anemia with marrow grafts from related donors other than HLA genotypically-matched siblings. Clin Transplant 1987;1:117.
118. Camitta B, Ash R, Menitove J, Murray K, Lawton C, Hunter J, Casper J. Bone marrow transplantation for children with severe aplastic anemia: use of donors other than HLA-identical siblings. Blood 1989;74:1852.
119. Bidwell JL, Bidwell EA, Savage DA, Middleton D, Klouda PT, Bradley BA. A DNA-RFLP typing system that positively identifies serologically well defined and ill defined HLA-DR and DQ alleles, including DRW10. Transplantation 1988;45:640–646.
120. Tiercy JM, Zwahlen F, Betuel H, Jeannel M, Mach B. Improved HLA class II matching in bone marrow transplantation with unrelated donors by DNA oligonucleotide probing. Exp Hematol 1989;17:705a.
121. Clay TM, Bidwell JL, Howard MR, Bradley BA, on behalf of collaborating centres in the IMUST study. PCR fingerprinting for selection of HLA matched unrelated donors. Lancet 1991;337:1049.
122. Hows JM, Anasetti C, Camitta BM, Gaijensky J, Gluckman E, Bacigalupo A. Unrelated donor transplant for severe acquired aplastic anemia (SAA). Bone Marrow Transplant (in press).
123. Speck B, Gratwohl A, Nissen C, et al. Treatment of severe aplastic anemia with antilymphocyte globulin or bone marrow transplantation. Br Med J 1981;282:860.
124. Champlin R, Ho W, Gale RP. Antithymocyte globulin treatment in patients with aplastic anemia. N Engl J Med 1983;308:113.
125. Camitta B, O'Reilly RJ, Sensenbrenner L, et al. Antithoracic duct lymphocyte globulin therapy of severe aplastic anemia. Blood 1983;62:883.
126. Marsh JC, Hows JM, Bryett KA, Al-Hashimi S, Fairhead SM, Gordon-Smith EL. Survival after lymphocyte globulin therapy for aplastic anemia depends on disease severity. Blood 1987;70:1046.
127. Young NS, Griffith P, Brittain E, et al. A multicentre trial of antithymocyte globulin in bone marrow failure. Blood 1988;72:1861.
128. Marsh JCW, Hows JM, Bryett KA, Gordon-Smith EC. Young age and outcome of treatment with antilymphocyte globulin for aplastic anemia. Bone Marrow Transplant 1988;3(suppl 1):238a.
129. Doney K, Kopecky K, Storb R, et al. Long-term comparison of immunosuppressive therapy with antithymocytic globulin to bone marrow transplantation in aplastic anemia. In: Shahidi NT, ed. Aplastic anemia and other bone marrow failure syndromes. Berlin: Springer, 1990:104–114.
130. Marin P, Schrezenmeier H, Bacigalupo A, Van Lint MT, for the EBMT SAA Working Party. Relapse of aplasia following ALG treatment: a report of the SAA working party. Bone Marrow Transplant 1990;28:48a.
131. Antin JH, Smith BR, Holmes, W Rosenthal DS. Phase I/II study of recombinant human granulocyte macrophage colony stimulating factor in aplastic anemia and myelodysplastic syndrome. Blood 1988;72:705.
132. Nissen C, Tichelli A, Gratwohl A, Speck B, Milne A, Gordon-Smith EC, Schaedelin J. Failure of recombinant human granulocyte-macrophage colony stimulating factor therapy in aplastic anemia patients with very severe neutropenia. Blood 1988;72:2045.
133. Vadhan-Raj S, Buescher S, Broxmeyer HE, et al. Stimulation of myelopoiesis in patients with aplastic anemia by recombinant human granulocyte macrophage colony stimulating factor. N Engl J Med 1988;319:1628.
134. Champlin RE, Nimer SD, Ireland P, Oette DH, Golde DW. Treatment of refractory aplastic anemia with recombinant human granulocyte macrophage colony stimulating factor. Blood 1989;73:694.
135. Guinan EC, Sieff CA, Oette DH, Nathan DG. A phase I/II trial of recombinant granulocyte-macrophage colony stimulating factor for children. Blood 1990;76:1077.
136. Morstyn G, Souza M, Keech J, et al. Effect of granulocyte colony stimulating factor on neutropenia induced by cytotoxic chemotherapy. Lancet 1988;1:667.
137. Bronchud, MH, Howell A, Crowther D, Hopwood P, Souza L, Dexter TM. The use of granulocyte colony stimulating factor to increase the intensity of treatment with doxorubicin in patients with advanced breast and ovarian cancer. Br J Cancer 1989;60:171.
138. Kojima S, Sukuda M, Miyajima Y, Matsuyama T, Horibe K. Treatment of aplastic anemia in children with recombinant human granulocyte colony stimulating factor. Blood 1991;77:937.
139. Ganser A, Lindemann A, Seipelt G, et al. Effects of recombinant human interleukin-3 in aplastic anemia. Blood 1990;76:1287.
140. deWitte T, Zwaan F, Herman SJ, et al. Allogeneic bone marrow transplantation for secondary leukemia and myelodysplastic syndrome: a survey by the Leukemia Working Party of the European Bone Marrow Transplantation Group (EBMTG). Br J Haematol 1990;74:151.
141. Freedman MG. Pure red cell aplasia in childhood and adolescence: pathogenesis and approaches to diagnosis. Br J Haematol 1993;85:246.
142. Nathan D, Oski I. Bone marrow failure syndromes. In: Nathan D, Oski I, eds. Hematology of infancy and childhood. 4th ed. Philadelphia: WB Saunders, 1993:270.

CHAPTER 11

Polycythemias

LEIF G. SUHRLAND

Of the diseases of the vein, and of the blood contained therein, there is a twofold cure: purging and blood-letting; but blood-letting is more necessary of the two in a plethora, either ad vala or ad vires; or in a plethoric Cacochymia, or in a very great and putrid Cacochymia, that a portion of the extremely corrupted blood may be taken away.
—Riolanus, *Physic and Chyrurgery* (1657)

What you thought you knew, you shall not know
And what you once thought best, you shall forego
—William Harvey, *De Motu Cordis* (1628)

Introduction

The polycythemias include a heterogenous group of conditions linked mainly by the laboratory finding of an elevated hemoglobin and hematocrit. In spite of the diversity of conditions giving rise to an elevated hemoglobin and hematocrit, it is possible to classify these laboratory findings into three main categories. When an elevated hemoglobin/hematocrit is associated with an increase in total red cell volume (TRCV), individuals have either (a) primary polycythemia, i.e., polycythemia vera or (b) secondary polycythemia. When there is no increase in TRCV, the term "relative," or "spurious polycythemia" is applied (table 11.1). Although this does not represent a true polycythemia, the clinical significance of relative polycythemia may be important and therefore will be included in the discussion of polycythemia.

Polycythemia vera was described by Osler in 1903 in the paper *Chronic cyanosis with polycythemia and enlarged spleen: a new clinical entity* (1). He included the case described by Vaquez (2), in addition to 8 other patients. Osler was unable to offer an explanation for the elevated red cell count, but stated that the "clinical picture was distinctive, the symptoms indefinite and the pathology obscure." Since then much has been learned about this clinical entity, yet many aspects of the pathogenesis still remain obscure. Accordingly, a case report has been selected to demonstrate the natural history of a disease modified by treatment, some of which is controversial.

The importance of well-controlled, randomized clinical trials through cooperative arrangements among several institutions will be emphasized. New information on the control of hematopoietic cell proliferation and differentiation in polycythemia will be presented where applicable or the reader may be referred to the appropriate sections in this book.

Case 1

F.C., a 63-year-old retired auto worker, was referred by a cardiologist who had followed the patient for 2 years for mild congestive heart failure and an elevated hemoglobin and hematocrit. Secondary causes for the polycythemia had been excluded and the patient was treated with periodic phlebotomies. However, the number of phlebotomies had increased over the past 12 months and a reevaluation was requested for possible treatment with ³²P. According to the patient, he could tell when his blood counts were high by the feeling of a "band around my head," dizzy spells, and worsening of his generalized pruritus. Past history revealed several operations over a 10-year period, beginning with a hiatus hernia repair in 1956, followed by a diagnostic thoracotomy for removal of a small granuloma from the left lung, and three later attempts to repair an inguinal hernia, the last in 1966. There were no postoperative complications. Physically, the patient was a well-developed, well-nourished white male with a ruddy complexion and the following vital signs: weight 156 pounds, height 5'8", blood pressure 122/64, T36⁸, P 82, R 18. Pertinent findings showed no evidence of clubbing and lungs that were clear to percussion and auscultation. The heart was not enlarged on percussion, and the rhythm was regular without murmurs. On abdominal examination the only abnormal finding was a spleen felt 1–2 cm below the left costal margin. The remainder of the physical examination was not remarkable.

Laboratory findings were as follows: red blood cell (RBC) count 8.0×10^{12}/L; hemoglobin 178 g/L; hematocrit 56%; white blood cell (WBC) count 10.2×10^9/L; platelets 833×10^9/L; differential normal.

Urinalysis and blood chemistry screen showed no abnormalities.

Table 11.1. Classification of Polycythemia

Primary polycythemia: polycythemia vera
Secondary polycythemia
    Secondary to tissue hypoxia with appropriate Epo secretion,
       lung disease, heart disease, or congenital heart disease,
       high altitudes, obesity
    Secondary to inappropriate Epo secretion, renal carcinoma,
       renal cysts, hydronephrosis, other tumors such as
       cerebellar hemangioblastoma, hepatomas, uterine
       fibroids
Familial polycythemia
Relative or spurious polycythemia

Discussion: *This patient with a previous history of elevated hemoglobin and hematocrit had been poorly controlled on phlebotomies in spite of an increasing frequency for this procedure. His symptoms included headache, a sense of fullness in the head, and dizziness. He was noted to have ruddy cyanosis, injected sclerae, an enlarged spleen, a normal-appearing heart and lung examination, with a high hemoglobin, hematocrit, red blood cell, and platelet count. These findings were compatible with the referral diagnosis of polycythemia vera, but the diagnosis needed to be more firmly established. Elevated hemoglobin, hematocrit, and RBC are not in themselves synonymous with an increased total red cell volume (TRCV), which is the sine qua non for the diagnosis of polycythemia. By definition, an increased TRCV is ≥ 36 ml/kg for males and ≥ 32 ml/kg for females. The ^{51}Cr-labeled red cell technique is a reliable, reproducible method for measuring TRCV (3) and was included in the laboratory workup.*

During the next 7 days the following tests and results were obtained:

Serum iron	*30 µg%*
Iron-binding capacity	*400 µg%*
Saturation	*8%*
Leukocyte alkaline phosphatase	*150 (normal 74–126)*
Chest x-ray	*Few calcified granulomatous lesions right upper lobe, postoperative changes left lower rib cage, normal heart size*
Intravenous pyelogram	*No evidence of tumors or cysts, normal calyceal system*
Bone marrow and biopsy	*60% Cellularity with a preponderance of myeloid elements, no stainable iron present*
Arterial oxygen saturation (SaO$_2$)	*90%*
Total blood volume	*86 ml/kg*
Red cell mass, TRCV	*44 ml/kg*
Liver/spleen scan	*Normal liver size with uniform uptake of radioactivity. Spleen is enlarged $3 \times$ without filling defects*

A diagnosis of polycythemia vera was confirmed by a TRCV of 44 ml/kg, an SaO$_2$ of 90%, a palpable spleen also enlarged by an isotope scan, an elevated leukocyte alkaline phosphatase, and a hypercellular bone marrow without stainable iron. These findings were consistent with the diagnostic criteria developed by the Polycythemia Vera Study Group (PVSG) for entry of patients into their study programs (table 11.2) (4, 5). The borderline SaO$_2$ of 90% most likely can be explained by previous thoracic surgery.

Based upon these data, the patient was scheduled for twice-weekly phlebotomies until the hematocrit was in the 45–47% range, at which time he was given 5.0 µCu of ^{32}P intravenously. The phlebotomies were performed to relieve the symptoms related to increased blood viscosity secondary to an elevated hematocrit and to reduce the risk of a thrombotic event.

Studies by Wells and Merrill (6) have shown that above a hematocrit of 50% the blood viscosity rises quite sharply. These observations have been verified many times with viscosity measured in a glass capillary tube viscosimeter (fig. 11.1). However, this may not reflect flow in the microvasculature of man (7). Blood viscosity is dependent not only upon hematocrit but upon shear rate as well, which for cylindrical vessels is a function of vessel radius and velocity flow. Within the vascular system of man, at any instant of flow there are an infinite variety of shear rates possible. In translating these observations to treatment, the hematocrit should be kept below 50% to relieve symptoms and decrease the risk of a thrombotic event (8). Yet, in the PVSG-01 study, a retrospective analysis of risk factors for thrombosis, neither elevations of the hematocrit or platelet count were associated with increased risk (9). The numbers of patients with hematocrits >52% were quite small in the analysis. In patients with a high phlebotomy requirement, a history of previous thrombosis and age appeared to be major risk factors for thrombotic events. In this same report the percentage of

Table 11.2. Diagnostic Criteria for Polycythemia Vera[°]

Category A	Category B
TRCF ♂ ≥ 36 ml/kg ♀ ≥ 32 ml/kg	Platelets >400,000 mm^3
Arterial O$_2$ saturation $\geq 92\%$	WBX >12,000 mm^3
Splenomegaly	LAP >100
	Serum B$_{12}$ >900 pg/ml
	UB$_{12}$ BC >2200 pg/ml

[°]Established by the Polycythemia Vera Study Group.
Diagnosis established if A1 + A2 + A3 or A1 + A2 + 2 from Category B

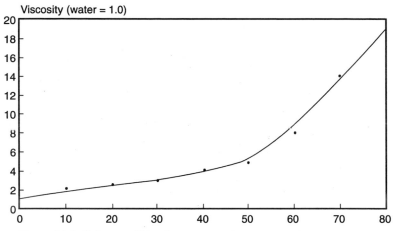

Figure 11.1. Relation of blood viscosity to hematocrit relative to water.

deaths due to thrombosis was 41% in patients treated by phlebotomy alone versus 26% in patients treated by phlebotomy plus chlorambucil, and 29% in patients treated by ^{32}P plus phlebotomy. These data demonstrate that some form of myelosuppression significantly reduces mortality from thrombosis. Prevention of thrombosis is of paramount importance since 26% of initial thrombotic events were fatal. In addition to the risk of thrombosis in polycythemia vera, hemorrhagic complications also occur. No consistent coagulation defects have been detected, but in uncontrolled polycythemia vera engorgement and distension of blood vessels renders hemostasis more difficult. A relative lack of fibrinogen secondary to a decrease in plasma volume may contribute to bleeding, especially when hemostasis is challenged with surgery. Major and fatal bleeding may occur if surgery is performed in uncontrolled polycythemia (10). When the hematocrit is <50% hemorrhagic episodes do not appear to be a major problem.

Over the next 4 years F.C. required 2 additional treatments with ^{32}P, supplemented with an occasional phlebotomy to maintain his hematocrit between 45–50%. Four years later he underwent a cholecystectomy for chronic cholecystitis and cholelithiasis without postoperative complications, and until 1978 he required only an average of two to four phlebotomies per year. At this time, due to poor control manifested by an increasing need for phlebotomy coupled with platelet counts of 600,000–800,000 mm[3], the patient was started on chlorambucil. After 4 months of intermittent chlorambucil therapy, the hematocrit and platelet count stabilized in the normal range. No supplementary phlebotomies were necessary and no further chlorambucil was required over an 18-month period. Generalized pruritus that had been an intermittent complaint for 10 years no longer was present. The spleen continued to be palpable 2–3 cm below the left costal margin (LCM).

In January 1980, F.C. felt well with no specific complaints; however, his hemoglobin was 117 g/L, hematocrit was 35%, and the platelet count had fallen to 80 × 10[9]/L.

Did the development of a mild anemia and thrombocytopenia herald a more ominous transition to postpolycythemic myeloid metaplasia (PPMM) (11)? A subsequent bone marrow biopsy demonstrated myelofibrosis with islands of hematopoietic cells, decreased megakaryocytes, and no stainable iron. This confirmed the diagnosis of PPMM. By March 1980, the patient's spleen had enlarged to 6–8 cm below the LCM, with laboratory findings as follows: hematocrit 29%; hemoglobin 90 g/L; WBC 8.2 × 10[9]/L; platelets 66 × 10[9]/L; peripheral blood film; no blasts or immature cells; frequent giant platelets; moderate anisocytosis; poikilocytosis; and rare nucleated RBCs (NRBCs).

Since these findings indicated a more progressive disease, the patient was given a trial of androgen therapy. When this failed, a course of corticosteroids was tried without benefit. Rapid, painful enlargement of the spleen occurred, necessitating the patient's hospital admission in May 1980. On examination, F.C. had massive splenomegaly extending into the pelvis, an enlarged liver, ascites, and pitting edema of the lower extremities with numerous scattered petechiae. His hemoglobin was now 83 g/L and his platelets had fallen to 15 × 10[9/L]. A bone marrow biopsy again revealed myelofibrosis, scattered areas of hematopoiesis with increased megakaryocytes in various stages of maturation, but no excess blasts. Deterioration of the patient with massive splenomegaly, portal hypertension, and severe thrombocytopenia without evidence of leukemic transformation made splenectomy a strong option. Review of the literature at this time revealed very limited data on the benefits of splenectomy for progressive PPMM. In view of the critical clinical condition of the patient, splenectomy was performed with appropriate red cell and platelet support. Postoperatively a gradual rise in platelets occurred and the patient was discharged from the hospital 8 days later with a hemoglobin of 105 g/L and platelet count of 85 × 10[9]/L. Pathologic finding demonstrated a 2660-g spleen with a red pulp that was diffusely infiltrated by myeloid and erythroid precursors with little evidence of maturation. The white pulp was mostly obliterated. A paraortic lymph node also showed myeloid metaplasia. A liver biopsy demonstrated a mixture of erythroid and myeloid elements in dilated hepatic sinusoids. Megakaryocytes were rare. A remarkable hematologic remission took place, and by October 1980, the patient was feeling quite well. On abdominal examination, the liver was only slightly enlarged and there was no evidence of ascites. Laboratory findings showed a hemoglobin of 132 g/L, WBC 22 × 10⁹/L uncorrected for nucleated RBCs, and a platelet count of 216 × 10⁹/L. However, over the next 18 months the patient's condition gradually deteriorated. His final admission in May 1982 was for a bilateral pulmonary infiltrate with no specific etiology established. Blood counts were as follows: hemoglobin 83 g/L; WBC 80 × 10⁹/L; 400 NRBCs/100 WBC; blast cells 15% with bizarre RBCs and giant platelets with megakaryocytic fragments.

He spiked daily fevers of 103–104°F and died on the 10th hospital day. His treatment consisted of blood transfusions, antibiotics, and oxygen. A bone marrow examination shortly after admission demonstrated marked dysplasia with myelofibrosis but no frank leukemia. Cytogenetic studies, which had been normal 10 months previously, were now abnormal with an interstitial deletion in the short arm of 7 chromosome, most likely related to a changing myeloproliferative process.

The final hematologic diagnosis was a PPMM in transition to an acute leukemia. His disease process evolved over more than 14 years from initial diagnosis to death, and was remarkable for the hematologic remission that followed a splenectomy for life-threatening thrombocytopenia. The course of his disease illustrates three phases that are found in many patients with polycythemia vera, representing the natural history modified by phlebotomy and myelosuppressive therapy.

Clinical Summation:

Phase 1 **Initial or proliferative phase**
Characterized by expansion of one or all of the hematopoietic elements, most frequently the erythroid compartment. In this phase, there is a need for phlebotomy as well as some myelosuppressive therapy. The usual duration is 2–8 years.

Phase 2 **Stable phase**
Little need for either phlebotomy or myelosuppression. The usual duration is 2–6 years.

Phase 3 **Anemic, terminal or final phase**
Characterized by myelofibrosis myeloid metaplasia (PPMM), transition to acute leukemia, evolution to a myelodysplastic syndrome, or all three conditions ending in acute leukemia. Duration 30 days to 4 years.

Polycythemia Vera

Pathophysiology

In the past, polycythemia vera has been described as a benign, chronic disease. It now is regarded as a hematologic malignancy of a clonal disorder of the pleuripotent hematopoietic stem cell, occurring predominantly in the older age group, with average age of diagnosis being 60 years. Although primary therapeutic efforts have focused on the expanded erythroid compartment, other cellular elements of the blood are involved, constituting a panmyelopathy. The myeloid and platelet components are increased and varying degrees of fibrosis are present. During the course of polycythemia vera, three major complications are encountered: (a) thromboembolic events, (b) bleeding, and (c) transition to a more malignant disorder.

The clonal origin of polycythemia vera was first demonstrated by Adamson and colleagues, who studied two female patients with polycythemia vera (12). These patients were also heterozygous for the x-linked chromosome for the isoenzymes of glucose-6-phosphate dehydrogenase (G-6-PD). An assay for type A and type B isoenzymes showed that both isoenzymes were present in the skin and fibroblasts, but only type A was found in the myeloid and erythroid elements. In 50 nonleukemic individuals who were heterozygous for G6PD, whenever both type A and type B were found in the skin and fibroblasts, both isoenzymes were always present in the hematopoietic cells. The relationship of the single isoenzyme present in the hematopoietic cells of patients with polycythemia vera to the abnormal proliferative process is unknown. It does, however, provide evidence of the clonal nature of the disease (13).

The inclusion of polycythemia vera under the umbrella of the myeloproliferative syndromes has led to investigation of cytogenetics in this disease to determine whether diagnostic or prognostic abnormalities may exist. In the PVSG-01 study, a number of abnormalities, such as aneuploidy and deletions, were found. Twenty-six percent of patients studied showed some definite abnormality. Deletion of the long arm of chromosome 20 (20q−) was noted with some consistency and generally has not been seen in other hematologic abnormalities (14). In another study performed at the Mayo Clinic, early in the disease only 15% of patients had abnormal results, whereas in the PPMM stage 78% were abnormal, and in leukemia or myelodysplastic syndrome (MDS) 100% of patients showed abnormalities (15). Smolin et al. (16) noted that if abnormalities were found at diagnosis these patients were not more prone to develop acute leukemia, and that the 20q- change was more common in patients treated with myelosuppression. A number of abnormalities that have been observed, especially trisomy of the C group of chromosomes, appear to be more related to the stage of the disease than to previous therapy (17).

Since expansion of the erythroid compartment is the most striking and consistent finding in early polycythemia vera, the role of the hormone regulating red cell production, erythropoietin (Epo), has been studied by a number of investigators (18–22). Comments in this chapter will emphasize only the part Epo plays in erythroid proliferation in the polycythemias.

In polycythemia vera, the progenitor cells BFU-E and CFU-E are of clonal origin and are independent of Epo control. These cells appear to act autonomously to produce an elevated hemoglobin, hematocrit, and TRCV. The interstitial renal cells responsible for secreting Epo are exposed to maximal tissue oxygen, which inhibits almost all Epo production. Measurement of plasma or urine Epo levels consistently shows a low or absent level. When normal or elevated levels of Epo are obtained (>3–5 million units/ml), the diagnosis of polycythemia vera should be questioned. The granulocytic and megakaryocytic elements in polycythemia vera also appear to be independent of normal control mechanisms responsible for cell proliferation and differentiation. This would be consistent with a clonal disorder and a panmyelopathy. The increased fibroblastic activity in the marrow during the course of polycythemia may represent reactive fibrosis or may also be part of an abnormal proliferative process.

The treatment of polycythemia vera first demands an accurate diagnosis to exclude the varied causes of secondary polycythemia. A careful history, physical examination, and the appropriate laboratory studies as outlined in table 11.2 are essential. The algorithm shown in figure 11.2 may be helpful in arriving at the correct diagnosis.

The options for initial treatment of the active proliferative phase are removal or reduction of the expanded red cell volume, some form of myelosuppression, or, more frequently, a combination of the two. Phlebotomy, or blood letting, has been used as a general therapeutic procedure for many centuries, and it was not until the early nineteenth century that it began to fall into disrepute (23). With few exceptions, the polycythemias are now perhaps the only conditions for which phlebotomy remains a clear therapeutic option. Once the diagnosis has been firmly established, phlebotomy should be performed one to two times per week until the hematocrit is in the low normal range (40–45%), then followed by a period of observation. The hematocrit range of 40–45% is lower then previously recommended. Presumably the lower maintenance hematocrit may decrease further the risk of thrombotic events. If more than 6 to 8 phlebotomies per year are required to keep the hematocrit in the low normal range, then a myelosuppressive agent should be considered (24).

During this period, complications of the initial phase such as gout, peptic ulcer, or gastrointestinal (GI) bleeding should be treated as necessary. The symptoms of generalized pruritus, possibly related to the release of histamine from granulocytes, can be relieved partially by antihistamines. Gouty arthritis and uric acid nephropathy can be prevented by the prophylactic use of allopurinol.

If some form of myelosuppression becomes necessary, preliminary data from the PVSG suggests that hydroxyurea will produce adequate control with minimal risk of acute leukemia developing (25). Treatment by phlebotomy alone resulted in a higher number of thrombotic episodes and early death, according to data from the PVSG (26). To avoid these untoward events, the same group investigated the effect of antiaggregating platelet therapy in polycythemia vera (27). The two-arm study compared phlebotomy plus daily aspirin and dipyridamole versus ^{32}P and phlebotomy as needed. After a median time of study of only 1.2 years, the aspirin-dipyridamole group had an overall failure rate due to thrombosis, hemorrhage, and death seven times greater than the ^{32}P group. The study was terminated at this time.

Prior to the PVSG programs, there were no data available from prospective, randomized, well-controlled, clinical trials. Evaluation of the effectiveness of various treatment programs was difficult, and the natural history of polycythemia vera was not well understood. In two separate reports (28, 29), the incidence of post-polycythemic myeloid metaplasia, PPMM, and acute leukemia (AL) were recorded, as well as the subsequent development of AL following PPMM (table 11.3). There was a significant risk for AL when preceded by PPMM. Furthermore, patients who have received myelosuppressive therapy and in whom PPMM develops are at even greater risk of AL's developing than patients treated by phlebotomy alone. Smolin et al. reported similar results in 57 patients who were also included in the PVSG study (29). The transition from PPMM to AL may be as short as 6 months or as long as 3–4 years. When PPMM becomes symptomatic secondary to an enlarged spleen, with pain, anemia, and thrombocytopenia, treatment is usually ineffective. Although splenectomy may be considered, it is hazardous and improvement is short-lived (30).

Table 11.4 summarizes data from four reports published between 1950 and 1986 (31–34). Only the European Organization for Research on Treatment of Cancer (EORTC) and PVSG studies were prospective randomized clinical trials, making comparisons to earlier retrospective observations difficult. When no ^{32}P is used, the incidence of acute leukemia is 1–2%. Survival times of the two later studies appear similar except for the group treated with chlorambucil. This drug was removed as a treatment option in 1981 (35). The incidence of AL in groups treated with ^{32}P was greater in the PVSG study and the EORTC. In the latter study the mean followup time was 8 years, which would account for the 5-fold disparity in findings.

Treatment options include a combination of some form of myelosuppression, with phlebotomy as necessary to maintain the hematocrit in 40–45% range. Because of the pressured increased frequency of acute leukemia, ^{32}P should be reserved for the older age group, >65 years. Busulfan or hydroxyurea are effective myelosuppressive agents and may prove to be less leukemogenic. When acute leukemia develops in the course of polycythemia, whether de novo or secondary to myelosuppression, treatment is rarely successful (36).

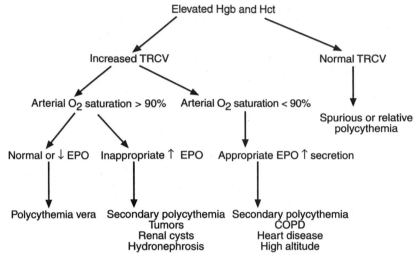

Figure 11.2. Algorithim for studying and elevated hemoglobin and hematocrit.

Table 11.3.

Therapy	No. of Patients	No. (%) of Patients with PPMM	No. (%) of Patients with PPMM + AL	Total No. (%) of Patients with AL
Phlebotomy°	134	16 (1.2)	1 (0.7)	2 (1.5)
³²p°	156	12 (7.7)	3 (1.9)	16 (10.3)
Chlorambucil°	141	11 (7.8)	5 (3.5)	19 (13.5)
³²p and/or x-ray†	181	45 (24)	16 (9.0)	26 (14.0)

°*Sources:* From PVSG-01 (29).
†From Lawrence (28).
Key: AL; acute leukemia; PPMM, postpolycythemic myeloid metaplasia.

Table 11.4.

Author or Group	Year of Report	No. of Patients	Treatment	No. (%) of Patient Deaths	No. (%) of Patients with AL	Median Survival (yr)
Videbaek (31)	1950	125	No ³²P°	76 (61)	2 (1.5)	M 4.5 F 8.5
Modan and Wienfeld	1965	512	³²P/x-ray	NA	51 (10)	NA
EORTC (33)	1981	140	³²P	47 (35)	2 (1.4)	>10
		145	Busulfan	28 (19)	3 (2.0)	>10
PVSG (34)	1986	134	Phlebotomy	43 (32)	2 (1.5)	13.9
		156	³²P	69 (44)	16 (10.3)	11.8
		141	Chlorambucil	71 (50)	19 (13.5)	8.9

°Included a small number treated with x-ray or nitrogen mustard.
EORTC, European Organization for Research on Treatment of Cancer; PVSG, Polycythemia Vera Study Group. NA, not applicable.

Secondary Polycythemia

Polycythemia has been defined as a condition when an elevated hemoglobin and hematocrit are accompanied by an increase in total red cell volume (TRCV). Measurement with ⁵¹Cr is accurate and reproducible. The classification is straightforward and most cases of secondary polycythemia are the result of tissue hypoxia. Cardiac and pulmonary diseases are the most common causes of low SaO_2, leading to increased production of Epo, which, in turn, stimulates erythropoiesis. Diagnosis usually can be made by careful history and physical examination, together with routine laboratory tests. Occasional conditions require more sophisticated techniques such as an Epo plasma or urine level. When increased Epo levels are found as a result of tissue hypoxia it is considered appropriate. If normal tissue oxygenation is present with increased Epo levels, then the secretion of Epo is *inappropriate*. An example of *appropriate* Epo secretion may be found in very obese individuals with low SaO_2 secondary to alveolar hypoventilation.

This so-called **Pickwickian Syndrome** improves with weight loss.

Most patients with polycythemia as a result of tissue hypoxia with an abnormally low SaO_2 demonstrate the "blue cyanosis" versus the "ruddy cyanosis" of polycythemia vera. In addition, there may be other clinical signs of impaired tissue hypoxia such as clubbing, spoon-shaped fingernails, increased anteroposterior diameter of the thorax, and heart murmurs. In patients with chronic obstructive pulmonary disease (COPD), hematocrits of >55–56% are generally not exceeded. Frequent bronchopulmonary infections may *inhibit* hematopoiesis, preventing erythrocytosis from developing. If symptoms of hyperviscosity are present, phlebotomy should be undertaken more slowly than in polycythemia vera.

The polycythemia found in individuals living at high altitudes can be diagnosed from history alone. As a result of decreased barometric pressure there is a reduction of partial pressure of arterial oxygen (p_aO_2) (arterial pO_2). When p_aO_2 falls below 65 mm Hg, the SaO_2 is also reduced and tissue hypoxia results. Stimulation of Epo secretion occurs, with a subsequent increase in TRCV. Such a chain of events has been observed at altitudes of >1550 m, in addition to a p_aO_2 <65 mm Hg (37). When individuals living at high altitudes with increased hemoglobin and hematocrit are brought to sea level, the elevated counts return toward normal over a period of time.

Reduced SaO_2 is found in moderate-to-heavy smokers. A study of carboxyhemoglobin levels in blood donors found 10–15 × normal levels in individuals who smoked an average of 1½ packs per day (38). Carboxyhemoglobin directly decreases SaO_2 by an amount equal to the carboxyhemoglobin present. In addition, carbon monoxide increases the affinity of hemoglobin for oxygen, making it less available to tissues (39). The elevations of hemoglobin and hematocrit are modest and *clinically* less significant than the direct effect of smoking on the pulmonary and cardiovascular systems.

Inappropriate production of Epo as a cause of an elevated total red cell volume is found in a variety of tumors both benign and malignant. The kidney is the most common site for tumors associated with an increased Epo urine or plasma level. Renal cell carcinoma, renal cysts, and hydronephrosis occasionally have been found in conjunction with increased production of Epo. In addition to the kidney, other tumor sites have been associated with elevated hemoglobin and hematocrit, as well as an increased TRCV and inappropriate Epo levels. These tumors include cerebellar hemangioblastoma, hepatoma, uterine fibroids, and tumors of the ovary, adrenals, thymus, and lung (40). Removal of the tumor usually results in a reduction in hemoglobin and hematocrit. Furthermore, tumor extracts have been found with Epo-like activity in addition to elevated Epo levels in urine or plasma. Other tumors of the ovary and adrenal may increase the TRCV secondary to androgen or cortisone secretion. Ingestion or injection of corticosteroids or androgens can also increase the TRCV.

Some athletes have sought to enhance their performance by these means.

Familial Polycythemia

The finding of polycythemia in multiple family members is rare, but has been reported sporadically. The erythrocytosis was mild to moderate, nonprogressive, and not associated with cyanosis. The obscure nature of this family syndrome was linked to an abnormal hemoglobin more than 25 years ago (41). Hemoglobin Chesapeake, an abnormally functioning hemoglobin found in three generations of family members, was associated with a mild but definite erythrocytosis. Since then a number of hemoglobin mutants, such as hemoglobin M, have been described in conjunction with an elevated hemoglobin and hematocrit (42). The amino acid substitution in these hemoglobin mutants results in an increased oxygen affinity of the molecule. The oxygen-hemoglobin dissociation curve is shifted to the left, making oxygen less available to the tissues. Epo secretion may then be stimulated leading to erythrocytosis. For the most part this type of erythrocytosis is well tolerated, but if symptoms of hyperviscosity are present, phlebotomy is the treatment of choice.

Spurious or Relative Polycythemia

Spurious or relative polycythemia, as the name implies, is not a true polycythemia, but a laboratory finding represented by an elevated hemoglobin and hematocrit without an increase in TRCV (42). It is not a primary diagnosis and there is no evidence of abnormal erythroid proliferation. In addition, the white blood cell (WBC) and platelet counts are usually not elevated. The bone marrow is not hyperplastic and there is no increase in reticulin. Transition to one of the myeloproliferative disorders is not part of the natural history of this laboratory finding. A reaction to stress has been implicated in the pathogenesis and has been termed *stress polycythemia*. There has been no consistent relationship between an elevated hematocrit and anxiety. On the other hand, a decreased or low normal plasma volume associated with such conditions as hypertension, smoking, obesity, or dehydration should be recognized and treated appropriately. The hematocrit and hemoglobin are found frequently to be within the extreme upper limits of normal. Treatment by phlebotomy or myelosuppression to lower the hemoglobin and hematocrit are to be avoided.

Summary

The polycythemias are a diverse group of conditions characterized by the laboratory findings of an elevated hemoglobin and hematocrit, and an algorithm has been presented to differentiate primary from secondary polycythemia. Polycythemia vera is a clonal panmyelopathy characterized by increased proliferation of erythroid, myeloid, and megakaryocytic elements. Early in the disease, an increase in the red cell compartment reflected by an elevated hemoglobin and hematocrit may be the initial presentation. Other causes of erythrocytosis must be considered. The Polycythemia Vera Study Group has established criteria for the diagnosis of polycythemia vera with an extremely low false-positive rate. Optimal treatment regimens have not been defined as yet, but include a combination of phlebotomy and myelosuppression. In spite of the many years that have elapsed since the disease was first described, the natural history is still unfolding (43, 44). The chronic course of polycythemia vera may be as long as two to three decades (45). Are the sequelae of postpolycythemic myeloid metaplasia, acute leukemia, and other nonhematologic malignancies avoidable? Preliminary observations by Silver (46) have shown control of the hematocrit in polycythemia vera by α-interferon for several months. α-Interferon also inhibits the action of platelet-derived growth factor (PDGF) which, in turn, suppresses fibroblastic activity. Some control of myelofibrosis may be possible through this mechanism. The answers to these questions, as well as determination of optimal therapy, will await data from prospective randomized clinical trials. With a chronic disease such as polycythemia vera, the investigators must be prepared to continue data collection throughout the life of enrolled patients that may span two to three decades.

Secondary polycythemia is usually distinguished from the polycythemia vera by a careful history and physical examination. Readily available laboratory and clinical tests separate those few patients in whom the diagnosis remains in question.

The term "relative" polycythemia should be replaced by the term "spurious," and is a nondiagnosis. An elevated hemoglobin and hematocrit is not synonymous with polycythemia, but should be investigated. Associated conditions, such as hypertension or dehydration, require treatment. Phlebotomy or the use of myelosuppressive agents should be avoided. Both primary and secondary polythermias require the presence of an elevated TRCV. Criteria have been established for the diagnosis of primary polycythemia with an extremely low false-positive rate. An optimal treatment regimen for primary polycythemia has not been defined as yet, but includes a combination of phlebotomy and myelosuppression. The natural history of primary polycythemia modified by treatment may extend over a period of two to three decades. If postpolycythemia myeloid metaplasia and its sequels can be avoided by timely intervention with certain cytokines, the ultimate course of primary polycythemia may be altered dramatically (46). Answers to these questions, as well as determination of optimal therapy, will need data from prospective randomized clinical trials collected over many years.

REFERENCES

1. Osler W. Chronic cyanosis and enlarged spleen: a new clinical entity. Am J Med Sci 1903;126:187–201.

2. Vaquez H. Sur une forme speciale de Cyanose s'accompanant d'hyperglobulie excessive et persistente. Compt Rend Soc Biol 1892;44:384–388.

3. Nathan DG. Comments on the interpretation of measurements of total red cell volume in the diagnosis of polycythemia vera. Semin Hematol 1966;3:216–219.

4. Berlin NI. Differential diagnosis of the polycythemias. Semin Hematol 1966;3:209–213.

5. Berlin NI. Diagnosis and classification of the polycythemias. Semin Hematol 1975;12:339–351.

6. Wells RE, Merrill EW. Influence of flow properties upon viscosity—hematocrit relationships. J Clin Invest 1962;41:1591–1598.

7. Castle WB, Jandl JH. Blood viscosity and blood volume: Opposing influences upon oxygen transport in polycythemia. Semin Hematol 1966;3:193–198.

8. Wasserman LR, Gilbert H. Complications of polycythemia vera. Semin Hematol 1966;3:199–208.

9. Wasserman LR, Balcerzak SP, Berk PD, Berlin NI, et al. Influence of therapy on cause of death in polycythemia vera. Trans Assoc Am Physicians 1981;94:30–38.

10. Wasserman LR, Gilbert HS. Surgical bleeding in polycythemia vera. Ann NY Acad Sci 1964;115:122–127.

11. Silverstein M. Postpolycythemia myeloid metaplasia. Arch Intern Med 1974;134:113–116.

12. Adamson JW, Fialkow PJ, Murphy S, Prchal JF, Steinmann L. Polycythemia vera: stem cell and probable clonal origin of the disease. N Engl J Med 1976;295:913–916.

13. Landaw SA. Polycythemia vera and other polycythemia states. Clin Lab Med 1990;10:857–871.

14. Wurster-Hill D, Whang-Peng J, McIntyre O, Hsu L, et al. Cytogenetic studies in polycythemia vera. Semin Hematol 1976;13:13–32.

15. Dietz-Martin JL, Graham DL, Pettit R, Dewald GW. Chromosome studies in 104 patients with polycythemia vera. Mayo Clin Proc 1991;66:287–299.

16. Smolin B, Weinfeld A, Westin J. A prospective long-term cytogenetic study in polycythemia vera in relation to treatment and clinical course. Blood 1988;72:386–395.

17. Testa J, Kanofsky JR, Rowley JD, Baron JM, Vardimen JW. Karyotypic patterns and their clinical significant in polycythemia vera. Am J Hematol 1981;11:29–45.

18. Zanjani E. Hematopoietic factors in polycythemia vera. Semin Hematol 1976;13:1–12.

19. Erslev AJ, Caro J, Kansu E, Miller O, Cobbs E. Plasma erythropoietin in polycythemia. Am J Med 1979;66:243–247.

20. Napier JA, Janowska-Wielzorek A. Erythropoietin measurements in the differential diagnosis of polycythemia vera. Br J Haematol 1981;48:393–401.

21. Erslev AJ, Caro J. Erythropoietin: from mountain top to bedside. Adv Exp Med Biol 1989;271:1–7.

22. Dudley JM, Westwood N, Leonard S, Eridani S, Pearson TC. Primary polycythemia positive diagnosis using the differential response of primitive and mature erythroid progenitors to erythropoietin interleukin-3 and alpha-interferon. Br J Haemat 1990;75:188–194.

23. Kluger MJ. The history of bloodletting. Nat History 1978;87:78–93.

24. Wasserman LR. The treatment of polycythemia vera. Semin Hematol 1976;13:57–78.

25. Kaplan ME, Mack K, Goldberg JD, Donovan PB, Berk PD, Wasserman LR. Long-term management of polycythemia

vera with hydroxyurea: a progress report. Semin Hematol 1986;23:167–171.

26. Wasserman LR. Polycythemia Vera Study Group: a historical perspective. Semin Hematol 1986;23:183–187.

27. Tartaglia AP, Goldberg JD, Berk PD, Wasserman LR. Adverse effects of antiagglutinating platelet therapy in the treatment of polycythemia vera. Semin Hematol 1986;23:172–176.

28. Lawrence JH, Winchell HS, Donald WG. Leukemia in polycythemia vera: relationship to splenic myeloid metaplasia and therapeutic radiation dose. Ann Intern Med 1969;70:763–771.

29. Ellis JT, Powers P, Geller SA, Rappaport H. Studies of the bone marrow in polycythemia vera and the evolution of myelofibrosis and second hematologic malignancies. Semin Hematol 1986;23:144–155.

30. Brenner B, Nagler A, Tatarsky I, Hashmonai M. Splenectomy in Agnogenic myeloid metaplasia and post polycythemic myeloid metaplasia. Arch Intern Med 1988;148:2501–2505.

31. Videbaek A. Polycythemia vera: course and prognosis. Acta Med Scand 1950;138:179–197.

32. Modan B, Wienfeld AM. Polycythemia vera and leukemia—the role of radiation treatment. Medicine 1965;44:305–344.

33. Haanen C, Mathe G, Hayat M. Treatment of polycythemia vera by radiophosphorus or busulfan: a randomized trial. Br J Cancer 1981;44:75–80.

34. Berk PD, Goldberg JK, Donovan PB, Fruchtman SM, Berlin NI, Wasserman LR. Therapeutic recommendations in polycythemia vera based on polycythemia vera: Study Group Protocols. Semin Hematol 1986;23:132–143.

35. Berk PD, Goldberg JD, Silverstien MN, Weinfeld A, et al. Increased incidence of acute leukemia in polycythemia vera associated with chlorambucil therapy. N Engl J Med 1981;304:441–447.

36. Landlow SA. Acute leukemia in polycythemia vera. Semin Hematol 1976;13:33–48.

37. Dainiak N, Spielvogel H, Sorba S, Cerdkowicz. Erythropoietin and the polycythemia of high altitude dwellers. Adv Exper Med Biol 1989;271:17 21.

38. Stewart RD, Baretta ED, Platte LR, et al. Carboxyhemoglobin levels in American blood donors. JAMA 1974;229:1187–1195.

39. Balcerzak SP, Bromberg PA. Secondary polycythemias. Semin Hematol 1975;12:353–382.

40. Hammond D, Winnick S. Paraneoplastic erythrocytosis and ectopic erythropoietin. Ann NY Acad Sci 1974;230:219–227.

41. Charache S. Weatherhall DJ, Clegg JB. Polycythemia and hemoglobinopathy. J Clin Invest 1966;45:813–822.

42. Adamson J. Familial polycythemia. Semin Hematol 1975;12:383–396.

43. Silverstein M. The evolution into and treatment of late stage polycythemia vera. Semin Hematol 1976;13:79–84.

44. Shamdos GJ, Speis CM, List AF. Myelodysplastic syndrome transformation of polycythemia vera: case report and review of the literature. Am J Hematol 1991;37:45–48.

45. Rosenthal N, Bassen F. Course of polycythemia. Arch Intern Med 1938;62:903–917.

46. Silver RT. Interferon in the treatment of myeloproliferative disease. Semin Hematol 1990;27:6–14.

EXERCISES AND TOOLS FOR RED CELL DISORDERS

The erythrocyte emerges from its gestation enucleated and programmed to carry out exquisite, albeit finite, processes before its 120-day sojourn comes to completion.

1. In normal erythropoiesis, 25% of the cells are in S phase, and nuclear and cytoplasmic protein syntheses are essentially synchronous. In megaloblastic states, as much as 50% of the cells may be in S phase, many of which, however, have ceased DNA synthesis (and thus the dysynchrony with cytoplasmic synthesis). These so-called U cells die because they are no longer involved in protein synthesis. Explain how this phenomenon may be an intracellular nutrient deficiency-induced death.

2. Develop a construct that identifies the molecular principles and time relationships involved in defective folate and cyanocobalamin metabolism. Include in this consideration of hematopoiesis the effects of defective folate and/or cobalamin metabolism on nonhematopoietic tissues. Include in the construct the enzymatic relationships between these agents and their respective roles in diet and digestion.

3. Develop a schema for megaloblastic transformation that incorporates environmental competition for foodstuffs or related material. In addition, explain the nature and underlying principles of megaloblastic maturation during the process of treating certain malignant disorders.

4. Review the roles of erythroid cell stimulating and inhibiting factors within the context of receptor biology and clinical expression. See Section I, Biological Control Mechanisms.

5. Review and develop a rationale for the sequential events of hemoglobin switching from intrauterine to postnatal life. Consider the time sequences of these events and examine the mechanism and significance of reverse-switching, i.e., from an alpha-beta chain complex to an alpha-gamma chain complex.

6. Construct a schema that encompasses the features of fetal hemoglobin as a hereditary state in codominant inheritance with sickle cell hemoglobin versus its presence with sickle hemoglobin as a separate gene-controlled chain complex. Consider similar constructs between a variety of alpha, beta, and gamma chain disorders.

7. Within the context of the material in Exercise 6, develop a series of globin chain relationships that address the inheritance of abnormally distributed amino acid hemoglobinopathies with those of impaired globin chain synthesis.

8. In Exercises 5, 6, and 7, develop a schema that includes the pattern of clinical responses that result from the underlying molecular defects.

9. Construct a paradigm that identifies the molecular bases of the various methemoglobinemias and their corresponding clinical manifestations.

10. Construct separate sickle cell disease and thalassemia paradigms that incorporate their distinct biological processes and determine if and how allogeneic and/or autologous bone marrow transplantation (stem cell infusion) can alter the clinical course of these disorders. See section on Tools for Transplantation.

11. Review the porphyrin pathway to heme synthesis and contrast it with the heme degradation pathway to bilirubin formation. Develop a schema that indicates the consequences of changes due to genetic or environmental influences.

12. Review the molecular biology of iron metabolism in order to construct an overview that addresses iron deficiency in the presence of iron abundance, iron lack states, mechanisms of iron transport, storage, utilization, and loss. Include in this schema factors that address abnormalities in any of these sequences.

13. Construct a schema that correlates the molecular biology of red cell skeletal deformability and stability with clinical abnormalities.

14. Develop a paradigm that encompasses knowledge of the supporting understructure of the red cell membrane, i.e., lipids and proteins (including in the latter glycophorins, spectrins, and ankrins) and their associated defects. Review appropriate chapter tables. The red cell antigens are discussed in the section on Tools for Transplantation.

15. Construct a schema that includes the consequences of defects in erythrocyte metabolism. Use as models deficiencies in glucose-6-phosphate dehydrogenase (G-6-PD) and pyruvate kinase (PK) and explain the striking clinical differences that result from deficiencies above and below the metabolism of trioses. Account for the clinical expression of G-6-PD polymorphism.

16. Based on a construct of the hexose monophosphate pathway, (a) develop a list of potential abnormalities other than those attributed to G-6-PD and PK and (b) theorize on their respective clinical severities.

17. Develop a schema that explains the nature of erythroid aplasia, hypoplasia, and dysplasia and relate it to the molecular bases of inherited and acquired defects. Outline a therapeutic plan based both on known and unknown etiologic events and include an assessment of transient self-limited events.

18. Distinguish between primary and secondary polycythemia and develop a construct that addresses oxygen tension, oxygen affinity, the role of 2-3 DGP (see hexose monophosphate metabolism), cardiovascular and renal diseases, erythropoietin (Epo) secreting tumors, autonomous Epo production, and the nature of secondary polycythemia. Note the reasons why these types of polycythemia have an associated red cell mass unlike the erythrocytosis secondary to hemoconcentration and develop a rationale to account for the clinical expressions of all of these events.

19. Provide a construct that explains (a) the nature of iron deposition in infection, (b) the role of foreign body invasion, alcohol consumption, endocrine dysfunction, aging, autoimmune disease and heat injury on marrow production and liver disease and (c) the effects of certain infectious agents on membrane integrity.

20. Develop a paradigm that explains the appearance and production status of the various inherited and acquired disorders. Use a schema based on hemoglobin content, cell size, and production activity.

SECTION II APPENDIX

Appendix 1. Morphology and Underlying Disorders

Normochromic, Normocytic with Reticulocytosis
  Hemolysis
  Hemorrhage
Normochromic, Normocytic with Reticulocytopenia
  Endocrine deficiency
  Endocrine excess
  Chronic renal disease
  Chronic liver disease
  Myelodysplasia
  Aplastic anemia
  Myelophthisic disorders
  Dyserythropoietic disorder
  Anemia of chronic disease
  Early iron deficiency
Macrocytic with Reticulocytosis
  Hemorrhage
  Hemolysis
  Marrow regeneration
Macrocytic with Reticulocytopenia
  Vitamin B_{12} deficiency
  Folate deficiency
  Drug effect
  Metabolic disease (orotic aciduria, etc.)
Hypochromic, Microcytic with Low Iron Levels
  Iron deficiency
Hypochromic, Microcytic with Normal-High Iron Levels
  Thalassemia
  Sideroblastic disorders

Appendix 2. Red Cell Disorders and Related Abnormalities

Disease	Appearance
Abetalipoproteinemia	Acanthocytes
Elliptocytosis	Elliptocytes
Phosphokinase/phosphoglycerate deficiencies	Echinocytes
Iron deficiency anemia	Hypochromia, Microcytes
Thalassemia	Hypochromia, Leptocytes, Anisocytes
Hb CC and EE diseases	Hypochromia, Targeting
Vitamin B_{12}/folic acid deficiency	Macrocytes, Ovalocytes
Hemoglobin SS disease	Sickled forms
Microangiopathies	Schistocytes
Uremia	
Hereditary/immune spherocytosis	Spherocytes
Stomatocytosis	Stomatocytes
Alcoholism	
Liver disease	
Myelofibrosis	Teardrop forms
Xerocytosis	Xerocytes

Appendix 3. Morphology of Hypochromic and/or Microcytic Anemias

Disorder	Microcytosis	Hypochromia	Anisocytosis	Basophilic Stippling	Target Formation
Severe iron deficiency	4	4	3	+/−	1
Anemia, chronic disease	1	0	1	0	1
Thalassemia major	4	4	4	3	3
HgB EE disease	3	0	2	2	3
HgB CC disease	2	0	2	2	3
Sideroblastic anemia	2	4	3	3	2
Refractory sideroblastic anemia	+/−	0	1	1	1

Absent, 0; mild 1–2; severe 3–4.

Appendix 4. Classification of Aplastic Anemias

Inherited
  Amegakaryocytic thrombopenia
  Dyskeratosis congenita
  Fanconi disease
  Reticular dysgenesis
  Splenic cysts
Acquired
  Chemical poisons: dose dependent and idiosyncratic
  Hypersplenism
  Idiopathic
  Immune-mediated (i.e., systemic lupus, etc.)
  Myesthenia (thymoma)
  Paroxysmal nocturnal hemoglobinuria
  Preleukemia
  Pregnancy
  Viral diseases
    Epstein-Barr
    Hepatitis A, B, ?C
    HIV
    Parvovirus
  Vitamin B_{12} or folate deficiency

Lymphocyte and Plasma Cell Disorders

CHAPTER 12

Nonmalignant Diseases of Lymphocytes: A Case-Study Approach

ARCHIE A. MACKINNEY JR., MD

The substance of the spleen is liable to all kinds of distemper, and to diverse swellings, especially that kind of hard swelling which is termed Scirrhus. Sometimes it is inflamed, and then the substance thereof is perceived to pant, by reaction of the Multitude of Arteries, of which it is full. It seldom impostumates. Its coat does often times grow thick and become cartilaginous.

It often grows great by abundance of Humors, and grows small again, sometime of itself, and sometime by use of medicines. It is better that the Spleen be small, than great.
—Riolanus, Physic and Chyrurgery 1657

Introduction

Suppressor/cytotoxic cells are a family of related cells, of which large granular lymphocytes, atypical lymphocytes, and natural killer (NK) cells are subsets. Immunofluorescent cell sorters, cell function, and molecular analysis rather than morphology are used for most of the discrimination between cell types. A glossary of markers is located at the end of the chapter.

Current interest centers around two syndromes: the mononucleosis syndrome (named after infectious mononucleosis) and the large granular lymphocyte syndrome. These syndromes involve CD8 (T8) cytotoxic/suppressor lymphocytes and related natural killer cells behaving in opposite ways. The mononucleosis syndrome is usually acute, and the suppressor/cytotoxic cells behave in a predictable and salutary way. The large granular lymphocyte syndrome is a chronic illness and cellular immunity appears to be deranged.

Comparable lymphoproliferative disorders of the CD4 (T4) lymphocytes have not emerged except for acute infectious lymphocytosis of childhood. This is an epidemic disease (1) characterized by rash, fever, diarrhea, and abdominal pain. Large numbers of small normal lymphocytes are found. Leukocytosis as high as 86 × 10⁹/L (2, 3) with 80% CD4 cells (4) has been reported. An impressive outpouring of small lymphocyte also accompanies pertussis.

Case 1

A 26-year-old single man was admitted to the hospital for elective achalasia repair. He related an incidental 10-day history of fever to 39°C, chills, myalgia, malaise, sore throat, and nonproductive cough. He had been seen at another hospital on the previous day, when penicillin and gentamycin were given. He denied headache, stiff neck, or photophobia. He had no shortness of breath or hemoptysis; no nausea, vomiting, diarrhea, or abdominal pain; no dysuria; and no rash, arthralgia, or lymphadenopathy. He denied recent travel.

Eleven years before admission, the patient had been involved in a motor vehicle accident that resulted in splenectomy for trauma, multiple blood transfusions, and a left femoral fracture. He had non-A, non-B hepatitis 10 years before admission, presumably related to transfusion. Osteomyelitis of the left femur developed 4 years after the fracture and 7 years before admission; it was adequately treated with antibiotics. His achalasia was being treated with nifedipine and ranitidine. He had a history of alcohol and drug abuse. Sexual history included contact with a girlfriend, who was also reputed to be alcoholic.

The physical examination revealed a young white male in no distress, except for malaise and weakness. His temperature was 39°C, pulse was 86, respiration was 16, and blood pressure was 120/70. The examination was otherwise normal. He had no pharyngitis or lymphadenopathy. The liver span was 12 cm. The spleen had been removed. There were no signs of osteomyelitis in the left femur.

Laboratory: The white cell count was 12.2 × 10⁹/L with 56% segs, 1 band, 27 lymphocytes, and 12 monocytes. Bacterial cultures of blood and other body fluids were negative. Serologic studies for hepatitis A, hepatitis

B surface antigen, and hepatitis B core antigen were negative for pathogens but were positive for hepatitis Bs antibody.

Fevers to 40°C continued despite multiple antibiotics. On the fifth hospital day, the white cell count rose to 34 × 10⁹/L with a striking change in the differential: 19 segs, 24 bands, 26 lymphs, 28 atypical lymphs. The SGOT was 66, the LDH was 303, peaking at 616; and the Alk phosphatase was 103, peaking at 151. Antibiotics, nifedipine, and ranitidine were stopped.

It was evident at this point that the patient had mononucleosis syndrome because of the unexpected appearance of atypical lymphocytes. The mononucleosis syndrome is a nonspecific immunologic response to viruses, especially the Epstein-Barr virus (EBV), and drugs as well as unknown stimuli.

Drugs

Among the diverse etiologies of the mononucleosis syndrome, drugs are the easiest to recognize and eliminate. Wood and Frenkel (5) reported that paraminosalicylic acid, diphenylhydantoin, and sulfasalazine were associated with a mononucleosis syndrome. Other cases of diphenylhydantoin (6–9) and sulfasalazine (10) mononucleosis have been described, as well as cases attributed to halothane (11) and dapsone (12). *We stopped nifedipine and ranitidine early in the course, although these drugs have not been implicated as a cause of the mononucleosis syndrome. The course of the illness was not altered.*

Viruses

The mononucleosis syndrome is most often associated with EBV infection. Horwitz, Henle, and co-workers reported that 89% of their patients with mononucleosis syndrome were diagnosed as having EBV infectious mononucleosis and 7.5% as having CMV infection (13). An infectious mononucleosis-like blood picture has been seen in a minority of cases of CMV, HIV (14), measles, mumps, hepatitis, and toxoplasmosis (15). Because these viruses cause mononucleosis less frequently, they are often neglected in the differential diagnosis. On the other hand, although the mononucleosis syndrome is a regular feature of EBV infection in adults, atypical lymphocytosis may not be as sensitive in diagnosing EBV infection, as most studies have suggested. In a group of 124 serologically confirmed cases, 61% did not meet the criteria of lymphocytosis >50% and atypical lymphocytes >10% (16).

The Atypical Lymphocyte

Distinction from Malignancy

The characteristic feature of the mononucleosis syndrome is the atypical lymphocyte. Atypical lymphocytes were first distinguished morphologically from malignant lymphoblasts of acute lymphocyte leukemia by Downey and McKinlay in 1923 (17). They described five types of atypical lymphocytes. It is possible to make a meaningful identification of at least four atypical lymphocytes, although these do not exactly correspond to Downey and McKinlay's categories. The large granular lymphocyte is a cytotoxic T cell or NK cell. The plasmacytoid lymphocyte is an activated B cell. The "typical" atypical lymphocyte is an activated CD8+ lymphocytes. The blastic lymphocyte may be any activated cell about to enter cell division.

Resemblance to Malignancy

Although Downey and McKinlay distinguished infectious mononucleosis from lymphoma or leukemia, other data emphasized malignant features. Studies showed that atypical lymphocytes in infectious mononucleosis were 10 times more likely to be in DNA synthesis than normal peripheral blood cells, (18, 19) with proportions comparable to acute leukemia or chronic myelocytic leukemia. In 1967, atypical lymphocytes from peripheral blood were observed to enter mitosis promptly in vitro (20). Hence, one aspect of their atypical morphology was the imminence of cell division, a finding expected of malignant cells.

Other aspects of infectious mononucleosis suggested malignancy. The virus that causes Burkitt's lymphoma (EBV) (21), was found to cause infectious mononucleosis in 1968 (22). EBV-infected B cells proliferate indefinitely in vitro and are, in that sense, immortal—another condition of malignancy (23). The pathology of infectious mononucleosis was sometimes confused with lymphoma (24). Reed-Sternberg cells were found in some cases, making the diagnosis of Hodgkin's disease a consideration (25, 26). Some patients died of the disease (27).

The concern about malignancy was quite real in this case. ENT examination showed hypertrophy of Waldeyer's ring suspicious for lymphoma. We believed it was necessary to resist the impulse of consultants to biopsy lymphoid tissue because its interpretation would likely be equivocal and would complicate rather than simplify our diagnostic approach. The bone marrow aspirate and biopsy were unremarkable.

Mononucleosis Syndrome As a Self-Limited Malignancy

In 1975, it was suggested that infectious mononucleosis was a self-limited lymphoma (28), but the restraining factor was not clear. When a sex-linked fatal form of infectious mononucleosis was discovered (29), an immune response that protected the normal host was proposed.

Early studies of infectious mononucleosis suggested that both humoral and cellular immunity were involved. In 1968, it was reported that peripheral blood infectious mononucleosis cells in vitro could synthesize heterophil antibody (30), and in 1973, an increase in thymically oriented lymphocytes (T cells) was found in the peripheral blood in this disease (31). These data suggested that one or more immunological reactions was represented in the atypical lymphocytes.

The next step was to analyze the atypical lymphocytes to determine whether a monoclonal population was present. Flow cytometry was performed on the twelfth hospital day, when the white cell count reached 51 × 10⁹/L and atypical lymphocytes were estimated at 62% (32 × 10⁹/L). The flow cytometer recognized 37,000/μL "small agranular" cells and gave the following data:

CD2	(T11)	(Sheep red blood cell receptor)	91%; 34,000	{nl 800–2500}
CD3	(T3)	(T cell receptor)	71%; 16,000	{nl 360–2100}
CD4	(T4)	(Helper/inducer)	12%; 4,400	{nl 400–1200}
CD8	(T8)	(Suppressor/cytotoxic)	63%; 23,000	{nl 180–830}
CD56	(NKH-1)	(Natural killer)	2%; 4,400	{nl 50–450}
CD57	(HNK-1)	(Natural killer)	17%; 6,000	{nl 220–960}
HLA-DR	(Ia)	(Activation antigen)	81%; 30,000	
CD20	(B1)	(B cell marker)	8%; 3,000	{nl 40–400}
CD29	(4B4)	(Helper, killer subsets)	96%; 36,000	
CD45RA	(2H4)	(Suppressor/killer subset)	40%; 15,000	{nl CD44+ 2H4 480–560}

These data were interpreted to show a 100-fold increase in CD8+ suppressor/cytotoxic cells, a reversed CD4/CD8 ratio of 0.2 {nl 1–2.4}, six- to 10-fold increase in natural killers (CD56, CD57) and B lymphocytes (B1; CD20), and activation of T cells (HLA-DR; Ia antigens). Helper T cells (CD4) were also increased six- to 10-fold.

To better understand these markers, we must explore cell-mediated immunity as expressed by T lymphocytes and related natural killer cells.

T-Cell Classification

T Cell vs. B Cell

The nature of thymically oriented lymphocytes (T cells) has been the subject of intense study for the past 30 years, and their physiology has proved much more complex than other cells in the blood. In 1962, it was perceived that there were two limbs to the immune system: thymic or cell-mediated immunity and the nonthymic or humoral immunity (32). The nonthymic lymphocytes were called B cells, first because they were found to originate in the Bursa of Fabricius in the chicken and later for the bone marrow, in which mammalian immunoglobulin-synthesizing cells originate. The T cells (thymocytes) were named for the thymus, in which cellular immunity is organized.

Thymectomy and autoradiography of DNA synthesizing cells were important early tools for studying thymus function. In the mouse, thymocytes were observed to replace their numbers every 3 to 5 days, but less than 10% were exported (33), the rest dying within the thymus. This strange phenomenon of high growth rate and efficient self-destruction is now believed to be central to the mechanism for tolerance so that thymocytes that react against self antigens are eliminated in the thymus before they enter the circulation.

B and T lymphocytes were found in peripheral blood of the mouse in 1970 using antigenic markers (34) and in man by immune adherence to sheep erythrocytes (35). About 70% of peripheral blood lymphocytes had receptors for sheep erythrocytes and had other markers for T cells as well; about 20% had B cell markers. In 1974, Waldmann and co-workers found that some peripheral blood leukocytes could suppress immunoglobulin synthesis of B cells and the suppressor T cell function was identified (36). Subsequently, cytotoxic T lymphocytes were described (37).

T4 vs. T8

In 1980, Schlossman and coworkers (38) separated the thymically oriented cells into two classes, T4 (CD4) and T8 (CD8). "CD" stands for "cluster distribution" and refers to a generally accepted cell surface antigen. The earliest, small (3%) group of subcortical thymocyte progeny are CD4 and CD8– and acquire one or the other of these antigens as they mature. CD8+ lymphocytes have receptors for HLA-A, B, C (Class I) and respond to peptide antigen on other cells coupled with Class I major histocompatibility complex (MHC) antigens. CD4+ lymphocytes have receptors for HLA-DP, DO, and DR (Class II) and respond to antigens complexed to these MHC antigens. CD4 cells promote immunoglobulin synthesis by B lymphocytes and assist CD8 cells. CD8 cells inhibit B-cell function by their ability to inhibit DNA synthesis or immunoglobulin production by B cells and perform other functions, including the killing of foreign cells.

Subtypes of T4 and T8

By 1990 (39), Schlossman and co-workers further separated the CD4 cells into inducer/suppressor and inducer/helper subsets and CD8 cells into three cell types: killer/effector, suppressor/effector, and natural killer subsets. It can be seen in Table 12.1 that CD29, CD45RA, and

Table 12.1. A Classification of T Lymphocytes

Cell Type	CD4	CD8	CD11b	CD29	CD45RA	CD45RO
Suppressor/inducer	X	0		0	X	0
Helper/inducer	X	0		X	0	X
Killer/effector	0	X	0	X	0	
Suppressor/effector	0	X	0	0	X	
Natural killer	0	X	X	X	X	
Natural killer	0	0	0	0	0	

CD45RO reciprocally define two CD4 cell types and that CD11b, CD29, and CD45RA similarly define three kinds of CD8 cells.

The CD4 suppressor/inducer cells secrete interferon-γ and IL-2, are cytotoxic, and inhibit immunoglobulin secretion (40); they can induce CD8+ cells to become suppressor/effectors. The CD_4 helper/inducer cells secrete IL-4 and assist specific antibody synthesis. The CD8+ CD11b+ killer subset suppresses B-cell immunoglobulin production independent of CD4 cells, whereas the CD8+CD11b-suppressor/effector cell requires the cooperation of suppressor/inducer (CD4+CD45RA+) cells to suppress B cells. Class-restricted cytotoxicity is a property of the CD8+CD11b+ (natural killer) cells.

There is also CD8− natural killer (NK) cell. Its origin has been controversial because it lacks the common T-cell antigens CD3, CD4, and CD8 while retaining CD2 (T11). It has been called a "null" cell or "L" cell. Evidence of its T-cell origin was the discovery of a truncated β transcript of the T-cell receptor (41). However, its lineage appears independent of the thymus. It has been defined variously by its ability to attack target cells, usually the cell line K562, without MHC class restriction, the presence of large lysosomal granules, and the antigen CD56 (NKH-1) or CD57 (HNK-1) (42). *The NK cell is currently defined as CD3−CD16+CD56+.* Four subsets of CD3−CD16+ NK cells have recently been described (43). Both killer/effector and natural killer cells appear to be large granular lymphocytes and cannot be distinguished from each other morphologically. Moreover, some small lymphocytes without granules are also NK cells (44). (For more on NK cells, see below under Large Granular Lymphocyte Syndrome.)

The "typical" atypical lymphocyte is different from the large granular lymphocyte. It has a polygonal nucleus and generous watery cytoplasm, which darkens where it contacts erythrocytes. Granules usually are not seen. Its immunologic identity has not been established, but it is an activated cell that may include several subtypes, such as CD3+CD19− and CD8+Cd11b−. Cell sorting studies of one patient with infectious mononucleosis showed that CD8+CD11b− (suppressor/effector) cells were atypical lymphocytes. Eventually, an immunologically based lymphocyte differential is expected to emerge from the combination of cell marker and morphologic studies. Figures 12.1 and 12.2 depict the large granular lymphocytes and atypical lymphocytes, respectively.

We continued to search for a viral cause of the patient's illness and obtained the following results: monospot test, negative; cold agglutinin titer, 1:32; repeat cold agglutinin, 1:256; cryoglobulin, positive; toxoplasma complement fixation, <1:16; CMV, 1:64, mumps comp. fix., <1:8; EBV IFC VCA IgG, 1:320, VCA IgM, <1:10; HIV, negative; Lyme titer, 1:128. We interpreted the data to show previous infection with EBV and hepatitis B. The Lyme titer was indeterminate. The rising cold agglutinin titer and positive cryoglobulin were compatible with a viral illness. After 3 weeks in the hospital, the patient had a repeat CMV serology that increased

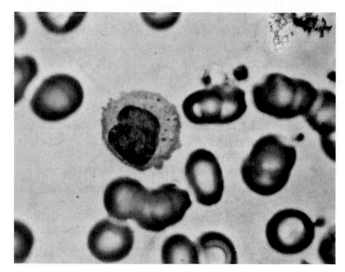

Figure 12.1. Large granular lymphocyte.

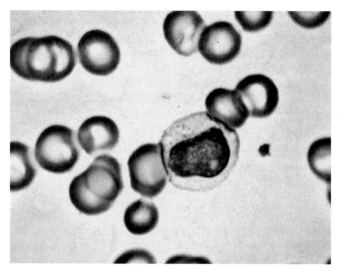

Figure 12.2. Atypical lymphocyte.

from 1:64 to 1:512. His fever broke and his symptoms subsided; atypical lymphocytes disappeared. Repeat ENT examination results were negative. We concluded that the patient had CMV mononucleosis. The achalasia was then repaired.

Virus Effects on Lymphocytes

Invasion

To describe the immune response that successfully resolves herpes-type virus infections, we rely on EBV mononucleosis rather than CMV infection because the former is better understood than the latter and the other herpesviruses. The EBV attaches to nasopharyngeal cells by the complement receptor, C3d. Virus is subsequently released to attach to B lymphocytes with the same receptor. Infected B cells express the Epstein-Barr nuclear antigen (EBNA) in10 hours and, by 40 hours, go into DNA synthesis. If allowed to grow unchecked, these B cells can destroy the host. The peak number of EBNA-positive cells in the blood of infectious mononucleosis patients varies from 0.03%[2] to 18%[3] in different studies. EBNA-positive cells are cleared from the blood over an 8-week period, but about 1×10^{-7} (0.00001%) cells in the blood remain virus-infected thereafter. Figure 12.3 depicts the clearance of EBNA-labeled cells from circulation.

Immune Reactions

The mechanism of attack on the virus-infected B cells, as noted above, involves both humoral and cellular immunity in vitro. Antibody reduces the transformation of infectious mononucleosis cells in vitro. Suppressor/cytotoxic activity has been shown in several tissue culture systems. Convalescent T cells can clear a culture of EBNA-positive cells (45). Suppressor T cells are active in killing EBNA-positive cells before they begin to proliferate while being stimulated to divide themselves. Thorley-Lawson (46) showed that T cells block proliferation of virus-infected B cells in vitro. Schooley and co-workers found that CD4 and CD8 cells inhibited EBV-transformed cells better than either cell type alone (47). Jondal and co-workers (48) extracted cells from a Burkitt lymphoma biopsy and demonstrated that T cells from the biopsy could kill EBV-containing cells lines. The antigen to which the T cells respond is not EBNA, however (or VCA or EA, which are commonly used to detect infectious mononucleosis clinically), but lymphocyte-detected membrane antigen (LYDMA), which can also stimulate the proliferation of killer cells in vitro (49).

The peripheral blood response to IM is incompletely understood with our present methods of analysis. Using antigenic markers with a flow cytometer is a significant technical advance, but there are few markers that are exclusive and identify a population precisely unless it is already clear that the population is monoclonal. Our case of CMV infection is illustrative of the complexity of analysis. We surmise that because 63% of the cells were CD8+, 96% were CD29+, and 40% were CD45RA+, the predominant cell would be CD8+CD29+CD45RA− (killer/effector), with the next most common cell being CD8±CD29+CD45RA+ (NK).

Two assumptions can be made. The first is that antibody against EBV is not present at the beginning of primary infection and will take 1–2 weeks to reach full strength. The second is that cells with detectors specific for LYDMA are not performed in quantity. Thus, we deduce that the NK cells are the first line of defense against EBV-infected, potentially malignant B cells.

Recent immunocytologic studies of infectious mononucleosis give us the outlines of the cellular response. Williams et al (50) found 1.8-fold increase in NK cells (CD57+ [HNK-1+]) in infectious mononucleosis, but decreased NK activity, perhaps due to temporary mononucleosis, but decreased NK activity, perhaps due to temporary depletion of lysosomal granules in the process of in vivo cell killing. A summary of this and five other studies (51–55) of immunologic markers shows that CD4 helper cells are increased 1.0- to 1.8-fold and CD8 cells are increased 2.5- to 10-fold during infectious mononucleosis. The CD4/CD8 ratio was reversed, but unlike the situation in AIDS, this reflects an increase in CD4 cells with a greater increase in CD8 cells. A recent publication finds that six classes of NK and suppressor/cytotoxic T cells are increased in infectious mononucleosis (56).

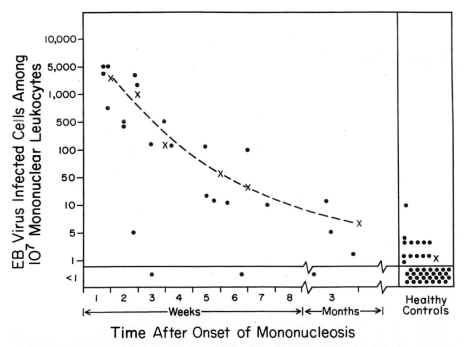

Figure 12.3. Clearance of Epstein-Barr nuclear antigen (EBNA)-labeled cells from circulation.

Clinical Scenario

The immune system does not kill the virus directly. NK cells, the first line of defense against virus-infected cells, detect newly infected B cells and kill them. NK cells proliferate briefly, but helper T cells also respond quickly and assist in the expansion of the population of suppressor/cytotoxic and suppressor/effector T cells. Cytotoxic T cells efficiently attack and kill most of the remaining EBV-infected cells. This effort is assisted by antibodies of various types. The virus remains at bay in a few infected cells for the rest of the person's life, and a continuing low level warfare is envisioned because antibody titers remain positive for life. But the immune system is so effective in this operation that only a grievous injury, such as is required to sustain a transplant, can allow the virus to escape from control (57). Figure 12.4 depicts the time course of T cell responses to IM.

CD4/CD8 Ratios in Disease

A reversed CD4/CD8 ratio may be mistaken as evidence for AIDS, but reversed ratios are quite common in other diseases. Blumberg and Schooley (58) reviewed lymphocyte markers in infectious disease and reported 10 diseases with reversed CD4/CD8 ratios, including leprosy, malaria, mumps, and varicella-zoster. Recently, patients with acute myocardial infarction (59) were shown to have reversed CD4/CD8 ratios that returned to normal after 2 days. Clearly, the T cell subpopulations are labile. Exercise in one patient with large granular lymphocyte syndrome induced a 40-fold, short-lived increase in CD8 lymphocytes

(60). Moreover, it has been found that migration of CD4, CD8, and NK cells was altered when lymph nodes in sheep were stimulated by antigen (61). Hydrocortisone has been shown to cause redistribution of NK cells in humans (62). Thus, decrease in peripheral blood CD4 or CD8 cells does not necessarily imply their death or immune impairment.

In summary, a young man with a history of drug abuse who had undergone a splenectomy had a severe, prolonged febrile illness with mild liver dysfunction and a blood clinical appearance strongly suggestive of EBV infectious mononucleosis. The illness differed from EBV infection because there was minimal pharyngitis or lymphadenopathy and the fever was severe. Our patient's illness was demonstrated to be due to CMV infection by four-fold rise in titer. The disease remitted spontaneously while the patient was under observation.

Immunosuppressive Effects of Viruses

It has been suggested that patients with viral infections are immunosuppressed by the virus. The issue is complex because the targets of the viruses vary in different diseases: EBV attacks B cells but does not kill them, instead immortalizing them until they are destroyed by the T cells. CMV infects both CD4 and CD8 cells (63). HIV attacks and destroys CD4 cells. Good and co-workers (64) investigated the immunosuppressive effects of HIV in view of the fact that as few as 1×10^{-5} lymphocytes may be infected, but the entire immune system is markedly suppressed. They found a viral transmembrane envelope protein that was immunosuppressive. A synthetic derivative of this envelope protein suppressed in-

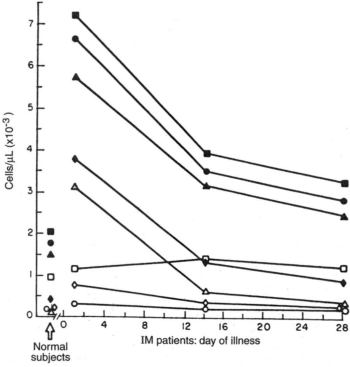

Figure 12.4. Time course of T-cell responses to IM.

terferon γ and IL-2 synthesis and inhibited generation of cytotoxic T cells.

Oldstone (65) reported that measles virus suppressed T- and B-cell function by arresting these cells in G1 (the resting phase before DNA synthesis begins) and that monkeys infected with measles have marked reduction in immunoglobulin production. His group also reported that CMV suppressed NK activity and T-cell proliferation (66). Goodenough (67) summarized the ways in which pathogens subvert the immune system by mimicry, parasitism, distraction, and camouflage.

Immunosuppression by the Immune System

It seems that the reactions of the immune system are also immunosuppressive. Rinaldo (68) reported that of the herpesviruses, CMV was most commonly associated with immunosuppression, probably because of increased numbers of suppressor cells. Less important changes were found in EBV, HSV1, HSV2, and varicella-zoster virus infections. These reactions are believed not to be important to the normal host but may be harmful in the immunosuppressed host. On the other hand, cytotoxic T cells specific for CMV are crucial to the survival of bone marrow transplant patients (69).

Immunosuppression by Splenectomy

The remaining question is whether our patient's previous splenectomy influenced the clinical course of his disease. The immune defect of splenectomy is expressed by increased susceptibility of encapsulated organisms such as *Streptococcus pneumoniae* and *Haemophilus influenzae*. No secondary infection occurred, and because the course of the disease was similar to that of others reported in the literature, we doubt that splenectomy had any significant impact on the disease.

Case 2

5/78: At 58 years of age, this retired garage mechanic presented to the hospital with fatigue, night sweats, and sore throats of 6 months' duration. He had fleeting arthralgia of the fingers and wrists. Splenomegaly, but no adenopathy (including negative lymphangiogram), was found.

Laboratory results were as follows: WBC count, 3.9 × 10⁹/L, with 99% lymphocytes; hematocrit 40%; and platelets, 200 × 10⁹/L. Bone marrow showed 40% lymphocytes and decreased nucleated red blood cells (RBCs). The lymphocytes had acid phosphatase-positive granules that were not tartrate resistant. The LDH was 299, and the rheumatoid factor was 1:640.

The patient was believed to have Felty syndrome (splenomegaly, neutropenia, and rheumatoid arthritis) or chronic lymphocytic leukemia. Felty syndrome, however, typically occurs after longstanding severe, erosive rheumatoid arthritis. Also, the patient had too few peripheral blood lymphocytes (<7 × 10⁹/L) and the wrong immunogenetic markers, as we shall subsequently see, to

meet the criteria for chronic lymphocytic leukemia (CLL) (CD5+CD19+, weak SIgM, SIgD).

The spleen was removed empirically to relieve symptomatic neutropenia. It weighed 1200 g and was infiltrated with lymphocytes. Liver biopsy also showed a lymphocytic infiltrate. After splenectomy, the absolute neutrophil count (ANC) rose to 1.6 × 10⁹/L, the platelets to 635 × 10⁹/L, and the hematocrit rose to 57%. But 5 months after splenectomy, the patient relapsed and the ANC fell to 0.59 × 10⁹/L.

3/81: The patient was admitted with recurrent symptoms of fatigue and inability to work. Laboratory values were as follows: hematocrit, 58%; absolute neutrophil count (ANC), 2.4 × 10⁹/L; absolute lymphocyte count, 4.4 × 10⁹/L; platelets, 309 × 10⁹/L. Bone marrow was unchanged. No treatment was given.

12/84: The patient was admitted with a transient ischemic attack. The hematocrit was again 58% and he was treated with phlebotomy.

12/85: The patient returned with fever, night sweats, and sore throat. Laboratory tests showed the following: hematocrit, 39%; WBC count, 6.7 × 10⁹/L with 91% lymphocytes; 4% monocytes; ANC, >0.5 × 10⁹/L; RF, 1:1280; antinuclear antibody (ANA), negative; lactic dehydrogenase (LDH), 467 units/L; IgG, 1346 mg/dL; IgA, 402; IgM, 137.

The flow cytometer analyzed 3.4 × 10⁹/L "agranular" cells.

CD2	(T11)	(T-cell marker; SRBC receptor)	80%; 2700	{nl 800–2500}
CD3	(T3)	(T-cell receptor)	74%; 2500	{nl 760–2100}
CD4	(T4)	(T-cell marker; class II receptor)	17%; 580	{nl 400–1200}
CD8	(T8)	(T-cell marker; class I receptor)	66%; 2200	{nl 180–860}
CD16	(Leu 11)	(NK cells; Fc receptor III)	2%; 70	
CD57	(Leu7)	(HNK1) (NK cells)	51%; 1700	{220–960}
CD19	(B4)	(B-cell marker)	8%; 270	
HLA-DR	(Ia)		47%; 1600	

The absolute number of suppressor/cytotoxic T cells (CD8) was increased more than three-fold. NK cells (CD57) were doubled. The CD4/CD8 ratio was 0.26 (nl 1–2.4). The predominant cell type would be read as CD2+CD3+CD8+CD16−CD57+. The low CD16 may represent saturation of this binding site (see below).

Bone marrow was hypercellular with GE ratio 0.6 and virtual absence of granulocytes beyond the promyelocyte. Bone marrow culture taken on 1/22/86 grew poorly, but granulocyte precursors were not inhibited by autologous T cells nor were erythrocyte precursors stimulated.

It was recognized that the patient fit the cases of large granular lymphocyte syndrome described by Wallis (29): arthralgias, positive rheumatoid factor, neu-

tropenia, and large granular lymphocytes. The cells met histochemical and immunologic criteria for suppressor/cytotoxic T cells, but the diagnosis was not made until these studies were done. Although the blood has been examined many times, large granular lymphocytes are in the minority (10–20%). The lymphocytosis is pleomorphic with a mixture of atypical large granular and small lymphocytes.

The Large Granular Lymphocyte

Considerable work has now been performed on what is called the large granular lymphocyte and its disorders because they were first described in 1975 (70, 71). The large granular lymphocyte is classically described as 12–15 m in diameter with red granules that are acid phosphatase and β-glucuronidase positive (72). The granules are frequently clustered close to an indentation in the nucleus. Some cells that meet the immunologic criteria do not show granules, but granules can be induced in short-term culture of lymphocytes by IL-2 and other stimuli. One criterion for the syndrome is $>2 \times 10^9$/L large granular lymphocytes (nl 0.25–0.46 × 10^9/L; about 15% of the lymphocytes) for 3 months without obvious cause (73, 74) but plainly immunologic criteria for suppressor/cytotoxic T cells must prevail.

Immunofluorescent Markers

Typical immunologic markers found in the large granular lymphocyte syndrome are CD3+ CD8+ CD16+ CD57+. However, in normal subjects, the CD3− CD8− CD16+ CD56+ cell is the predominant NK with large granular lymphocyte morphology and a CD3+ CD8+ CD16− CD56+, IL-2 dependent cell is the next most common (75). Because we know that there are at least six kinds of suppressor/cytotoxic/NK cells in normal blood, we may expect heterogeneity in cell markers, and if we are dealing with abnormal cells, the markers may vary further. For example, an AIDS patient had a large granular lymphocytosis with CD3− CD16+ CD56− cells (76).

After his relapse after splenectomy, our patient was treated successfully with prednisone until low back pain and L3 compression fracture developed. Cytoxan was started in 500–600 mg pulses as needed to keep the ANC above 1 × 10^9/L. The patient has tolerated two major abdominal surgeries and various minor procedures without significant infections.

Predictions of Behavior

Some attempts have been made to relate clinical behavior to the immunogenetic markers. One group (77) found that patients with CD3+ cells (i.e., T cells) had stable clinical situations and expressed no natural killer activity, whereas those with CD3− cells had aggressive disease and ¾ died within 3 months. Another group (78) studied 9 patients with CD3+ cells and found that they had frequent autoimmune phenomena, whereas two patients with CD3− cells did not. Even within patient populations, there is het-

erogeneity of clinical and antigenic expression. A patient with rare CD4+ large granular lymphocytosis has been described.

Cytotoxic Cell Physiology

The physiology of cytotoxic T cells and NK cells is complex. Growth of cytotoxic T cells is enhanced by IL-3, IL-4, and IL-6 (79, 80), and is down-regulated by IL-7 (81). Of peripheral CD8+ cells, 90% have cytotoxic potential. A minority (2.5%) of CD4+ cells are also cytotoxic.

There are three kinds of cytotoxic T-cell functions.

I. Those That Are Cytolysis Specific for Peptides Presented with HLA Alloantigens.

These killer cells require the CD8 marker and the presence of class I HLA antigens (HLA-A, B, C) on the target cell to initiate cell killing.

2. Cytolysis Not Restricted By HLA Antigens (The Natural Killer [NK] Function).

The system typically used to assay this function is the K562 cell line, because this target cell lacks both CD4 and CD8 antigens.

3. Antibody-Dependent Cytotoxicity (ADCC).

These killer cells carry the Fc receptor for g (IgG) chains (CD16) and may require antibody-coated cells for killing. Chicken RBCs coated with erythrocyte-specific antibody are used as target cells.

Neutrophils and monocytes also have ADCC. In addition, NK cells (CD3−CD16 ± CD56+) were recently reported to process antigen (82) and kill both Gram-negative and Gram-positive bacteria (83).

NK cells (CD3−CD16+CD56+) can be generated directly from bone marrow, suggesting that they had a lineage independent of conventional T cells (84, 85) or that they at least do not require the thymus for their maturation. Figure 12.5 depicts the lineage of the NK cell versus the T and B cells.

"Suppressor" function, as distinct from cytotoxic function, usually refers to the suppression of immunoglobulin synthesis, using peripheral blood lymphocytes driven by pokeweed mitogen. In addition, NK (CD57, HNK−1+) cells can suppress human erythroid stem cell proliferation in tissue culture (86). Inhibition of granulopoiesis is a prominent feature of the large granular lymphocyte syndrome.

Killer Cell Function

The red granules that characterize these lymphocytes contain a pore-forming protein, porphyrin, at least seven serine esterases (granzymes A–G), a tumor necrosis factor (TNF)-like molecule, and a variety of other enzymes. When the T-cell receptor is engaged by a target cell, porphyrin, a protein homologous with complement components, especially C9, forms a polymer at the cell surface.

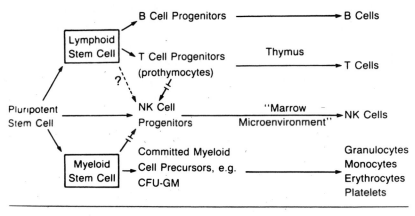

→/→ Pathways of Differentiation Ruled Out

Figure 12.5. Lineage of the NK cell vs. T and B cells.

This ring-like structure makes a hole in the target cell membrane. However, unlike complement, which causes similar cytoplasmic damage but leaves the nucleus intact, killer cells also activate host cell endonucleases, perhaps by a TNF-like molecule, so that the nucleus is destroyed—a phenomenon called apoptosis (87). In experimental conditions, the cytoplasmic damage—necrosis— and the nuclear damage—apoptosis—can be dissociated. The target cell's own enzymes are involved, because metabolic inhibitors applied to a target cell prevent nucleolysis (88). Other work indicates that the serine esterases of the cytotoxic T cell are also critical to the nucleolysis (89). DNA damage varies with the target (90) and the biochemistry of cytolysis varies with different cytotoxic subsets (91).

Modulation of NK Cells

NK cells are subject to modulation of their functional groups. IL-2 induces CD56 (NKH-1) in fresh thymocytes (92). CD39, an activation antigen, is induced in NK cells by several mitogens (93). C-reactive protein activates NK cells (94). Defective NK cells in hairy cell leukemia can be induced to function by interferon-α (95). Rheumatoid factor activates CD16 and exhausts NK cytolytic activity (96). GM-CSF suppresses the generation of NK cells in vitro (97). For a comprehensive review of NK cells, see Trinchieri (98).

Cell Functions in Large Granular Lymphocyte Syndrome

The functions of lymphocytes from 35 patients with large granular lymphocyte syndrome were studied by Reynolds and Foon (99). They found that cells from 9 of 21 patients suppressed immunoglobulin synthesis, four of four patients with RBC aplasia expressed erythroid stem cell (CFUe/BFUe) growth inhibition, 21 of 28 patients expressed ADCC, and 9 of 20 patients showed NK activity. Similarly, Loughran and Starkebaum (100) estimated that 14 of 45 patients in their review showed NK activity, 33 of 45 patients showed ADCC, and 10 of 27 patients suppressed B-cell immunoglobulin synthesis. One explanation for the failure of suppressor/cytotoxic T cells to express uniform properties is the variety of cell types involved and the lability of their antigens and functions.

In summary, a patient with neutropenia, large granular lymphocytosis, and arthralgias with positive rheumatoid factor has been followed more than 13 years. This patient also had symptomatic erythrocytosis requiring at least 22 phlebotomies. We have not found erythrocytosis complicating other cases in the literature, although there is one report of normal large granular lymphocytes stimulating primitive erythroid cells (101) in vitro. That patient responded successively to splenectomy and administration of corticosteroids and of cytoxan by intermittent pulses. The rationale for the use of low-dose cyclophosphamide is that suppressor cells are selectively sensitive to doses <500 mg/m² (102, 103).

Suppressor/Cytotoxic Cells in Infectious Disease

Because we do not understand the pathophysiology of the large granular lymphocyte syndrome, we may learn about it from the behavior of such cells in other diseases. As noted above, cytotoxic T cells are important in the defense against EBV and CMV. In one case, a child with no detectable cytotoxic T cells had life-threatening infections with varicella, CMV, and herpes simplex (104). However, one healthy adult has been described who had only 7% T cells during acute infection with CMV, but who nevertheless had a normal course of illness and effective titers of antibody (105). CD8+ cells are important in defense against measles (106). In mice, cytotoxic T cells are part of the early line of defense against mycobacteria (107). Cytotoxic T lymphocytes respond vigorously in early HIV infection (108), but NK cells cannot kill retrovirus-infected cells in vitro (109). Patients who are seropositive for *Toxoplasma* can generate cytotoxic lymphocyte clones in vitro (110).

Suppressor/Cytotoxic Cells in the Pathophysiology of Malignancy and Other Chronic Diseases

Suppressor/cytotoxic cells are increased in advanced CLL (111, 112) and can suppress immunoglobulin synthesis (113). Suppressor/cytotoxic cells are increased in lymphoma (114) and Hodgkin's disease (and can be blocked by prostaglandin inhibitors) (115). NK activity is increased in early myeloma and decreased in later stages (116, 117). Cytolytic cells infiltrate nasopharyngeal carcinoma (118). Depletion of host NK cells enhances engraftment of bone marrow in animals (119). NK cell activity is decreased in juvenile rheumatoid arthritis (120). T cells have been shown to suppress granulopoiesis in vitro in Felty syndrome (121) and other rheumatic diseases (122). Suppressor cell function is markedly depressed in Chediak-Higashi disease (123), perhaps because the granules are defective. One type of adult-onset cyclic neutropenia is associated with large granular lymphocytes (124).

Thus, cytotoxic T cells can kill tumor cells, virus-infected cells, and bacteria; process antigen; and modulate lymphoid and myeloid functions. When we see them in the infectious diseases of the normal host, their benefits are obvious. But when they are responding to malignancy or acting in the chronically ill host, their effects may complicate the disease by suppressing granulocyte production, red cell production, or immunoglobulin synthesis and add to the morbidity.

Prognosis in Large Granular Lymphocyte Disease

As the biologic data suggest, patients with large granular lymphocyte syndrome have variable clinical syndromes and prognoses. Pandolfi and co-workers (74) collected 151 cases with ages ranging from 5–88 years (mean age, 55). Of these, 20% died in 4 years and 12 had splenectomy with only one favorable result. Loughran and Starkebaum (125) described 38 cases and reviewed 76 others. Of these, 24 of 38 patients had severe neutropenia (<500/mL) and 15 of 38 patients had rheumatoid arthritis. Autoantibodies were found in >50%. Oshimi (126) described 12 patients in detail and found wide variation in granule size and frequency, immunologic markers, and suppressor function.

Three Prognostic Classes

Semenzato and co-workers (127) concluded that the large granular lymphocyte syndrome is a continuum of patients with reactive processes (responding to known antigens), an unknown middle group, presumably expressing autoimmune phenomena, and a malignant group. Of their 34 patients, 28 were in a steady state, two seemed to go into spontaneous remission, and five had a progressive course.

A Case of Reactive Disease

Agostini and co-workers (128) described a remarkable case of large granular lymphocyte syndrome (33 × 10⁹/L {CD3+CD8+CD57+[HNK1]}) lasting 2 years due to hepatitis B (HBV). In this case, the patient was and remained seronegative for HBV and had normal liver functions, but HBV DNA was found fortuitously in CD4 lymphocytes. The patient cleared the blood of infected CD4 cells after 2 years. The autologous cytotoxicity assay against CD4 cells was negative at the beginning of illness but was positive at 24 months, when the process subsided and the large granular lymphocytes disappeared.

It is interesting to speculate that other viruses and foreign antigens, perhaps still unknown, could generate similar responses. We have found large granular lymphocytosis in one patient with large cell lymphoma and in a patient with relapsing acute myelomonocytic leukemia; we believe that these were reactive processes. Our case study falls in the middle group of patients with a low-grade lymphocytosis and an indolent but symptomatic course of what we believe to be an autoimmune disease.

Leukemia vs. Benign Process

Loughran and Starkebaum (125) argue the large granular lymphocyte syndrome is a leukemia on the basis of abnormal cytogenetics in 3 of 13 patients and TCRb gene rearrangement in 11 of 11 patients. There are other criteria of malignancy: cell mass, growth fraction, and karyotype. Some cases show ungovernable lymphocytosis and rapid death, leaving no doubt about the aggressiveness of the disease, irrespective of laboratory criteria.

The T-cell receptor

To further evaluate the question, we will need to learn more about the T-cell receptor (TCR), its organization, and genetics. B cells undergo somatic rearrangement of D, J, and V genes, which combine with a constant region gene, C, to make a complete new immunoglobulin. The T cell achieves diversity in a manner similar to the B cell, by rearrangement of its TCR genes. These genes have considerable homology with immunoglobulin genes, with constant and variable regions, and rearrange in a similar fashion (fig. 12.6).

There are seven genes so far described: a, b, g, d, e, z, and h (129). Of these, g and d genes are rearranged first, followed by b and a (fig. 12.7). The genetic events and their effect on cell function are the subject of intense study. Although the finding of monoclonal arrangement of these genes may be helpful to the diagnosis of neoplasia, it is not sufficient, as Gresser and co-workers have pointed out (130). It seems unlikely that any single criterion will suffice to establish the diagnosis in this intriguing new group of diseases.

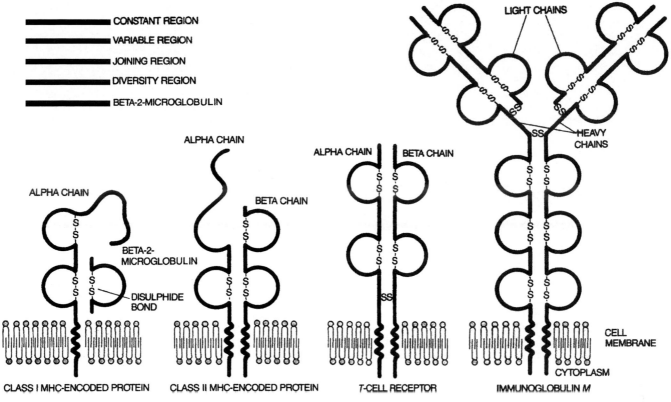

Figure 12.6. Rearrangement of B- and T-cell receptors.

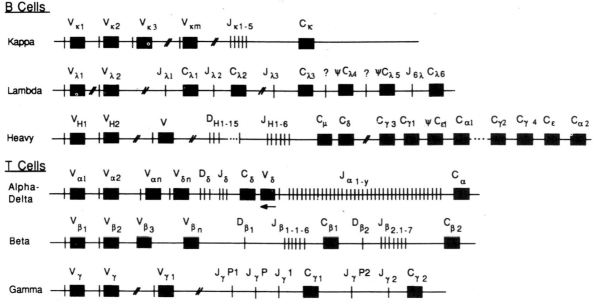

Figure 12.7. Diagram of the T-cell receptor.

REFERENCES

1. Sumaya CV, Ench Y. Epstein-Barr virus infectious mononucleosis in children. I. Clinical and general laboratory findings. Pediatrics 1985;75:1003.

2. Horowitz CA, Henle W, Henle G, et al. Clinical and laboratory evaluation of elderly patients with heterophile-antibody positive infectious mononucleosis. Am J Med 1976;61:333.

3. Tosato G, Magrath I, Kiski I, et al. Activation of suppressor T cells during Epstein-Barr induced infectious mononucleosis. N Engl J Med 1979;301:1133.

4. Strauss S, Cohen JI, Tosato G, Meier J. Epstein-Barr virus infections: biology, pathogenesis, and management. Ann Intern Med 1993;118:45.

5. Wood TA, Frenkel EP. The atypical lymphocyte. Am J Med 1967;42:923.

6. Weedon AP. Diphenylhydantoin sensitivity: a syndrome resembling infectious mononucleosis with a morbilliform rash and cholestatic hepatitis. Aust NZ J Med 1975;5:561.

7. Brown M, Schubert T. Phenytoin hypersensitivity to hepatitis and mononucleosis syndrome. J Clin Gastroenterol 1986;8:469.

8. Gropper AL. Diphenylhydantoin sensitivity. Report of a fatal case with hepatitis and exfoliative dermatitis. N Engl J Med 1956;254:522.

9. Siegal S, Berkowitz J. Diphenylhydantoin hypersensitivity with infectious mononucleosis-like syndrome and jaundice. J Allergy 1961;32:447.

10. Poland GA, Love KR. Marked atypical lymphocytosis, hepatitis and skin rash in sulfasalazine drug allergy. Am J Med 1986;81:707.

11. Flaherty G. Halothanitis or glandular fever. Anaesth Intensive Care 1975;3:162.

12. Gan TE, Martin BVW. Dapsone-induced mononucleosis-like syndrome. Med J Aust 1982;1:350.

13. Horwitz CA, Henle W, Henle G, Polesky H, Balfour HH Jr, Siem RA, et al. Heterophil-negative mononucleosis and mononucleosis-like illness. Am J Med 1977;83:947.

14. Steeper TA, Horwitz CA, Hanson M, Henle W, Henle G, Rosenstein H, et al. Heterophil-negative mononucleosis and mononucleosis-like illness with atypical lymphocytosis in patients undergoing seroconversion to the human immunodeficiency virus. Am J Clin Path 1988;90:169.

15. Beverly JKA, Beattie CP. Glandular toxoplasmosis Lancet 1958;ii:379.

16. Fleisher GR, Collins M, Fager S. Limitations of available tests for diagnosis of infectious mononucleosis. J Clin Microbiol 1983;17:619.

17. Downey H, McKinlay CA. Acute lymphadenosis compared with acute lymphocyte leukemia. Arch Int Med 1923;32:82.

18. Gavosto F, Pileri A, Maraini G. Incorporation of thymidine labeled with tritium by circulating cells of infectious mononucleosis. Nature 1959;183:1691.

19. MacKinney AA Jr. Tissue culture of cells already in DNA synthesis from patients with infectious mononucleosis. Blood 1965;26:36.

20. MacKinney AA Jr. Division of leukocytes already in DNA synthesis from patients with acute leukemia and infectious mononucleosis. Acta Haematol 1967;38:163.

21. Epstein MA, Achong BG, Barr YM. Virus particles in cultured lymphocytes from Burkitt's lymphoma. Lancet 1964;I:702.

22. Henle G, Henle W, Diehl V. Relation of Burkitt's lymphoma-associated Herpes-type virus to infectious mononucleosis. Proc Nat Acad Sci 1968;59:94.

23. Glade RP, Kasel JA, Moses HL, Whang-Peng J, Hoffman PF, Kammermeyer JK, et al. Infectious mononucleosis: continuous suspension culture of peripheral blood leucocytes. Nature 1968;217:564.

24. Salvador AH, Harrison EG Jr, Kyle RA. Lymphadenopathy due to infectious mononucleosis:its confusion with malignant lymphoma. Cancer 1971;27:1029.

25. Lukes RJ, Tindle BH, Parker JW. Reed-Sternberg-like cells in infectious mononucleosis. Lancet 1969;ii:1003.

26. McMahon NJ, Gordon HW, Rosen RB. Reed-Sternberg cells in infectious mononucleosis. Am J Dis Child 1970;120:148.

27. Custer RP, Smith EB. The pathology of infectious mononucleosis. Blood 1948;3:830.

28. Carter RL. Infectious mononucleosis: model for self-limiting lymphoproliferation Lancet 1975;i:846.

29. Grierson H, Purtilo DT. Epstein-Barr virus infection in males with the X-linked lymphoproliferative syndrome. Ann Int Med 1987;106:538.

30. MacKinney AA Jr. Studies of plasma protein synthesis by peripheral cells from normal persons and patients with infectious mononucleosis. Blood 1968;32:217.

31. Virolainen M, Anderson LC, Lalla M, Von Essen R. T-lymphocyte proliferation in mononucleosis. Clin Immunol Immunopath 1973;2:114.

32. Good RA, Dalmasso AP, Martinez C, Archer OK, Pierce JC, Papermaster BW. The role of the thymus in development of immunologic capacity in rabbits and mice. J Exp Med 1962;116:773.

33. Matsuyama M, Wiadrowski MN, Metcalf D. Autoradiographic analysis of lymphopoiesis and lymphocyte migration in mice bearing multiple thymus grafts. J Exp Med 1966;124:559.

34. Raff MC. Two distinct populations of peripheral lymphocytes in mice distinguishable by immunofluorescence. Immunol 1970;19:637.

35. Bach JR, Muller J-Y, Dardeune M. In vivo specific antigen recognition by rosette-forming cells. Nature 1970;227:1251.

36. Waldmann TA, Duren M, Broder S, Blackman M, Blaese RM, Strober W. Role of suppressor T cells in pathogenesis of common variable hypogammaglobulinaemia. Lancet 1974;ii:609.

37. Allison AC, Ferluga J. How lymphocytes kill tumor cells. N Engl J Med 1976;295:165.

38. Reinherz EL, Kung PC, Goldstein G, Levey RH, Schlossman SF. Discrete stages of human intrathymic differentiation: analysis of normal thymocytes and leukemic lymphoblasts of T-cell lineage. Proc Nat Acad Sci 1980;77:1588.

39. Sohen S, Rothstein DM, Tallman T, Gaudette D, Schlossman SF, Morimoto C. The functional heterogeneity of CD8+ cells defined by anti CD45RA (2H4) and CD29 (4B4) antibodies. Cell Immunol 1990;128:314.

40. Bottomly K. A functional dichotomy in CD4+ T lymphocytes. Immunology Today 1988;9:268.

41. Ritz J, Campen TJ, Schmidt RE, Royer HD, Hercend T, Hussey RE, Reinherz EL. Analysis of T-cell receptor gene rearrangement and expression in human natural killer clones Science 1985;228:1540.

42. Abo R, Cooper MD, Balch CM. Characterization of HNK-1 (leu 7) human lymphocytes. J Immunol 1982;129:1752.

43. Moretta A, et al. Identification of four subsets of human CD3-CD16+ natural killer cells by the expression of clonally distributed functional surface molecules: correlation between subset assignment of NK clones and ability to mediate specific alloantigen recognition. J Exp Med 1990;172:1589.

44. Inverardi L, Watson JC, Fuad SA, Winkler-Picket RT, Ortaldo JR, Bach FH. CD3 negative "small agranular lymphocytes" are natural killer cells. J Immunol 1991;146:4048.

45. Rickinson AB, Moss DJ, Wallace LS, et al. Long term T cell mediated immunity to Epstein-Barr virus. Cancer Res 1981;41:4216.

46. Thorley-Larson DA. The suppression of Epstein-Barr virus infection in vitro occurs after infection but before transformation of the cell. J Immunol 1980;124:745.

47. Schooley RT, Arbit DI, Henle W, Hirsch MS. T-lymphocyte subset interactions in the cell-mediated immune response to Epstein-Barr virus. Cell Immunol 1984;86:402.

48. Jondal M, Svedmyr E, Klein E, Singh S. Killer T cells in a Burkitt's lymphoma biopsy. Nature 1975;255:405.

49. Epstein MA, Achong BG. Pathogenesis of infectious mononucleosis. Lancet 1977;2:1270.

50. Williams NL, Loughran TP Jr, Kidd PG, Starkebaum GA. Polyclonal proliferation of activated suppressor/cytotoxic T cells with transient depression of natural killer cell function in acute infectious mononucleosis. Clin Exp Immunol 1989;77:71.

51. Verucci G, Attard L, Maldini M, et al. Cell-mediated immunity in infectious mononucleosis. Adv Exp Med Biol 1989;257:279.

52. Tomkinson BE, Wagner DK, Nelson DL, Sullivan JL. Activated lymphocytes during acute Epstein-Barr virus infection. J Immunol 1987;139:3802.

53. Reinherz EL, O'Brien C, Rosenthal P, Schlossman SF. The cellular basis for viral-induced immunodeficiency analysis by monoclonal antibodies. J Immunol 1980;125:1269.

54. DeWaele M, Thielemans C, VanCamp BKG. Characterization of immunoregulatory T cells in EBV-induced infectious mononucleosis by monoclonal antibodies. N Engl J Med 1981;304:460.

55. Haynes BF, Schooley RT, Grouse JE, Payling-Wright CR, Dolin R, Fauci AS. Characterization of thymus-derived lymphocyte subsets in acute Epstein-Barr virus-induced infectious mononucleosis. J Immunol 1979;122:699.

56. Furukawa S, et al. Comparison of Kawasaki disease and infectious mononucleosis in terms of natural killer cell and CD8+ subsets. J Infect Dis 1991;163:417.

57. Ho M, et al. Frequency of Epstein-Barr virus infection and associated lymphoproliferative syndrome after transplant and its manifestation in children. Transplantation 1988; 45:719.

58. Blumberg RS, Schooley RF. Lymphocyte markers and infectious disease. Semin Hematol 1985;22:81.

59. Syrjala H, Surcel H-M, Ilonen J. Low CD4/CD8 T lymphocyte ratio in acute myocardial infarction. Clin Exp Immunol 1991;83:326.

60. Mulligan SP, Wills EJ, Young GAR. Exercise-induced CD8 lymphocytosis: a phenomenon associated with granular lymphocyte leukemia. Br J Haematol 1990;75:175.

61. Kempton WG, Washington EA, Cahill RNP. Nonrandom migration of CD4+, CD8+ and gd T19+ lymphocyte subsets following in vivo stimulation with antigen. Cell Immunol 1990;130:236.

62. Onsrud M, Thorsby E. Influence of in vivo hydrocortisone on some human blood lymphocyte subpopulations. Scand J Immunol 1981;13:573.

63. Schrier RD, Nelson JA, Oldstone MBA. Detection of human cytomegalovirus in peripheral blood lymphocytes in a natural infection. Science 1985;230:1048.

64. Good RA, Ogasawara M, Liu WT, Lorenz E, Day NK. Immunosuppressive actions of retroviruses. Lymphology 1990; 23:56.

65. Oldstone MBA. Viral persistence and immune dysfunction. Hosp Pract 1990;25:81.

66. Schreier RD, Rice GPA, Oldstone MBA. Suppression of natural killer cell activity and T cell proliferation by fresh isolates of human cytomegalovirus. J Infect Dis 1986; 153:1084.

67. Goodenough UW. Deception by pathogens. Am Scientist 1991;79:344.

68. Rinaldo CR Jr. Immune suppression by herpesviruses. Ann Rev Med 1990;41:331.

69. Reusser P, Riddell SR, Meyers JD, Greenberg PD. Cytotoxic T-lymphocyte response to cytomegalovirus after human allogeneic bone marrow transplantation: pattern of recovery and correlation with cytomegalovirus infection and disease. Blood 1991;78:137.

70. Wallis JW, Loughran TP Jr, Kadin ME, Clark EA, Starkebaum GA. Polyarthritis and neutropenia associated with circulating large granular lymphocytes. Ann Intern Med 1985;103:357.

71. Brody JL, Burningham RA, Nowell PC, Rowlands DT, Freiberg P, Daniele RP. Persistent lymphocytosis with chromosomal evidence of malignancy. Am J Med 1975; 58:547.

72. Brouet JC, Flandrii G, Sasportes M, Gajl-Peczalska KJ, Seligmann M. Chronic lymphocytic leukemia of T-cell origin. Lancet 1975;2:890.

73. Reynolds CW, Foon KA. Tg-lymphoproliferative disease and related disorders in human and experimental animals: a review of the clinical, cellular and functional characteristics. Blood 1984;64:1146.

74. Pandolfi F, et al. Clinical course and prognosis of the lymphoproliferative disease of granular lymphocytes. Cancer 1990;65:341.

75. Lanier LL, Le AM, Civin CI, Loken MR, Phillips JH. The relationship of CD16 (Leu 11) and Leu 19 (NKH-1) antigen expression on human peripheral blood NK cells and cytotoxic lymphocytes. J Immunol 1986; 136:4480.

76. Ghali V, Castella A, Louis-Charles A, Agranosky E, Croxson ST. Expansion of large granular lymphocytes (natural killer cells) with limited antigen expression (CD2+, CD3−, CD4−, CD16+, NKH-1-) in a human immunodeficiency virus-positive homosexual man. Cancer 1990;65:2243.

77. Taniwaki M, et al. Chromosomal abnormalities define clonal proliferation in CD3− large granular lymphocyte leukemia. Am J Hematol 1990;33:32.

78. Chan WC, Link S, Mawle A, Check I, Byrnes RK, Winton EF. Heterogeneity of large granular lymphocyte proliferations: delineation of 2 major subtypes. Blood 1986; 68:1142.

79. Holda JH, Maier T, Claman HN. IL-3, IL-4, and IL-6 enhance IFN-g dependent bone marrow natural suppressor activity. Cell Immunol 1990;125:459.

80. Ming JE, Cernetti C, Steinman RM, Granelli-Piperno A. Interleukin 6 is the principal cytolytic T lymphocyte differentiation factor for thymocytes in human leukocyte conditioned medium. J Mol Cell Immunol 1989;4:203.

81. Hickman CJ, Crim JA, Mostowski HS, Siegel JP. Regulation of human cytotoxic T lymphocyte development by IL-7. J Immunol 1990;145:2415.

82. Roncarolo M-G, Bigler M, Haanen JBA, et al. Natural killer cell clones can efficiently process and present protein antigens. J Immunol 1991;147:781.

83. Garcia-Penarrubia P, Koster FJ, Kelley RO, McDowell TD, Bankhurst AD. Antibacterial activity of human natural killer cells. J Exp Med 1989;169:99.

84. Hackett J, Bosma GC, Bosma MJ, Bennett M, Kumar V. Transplantable progenitors of natural killer cells are distinct from those of T and B lymphocytes. PNAS 1986; 83:3427.

85. Lotzova E, Savary CA. Generation of NK cell activity from human bone marrow. J Immunol 1987;139:279.

86. Mangan KF, Hartnett ME, Matis SA, Winkelstein A, Abo A. Natural killer cells suppress human erythroid stem cell proliferation in vitro. Blood 1984;63:260.

87. Tschopp J, Nabholz M. Perforin-mediated target cell lysis by cytolytic T lymphocytes. Ann Rev Immunol 1990; 8:279.

88. Zychlinsky A, Zheng LM, Liu C-C, Young JD. Cytolytic lymphocytes induce both apoptosis and necrosis of target cells. J Immunol 1991;146:393.

89. Welsh RM, Nishioka W, Antia R, Dundon PL. Mechanism of killing by virus-induced cytotoxic T lymphocytes elicited in vivo. J Virol 1990;64:3726.

90. Sellins KS, Cohen JJ. Cytotoxic T lymphocytes induce different types of DNA damage in target cells of different origins. J Immunol 1991;147:795.

91. Hengel H, Wagner H, Heeg K. Triggering of CD8+ cytotoxic T lymphocytes via CD3-e differs from triggering via a/b T cell receptor. CD3-e-induced cytotoxicity occurs in the absence of protein kinase C and does not result in exocytosis of serine esterases. J Immunol 1991;147:1115.

92. Caliguiri MA, Murray C, Levine H, Longtine JA, Ritz J. Clonal evidence for the induction of NKH-1 on activated human thymocytes. Eur J Immunol 1989;19:1735.

93. Kansas GS, Wood GS, Tedder TF. Expression, distribution and biochemistry of human CD39. J Immunol 1991; 146:2235.

94. Hamoudi WH, Baum LL. Anti-C-reactive protein inhibits the calcium-dependent stage of natural killer cell activation. J Immunol 1991;146:2873.

95. Trentin L, et al. Mechanisms accounting for the defective natural killer activity in patient with hairy cell leukemia. Blood 1990;75:1525.

96. Hendrich C, Kuipers JG, Kolanus WS, Hammer M, Schmidt RE. Activation of CD16+ effector cells by rheumatoid factor complex. Arthr Rheum 1991;34:423.

97. Taguchi K, Shibuya A, Inazawa Y, Abe T. Suppressive effect of granulocyte-macrophage colony-stimulating factor on the generation of natural killer cells in vitro. Blood 1992; 79:3227.

98. Trinchieri G. Biology of natural killer cells. Adv Immunol 1989;47:187.

99. Reynolds CW, Foon KA. Tg-lymphoproliferative disease and related disorders in human and experimental animals: a review of the clinical, cellular and functional characteristics. Blood 1984;64:1146.

100. Loughran TP Jr, Starkebaum G. Large granular lymphocyte leukemia. Medicine 1987;66:397.

101. Pistoia V, Ghio R, Nocera A, Leprini A, Perata A, Ferrarini M. Large granular lymphocytes have a promoting activity on human peripheral blood erythroid burst-forming units. Blood 1985;65:464.

102. Fahey JL, Sarna G, Gale RP, Seeger R. Immune interventions in disease. Ann Intern Med 1987;106:257.

103. Hoover SK, Barrett SK, Turk TMT, Lee L-C, Bear HD. Cyclophosphamide and abrogation of tumor-induced suppressor T cell activity. Cancer Immunol Immunother 1990; 31:121.

104. Biron CA, Byron KS, Sullivan JL. Severe herpes virus infections in an adolescent without natural killer cells. N Engl J Med 1989;320:1731.

105. Oill PA, Fiala M, Schofferman J, Byfield PE, Guze LG. Cytomegalovirus mononucleosis in a healthy adult. Am J Med 1977;62:413.

106. Van Dinnendijk RS, et al. The predominance of CD8+ T cells after infection with measles virus suggests a role for CD8+ class I MHC-restricted cytotoxic T lymphocytes (CTL) in recovery from measles. J Immunol 1990; 144:2394.

107. Inoue T, Yoshikai Y, Matsuyaki G, Nomoto K. Early appearing g/d bearing T cells during infection with Calmette Guerin bacillus. J Immunol 1991;146:2454.

108. Walker BD, Plata F. Cytotoxic T lymphocytes against HIV. AIDS 1990;4:177.

109. Zheng Z-Y, Zucker-Franklin D. Apparent ineffectiveness of natural killer cells vis-a-vis retrovirus-infected targets. J Immunol 1992;148:3679.

110. Khan JA, Smith KA, Dasper LH. Induction of antigen-specific human cytotoxic T cells by Toxoplasma gondii. J Clin Invest 1990;85:1879.

111. Terstappen LWMM, deGrooth BG, Segers-Nolten I, Greve J. Cytotoxic lymphocytes in B-cell chronic lymphocytic leukemia. Blut 1990;60:81.

112. Lauria F, Catovsky D. Increase in T gamma lymphocytes in B-cell chronic lymphocytic leukemia. Scand J Haematol 1980;24:187.

113. Kay NE, Perri RT. Evidence that large granular lymphocytes from B-CLL patients with hypogammaglobulinemia down-regulate B-cell immunoglobulin synthesis. Blood 1989;73:1016.

114. Hawrylowicz CM, Rees RC, Hancock BW, Potter CW. Depressed spontaneous natural killing and interferon augmentation in patient with malignant lymphoma. Eur J Cancer Clin Oncol 1982;18:1081.

115. Goodwin JS, Messner RP, Bankhurst AD, Peake GT, Saiki JH, Williams RC Jr. Prostaglandin-producing suppressor cells in Hodgkin's disease. N Engl J Med 1977; 297:963.

116. Osterborg E, Nilsson B, Bjorkholm M, Holm G, Mellstedt H. Natural killer cell activity in monoclonal gammopathies: relation to disease activity. Eur J Haematol 1990;45:153.

117. Ogmundsdottir HM. Natural killer cell activity in patients with multiple myeloma. Cancer Detect Prevent 1988; 12:143.

118. Takhdar M, Aribia B, Maalej M, Ladgham A. Selective homing of phenotypically lytic cells within nasopharyngeal carcinoma biopsies: numerous CD8− and CD16+ cells in the tumor. Int J Cancer 1991;48:57.

119. Tiberghien P, Longo DL, Wine JW, Alvord WG, Reynolds CW. Anti-sialo GM1 antiserum treatment of lethally irradiated recipients before bone marrow transplant: evidence that recipient natural iller depletion enhances survival, engraftment and hematopoietic recovery. Blood 1990; 76:1419.

120. Strelkauskas AJ, Callery RT, McDowell J, Borel Y, Schlossman SF. Direct evidence for loss of human suppressor cells during active auto-immune disease. PNAS 1978; 75:5150.

121. Abdou NI, NaPombejara C, Ballentine L, Abdou NL. Suppressor cell-mediated neutropenia in Felty's syndrome. J Clin Invest 1978;61:738.

122. Bagby GC Jr, Gabourel JD. Neutropenia in three patients with rheumatic disorders. J Clin Invest 1979;64:72.

123. Haliotis T, Roder J, Klein M, Ortaldo J, Fauci AS, Herberman RB. Chediak Higashi gene in humans; I, impairment of natural killer function. J Exp Med 1980; 151:1039.

124. Loughran TP Jr, Clark EA, Price FH, Hammond WP. Adult-onset cyclic neutropenia is associated with increased large granular lymphocytes. Blood 1986;68:1082.

125. Loughran TP Jr, Starkebaum G. Large granular lymphocyte leukemia. Medicine 1987;66:397.

126. Oshimi K. Granular lymphocyte proliferative disorders: report of 12 cases and review of the literature. Leukemia 1988;2:617.

127. Semenzato G, et al. The lymphoproliferative disease of granular lymphocytes. Cancer 1987;60:2971.

128. Agostini et al. Lymphoproliferative disease of granular lymphocytes in a patient with concomitant hepatitis B virus infection of CD4 lymphocytes. J Clin Immunol 1989; 9:401.

129. Clayton LK, Bauer A, Jin Y-J, D'Adamio L, Koyasu S, Reinherz EL. Characterization of thymus-derived lymphocytes expressing Tia-bCD3gdez-z, Tia-bCD3gdeh-h or Tia-bCD3 dez-z/z-h antigen receptor isoforms: analysis by gene transfection. J Exp Med 1990;172:1243.

130. Gresser H, Tkachuk D, Reis MD, Mak TW. Gene rearrangements and translocations in lymphoproliferative diseases. Blood 1989;73:1402.

GLOSSARY OF PERTINENT CLUSTER DISTRIBUTION (CD) ANTIGENS

"Cluster distribution" refers to groups of monoclonal antibodies that recogize the same antigen. When the molecular weight of this antigen is known and the identity of a group of monoclonal antibodies is established by an international workshop, a CD number is given. In some cases, the CD number corresponds to another designated number (e.g., T4 = CD4; T8 = CD8), but in most other cases the number is arbitrary.

CD2. Sheep red blood cell (E) receptor. Leu 5b. This was the original mark that identified the T cell.

CD3. T-cell antigen receptor complex. Leu 4.

CD4. T helper/inducer cell marker. Leu 3a, 3b. Recognizes HLA class II antigens. HIV receptor.

CD8. T cytotoxic/suppressor cell marker. Leu 2a, 2b. Recognizes HLA class antigens.

CD11b. Adhesion molecule (Mac. 1). Complement receptor III.

CD16. IgG Fc receptor III (low affinity). Leu 11. Marker for natural killer (NK) cell.

CDw29. 4B4. VLA β-chain. Marker for subset of CD4 helper cells.

CD39. An activation enzyme inducible in NK cells, endothelial cells, etc.

CD45RA. Leu 18; 2H4. Leukocyte common antigen, marking a subset of CD4 helper cells.

CD45RB. Antigen marker for CD4 subset.

CD45RO. UCHLI. Antigen marker for CD4 subset.

CD56. NKH-1; Leu 19. Adhesion molecule: N-CAM. Marker for NK cells.

CD57. HNK-1; Leu 7. Marker for NK cells.

CHAPTER 13

Inherited Disorders of B-Lymphocytes

MARTIN R. KLEMPERER

Half of the secret of resistance to disease is cleanliness; the other half is dirtiness.
—Anonymous

Deficiencies of the antibody-producing cells are characterized in the laboratory by a decreased level of one or more of the immunoglobulins, or a decrease in the rate or the degree of response to a defined antigen. Clinically, antibody-deficiency states are characterized by prolonged infectious episodes, repeated infections, or infections caused by unusual microorganisms. This chapter will discuss the clinical and pathophysiologic aspects of primary deficiencies of the antibody response.

Case 1

The patient was a 4-month-old biracial male infant who was hospitalized because of a history of difficulty breathing of 1 week's duration. He had no history of previous prolonged infections. He had received diphtheria, pertussis, tetanus (DPT), and oral polio vaccine at 2 and 4 months of age. However, at 3 months of age he had been hospitalized with a diagnosis of Pseudomonas aeruginosa sepsis and neutropenia. The infant was born at full term. Labor, delivery, and postnatal course were unremarkable. The mother had received treatment for a chlamydial infection during the first trimester. She had had gonorrhea 2 years earlier and had multiple sexual partners, but had no history of intravenous drug abuse. There was no maternal family history of fetal deaths or of infant deaths. The father's history was unknown.

On physical examination, the patient was afebrile, his respirations were 64 breaths/minute, and an apical rate was 140 beats/minute. His weight and height were between the 10th and 20th percentiles. He had substernal and intercostal retractions and flaring of the alae nasae. Head, eyes, ears, nose, and throat (HEENT) examination was unremarkable except for very small tonsils. The lungs were clear with good air exchange. The remainder of the examination was within normal limits.

Chest x-ray was consistent with diffuse bilateral infiltrates. Oxygen saturation in room air was 87%. After increasing respiratory distress developed, the baby was transferred to the medical intensive care unit and intu-

bated. The patient initially was treated with cefotaxime to which sulfamethoxazole was added after intubation.

Assessment: The patient was initially seen at an early age with a history of previously documented sepsis in which *P. aeruginosa* was identified. One month later, he was examined for the signs of respiratory distress. A chest film was consistent with a diffuse bilateral pneumonia. The patient's history is consistent with a basic defect in host defense, because *Pseudomonas* sepsis is unusual in a normal infant and the patient presented with diffuse bilateral pneumonia. The pathologic process could be defined by: (a) defective neutrophil function, due to number, defective killing, or defective chemotaxis or adherence; (b) defective cell-mediated immunity; (c) defective opsonic function due to a lack of immunoglobulin synthesis, an absence of a complement component such as C3, or an inhibitor of complement activation such as factor H. Although the occurrence of two significant infections might be due to chance, the question of an underlying defect in the immunity system must be raised. The identification of an infectious agent associated with the pneumonia might be of use in defining any possible immunologic defect.

Immune Deficiency Disease

Bronchoalveolar lavage was performed and demonstrated the cysts of Pneumocystis carinii. On the 8th day of therapy, hives developed in the patient, and after his medication was changed to intravenous pentamidine he steadily improved. At the time of discharge, his chest film was normal with a normal thymic silhouette.

The identification of Pneumocystis carinii in the bronchial washings must direct one's diagnosis to a significant immune deficiency state. A diagnostic workup was initiated. Laboratory findings are given in table 13.1.

With polymerase chain reaction (PCR), mRNA for μ-heavy chains and for CD2O was identified (1). T-Cell functions, including quantitative lymphocyte transforma-

Table 13.1. Laboratory Studies: Case 1

Hemoglobin	11.5 g/L
Hematocrit	0.35
White blood cell count	14.4×10^9/L
Band forms	0.02
Segmented neutrophils	0.48
Lymphocytes	0.48
Eosinophils	0.02
Platelets	623×10^9/L
T-cell and B-cell determinations	
T-3	93% (normal 63–85%)
T-4	71% (normal 37–51%)
T-8	26% (normal 18–36%)
T-11	94% (normal 71–89%
T-4/T-8	2.73 (normal 1.0–3.2)
Natural killer (NK) cells	25% (normal 2–14%)
T-3/I-3 (activated T-cells)	2 (normal 1–8)
B-1	<1% (normal 7–19%)
Immunoglobin G (IgG)	20 mg/dl (normal 244–663 mg/dl)
Immunoglobin M (IgM)	22 mg/dl (normal 33–131 mg/dl)
Immunoglobin A (IgA)	Undetectable (normal 3–42 mg/dl)
Complement studies	CH50 = 80 (normal 65–95)
Antibody studies	
Diptheria	Undetectable
Tetanus	Undetectable
Anti-B	Undetectable
Bone marrow biopsy[a]	No plasma cells
Rectal biopsy[a]	No plasma cells
B-cell markers	1% SIg, κ or λ B-4, or B-6 antigen
	No intracytoplasmic μ heavy chains

[a]No plasma cells present.

tion to mitogens and to specific antigens, were within normal limits.

Karyotype was normal XY. Human immunodeficiency virus (HIV) studies in the mother and the patient with PCR and culture were negative.

The patient's history and the isolation of P. aeruginosa *and* Pneumocystis carinii *at the times of his acute illness are consistent with an underlying immunodeficiency. The majority of tests were obtained simultaneously. However, for discussion purposes the test results and their importance will be discussed sequentially.*

The white blood cell (WBC) count and differential were unremarkable for a 4-month-old baby. The absolute neutrophile count was 7,200/mm³. Therefore, we ruled out neutropenia. However, neutrophile functional defects such as glucose-6-phosphate dehydrogenase (G-6-PD) deficiency or chronic granulomatous disease could still be considered in a male infant. Specific enzyme assays, nitro blue tetrozolium reduction, and spontaneous chemiluminescence were not performed. Such assays would be required if a defect in other immunologic systems could not be identified.

When serum immunoglobulins were determined, all were found to be significantly deficient. IgG, IgA, and IgM were significantly below the normal range for the

patient's age. The low absolute value of IgG, 20 mg/dl, made the quantitation of IgG subclasses impossible.

The virtual absence of serum immunoglobulins does not absolutely establish a diagnosis of isolated hypogammaglobulinemia, because infants with combined T-cell and B-cell defects may be initially seen with hypogammaglobulinemia. Secondary deficiencies due to loss in the urine, stools, or ascitic fluid must be investigated if appropriate. Therefore, the peripheral blood T-cells were evaluated. Mature T-cells, as defined by expression of the surface antigen CD3, were increased relatively because of the lack of circulating B-cells. However, in their major subset distribution, the T-cells were normal. Results of classic studies of T-cell function were normal. Since the majority of infants with combined immunodeficiency or with hypogammaglobulinemia are male, the sex of the patient was not useful in narrowing the diagnostic possibilities. The presence of an adequate number of T-cells and their being functionally normal does rule out the possibility of a severe combined immunologic deficiency state.

The B-Cell System

In order to clarify the nature of the patient's immune deficiency, an overview of the nature and function of the antibody-producing system is presented. The B-cell system includes those cells capable of immunoglobulin synthesis. When immunoglobulin production is provoked by specific chemical configurations, the specifically evoked immunoglobulin molecules are termed "antibody." Whether or not all immunoglobulins generated by a normally functioning B-cell system have demonstrable antibody specificity is conjectural. However, through usage the terms "immunoglobulins," "γ-globulins," "immune serum globulins," and "antibodies" are used interchangeably. Although, immunoglobulins are thought of mainly in the context of serum proteins, they are found in the extracellular fluids, secretions of exocrine glands and mucosal cells, and as a component of the cell membrane of B-cells and tissue mast cells. The biologic functions of immunoglobulins are dependent upon the structure of the constant regions of the heavy chain Fc fragments, while antibody specificity is governed by the variable and hypervariable regions of the heavy chain and the light chain that constitute the Fab fragment (fig. 13.1, table 13.2).

The immunoglobulins constitute a heterogenous array of proteins that are made up of light chains and heavy chains. Although the basic structure of IgG, IgA, and IgM has many similarities, variations in the constituent amino acids give rise to differences that modify their electrophoretic mobility (2). When serum is subjected to electrophoresis, the immunoglobulins migrate as γ-, β-, and α-2 proteins. Because the α-globulin moiety constitutes the largest fraction, α-globulin is used frequently synonymously with immunoglobulin. All immunoglobulins have a similar basic structural unit composed of two light

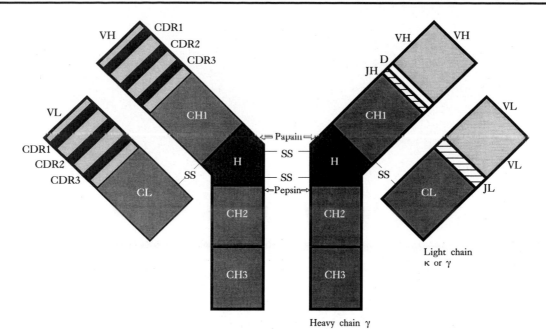

Figure 13.1. The basic structure of the human IgG molecule. The constant regions of the light and heavy chains, respectively, are CL and CH1,2,3. The hinge region is designated as *H*. The variable regions of the light and the heavy chains are *VL* and *VH*. The hypervariable regions of the light and the heavy chains that govern antibody specificity are termed "complementarity-determining regions" (CDR1,2,3).

Segments encoded by the junctional gene sequences are designated as *J* and those of the diversity gene sequences are designated *D*. Constant domains of the light chain are designated *CL*. Constant domains of the heavy chains are designated *CH1*, *CH2*, and *CH3*. Interchain disulfide bonds are designated -SS-. This basic structure is common to all immunoglobulins, but IgA is present primarily in a dimeric configuration and IgM in a pentaneric configuration is depicted in figure 13.2. When IgG is exposed to papain it is cleaved at the hinge region so that two Fab fragments consisting of a light chain joined to the V, D, J, and Ch1 regions of the heavy chain are formed. A single Fc fragment, crystalizable fragment, is formed by the joined remainders of the heavy chains. Exposure to pepsin cleaves IgG into a fragment formed by the light chains joined to a portion of the heavy chains by intact disulfide bonds, F(abó)2.

The remainder of the heavy chains undergo digestion and serve no biologic function.

Table 13.2. Immunoglobulin Values in Children and Adults

	IgA	IgG	IgM	IgE	IgD
Molecular weight (kd)	150	150	950	190	185
Heavy chain	α	Y	μ	ϵ	λ
Light chain					κ, λ
Biologic life (T½d)	6	21	5	2	3
Serum concentration	2.5	11.0	1.5	<.05	<.05
distribution (%)	15	80	5		

chains linked to two heavy chains (3). Each immunoglobulin molecule consists of two identical light chains and two identical heavy chains. There are two types of light chains, kappa, κ, and lambda, λ, and five types of heavy chains: gamma, α; mu, μ; alpha, α; epsilon, ϵ; and delta δ. Therefore, the paired heavy chains determine the class of immunoglobulin. The light chains are common to all immunoglobulins chains, but each immunoglobulin molecule has only paired κ- or λ-chains. Generally, each light chain couples to a heavy chain through disulfide bonds. Disulfide bonds also couple the heavy chain pairs.

In plasma IgG, IgA and IgE are present as a monomeric unit of two light chains and two heavy chains. IgM is present almost exclusively as a pentamer of five monomeric units joined by a polypeptide molecule, the J, or joining, chain (fig. 13.2). Minute quantities of monomeric IgM can be detected in normal individuals. Secretory IgA is produced by IgA-secreting plasma cells in the lamina propria of mucosally lined tissues such as the gastrointestinal tract, respiratory tract, and urogenital system. Secretory IgA is composed of two monomeric units joined by a J chain and a secretory component (SC), which is necessary for its transport across surface epithelial cells and is synthesized by those cells (4) (fig. 13.2).

Immunoglobulins G and A can be further categorized by antigenic differences of their heavy chains. These antigenic differences give rise to four IgG subclasses termed "IgG1," "IgG2," "IgG3," and "IgG4" (4). There are two IgA subclasses: IgA1 and IgA2 (5). Although subgroups of immunoglobulin λ-light chains have been identified, these have not been systematized as have those of the heavy chains.

The introduction of bacterially derived restriction endonucleases that cleave DNA or RNA at specific sites and "excise" fragments of genetic material has greatly increased the sophistication and the accuracy of analysis of immunoglobulin structure and antibody diversity. In man the chromosomal locations of the genes encoding the light and the heavy chains of immunoglobulins have been identified. The heavy chains are encoded by genes on chromosome 14

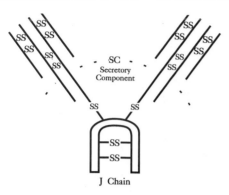

Secretory IgA

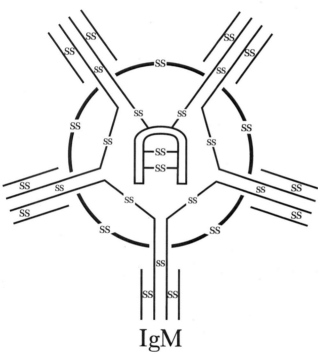

IgM

Figure 13.2. The basic structures of IgA and IgM. Secretary IgA is formed by the joining of two monomeric IgA units by a J chain. The secretory component SC binds to this dimer and protects it from proteolysis by digestive enzymes. Serum IgM is formed by the joining of five monomeric units by a single J chain. In both immunoglobulins, light chains and heavy chains of the monomeric units are joined by disulfide bonds.

at band 832. κ-Light chains are encoded by genes on chromosome 2 at band p11. λ-Light chains are encoded by genes on chromosome 22 at band q11 (6). The precise arrangement of the DNA sequences which determine the structure of the heavy chains and the light chains has been identified. When used in conjunction with bacterial endonucleases, the polymerase chain reaction has enabled investigators to replicate, in quantity, DNA fragments of the constant domains, and the variable and the hypervariable regions of immunoglobulins. This development has permit-

ted the amino acid sequencing of immunoglobulin fragments and the identification of the specific amino acid sequences that affect antibody idiotypic specificity in isolated monoclonal antibodies.

DNA analysis has demonstrated that the primordial cells that give use to the cellular components of the B-cell system have the genes, "exons," and intervening DNA sequences, "introns," arranged in germ line configuration. In the germ line state, the light chain exons and introns, "domains," are grouped in a specific sequence. In κ-light chains, the variable (V) domains are separated from the joining (J) domains, which in turn are separated from the constant (C). The variable locus has 30–100 gene segments that govern the sequence of amino acids 1–95 of the variable region of the κ-light chain. The joining segment has five exons, one of which will encode the next 13 amino acids of the light chain. The κ-chain has only one constant (C) domain in germ line configuration. The λ-light chain has a different germ line configuration. The exons governing the variable region are separated from six paired J and C regions. Complementary J and C regions are always selected as a unit, $J\lambda 1, C\lambda 1$, through $J\lambda 6, C\lambda 6$. The IgG heavy chain is arranged similarly, but has a series of diversity (D) gene segments separating the V and J domains. There is a series of functional constant domain gene sequences that by selective deletion and recombination will determine the class of immunoglobulin IgM, G, A, D, or E produced by each cell. Two pseudogenes, ψ and $\psi\gamma$, are also located in this sequence. This process is termed "immunogloblin class switching" (7) (fig. 13.3). In the cell, heavy chain recombination antedates light chain recombination.

The process of immunoglobulin class switching is effected through a series of steps, culminating in the fully differentiated plasma cell that synthesizes antibody, of a single isotype and specificity. The pluripotential stem cells that initially become committed to B-cell differentiation do so through the action of a DNA recombinase, which in a κ-light chain B-cell results in the close approximation of one $V\kappa$ segment to one of the five J segments. The specific VJ combination is then approximated to the constant region. The intervening introns are still in place. These are excised by RNA recombinases, which leads to the creation of specific messenger RNA, mRNA. The heavy chain is generated through a similar series of recombinational steps (fig. 13.3). These gene rearrangements lead to the expression of primitive λ-5-genes and V pre-B-light chain genes, and can be used to define these early pre-B-cells by molecular techniques. Cytologically, the earliest pre-B-cell is defined by the presence of intracytoplasmic μ-chains that are demonstrated through the use of fluorescein-labeled specific anti-μ-antibodies or (Fab')2-fragments. The process of light chain gene rearrangement antecedes the appearance of membrane IgM (mIgM), which only occurs with the generation of paired heavy and

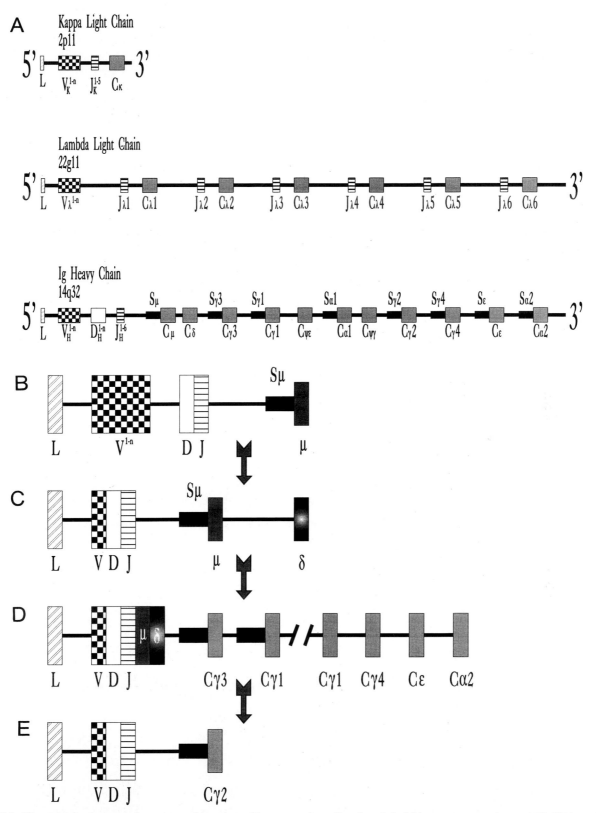

Figure 13.3. The organization and chromosomal location of immunoglobulin heavy chain and light chain genes. The germ line configuration is depicted (a). Antibody diversity is generated through the random joining of one D_H gene sequence with a JH sequence. The cleavage of the exons is not precise, so that there is variation in the DJ fusion products (b). The VH gene sequence is then joined to the DJ sequence. There is variability in the splice site of the VH sequence, so that variable VDJ combinations are formed (c). Initially, the rearranged VDJ gene DNA leads to the selection of Cμ and C-∣ genes segments (d). Further B-cell development levels to isotype switching by splicing at the switch region, S, of the final immunoglobulin class IgG2 is represented (e).

light chains. These membrane immunoglobulin-positive cells are already committed to the specificity of antibody that they and their progency will produce. The majority of these cells will generate membrane IgD (mIgD) early during their maturation and coexpress IgM and IgD on their surface membranes. When these cells are exposed to and respond to specific antigens, further maturation occurs in which subclass or isotypic specificity becomes fixed, and mIgM and mIgD can no longer be detected. The exons coding for M and D are downstream, nearer the 5′ terminus, from the heavy chain constant region. Such B-cells, although morphologically not plasma cells, are capable of secreting specific antibody. The generation of membrane-bound antibody or secreted antibody is the result of mRNA splicing that results in differing mRNAs governing the synthesis of secreted or membrane immunoglobulin structure. Associated with the process of isotypic diversification, B-cells express surface receptors that enable interactions with T-cells secreting IL2 through 7, and macrophages secreting IL-1 (fig. 13.4). In addition, complement receptors (CR1 and CR3) Fc receptors, Epstein-Barr virus (EBV) receptor, and human lymphocyte antigen (HLA)-DR antigens influence B-cell proliferation and maturation. Such differentiated B-cells are capable of responding to activation by dif-

ferentiating into plasma cells or memory B-cells. It is the memory B-cells that, when restimulated by specific antigen, can give rise to plasma cells that produce greatly increased amounts of high-affinity antibody, the secondary or "anamnestic" immune response.

The maturational process occurs in tandem with a proliferation of B-cells in each stage of development. It is during these proliferative phases that diversification occurs. The precise mechanism for diversification in man is not known. The principal sites of the B-cell system are the spleen, the lymph nodes, the lymphoid tissue of the gastrointestinal tract, and the respiratory tract, the liver, bone marrow, and the exocrine glands. In the chicken, B-cell formation is limited to the bursa of Fabricius during embryogenesis and early posthatching life (8). In mammalian species, no localized structure such as the bursa exists as a site for B-cell development. The most accepted concept is that during fetal development the liver, and later in life the liver and bone marrow, are the mammalian "bursal-equivalent" (9, 10). Anatomically in mammals, the Peyer patches of the ileum and the gut-associated lymphoid tissue (GALT) most resemble the bursa of Fabricius (11). In sheep, at 2–3 months of age when the ileal Peyer patches are at their maximal size, up to 3×10^9 surface IgM-positive B-cells are produced per hour. This high rate of

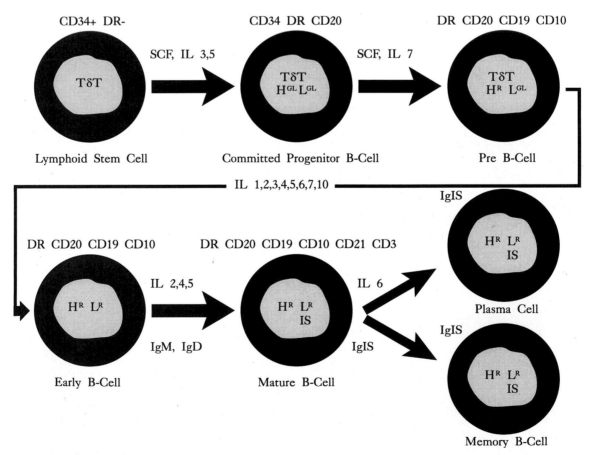

Figure 13.4. B-cell maturation. Immunoglobulin rearrangement and isotype switching is paralleled by changes in surface number, CD and DR, which identify the maturation of B-lineage cells. Cluster diversity, CD; major histocompatible complex antigen, DR; and light chains in germ line configuration, H^{GL} and L^{GL}; rearranged heavy and light chains, H^R and L^R isotype-specific heavy chians, IS; immunoglobulin, Ig; interleukin, IL.

production, most probably driven by exposure to food and bacterial antigens, is accompanied by an increasing diversity in the DNA's encoding for the V regions of the light and heavy chains. This hypermutation is not achieved by gene conversion as in the rabbit (12), but by untemplated somatic mutation (13). Which mechanism is at work in man is as yet unknown, possibly a combination of both.

The Histology of the B-Cell System

The B-cell system in man can be subdivided into two major functional units: (a) the bone marrow, and to some degree, the thymus and liver, which at some time in ontogeny contain pluripotent stem cells, and (b) the structural lymphoid follicles of the lymph nodes, gastrointestinal tract, tonsils, spleen, and the lymphocytes present in the gastrointestinal lamina propria, the exocrine glands, and the blood. The bone marrow and liver constitute the central B-cell organ. The other lymphoid tissues constitute the peripheral B-cell organ. After birth and throughout life, the bone marrow is the principal source of pluripotential B-cells.

The bone marrow has no circumscribed B-cell structure. However, there is an organization to B-cell maturation. Immature B-cells are located marginally at the endothelial surface of the cortex. As these cells proliferate and mature, they migrate centrally and are released into the venous sinuses of the marrow (14). The B-cells develop in contact with bone marrow stromal cells which supply cytokines such as IL-7 that are necessary for proliferation and maturation. In mice, approximately 75% of the B-cells are selectively destroyed during maturation in the marrow (15).

In lymph nodes, B-cells are located in the primary follicles and secondary germinal centers of the cortex. These are surrounded by the T-cell-rich paracortical area. It is in the follicles of the cortex that B-cells proliferate in response to antigen provocation. Antigens access lymph nodes via the afferent lymphatics, are processed by macrophages and rendered antigenic to T-cells and B-cells, and are then presented by the follicular dentritic cells (FDCs). In the follicle cell-dense "dark zone," apoptotic selection occurs in the adjacent basilar "light zone," and further differentiation into memory cells and plasma cells takes place in the apical light zone. Mature B-cells then migrate to the surrounding follicular mantle and B-cells proliferate and mature in response to processed antigen and T-cell-soluble cytokines. The resulting plasma cells migrate and are concentrated in the medulla of the node (fig. 13.5).

In the spleen, B-cells are located in the periarterial white pulp, marginal to the periarterial cuff of T-cells. As a mirror image of the follicular organization in lymph nodes, plasma cells are concentrated at the periphery of the B-cell follicles and distributed in the red pulp. The tonsils and the lymphoid follicles of the gut, e.g., Peyer patches, are the equivalent of the lymphoid tissues of the lymph nodes and the spleen (figs. 13.6 and 13.7).

The majority of B-cell antigen interactions that evoke an antibody response are the result of B-cell/T-cell interaction, i.e., T-cell-dependent antibody responses. In the unstimulated primary lymph node follicle, follicular dendritic cells (FDCs) form an interdigitating network that is filled with recirculating SIgD$^+$ B-cells. There are also a few CD4$^+$ T-cells and macrophages (16). When B-cell proliferation ensues as a result of antigenic stimulation, secondary follicles are formed. Initially, small follicular B-cells undergo blastic transformation and proliferate rapidly in the primary follicle center. Nonreacting small follicular B-cells are forced to the periphery and form the mantle. The next phase leads to the formation of the classical germinal center in which there is a rapid expansion of blastic cells derived from the initially proliferating cells. This progeny undergoes further expansion, migrates to the medullary cords, and differentiates into the IgM-secreting plasma cells of the primary immune reaction (17). The majority of cells involved in this process do not mature, but are subject to apoptosis, a programmed and selective death. The resulting nuclear detritus forms the densely basophilic "tingible" bodies seen in the macrophages of the germinal center. This process limits the number of B-cell clones that will generate a secondary immune response (18).

The dendritic cells of the follicle serve as antigen-presenting cells binding antigen for both B- and T-lymphocytes. Their dendritic processes make direct contact with each reatice lymphoid cell. Antigen presentation is required for both the primary and the secondary immune responses. If a secondary antigenic stimulus is not given, the germinal center involutes so that only a central core of B-blasts remains. If antigenic stimulation recurs, under T-cell control renewed proliferation ensues, resulting in B-cells with sIgM. These cells undergo further differentiation, lose their sIgM, and are programmed to produce antibodies of IgG or IgA class (19, 20).

The interaction of T-cells and B-cells that leads to maximal antibody synthesis is complex and incompletely understood. Cell-to-cell or intercellular communication is dependent upon the capacity of cells to make contact and adhere to one another (21). Cytoadhesion molecules such as LFA1 and ICAM1 and intercellular adhesion molecule are present on the surfaces of both T-cells and B-cells. Adhesion molecules also play a role in the trafficking of lymphocytes from the bone marrow to the peripheral lymphoid tissues and between lymphoid tissues (22). For most antigens, T-cell competence is required for effective antibody production by B-cells. The interaction of antigen-processing cells, T-cells, and B-cells is governed by identity of the major histocompatibility complex (MHC) antigens, termed "MHC restriction." For helper, CD4$^+$ T-cells, it is the D series of antigens, class II antigens, that must be identical, and for suppressor CD8$^+$ T-cells, it is the Class I antigens that must be identical. Antigen-bearing macrophages and B-cells interact with MHC restricted T-cells.

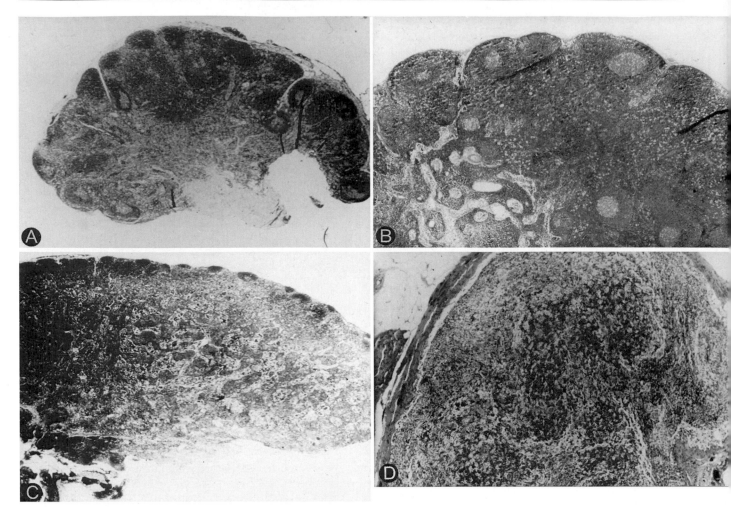

Figure 13.5. Lymph node—normal and X-linked a-γ-globulinemia. **A. Normal-low power.** The cortical and medullary areas are densely populated. The cortical area has numerous primary follicles with light central areas and germinal centers more homogeniously dark. These areas are composed primarily of B-cells. The medulla and medullary cords between the follicles are densely populated with T-cells. **B. Normal-high power.** The germinal centers are well demarcated. The areas in between are populated primarily with T-cells. **C. X-linked a-γ-globulinemia-low power.** The cortical areas are hypocellular. No primary follicles or germinal centers are seen clearly. The medulla is normally cellular. **D. X-linked hypo-γ-globulinemia-high power.** The cortical B-cell areas are hypoplastic. The medullary cords have a normal number of cells. (Courtesy of F. A. Good.)

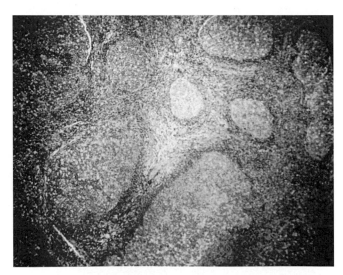

Figure 13.6. Normal tonsil. The B-cell risk follicles are well demaricated and highly cellular. (Courtesy of R. A. Good.)

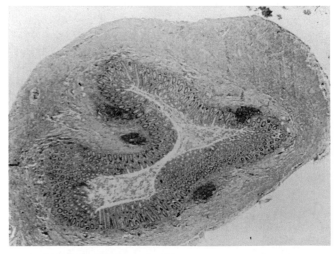

Figure 13.7. Normal appendix. The laminar propria contains richly populated follicles containing B-cells, characteristic of the gut-associated lymphoid tissue (GALT). (Courtesy of R. A. Good.)

Antigens can be "recognized" effectively only in conjunction with MHC restriction. This recognition activates T-cells and macrophages to synthesize and secrete soluble growth factors called "lymphokines" or "cytokines," which results in ampliation of both the T-cell and B-cell response (23). In addition to their proliferative and activating effects, lymphokines can also have suppressive activities, and through these can balance the immune response (24). This T-cell/B-cell interaction evokes mutual activation and proliferation. B-Cells also act as antigen-presenting cells for T-cells that respond and secrete growth and maturational factors further enhancing B-cell activation and proliferation.

B-Cells can respond to a limited array of antigens without interaction with T-cells. These T-cell-independent immune reactions are generally stimulated by exposure to complex repetitive structures such as polysaccharides, endotoxin, and aggregated protein. The resulting antibodies are exclusively of IgM class, since T-cell interaction is required for B-cells to switch antibody type from IgM to IgG, IgA, or IgE.

Immune regulation on a cellular basis is effected through the helper/inducer CD4$^+$ and suppressor/cytotoxic CD8$^+$ T-cell populations, and through the secretion into the fluid phase of cytokines by these cells. Antibodies produced to a specific antigenic determinant or "epitope" have a specific amino acid sequence in the hypervariable region of the heavy chains and the light chains. This structural unit is termed an "idiotype." Because of this unique amino acid sequence, idiotypic antibodies can stimulate the production of antiidiotypic antibodies. This reciprocal production is another mechanism for controlling the antibody response. The dynamic balance between idiotypic antibody and antiidiotypic antibody has been termed the network theory by Jerne (25). Depending upon the interaction with antibody and specific T-cells, antiidiotypic antibodies can stimulate or inhibit specific antibody production. The demonstration of antiidiotypic antibody in commercially available pooled intravenous α-globulin supports the notion that such antibodies do occur as a consequence of the normal immune response (26).

Immunoglobulin Structure and Function

The B-cell system subserves a single function: the production of antibodies in response to immune provocations. It is these antibodies of differing specificities that are the effector molecules of the humoral immune system. Immunoglobulins have a basically similar structure that endows each molecule with the separate properties of antibody specificity and of biologic function. Antibody specificity is determined by the antibody-combining site of the variable regions of the light and the heavy chain,

the Fab or F(ab')$_2$ fragment. Biologic activity is determined solely through the structure of the constant regions of the heavy chain, which comprise the Fc fragment.

The separation of plasma or serum proteins entered the modern era through the development of electrophoresis in 1937. In this procedure, the migration of proteins is effected by placing serum in a buffered electric field. The proteins' migration is dependent upon their charge at a given pH. The original procedure was cumbersome, but did identify the five protein fractions that are still defined presently: the α-, β-, α-2- and α-1 globulins, and albumin.

Immunoglobulins are quantitatively greatest in the α-globulin fraction, but have broad electrophoretic mobility and are present also in the β- and α-2-globulin fractions. If used, serum electrophoresis primarily serves only as a screening procedure since it is not selective for immunoglobulins. The most useful nonquantitative technique for detecting abnormalities of serum immunoglobulins is immunoelectrophoresis. In this procedure, serum is placed in a well cut in an agar-coated slide on an acrylamide strip. After electrophoresis has been completed, a trough is cut parallel to the direction of protein migration. The trough is filled with an antiserum to whole human serum or to selected serum proteins. The antiserum and the electrophoresed serum proteins diffuse through the gel and form precipitates in the gel. Each preciptin line defines a specific serum protein class. Immunoelectrophoresis permits the qualitative identification of IgG, IgM, and IgA, and is of use in detecting globulins of restricted mobility. The latter are termed "paraproteins" and are the products of a single clone of cells as is seen in multiple myeloma. The quantification of specific immunoglobulins is best accomplished by the use of radial immunodiffusion, enzyme-linked immunosorbent assays (ELISA), or nephelometric techniques.

The structure of the immunoglobulins has been well defined and has been codified by the World Health Organization (2, 3). Five classes of immunoglobulin (Ig) have been recognized: IgG, IgM, IgA, IgD, and IgE. IgG has been subdivided further into four subclasses: IgG1, IgG2, IgG3, and IgG4 (4). The subdivision has been based on antigenic differences of the heavy chains. Similar differences are present in the heavy chains of IgA. These have two identified subclasses, IgA1 and IgA2 (5). A further delineation of IgG diversity is the allotype differences of the Gm antigens of the heavy chains. The Gm allotypes are inherited as codominant allelic gene products and are usually defined by hemagglutination inhibition of Rh+ erythrocytes coated with IgG anti-D of known Gm specificity (indicator). The antibody-coated red cells are agglutinated by human serum-containing antiallotypic antibody for the specific Gm type of the anti-D. If serum contains IgG of the same allotype as that of the indicator, it will inhibit agglutination when the specific antiallotype antibody is added. By use of this technique, allotypic markers have been identified in IgG1, IgG2, IgG3, IgG4, IgA₂, and IgE (27). Allotypic differences in Gm types are associated with differences in the levels of IgG1, IgG2, and IgG3 (28). κ-Chain allotypes (Km) have also been identified with this technique. Antibody responses to *Haemophilus influenzae* polysaccharide vaccine have been associated with differences in Km allotypes (29).

Structural and Metabolic Properties of the Immunoglobulins

The genetic information for encoding the immunoglobulins is distributed on three chromosomes: the heavy chains on chromosome 14, κ-light chains on chromosome 2, and λ-light chains on chromosome 22. Individual immunoglobulin molecules are assembled intracellularly after the heavy and light chains have been synthesized on the endoplasmic reticulum of the ribosomes. The diversity of antibodies is generated through combination differences between the V and J regions of the light chains and the V, D, and J regions of the heavy chains and also through the C regions of the heavy chains generated through isotype switching. To date, 300 V region, 30 D region, and 6 functional J region heavy chain genes have been identified (30) (fig. 13.1).

Antibody specificity is established through the pairing of heavy chains and light chains. The specificity is determined primarily by the V_H domain since antibodies of differing specificities rarely have the same V_H domain. However, antibodies of differing specificities may contain identical V_L domains (31). The association between light chains and heavy chains is not random. The binding affinities for complementary heavy chains and light chains are greater than that of randomly paired chains. The diversity of antibodies is created primarily through the process of somatic joining of different V segments, D and J segments of the heavy chain, and V and J segments of the light chain, and not through multiple gene products. The number of permutations is increased through imprecise excision of the V, D, J segments prior to assembly so that minor amino acid sequence differences in the leader, i.e., the upstream portion of the V, D, and J segments (32). These variations underlie the estimated 10^{10} distinct specificities present in humans.

The paired light and heavy chains are joined by disulfide bonds forming a unit. The heavy chains of two identical units are then joined by disulfide bonds forming an immunoglobulin molecule (fig. 13.8). IgA2 molecules lack the disulfide bonding of heavy and light chains. In this subclass, the light chains are joined by covalent disulfide bonds, while the heavy and light chains are joined together by non-covalent bonds. The paired light chains and heavy chains are fundamental to the structure of the immunoglobulin molecule. All IgG antibodies consist of two

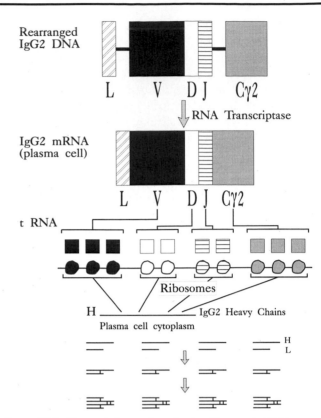

Figure 13.8. Transcription and synthesis of human IgG2. The specifically rearranged IgG2 DNA is transcribed through the enzymatic action of RNA transcriptasce to IgG2 messenger RNA (mRNA). Through the activity of transfer RNA (tRNA), the IgG2 transcript is incorporated into ribosomes from which nascent IgG2 heavy chains κ-light chains are synthesized, undergo similar processing, and are synthesized independently. Complimentary heavy chains and light chains are joined intracellularly, forming IgG2 molecules of given specificity.

α-heavy chains and two identical κ- or λ-light chains. Antibodies of the IgM class consist of five identical molecules of paired μ-heavy chains and light chains joined by the J (joining) piece. IgA molecules are composed of two or three identical molecules of paired α-heavy chains and light chains joined by a J piece. Secretory IgA has, in addition, a protective secretory component (SC) (fig. 13.2). The secretory component is synthesized by epithelial cells in proximity to the IgA-producing plasma cells. The binding of the SC to IgA molecules occurs extracellularly prior to transport of IgA through mucosal epithelial cells. IgE and IgD are similarly comprised of paired ϵ- or δ-heavy chains and κ- or λ-light chains. When molecules of IgG are exposed to reducing agents in urea-containing buffers, the interchain disulfide bonds are cleaved, releasing light chains and heavy chains. The light chains and heavy chains subsequently can be separated by chromatography on gel filtration columns.

Two other degradative procedures employed to derive fragments from IgG have yielded important information about the structure and function of IgG and, by extension, to the other classes of immunoglobulins. When IgG is exposed to the enzyme papain in a cysteine-containing buffer, it is cleaved into three fragments. A crystallizable fragment composed of portions of the heavy chain, the Fc fragment, and two Fab fragments that contain the antibody-combining region of the light chain and the heavy chain. The Fab fragments are univalent and have the capacity to bind antigen, but not to form precipitates. The Fab and the Fc fragments can be separated by employing column chromatography or block electrophoresis. IgG is also subject to degradation when exposed to the action of the enzyme pepsin in buffered solution. Pepsin cleaves the molecules yielding a retrievable (Fab′)2 fragment that consists of the antibody-combining sites of paired light chains and a portion of the heavy chain. The fragment retains an interheavy chain disulfide bond. Therefore, it is bivalent and can form precipitates with specific antigen. The portion of the heavy chain not contained in the F(ab′)2 fragment is cleaved into multiple fragments so that no heavy chain functional unit corresponding to the Fc fragment is formed. The disulfide bonds of the Fab fragment, F(ab′)2 or the Fc fragment can be cleaved by exposure to reducing agents yielding the individual constituent light chain (fig. 13.1).

Investigations of the subunits of IgG have furthered understanding of the basic structure and function of the immunoglobulins. Light chains consist of a variable domain, a junctional domain, and a single constant domain or region. Heavy chains of the immunoglobulins contain three variable domains that are determined by the V, D, and J gene product alignments. These inconstant domains are linked to the constant region domains that differ in number in the different immunoglobulin classes. IgG, IgA, and IgD heavy chains each have three constant domains, C1–C3. IgM and IgA heavy chains each have four constant domains, C1–C4.

The antibody-combining site is determined by the amino acid sequences of the V region of the light and heavy chains. The amino acid sequences of the first 95 amino acids of the light chain and 94 amino acids of the heavy chain govern antibody specificity. It must be noted, however, that antibodies of different specificities may have identical amino acid sequences in the VH and the VL domains (31). Antibody specificity may be influenced by subtle configurational variations that permit alterations in electrical charge of the combing site (33). If Fab light chains and heavy chain moieties of a given antibody are separated by reductive cleavage, weak binding of the heavy chain to the antigen can be demonstrated. However, binding to antigen is optimal only when specific light chains and heavy chains are joined.

The biologic properties of immunoglobulins are determined by the constant regions of the heavy chains and reside within the Fc fragment (table 13.3). The level of IgG in the newborn is governed by placental transport of maternal IgG. This active transport is specifically dependent upon the Fc fragment. The level of IgG at birth is therefore dependent upon the mother's IgG level. Not all subclasses of IgG are transported equally. In the newborn, the level of IgG2 is lower than that of the mother. Immunoglobulins of IgA, IgM, and IgE classes are not transported transplacentally. The presence of significant levels of IgM or IgA in the newborn is evidence of intrauterine infection, e.g., rubella, cytomegalovirus, HIV. Elevated levels of IgE in the newborn may predict atopy in later life.

Complement activation is one of the principal immunologic amplification systems effected primarily by antibodies of IgG or IgM class. Complement activation products enhance phagocytosis of particulate antigens, influence the binding of antibody to antigens and modify both T-cell and B-cell responses to antigens. Variability exists among the IgG subclasses in their capacity to activate the classical complement pathway. Antibodies of IgG1 and IgG3 subclasses are potent activators; IgG2 antibodies have less capacity to activate complement and IgG4 antibodies lack the capacity to activate complement. The pentameric form of IgM antibodies are the most effective activators of the classical complement pathway. Antibodies of the IgA class do not activate complements via the classical pathway, but can activate complement via the alternative pathway. The classical pathway is activated when antibody-antigen complexes bind C1. After binding C1 cleaves C4 and C2, which in turn results in

Table 13.3. Biologic Functions of Immunoglobulins IgG, M, A, and E

Function	IgC1	IgG2	IgG3	IgG4	IgM	IgA	IgA (secretory)	IgE
Transported across placenta	+	±	+	+	−	−	−	−
Associated with primary response	−	−	−	−	+	−	−	−
Associated with secondary response	+	+	+	+	−	+	+	+
Present in exocrine secretions	+	+	+	−	+	+	−	−
Complement activation	+	±	+	−	+	+[a]	+[a]	−
Opsonization	+	+	+	+	+	−	−	−
Agglutination	+	+	+	+	+	−	−	−
Hemolysis	+	+	+	+	+	±	−	−
Mast cell degranulation	−	−	−	−	−	−	−	+
Passive cutaneous anaphylaxis	−	−	−	−	−	−	−	+
Virus neutralization	+	+	+	+	+	−	+	−

[a]Activation via the alternative pathway.

activation/cleavage of C3 and the late complement components, C5–C9. The alternate pathway is a non-antibody-dependent mechanism of cleaving C3 and the late components and does not require the activation of C1, C4, or C2.

The classes of immunoglobulins vary significantly in their distribution in the body. This distribution influences the broad biologic role subserved by each immunoglobulin class. IgG is the major immunoglobulin of the intravascular and extravascular fluid compartment and constitutes the major immunoglobulin of the secondary response. It constitutes approximately 75% of the plasma immunoglobulins and almost all of the immunoglobulins of the interstitial fluids. Approximately 55% of the total body IgG is intravascular. Because of their distribution and their capacity to activate complement, antibodies of IgG class are the major effector molecules of the host's defense against microorganisms and virus. The antibody repertoire of each subclass of IgG varies in its broad specificities. Antibodies of IgG1 subclass have antiprotein specificity. IgG2 antibodies possess anticarbohydrate specificity. IgG3 antibodies have antiviral activity. Antibodies of IgG4 subclass have been associated with antifactor VIII activity, but their principal antigen targets have not been identified. The Fc portion of IgG antibodies subserves their binding to many differing cell types, neutrophils, macrophages, T-cells, and platelets, and facilitates phagocytosis and intracellular killing by neutrophils and macrophages and antibody-dependent cell-mediated cytotoxicity by T-cells. Clinically, significant susceptibility to bacterial infection has been associated with a deficiency of one or more IgG subclasses or an IgG subclass and IgA deficiency (34). Many of these patients may have total serum IgG in the normal range and therefore require quantitation of the individual subclasses to define their immunodeficiency.

IgM antibodies are the antibodies produced initially in the primary response to antigenic stimulation. This IgM response characteristically is short-lived and in most instances decreases as mature B-cells switch to the specific antibody class affecting more durable immunity. Certain antigens, the T-cell independent antigens, do not result in isotype switching, and persistence of IgM antibodies results. Such antigens are frequently polysaccharide antigens such as the A and B blood group substances, P antigens, and cardiolipin or endotoxin. Antibodies to Gm allotypes found in the serums of many individuals with rheumatoid arthritis and rheumatoid factor are of IgM class.

Since agglutination occurs when antigens present on a particular surface are in close approximation and are linked by antibody of multiple valance, the pentameric form of IgM is the most potent agglutinating antibody. Complement activation is most effective when at least two heavy chain Fc fragments of antigen-bound antibody are in close approximation. Such a configuration is most frequently observed in the interaction of pentameric IgM with antigen. Therefore, IgM antibodies are the most effective activators of the classical complement system.

Because of its large size (900 kd molecular weight), IgM is restricted primarily to the intravascular space. Since it agglutinates particles and is an efficient activator of complement, IgM is a major immunoglobulin involved in specific host defense to intravascular bacterial infection. Agglutinated and opsonized antibody plus complement-coated particles are efficiently phagocytosed by the fixed macrophage system of the spleen and the liver. IgM also exists in monomeric form, and IgM monomers are present in serum from cord blood. However, in immunologically mature individuals, IgM monomers have been found primarily in individuals with immunodeficiencies such as ataxia-telangeletasia and dys-γ-globulinemia, and in perturbed immunologic states such as rheumatoid arthritis, Waldenstrom macroglobulinemia, and systemic lupus erythematosus.

IgA is the major antibody class found in secretions of the gastrointestinal tract, the respiratory tract, and the genitourinary tract. In these secretions, IgA is present primarily in its dimeric form containing the J piece and the secretory component. The majority of secretory IgA is of IgA2 subclass. Within the intravascular compartment, IgA is monomeric, lacks the J and SC portions of the molecule, and is primarily of IgA1 subclass. IgA antibodies are effective in host defense by their specific binding at mucosal surfaces to bacteria, parasites, and virus. IgA in the plasma is reflective of secretory IgA, and much intravascular IgA is produced by exocrine glands. Physiologically, IgA2 is resistant to bacterial IgA proteases, whereas IgA1 is cleaved by these enzymes. Because absence of secretory IgA is associated with absent serum IgA, screening for IgA deficiency is performed on serum. Secretory IgA can be collected with relative ease by stimulating the secretion of saliva by having the patient chew wax. The use of a Kirby parotid cap provides a noninvasive means of obtaining salivary IgA directly from the parotid gland. Individuals with IgA deficiencies have an increased frequency of acute and chronic sinopulmonary infections, demonstrating the unique role of this immunoglobulin in the host's mucosal defense.

The precise role of IgE in host defense has not been defined. This immunoglobulin is known through its role in type I anaphylactic reactions. These reactions are mediated through the release of vasoactive substances, which occurs when tissue mast cells or basophiles are activated through the binding of specific antigens by membrane bound IgE. The interaction of membrane bound IgE with antigen and the release of vasoactive peptides enhances vascular permeability which may permit more intravascular IgG to diffuse into a specific tissue site. Deficiencies of serum IgE have not been associated with any clinical syndrome of immune deficiency.

The biologic importance of IgD most probably is related to its presence on the cell surface of early B-cells where it serves as an antigen receptor. IgD constitutes <1% of intravascular immunoglobulin, but constitutes a significantly greater presence on B-cell membranes and is involved in the cellular generation of the antibody response.

The early diagnosis of an immunodeficiency disorder is based on the recognition that a patient's infectious history differs from what is to be expected in a normal individual of comparable age. Since the majority of defined immunodeficiencies in childhood occur in boys, an accurate family history with emphasis on the maternal pedigree is valuable. Family history is also important in order to define inbreeding, e.g., first cousin marriages in which offspring have an 8-fold increase in autosomal recessive inherited diseases above that of the general population. An infectious disease history of the parents, especially with regard to factors associated with an increased risk of HIV infection, e.g., multiple sex partners, high-risk sexual practices, intravenous blood products, and the birth of a child with documented HIV infection must be obtained, since the associated immunodeficiency has become the most frequent identifiable immunodeficiency state.

Case 1 (continued)

The subject was initially seen clinically at 3 months of age with P. aeruginosa *sepsis and neutropenia. His clinical course during this episode was not remarkable. The occurrence of* Pseudomonas *sepsis in an infant of this age certainly could be viewed with interest since this bacterium is an unusual cause of sepsis in infancy. However, the rapid improvement of the patient and his normal growth did not prompt further investigation. We believed that his sepsis might have been a chance event. Furthermore, the patient received DPT immunization, which is ineffective in severe immunologic-deficient patients, and oral polio vaccine, which is contraindicated in such patients, because of the risk of paralytic disease in immunocompromised infants.*

A list of probable immunodeficiencies that could be the base for infections at 3 months of age would include HIV infection, severe combined immunodeficiency disease, or other significant T-cell deficiency states and defects of the phagocytic system. Unusual infections in full-term infants with primary B-cell deficiencies are infrequent before 6 months of age because of protection afforded by transplacentally transported maternal IgG. At birth, infants' IgG levels are equal to or higher than their mothers'. If a mother has low IgG, the newborn will have a low level.

At 4 months of age, the patient was found to have Pneumocystis carinii *pneumonia. The isolation of this protozoa by bronchoalveolar lavage or open-lung biopsy is prima facie evidence of significant immunodeficiency essentially in the host. When this event is coupled with the episode of* Pseudomonas *sepsis at the age of 3 months, a clinical diagnosis of immunodeficiency essentially is established. The problem facing the clinician is to define precisely the basis of the immunodeficiency.*

Classically, an unusual history of infections in the first 4 months of life is characteristic of T-cell deficiencies or of combined T-cell and B-cell deficiencies. Such immunodeficiencies are characterized more by fungal infections and opportunistic infections, such as *Pneumocystis carinii*, than by bacterial infections. Many affected infants also suf-

fer from chronic diarrhea and failure to thrive. Although useful, these parameters are not precise enough to distinguish cellular from humoral immunodeficiencies. It is through laboratory determinations of the cellular and the humoral components of the immune system that a defect can be categorized (fig. 13.9).

Absolute Lymphocyte Count

The absolute lymphocyte count, WBC $\times$ percentage of lymphocytes, may be decreased in T-cell deficiencies, in severe combined immunodeficiency states, and in advanced HIV infections, but not in restricted antibody deficiency states. Since only 15–20% of circulating lymphocytes are of B-cell lineage, even their complete absence will not decrease the lymphocyte count $<1.5 \times 10^9/L$. The patient discussed had an absolute lymphocyte count of $(64,000 \times 0.48)$, $6.912 \times 10^9/L$. This finding excludes the majority of T-cell deficiencies or combined immunodeficiencies as probable diagnostic possibilities, but does not rule them out entirely.

T-Cell and B-Cell Determinations

The availability of monoclonal antibodies has enabled the ready laboratory characterization of the broad classes of T-cells and B-cells and the specific developmental stages and subsets that identify their maturational stage and physiologic roles. The patient had increased percentages of mature, T-3 positive and T-11 positive, T-lymphocytes and the virtual absence of mature B-lymphocytes identified as B positive. Further evidence consistent with a profound B-cell deficiency was the lack of surface immunoglobulin, κ- or λ-chains, and the lack of demonstrable intracytoplasmic μ-chains. Biopsy specimens of the bone marrow and rectal mucosa lacked any identifiable plasma cells. In terms of cellular constituents, the patient suffered from an apparent pure B-cell deficiency. The absence of expression of intracytoplasmic chains identifies the defect as occurring earlier in B-cell maturation than the pre-B cell that is the maturational stage noted in patients with classical X-linked a-γ-globulinemia. In vitro assays of T-cell function, responses to mitogens such as PHA, ConA, and tetanus were within the normal range. These findings effectively rule out severe T-cell or severe combined immunodeficiencies as the cause of the patient's immune defect. Since profound T-cell deficiency seems an unlikely cause for the patient's infections, investigation should be directed towards the B-cell or antibody deficiency diseases.

Quantification of Serum Immunoglobulins and Antibodies

Immunoglobulins were assayed by single radial immunodiffusion. In this technique, a precise amount of serum, 10 μl, is placed in a well cut in a gel containing specific antibody to the protein to be quantified. As the serum dif-

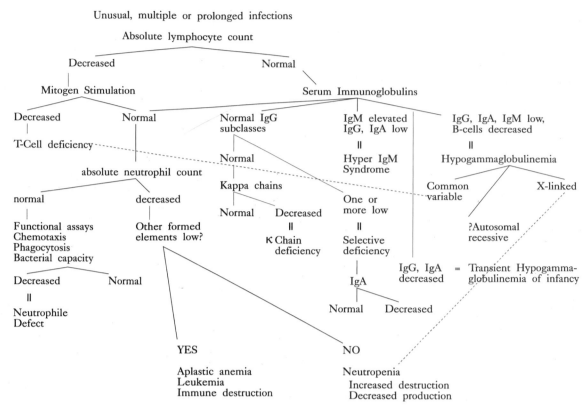

Figure 13.9. Algorithm for the diagnosis of the patient with B-cell deficiency.

fuses into the gel, a circular area of precipitation appears. After overnight incubation, the diameter of the circle is measured. A number of standard concentrations of the specific protein are assayed with each lot of sera to be quantified. The concentration of the protein is proportioned to the $\log_{10}$ of the diameter of the precipitin reaction. The diameters of the precipitates of the standards are plotted on semilogarithmic paper, and from the lines constructed the concentrations of the unknown samples are determined. The patient's immunoglobulins G, M, and A were significantly below the levels of normal infants of the same age. Since the patient had received two immunizations with DPT, detectable antibody levels to diphtheria and tetanus would be expected, but none were demonstrated. Detectable anti-A or anti-B isohemagglutinins would be expected in an infant of 4 months of age. The patient was of blood group A, but had no detectable anti-B. Therefore, by these parameters, the patient lacked the ability to respond to specific antigen challenge.

Patients may have low immunoglobulin levels and borderline specific antibody responses, but not suffer from a primary antibody deficiency. Such low levels may be found in patients with significant protein loss, e.g., patients with exudative enteropathy or the nephrotic syndrome. In such individuals, the protein loss is generalized and not restricted to immunoglobulins. This loss would be manifest by a low serum albumin. The patient's serum albumin was normal, 3.8 g/dl. Therefore, since no evidence for immunodeficiency secondary to HIV infection was identified, the patient suffers from a primary antibody deficiency.

The primary antibody deficiency states have been classified recently by a scientific group of the World Health Organization (6). Table 13.4 lists the major features of the antibody deficiency states. The investigation of these "experiments of nature" has provided vital information about normal B-cell function and its role in normal host defense mechanisms. Although as tabulated, each entity appears to be clearly delineated, there is a continuum of pathogenetic mechanisms, so that the intrinsic defects are not always clearly defined. Therefore, categorization may depend on the clinical course of the individual patient.

Specific Deficiency States (Fig. 13.9)

X-Linked A-γ-globulinemia

The initial report by Bruton of a boy with repeated infections and absent serum γ-globulins as defined by serum electrophoresis (35) established the identity and the concept of an inborn defect of antibody production. Classical X-linked a-γ-globulinemia is inherited as a Mendelian X-linked trait, and only males are affected.

It must be remembered that the genes encoding the heavy chains are located on chromosome 14_q32, the κ-chain on chromosome 2p11 and the λ-chain on 22_q11. The genes associated with classical X-linked a-γ-globulinemia are located at $X_q21.2\text{-}22$ (36). Since this molecular genetic finding defines X-linked a-γ-globulinemia, the effect cannot determine heavy or light chain synthesis, but must in some manner influence B-cell maturation. Consistent with this chromosomal finding is the "arrest" of B-cell maturation at the pre-B-lymphocyte stage. There is a virtual absence of surface immunoglobulin bearing B-cells in the peripheral blood of patients with classical X-linked disease (37). However, pre-B-cells can be identified in the bone marrow (38). The early B-cells of mothers who are obligate carriers have been reported to have abnormal development of immunoglobulin secretion (39). There appears to be a nonrandom inactivation of the X-chromosome in the B-cell line of obligate carriers, since B-cell lines "immortalized" by Epstein-Barr virus

(EBV) transformation have only the normal X pattern rather than the 1:1 ratio of normal and abnormal X patterns anticipated by the Lyon hypothesis (40). This unique lyonization permits the detection of female carriers of the classic disease.

There can be no doubt that X-linked a-γ-globulinemia is the quintessential example of an antibody deficiency state. When restricted in its definition to (a) males, (b) a lack of circulating B-cells, (c) the presence of pre-B-cells, (d) absence of immunoglobulins and lack of specific antibody responses to potent antigens, (e) normal cell-mediated immunity, (f) a demonstrated genetic variant at X_q 21.3-22,

Table 13.4. Primary Antibody Deficiencies States[a]

Designation	Serum Ig	Circulating B-cells	Presumed Pathogenesis	Inheritance	Associated Features
X-linked agammaglobulinemia	Al isotypes decreased	Profoundly decreased	Intrinsic defect pre-B- to B-cell differentiation	XL	
Ig deficiency with increased IgM (hyper-IgM syndrome)	IgM increased and IgD increased or normal other isotypes decreased	IgM and IgD bearing cells normal; others absent	Isotype switch defect	Various; XI, AR, unknown	Autoimmune neutropenia, thrombocytopenia, hemolytic anemia
Ig heavy chain gene deletions	IgG1 or IgG2, IgG4 absent and in some cases IgB and IgA2 absent	Normal	Chronfosomial deletion at 14q32	AR	
κ-Chain deficiency	Ig(k) decreased; antibody response normal or decreased	Normal or decreased κ-bearing B-cells	Point mutations at chromosome 2p11 in some patients	AR	
Selective deficiency of IgG subclasses (with or without IgA deficiency)	Decrease in one or more IgG isotypes	Unknown	Defects or isotype differentation	Unknown	Recurrent sinopulmonary infections
CVID	Various decreases of multiple isotypes	Normal or decreased	Failure of terminal differentiation in B-cells of multiple isotypes; low B-cell unknown numbers; defective T helper function; antibodies to B-cells; augmented suppressor function	Various: AR, AD, or unknown	Recurrent sinopulmonary infections, chronic lung disease, increased lymphoreticular malignancies
IgA deficiency	IgA and IgA2 decreased	Normal	Failure of terminal differentiation in IgA B-cells	Various; AR, unknown	Autoimmune and allergic disorders
Transient hypo-γ-globulinemia of infancy	IgG and IgA decreased	Normal	Differentiation defect: delayed maturation of helper function in some patients	Unknown	Frequent in families with other IDS

[a]Adapted from reference 6, by permission. CVID, common variable immunodeficiency; IDS, immune deficiency states.

and (g) a lack of normal lyonization of the X-chromosomes, classical X-linked a-γ-globulinemia becomes a specific disease entity (41). The recent delineation of a specific gene mutation is a significant advance in the diagnosis of this deficiency state (42). However, there are several entities which, although clinically identical, because lack of immunoglobulins, antibody synthesis, and by histologic appearance must be excluded from this diagnosis. The patient in case 1 had no identifiable pre-B-cells in the bone marrow and no family history consistent with X-linked disease. Studies are under way to define nonrandom X-inactivation and the gene abnormality. At least two families have been reported to have X-linked hypo-γ-globulinemia and isolated growth hormone deficiency (43, 44). When genetic studies were performed on the first families, no localization to X_q 21:3-22 could be defined (43). Female siblings with laboratory and clinical findings virtually indistinguishable from the X-linked disease have also been reported, which raises the possibility of a variant that has an autosomal recessive mode of inheritance (45).

The clinical course of children with X-linked a-γ-globulinemia is remarkably homogeneous. Usually, affected individuals begin to have recurrent pyogenic bacterial infections in infancy. Infections before 6–12 months of age are unusual because of the protection afforded the infant through the placental transport of maternal IgG. The most frequent sites of infection during early life are the middle ear, the sinuses, the lungs, and the skin. The infections, particularly of the ears and lungs, tend to be repetitive while the sinus infections are frequently chronic in nature. The majority of the ear and respiratory tract infections are found to be caused by *H. influenzae, Micrococcus aureus,* and *Streptococcus pneumoniae.* Infections with β-hemolytic *Streptococcus* and with *Pseudomonas* species are relatively infrequent (46). Gastrointestinal infections may be bacterial in origin, but opportunistic organisms such as *Giardia lamblia,* although infrequent, must be considered, particularly in patients with chronic diarrhea and weight loss. Pulmonary infections with *Pneumocystis carinii* do occur and attempts should be made to isolate this organism directly from the lungs in patients who suffer oxygen desaturation or appear to have an atypical course. In contrast to a preponderance of pyogenic bacterial infections, disease is infrequently associated with enteric Gram-negative bacteria.

The clinical course of most viral infections does not differ significantly from that of immunologically normal individuals, evidence that the immune response to viral infections is usually effective. However, a possibly increased incidence of paralytic disease has been reported to be associated with live polio vaccine (47). Therefore, immunization with any live viral vaccine must be avoided. Most patients have uncomplicated infections with varicella zoster and herpes simplex, but chronic cutaneous herpes simplex has been reported (48). Patients are susceptible to chronic enteroviral meningoencephalitis. Echovirus is the most frequently isolated agent, 37 of 41 cases, and X-linked a-γ-globulinemia was the most common antibody deficiency, 18 of 42 patients (49). Several patients have suffered from more than a single episode of enteroviral central nervous system (CNS) infections and 2 patients had paralytic polio prior to their echoviral infections. In patients with X-linked disease, echovirus infection is frequently associated with hepatitis, and a dermatomyositis-like syndrome, with large joint involvement, edema, and rashes. These nonneurologic findings are usually associated with disseminated disease or with chronic disease. The large joint arthritis is difficult to distinguish from a nonviral arthritis involving the large joints. Boys whose diagnosis has been delayed or who have been given inadequate doses of immunoglobulin frequently present with bronchiectasis caused by smoldering repeated episodes of pneumonia or with the nonviral arthritis which improves when adequate doses of γ-globulin are administered.

Bacterial meningitis has been reported to be the presenting illness in 10% of patients with X-linked disease. Septicemia is unusual and may reflect the adequacy of the nonspecific immune system, complement activation via the alternative pathway, in preventing bacterial dissemination through the generation of heat-labile opsonins.

Neutropenia is frequently associated with X-linked a-γ-globulinemia. It has been reported to occur in one-third of patients during the cause of their disease (50) and is frequently seen in association with pyogenic infections (51). Inspection of the bone marrow usually reveals normal myeloid maturation or a marrow "arrest" at the promyelocyte/myelocyte stage. The precise cause of the neutropenia remains ill defined. In most cases, the neutrophil count becomes normal when γ-globulin therapy is instituted. Autoimmune hemolytic anemia has been described in a child with X-linked disease (52).

The variability of the immunologic defect in patients with X-linked a-γ-globulinemia is perplexing and possibly will be resolved with modern molecular genetic techniques. As stated earlier, the definition of the disease may be restricted to individuals with the X_q 21.3-22 specific restriction length fragment polymorphism (RLFP). Even with this caveat, variability may be observed due to a "leaky gene effect." Such findings eventually may explain variants such as patients with X-linked a-γ-globulinemia in whom monoclonal IgG production develops (53) or whose B-cells contain intracytoplasmic IgG, but not surface IgG (54).

Physical Findings

The single physical finding common to individuals with X-linked a-γ-globulinemia is hypoplastic or absent tonsils, since tonsils contain primarily B- and not T-cells. The lymph nodes frequently are small and all B-cell-containing tissues are hypocellular (figs. 13.5–7). Plaque-like indurated skin lesions have been noted that consist of lymphohistiocytic cells (55). Hives developed in the patient in case 1 trimethaprim-sulfa methoxazole was administered. Urticarial reactions, while frequently associated with IgE-mediated mast cell degranulation, can be caused by non-immunologic mediators of mast cell histamine release, which may explain the nature of the patient's rash.

Laboratory Diagnosis

The diagnosis is dependent on the demonstration of markedly decreased levels of all serum immunoglobulin classes. In most individuals, IgG is <200 mg/dl. Antibody responses to specific antigens such as tetanus and diphtheria antigens are virtually absent after three challenges. Isohemagglutinins are usually undetectable. Investigations employing bacteriophage $\phi\xi$174 as a specific immunogen are particularly revealing. When this agent is administered to normal individuals, it is cleared from the blood within 3–4 days and is followed by an IgM primary response. A second dose will provide a secondary IgG antibody response and rapid clearance in the blood. In individuals with X-linked a-γ-globulinemia, antigen persists for weeks and no specific antibody IgM or IgG can be detected (56). However, this agent is available for investigational use only.

Transient Hypo-g-globulinemia of Infancy

Transient hypo-γ-globulinemia of infancy is seen at an early age with repeated pyogenic bacterial infections. Both sexes are affected. When this entity occurs in males, it must be distinguished from X-linked a-γ-globulinemia and from the physiologic hypo-γ-globulinemia of infancy, which characteristically occurs between the 3rd and 6th month of life (57). In its classical form, this syndrome clinically appears to be a prolongation of the physiologic state in which most patients become completely immunocompetent by 18–36 months of age. Common to all forms of this immunodeficiency is a decreased level of IgG. However, it must be noted that IgG levels in premature infants may be below the normal range for age, since the levels of IgG in infancy are influenced by the placental transfer of maternal IgG. This active transport begins at about 30 weeks of gestation and increases to term. Decreased levels of IgM or IgA or both may be associated with low IgG. Among the variants of this syndrome are infants who have a family history of immunodeficiency, especially severe combined immunodeficiency (58), or patients in whom IgA deficiency develops in later life (59). There is a significant variation in the ability to mount specific antibody responses to specific antigens such as diphtheria, tetanus, or bovine serum albumin. Isohemagglutinins are present, but may be reduced in titer (60). Patients must be followed over the long term in order to define the specific nature of their immunodeficiency.

Studies of lymphocyte populations invariably demonstrate the presence of membrane immunoglobulin-positive B-cells. These may be normal or even elevated in number. T-Cells are normal in number but may have an absolute decrease in the T4 subset. The response to mitogens is frequently normal; it may be reduced but not absent. In vitro studies of B-cell/T-cell interaction have demonstrated normal B-cell function but, in some patients, a lack of T-cell helper function (61). The decreased T-helper cell function becomes normal as the immunodeficiency abates. Lymph nodes, when biopsied, reveal abortive or absent germinal centers with a marked decrease in plasma cells.

Common Variable Immunodeficiency or Late Onset Hypo-γ-globulinemia

Common variable immunodeficiency is a classification applied to a diverse group of patients who have manifestations primarily of impaired B-cell function, but who most frequently have normal numbers of B-lymphocytes and subtle abnormalities of T-cell function. Although there is no single identifiable defect, all patients manifest abnormalities of antibody production and have a decrease in, or absence of, mature plasma cells in their lymphoid tissues. The abnormality is therefore defined by a lack of B-cell maturation at different stages of differentiation (62–64). A variety of causes for the perturbation of B-cell function have been reported: (a) the presence of serum-suppressive activity on B-cells (65); (b) suppressor T-cell activity (66); (c) absence of functional helper T-cell activity (67); (d) decreased of natural killer (NK) cell activity (68); and (e) autoantibodies directed against B-lymphocytes (69, 70). The spectrum of pathogenesis and the degree of immunologic heterogeneity reported in patients supports the postulate that common variable immunodeficiency is a group of immunodeficiencies that does not have a single cause, but does have a common clinical appearance—i.e., multiple infections with the laboratory findings of decreased IgG usually in association with decreased IgA and IgM. However, the levels of all immunoglobulins may vary and, with the exception of IgM, may be in the normal range. In vitro correction of IgG and IgM production has resulted from exposing autologous T-cells to the stimulating affect of a mitogenic monoclonal anti-CD3 antibody (71). Approximately 50% of affected individuals have defective T-cell function (72) and the degree of T-cell function appears to increase with the age of the patient (73). This implies that aberrations of T-cell function may have a significant pathogenic role in the genesis of this apparent B-cell deficiency.

Clinical Manifestations

The age at diagnosis of patients with common variable immunodeficiency varies widely. Although it occurs most frequently in the second and third decades of life, patients range from 3–71 years of age (74). Males and females are affected equally. Patients with common variable immunodeficiency invariably present with a history of recurrent bacterial sinopulmonary illness. These episodes are usually associated with infection by *M. pyogenes, H. influenzae,* and *S. pneumococcus.* Pulmonary infections with *Mycoplasma pneumoniae* and other

Mycoplasma species are also frequent, and if left untreated may result in chronic lung disease with bronchiectasis (74). At the time of diagnosis, chronic lung disease is a prominent and frequent physical finding in patients with common variable immunodeficiency. Therefore, cystic fibrosis is a frequent differential diagnosis. Documented episodes of pneumonia occur in at least 75% of patients (75). Other major sites of infection are the conjunctiva, liver, and meninges. Infrequently, infectious agents such as *H. zoster* and *P. carinii* that are associated with T-cell deficiency do cause disease.

Gastrointestinal disease characterized by recurrent or intractable diarrhea is also frequent in patients with common variable immunodeficiency. An incidence of 60% has been reported (76) in one series, but is significantly lower in the series of Cunningham-Rundles (74). The incidence of malabsorption in these two reports is 40% and 9%, respectively. *G. lamblia* has been the most frequently isolated organism in patients with gastrointestinal disease. Other identified causative agents include *Campylobacter* and *Cryptosporidum*. In the majority of cases, no causative agent is isolated from the stool or from biopsy specimens. Specific treatment for the isolated organism frequently results in abatement of the symptoms. Empiric therapy is rarely successful.

The targeted gastrointestinal tract usually demonstrates one of two forms of pathologic change: atrophy or nodular hyperplasia. Gastric atrophy may be associated with pernicious anemia (77). Villus atrophy of the bowel is associated with a protein-loosing enteropathy and a sprue-like syndrome with increased loss of fecal fat and decreased absorption of folic acid, vitamin B_{12}, and carotenes. Treatment of the sprue-like syndrome with elimination of gluten-containing foods rarely results in clinical improvement. Nodular lymphoid hyperplasia of the small or the large bowel may be seen in association with or independent from villus atrophy. The lymphoid nodules appear to be reactive and resemble Peyer patches. The follicular cells may consist of IgM-bearing lymphocytes or contain no detectable immunoglobulin, but do not have demonstrable IgG- or IgA-positive cells or plasma cells. The cellular constituents of follicles may represent an abortive response to antigenic stimulation that cannot progress due to the lack of an effective switch to IgG or IgA production (77).

Common variable immunodeficiency represents an aberration of the immune system in which patients are not completely devoid of the capacity to respond to antigens. It may be characterized by a state of immune dysregulation in which patients suffer from autoimmune disorders. The most frequent autoimmune diseases are immune thrombocytopenia and autoimmune hemolytic anemia, which may be fatal (78). Immune neutropenia and pernicious anemia have been reported (79). The development of anti-IgA antibodies in affected individuals is clinically manifested by anaphylactoid reactions to intravenous γ-globulin. Classical rheumatoid arthritis, juvenile-onset rheumatoid arthritis, scleroderma, sicca syndrome,

dermatomyositis, and systemic lupus erythematosus may develop in patients. In rare instances, classical systemic lupus erythematosus antedates common variable immunodeficiency (80). Abnormalities of the immune system are noted with increased frequency in the families of individuals with common variable immunodeficiency. In these family members, selective IgA deficiency is most frequently found and hypo-γ-globulinemic individuals have been identified. However, the haplotype HLA A1,B8,DR3 is increased only infrequently in these family members. No consistent mode of inheritance has been identified in such families.

The incidence of malignancy has been reported to be increased in patients with common variable immunodeficiency. Non-Hodgkin lymphoma occurs most frequently (72). Other malignancies include Waldenstrom macroglobulinemia, adenocarcinoma of the gastrointestinal tract and ovaries, and epithelial malignancies of the skin, cervix, and vagina. Malignancy was the cause of death in 7 of 15 patients and accounted for 30% of deaths in one longitudinal series (72). In this study, the average age at death for females was 55.4 years and that of males was 28.8 years.

Physical Findings

The physical findings are similar to those noted in X-linked a-γ-globulinemia. The tonsils usually are small, but not absent, and the lymph nodes are not enlarged in the majority of individuals. However, significant lymphadenopathy and splenomegaly may be noted. Presumably, this is result of an aberrant, nonmalignant, lymphocyte proliferation to immunologic stimulation. Most individuals will have abnormal physical findings when their lungs are examined. Rales, coarse inspiratory and expiratory breath sounds, and a prolonged expiratory phase are frequent. Clubbing of the fingers is observed in individuals with chronic lung disease. Individuals with significant malabsorption may have trophic changes of the mucous membranes of the mouth and tongue.

Laboratory Findings

The diagnosis cannot be established until the patient is >2 years of age. By that age, most individuals with transient lypo-γ-globulinemia of infancy will have normal immunologic studies. The distinction may not always be clear cut, since some children who are initially seen with apparent transient hypo-γ-globulinemia manifest a more profound immunodeficiency at a later age.

Quantification of serum immunoglobulins most frequently reveals a decrease in IgG, IgA, and IgM. The levels of IgG are usually higher than those seen in individuals with classic X-linked a-γ-globulinemia. However, there is great variation and one or more immunoglobulins may fall within the normal range for age and may vary during the course of the disease. Generally, there is a high correlation between the serum levels of IgG and IgA. Isohemagglutinins may be present in low titers. Circulating B-cells are present and most frequently are quantitatively normal. This situation distinguishes this entity from classic a-γ-globulinemia. Only rarely are circulating B-cells absent. The response to antigens frequently is blunted and the switching from IgM to IgG on repeat challenge does not occur.

Assessment may show T-cell function to be normal. However, a significant number of individuals have a definably decreased response to one or more mitogens or to allogeneic cell stimulation as defined by mixed lymphocyte culture (73). T-Cell subset analysis may reveal a decrease in the T4/T8 ratio. Assays of B-cell proliferation are depressed. These may reflect suboptimal B-cell/T-cell interaction, lack of T-cell production of IL-4 or IL-6, or T-cell inhibition of B-cell differentiation. Results of in vivo skin tests for delayed-type hypersensitivity, e.g., tuberculin, tetanus toxoid, and *Candida* are most frequently normal.

Immunoglobulin Deficiency with Increased IgM: The Hyper-IgM Syndrome

This syndrome is clinically manifested by repeated pyogenic bacterial infections beginning in early childhood. Most of the reported cases are in males and are consistent with an X-linked recessive mode of inheritance (81). Females may be affected and family studies may be consistent with an autosomal recessive mode of inheritance (82). The syndrome is characterized by a failure of isotype switching from IgM to the other classes of immunoglobulins. Therefore, B-cells express surface IgM, but B-cells expressing surface IgG or IgA are markedly decreased or absent. The maturational "arrest" appears to reside exclusively in the B-cells and results in IgM production exclusively (83).

Clinical Manifestations

Bacterial infections of the respiratory tract, tonsils, and ears begin in early childhood. Patients who have episodic neutropenia will have recurrent mouth ulcers and stomatitis. Autoimmune diseases such as thrombocytopenia, hemolytic anemia, and possibly neutropenia have been reported in patients and presumably are the result of immune deregulation. Other manifestations of immune disregulation are arthritis and nephritis.

Physical Findings

In contrast to patients with other B-cell deficiencies, individuals with this syndrome have markedly enlarged tonsils and lymph nodes. Significant splenomegaly is a frequent finding. Patients with neutropenic episodes, particularly those with chronic neutropenia, will frequently have gingivitis.

Laboratory Findings

The syndrome is characterized by the presence of elevated serum IgM which is polyclonal. Monoclonal IgM may be present and IgG and IgA are decreased or absent. Antibodies of IgM class, e.g., isohemagglutinins, heterophile antibodies may be present and appropriate IgM secondary responses are evoked with antigen challenge. Lymphoid organs do not contain germinal centers. However, plasma cells are seen but are present in decreased number. Since the subpopulations of T-cells are normal, T-cell function is normal by in vitro assays and delayed type hypersensitivity to intradermal challenge is intact.

Selective IgG Subclass Deficiency with IgA Deficiency

Characterized by a decreased level of one or more of the IgG subclasses, this heterogeneous group of immunodeficiencies is frequently associated with a decreased serum level of IgA. Serum IgG levels are normal except in individuals who have a deficiency in the subclass IgG1. Because there is no standard assay for the IgG subclasses and the normal age-adjusted levels for each has not been defined, it is difficult to categorize specific disease states with each subclass deficiency.

The pathogenesis of the syndrome is based on defective switching of the constant region of the IgG heavy chain. In general, IgG1 antibodies are generated in response to protein antigens and IgG2 to polysaccharide antigens. IgG3 antibodies are evoked by viral antigens, and IgG4 antibodies may be associated with intestinal parasites and reactions to IgA. Significant decreases or absence of IgG1, IgG2, and IgG3 have been associated with recurrent infections. However, many individuals with isolated subclass deficiencies have not suffered an increased incidence of infections. Those individuals who have IgG subclass deficiencies, especially IgG2, associated with an absence of serum IgA appear to have an increased incidence of pyogenic respiratory tract infections (84). Deficiencies of IgG subclasses are increased in relatives of patients with common variable immunodeficiency and with apparent isolated IgA deficiency. In the pediatric age group, IgG subclass deficiency is more prevalent among males than females, a 3:1 ratio. This is reversed in adults (85).

Clinical Manifestations

The major consequences attributable to subclass deficiency are recurrent and chronic pyogenic pulmonary tract infections. Other infections include otitis media, sinusitis, and meningitis.

Laboratory Findings

Immunoglobulin subclasses are generally quantified by employing the techniques of radial immunodiffusion, radioimmunoassay, or ELISA. Each of these techniques requires the use of specific monoclonal antibodies. In adults IgG1 is the major serum component, constituting >60% of the total serum IgG. IgG2 constitutes approximately 25%, IgG3 approximately 5–10% and IgG4 <5%. In children, the levels vary with age, with IgG1 and IgG3 reaching adult values by 6 years of age and IgG2 and IgG4 reaching adult values by 8–10 years of age. Because of the great range in subclass levels at any age, discretion must be used in interpreting the clinical relevance of the reported values. In vitro assays have demonstrated T- or B-cell dysfunction in 75% of individuals (86).

Selective Immunoglobulin A (IgA) Deficiency

A decreased level of serum IgA is the most frequently detected "immunodeficiency" among the white population, in which 1 of 700 individuals is affected. In contrast, the incidence is 1 of 12,500 individuals in the Japanese population. Many individuals lacking serum IgA appear to be normal; however, when investigated intensively, such individuals have an increased incidence of sinopulmonary infections, chronic diarrhea, and autoimmune disorders (87). Most individuals with selective IgA deficiency lack both serum IgA, IgA1, and secretory IgA, IgA2. Individuals who are totally deficient in IgA usually have normal T-cell function. A small subpopulation has a more severe immunologic deficit with associated T-cell abnormalities as defined by defects in the response to mitogens (88) or increased IgA- specific T-cell suppressor activity (89). Analysis of the B-cell population of the gastrointestinal mucosa in IgA-deficient individuals has demonstrated only a slight decrease in number. This is attributed to a compensatory increase of IgG+ and IgM+ immunocytes. IgA+ cells were not observed (90). A small population of patients lack IgA1, but have normal levels of serum secretory IgA2. These individuals have a normal number of IgA secretory cells on intestinal biopsy (91).

The heterogeneity of immunologic findings among individuals with IgA deficiency implies that there are diverse causes. Inheritances of IgA deficiency has been consistent with an autosomal recessive mode of inheritance, an autosomal dominant mode of inheritance, or, most frequently, no definable mode of inheritance (92). IgA deficiency has been associated with abnormalities of chromosomes 18, 14, and 6, but this is not consistent and there are no common definable patterns. Other evidence for an heritable basis for IgA deficiency is the identification of rare major histocompatibility complex (MHC) class III haplotypes involving C4 or C2 such as A1, B8, C4AQO, C4B1, BfS, DR3 (93, 94).

IgA deficiency has been associated frequently with autoimmune disorders and these disorders are associated with the MHC haplotypes which have an increased frequency in individuals with selective IgA deficiency or IgA deficiency and IgG subclass deficiency (95). Among these diseases are juvenile rheumatoid arthritis, systemic lupus erythematosis, Sjorgren syndrome, multiple endocrinop-

athies, pernicious anemia, and immune hemolytic anemia (96). It has been postulated that the mechanism for autoimmunity is based on the pathophysiologic role of the IgA of the mucosal immune system in acting as a barrier to the entrance of ingested antigens into the circulation. IgA antibody-antigen complexes would be cleared locally or by the liver if access were gained to the portal venous system. Supporting evidence for this concept is the observation that IgA- deficient individuals have food antigen containing circulating immune complexes as well as precipitins against food proteins (97). The incidence of atopic disease also has been reported to be increased in selective IgA deficiency (98). The underlying mechanism has been postulated to be the same as that for autoimmune disease.

κ-Chain Deficiency

This exceedingly rare defect has been reported in two kindreds (99, 100). Affected individuals may have no increased susceptibility to infections despite the lack of κ-chain bearing immunoglobulins are present. In one kindred, point mutations in the κ-chain gene at 2p11 have been reported (101).

Treatment of B Cell Deficiencies

All of the B-cell deficiency states are characterized by significant impairments or total absence of the antibody response to immunogens. It is this defective response that underlies the infectious complications of these disorders. Although meningitis and sepsis constitute the most spectacular and acute life- threatening events, it is the recurrent and chronic pulmonary infections that ultimately result in the most frequent nonmalignant cause of morbidity and mortality, chronic lung disease, pulmonary insufficiency, and consequent cor pulmonale. These are the results of indolent unrecognized infection, which must be recognized and treated effectively. Therefore, thorough examination of the lungs is a vital part of the physical examination, and when the patient becomes cooperative enough, pulmonary function tests should be performed annually or as frequently as indicated clinically.

The availability of commercially available preparations of IgG for intravenous administration has simplified and increased the effectiveness of γ-globulin replacement therapy (102). Patients should be treated with monthly doses of intravenous γ-globulin in amounts to necessary maintain the serum IgG level >500 mg/dl. The dose required varies among patients, but the usual required dose range is 400–600 mg/kg every 4 weeks. If patients have breakthrough sinopulmonary infections, γ-globulin may be more effective if given at a lower dose, i.e., 300–500 mg every 3 weeks. Patients with IgG subclass deficiencies or common variable immunodeficiency whose serum IgG is >500 mg/dl should be treated at a dose of 200–400 mg/kg every 4 weeks in order to maintain the serum IgG level >600 mg/dl. In most instances, priming doses of γ-globulin are not required. Therefore the serum IgG level will increase >3–4 months before it reaches a plateau level. If infections occur, appropriate antibiotic therapy must be given for a minimal period of 2 weeks for respiratory tract infections and 4 weeks for sinus infections. The most frequently used agents are ampicillin with clavulinic acid, trimethoprim sulfamethoxazole, and oral cephalosporins closporins or tetracycline derivatives in adults. In addition, patients with evidence of bronchiectasis should have adequate maintenance postural drainage.

Patients with selective IgA deficiency may suffer anaphylactic reactions when blood products or intravenous IgG is administered. In some patients, IgG and IgE antibodies to IgA have been demonstrated (103). Therefore, it is urged that γ-globulin preparations free of trace amounts of IgA be used in all patients with selective IgA deficiency, e.g., Gammagard, Cutter.

Patients with immunodeficiency who suffer from chronic gastrointestinal symptoms and diarrhea should be evaluated for the presence of enteric parasites, particularly *G. lamblia*. If organisms or cysts are not observed in fresh stool samples, small bowel biopsy should be obtained for a more definitive diagnosis. If positive for *G. lamblia* therapy with metronidazole or chloroquin should be instituted.

The objectives of all therapy in immunodeficient patients are to prevent infection and eradicate existing chronic infections. Aggressive therapy will not only prolong life, but will decrease the incidence of chronic debilitating disease and effect a more normal life for afflicted individuals.

REFERENCES

1. Haire R. Personal communications, 1992.
2. World Health Organization. Nomenclature for human immunoglobulins. Bull WHO 1964;30:447–450.
3. World Health Organization. An extension of the nomenclature for immunoglobulins. Immunochemistry 1970;7:497–500.
4. World Health Organization. Notation for human immunoglobulin subclasses. Bull Who 1966;35:953.
5. Kunad HG, Young WG. Heavy chain subgroups of IgG and IgA globulins In Merler E, ed. Immunoglobulins: biologic aspects and clinical uses. Washington, DC: National Academy of Sciences, 1970:137–144.
6. World Health Organization. Primary immunodeficiency diseases: report of a WHO scientific group. Immunodef Rev 1992;3:195–236.
7. von Schwedler U, Jack HM, Wabl M. Beswitched: the looping out model for immunoglobulin class switching: the Biologist 1990;2:657–662.
8. Cooper MD, Peterson RDA, Good RA. Delineation of the thymic and bursal lymphoid systems in the chicken. Nature 1965;205:143–145.
9. Owen JJT, Cooper MD, Raff MC. In vitro generation of B lymphocytes in mouse foetal liver, "mammalian" bursa equivalent." Nature 1974;249:361–363.
10. Reyser JE, Vassalli P. Mouse bone marrow lymphocytes and their differentiation. J Immunol 1974;173:719–729.
11. Good RA. Immunodeficiency in developmental perspective. Harvey Lect 1973;67:1–107.
12. Becker RS, Knight KL. Somatic diversification of immunoglobulin heavy chain VDJ genes: evidence for somatic gene conversion in rabbits. Cell 1990;63:987–997.
13. Reynaud CA, MacKay CR, Muller RG, Weill JC. Somatic generation of diversity in a mammalian primary lymphoid organ: the sheep ileal Peyer's patches. Cell 1991;64:995–1005.
14. Jacobsen K, Osmond DG. Microenvironmental organization and stromal cell associations of B lymphocyte precursor cells in mouse bone marrow. Eur J Immunol 1990;20:2395–404.
15. Gallagha RB, Osmond DG. To B or not to B: that is the question. Immunol Today 1991;12:1-3.
16. MacLennan ICM, Liu YJ, Oldfield S, Zhang J, et al. The evaluation of B-cell clones. Curr Top Microbiol Immunol 1990;159:37–63.
17. Dobashi M, Terashima K, Imai Y. Electron microscopic study of differentiation of antibody-producing cells in mouse lymph nodes after immunization with horseradish peroxidase. J Histochem Cytochem 1982;30:67–74.
18. Blier PR, Bothwell A. A limited number of B cell lineages generates the heterogeneity of a secondary immune response. J Immunol 1987;139:3996-4006.
19. Klaus GGB, Kunkl A. The role of germinal centers in the generation of immunological memory. In: Microenvironments in hematopoietic and lymphoid differentiation. London: Pitman Medical 1981:265–280.
20. Kraal G, Weissman IL, Butcher EC. Germinal centre B cells: antigen specificity and changes in heavy chain class expression. Nature 1982;298:377–379.
21. Long MW. Review: blood cell cytoadhesion molecules. Exp Hematol 1992;20:288–301.
22. Abernathy NJ, Hay JB, Kimpton WG, Washington E, et al. Lymphocyte subset-specific and tissue-specific lymphocyte-endothelial cell recognition mechanisms independently direct the recirculation of lymphocytes from blood to lymph in sheep. Immunology 1991;72:239–245.
23. Aggarwhal BB, Gutterman JU, eds. Human cytokines. Oxford: Blackwell 1991:1–191.
24. Halpern MT. Human nonspecific suppressive lymphokines. J Clin Immunol 1991;11:1–12.
25. Jerne NK. Towards a network theory of the immune system. Ann Immunol (Paris) 1974;125C:373–389.
26. Evans MJ, Suenaga R, Abdou NI. Detection and purification of anti-idiotypic antibody against anti-DNA in intravenous gamma globulin. J Clin Immunol 1991;11:291–295.
27. Schonfield MS, van Loghem E. Human immunoglobulin allotypes. In: Weir DM, et al. eds. Handbook of experimental immunology. Oxford: Blackwell, 1986;94.1–94.18.
28. Sarvas H, Rautonen N, Makela O. Allotype associated differences in concentrations of human IgG subclasses. J Clin Immunol 1991;11:39–45.
29. Granoff DM, Pandey JP, Boies E, Squires J, et al. Response to immunization with *Haemophilus influenzae* type b polysuccharide-pertussis vaccine and the risk of *Haemophilus* meningitis in children with Km(1) immunoglobulin allotype. J Clin Invest 1984;74:1708–1714.
30. Pascual V, Capra JD. Human immunoglobulin heavy chain variable region genes: organization, polymorphism, and expression. Adv Immunol 1991;49:1–74.

31. Kabat EA, Wu TT. Indentical V region amino acid sequences and segments of sequences in antibodies of different specificities: relative contributions of V_H and V_L genes, minigenes and complementarity—determining regions to binding of antibody-combining sites. J Immunol 1991;147: 1709–1719.

32. Alt FW, Baltimore D. Joining of immunoglobulin heavy chain gene segments: implications from a chromosome with evidence of three D-JH fusions. Proc Natl Acad Sci USA 1982;79:4118–4122.

33. Heidelberger M. Precipitating cross reactions among pneumococcal types. Infect Immunol 1983;41:1234–1244.

34. Oxelius VA, Laurell AB, Lindquist B, Golebiowska H, et al. IgG subclasses in selective IgA deficiency: importance of IgG2-IgA deficiency. N Engl J Med 1981;304:1476–1477.

35. Bruton OC. Agammaglobulinemia. Pediatrics 1952;9: 722–728.

36. Kwan SP, Kunkel L, Bruns G, Wedgwood RJ, et al. Mapping of the X-linked agammaglobulinemia locus by use of restriction length polymorphism. J Clin Invest 1986;77: 649–652.

37. Cooper MD, Lawton NR. Circulating B-cells in patients with immunodeficiency. Am J Pathol 1972;69: 513–528.

38. Pearl ER, Vogler LB, Okos AJ, Crist WM, et al. B lymphocyte precursors in human bone marrow: an analysis of normal individuals and patients with antibody deficiency states. J Immunol 1978;120:1169–1175.

39. Schwaber J, Payne J, Chen RB. Lymphocytes from X-linked agammaglobulinemia: delayed expression of light chain and demonstration of Lyonization in carriers. J Clin Invest 1988;81:514–522.

40. Fearon E, Winkelstein J, Civin C, Pardoll DM, et al. Carrier detection in X-linked agammaglobulinemia by analysis of x-chromosome inactivation. N Engl J Med 1987;316: 427–431.

41. Rosen FS. Genetic deficiencies in specific immune responses. Semin Hematol 1990;27:333–341.

42. Vetrie D, Vorechovsky I, Sideras P, Holland J, et al. The gene involved in X-linked agammaglobulinaemia is a member of the src family of protein-tyrosine kinases. Nature 1993;361:226–233.

43. Sitz KV, Burks AW, Williams LW, Kamp SF, et al. Confirmation of X-linked hypogammaglobulinemia with isolated growth hormone deficiency as a disease entity. J Pediatr 1990;116:292–294.

44. Fleisher TA, White RM, Broder S, Nissley SP, et al. X-linked hypogammaglobulinemia with isolated growth hormone deficiency. N Engl J Med 1980;302:1429–1434.

45. Hoffmann T, Winchester R, Schulkind M, Frias JL, et al. Hypoimmunoglobulinemia with normal T cell function in female siblings. Clin Immunol Immunopathol 1977;7: 364–371.

46. Lederman HM, Winkelestein JA. X-linked agammaglobulinemia: an analysis of 96 patients. Medicine 1985;64: 145–156.

47. Wright JJ, Hatch MH, Kasselberg AG, Lowry SP, et al. Vaccine-associated poliomyelitis in a child with sex-linked agammaglobulinemia . J Pediatr 1977;91:408–412.

48. Olson NY, Hall JC. Chronic cutaneous herpes simplex and X-linked hypoagammaglobulinemia. Pediatr Dermatol 1987;4:225–228.

49. McKinney RE, Jr, Katz SL, Wilfert CM. Chronic enteroviral meningoencephalitis in agammaglobulinemic patients. Rev Infect Dis 1987;9:334–356.

50. Buckley RH, Rowlands DT. Agammaglobulinemia, neutropenia, fever and abdominal pain. J Alllerg Clin Immunol 1973;51:308–318.

51. Kozolwski C, Evans DIK. Neutropenia associated with X-linked agammaglobulinemia. J Clin Pathol 1991;44: 388–390.

52. Robbins JB, Skinner RG, Pearson HA. Autoimmune hemolytic anemia in a child with congential X-linked hypogammaglobulinemia. N Engl J Med 1969;280:75–79.

53. Gemke RJBJ, Haasnoot K, Veerman AJP. Early onset agammaglobulinemia with monoclonal IgG production. Eur J Pediatr 1989;148:755–757.

54. Schutt C, Eggers G, Wegener S, Seyfarth M, et al. X-linked hypoagammaglobulinemia with a late secretion defect: a family study. Fol Haematol (Leipeiz) 1987;114:382–389.

55. Bentur L, Shear N, Roifman CM. Cutaneous lymphohistocytic infiltrates in patients with hypogammaglobulinia. J Pediatr 1990;116:68–72.

56. Wedgwood RJ, Ochs HD, Davis SD. The recognition and classification of immunodeficiency diseases with bacteriophage fc174. In: Bergma D, ed. Immunodeficiency in man and animals: birth defects. Sunderland, MA: Sinaur, 1975; 11:331–338.

57. Gitlan D, Janeway CA. Agammaglobulinemia: congenital, acquired, and transient forms. Prog Hematol 1956;1: 318–329.

58. Priger CHL, Nelson LA, Peri BA, Lustig JV, et al. Transient hypogammaglobulinemia of infancy. J Pediatr 1977;91: 601–603.

59. Tiller TL, Jr, Buckley RH. Transient hypogammaglobulinemia of infancy: review of the literature, clinical and immunological features of 11 new cases and long-term follow-up. J Pediatr 1978;92:347–353.

60. Dressler F, Peter HH, Muller W, Riegler CHL. Transient hypogammaglobulinemia of infancy: five new cases, review of the literature and redefinition. Acta Paediatr Scand 1989; 78:767–774.

61. Siegel RL, Isse Kutz T, Schwaber J, Rosen FS, et al. Deficiency of T helper cells in transient hypogammaglobulinemia of infancy. N Engl J Med 1981;305:1307–1313.

62. Rodriquez MA, Bankhurst AD, Williams RC. Characterization of the suppressor activity in lymphocytes from patients with common variable hypogammaglobulinemia: evidence for an associated primary B-cell defect. Clin Immunol Immunopath 1983;29:35–50.

63. Duggan-Keen MF, Bird AG, Bird P, Smith SWG, et al. B-cell differentiation and lymphocyte surface phenotype in late onset hypogammaglobulinemia. Dis Markers 1990;8: 69–83.

64. Saiki O, Ralph P, Cunningham-Rundles C, Good RA. Three distinct stages of B-cell defects in common variable immunodeficiency. Proc Natl Acad Sci (USA) 1982;79: 6008–6012.

65. Geha RS, Schneeberger E, Merler E, Rosen FS. Heterogeneity of "acquired" or common variable agammaglobulinemia. N Engl J Med 1974;291:1–6.

66. Waldman TA, Durm M, Broder S, Blackman M, et al. Role of suppressor T cells in the pathogenesis of common variable hypogammaglobulinemia. Lancet 1974;2:609–613.

67. Reinheiz EL, Geha R, Wohl ME, Morimato C, et al. Immunodeficiency associated with loss of T4+ inducer T-cell function. N Engl J Med 1981;304:811–816.
68. Aparicio-Pages MN, den Hartog G, Verspaget HW, Pena S, et al. Decreased natural killer cell activity in late-onset hypogammaglobulinemia. Clin Sci 1990;78:133–137.
69. Gelfand EW, Borel H, Berkel AI, Rosen FS. Auto-immunosuppression recurrent infections associated with immunologic unresponsiveness in the presence of an autoantibody to IgG. Clin Immunol Immunopath 1972;1:155–163.
70. Tuez T, Preud'Homme JL, Laboume S, Matuchansky C, et al. Autoantibodies to B lymphocytes in a patient with hypogammaglobulinemia: characterization and pathogenic rate. J Clin Invest 1977;60:405–410.
71. Stahl W, Cunningham-Rundles C, Maeger L. In vitro induction of T cell-dependent B cell differentiation in patients with common varied immunodeficiency. Clin Immunol Immunopath 1988;49:273–289.
72. Cunningham-Rundles C, Siegal EP, Cunningham-Randles C, Lieberman P. Incidence of cancer in 98 patients with common varied immunodeficiency. J Clin Immunol 1987;7:294–299.
73. Reinherz EL, Rubinstein A, Geha R, Strelbaushas AJ, et al. Abnormalities of immunoregulatory T cells in disorders of immunofunction. N Engl J Med 1979;301:1018–1021.
74. Cunningham-Rundles C. Clinical and Immunologic analysis of 103 patients with common variable immunodeficiency. J Clin Immunol 1989;9:22–23.
75. Dukes RJ, Rosenow EC, Hermans PE. Pulmonary manifestations of hypogammaglobulinemia. Thorax 1978;33:603–607.
76. Hermans PE, Diaz-Buxo JA, Stobo JD. Idiopathic late-onset immunoglobulin deficiency: clinical observations in 50 patients. Am J Med 1976;61:221–237.
77. Ochs HD, Ament ME. Gastrointestinal tract and immunodeficiency. In: Ferguson A, MacSween RNM, eds. Immunological aspects of the liver and gastrointestinal tract. Lancaster, England: MTP Press, 1976:83–120.
78. Boyd AS, Kennedy DH, Boyd JF. Fatal haemolytic anemia complicating a case of common variable hypogammaglobulinemia. Scot Med J 1990;35:147–148.
79. Conley ME, Park CL, Douglas SD. Childhood common variable immunodeficiency with autoimmune disease. J Pediatr 1986;108:915–922.
80. Baum CG, Chiorazzi N, Frankel S, Shepherd GM. Conversion of systemic lupus erythematosus to common variable hypogammaglobulinemia. Am J Med 1989;87:449–456.
81. Rosen FS, Kevy SV, Merler E, Janeway CA, et al. Recurrent bacterial infection and dysgammaglobulinemia: deficiency of 7S gamma-globulins. Pediatrics 1961;28:182–195.
82. Rosen RS, Bougas JA. Acquired dysgammaglobulinemia elevation of the 19S gammaglobulin and deficiency of the 7S gamma-globulin in a woman with chronic progressive brochiatasis. N Engl J Med 1963;269:1336–1340.
83. Brahmi Z, Lazarus KH, Hodes ME, Baehner RL. Immunologic studies of three family members with the immunodeficiency with hyper-IgM syndrome. J Clin Immunol 1983;3:127–134.
84. Oxalius VA, Laurell AB, Lindquist B, Galebiowha H, et al. IgG subclasses selective IgA deficiency: Impor-

85. Hansen LA, Soderstrom R, Avanzini A, Bergtason U, et al. Immunoglobulin subclass deficiency. Pediatr Inf Dis J 1988;7(5 Suppl):s17–21.
86. Soderstrom T, Soderstrom R, Avanzini A, Brandtzaeg P, et al. Immunoglobulin G subclass deficiencies. Int Arch Allergy Appl Immunol 1987;82:476–480.
87. Hanson LA. Aspects of the absence of the IgA system. In: Bergsma D, Good, RA, eds. Immunologic diseases of man. National Foundation: Birth Defects Original Article Series: 4:No. 1. Battman. Baltimore: Williams & Wilkins, 1968:292–297.
88. Epstein LB, Ammann AJ. Evaluation of T lymphocyte effector function in immunodeficiency diseases: abnormality in mitogen-stimulated interferon in patients with selective IgA deficiency. J Immunol 1974;112:617–626.
89. de Laat PC, Weemaers CM, Bakkeren JA, von den Brandt FC, et al. Familial selective IgA deficiency with circulating anti-IgA antibodies: a distinct group of patients? Clin Immunol Immunopath 1991;58:92–101.
90. Nilssen DE, Brandtzaeg P, Froland SS, Fausa O. Subclass composition and J-chain expression of the "compensatory" gastrointestinal IgG cell population in selective IgA deficiency. Clin Exp Immunol 1992;87:237–245.
91. Hazenberg BP, Hodemaker PJ, Niewenhuis P, Mandema E. Source of IgA in intestinal secretions. In: Peeters H, ed. Protides of the biological fluid. Proceedings of the Sixteenth Colloquium, Oxford: Pergamano, 1968:491–497.
92. Cunningham-Rundles C. Genetic aspects of immunoglobulin A deficiency. Adv Hum Genet 1990;19:235–266.
93. Keyeux G, Lefranc MP, Chevailler A, Lefranc G. Molecular analysis of the IGHA and MHC Class III region genes in one family with IgA and C4 Deficiencies. Exp Clin Immunogenet 1990;7:170–180.
94. Schaffer FM, Palermos J, Zhu ZB, Barger BO, et al. Individuals with IgA deficiency and common variable immunodeficiency share polymorphisms of major histocompatibility complex class III genes. Proc Nat Acad Sci (USA) 1989;86:8015–8019.
95. French MA, Dawkins RL. Central MHC genes, IgA deficiency and autoimmune disease. Immunol Today 1990;11:271–274.
96. Dalton TA, Bennet JC. Autoimmune disease and the major histocompatibility complex: therapeutic implications. Am J Med 1992;92:183–188.
97. Cunningham–Rundles C, Brandies WE, Good RA, Day NK. Bovine antigens and the formation of circulating immune complexes in selective immunoglobulin A deficiency. J Clin Invest 1979;64:272–279.
98. Plebani A, Monafo V, Ugazio AG, Monti C, et al. Comparison of the frequency of atopic diseases in children with severe and partial IgA deficiency. Int Arch Allergy Appl Immunol 1987;82:485–486.
99. Bernier GM, Gunderman JR, Ruymann FR. Kappa chain deficiency. Blood 1972;40:795–805.
100. Zegers BJM, Maertzdorf WJ, Van Loghem E, Mul NAJ, et al. Kappa-chain deficiency. An immunoglobulin disorder. N Engl J Med 1976;294:1026–1030.

101. Stavnezer J, Zegers BJM. Aberrant kappa constant region genes in a patient lacking type kappa immunoglobulins. In: Eibl MM, Rosen FS, eds. Primary immunodeficiency diseases. Amsterdam: Elsevier Science Publishing, 1986:55–59.

102. Roifman CM, Gelfand EM. Replacement therapy with high dose intravenous gamma-blobulin improves chronic sino-pulmonary disease in patients with hypogammaglobulinemia. Pediatr Infect Dis J 1988;7:S92–S96.

103. Ferreira A, Garcia-Rodriquez MC, Lopez-Trascasa M, Pascual Salcedo D, et al. IgA antibodies in selective IgA deficiency and in primary immunodeficient patients treated with gamma-globulin. Clin Immunol Immunopath 1988;47:199–207.

CHAPTER 14

Inherited Disorders of T-Lymphocytes

TALAL CHATILA, RICARDO SORENSON

We've made great medical progress in the last generation. What used to be merely an itch is now an allergy.
—Anonymous

T-Lymphocytes and Their Disorders

Thymus-derived (T) lymphocytes are an essential component of the immune system. They are the primary orchestrators of immune responses, being endowed with several characteristics that enable them to regulate the functions of other components of the immune system. T-Lymphocytes are immunologically specific. They recognize unique peptide antigens presented by major histocompatibility complex (MHC) molecules by virtue of clonally restricted antigen receptors expressed on the surface of T-lymphocytes and specific for peptide/MHC complexes. They mount antigen-specific cellular immune responses such as those directed against intracellular pathogens. They discriminate between self- and nonself-antigens, and play a leading role in the rejection of foreign, transplanted tissues and in the lysis of tumor cells. They direct the generation of antigen-specific antibodies by B-cells, and act to activate phagocytic cells and natural killer (NK) cells by secreted lymphokines. T-Lymphocytes are also endowed with immunologic memory. The function of T-lymphocytes extends to the regulation of erythroid cell maturation in the bone marrow.

A large number of defects that affect the development and/or function of T-lymphocytes both in humans and in experimental animals have been described. These defects have served as experiments of nature to unravel the complexities of T-cell development and function. The impact of these defects can spread beyond T-lymphocytes to affect the function of several limbs of the immune system. Abnormalities affecting T-cells frequently lead to states of combined immunodeficiency, the severity of which depends on the extent of the T-cell defect.

In this chapter, we will examine the clinical presentation and management and the underlying pathophysiology of some of the common, inherited T-cell deficiencies by means of model case studies. These case histories will also serve to illustrate the development and function of T-cells in the normal host.

T-Cell Immunodeficiencies: Clinical Considerations

Case 1

T.G. was a 5-month-old infant boy who presented with respiratory distress, severe diarrhea, and failure to thrive. Born following full-term gestation and normal vaginal delivery, he did relatively well for the first 3 weeks of life. Thereafter he had recurrent bouts of diarrhea and severe oral thrush. At 2 months of age otitis media developed, which recurred soon after the cessation of a standard 10-day course of antibiotic therapy and again 1 month after a second round of antibiotic treatment. One week prior to his presentation, progressive respiratory distress developed, with tachypnea and fever. A chest x-ray revealed the presence of diffuse interstitial infiltrates. Bronchoscopy was undertaken, and a diagnosis of Pneumocystis carinii *pneumonia was made based on the identification of the pathogen in bronchioalveolar lavage fluid. Investigation of his family history revealed healthy, nonconsanguinous parents and 2 healthy female siblings. A paternal uncle died in infancy with an unknown, overwhelming infection.*

Clinical examination revealed a sick-looking, tachypneic child who was below the 5th percentile for both weight and height. He had oral thrush and his tonsils were severely atrophied. The baby had diffuse bilateral rales detected on chest examination. He had no palpable lymph nodes, and on abdominal examination his liver and spleen were not enlarged.

Repeated investigation of his immune function identified lymphopenia (lymphocyte count 730×10^9/L). Analysis of lymphocyte subsets revealed that only 10% of his peripheral blood lymphocytes expressed the pan T-cell marker CD-3 (normal 65–75%); 81% of his lymphocytes expressed the pan B-cell surface marker, CD-19 (normal 5–15%). The remaining 9% of his lymphocytes expressed the NK cell markers, CD-56 and/or CD-16.

Karyotype analysis of his T-lymphocytes revealed a 46,XX phenotype, indicative of maternal origin. He failed to mount delayed-type hypersensitivity responses upon intradermal skin testing with a battery of antigens that included tetanus toxoid, to which he had been twice previously vaccinated, and Candida albicans. His lymphocytes failed to proliferate in vitro in response to mitogen stimulation including lectins such as phytohemagglutinin (PHA), concanavalin A, and pokeweed. Investigation of his humoral immunity revealed decreased immunoglobulin levels: IgG 235 mg%, IgM 22 mg%, and IgA 7 mg%. His antigen-specific antibody responses, as measured by his response to tetanus toxoid vaccination, were either low or absent. The peripheral blood cell activity of purine salvage pathway enzymes, adenosine deaminase and purine nucleoside phosphorylase, the deficiency of which results in severe combined immunodeficiency, were normal. Tests for infection with HIV were negative. A clinical diagnosis of X-linked **Severe Combined Immunodeficiency (SCID)** *was made, and the child was started on specific P. carinii therapy, as well as intravenous immunoglobulin replacement therapy (IVIG) at 400 mg/kg every 3 weeks.*

In view of the dire prognosis of his underlying immunodeficiency and the pace at which his medical condition was worsening, we decided that the child's best chance for survival lay in a bone marrow transplant (BMT) to be given as soon as his medical condition stabilized. Human lymphocyte antigen (HLA) typing of his family members failed to reveal histocompatibility with either parent or siblings. It was therefore decided that he would receive a haploidentical bone marrow graft from his mother. In preparation for the transplant, the child received preBMT cyclophosphamide and antilymphocyte antiserum to remove any immunocompetent cells capable of rejecting the graft. On the day of the BMT, his mother's bone marrow was modified to deplete it of T-cells (to prevent severe graft-versus-host disease [GVHD]) by incubation of the graft with a pan anti-T-cell antibody and complement. Cyclosporine A therapy was administered orally post-BMT for the same purpose of preventing GVHD. At 14 days post-BMT, the baby had a white blood cell (WBC) count of .750 × 10⁹/L with 40% granulocytosis and a platelet count of 30 × 10⁹/L. Three weeks post-BMT, a measles-like skin rash (consistent with early GVHD), diarrhea, eosinophilia, and mild elevation of liver function tests developed. Prednisone was added to the therapy. He was diagnosed with grade II GVHD, which was successfully treated with a short course of steroids. At week 6 post-BMT, the lymphocyte count started increasing steadily, and the baby's lymphocyte proliferation in response to the T-cell mitogen phytohemagglutinin normalized by week 12 post-BMT. The child was discharged from the hospital at week 16 posttransplant on a regimen of cyclosporine A and intravenous immunoglobulin (IVIG) therapy. Cyclosporine A was discontinued 6 months post-BMT, but the child's B-lymphocyte function did not improve in 1 year, thereby necessitating maintenance of IVIG therapy.

Presentation and Management of T-Cell Immunodeficiencies

T-Cell immunodeficiencies occur either as primary or as secondary disorders. Primary T-cell immunodeficiency diseases are inherited defects that typically manifest soon after birth, although some become evident later in life. Secondary immunodeficiencies may be acquired as a consequence of treatment with immunosuppressive agents, nutritional deficiencies, or certain pathogens such as HIV. Frequent infections are the hallmark of immune system defects, and T-cell immunodeficiencies are no exception. The diversity of infections affecting patients with T-cell immunodeficiencies is a reflection of the myriad roles played by T-cells both as effectors of cellular immunity and as regulators of diverse limbs of the immune system, including the B-cell and the phagocytic compartment. Patients with severe T-cell immunodeficiencies often have recurrent fungal, viral, opportunistic and parasitic infections, and recurrent bacterial infections commonly associated with B-cell defects. These patients are at an increased risk for malignancies both of lymphoreticular organs and of other tissues. More moderate defects in T-cell function may present with discrete abnormalities in cell-mediated immunity with or without accompanying humoral immunodeficiency. At times, specific T-cell defects may be seen primarily as antibody deficiency syndromes, as seen in the hyper-IgM-immunodeficiency syndrome. This disease results from defects in gp39, a T-cell surface protein that serves as a counter-receptor for the B-cell surface protein CD-40. Interaction of this ligand pair is required for B-cells to switch isotypes from IgM to IgG, IgA, or IgE.

The diagnosis of immunodeficiency, including disorders of T-cell function, can be deduced from careful history taking and from findings on physical examination. *In the child described above, elements in his history point to the presence of an underlying immunodeficiency. First, he suffered from recurrent infections, including severe oral thrush, recurrent ear infections, and P. carinii pneumonia early in life.* Recurrent infections are the hallmark of defective immune function. Some of the infections are commonly encountered in immunocompetent, age-matched peers. For example, an ear infection at 2 months of age, while uncommon in healthy infants, certainly does occur. Mild cases of thrush are frequently seen in this age group only to disappear as the patient grows older. However, the confluence of these infections, their persistence and their recurrence, and the occurrence of an unusual, opportunistic infection clearly distinguished our immunodeficient child from his immunocompetent peers.

Another element in this child's history that points to an underlying immunodeficiency is his family history, notable for the death of a maternal uncle in infancy due to an overwhelming infection. This suggests that we may be dealing with an inherited, X-linked immunodeficiency disease. This is particularly relevant as many of the primary disorders of both cellular and humoral immunity are inherited in an X-linked pattern.

There were several findings in the clinical examination that are consistent with the presence of an immunodeficiency. The first is the infant's growth retardation; this is a cardinal manifestation of severe immunodeficiency states. Another is the presence of oral thrush, which has persisted despite therapy. A third finding is the presence of severely atrophied tonsillar tissue and the inability to detect any lymph nodes despite the history of recurrent infections.

The presence of an underlying immunodeficiency was confirmed by laboratory investigation. The patient had severe absolute lymphopenia, a finding commonly encountered in immunodeficiency diseases, and he failed to mount either a delayed-type hypersensitivity reaction to Candida albicans despite his chronic infection with thrush or to tetanus toxoid despite prior inoculations with this vaccine. He also had humoral immunodeficiency evidenced by low immunoglobulin levels and by absent specific antibody responses to tetanus. The finding of a very small number of maternal T-cells in his circulation indicated the presence of a severe host T-cell depletion that prevented his immune system from otherwise attacking and destroying foreign cells. Impairment of his cellular immunity also underlies the poor proliferative responses observed in vitro with classical T-cell mitogens.

*In summary, this child had clinical and laboratory findings suggestive of severe combined immunodeficiency (SCID), a disorder at the extreme end of the spectrum of immunodeficiency states. It is characterized by the breakdown of adaptive immune function, both cellular and humoral. This can be the result of severe T-cell depletion (or dysfunction) with secondary B-cell dysfunction or may be due to abnormalities equally affecting both compartments. When fully manifested, SCID poses the risk of imminent death to its victims. It is caused by a heterogenous group of genetic abnormalities afflicting the immune system (1, 2). As demonstrated in this child, patients with SCID are susceptible to infections by any of the known pathogenic microorganisms, including bacteria, viruses, fungi, and protozoa. Persistent infections of the lung, chronic diarrhea, and wasting dominate the clinical picture. Monilial infections of the oropharynx, esophagus, and skin are common and are among the early manifestations of the disease. Infections with rotavirus can be persistent and may spread to extraintestinal sites (3), while respiratory syncytial virus infections often result in giant cell pneumonia (4). Varicella, herpes, measles, and adenoviruses may result in progressive, ultimately fatal infections. Infection with **Pneumocystis carini** (5) and/or cytomegalovirus can lead to chronic, progressive pneumonitis, and patients with SCID frequently*

*fall victim to inadvertent inoculation with live, attenuated organisms. Fatal infections have been reported following vaccination of SCID patients with either live viral vaccines such as that of measles (6) or with the mycobacterium **Bacillus Calmette-Guerin (BCG)** (7). Transfusion with blood products that contain T-lymphocytes and that have not been irradiated may lead to severe GVHD (8). A form of GVHD that is usually milder may result from maternal T-cells that have crossed the placenta. Pathologically, the thymus in SCID patients is usually small and depleted of thymocytes and Hassall corpuscles. Peripheral lymphoid tissues are also commonly atrophied and depleted of lymphocytes.*

Most patients with SCID become acutely sick and require urgent medical attention within a few months after birth. However, the age at presentation and the clinical manifestations of SCID can vary widely among different patients, including those with the same disease etiology and even among affected members of the same family. Moreover, depending on the underlying abnormality, many patients with SCID can start life with seemingly normal immune function only to have progressive immunodeficiency develop over a period of several years.

In contrast to patients with florid SCID diseases, those with less severe defects of cellular immunity may present with more subtle findings. Patients with a partial or incomplete form of the DiGeorge syndrome may be seen clinically with few infections or none at all. Patients with defective expression of MHC class I molecules may not present until early adolescent years with chronic lung disease. As will be discussed, many patients with T-cell defects are also at increased risk of autoimmune diseases developing. Also, because of failure of immune surveillance, these patients are often at increased risk for development of malignancies.

The diagnosis of a T-cell immunodeficiency is confirmed by appropriate laboratory investigation. In most cases, simple tests can provide clues to the presence of T-cell immunodeficiency. These tests include a complete blood count (CBC) with a white blood cell (WBC) differential, erythrocyte sedimentation rate (ESR), delayed type hypersensitivity by skin testing, and a chest x-ray. The WBC and differential may reveal the presence of absolute lymphopenia, a finding frequently present in SCID patients (9), but a normal lymphocyte count does not exclude T-cell defects or SCID. Many other patients actually present with normal lymphocyte counts. In other cases, decreased cell counts of other blood components may point to specific immunodeficiency disorders such as the thrombocytopenia in the Wiskott-Aldrich syndrome and the granulocytosis/neutropenia in reticular dysgenesis. The finding of an elevated ESR would provide support for a history of recurrent infections. Examination of delayed-type hypersensitivity responses to a battery of recall antigens (tetanus toxoid, monilia) by intradermal skin testing is a cheap and simple method to screen for T-cell dysfunction. While intradermal skin testing is frequently negative in young infants, in the wake of acute infections, or during therapy with immunosuppressive agents, a positive skin test result would be effective in ruling out a significant T-cell abnormality. Chest films may reveal an absent thymic shadow, as seen in the DiGeorge syndrome and in most of the SCID patients.

Antibody deficiency syndromes frequently accompany T-cell immunodeficiencies (combined immunodeficiencies) either as a consequence of T-cell dysfunction or due to the involvement of B-cells by the same disease process. Because the clinical history alone may not differentiate between isolated antibody deficiency syndromes and disorders of T-cell function, evaluation of humoral immunity should be carried out in cases of suspected T-cell dysfunction. This can be achieved by quantitation of serum immunoglobulin levels and measurement of specific antibody titers to one of the childhood vaccines such as tetanus toxoid. The latter test provides for a particularly sensitive measure of T-cell help for antigen-specific antibody production. Elevated specific titers would indicate adequate T-cell helper function while a low titer would be compatible with either T- or B-cell immunodeficiency.

Detailed immunologic investigation is usually required to confirm the diagnosis of specific T-cell immunodeficiency syndromes. Key among the investigative procedures employed are lymphocyte phenotyping by flow cytometry and in vitro functional T-cell studies. Lymphocyte phenotyping frequently provides the diagnosis in suspect cases. It may reveal depletion or absence of both T- and B-cells, a finding that would suggest a defect affecting lymphoid stem cell development, such as that seen in Swiss-type SCID, or a severe metabolic abnormality adversely affecting the survival of lymphocytes such as the adenine deaminase deficiency state. In other cases, the T-cells are the major cell type affected. Selective depletion of T-cells or subsets thereof would suggest a defect affecting T-cell development (e.g., X-linked SCID). Specific T-immunodeficiency syndromes resulting from deficient expression of specific cell surface molecules such as MHC molecules or the T-cell receptor (TCR)/CD-3 complex (TCR)/CD-3 are readily diagnosed by flow cytometry. Finally, SCID syndromes with normal lymphocyte numbers and phenotype would suggest a defect in T-cell function (e.g., defective production of key T-cell lymphokines such as IL-2).

Defective in vitro functional T-cell studies provide strong evidence for a T-cell abnormality. These studies include testing for proliferation to classical T-cell mitogen such as the lectins phytohemagglutinin, concanavalin A, and pokeweed mitogen. They also include proliferation to recall antigens such as tetanus toxoid (ideally after booster vaccination) and to alloantigens (allogenic lymphocytes in a mixed lymphocyte reaction). Measurement of lymphokine production by mitogen-activated T-cells provides screening for lymphokine deficiency states underlying some cases of SCID.

Any patient suspected of having severe combined immunodeficiency is usually tested for enzymatic defects in the purine salvage pathway (adenine deaminase [ADA] and purine nucleoside phosphorylase [PNP]) because deficiency in these enzymes is the underlying etiology in up to 15% of SCID cases. Also, infection with HIV should be considered in the differential diagnosis of all cases of immunodeficiency. When clinically appropriate, this latter diagnosis should be investigated by standard enzyme-linked immunosorbent assay (ELISA) and Western blotting tests on both the child and the mother. Direct detection of viral genome can be carried out by using the polymerase chain reaction technique and/or by viral cultures.

T-Cell Immunodeficiencies: Pathogenic Considerations

T-Cell immunodeficiencies may arise out of a number of diverse defects. Some of these defects result in partial or complete depletion of T-lymphocytes due to developmental failure or to metabolic toxicity. Included in this group are a number of intrinsic stem cell abnormalities which interrupt the development of T-cells, thymic hypoplasia which leads to disruption of the environment in which T-cell development takes place, and metabolic abnormalities of the purine salvage pathway which act to compromise the viability of both developing and mature lymphocytes. Another set of defects acts to interfere with the differentiated function of T-lymphocytes such as antigen recognition or the ensuing processes of T-cell activation and lymphokine production.

The patient in case 1 had selective depletion of T-lymphocytes in the presence of increased numbers of circulating B-cells. His condition suggests abnormal T-cell development perhaps due to a stem cell defect or to an unknown metabolic toxicity. In approaching his disorder, it is useful to have a thorough understanding of the normal process of T-cell development, as detailed below.

T-Cell Development and Its Disorders

T-Cell development proceeds through a series of well-defined developmental steps that occur primarily in the thymus and are schematically illustrated in figure 14.1 (for a general review on thymic development, see Sprent [10]). It is initiated upon the migration into the thymus of precursor cells committed to the T-cell lineage. The most immature thymocytes reside in the subcapsular region of the thymic cortex and can be identified by their reactivity with monoclonal antibodies directed against the T-cell surface markers CD-7 and CD-2 (see The Cluster of Differentiation [CD] System). They do not express TCR molecules, CD-3, CD-4, or CD-8 surface antigen. The next stage in thymic development involves the rearrangement of TCR genes, giving rise to heterodimers composed of ab and gd subunits. All four

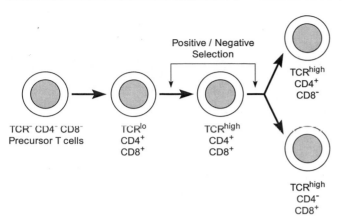

Figure 14.1. Development of T-lymphocytes in the thymus. Precursor T-cells (TCR-CD-4-CD-8-) acquire the expression of both CD-4 and CD-8 and of T-cell receptor (TCR) molecules as they mature in the thymus. These double-positive thymocytes give rise to mature, single-positive T-lymphocytes. Thymocytes undergo positive and negative selection, as detailed in the text. Selection is thought to take place in the double-positive stage, although the exact step(s) at which the selection processes operate is still a topic of debate.

chains—α-, β-, γ-, and δ-—are composed of variable regions and constant regions. The TCR β- and δ- chains are encoded by three variable genetic elements termed *V* (variable), *D* (diversity), and *J* (joining), and a constant region termed *C*. Similarly, the α and γ are encoded by two variable genetic elements: *V* and *J*, and a constant region termed *C*. For each chain, there exists in the genome a large number of variable region elements. These elements, which are separated in the genome by large stretches of DNA, are brought together by DNA rearrangement. The large numbers of potential *VDJ* or *VJ* recombinations account for the diversity in T-cell receptor (TCR) molecules. Each T-cell expresses either one ab heterodimer or one gd heterodimer. The majority (>90%) of developing thymocytes and peripheral blood T-lymphocytes express the ab TCR, while the remaining minority express the gd TCR. Both types of TCR heterodimers are expressed on the cell surface only in association with subunits of the CD-3 complex (CD-3g, d, and e) and dimeric products of the z gene (z and/or the closely related h).

The T-cell receptor is the singular tool by which T-cells recognize and respond to antigens. T-Cells do not recognize native proteins, nor do they recognize polysaccharides or lipids. They only recognize small peptide fragments, 9–15 residues long, that are presented by MHC molecules of antigen-presenting cells. These peptides are derived from intracellular processing of native self- or foreign proteins. Each TCR molecule has a unique specificity for a peptide/MHC combination that is determined by the variable regions of the heterodimeric pair. The sum of all TCR specificities found in the immune system represents the T-cell repertoire of that immune system. Disruption of T-cell repertoire formation in the thymus due to abnormal recombination of gene elements that constitute the TCR

underlies some forms of human and experimental SCID diseases. Failure of T-cell receptor recombination would block further thymocyte maturation and would result in a clinical picture of SCID.

Expression of TCR/CD-3 complexes is closely coupled in most developing thymocytes with expression of both CD-4 and CD-8 on the cell surface, resulting in a "double-positive" phenotype. Double-positive thymocytes constitute the majority of thymocytes (75–85%), and they characteristically express the cell surface antigen CD-1a. Their further development in the medulla results in the generation of the single positive (CD-4+CD-8- or CD-8+CD-4-) phenotype characteristic of peripheral blood T-cells.

The T-cell repertoire of developing thymocytes is shaped by two selection processes that ensure the capacity of TCR molecules to recognize peptides presented by self-MHC complexes and yet allow for the discrimination between peptides derived from self-proteins versus those derived from foreign proteins. The first of the processes, termed "positive selection," allows the further development of only those thymocytes whose surface TCR displays some affinity for self-MHC molecules. This ensures the capacity of mature T-cells to recognize foreign peptides when presented with the body's own MHC molecules. A second process of negative selection ensures, however, that these same thymocytes do not have too high an affinity for their own self-peptide/MHC complexes lest autoreactive T-cells are generated. The overall result of these two selection processes is to generate self-tolerant T-cells whose TCR exhibits low affinity of interaction with self-peptide/MHC complexes but still retains the capacity to recognize with high affinity self-MHC complexes bearing foreign peptides leading to T-cell activation. Those thymocytes that do display heightened affinity for self-peptide/MHC complexes are deleted by a process of TCR-triggered programmable cell death.

Only a small percentage (<5%) of thymocytes successfully undergo positive and negative selection, with the remaining thymocytes dying in the thymus within a few days. The processes of positive and negative selection in the thymus can be readily disrupted by a variety of clinically relevant defects. One particular consequence of abnormal thymic development that is uniquely encountered in partial T-cell defects is a propensity for autoimmune disorders. This may be due to inefficient negative selection of autoreactive T-cells, allowing for their escape into the periphery.

The Cluster of Differentiation (CD) System

The biochemical characterization and cloning of scores of molecules expressed on the surface of immune cells and the availability of numerous monoclonal antibodies against these molecules has allowed for an unparalleled capacity to identify and track various subsets of immune cells during their development, activation, and differentiation. This process has been facilitated by the adoption of the cluster of differentiation (CD) designation as a unified nomenclature system for leukocytes' surface molecules. In this system, cell surface molecules (also referred to as antigens or markers), whose structure is well defined as recognized by a group (cluster) of monoclonal antibodies (mAbs), are given a CD number, such as CD-1, CD-2, etc. CD designation is determined by international workshops, and molecules recently identified by newer mAbs are assigned a new designation number and introduced as regular members to the list of CD molecules or are introduced with the qualification of being new "workshop" candidates (CDw), pending final approval. While originally developed for human leukocyte surface molecules, the same CD designation is now applied to homologous molecules found in other species.

CD antigens are grouped into categories that include T-cell antigens, B-cell antigens, NK cell antigens, myeloid antigens, platelet antigens, antigens not restricted to any lineage, and activation antigens. It is important to realize that many CD antigens usually thought of as being restricted to a particular lineage may be expressed on different lineages either constitutively or in a developmental or activation stage-dependent manner (e.g., CD-5, which is expressed on all mature T-cells and a subset of B-cells, and CD-8, which is expressed on subsets of T- and NK cells). It follows that a particular lineage or subsets thereof can be better defined by using combinations of mAb (e.g., CD-3/CD-8 for CD-8+ T-cells).

Stem Cell Defects

There are several forms of SCID that result from lesions that disrupt different steps along the T-lymphocyte developmental pathway (fig. 14.2). One form of SCID resulting from disruption of a very early step in lymphoid development is **Reticular Dysgenesia**. This congenital disease is characterized by defective maturation of lymphoid (T- and B-cells) and myeloid precursors in the presence of normal erythroid and megakaryocytic development (11, 12). Developing lymphoid and myeloid precursors are progressively depleted as they mature into effector cells (13). This raises the possibility that a growth factor necessary for the development of lymphoid and

myeloid lineages is deficient or cannot signal the cells of these patients. The affected neonates are susceptible to recurrent infections with a wide variety of bacterial, fungal, and viral organisms. The disease is fatal unless treated with bone marrow transplantation, which is curative.

Failure of lymphoid stem cell development is the hallmark of the **Swiss-Type SCID**. This is the first SCID condition ever described. It is an autosomal recessive disorder characterized by fatal infections associated with severe lymphopenia (14). The net biologic effect is the lack of both T- and B-cells at all stages of development. Other hematopoietic cell lineages are spared. Bone marrow transplantation is potentially curative. While the cause of Swiss-type SCID is unknown, insight into potential etiologic mechanisms has been provided by "SCID mouse" model, which features selective depletion of T- and B-cell lineages at all stages of development. The defect in the SCID mouse resides in the inability to achieve successful *VDJ* rearrangement in both T-cell receptor and immunoglobulin genes due to abnormal recombinase activity (15). Fibroblasts of SCID mice exhibit heightened radiosensitivity, indicating that the underlying defect may be a disorder of DNA repair leading to failure of TCR and immunoglobulin gene recombination. It has also been shown that some patients with Swiss-type SCID have an abnormal recombination pattern of the *DJ* elements of their immunoglobulin heavy chain gene locus (16), suggesting that they have a defect related to that of the SCID mouse.

The **Omenn Syndrome** may represent a variant form of T-B-SCID. This disease is characterized by eosinophilia with T-cell infiltration of several organs, including the skin, gut, liver, and spleen (17). It is associated with a clinical appearance that approximates GVHD and includes intense erythroderma, protracted diarrhea, hepatosplenomegaly, and failure to thrive. There is severe lymphocyte depletion from the thymus and other lymphoid organs. B-Cell numbers are either markedly depressed or totally lacking, and the T-cells are severely restricted in their heterogeneity (18). Both fibroblasts and granulocyte macrophage colony-stimulating units of patients with Omenn syndrome show heightened radiosensitivity, reminiscent of the SCID mouse model (19). Additionally, siblings of patients with Omenn syndrome may present with a lymphocytosis (Swiss-type SCID clinical appearance). Overall, these findings indicate that Omenn syndrome may represent a leaky phenotype of the T-B-SCID that results from failure of TCR immunoglobulin gene rearrangement. Some cells appear to escape this defect only to become highly autoreactive, leading to an appearance of autoimmunity with eosinophilia.

The presence of a high number of B-lymphocytes in the patient's circulation together with his normal myeloid development effectively ruled out reticular dysgenesia and Swiss-type SCID as the underlying abnormality.

The finding of isolated failure of T-cell development in the presence of apparently normal B-cell develop-

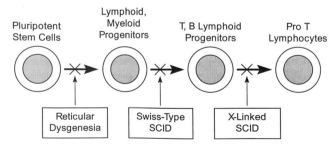

Figure 14.2. SCID diseases resulting from stem cell defects. In reticular dysgenesia, a lesion early in stem cell maturation affects both lymphoid and myeloid development. The Swiss-type severe combined immunodeficiency (SCID) mutation selectively affects commitment to lymphoid lineage, while X-linked SCID selectively affects commitment to a T-cell lineage.

ment is the hallmark of X-linked SCID (20). This disease accounts for up to 25% of all SCID cases. Family history of X-linked disease can be elicited in one-third of the patients. The rest of the cases result from an unrecognized carrier state. As noted, it is characterized by the failure of T-cell development, absence of host T-cells from both circulation and lymphoid organs, and a hypoplastic thymus devoid of thymocytes and Hassall corpuscles. While transplacental engraftment of maternal lymphocytes frequently results in the presence of significant numbers of circulating T-cells, the maternal T-cells are poorly functional (20). The numbers of circulating B-cells are usually increased and have a normal phenotype but abnormal function. They produce reduced amounts of immunoglobulins in vitro and appear to have a block affecting their terminal differentiation. T-Cells of female carriers display nonrandom inactivation of their X-chromosome. All examined T-cells appear to retain the X-chromosome carrying the wild type but not the defective X-linked-SCID allele, indicating an essential role for this allele in T-cell survival. Interestingly, although female carriers exhibit a random pattern of X-chromosome inactivation in their immature, surface Igm positive B-cells, they exhibit a nonrandom inactivation pattern in their mature, surface IgM negative B-cells, indicative of a requirement from the X-linked SCID allele for terminal B-cell maturation.

X-Linked patients carry mutations in a cytokine receptor subunit, termed common g-chain or gc, whose gene was found to map in the region on the X-chromosome (Xq13.1) previously determined to be the locus for X-linked SCID (21). gc is a component of IL-2, IL-4, and IL-7 receptors, and is thought to play an essential role in signaling via these receptors (22). While IL-2 deficiency can result in a SCID phenotype, patients suffering from IL-2 deficiency display normal numbers of circulating T-lymphocytes (see section on T-Cell Activation Defects). Similarly, normal T-cell development is observed in mice rendered deficient in IL-2 or IL-4 by targeted gene disruption. Thus, failure of T-cell development in X-linked SCID is unlikely to be due to dysfunctional IL-2 or IL-4 receptors. In contrast, treatment of mice with an IL-7 monoclonal antibody results in failure of both T- and B-cell development, suggesting that disruption of the IL-7 receptor function may underlie the failure of T-cell development in X-linked SCID. Abnormal IL-4 receptor function may additionally impair the maturation of B-cells in view of the important role played by IL-4 in B-cell activation and differentiation.

Diagnosis of X-linked SCID has been accomplished by examining T-lymphocytes of carrier females for nonrandom X-chromosome inactivation pattern (23, 24). Bone marrow transplantation restores normal T-cell development and function. However, it frequently fails to correct the impaired B-cell function due to aborted engraftment of transplanted B-cells leaving the patients with their own B-cells. In such cases, intravenous immunoglobulin therapy is maintained indefinitely.

A very few cases of SCID with selective failure of T-cell development and autosomal recessive inheritance have been described, the molecular basis of which remains unknown.

The DiGeorge Syndrome

In contrast to the aforementioned diseases, the DiGeorge syndrome represents a prime example of aborted T-cell development due to the absence or disruption of the thymic microenvironment. In contrast to X-linked SCID and other disorders of lymphoid stem cells, in which the lymphoid lineages are the only tissues affected, the DiGeorge syndrome exhibits aberrant development of several tissues, including thymic, craniofacial, cardiac and parathyroid (25). It results from the disruption in normal embryogenesis of a group of cephalic neural crest cells. Conditions associated with the DiGeorge syndrome include chromosome 22 aneuploidy (monosomy 22 or deletions of the long arm of chromosome 22) (26), fetal alcohol syndrome (27), and retinoic acid embryopathy (28). While most cases are not inherited, both autosomal dominant (29) and autosomal recessive (30) forms of the anomaly have been reported. In recent years, several studies have demonstrated hemizygous deletions of chromosome 22q11 in the overwhelming majority of patients with the DiGeorge syndrome (31). Deletions in the same locus are also present in the closely related velocardiofacial syndrome. Prenatal diagnosis is possible by fluorescent in situ hybridization using appropriate DNA probes.

The clinical manifestations of the DiGeorge syndrome can be mild and isolated or more severe and widespread, depending on the severity of the underlying insult. Commonly encountered craniofacial findings include micrognathia, hypertelorism, shortened philtrum, and low-set, dorsally rotated auricles with or without malformations. Cardiac anomalies include conotruncal defects, such as tetralogy of Fallot, transposition of the great vessels, double-outlet right ventricle and ventricular septal defects, and branchial arch defects such as interrupted or hypoplastic aortic arch. The parathyroid glands may be absent or reduced in number, and subclinical hypoparathyroidism is frequently present (32). Major congenital anomalies involving the diaphragm, the eyes, the kidneys, and the central nervous system also abound (33). Moderate-to-severe mental retardation is seen in most patients (34).

The thymus in the DiGeorge syndrome may be absent or, more commonly, hypoplastic (33). The spectrum of immune dysfunction observed in this condition ranges from the severe (so-called "complete" DiGeorge syndrome) to the subtle (partial DiGeorge syndrome) (34, 35). In the complete form of the DiGeorge syndrome there exists a picture of combined T- and B-cell immunodeficiency. The T-cells may be depleted and their function is severely depressed. B-Cell numbers are usually elevated, but hypo-γ-globulinemia and absent antigen-specific antibody responses are prevalent. Far more common is the picture of partial DiGeorge syndrome, where T-cell dysfunction is moderate to minimal and B-cell number and function are normal. NK cell activity is generally unaffected in both forms of the disease. Defective thymic selection processes may predispose patients to autoimmune diseases, and at least 2 cases of autoimmunity associated with the DiGeorge syndrome have been reported to date (36).

In most cases, the immunologic deficit ameliorates with time. This may be accounted for by functioning residual thymic tissue or by extrathymic maturation of T-cells. This severe immunologic deficit has been successfully managed with fetal thymic transplants (37, 38). However, the spontaneous improvement in immunologic function noted in most patients renders this type of therapy moot. IVIG therapy can be of some benefit in cases with severe immunologic deficit.

SCID with Metabolic Defects

Metabolic abnormalities that result in forms of SCID include two disorders of the purine salvage pathway, ADA and purine nucleoside phosphorylase (PNP) deficiency, which in turn account for 15–20% of all SCID cases in North America (39, 40). ADA deficiency compromises the viability of both T- and B-cells, and is particularly toxic to developing thymocytes. In contrast, PNP deficiency more selectively impacts T-cells and their progenitors, although in some patients B-cells may also be affected. Both conditions are inherited as autosomal recessives of ADA deficiency, and most cases are caused by point mutations and deletions affecting the ADA gene or chromosome 20 (41) that result in either loss of enzyme expression or in the production of an unstable or inactive protein (42–48). Partial ADA deficiency resulting from mutations affecting the stability and/or the activity of the enzyme has been reported (49). However, most were healthy individuals and did not demonstrate the gross biochemical abnormalities seen in SCID patients (50).

While ADA is expressed by all cell types, ADA deficiency per se selectively affects the immune system. This is due to unique attributes of purine metabolism in lymphoid cells (51) (fig. 14.3). ADA catalyzes the deamination of adenosine and deoxyadenosine to inosine and deoxyinosine, respectively (fig. 14.3). In ADA deficiency, the chief abnormality relates to deoxyadenosine metabolism. Deoxyadenosine accumulates in ADA-deficient lymphocytes, predominantly in thymocytes, due to the high turnover rate of the latter cells. Toxic metabolites, particularly deoxyadenosine triphosphate (dATP), are selectively entrapped, because deoxyadenosine kinase, an enzyme that phosphorylates the accumulating deoxyadenosine into dATP, is highly expressed in lymphoid tissue (52). Conversely, lymphocytes express very low levels of the enzyme 5'-nucleotidase, which catalyzes the de-

phosphorylation of nucleotides and deoxynucleotides. The net effort is selective accumulation of dATP in lymphoid tissues to levels 50- to 1000-fold higher than those normally found. High levels of dATP are toxic to lymphocytes, and especially to thymocytes. Several mechanisms account for this toxicity. First, dATP inhibits the interconversion of ribonucleotides to deoxyribonucleotides catalyzed by the enzyme ribonucleotide reductase by a feedback mechanism. This deprives lymphocytes of deoxyribonucleotides (other than dATP) that are necessary for DNA synthesis and results in cell cycle arrest. High levels of dATP also inhibit RNA synthesis, disrupt DNA repair mechanisms (53), and interfere with DNA methylation by blocking the activity of the enzyme S-adenosylhomocysteine hydrolase.

Within months after birth, patients with ADA deficiency usually present with recurrent infections associated with profound lymphopenia and hypo-γ-globulinemia. However, ADA deficiency may also present as a slowly progressive immunodeficiency with initial studies showing normal or near-normal immune parameters. Skeletal abnormalities, including cupping and flaring of the costochondral junctions and dysplasia of the pelvis, are frequently encountered but are not pathognomonic. The thymus is depleted of thymocytes, though changes suggestive of early thymocyte differentiation and rare Hassall corpuscles may occasionally be seen. Diagnosis is established by demonstrating low ADA activity in blood cells in conjunction with elevated levels of deoxyadenosine and dATP in blood and urine. Prenatal diagnosis can be made on fetal blood samples. In all cases, the outcome is fatal unless treated with bone marrow transplantation, which currently is the only therapy that provides permanent cure for this disease (54–57). However, the peculiarly high incidence of graft failure in these patients makes such efforts tenuous (57). Enzyme replacement therapy with ethylene glycol-modified ADA provides an alternative, ongoing treatment modality that is safe but only moderately effective for patients lacking a suitable bone marrow donor (58). Gene replacement modalities may, in the foreseeable future, provide lasting therapy for ADA-deficient patients.

Unlike ADA deficiency, PNP deficiency, which results in accumulation of inosine and guanosine, is frequently associated with relatively normal B-cell numbers and immunoglobulin levels in the presence of profoundly depressed T-cell numbers and function (40). PNP is coded by a single gene located on chromosome 14 (59) and the enzyme catalyzes the conversion of inosine to hypoxanthine and guanosine to guanine (fig. 14.3). PNP deficiency may result from point mutations or deletions affecting the PNP gene (60). As in ADA deficiency, the deleterious effects of PNP deficiency on T-lymphocytes is related to the way the cells handle the accumulating substrates of PNP. T-Cells have the highest activity of deoxyguanosine and deoxyinosine kinase, but, as previously pointed out, little

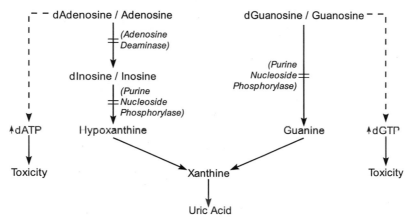

Figure 14.3. Purine metabolism and its disruption in adenosine deaminase (ADA) and purine nucleoside phosphorylase (PNP) deficiency. ADA results in failure of conversion of adenosine and deoxyadenosine to inosine and deoxyinosine. PNP deficiency in-terrupts the conversion of inosine/deoxyinosine and guanosine to hypoxanthine and guanine, respectively. The accumulation of toxic metabolites (*dashed lines*) leads to lymphocyte depletion and immunodeficiency.

5'-nucleotidase activity. Consequently, the accumulating guanosine and inosine are selectively metabolized to deoxyguanosine triphosphate (dGTP) and to deoxyinosine triphosphate, respectively, leading to inhibition of ribonucleotide reductase activity and cessation of DNA synthesis. Clinically, the patients have recurrent severe bacterial and viral infections. Additionally, neurologic abnormalities are seen in upwards of two-thirds of the patients; and autoimmune diseases, including autoimmune hemolytic anemia and thrombocytopenia, occur in about a third of the cases. The thymus is severely depleted of developing T-cells. Bone marrow transplantation is currently the only therapeutic modality available for these children. As for ADA deficiency, diagnosis is established by demonstrating low PNP activity in blood cells in conjunction with elevated levels of deoxyguanosine and dGTP in blood and urine.

Differentiated Functions of T-Lymphocytes and Their Disorders

As noted previously, the immunologic specificity of T-cells is determined during their development in the thymus by the recombination of the variable elements of their T-cell receptor chains. It predates the encounter of T-cells with foreign peptide antigens, with the result that T-cells emerge from the thymus as virgin cells. The process of turning a single virgin T-cell into an expanded population of effector memory cells is complex and has many steps. It takes place in peripheral lymphoid tissues and is initiated upon the engagement of T-cell receptor molecules by foreign peptides presented in the context of MHC molecules of "professional," antigen-presenting cells. This triggers a series of biochemical events in T-cells that lead to activation, proliferation, and eventually to their maintenance as memory cells. It is implicit in the complexity of the system that defects in any one of the several steps involved in T-cell activation and differentiation into effector memory cells could render the

host immunodeficient. An example illustrative of this is given below.

Case 2

R.C., a 5-year-old girl of North African descent, presented with a history of recurrent infections since birth. The child, the product of a consanguineous marriage, was born following a full-term pregnancy and an uneventful delivery. Her problems started soon after birth with the onset of thrush and diarrhea. Recurrent, incessant sinopulmonary infections ensued. Investigation of her immune function revealed a total lymphocyte count of 2.4 × 10⁹/L. Her lymphocyte phenotyping revealed a total of 63% of her peripheral blood lymphocytes expressed as the pan T-cell marker CD3. Moreover, 48% of her T-cells expressed the ab TCR heterodimer, 8% of which were CD4+ and 40% CD8+. The remaining 15% of her T-cells expressed the gd TCR heterodimer and were CD4-CD8-. Examination of her lymphocytes for expression of MHC molecules revealed normal expression of MHC class I molecules on all of the lymphoid cells. In contrast, no MHC class II expression was detectable on either B-lymphocytes or monocytes. Also, unlike normal T-cells, her T-lymphocytes failed to express MHC class II molecules following activation with mitogen. Finally, her peripheral blood mononuclear cells failed to express MHC class II molecules following treatment with interferon-γ, a cytokine that normally upregulates MHC class II expression. The child was diagnosed with MHC class II deficiency, and was referred to the bone marrow transplant service for therapy.

TCR/MHC Interactions and Their Disorders

The vast majority of circulating T lymphocytes are either CD4+or CD8−. The double-positive phenotype

(CD−4+ CD−8+) which predominates in the thymus is either extremely rare or absent, while a small percentage of T lymphocytes exhibit a CD-4-CD-8- phenotype and are mostly TCRgd+. The fundamental distinguishing feature between CD-4+ and CD-8+ T-cells is that CD-4+ T-cells recognize peptide antigens presented in association with MHC class II molecules while CD-8+ T-cells recognize peptide antigens in the context of MHC class I molecules (61). This strict dichotomy in MHC recognition accounts for the differences in function observed between CD-4+ and CD-8+ T-cells. By and large, MHC class I molecules present peptides derived from cytosolic proteins transported into the endoplasmic reticulum by specialized peptides to combine with nascent MHC class I molecules. This accounts for the preponderance of CD-8+ responses to intracellular pathogens (bacterial, viral, protozoan) and to transformed or allogenic cells. MHC class II molecules specialize in presenting peptides derived from soluble proteins that have been internalized by the antigen-presenting cells. This accounts for the dominance of CD-4+ responses to soluble protein products such as tetanus toxoid. The function of CD-4+ in helping B-cells secrete immunoglobulins relies in part on the capacity of B-cells to capture circulating protein antigens via their surface immunoglobulins and to present peptides derived from these proteins complexed with MHC class II molecules to antigen-specific CD-4+ T-lymphocytes.

The molecular basis for the strict specialization of MHC recognition by the respective T-cell subset lies in the capacity of the CD-4 molecules to physically interact with MHC class II gene products and CD-8 with MHC class I gene product. These interactions facilitate the cognate recognition of peptide/MHC complexes by TCR molecules. As alluded to above, CD-4+ T-cells are frequently referred to as helper T-cells because of their capacity to support immunoglobulin production by B-cells. In turn, CD-8+ T-cells have been referred to as suppressor/cytotoxic T-cells because of their capacity to lyse target cells and to suppress immune responses. It should be noted that these terms, while useful, are less accurate in portraying the function of CD-4+ and CD-8+ subsets compared with a definition based on dichotomy in MHC recognition. Thus, CD-4+ T have been reported to occasionally exhibit cytotoxic and suppressor function. While the predominantly cytotoxic function of CD-8+ T-cells is undisputed, the concept of a suppressor function for CD-8+ T-cells has been held in question.

CD-4/MHC class II and CD-8/MHC class I interactions are critical to the processes of positive and negative selection of T-lymphocytes in the thymus. Both CD-4 and CD-8 molecules enhance the avidity of interaction of TCR of developing thymocytes with MHC molecules. Lesions that disrupt these interactions may result in the depletion of CD-4 or CD-8 T-lymphocytes, seemingly due to the abrogation of positive selection in the thymus. This was elegantly demonstrated in MHC class I or MHC class II

molecule deficient mice, who were found to suffer from severe failure of development of CD-8+ or CD-4+ T-cells (62–65). The same interactions allow for potential autoreactive TCR specificities to be uncovered, leading to the deletion of self-reactive T-cells in thymus. As will be discussed below, lesions that interfere with these interactions are associated with enhanced incidence of autoimmune disorders.

It can be appreciated from this discussion that patients lacking in the expression of MHC class I or class II molecules would present with specific abnormalities affecting the development and functioning of CD-8+ and CD-4+ cells. As can be seen in our patient, who lacked in MHC class II expression, the development of CD-4+ T-cells in thymus is markedly impaired, although not totally aborted. This is a direct consequence of the failure of CD-4+ thymocytes to undergo positive selection (66). More importantly, because CD-4+ T-cells are restricted in their responses to antigens presented in the context of MHC class II molecules, MHC class II deficiency results in the failure of immune recognition by CD-4+ T-cells. The available CD-4+ T-lymphocytes cannot mount delayed type hypersensitivity responses nor can they provide help to B-cells to generate antigen-specific humoral responses, resulting in a combined immunodeficiency. Responses to mitogenic lectins and to allogeneic cells are usually preserved. Patients with MHC class II deficiency are prey to recurrent infections not unlike those seen in other forms of SCID. Chronic diarrhea and malabsorption are very common, and recurrent severe viral infections can be fatal. Bone marrow transplantation corrects the immune deficit. The clinical and immunologic findings in MHC class II-deficient children have been recently reviewed (67).

A reciprocal scenario of failure of CD-8+ T-cell development and function attends cases of MHC class I deficiency. These patients suffer from recurrent viral infections, and some are particularly prone to chronic lung disease. In these patients, CD-8 development is impaired, and those circulating CD-8+ T-cells may fail to recognize antigens due to the lack of peptide antigen-presenting MHC class I molecules.

The molecular basis of MHC deficiency syndromes has been well worked (68). SCID with MHC class II deficiency is autosomal recessive, which accounts for 5% of all SCID cases and which results from the failure to express MHC class II molecules, including HLA-DP, HLA-DQ, and HLA-DR (69). It is most prevalent in patients of Mediterranean ancestry. The underlying abnormalities reside not in the MHC genes but in transacting regulatory factors that control the expression of these genes. At least two distinct molecular defects have been identified. The first is a transcriptional factor termed "CIITA," which is a general regulator of MHC class II gene expression and which mediates the induction of these genes by interferon-γ. Some patients with MHC class II deficiency appear to have deletions that disrupt CIITA messenger RNA or that alter its processing. Another defect affects a factor termed RF-X that binds a conserved response element (X box) in the MHC class II promoter region.

MHC class I deficiency is another autosomal recessive, albeit much rarer. The MHC class I genes in this disease are also unaffected. In one well-characterized family, the defect was found to reside in one subunit (TAP1) of a heterodimeric transporter protein formed by two homologous proteins known as TAP1 and TAP2 (70). This transporter acts to transport peptides from the cytosol to the endoplasmic reticulum where they associate with MHC class I molecules. Failure to transport peptides results in the formation of MHC class I/b2 microglobulin complexes that do not carry any peptides. These complexes are not stable

and are not efficiently transported to the surface (fig. 14.4).

Impairment of TCR/MHC recognition can also result from defects affecting TCR expression. At least two kindred have described in which TCR receptor expression has been severely impaired due to point mutations in the TCR-associated CD-3 subunits g (71, 72) and e (73). These mutations impair the assembly and the export of TCR chains to the cell surface. The patients' T-cells have decreased responses to mitogen that act via the TCR/CD-3 such as MHC-restricted antigens, lectins, or monoclonal antibodies to the various subunits of TCR/CD-3. Clinically, the patients have severe recurrent infections with bacteria and viruses, as well as intractable diarrhea and failure to thrive.

As alluded to above, an important consequence of impairment of TCR/MHC interaction in the thymus is the development of enhanced propensity for autoimmunity. This is a direct consequence of derangement of negative selec-

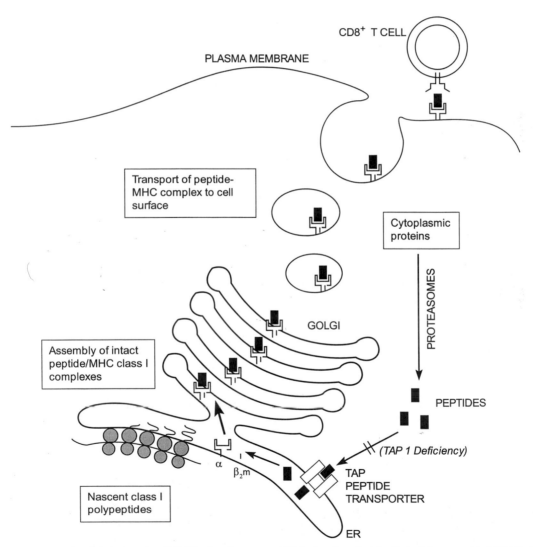

Figure 14.4. Major histocompatibility complex (MHC) class I assembly and its disruption in TAP1 deficiency. MHC class I binding peptides are generated from cytoplasmic proteins, which are generated by proteolysis by specialized particles (proteosomes). These peptides are then translocated into the endoplasmic reticulum by TAP proteins, where the peptides combine with nascent MHC class I chains and β2 microglobulin to form a functional MHC class I molecule. Only fully assembled MHC class I molecules can leave the endoplasmic reticulum to the cell surface. TAP1 deficiency results in failure of peptide transport into the endoplasmic reticulum. This leads to the assembly of MHC class I molecules lacking in peptide antigens. Such empty molecules are retained in the endoplasmic reticulum leading to failure of MHC class I surface expression and consequent immunodeficiency.

tion in the thymus, leading to the export of autoreactive T-cells to the periphery. Both MHC and TCR deficiency syndromes are associated with autoimmune phenomena (hemolytic anemia, enteropathy, and autoantibody production). This association extends to include other T-cell immunodeficiencies in which the underlying pathology may impair processes of thymic selection. Included in this group are ADA and PNP deficiency, the DiGeorge syndrome, and a host of other less common T-cell defects.

T-Cell Activation and Its Disorders

Engagement of the TCR by foreign peptide/MHC complexes results in the transmission to T-cells of activation signals leading to their proliferation and differentiation into effector cells (fig. 14.5). These signals are generated by several distinct, surface receptor–associated tyrosine kinases. Some of these kinases, such as the protein tyrosine kinases p59fyn and ZAP 70, associate directly with the TCR/CD-3 complex, while another, p56lck, is found associated with CD-4 and CD-8 molecules. Once activated, these protein tyrosine kinases act to trigger a rise in free intracellular calcium concentrations and to activate other intracellular protein kinases including the serine/threonine-specific protein kinase C. These biochemical events culminate the initiation of transcription of a number of genes encoding activation products including lymphokines and their receptors and the progression of T-lymphocytes through the cell cycle leading to their proliferation.

Several forms of T-cell immunodeficiency have been determined to result from defects affecting T-cell activation. Unlike SCID resulting from disorders of T-cell development and/or from metabolic defects, the number of circulating T-cells in these disorders is either normal or only mildly reduced. In many cases, the phenotype of these circulating lymphocytes is normal. However, functional studies reveal profound abnormalities in the cellular and, frequently, the humoral compartments.

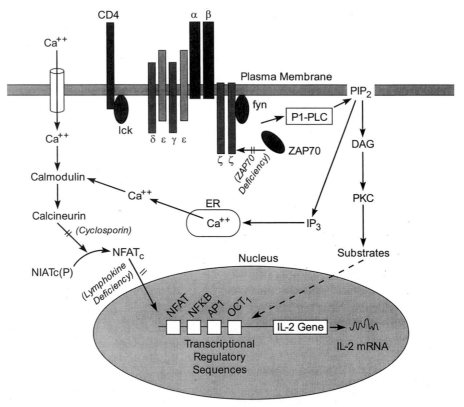

Figure 14.5. Signal transduction pathways mediating T-cell activation. Engagement of TCR/CD-3 by MHC/peptide complexes activates intracellular tyrosine kinases, including p56lck, p50fyn, and ZAP 70, which in turn phosphorylate and activate target proteins such as phospholipase C-g1. This enzyme breaks down membrane phosphoinositides, such as phosphatidylinositol 4,5 bisphosphate, to generate intracellular second messengers. These include diacylglycerol, a second messenger that activates protein kinase C, and inositol 1, 4, 5-triphosphate, which mediates the release of Ca+2 from intracellular stores. These biochemical signals activate transcriptional factors that initiate the transcription of target genes such as IL-2. Ca+2 signaling, mediated by the Ca+2/calmodulin-dependent phosphatase calcineurin, acts on the nuclear factor of activated T-cells (NFAT) to induce its translocation to the nucleus. Protein kinase C activation induces the transcription and assembly of protein components of the transcriptional AP1. The assembly of these and other factors such as NF-kB and OCT1 allows for the transcription of cytokine genes such as IL-2. In ZAP 70 deficiency, there is failure of signaling via the T-cell receptor leading to immunodeficiency. The immunosuppressive drug cyclosporin A acts to inhibit calcineurin and consequently NFAT activation. Primary defects affecting NFAT may also result in cytokine deficiency, as seen in some patients with immunodeficiency.

A prominent example of the essential role played by receptor-associated protein tyrosine kinases in T-cell development and in the initiation of T-cell activation came from the discovery of a SCID form associated with deficiency in the protein tyrosine kinase ZAP 70 (74–76). Patients suffering from this autosomal recessive disease present with recurrent infections with evidence of impairment of both cellular and humoral immunity (77, 78). These patients display virtually no CD-8+ T-cells in their circulation, and examination of their thymuses revealed the presence of CD-4+CD-8+ immature thymocytes but no CD-8+ single positive mature thymocytes. This indicated a vital role played by ZAP 70 in the development of CD-8+ T-lymphocytes. While the patients have normal numbers of CD-4+ T-cells, these cells do not respond to T-cell mitogen that acts by engaging the T-cell receptor. However, they do undergo activation and proliferation in response to mitogen that bypasses surface receptors and directly activates intracellular signaling pathways. The latter observation provided a clue to the presence of a T-cell abnormality, which was confirmed by the discovery of ZAP 70 deficiency. These patients have been found to suffer from insertions and mutations affecting the kinase DNA. Bone marrow transplantation is the only curative approved.

Defective signaling via TCR/CD-3 has also been observed in another patient who suffered from SCID despite the presence of normal numbers of both circulating CD-4+ and CD-8+ T-cells (79). Surface expression of TCR/CD-3 was normal. However, engagement of TCR/CD-3 on the patient T-cells did not result in the induction of early activation events associated with T-cell activation. The defect could be corrected in vitro by stimulation with agents that bypass the TCR/CD-3 to directly activate the intracellular activation pathways. While the phenotype is distinct from that of ZAP 70 deficiency, it points to the presence of a host of heterogenous defects which derange signaling via the T-cell receptor and lead to immunodeficiency.

Another group of SCID patients whose circulating lymphocytes are normal in number and in phenotype appear to suffer from defects in the production of T-cell lymphokines. Several cases of SCID with defective production of IL-2 have been described (80–83). The patients exhibit a normal or mildly reduced number of circulatory T-cells with severely defective proliferative responses to mitogen. Supplementation with IL-2 restores the proliferative responses to normal levels, thus confirming the existence of an IL-2 deficiency state. The defects resulting in IL-2 deficiency are likely to be heterogeneous and may include deletions or mutations affecting the IL-2 gene, its 5′ regulatory region, or in transacting regulatory factors. Some of the transacting factors that regulate IL-2 are also involved in the regulation of other lymphokines such as IL-3, IL-4, IL-5 and interferon-γ and are the target of action of the immunosuppressive agents, cyclosporine and FK506. Indeed, a cyclosporine-like defect resulting from defective transcription of multiple lymphokines and presenting as an IL-2 deficiency has been described and traced to a defect in a transacting factor termed NFAT that acts to activate lymphokine gene transcription (fig. 14.5). This factor is itself a target for immunosuppressive drugs such as cyclosporine, and FK506, both of which act to inhibit its assembly in the nucleus (83, 84). In this case, IL-2 replacement therapy has been successfully applied when repeated bone marrow transplantation failed (80). The future role of IL-2 replacement therapy in these children remains to be determined.

Combined Immunodeficiencies Associated with Other Defects

In addition to T-cell development and activation disorders, there are a host of other diseases associated with T-cell dysfunction, two of which, **Ataxia Telangiectasia** and **Wiskott-Aldrich Syndrome,** are especially pertinent.

Ataxia Telangiectasia

Ataxia telangiectasia (AT) is an autosomal recessive disease characterized by progressive cerebellar ataxia, occulocutaneous telangiectasia, immunodeficiency, and increased cellular sensitivity to ionizing radiation (85–87). Heterozygote carriers are estimated to constitute as many as 1.4% of the United States population (88, 89). A hallmark of this disease is the heightened sensitivity of tissues of AT patients to ionizing radiation and radiomimetic agents (90, 91), suggesting a defect in DNA repair as the underlying abnormality in this disease.

Ataxia usually manifests first. It presents as a staggering gait in infancy and is followed by other manifestations of neurologic dysfunction, including ocular apraxia and choreoathetosis. Telangiectasias are first apparent as dilations of small blood vessels in the bulbar conjunctivae and then become visible in the skin, most notably around the ears, the neck, and antecubital and popliteal fossae, at the age of 5 years. Endocrine abnormalities, including gonadal dysgenesis and insulin-resistant diabetes mellitus, are frequently encountered. Recurrent sinopulmonary infections leading to bronchiectasis are notable features of the disease and reflect the underlying immunodeficiency. Serum levels of oncofetoproteins, including serum α-1-fetoprotein (92) and carcinoembryonic antigen (93) are elevated. For children ≥1 year of age, elevated α 1 fetoprotein determination coupled to a clinical picture of AT confirms the diagnosis (89).

Immunodeficiency in AT is the result of defects in both cellular and humoral immunity. The thymus is abnormally small, sparsely populated, and poorly demarcated between the cortex and the medulla. Hassall corpuscles are diminuted or absent (94, 95). While the number of circulating T-cells in most patients is normal or near normal, examination of peripheral lymphoid tissues frequently reveals depletion of resident T-cells. The number of circulating CD-4+ T-cells may be reduced, while the population of circulating gdTCR+ T-cells may be expanded (96). Parameters of T-cell function such as proliferation in response to mitogens, ability to reject an allograft, and delayed-type hypersensitivity reactions are usually defective. B-Cells are usually normal in numbers. However, there is a high frequency of immunoglobulin isotype deficiency. This is the result of an isotype switch defect precipitated by the impairment in DNA repair mechanism. Those isotypes whose heavy chain constant region genes are located further downstream (3′) from the variable genes are most severely affected (5′ VDJ χm, d, g3, g1, a1, g2, g4, e, a2 3′). The products of the most proximally located genes, IgM and IgD, are unaffected. In contrast, IgA deficiency is encountered in as many as 70% of the affected persons and may precede the clinical manifestation of immunodeficiency by many years (95). IgE deficiency is similarly prevalent (97, 98). IgG deficiency, which is found in up to one-half of all patients, most frequently reflects a selective decrease in the levels of IgG2 and IgG 4 subclasses (99, 100).

Patients with AT are at a high risk for developing malignancies, particularly those of the lymphoid system (101). Over 85% of the tumors reported in affected children are acute lymphocytic leukemias or lymphomas. The incidence of tumors of epithelial origin increases progressively with age. The increased frequency of tumors in this syndrome extends to include relatives of affected patients (102–105). Chromosomal abnormalities abound, and are thought to contribute to the increased tumorigenicity in this disease. Loci of recombining immunoglobulin and T-cell receptor genes are particularly affected. Most of the chromosomal breaks are found in chromosomes 7 and 14 at sites of rearranging immunoglobulin superfamily genes (106): at chromosome 14q11-q12, site of TCR α- and δ-chain loci; at 7q35, in the TCR β-chain locus; at 7p15, site of the TCR γ-chain locus, and at 14q32, site of the IgG heavy chain locus. In light of heightened sensitivity to ionizing radiation and increased risk for developing malignancies, it is imperative to curtail exposure of AT patients to x-rays. Similarly, radiomimetic agents should be avoided when treating malignancies in these patients.

The AT locus has been mapped on the long arm of chromosome 11 at 11q22-23 (89, 107, 108). The disease is probably the result of heterogenous mutations affecting the locus. When fused, fibroblasts from different patients are found to cross-correct the defects in x-ray hypersensitivity, suggesting that AT is a heterogenous disorder (109–111). The finding of heightened radiation sensitivity pointed to a defect in DNA repair as the underlying abnormality. This hypothesis is bolstered by the discovery of DNA ligase I deficiency in Bloom syndrome, a disease that also features telangiectasia, immunologic and central nervous system abnormalities, and a high incidence of leukemia (112, 113).

Wiskott-Aldrich Syndrome (WAS)

This disease, first described by Wiskott in 1937 (114) and later by Aldrich and colleagues in 1954 (115) is an X-linked immunodeficiency state. In its "classical" form, affected males have thrombocytopenia with a severe bleeding tendency, eczema, and increased susceptibility to pyogenic and opportunistic infections (116). "Attenuated" forms of WAS exist in which the bleeding tendency is less severe, and eczema and immunodeficiency are variably expressed (117–120).

The first symptoms of WAS occur early in infancy, and the defect becomes manifest as gastrointestinal bleeding and bloody diarrhea or excessive bleeding following circumcision. Eczema is frequently accompanied by eosinophilia, elevated IgE, and positive prick tests to common allergens, suggesting an underlying allergic etiology. The eczematous skin becomes infected, usually with *Staphylococcus* organisms, due to pruritus and excessive scratching. Persistent otitis media and rhinorrhea are usually noted. Varicella and other childhood viral infections may be unusually severe. Death from bleeding or infection usually occurs in the first decade of life. WAS patients are at high risk of malignancies developing. In a study of 301 patients, malignancies, the majority of which were lymphomas and leukemias, developed in 12% of the group (121). Lymphomas commonly develop at extranodal sites, particularly in the brain and in the gastrointestinal tract.

WAS is associated with abnormalities in lymphocytes, platelets, and phagocytic cells. The platelets are invariably low in number, are small in size, volume being one-half that of normal platelets (122), and display impaired aggregation in response to ADP, epinephrine, ristocetin, and collagen (123, 124). The thrombocytopenia results from both ineffectual thrombocytosis and enhanced sequestration (125). Although megakaryocytes are normal in number, the production of viable platelets is generally decreased (125). Splenectomy helps to ameliorate the thrombocytopenia, suggesting a splenic sequestration effect (126). A role for an immune-mediated mechanism has been suggested by the observation that WAS platelets, when compared with normal platelets, are coated with increased amounts of immunoglobulins and that platelet-associated immunoglobulins return to normal postsplenectomy (122). It is not clear whether increased levels of platelet-associated immunoglobulins result from nonspecific or specific deposition of antiplatelet antibodies. However, autoimmune thrombocytopenia may account for sudden, rapid onset of postsplenectomy thrombocytopenia in some WAS patients (122, 126), in which elevated levels of platelet-associated immunoglobulins can be demonstrated (122).

Immunodeficiency in WAS results from impairment of both cellular and humoral immunity. T-Cell responses to mitogens and specific antigens may be normal at first but become progressively diminished with age (119, 127). Lymphocyte proliferative responses to irradiated allogeneic cells are also reduced, while cutaneous anergy is commonly encountered. Lymphopenia also develops with age, and the ratio of CD-4 to CD-8 cells is frequently inverted. T-Lymphocytes have a characteristic morphologic abnormality; they appear to be relatively devoid of microvilli when examined by electron microscopy (120, 128). Humoral abnormalities abound and may, in part, reflect the abnormalities in T-cell function. There is increased catabolism of serum immunoglobulins, whose levels have a regular pattern: the IgA and IgE are elevated, the IgM decreased, and the IgG normal. The response to polysaccharide antigens is absent or very diminished; isohemagglutinins are absent and the response to polysaccharide vaccines of *Haemophilus influenzae* type B (Hib) and *Pneumococcus* is very poor (129). Response to protein antigens is also defective, reflecting abnormal T-helper cell function. The chemotactic response of neutrophils to chemoattractants is defective (119).

The WAS gene has been mapped to the proximal short arm of the X-chromosome, at Xp11.2 (130, 131). The nature of the defect in WAS is not clear. Previous studies have demonstrated several phenotypic abnormalities affecting WAS blood elements. For example, WAS cells have been shown to defectively express several surface sialoglycoproteins, most prominently the cell surface glycoprotein sialophorin (CD-43) (132). It has been suggested that this abnormality may reflect a defect in *O*-glycosylation (133). Other abnormalities include the aforementioned lack of microvilli in WAS blood lymphocytes (which is indicative of abnormal cytoarchitecture), defective signaling, and failure of proliferation in response to mitogens (134).

Recently, a candidate WAS gene was isolated (135). The gene, termed "WASP," which maps to the same locus of the WAS allele, is expressed in lymphocytes, spleen, and thymus. It encodes a proline-rich, 501-peptide amino acid that has a predicted molecular mass of 54 kd. Importantly, unrelated patients with WAS have been demonstrated to suffer from deletions and mutations affecting the WASP gene. The presence of classical and variant forms of the disease suggests the presence of different mutations affecting the WAS gene and giving rise to distinct clinical manifestations. Although the function of this protein remains unknown at this time, it is expected to be an important regulator of lymphocyte and platelet function. This is supported by the finding that obligate female heterozygotes exhibit nonrandom X-chromosome inactivation in all blood cell lines but not in other tissues such as fibroblasts. As in the case of X-linked SCID and other X-linked immunodeficiency diseases, this finding indicates that hematopoietic cells carrying the inactive WAS alleles are impaired in their development and/or survival relative to their normal counterparts (136–138).

The nonrandom X-chromosome inactivation in WAS female heterozygotes has allowed for screening of carrier state and for prenatal diagnosis of the disease, as detailed previously for X-linked SCID. Other methods useful for prenatal diagnosis include examination of fetal blood for platelet number and size and for decreased microvilli on fetal blood T-cells. The last two tests are not useful for detecting carrier states, as the platelets and lymphocytes of female carriers are normal in number, morphology, and function. The identification of the WAS gene will now allow for development of improved screening methods.

The treatment of choice in WAS is a bone marrow transplant when a histoidentical donor is available (139). Transplants from haploidentical donors have met with limited success. In such situations, when an identical donor is not available splenectomy often has a satisfactory outcome in improving the platelet count and normalizing platelet size (126). However, splenectomy compounds the immunologic defect in this syndrome because of the enhanced risk of overwhelming infections with encapsulated organisms. Intravenous γ-globulin administered at intervals of 2–3 weeks is beneficial in preventing pyogenic infections and is mandatory after splenectomy to counter the added risk of infections, particularly when prophylactic antibiotics are not administered. By and large, intravenous γ-globulin does not improve the thrombocytopenia of WAS.

Treatment of T-Cell Disorders

The first element of treatment in any disease is to avoid doing further harm to the patient. It is imperative to remember that innocuous ailments such as the common cold can prove deadly to patients with SCID. Therefore, SCID patients should be placed in a protective environment where isolation procedures are enforced. Blood products should be irradiated to prevent the onset of transfusion-associated graft-versus-host disease (GVHD). All patients with SCID and patients with less severe forms of T-cell dysfunction who nevertheless display defective humoral immunity should receive intravenous immunoglobulin therapy. Prophylaxis against bacterial and opportunistic infections, particularly *P. carinii*, should be initiated. For this purpose, daily therapy with trimethoprim-sulfamethoxazole is appropriate. Patients with significant T-cell defects should avoid vaccination with live viral vaccines or with bacillus Calmette-Guerin (BCG). These attenuated organisms, which are usually benign for the immunocompetent host, can prove deadly for patients with T-cell immunodeficiency.

Bone marrow transplantation (BMT) is, at present, the only curative treatment available for T-cell immunodeficiencies (55, 57). It is a life-saving procedure for patients with SCID, and is also recommended for patients with more restricted abnormalities including those with WAS and abnormalities of T-cell activation. BMT is also useful for patients with ill-defined functional T-cell abnormalities whose immune defect results in severe infections without or with autoimmunity (140).

Histocompatible BMT provides an excellent prospect of immune reconstitution with a low profile of toxicity. Matched donor marrows are not manipulated and usually no pretransplant chemotherapy is necessary in those cases marked by absent T-cells. In SCID cases where residual T-cell function is present (especially in ADA- or CK-deficient patients), a conditioning pretransplant regimen is given. A state of mixed chimerism is frequently noted in

SCID patients receiving a matched marrow: the T-cells are of donor origin while other hematopoietic elements, including (at times) the B-cells, are of recipient origin. T-Cells of donor origin can be detected as early as 1–2 weeks posttransplant. These cells are probably derived from mature T-cells present in the graft that have expanded following marrow transplantation. Precursor T-cells of graft origin also migrate to the host thymus and reestablish the normal course of thymic development. Evidence of reconstitution of T- and B-cell function is noted as early as 2–4 weeks posttransplant. T-Cell function becomes normal by 4 months posttransplant. Survival in matched marrow transplants is excellent, and >97% cure rate has been achieved in European studies (55).

For those patients who lack a fully matched donor, as was the case with our child with X-linked SCID, therapy is indicated with lymphocyte-depleted halploidentical bone marrow grafts (55, 57). Depletion of donor T-lymphocytes from the graft is required to avoid fatal GVHD. GVHD prophylaxis with immunosuppressive agents is also required. Depletion of T-cells has its own risk: it takes longer for engraftment to occur, and there is a higher rate of graft failure. Patients with increased NK cell function prior to transplant are at a higher risk of graft failure. Therefore, pretransplant chemotherapy has to be provided to ablate these cells and to mitigate the occurrence of GVHD by ablating all donor hematopoietic and lymphoid elements.

Immune reconstitution is delayed in recipients of haploidentical marrows. The delay reflects, at least in part, the time required for lymphoid precursor cells to develop in host tissues (thymus for T-cells; bone marrow for B-cells). Functional responses of engrafted T-cells start to appear 6–8 weeks posttransplant, and T-cell function may take up to 7 months to normalize. The delay in reconstitution of T-cell function after haploidentical transplantation with T-cell depleted marrow may reflect the time required for precursor cells to recapitulate lymphoid cell ontogeny. This means that precursor cells committed to T-cell lineage have to migrate to the thymus and undergo thymic development leading to the production of mature T-cells. This process also occurs in the case of fully matched transplants. However, matched, unmanipulated marrows also carry mature T-cells that expand quickly and result in earlier recovery. The requirement for an intact thymus for successful engraftment precludes using BMT as an option for patients with thymic aplasia (e.g., the DiGeorge syndrome).

GVHD represents a potential problem in BMT performed for SCID patients. Factors that affect the incidence of GVHD after BMT include the degree of genetic disparity between the graft and the host, the cellular composition of the graft recipient (particularly T-cells), recipient and donor age, and posttransplant immune suppression. The use of HLA-identical sibling grafts results in the recovery of immune function in the vast majority of patients (>90%) with little or no GVHD. The use of T-cell-depleted haploidentical grafts has greatly reduced the incidence of GVHD that would have otherwise resulted from using these HLA-disparate marrows. In the majority of cases, GVHD developing in SCID patients following haploidentical marrow transplants can be overcome with appropriate immunosuppressive therapy.

Reported survival in SCID patients receiving haploidentical marrow transplants has ranged from around 55–75%. The lower incidence of survival in haploidentical marrow recipients as compared with those receiving HLA-identical marrows (>80%) is due to a high incidence of graft failure and to infections that frequently develop in haploidentical marrow recipients because of the longer time required for gaining immunocompetence. Some continuing problems in haploidentical marrow transplants include the frequent failure to develop humoral immunity and a significant increase in the risk of developing autoimmunity and lymphoreticular malignancies. In fully as many as one-half of transplanted patients, especially those suffering from X-linked SCID, functional humoral immunity fails to develop. Mainly, this is due to failure of donor B-cell engraftment. Presence of donor, but not recipient B-cells correlates with recovery of humoral immunity. In these cases where humoral immunity fails to be established, therapy with intravenous γ-globulin is required. Autoimmunity, most frequently to blood elements, represents another commonly encountered problem. It correlates with the persistence of poor B-cell function in marrow recipients and may decline upon complete reconstitution of T-cell immunity. Lymphomas have been observed in a few SCID patients with haploidentical grafts. In most cases the cells are B-lymphocytes of donor origin that are infected with EBV. Incidence of these lymphomas correlates with incomplete or declining reconstitution of T-cell function, and their course is unfortunately fulminant.

REFERENCES

1. Rosen FS, Cooper MD, Wedgewood RJ. The primary immunodeficiencies. Parts I and II. N Engl J Med 1984; 311:235.
2. Wedgewood RJ, Rosen FS, Paul NW. Primary immunodeficiency diseases. March of Dimes Birth Defects Foundation. New York: Alan R. Liss, 1983.
3. Gilger MA, et al. Extraintestinal rotavirus infections in children with immunodeficiency. J Pediatr 1992;120:912.
4. Hall CB, et al. Respiratory syncytial viral infection in children with compromised immune function. N Engl J Med 1986;315:77.
5. Leggiadro RJ, Winkelstein JA, Hughes WT. Prevalence of *Pneumocystis carinii* pneumonitis in severe combined immunodeficiency. J Pediatr 1981;99:96.
6. Monafo WJ, et al. Disseminated measles infection after vaccination in a child with a congenital immunodeficiency. J Pediatr 1994;124:273.
7. Gonzales B, et al. Clinical presentation of bacillus Calmette-Guerin infections in patients with immunodeficiency syndromes. Pediatr Infect Dis J 1989;8:201.
8. Anderson KC, Weinstein HJ. Transfusion-associated graft-versus-host disease. N Engl J Med 1990;323:315.

9. Gossage DL, Buckley RH. Prevalence of lymphocytopenia in severe combined immunodeficiency. N Engl J Med 1990;323:1422.

10. Sprent JT. Lymphocytes and the thymus. In: Paul WE, ed. Fundamental immunology. 3rd ed. New York: Raven Press, 1993.

11. de Vaal OM, Seynhaeve V. Reticular dysgenesis. Lancet 1959;2:1123.

12. Gitlin D, Vawter G, Craig MM. Thymic alymphoplasia and congenital aleukocytosis. Pediatrics 1964;33:184.

13. Roper MA, et al. Severe congenital leukopenia (reticular dysgenesis): immunologic and morphologic characterization of leukocytes. Am J Dis Child 1985;139:832.

14. Hitzig WH, Willi H. Hereditare lymphoplasmocytase dysginesie. Schweiz Med Wochenschr 1961;91:1625.

15. Schuler W, et al. Rearrangement of antigen receptor genes is defective in mice with severe combined immunodeficiency. Cell 1986;46:963.

16. Schwarz K, et al. Severe combined immunodeficiency (SCID) in man, B cell negative (B−) SCID patients exhibit an irregular recombination pattern at the Jh locus. J Exp Med 1991;174:1039.

17. Omenn G. Familial reticuloendotheliosis with eosinophilia. N Engl J Med 1965;273:427.

18. de Saint-Basile G, et al. Restricted heterogeneity of T lymphocytes in combined immunodeficiency with hypereosinophilia (Omenn's syndrome). J Clin Invest 1991; 87:1352.

19. Cavazzana-Calvo M, et al. Increased radiosensitivity of granulocyte macrophage colony-forming units and skin fibroblasts in human autosomal recessive severe combined immunodeficiency. J Clin Invest 1993;91:1214.

20. Conley MA, et al. X-linked severe combined immunodeficiency. Diagnosis in males with sporadic severe combined immunodeficiency and clarification of clinical findings. J Clin Invest 1990;85:1548.

21. Noguchi M, et al. Interleukin-2 receptor g chain mutation results in X-linked severe combined immunodeficiency in humans. Cell 1993;73:147.

22. Leonard WJ. The defective gene in X-linked severe combined immunodeficiency encodes a shared interleukin receptor subunit: implications for cytokine pleiotropy and redundancy. Curr Opin Immunol 1994;6:631.

23. Puck JM, Nussbaum RL, Conley MA. Carrier detection in X-linked severe combined immunodeficiency based on X chromosome. J Clin Invest 1987;79:1395.

24. Puck JM, et al. Prenatal test for X-linked severe combined immunodeficiency by analysis of material X-chromosome inactivation and linkage analysis. N Engl J Med 1990; 322: 1063.

25. Lammer EJ, Opitz JM. The DiGeorge anomaly as a developmental field defect. Am J Med Genet 1986; (suppl 2):113.

26. De la Chapelle A, et al. A deletion in chromosome 22 can cause DiGeorge syndrome. Hum Genet 1981;57:253.

27. Ammann AJ, et al. The DiGeorge syndrome and the fetal alcohol syndrome. Am J Dis Child 1982;136:906.

28. Lammer EJ, et al. Retinoic acid embryopathy. N Engl J Med 1985;313:837.

29. Steele RW, et al. Familial thymic aplasia: attempted reconstitution with fetal thymus in a millipore diffusion chamber. N Engl J Med 1972;287:787.

30. Raatika M, et al. Familial third and fourth pharyngeal pouch syndrome with truncus arteriosus: DiGeorge syndrome. Pediatrics 1981;67:173.

31. Driscoll DA, et al. Prevalence of 22q11 microdeletions in DiGeorge and velocardiofacial syndromes: implications for genetic counseling and prenatal diagnosis. J Med Genet 1993;30:813.

32. Gidding SS, Miniciotti AL, Langman CB. Unmasking of hypoparathyroidism in familial partial DiGeorge syndrome by challenge with disodium edetate. N Engl J Med 1988; 319: 1589.

33. Conley MA, et al. The spectrum of the DiGeorge syndrome. J Pediatr 1979;94:883.

34. Muller W, et al. The DiGeorge syndrome; I, clinical evaluation and course of partial and complete forms of the syndrome. Eur J Pediatr 1988;147:496.

35. Muller W, et al. The DiGeorge sequence: II, immunologic findings in partial and complete forms of the disorder. Eur J Pediatr 1989;149:96.

36. Urval KR, et al. Partial DiGeorge anomaly—a review of immunologic parameters. Pediatr Res 1990;27:162.

37. Cleveland WW, et al. Foetal thymic transplant in a case of DiGeorge's syndrome. Lancet 1968;2:1211.

38. August CS, et al. Establishment of immunological competence in a child with congenital thymic aplasia by a graft of fetal thymus. Lancet 1970;1:1080.

39. Hirschhorn R. Adenosine deaminase deficiency. Immunodef Rev 1990;2:175.

40. Markert ML. Purine nucleoside phoysphorylase deficiency. Immunodef Rev 1991;1;3:45.

41. Creagen RP, et al. Autosomal assignment of the gene for the form of adenosine deaminase which is deficient in patients with combined immunodeficiency syndrome. Lancet 1973;2:1449.

42. Adrian GS, Wiginton DA, Hutton JJ. Structure of adenosine deaminase mRNAs from normal and adenosine deaminase-deficient human cell lines. Mol Cell Biol 1984;4:1712.

43. Bonthorn DT, et al. Identification of a point mutation in the adenosine deaminase gene responsible for immunodeficiency. J Clin Invest 1985;76:894.

44. Valerio D, et al. One adenosine deaminase allele in a patient with severe combined immunodeficiency contains a point mutation abolishing enzyme activity. EMBO 1986; J5: 113.

45. Akeson AL, et al. Mutations in the human adenosine deaminase gene that affect protein structure and RNA splicing. Proc Natl Acad Sci USA 1987;84:5947.

46. Berkvens TM, et al. Severe combined immune deficiency due to a homozygous 3.2-kb deletion spanning the promoter and first exon of the adenosine deaminase gene. Nucleic Acids Res 1987;15:9365.

47. Markert ML, et al. Adenosine deaminase (ADA) deficiency due to deletion of the ADA gene promoter and first exon by homologous recombination between two Alu elements. J Clin Invest 1988;81:1323.

48. Markert ML, Norby-Slycord C, Ward FE. A high proportion of ADA point mutations associated with a specific alanine to valine substitution. Am J Hum Genet 1989; 45:354.

49. Hirshhorn R. Genetic deficiencies of adenosine deaminase and purine nucleoside phosphorylase: overview, genetic heterogeneity, and therapy. In: Wedgewood RJ, Rosen FS, Paul NW, eds. Primary immunodeficiency diseases. New York: Alan R. Liss, 1983.

50. Morgan G, et al. Heterogeneity of biochemical, clinical and immunological parameters in severe combined immunode-

ficiency due to adenosine deaminase deficiency. Clin Exp Immunol 1987;70:491.

51. Polmar SH. Metabolic aspects of immunodeficiency disease. Semin Hematol 1980;17:30.

52. Carson DA, Kaye J, Seegmiller JE. Lymphospecific toxicity in adenosine deaminase deficiency and purine nucleoside phosphorylase deficiency: possible role of nucleoside kinases. Proc Natl Acad Sci USA 1977;74:5677.

53. Seto S, et al. Mechanism of deoxyadenosine and 2-chlorodeoxyadenosine toxicity to non dividing T lymphocytes. J Clin Invest 1985;75:377.

54. Fischer A, et al. Bone marrow transplantation for immunodeficiencies and osteopetrosis: European survey, 1968–1985. Lancet 1986;2:1080.

55. Fischer A, et al. European experience of bone-marrow transplantation for severe combined immunodeficiency. Lancet 1990;2:850.

56. Good RA. Bone marrow transplanation for immunodeficiency diseases. Am J Med Sci 1987;294:68.

57. O'Reilly RJ, et al. The use of HLA-non identical T cell depleted marrow transplants for correction of severe combined immunodeficiency diseases. Immunodef Rev 1989; 1: 273.

58. Hershfield MS, et al. Treatment of adenosine deaminase deficiency with polyethylene glycol-modified adenosine deaminase. N Engl J Med 1987;316:589.

59. Ricciuti F, Ruddle FH. Assignment of nucleoside phosphorylase to D14 and localization of X-linked loci in man by somatic cell genetics. Nature 1973;214:180.

60. Williams SR, et al. A human purine nucleoside phosphorylase deficiency caused by a single base change. J Biol Chem 1987;262:2332.

61. Swain S. T cell subsets and the recognition of MHC class. Immunol Rev 1983;74:129.

62. Koller BH, et al. Normal development of mice deficient in b2M, MHC class I proteins, and CD-8+T cells. Science 1990;248:1227.

63. Zijlstra M, et al. b2-Microglobulin-deficient mice lack CD-4-CD-8+ cytolytic T cells. Nature 1990;344:742.

64. Grusby MJ, et al. Depletion of CD-4+ T cells in MHC class II-deficient mice. Science 1991;253:1417.

65. Cosgrove D, et al. Mice lacking MHC class II molecules. Cell 1992;66:1051.

66. Clement L, et al. Abnormal differentiation of Immunoregulatory T lymphocytes subpopulations in the major histocompatibility complex (MHC) class II antigen deficiency syndrome. J Clin Immunol 1988;8:503.

67. Klein C, et al. Major histocompatibility complex class II deficiency: clinical manifestations, immunologic features and outcome. J Pediatr 1993;123:921.

68. Mach B, Steimle V, Reith W. MHC class II-deficient combined immunodeficiency: a disease of gene regulation. Immunol Rev 1994;138:207.

69. Lisowska B, et al. Defect of expression of MHC genes responsible for an abnormal HLA class I phenotype and the class II phenotype of lymphocytes from patients with combined immunodeficiency. In: Albert ed, Bant MP, Mayr WR, eds. Histocompatibility testing. Berlin: Springer, 1984:650.

70. de la Salle H, et al: Homozygous human TAP peptide transporter mutation in HLA class I deficiency. Science 1994; 265: 237.

71. Alarcon B, et al. Congenital T cell receptor immunodeficiencies in man. Immunodef Rev 1990;2:1.

72. Arnaiz-Villena A, et al. Brief report: primary immunodeficiency caused by mutations in the gene encoding the CD-3-g subunit of the T-lymphocyte receptor. N Engl J Med 1992;327:529.

73. Soudais C, et al. Independent mutations of the human CD-3-epsilon gene resulting in a T cell receptor/CD-3 complex immunodeficiency. Nature Genetics 1993;3:77.

74. Arpaia E, et al. Defective T cell receptor signaling and CD-8+ thymic selection in humans lacking ZAP-70 kinase. Cell 1994;76:947.

75. Elder ME, et al. Human severe combined immunodeficiency due to a defect in ZAP-70, a T cell kinase. Science 1994;264:1596.

76. Chan AC, et al. ZAP-70 deficiency in an autosomal recessive form of severe combined immunodeficiency. Science 1994;264:1599.

77. Roifman CM, et al. Deletion of CD-8+ cells in human thymic medulla results in selective immune deficiency. J Exp Med 1989;170:2177.

78. Monafo WJ, et al. A hereditary immunodeficiency characterized by CD-8+ T lymphocyte deficiency and impaired lymphocyte activation. Clin Exp Immunol 1992;90:390.

79. Chatila T, et al. An immunodeficiency characterized by defective signal transduction in T lymphocytes. N Engl J Med 1989;320:696.

80. Pahwa R, et al. Recombinant interleukin 2 therapy in severe combined immunodeficiency. Proc Natl Acad Sci USA 1989;86:5069.

81. Disanto JP, et al. Absence of interleukin 2 production in a severe combined immunodeficiency disease syndrome with T cells. J Exp Med 1990;171:1697.

82. Weinberg K, Parkman R. Severe combined immunodeficiency due to a specific defect in the production of interleukin-2. N Engl J Med 1990;322:1718.

83. Chatila T, et al. Primary combined immunodeficiency resulting from defective transcription of multiple T-cell lymphokine genes. Proc Natl Acad Sci USA 1990;87:10033.

84. Castigli E, et al. Molecular basis of a multiple lymphokine deficiency in a patient with severe combined immunodeficiency. Proc Natl Acad Sci USA 1993;90:4728.

85. Bridges BA, Harnden DG. Ataxia telangiectasia: a cellular and molecular link between cancer, neuropathology and immune deficiency. Chichester: John Wiley, 1982.

86. Gatti A, Swift M. Ataxia-telangiectasia: genetics, neuropathology, and immunology of a degenerative disease of childhood. New York: Alan R. Liss, 1985.

87. Gatti RA, et al. Ataxia-telangiectasia: an interdisciplinary approach to pathogenesis. Medicine 1991;70:99.

88. Swift M, et al. The incidence and gene frequency of ataxia telangiectasia in the United States. Am J Hum Genet 1986;39:573.

89. Swift M. Genetic aspects of ataxia telangiectasia. Immunodef Rev 1990;2:67.

90. Gotoff SP, Amirmokri E, Liebner EJ. Ataxia telangiectasia: neoplasia, untoward response to x-irradiation and tuberous sclerosis. Am J Dis Child 1967;114:617.

91. Taylor AM, et al. Ataxia telangiectasia: a human mutation with abnormal radiation sensitivity. Nature 1975; 258:427.

92. Waldmann TA, McIntire KR. Serum-alpha-fetoprotein levels in patients with ataxia telangiectasia. Lancet 1972; 2:1112.

93. Sugimoto T, et al. Plasma levels of carcinoembryonic antigen in patients with ataxia telangiectasia. J Pediatr 1978; 92: 436.

94. Peterson RDA, Blaw M, Good RA. Ataxia telangiectasia: a possible clinical counterpart of the animals rendered immunologically incompetent by thymectomy. J Pediatr 1963;63:701.

95. Peterson RDA, Cooper MD, Good RA. Lymphoid tissue abnormalities associated with ataxia telangiectasia. Am J Med 1966;41:342.

96. Carbonari M, et al. Relative increase of T cells expressing the gamma/delta rather than the alpha/beta receptor in ataxia-telangiectasia. N Engl J Med 1990;322:73.

97. Ammann AJ, et al. Immunoglobulin E deficiency in ataxia Telangiectasia. N Engl J Med 1969;281:469.

98. Polmar SH, et al. Immunoglobulin E in immunologic deficiency diseases: I, relation of IgE and IgA to respiratory tract disease in isolated IgE deficiency, IgA deficiency and ataxia telangiectasia. J Clin Invest 1972;51:326.

99. Oxelius VA, Berkel AI, Hanson LA, IgG2 deficiency in ataxia telangiectasia. N Engl J Med 1982;28:515.

100. Aucouturier P, et al. Serum IgG subclass deficiency in ataxia telangiectasia. Clin Exp Immunol 1987;68:392.

101. Morrell D, Cromartie E, Swift M. Mortality and cancer incidence in 263 patients with ataxia telangiectasia. J Natl Cancer Inst 1986;77:87.

102. Swift M, et al. Malignant neoplasms in the families of patients with ataxia telangiectasia. Cancer Res 1976;36:209.

103. Swift M, et al. Breast and other cancers in families with ataxia-telangiectasia. N Engl J Med 1987;316:1289.

104. Pippard EC, et al. Cancer in homozygotes and heterozygotes of ataxia telangiectasia and xeroderma pigmentosum in Britain. Cancer Res 1988;48:2929.

105. Swift M, et al. Incidence of cancer in 161 families affected by ataxia telangiectasia. N Engl J Med 1991;325:1831.

106. Aurias A, Dutrillaux B. Probably involvement of immunoglobulin superfamily genes in most recurrent chromosomal rearrangements from ataxis telangiectasia. Hum Genet 1986;72:210.

107. Ziv Y, et al. The ATC (ataxia telangiectasia complementation group C) locus localizes to 11q22-23. Genomics 1991;9: 373.

108. Foroud T, et al. Localization of an ataxia telangiectasia locus to a 3-cM interval on chromosome 11q23: linlage analysis of 111 familes by an international consortium. Am J Hum Genet 1991;49:1263.

109. Murnane JP, Painter RB. Complementation of the defects in DNA synthesis in irradiated and unirradiated ataxia-telangiectasia cells. Proc Natl Acad Sci USA 1982; 79:1960.

110. Jaspers NGJ. Bootsma genetic heterogeneity in ataxia telangiectasia studied by cell fusion. Proc Natl Acad Sci USA 1982;79:2641.

111. Jaspers NG, et al. Genetic complementation analysis of ataxia telangiectasia and Nijmegen breakage syndrome: a survey of 50 patients. Cytogenet Cell Genet 1988; 49:259.

112. Willis AE, Lindahl T. DNA ligase I deficiency in Bloom's syndrome. Nature 1987;324:355.

113. Chan JYH, et al. Altered DNA ligase I activity in Bloom's syndrome. Natuer 1987;324:357.

114. Wiskott A. Familiaerer, angeborener Morbus werlhofi? Monatsschr Kinderheikd 1937;68:212.

115. Aldrich RA, Steinberg AGI, Campbell DC. Pedigree demonstrating sex-linked recessive condition characterized

116. Standen GR. Wiskott-Aldrich syndrome: new perspectives in pathogenesis and managment. J R Coll Physicians Lond 1988;22:80.

117. Canales L, Mauer AM. Sex-linked hereditary thrombocytopenia as a variant of Wiskott-Aldrich syndrome. N Engl J Med 1967;277:899.

118. Amaya CA, et al. Attenuated form of Wiskott-Aldrich syndrome. J Pediatr 1973;82:175.

119. Ochs HD, et al. The Wiskott-Aldrich syndrome: studies of lymphocytes and platelets. Blood 1980;55:243.

120. Kenney D, et al. Morphologic abnormalities in the lymphocytes of patients with the Wiskott-Aldrich syndrome. Blood 1986;68:1329.

121. Perry GS, et al. The Wiskott-Aldrich syndrome in the United States and Canada. J Pediatr 1980;97:72.

122. Corash L, Shafer B, Blaese M. Platelet-associated immunoglobulin, platelet size, and the effect of splenectomy in the Wiskott-Aldrich syndrome. Blood 1985; 65:1439.

123. Grottum KA, et al. Wiskott-Aldrich Syndrome: qualitative platelet defects and short survival. Br J Hematol 1969; 117:373.

124. Parkman R, et al. Surface protein abnormalities in lymphocytes and platelets from patients with Wiskott-Aldrich syndrome. Lancet 1981;2:1387.

125. Ochs HD, et al. The Wiskott-Aldrich syndrome: studies of lymphocytes, granulocytes and platelets. Blood 1980; 55:243.

126. Lum LG, et al. Splenectomy in the management of the thrombocytopenia of the Wiskott-Aldrich syndrome. N Engl J Med 1980;302:892.

127. Oppenheim JJ, Blaese RM, Waldmann TA. Defective lymphocyte transformation and delayed hypersensitivity in Wiskott-Aldrich-syndrome. J Immunol 1970; 101:835.

128. Moline IJ, et al. T cell lines characterize events in the pathogenesis of the Wiskott-Aldrich syndrome. J Exp Med 1992; 176:876.

129. Blaese RM, et al. The Wiskott-Aldrich syndrome: a disorder with a possible defect in antigen recognition. Lancet 1968; 1:1056.

130. Peacocke M, Siminovitch KA. Linkage of the Wiskott-Aldrich syndrome with polymorphic DNA sequences from the human X chromosome. Proc Natl Acad Sci USA 1987; 84:3430.

131. Kwan S-P, et al. Genetic mapping of the Wiskott-Aldrich syndrome with two highly-linked polymorphic DNA markers. Genomics 1988;3:39.

132. Remold-O'Donnell E, Rosen FS. Sialophorin (CD-43) and the Wiskott-Aldrich syndrome. Immunodef Rev 1990; 2:151.

133. Greer WL, et al. Altered expression of leukocyte sialoglycoprotein in Wiskott-Aldrich syndrome is associated with a specific defect in O-glycosylation. Biochem Cell Biol 1989; 67:503.

134. Moline IJ, et al. T cells of patients with the Wiskott-Aldrich syndrome have a restricted defect in proliferative responses. J Immunol 1993;151:4383.

135. Derry JM, Ochs HD, Francke U. Isolation of a novel gene mutated in Wiskott-Aldrich syndrome. Cell 1994; 78:635.

136. Fearon ER, et al. Carrier detection in the Wiskott-Aldrich syndrome. Blood 1988;72:1735.

137. Greer WLM, et al. X-Chromosome inactivation in the Wiskott-Aldrich syndrome: a marker for detection of the carrier state and identification of cell lineages expressing the gene defect. Genomics 1989;4:60.

138. Puck JM, et al. Atypical presentation of Wiskott-Aldrich syndrome: diagnosis in two unrelated males based on stud ies of maternal T cell X chromosome inactivation. Blood 1990;75:2369.

139. Parkman R, et al. Complete correction of the Wiskott-Aldrich syndrome by allogeniec bone marrow transplantation. N Engl J Med 1978;298:921.

140. Berthet FB, et al. Clinical consequences and treatment of primary immunodeficiency syndromes characterized by functional T and B lymphocyte anomalies (combined immunodeficiency). Pediatrics 1994;93:265.

CHAPTER 15

Genetics of Hematopoietic Malignancies

ANTHONY A. MELUCH, DONALD M. MILLER

The madness of King George
—Anonymous

Introduction

Recent developments in molecular and cellular genetics have unraveled some of the mysteries surrounding the initiation and proliferation of hematologic malignancies. Our current capability to detect genetic abnormalities, isolate specific genomic fragments, and analyze their ability to transform normal cells has provided us with invaluable instruments for understanding the processes of malignant transformation involved in clinical diseases. The current concepts and tools of molecular biology are just beginning to elucidate the genetic mechanisms involved in the pathophysiology of neoplastic diseases, and more importantly, are offering new approaches for diagnosis and therapy.

Cancer has classically been defined as the potential for invasion and/or metastasis, resulting in organ damage or failure and sometimes death (1). Until recently, the molecular mechanisms of human myeloid and lymphoid leukemogenesis were unknown. Historically, the increased incidence of acute myelogenous leukemia noted in individuals with a history of previous exposure to benzene, chemotherapeutic alkylating agents, and high doses of γ-irradiation suggested an etiologic association between these entities and the development of leukemia (2). Cytogenetic analysis of leukemic cells, as well as those of other hematologic malignancies, demonstrated characteristic chromosomal abnormalities. More recently, the discovery of the t(9;22) translocation in human chronic myelogenous leukemia, popularly known as the Philadelphia chromosome, along with the identification of the c-abl oncogene as a part of this specific chromosomal alteration, has led to a flurry of investigation into the genetic mechanisms of malignancy (3, 4).

Nearly 100 protooncogenes have been identified, many of which have well-defined homologs among viral oncogenes (5). The association of many of these protooncogenes in nonrandom chromosomal translocations found in lymphoid and myeloid neoplastic disorders provides some of the strongest indirect evidence identifying genetic alterations of oncogenes as both initiators and promoters of neoplastic disorders. The demonstration of a single isoform of glucose-6-phosphate dehydrogenase (G-6-PD) in

the hematologic precursor cells of chronic myelogenous leukemia patients, who otherwise were heterogenous for this enzyme, proved the clonal nature of this particular neoplasm (5). Our current level of understanding of the etiology of human and animal malignancies suggests an alteration of our definition of malignancy, to now include demonstration of genetic clonality as confirmatory evidence of a neoplastic process.

Numerous discoveries have helped bridge the gap between chromosomal abnormalities and physiologic phenomena. The demonstration of the involvement of a transmissible virus as the cause of certain animal tumors, followed by the discovery in 1970 that the enzyme reverse transcriptase, which is found in certain RNA tumor viruses, could transcribe a coded DNA sequence from an RNA template, and the subsequent discovery of the first human retrovirus in 1980 eventually led to the recognition of the role of viral oncogene expression in malignant transformation in certain neoplastic processes (7–11).

The normal human genome is comprised of over 100,000 genes, among which are the human homologs of viral oncogenes, protooncogenes (c-onc). Protooncogenes are defined as genes that encode for products involved in the control of normal cellular growth and differentiation (12). The incorporation of a portion or all of a cellular protooncogene into a host genome of a retrovirus can result in altered expression of this normal cellular gene, now termed a viral oncogene (v-onc), and subsequent malignant transformation. Many retroviral oncogenes and their associations with leukemias and lymphomas as well as other cancers have now been identified.

In contrast to these dominantly transforming oncogenes, tumor suppressor genes, termed anti-oncogenes, i.e., the retinoblastoma (RB) and P53 gene products, have also recently been identified. Current knowledge of antioncogenes indicates that they function by repressing or negatively regulating cellular proliferation. Both the P53 and the RB gene products function in a recessive manner requiring the functional loss of both normal alleles for the lack of suppression of tumorigenesis (6, 12).

Exploring the mechanisms by which protooncogenes can be activated has provided important new information about the basic biology of cancer. The current evidence supports a model of normal cellular growth governed by multiple interacting regulatory pathways involving nuclear, cytoplasmic, and extracytoplasmic factors (fig. 15.1). Protooncogenes have been classified according to the location or biologic function of their gene products (table 15.1). Secretory proteins, such as epidermal growth factor (EGF) and platelet-derived growth factor (PDGF) for which the B-chain of the parent polypeptide is encoded by the c-sis oncogene, function as intercellular growth factors. These regulatory proteins bind to cell surface molecules known as growth factor receptors initiating cytoplasmic events. Several growth factor receptors have been well characterized: c-Erb-B1, which encodes the receptor for EGF, and c-fms, which codes for the receptor for colony-stimulating factor 1 (CSF-1). Once a cell is stimulated, cytoplasmic proteins such as protein kinases and G-proteins, gene products of src and ras protooncogene families, respectively, are activated; and through currently unknown mechanisms, information penetrates the nuclear envelope. The last category of protooncogene products are nuclear proteins, which can function as DNA-binding proteins, i.e. myc, fos, and jun, influencing transcriptional control. The complexity of this regulatory

cascade provides multiple opportunities for genetic alterations (13, 14).

The early discovery of the transforming capability of the retroviruses led to a variety of potential mechanisms of transformation, which can be divided into three subgroups: (a) random insertion of the retroviral genome near regulatory gene sequences of the host genome resulting in turning on of the cellular gene in uncontrolled proliferation; (b) transcription of an oncogene within the genome of a retrovirus that has been inserted into the DNA of a host cell exhibiting transforming capabilities; (c) finally, products of retroviral genes, such as the tat gene, can transregulate viral, as well as host, genes involved in cellular growth (11, 12) (fig. 15.2).

It is clear that although retroviruses play a role in the malignant transformation of some neoplasms, the majority of neoplastic events are initiated by mutations within the normal eukaryotic genome. Genetic changes of normal human protooncogenes can arise by a variety of mechanisms without the involvement of retroviruses. Expression of genetic mutations, which are often chromosomal rearrangements but may also be smaller point mutations or deletions, can generate a protein with altered properties resulting in transforming potential. The hap-

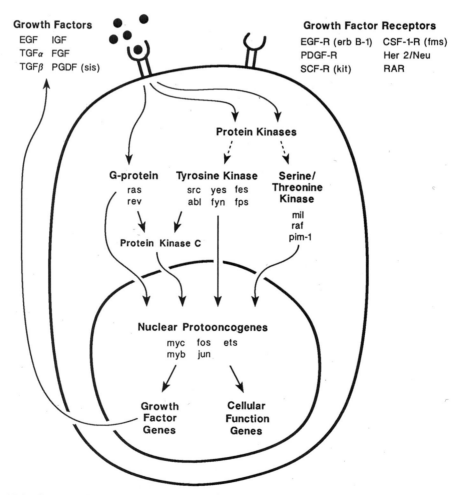

Figure 15.1. Cascade of signal transduction and cellular growth regulation. Representative protooncogene (*small letters*) and protooncogene products (*capitalized letters*) are listed at their cellular locations.

Table 15.1 Classes of Protooncogene

Classes	Examples	Activity	Cellular Location
Growth factors	c-sis	B-chain PDGF	Secreted
	int-2	Fibroblast growth factor related	
	hst		?
Growth factor receptors	c-kit	Receptor stem cell factor	Membrane
	c-erbB-1	Receptor EGF	Membrane
	c-erbA	Receptor thyroid hormone	Membrane
	c-fms	Receptor for CSF-1	Membrane
	c-met, c-ros1	Probable receptors	?
	Her2/neu	Receptor for ?	Membrane
Protein kinases	c-Abl, src, fyn,	Protein kinases	Inner membrane/cytoplasm
	hck, lck, fgr,	(Tyrosine)	
	blk, yes, fes, fps,		
	c-mil, raf, pim-1,	Protein kinases	
	mos	(Serine/tyrosine)	
G-Proteins	c-Ha-ras	Signal transduction	Cytoplasm
	c-Ki-ras	GTP-binding, GTPase	
	N-ras	G-protein-like	?
	c-rev	G-protein-like	?
Nuclear	c-myc	DNA-binding	Nucleus
	c-fos	Transcription regulation	Nucleus
	c-jun	Transcription regulation	Nucleus
	p53 gene	? Regulator DNA polymerase α	Nucleus
	c-myb	?	Nucleus
	c-ets-1, ets-2,	Transcription regulation	Nucleus
	elk-1, elk-2		
	egr, rel		
	RAR-α RAR-ß,	DNA binding	Cytoplasm/nucleus
	RAR-γ, RAR-χ		

*These cytogenic abnormalities are the most common recurring structural abnormalities observed in de novo acute myeloid leukemia (AML) although they may also be seen in myelodysplastic syndrome (MDS) and myeloproliferative (MPD).

loid human genome contains only a single copy of a protooncogene. Duplication, and more often amplification, of a protooncogene can confer the potential for increasing the level of expression of a specific gene. Other transforming mechanisms include rearrangement of chromosomal sequences, such as inversions and translocations, which can result in the formation of altered forms or quantities of the normal protein gene products (15) (fig. 15.3). For example, the translocation involving the c-myc protooncogene located on chromosome 8 with the immunoglobulin heavy chain gene locus (IgH) located on chromosome 14, or the κ- or λ-light chain genes located on chromosome 2 and 22, respectively, produces an abnormally regulated c-myc gene product in Burkitt lymphoma (16).

The focus of this chapter is to consolidate the current knowledge and techniques of molecular biology that have provided dramatic improvements in our understanding of hematopoietic abnormalities and malignancies. Through the use of a clinical case presentation, we will illustrate some important historic milestones in the developments of molecular biology, discuss the biologic significance and mechanisms of genetic changes in hematologic malignancies, and provide insight into the current and future roles

of molecular biology in the diagnostic, prognostic, and therapeutic aspects of hematology.

Clinical Case Presentation

The clinical case history will provide a springboard from which to explore the molecular alterations of hematologic disorders and their physiologic consequences. This produces a framework from which one can explore the field of molecular biology. Following the case history, the reader will be introduced to the common chromosomal changes and then the more basic molecular abnormalities found in hematologic disorders, as well as the tools that have allowed for these discoveries.

Case 1

The patient, a 46-year-old white man, was referred for evaluation of abdominal pain and leukocytosis. He initially presented to his local physician approximately 4 weeks prior to admission with complaints of intermittent left lower quadrant abdominal pain. The pain was not associated with oral intake, changes in bowel habits, including diarrhea and constipation, or fevers, chills, and other infectious-type symptoms. Results of physical

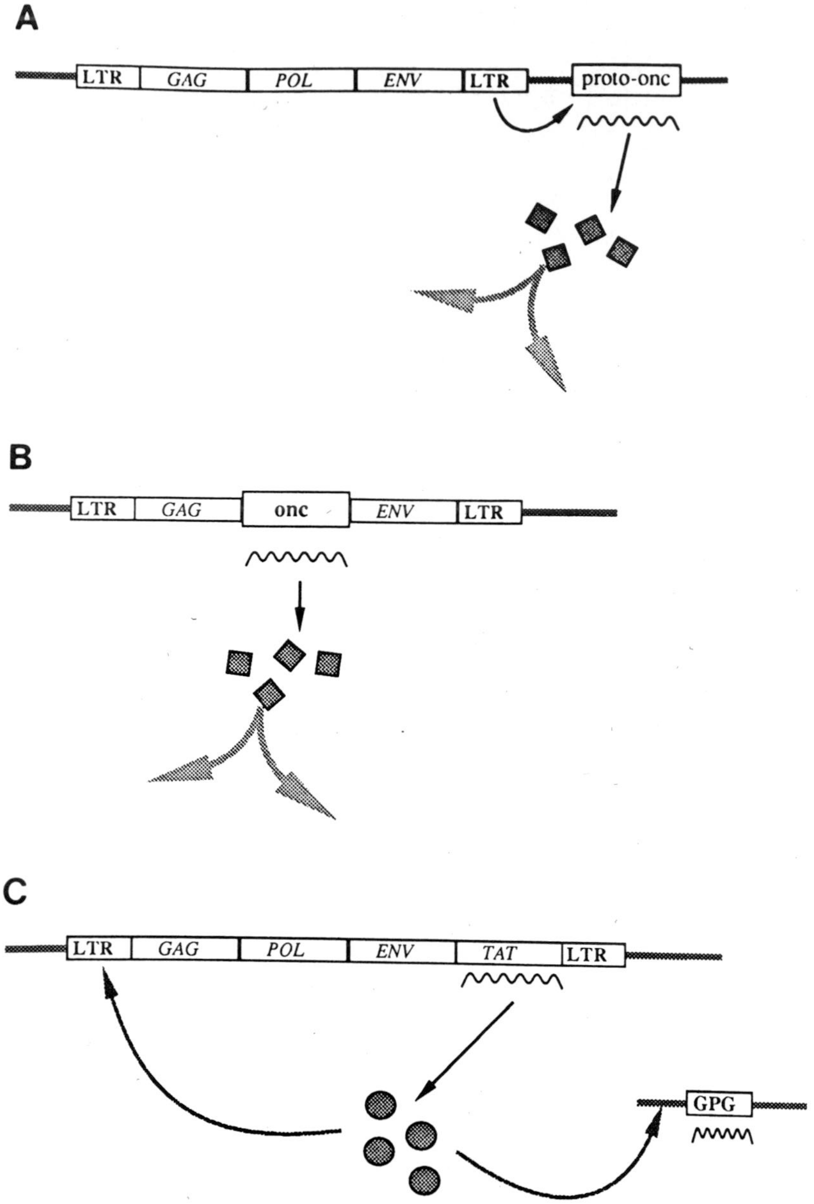

A

B

C

Figure 15.2. Leukemia retrovirus genomes and mechanisms of leukemogenesis. Retroviruses containing the "prototype" genes gag, pol, and env flanked by the long terminal repeat (LTR) regions can initiate cell transformation by various mechanisms. **A.** Insertion of the provirus in close proximity to a cellular gene (e.g., pro-tooncogene) activates it in cis, stimulating the cell to unrestricted growth. **B.** An oncogene can be inserted in place of a retroviral gene. Insertion of the provirus anywhere in the host genome can lead, upon activation, to production of the oncogene products. **C.** Transregulating retroviruses carry additional genes that regulate provirus transcription. (Reprinted from reference 11.)

examination were nonrevealing. The patient was thought to have gastritis and was treated with antacids on an as-needed basis. Four weeks later, he returned to the same physician complaining of continued, worsening abdominal discomfort. His pain was associated with decreased energy level and increasing fatigue. He had noted a 12-pound weight loss.

When examined physically, he was afebrile with a regular pulse of 74 beats/minute and blood pressure of 120/74. He was slightly pale and had a palpable spleen tip. Initial laboratory evaluation disclosed a white blood cell (WBC) count of 93 × 10⁹/L, the majority of which were myeloid forms. His hematocrit was 34 with a mean

corpuscular volume (MCV) of 89, and his platelet count was 395 × 10⁹/L. The physician was concerned that the patient might have a leukemia and referred him to a local university hospital.

On admission, the patient complained of continued abdominal pain, diffuse weakness, and new left shoulder pain. A review of his past medical history revealed that he had no other known medical problems or known allergies. His only medication was an over-the-counter antacid. Social history was notable for a 20 pack per year history of tobacco use and an alcohol intake that included approximately 3–6 beers per week. The patient denied any exposure to any drugs, toxins, or infectious

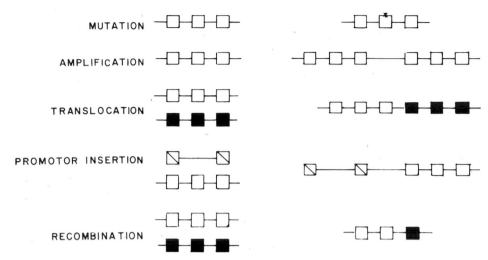

Figure 15.3. Possible mechanism of oncogene activation. The *boxes* indicate exons; the *lines* indicate introns; the *open boxes* indicate a protooncogene; the *closed boxes* indicate a second gene. Normal configuration is shown on the *left*, activated gene on the *right*. (Reprinted from reference 15.)

diseases and claimed to have a monogamous heterosexual relationship with his wife. His family history was noncontributory. Review of systems disclosed occasional seasonal allergies, but was otherwise unremarkable.

Physically, his vital signs included a temperature of 98.6°F, pulse of 104 beats/minute, respiration rate of 12 breaths/minute, and a blood pressure of 128/82. He was a pale-appearing, somewhat lethargic white male who was in no acute distress. His skin was warm and moist throughout the examination and he had several acneiform lesions located on both cheeks and his back. Pupils were equal, round, and reactive to light. Extraocular muscles were intact. Sclera were clear and conjunctiva were pink. Fundoscopic examination results were within normal limits. His neck was supple and nontender, without evidence of thyroidomegaly or palpable lymphadenopathy. Auscultation of the lungs disclosed a few bibasilar rales that cleared with coughing. Cardiovascular examination revealed mild tachycardia, but no evidence of murmurs, gallups, or jugular venous distension. Pulses were +2/+4 throughout without bruits. Evaluation of the abdomen revealed mild tenderness in the left upper quadrant, but no evidence of rebound or guarding. Bowel sounds were positive and the liver size was about 12 cm by percussion. A palpable tender spleen extended 8 cm below the left costal margin at the midclavicular line. Rectal examination revealed normal sphincter tone and no evidence of masses or abnormalities of the prostate. His overall neurologic examination results were grossly nonfocal.

His laboratory evaluation included a WBC count of 104×10^9/L cells, which included 19% segmented neutrophils, 16% bands, 17% metamyelocytes, 6% myelocytes, 3% promyelocytes, 1% blast form, 21% lymphocytes, 8% monocytes, 2% eosinophils, and 7% basophils. Hemoglobin was 130 g/dl with a hematocrit of 34% and a platelet count of 412×10^9/L. Evaluation of a peripheral smear demonstrated some mild anisocytosis and poikilo-

cytosis of the red blood cells (RBCs). There was a marked increase in the number of leukocytes, the majority of which were myeloid forms of various stages of maturation that morphologically appeared normal. A rare blast form was also identified. Several large platelets were noted. Serum electrolytes were normal, creatinine 1.0 mg/100 μl, blood sugar 65 mg/100 μl, total bilirubin 0.2 mg/100 μl, direct bilirubin 0.1 mg/ 100 μl, alkaline phosphate 92 U/L, serum glutamic oxaloacetic transaminase (SGOT) 21 U/L, serum glutamic pyruvic transaminase (SGPT) 15 U/L, GGT 23 U/L, lactic dehydrogenase (LDH) 378 U/L, serum calcium 8.9 mg/100 μl, phosphorus 3.4 mg/100 μl, total protein 6.8 U/L, albumin 3.4 U/L, uric acid 8.3 mg/100 μL. Chest x-ray and electrocardiogram were normal. Other laboratory data obtained in the initial evaluation included a vitamin B_{12} level that was elevated at 1,500 pg/ml and a neutrophil alkaline phosphatase level that was undetectable.

A bone marrow aspiration biopsy revealed a hypercellular marrow (overall cellularity 90%) composed predominately of myeloid precursors of variable developmental stages, including approximately 3% blasts. Numerous bands and segmented neutrophils were noted. The myeloid-erythroid ratio was approximately 20:1 with an overall decrease in erythropoiesis. The specimen was sent for cytogenic evaluation and the following karyotypic analysis was obtained (fig. 15.4). The genetic abnormalities present, commonly known as the Philadelphia (PH) chromosome, consist of a translocation of a portion of the long arm of chromosome 9, beginning at band 34 (q34) with the long arm of chromosome 22, beginning at band 11 (q11).

*A diagnosis of **Chronic Myelogenous Leukemia (CML)** was made. The initial management of this patient included the administration of oral hydroxyurea, intravenous fluids, and allopurinol. Over the next several days a marked decrease in his leukocytosis was noted and the chemotherapy was tapered accordingly. Con-*

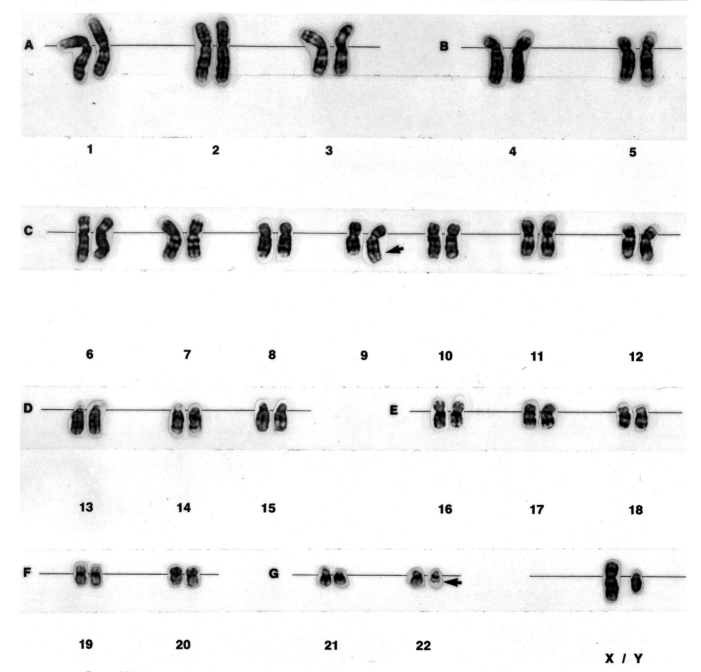

Figure 15.4. A complete karyotype showing the 9;22 translocation associated with Philadelphia chromosome position, chronic myelogenous leukemia (CML). *Arrows* indicate the approximate position of the breakpoints (9q34 and 22q11) on the derivative chromosomes.

currently, his symptoms resolved and there was a marked reduction in his splenomegaly. Overall, this patient is a fairly typical example of some of the common clinical and laboratory manifestations of CML. Over the last several decades, discovery of the Philadelphia chromosome and its role in this disease has linked the minute world of the cytogeneticists and molecular biologists with the ever-evolving clinical expertise of hematologists and oncologists.

Karyotype: The Philadelphia chromosome was first identified as a minute chromosome found in specimens of bone marrow from patients with CML by Nowell

and colleagues in 1960 (3). Since then, it has become almost synonymous with this leukemic disorder. It is routinely found on the karyotype (a full complement of chromosomes from a particular cell that are arranged for analysis according to size from the largest to the smallest of these patients). Specific chromosomes are identified by their banding patterns, as well as their short (p) and long (q) arms, which are biologically determined by the location of the centromere. Karyotypic patterns are labeled according to the international system for human cytogenetic nomenclature (17). A patient with a Philadelphia chromosome would be labeled

46,XY,t(9;22), (q34.1;q11.21). Thus, the chromosomal content of a particular cell can be characterized according to its gross morphology and compared with normal and known abnormal karyotypic patterns or classified as a new variant.

Following the initial description by Nowell et al. in 1960, Caspersson and colleagues identified a significant deletion of chromosome 22 in the Philadelphia chromosome using quinacrine fluorescence (18). With giemsa banding, in 1973 Rowley accurately described the Philadelphia chromosome as the result of a reciprocal translocation involving both long arms of chromosomes 9 and 22 (19) (fig. 15.5). Subsequent karyotypic analysis of CML patients led to the finding of the Philadelphia chromosome in nearly 95% of patients. Interestingly, this chromosomal marker is also found in cells of the myeloid, megakaryocytic, and erythroid lineages, providing compelling evidence that this disease initiated from the neoplastic transformation of a very early hematopoietic stem cell (20). The clonal nature of this disorder was demonstrated by Fialkow et al., who observed only a single glucose-6-phosphate dehydrogenase (G-6-PD) isoform in the bone marrow of cells of CML patients who were otherwise heterozygous for this enzyme (6). Although the Philadelphia chromosome was the first chromosomal abnormality linked to a neoplastic process, it is not alone in this relationship, nor is it specific to CML. The Philadelphia chromosome has been found in about 15–20% of adult patients and 10% of children with acute lymphocytic leukemia (ALL) and <5% of adults with acute myelogenous leukemia (AML) (20). There have been numerous karyotypic abnormalities with increased incidence in other hematologic disorders, although these do not occur with the same prevalence of the Philadelphia chromosome with CML (tables 15.2–15.5) (5, 21). The karyotypic pattern of Burkitt lymphoma demonstrates the chromosomal translocation t(8;14)(q24.1;q32) in the majority of cases and, less often, t(2;8) (p12;q24) and t(8;22) (q24;q11). Some recurring abnormalities in other B-cell lymphomas include a t(14;18) (q32;q21) found in increased numbers in follicular lymphomas and t(11;14) (q13;q32) found in small and intermediately differentiated lymphomas along with chronic lymphocytic leukemia. Numerous chromosomal rearrangements have also been discovered in T-cell lymphomas and in various leukemias. Some of the more common chromosomal changes appearing in myelodysplastic syndromes include: +8, −5, −7, and del (deletion) 20q. The most recurring chromosomal abnormality in acute myelogenous leukemia is the t(15;17) translocation found in acute promyelocytic leukemia (APL) (6, 14–16, 21–23). The high incidence of chromosomal abnormalities found in

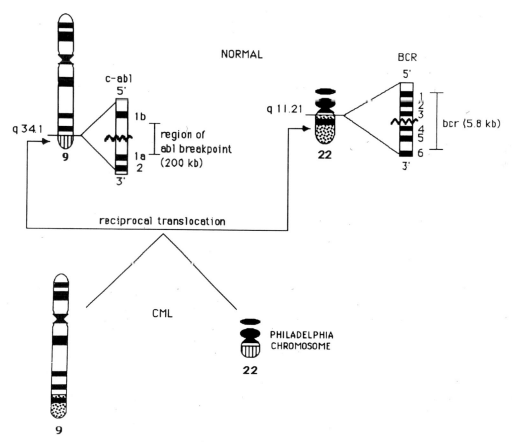

Figure 15.5. Involvement of c-abl and BCR genes in the Philadelphia chromosome translocation. The Philadelphia chromosome is produced by a reciprocal translocation of the long arm of chromosome 9 (hatched area) and the long arm of chromosome 22 (speckled area) during which 3' segments of the c-abl gene are juxtaposed to 5' segments of the BCR gene. (Reprinted from reference 20.)

malignant hematologic disorders, clonality studies demonstrating the origin of neoplastic cells from a single cell, and the prognostic significance associated with some of these karyotypic phenomenon have led many scientists to attempt to relate the nature and implications of these genetic changes.

Introduction to Molecular Biology

The relationship between the basic structure of a chromosome and the phenotypic expression of neoplastic disease is complex. It is easy to conceptualize how the deletion or movement of a portion of a chromosome from one chromosome to another can result in the loss or alteration of a protein product. In order to help elucidate the possible relevance of some of the molecular events that occur in hematologic malignancies, we will briefly review current knowledge of molecular biology.

The human genome is comprised of deoxyribonucleic acid (DNA). DNA is a highly dynamic substance that undergoes amplifications, mutations, insertions, translocations, and deletions. Current evidence strongly implies that all neoplastic processes, as well as many nonneoplastic disorders, are the result of an alteration in DNA content or the processes that transcribe this information into functional proteins. Watson and Crick proposed a double-helical model for the three-dimensional structure of DNA in 1953 that exists today: two strands of DNA, running in opposite directions (antiparallel) in the shape of a double helix (24). All organisms have the necessary machinery to replicate DNA, as well as to transcribe it into ribonucleic acid (RNA) that can then be translated into functional proteins. Each strand of DNA is composed of a sequence of nucleotide bases that differ only in the nitrogen-based side chain they contain. These four bases consist of two purines, adenine (A) and guanine (G), and two pyrimidines, cytosine (C) and thymidine (T). The nucleotide bases in sequence are bound together along a phosphate and deoxyribose-sugar backbone and held to complementary bases on the opposing strand by hydrogen bonds. The nucleotides have a strict complementary code for binding: adenine with thymine and guanine with cytosine. Each chromosome is comprised of thousands of genes and it is this specific nucleotide sequence within the gene that confers the genetic code ultimately responsible for presenting phenotypes. Of the two stands, the "sense" strand runs in a 5'–3' direction, while the "antisense" strand runs in a 3'–5' direction (fig. 15.6). The actual encoded information of an individual gene is only a small fraction of the genetic sequence. It is conferred by segments known as "exons" that are separated from each other by intervening sequences termed "introns" (17, 25) (fig. 15.7).

Nucleotide sequences 5' to the first exon of the gene are referred to as promoter sequences and are integrally involved in regulating genetic transcription. Terminal 3' sequences can also be involved in transcriptional regulation,

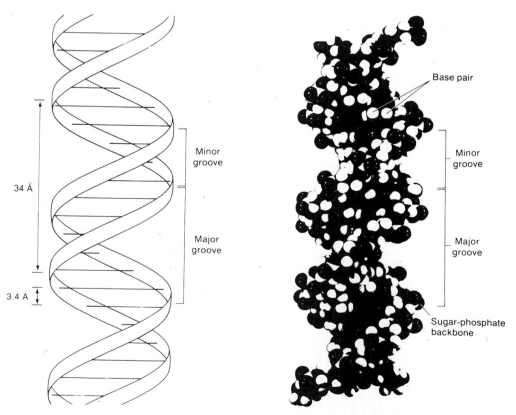

Figure 15.6. **A.** Diagram of the DNA double helix. **B.** Space-filling sphere model of DNA.
(Reprinted from reference 25.)

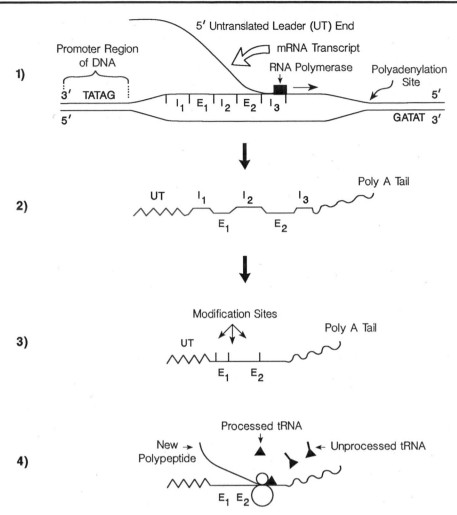

Figure 15.7. Gene transcription and translation. Introns (*I*), exons (*E*), important nucleotide regions, and modification sites have been identified. **A.** Transcription. Messenger RNA (mRNA) is synthesized in a 5′→3′ direction by the action of RNA polymerase II on a single strand of DNA. Transcription is initiated at a promoter site and occurs in antiparallel fashion (3′ → 5′ orientation) along the DNA template. **B.** Nascent mRNA containing untranslated leader (*ut*) polyadenylated tail (poly A tail) and introns ($I_1 - I_3$). **C.** Processed mRNA. Introns have been removed (spliced) and individual nucleotides modified. **D.** Translation. The information contained in mRNA is translated on polyribosomes with the assistance of transfer RNA (tRNA) into polypeptide chains. (Reprinted from reference 26.)

as well as modification that may occur with RNA processing. Within each exon, consecutive sequences of three nucleotides, termed "codons" encode for specific amino acids whose sequence determines the functional properties of the resultant proteins (table 15.2). Structurally, the two stands of DNA wound in a double-helix actually exist in the nucleus in a tertiary, supercoiled arrangement.

DNA has two very important primary functions. The first is to retain the information necessary to maintain the biologic properties of a functional organism so that it is transmissible to future progeny both on a cellular and organ level. This is accomplished by the process of replication. The actual separation and subsequent replication of each individual DNA strand into a complimentary strand requires several enzymatic proteins, including: gyrases, which unwind DNA; DNA polymerases, which function by copying the nucleotide sequence; and DNA ligases, which link strands of nucleotides together. Replication always oc-

curs in a 5′–3′ direction. Short segments of RNA are usually required as primers to initiate the replication process. Eukaryotic cells have a number of enzymatic processes capable of correcting any abnormalities that may have occurred during the replication processes (17, 25).

Yet another important function of DNA is the ability to control the physiologic properties of the cell. Each cell has a complement of enzymes, such as RNA polymerases, which transcribe the DNA sequences into a specific form of nucleic acid, messenger RNA (mRNA), which is complimentary in base sequence to the parent DNA. RNA differs from DNA by the replacement of the sugar moiety deoxyribose with ribose, and use of the pyrimidine uridine in place of thymidine. Once transcribed, mRNA is further processed by deletion of intron sequences, capping of the 5′ end, addition of a "poly-A-tail" to the 3′ end, and varying amounts of modification such as methylation and phosphorylation of the individual nucleotide basis. Transcrip-

Table 15.2. Chromosomal Rearrangements Associated with de novo AML°

Chromosomal Rearrangement	Clinical Association
t(15;17)(q22:q11)	AML FAB M3, M3m
t(8;21)(q22:q22)	AML FAB M1, M2; Auer rods
inv(16)(p13q22)	AML FAB M4, M4eo; abnormal
t(16;16)(p13;q22)	eosinophils
del(16)(q22)	
del(5q)	AML, MDS
del(7q)	AML, MDS, MPD
t(9;11)(p21;q23)	AML M4, M5
del(12)(p11-p13)	AML; panmyelosis; marrow basophilia
del(9)	AML, MPD
del(20q11)	AML, MDS, PV
inv(3)(q21q26)	AML, MDS, MPD
t(3;3)(q21;q26)	Thrombocytosis; abnormal platelets
ins(3;3)(q21;q21q26)	
t(6;9)(p23:q34)	AML; Marrow Basophilia
del(13)(q21-q22)	AML; MDS; MPD

°These cytogenic abnormalities are the most common recurring structural abnormalities observed in de novo acute myeloid leukemia (AML) although they may also be seen in myelodysplastic syndrome (MDS) and myeloproliferative disease (MPD).

tion also always occurs in a 5′–3′ direction (fig. 15.7). Another form of RNA, transfer RNA (tRNA), is adjoined to the mRNA by ribosomes according to the specific nucleotide sequence. Structurally, tRNA carries a specific three- nucleotide sequence termed "anti-codon," which recognizes a specific codon of mRNA on one end and a corresponding amino acid adjoined to the other (fig. 15.8). The alignment of specific tRNAs to mRNA allows ribosomes to appropriately align amino acids in sequence for adjoining and eventually release a newly formed polypeptide (fig. 15.7). Further modification by various enzymes including phosphorylases, kinases, etc., eventually result in a functioning protein (17, 25, 26).

DNA Sequence Involved in the Philadelphia Chromosome

The very high prevalence of the t(9;22) translocation in patients with CML makes it a quite sensitive diagnostic test. However, the association of this translation with other disorders lowers its specificity. Such a high prevalence rate found predominately within CML patients led previous investigators to also question its functional significance in this hematologic disorder. In order to unravel the mysteries surrounding the Philadelphia chromosome it was important to determine the actual alterations of the nucleotide sequences involved in the translocation.

The localization of the c-abl oncogene to chromosome 9q and the c-sis oncogene to chromosome 22q aroused the interest of investigators exploring the nature of Philadelphia chromosome (4, 27, 28). V-abl was first

discovered in 1970 by Abelson and Rabstein who noted that a mouse strain inoculated with the Moloney murine leukemia retrovirus (M-MuLV) developed an acute B-cell leukemia that was quite different from the usual T-cell leukemia induced by this virus (29). This virus was initially termed the "Abelson murine leukemia virus" (A-MuLV) and was eventually found to contain a genetic recombination product of the N-terminal gag sequences of M-MuLV with C-terminal sequences of a normal host cellular gene, eventually named c-abl. In vitro studies of A-MuLV demonstrated its ability to transform both murine lymphoid and fibroblast cell lines (20, 29). Subsequent analysis has demonstrated that this abnormal homolog of c-abl, v-abl, lacked coding information present in both the 5′ and 3′ end of the normal murine c-abl, and that it encoded for a 160-kd (P160) protein. Interestingly, this new polypeptide was slightly larger than the 150-kd (P150) murine c-abl gene product and had an enhanced ability to autophosphorylate tyrosine residues (20, 30–32). Based on its physiologic properties, the abl oncogene has been grouped with other oncogenes encoding tyrosine kinase activity. The group is referred to as the "src" family based on the original isolation of this oncogene from the Rous sarcoma virus. It includes the erb-B oncogene that encodes for a portion of the epidermal growth factor receptor, the fms oncogene that encodes for CSF-1, as well as fes, fps, fgr, and lyn (5, 33). The altered ability of these transforming oncogenes to autophosphorylate tyrosine residues suggests an important role for this process in the proliferative response. The analysis of the c-sis protooncogene has shown that it encodes the β-chain of the platelet-derived growth factor (PDGF). v-sis was first discovered as the acute transforming gene of the simian sarcoma virus (12, 23, 34). The association of these two potentially transforming oncogenes, abl and sis, with the translocated regions of the Philadelphia chromosome inspired investigators to look more closely at this genetic sequence.

The identification of specific DNA sequences contained within the large quantity of genetic information in the human genome is a monumental task. A phenomenal breakthrough that allowed for the dissection of DNA into smaller, more discreet fragments was the discovery of bacterial restriction endonucleases. These enzymes, primarily named for the species of bacteria in which they were discovered, recognize specific nucleotide sequences and are able to create a double-stranded break at that particular site. The recognizable break site of DNA is usually a six-base sequence, but may be more or less. Many of these enzymes have been identified and purified for utilization in vitro studies (23, 25, 35). Examples of specific restriction endonucleases and the specific sequence they recognize are listed in table 15.3. Since these recognizable nucleotide sequences occur at multiple sites within the given DNA of an organism, exposure to a particular restriction endonuclease will result in a reproducible array of discretely sized fragments. These fragments can be separated according to size by gel electrophoresis (23, 25, 35). Typical gels for separating DNA fragments are composed of a

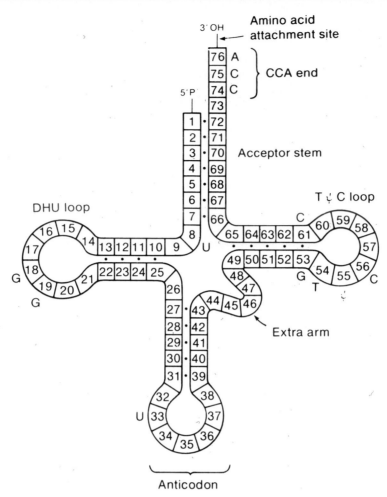

Figure 15.8. The currently accepted "standard" tRNA cloverleaf with its bases numbered. A few bases present in almost all tRNA molecules are indicated. Codon and anticodon regions are noted. (Reprinted from reference 25.)

Table 15.3. Chromosomal Rearrangements Associated with Secondary Acute Myeloid Leukemia (AML)°

Chromosomal Rearrangements	Clinical Association
del(5q)	AML, MDS
del(7q)	AML, MDS, MPD
t(1;3)(p36;q21)	AML, MDS, MPD
t(1;7)(p11;p11)	AML, MDS, MPD
t(2;11)(p21;q23)	MPD, MDS, AML

°These cytogenetic abnormalities are the most common recurring abnormalities observed in secondary AML following an antecedent hematologic disorder or prior therapy. MDS = Myelodysplastic syndrome, MPD = Myeloproliferative Disease.

semisolid agarose matrix, the concentration of which determines the pore size that DNA fragments must traverse. This technique allows one to separate DNA fragments ranging from 500 to approximately 30,000 bp. Smaller DNA fragments can also be separated in a similar manner using polyacrylamide gels. The individual gel-separated DNA segments can then be cut out from the gel, biochemically removed from the matrix, and used for subsequent investigations. Alternatively, the DNA fragments can be transferred to a solid matrix (i.e., nitrocellulose filter).

Exposing a nitrocellulose filter impregnated with DNA fragments to a radiolabeled segment of DNA that is complementary to a particular nucleotide sequence of interest (probe) under appropriate conditions will result in hybridization (binding). Autoradiography of the hybridized product will identify a particular sized segment of DNA based on the initial restriction endonuclease. This technique was first described by E. M. Southern in 1975 and hence the name "Southern blotting" (23, 25, 36) (fig. 15.9). A restriction endonuclease "map" is created by hybridization of a specific probe to multiple sets of DNA segments, each of which was enzymatically generated by a different restriction endonuclease (23). Unless some form of genetic alteration has occurred, the Southern blot or restriction endonuclease map for a particular DNA segment of a specific cell will always be the same. A change in one or more nucleotides may disrupt the particular recognizable sequence of an endonuclease enzyme and thus produce a variant Southern blot pattern. Southern hybridization can detect an abnormal clone when present in 0.5–1% of a given population of cells.

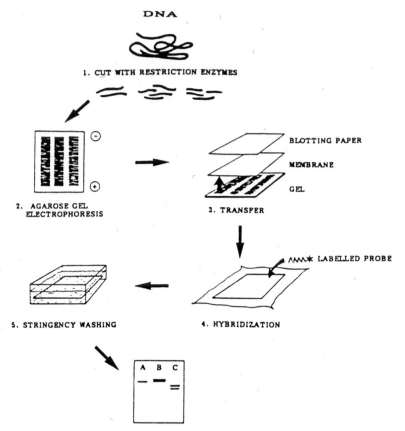

Figure 15.9. Schemata of Southern blotting. Step 1—genomic DNA cut with restriction endonucleases; step 2—DNA restriction fragments separated by molecular weight; step 3—DNA fragments transferred from gel to fixed membrane by capillary action; step 4—membrane-bound DNA hybridized to radiolabeled DNA probe that contains DNA sequence being assayed; step 5—posthybridization membrane stringently washed to remove unbound graphic film exposed to posthybridization membrane reveals radioactivity where probe stringently bound to areas of high homology. Lane A—gene complement in normal DNA; lane B—demonstrates amplified gene copy number; lane C—rearranged gene structure.

The first step in the identification of an abnormal or translocated normal abl oncogene was to obtain probes from the region of the normal c-abl oncogene on chromosome 9. In 1983, Heisterkamp used a v-abl probe to screen a recombinant DNA library. Through these hybridization experiments he was initially able to isolate five clones that encoded the entire normal c-abl gene sequence (27, 33, 37) (fig. 15.10). A typical DNA library is created by inserting a series of DNA clones created by restriction endonuclease digestion into a plasmid vector that is then introduced into a host of bacterial cells, such as *Escherichia coli*. It can then be purified in large quantaties for further investigation (23, 35). The size and amount of the particular DNA needed to be cloned for making a library or for cloning purposes in general determines which type of vector can be used.

Plasmids are circular self-replicating extrachromosomal double-stranded DNA molecules that contain a replication site, a cloning site, and a selectable marker, such as sensitivity or resistance to a particular antibiotic or mutagen. They are mainly used to clone smaller pieces of DNA measuring <10 kb. In vitro techniques have been developed to insert plasmids into bacterial cells (transfection) where they are then capable of self-replication and transcription independently of the cell cycle. Lambda (λ) phage vectors are more suitable for larger particles of cloned DNA measuring approximately 10–20 kb. Infection of a cell by λ-phage results in the lysis of the cell as a consequence of the injection of numerous toxic phage particles, each containing its own genomic copy, or lysogenic growth within the cell, which occurs after incorporation of the λ-phage DNA into the chromosomes of the host cell. A large portion of the λ-phage genome is dispensable and thus available for insertion of cloned DNA. Larger cloned DNA fragments >20 kb can be accommodated by cosmids, which contain a replication site and selectable marker(s) of plasmid origin combined with the insertion (cos) site and packaging information from a λ-phage (25, 35) (fig. 15.11). In general, the insertion of a desired DNA fragment into the vector genome requires isolation of the genetic sequences of interest, often by restriction endonucleases. After isolating the initial 5′ clones of c-abl, Heisterkamp characterized the genomic sequence of c-abl by screening a genomic library with the extreme 5′ and 3′ ends of the cDNA clone, thus identifying approximately a 40-kb region of the normal c-abl oncogene (37, 38). This procedure is termed "chro-

c-abl Map

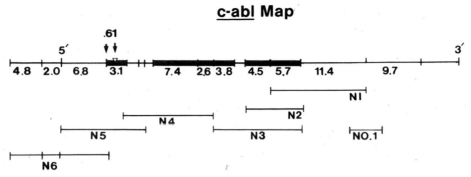

Figure 15.10. Restriction map of the human c-abl locus showing the phage clones isolated. The *vertical lines* denote EcoRI restriction sites, the *inverted triangle* indicates a BamHI site. The EcoRI fragments indicated by the *thicker horizontal line* are the fragments that hybridize to a v-abl probe (the v-abl homologous region). Numbers indicate the size of the restriction fragments in kilobase. Clones N1 through N5 were isolated using a cloned fragment of v-abl as probe; then the 5′ end of clone N5 and the 3′ end of clone N1 were used to isolate clones N6 and N1, which extended further from the v-abl homologous region. (Reprinted from reference 33.)

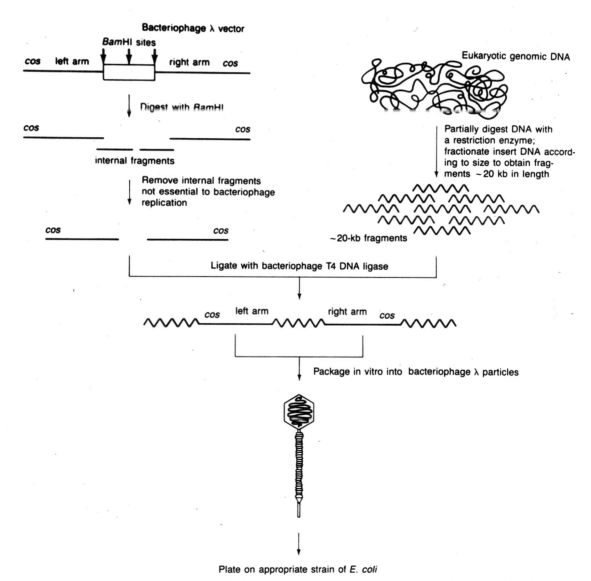

Figure 15.11. Construction of eukaryotic DNA library. Genomic bacteriophage λ-vector segments (*left*) are ligated to previously digested eukaryotic DNA fragments (*right*) under appropriate conditions by bacteriophage T₄ DNA ligase. Newly formed recombinant DNA molecules are individually inserted into separate bacteriophage λ-particles and then amplified by growth in *Escherichia coli*. Bacterial lysates contain a library of recombinant clones representing the majority of the initial digested eukaryotic genome. (Reprinted from reference 35.)

mosome walking" (23, 38). Restriction mapping using clones of the normal c-abl oncogene, initially performed by Heisterkamp, Leibowitz, and, subsequently, others, produced abnormal Southern blots, which identified numerous translocation breakpoints occurring along a 200-kb sequence of the first intron of c-abl (20, 33, 38–40) (fig. 15.12). Several investigators using fragments containing c-abl translocation breakpoints constructed λ-phage recombinant DNA libraries from patients with CML, and then screened these libraries with a radiolabeled copy of the same fragment of the DNA clone. It was at this point that fragments containing portions of chromosome 22 connected to portions of the c-abl oncogene were discovered (33, 38, 41). This important discovery enabled investigators to screen a recombinant DNA library from a normal chromosome 22 with probes that recognized the junctional fragment. This and the technique of chromosomal walk-

ing, followed by further restriction endonuclease mapping, isolated a small 6-kb region located on chromosome 22 that contained the breakpoints found in various patients with CML. This region was termed the "breakpoint cluster region" (bcr) (20, 33, 40, 42) (e.g., fig. 15.13).

The discovery of the molecular changes underlying the formation of the Philadelphia chromosome was a major breakthrough in understanding the relationship between molecular alterations and clinical manifestations. It was further analyzed by a more refined diagnostic technique, chromosome in situ hybridization. With this technique, the DNA of a cell is fixed as in a karyotypic analysis. Following denaturing into single-strand isoforms, the chromosomes are hybridized to a radiolabeled genetic sequence (probe) of interest under annealing conditions. Hybridization to a homologous area can be detected by autoradiography, providing a specific imprint. Subsequent analysis of the

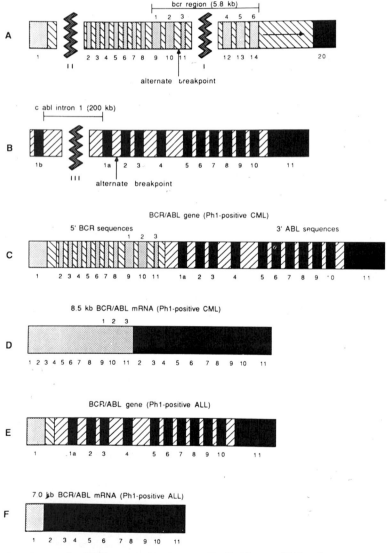

Figure 15.12. BCR/ABL translocations and mRNA transcripts in Ph-positive chronic myelogenous leukemia (CML) and acute lymphocytic leukemia (ALL). Introns (*hatched areas*) BCR exons (*shaded areas*) c-abl exons (*black areas*) and breakpoints have been depicted. **A.** BCR gene. I. Breakpoint region (bcr) in classic pH-positive CML. II. Breakpoint region in pH-positive ALL. **B.** C-abl gene. III. Breakpoint areas within 200-kb region of intron I. **C.** Hybrid BCR/ABL gene in classic pH-positive CML. **D.** 8.5-kb mRNA transcript of part **C** lacking exon 1a of BCR (spliced out due to lack of 5′ acceptor site). **E.** Hybrid BCR/ABL gene in pH-positive ALL. **F.** 7-kb mRNA transcript of part **E.** (Reprinted from reference 20.)

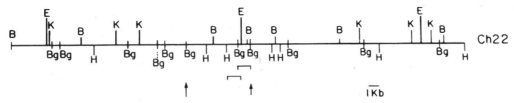

Figure 15.13. Restriction endonuclease map of a portion of chromosome 22 containing the BCR gene (outlined on each end by the two vertical arrows). The small horizontal bars represent two of the initial cloned probes that were used for analyzing the genomic rearrangements involved in the pH chromosome. (Reprinted from reference 33.)

chromosomal pattern with usual staining techniques and comparison to the autoradiography print will allow for localization of the gene of interest (24, 25). This method not only led to further clarification of the translocation involving bcr/abl, but also identified other patients with CML, as well as chromosomal abnormalities in other hematologic disorders such as the t(15;17) of APL and the t(8;14) in Burkitt lymphoma (5, 14–16, 22, 43).

The final elucidation of the exact nucleotide changes that occur in specific chromosomal aberrations such as the Philadelphia chromosome was made possible by the development of techniques for determining the nucleotide sequence of DNA. Both of the popular sequencing techniques randomly create variable sized radiolabeled oligonucleotides that originate at a particular point and terminate for a specific nucleotide(s) of interest. The procedures are performed so that the multiple locations of a nucleotide, e.g., guanine, results in a generation of DNA fragments accounting for all of its positions. The chemical sequencing technique, first described in 1977 and later modified in 1980 by Maxam and Gilbert, involves subjecting a single-stranded DNA fragment of interest to several chemical treatments (each of which is specific for a given nucleotide) under conditions that modify a "single" nucleotide in the sequence, making it susceptible to cleavage. By radiolabeling the 5' phosphate end with polynucleotide kinase and performing the procedures under conditions in which each of the reactions cleaves at a specific oligonucleotide, the entire sequence of a DNA fragment can be elucidated (25, 35, 44) (fig. 15.14). In 1977, Sanger and colleagues developed a similar enzymatic-based chain-termination procedure to sequence DNA (45). The process involved annealing a small oligonucleotide primer to the DNA segment, then adding DNA polymerase, which normally would result in the synthesis of the complimentary strand. The addition of a dideoxynucleoside triphosphate (ddNTP), which lacksa hydroxyl moiety on the 3' position of deoxyribose, results in random termination of elongation of the oligonucleotide sequence at each ddNTP. Using ddNTPs for each of the four nucleosides, under similar conditions a series of oligonucleosides can be generated for each A, G, C, or T position in the template strand. In situations where the template of interest is unknown, a universal primer complementary to a vector sequence added to the 3' end of the template can be used (35, 45).

Each of these techniques generates four sets of oligonucleotides specific for each of the particular nucleotides, i.e., A, G, C, or T, which can be separated by polyacrylamide gel electrophoresis. Autoradiography of the product allows one to determine the nucleotide sequence by reading the position of the radioactive imprint in the lanes from bottom to top. Variations of these techniques, including one-lane methods that identify nucleotides by varying intensities of radioactivity, have also been developed for use in certain circumstances (25, 35).

Another technique that has greatly simplified the task of isolating and analyzing DNA sequences is the polymerase chain reaction (PCR). The process of cloning a particular DNA sequence of interest (identification and isolation of a DNA sequence of interest followed by insertion into a vector that is then incorporated into a bacterial or mammalian cell line) is both time consuming and laborious. Additionally, cloning requires a large number of cells for DNA analysis. Similarly, the isolation of DNA for Southern blot analysis to identify genetic alterations in patients with hematologic disorders such as CML requires from 10^7–5×10^7 peripheral blood or bone marrow cells. The development of PCR significantly reduces the quantity of DNA required for these studies, as well as reducing the necessary expenditures of time and effort. In the polymerase chain reaction, a DNA template of interest, either DNA or cDNA (the enzymatic product of exposing RNA templates to reverse transcriptase) (fig. 15.15), is first denatured, and then oligonucleotides that are complimentary to regions 5' and 3' of the desired sequence are annealed to these opposing strands. These oligonucleotides can serve as primers in the presence of a unique heat-stable DNA polymerase (isolated from a retrovirus found in natural hot springs) to copy both the sense and antisense strands. By using identical cycles of varying temperatures, the newly formed double-stranded DNA complexes are denatured into single strands and reannealed to the oligonucleotide primers, which allows for repeated replication of the DNA sequence of interest to result in an exponential amplification of the original template that can approach a million-fold. The process can be accomplished in less than a day and allows for the detection of a specific nucleotide sequence in as few as 10^{-5}–10^{-6} cells (23, 35, 46) (fig. 15.16).

The use of PCR and DNA sequencing techniques has greatly facilitated the analysis of the nucleotide content in genetic rearrangements found in the Philadelphia chromosome, as well as genetic alterations noted in other hemato-

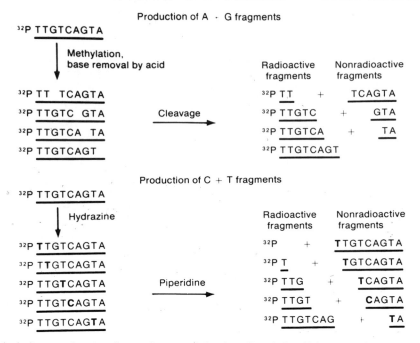

Figure 15.14. A diagram showing the production of the A + G and C + T fragments by the Maxam-Gilbert sequencing procedure. In the hydrazine-treated molecules the *bold-faced letters* indicate the affected bases. The generation of the G-only and C-only fragments is not shown. (Reprinted from reference 25.)

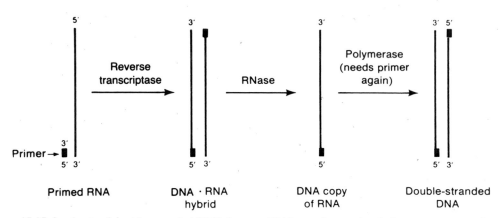

Figure 15.15. Synthesis of double-stranded DNA from an RNA template molecule by reverse transcriptase. A primer that could be either RNA or DNA is shown. (Reprinted from reference 25.)

logic malignancies. The structure of the Philadelphia chromosome has now been well characterized and, as mentioned earlier, consists of a t(9;22) (q34.1; q11.21). Translocation, the majority of the translocation breakpoints associated with the c-abl gene of chromosome 9, occur at random positions located along a 200-kb sequence of intron 1 located between exon 1b and 1a (fig. 15.12). The variability of the breakpoints is related to the extreme length of the first intron. The translocation connects 3' c-abl sequences starting with either exon 1a or 2 through 11 to 5' breakpoint cluster region sequences on chromosome 22. Unlike the normal human c-abl gene of chro-mosome 9, which consists of 11 exons and 250-kb nucleotide pairs, the normal bcr gene consists of 20 exons and spans only 70-kb pairs. A small 5.8-kb area centered between exon 9 and exon 14, termed the "breakpoint cluster region" (bcr), contains the usual translocation breakpoint of chromosome 22. More often than not, the breakpoint occurs 3' to exon 11. During translocation, the last 10 or 11 exons of the c-abl gene are exchanged with the last 6–10 exons of the bcr gene, resulting in the common karyotypic abnormality (20, 33, 40) (fig. 15.12).

These molecular techniques have also come to play an important role in diagnostic management. The use of PCR with Southern blot hybridization can clearly identify the bcr-abl rearrangement in CML patients with the Philadelphia chromosome. It has also helped to identify bcr rearrangements in patients who lack the Philadelphia chromosome but demonstrate the appropriate phenotype for the disease, as well as in the 20% of adult patients with

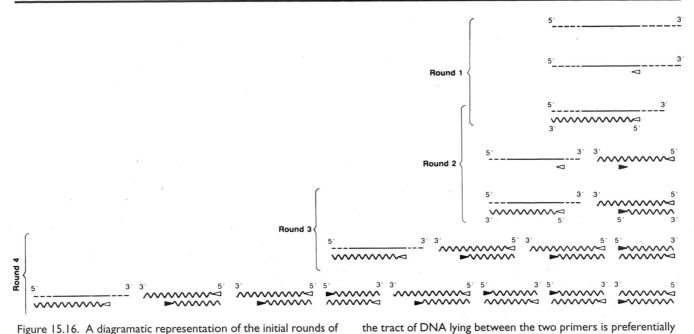

Figure 15.16. A diagramatic representation of the initial rounds of a polymerase chain reaction. The original template (*top line*) is single-stranded DNA and the leftward and rightward oligonucleotide primers are shown as ◄ and ►, respectively. The initial products of the amplification reaction are heterogeneous in size. However, the tract of DNA lying between the two primers is preferentially amplified and quickly becomes the dominant product of the amplification reaction. If the original template is double stranded, an equivalent set of reactions will take place using the complementary strand as template. (Reprinted from reference 35.)

Table 15.4. Chromosomal Rearrangements Associated with Acute Lymphocytic Leukemia (ALL)

Chromosomal Rearrangements	Clinical Association
t(8;14)(q24:q23)	B-cell ALL
t(2;8)(p11-12;q24)	B-cell ALL
t(8;22)(q24;q11)	B-cell ALL
t(5;14)(q31;q32)	B-cell ALL
t(1;19)(q23;p13)	Pre-B-cell ALL
t(9;22)(q34;q11)	Early pre-B-cell ALL
t(8;14)(q24;q11)	T-cell ALL
t(11;14)(p15;q11)	T-cell ALL
t(1;14)(p32;q11)	T-cell ALL
t(7;19)(q35;p13)	T-cell ALL
t(1;7)(p32;q35)	T-cell ALL

Table 15.5. Chromosomal Associations with Other Hematologic Disorders

Chromosomal Rearrangements	Clinical Association
t(8;14)(q24;q32)	Burkitt lymphoma
t(2;8)(p12;q24)	
t(8;22)(q24;q11)	
t(11;14)(q13;q32)	Diffuse small cleaved cell lymphoma
(bcl-1)°	B-cell CLL
	Multiple myeloma
t(14;18)(q32;q21)	Follicular lymphoma
(bcl-2)°	Diffuse large cell lymphoma
	Hodgkin disease
t(14;19)(q32;q13)	CLL
(bcl-3)°	
+12 11q, 6q, 14q+, 13q	CLL
t14(q11;q32)	Ataxia telangiectasia

°Characterized genes associated with translocations in various B-cell disorders with involve 14q32. CLL = Chronic lymphocytic leukemia.

ALL, and the lesser percentages of childhood patients with ALL and AML who also have chromosomal abnormality (20, 21, 46–48). Thus, >95% of patients presenting with CML can be identified by demonstration of rearrangement of the bcr region. Approximately one-half of Philadelphia chromosome–positive ALL adult patients actually represent CML in blast crisis. The other half have been shown to have a translocation of exons 2 through 11 of the c-abl gene to a different area of the bcr gene of chromosome 22 located within the first intron, approximately 50-kb 5′ of the usual bcr region (20, 47, 48) (fig. 15.12). More recently, these techniques have characterized other rearrangements in various hematologic malignancies: a t(15;17)(q22;q12-q21) translocation in approximately 92% of patients presenting with APL, a t(8;14) (q24;q32) translocation in 80% of patients with Burkitt lymphoma or either a T(2;8) (p11;q24) translocation or a t(8;22) (p11;q24) translocation in the remaining 20%, a t(14;18) (q32;q21) translocation in >85% of patients with follicular lymphomas, and numerous other abnormalities (5, 16, 21, 23, 43, 46) (tables 15.4–15.7). The majority of these genetic alterations cannot be visualized on a typical karyotype.

The clinical relevance of this technology is now evident. It has already demonstrated its usefulness. However, the

Table 15.6. The "Universal" Genetic Code°

First Position (5' end)	Second Position				Third Position (3' end)
U	U	C	A	G	U
	Phe	Ser	Tyr	Cys	C
	Phe	Ser	Tyr	Cys	A
	Leu	Ser	Stop	Stop	G
	Leu	Ser	Stop	Trp	
C	Leu	Pro	His	Arg	U
	Leu	Pro	His	Arg	C
	Leu	Pro	Gln	Arg	A
	Leu	Pro	Gln	Arg	G
A	Ile	Thr	Asn	Ser	U
	Ile	Thr	Asn	Ser	C
	Ile	Thr	Lys	Arg	A
	Met	Thr	Lys	Arg	G
G	Val	Ala	Asp	Gly	U
	Val	Ala	Asp	Gly	C
	Val	Ala	Asp	Gly	A
	Val	Ala	Asp	Gly	G

°Note: The italicized codons are initiation codons. GUG is very rare.

development of the molecular understanding of the Philadelphia chromosome has raised this question: does the Philadelphia chromosome bear functional significance in the pathology of CML?

The RNA Message

The normal process by which the information contained within DNA controls the phenotype of individual cells involves transcription into mRNA. Determining whether the Philadelphia chromosome in our patient with CML is transcribed into a functioning protein requires the demonstration of bcr/abl mRNA in his leukemic cells. Several groups of investigators sought to find this mRNA product in 1984 and 1985. After first isolating total RNA from several CML patients, as well as a CML-derived cultured cell line, K562, the RNA was separated according to size by gel electrophoresis and then transferred onto a solid phase matrix for hybridization (33, 49–51). This process, called "Northern hybridization," is quite similar to that described for Southern blotting (23, 35) (fig. 15.17). Exposing these blots to a radiolabeled DNA probe complimentary to the normal abl gene sequence has yielded interesting results. The normal mRNA product of the c-abl gene is a 7-kb mRNA transcript. Interestingly, the investigators not only found these normal-sized abl transcripts, but in addition, a new 8.5-kb mRNA transcript (49). The finding of the normal transcripts was not surprising since many CML patients retain an unaltered chromosome 9. The discovery of the larger bcr/abl mRNA was the first clue that an altered genomic sequence, bcr/abl, may participate in the pathophysiology of CML. The hybrid bcr/abl mRNA transcript is formed by

the joining of the products of the first 10 or so exons of the bcr gene at the 5' end and the products of exons 2–11 of c-abl at the 3' end. Upon processing, the introns, as well as exon 1A of c-abl, are removed, resulting in the final 8.5-kb species (fig. 15.12). In a similar fashion, patients with Ph1-positive ALL who lack the typical bcr/abl rearrangement were found to have an abnormal 7-kb RNA transcript that is complementary to exon 1 of the bcr gene at the 5' end connected to exons 2–11 of the abl gene on the 3' end (20, 33, 47, 48) (fig. 15.12).

The characterization of the bcr/abl translocation in CML has stimulated the search for transcriptional changes in other hematologic disorders with known genetic abnormalities. Alterations in the transcription of the c-myc protooncogene were found by examining RNA of cells from patients with Burkitt lymphoma [t(8;14) (q24;q32.3), t(2;8) (p11;q24), t(8;22) (q24;q11)], and other disorders such as T-cell ALL [t(8;14) (q24;q11)], which contained known rearrangements of the c-myc protooncogene. This gene, which is located on chromosome 8 and encodes for a DNA-binding protein, functions by regulating DNA transcription. Positioning of the myc sequence close to areas of enhanced gene expression, such as the highly transcribed immunoglobulin gene sequences of Burkitt lymphoma, has been hypothesized to play an important role in malignant transformation (14–16, 21). More recently, De The et al. identified a new fusion messenger RNA, PML-RAR-α, composed of a portion of the retinoic acid receptor α (RAR-α) gene on chromosome 17 and the myl gene (now referred to as the PML gene) on chromosome 15 in patients with APL [t(15;17) (q22) (q12-q21)] (53). This rearrangement, unique to APL, involves the translocation of a truncated portion of the genetic sequence (encoding the B through F regions) of RAR-α to the promyelocyte (PML) gene located on chromosome 15 (21, 43, 52–54). The demonstration of these genetic abnormalities has opened the possibility that these changes led to the formation of an altered protein product.

The Abnormal Protein

The ultimate expression of a cell's phenotype is directly related to the type and quantity of proteins it produces. In other words, the clinical appearance and activity of a typical malignant cell in our patient with CML is dictated by its DNA content, but is expressed as the proteins that create the cell's unique qualities. The primary structure of a protein is the sequence of amino acids that compose the polypeptide chain. Based upon the intramolecular electrostatic forces of the individual amino acids and their side chains, the polypeptide chain assumes a secondary structure, which is manifested as various folded or coiled configurations. Other interactions among folded or coiled polypeptide sections of one or more proteins dictate the final tertiary structure of the protein (fig. 15.18). The electrostatic charge, various binding affinities, and antigenicity of a protein are all integrally related to the formation of this structure, which is highly dependent on the sur-

Table 15.7. Some Restriction Endonucleases and Their Cleavage Sites°

Microorganism	Name of Enzyme	Target Sequence and Cleavage Sites
Microorganisms that generate cohesive ends		
Escherichia coli RY13	EcoRI	G↓A A | T T C
		C T T | A A↑G
Bacillus amyloliquefaciens H	BamHI	G↓G A | T C C
		C C T | A G↑G
Bacillus globigii	BglII	A↓G A | T C T
		T C T | A G↑A
Haemophilus aegyptius	HaeII	PuG C | G C↓Py
		Py↑CG | C G Pu
Haemophilus influenza R_d	HindII	A↓A G | C T T
		T T C | G A↑A
Providencia stuartii	PstI	C T G | C A↓G
		G↑A C | G T C
Streptomyces albus G	SalI	G↓T C | G A C
		C A G | C T↑G
Xanthomonas badrii	XbaI	T↓C T | A G A
		A G A | T C↑T
Thermus aquaticus	TaqI	T↓C | G A
		A G | C↑T
Microorganisms that generate flush ends		
Brevibacterium albidum	BalI	↓
		T G | C A
		A C | G G T
		↑
Haemophilus aegyptius	HaeI	↓
		(A)G G | C C(T)
		(T)C C | G G(A)
		↑
Serratia marcescens	SmaI	↓
		C C'C | G G G
		G G G | C C C
		↑

Note: The *vertical dashed line* indicates the axis of dyad symmetry in each sequence. *Arrows* indicate the sites of cutting. The enzyme Taq1 yields cohesive ends consisting of two nucleotides, whereas the cohesive ends produced by the other enzymes contain four nucleotides. The enzyme HaeI recognizes the sequence GGCC whether the adjacent base pair is A · T or T · A, as long as dyad symmetry is retained. Pu and Py refer to any purine and pyrimidine, respectively.

rounding environment (18, 25). Proteins may be separated by size, using techniques such as chromatography or gel electrophoresis. Denaturing proteins by exposure to various detergents (i.e., SDS and NP-40) eliminates secondary and tertiary structures and alters their charge to the individual size of the particular protein and its primary structure to become the separating determinant. Proteins separated on acrylamide gel electrophoresis can be electrophoretically transferred to solid matrices such as nitrocellulose filter or Whatman filter paper. Exposure of these fixed proteins to antigen-specific antibodies followed by colorometric enzyme or radiolabeled protein A analysis (protein A has strong affinity for IgG) enables one to identify proteins of interest. This process is called Western blotting (5, 25, 35). The antigenicity of protein also allows for a particular protein to be immunoprecipitated by an antigen-specific antibody that can be further analyzed by using some of the techniques mentioned above. Characterizing competition among various proteins for particular binding sites enables one to estimate relative affinity strength. Scientists utilized these techniques to detect a protein encoded by the bcr/abl genetic rearrangement.

The normal murine c-abl gene product, P150, is similar to the 145-kd normal human c-abl gene product (P145). In comparison, the protein product of v-abl in A-MuLV, P160, was discovered to be larger and to cause extensive autophosphorylation of tyrosine moieties, some of which were not phosphorylated by the normal gene product. In addition, unlike the normal human and murine gene products, this tyrosine kinase activity was detectable in vitro and, in subsequent studies, in vivo (20, 30–32, 55–57). Tyrosine kinases are important regulators of metabolic pathways. Increased activity has been well documented with other transforming oncogenes such as v-src, v-erb, and v-fms. These and other growth factor receptors with inherent tyrosine kinase activity have been shown to confer growth factor independence to various cultured cell lines (5, 20, 33, 40, 57–59). Tyrosine phosphorylation can be characterized by thin layer chromatography, or by two-

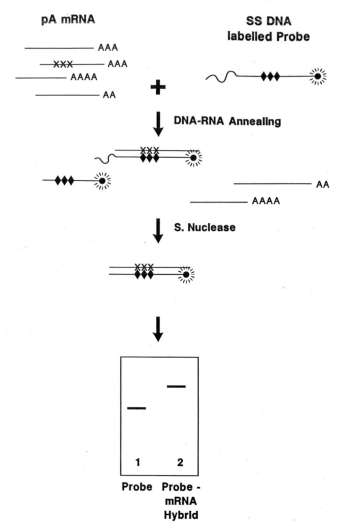

Figure 15.17. S1 nuclease northern blot analysis. Polyadenylated (pA) mRNA of interest has been marked with x's. A radiolabeled complementary single-stranded DNA probe is denatured and mixed with a population of mRNAs, resulting in hybridization (annealing) of complementary regions. Addition of S1 nuclease degrades all single-strand DNA and RNA. The resistant DNA-RNA hybridized product is analyzed by gel electrophoresis and autoradiography. (Reprinted from reference 26.)

dimensional gel electrophoresis (20, 35). Using the above information, Konopka et al. immunoprecipitated a 210-kd (P210) protein by using antigen-specific antibodies for the murine v-abl protein in K562 cells, and then from a patient with CML (56, 60). Subsequent investigations by Witte's and Baltimore's labs demonstrated that not only was this protein considerably larger than normal human c-abl gene product (P145), it was also recognizable by antiserum prepared against both human c-abl and bcr protein determinants (61). They also discovered that it contained a very high level of tyrosine kinase activity. Previous experiments have documented a relatively weak in vitro autophosphorylation ability of the normal P145 on a single peptide moiety. Additional experiments confirmed the presence of P210 and showed that it was capable of phosphorylating tyrosines on at least three major and several minor peptide

domains of the protein in a pattern similar to that of transforming v-abl P160 (33, 56, 62–64). A similar analysis performed on pH-positive ALL cells with the abnormal complementary 7-kb RNA transcript identified an abnormal 185–190-kd (P190) size protein (20, 40, 63, 65, 66). Its in vitro tyrosine autophosphorylation capabilities were also found to be quantitatively increased. However, the phosphorylated target peptide sequence was identical to that for the normal P145 (63).

Other chimeric protein products produced by genetic rearrangements have also been identified. Reflecting back on the t(15;17) translocation found in patients with APL, a protein composed of PML sequences joined to portions of the normal RAR-α protein was isolated and demonstrated to be complementary to its translocated nucleic acid derivative (43, 67, 68). The new protein lacks the "A region" responsible for activation of adjacent genes that occurs upon binding of the normal RAR-α to appropriate promoter regions (43, 46, 68). These discoveries confirm the capabilities of genetic rearrangements and alterations to alter cellular phenotype.

The Effect of the Abnormal Protein

Following up on their earlier observations, Witte et al. demonstrated that the loss of the tyrosine kinase activity of the v-abl protein in A-MuLV resulted in the disappearance of its transforming capabilities (32). The development of transfection and transformation assays dramatically improved our ability to analyze mutagenic properties. A transfection assay is an in vitro analysis of the effect of the insertion of a DNA sequence of interest into a mutagensensitive cell line, for example, the premalignant NIH-3T3 fibroblast cell line. Transformation assays involve insertion of a DNA sequence capable of inducing transformation

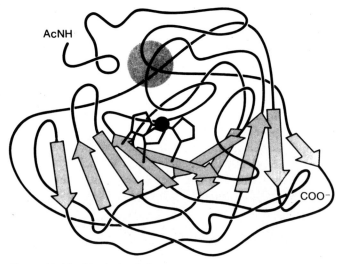

Figure 15.18. An idealized drawing of the tertiary structure of a protein human carbonic anhydrase. The peptide chain (*line*), zinc ion (*sphere*), three histidines (*pentagons*), individual β-sheet peptide configurations (*arrows*), amino and carboxy terminal ends are indicated. (Reprinted from reference 25.)

into a host or host cell line, either by precipitation or by infecting the target with a retrovirus carrying the DNA fragment (12, 15, 25). By infecting BALB/c mice bone marrow cells with a M-MuLV retrovirus that contained a bcr/abl cDNA insert, Kelliher et al. produced a clonal population of pre-B-cells that expressed P210 and were phenotypically similar to chronic phase CML cells (69). Subsequent experiments by Baltimore et al. and Witte and Rosenberg documented the ability of murine bone marrow cells infected with retroviruses containing v-abl, and more importantly, bcr/abl cDNA inserts, to induce a myeloproliferative syndrome consistent with the chronic phase of chronic myelogenous leukemia in lethally irradiated mice. The investigators were able to demonstrate not only the provirus, which encoded for bcr/abl, but the expression of P210 in the bone marrow of the adult animals (69, 70). More recently, the ability of the P190$^{bcr/abl}$ DNA construct to transform murine bone marrow cells and induce an acute leukemia, either myeloid or lymphoid, has been demonstrated (71, 72). Thus, a direct causal link between the Philadelphia chromosome identified in our patient and his leukemic condition, CML, has been established.

Although these discoveries have dramatically improved our understanding of CML, they by no means provide a complete story. The primary malignant progenitor cell in CML is believed to be a pluripotent hematopoietic stem cell, and although other factors in addition to the bcr/abl gene products are important for its malignant potential, they remain unidentified.

Evaluation of pluripotent hematologic precursors is quite complex. Our current means of identifying these cells by in vitro cell culture and flow cytometry for early developed antigens such as CD34 remain inadequate for routine analysis. In addition, the genotypic characteristics of CML are not completely homogenous. As noted earlier, about 10% of patients with CML lack the Philadelphia chromosome on karyotypic analysis. Of these patients, ≤5% are presumed to have another myeloproliferative or a myelodysplastic syndrome. The other 5% can be identified as having a genetic insertion of abl into the bcr segment or a bcr/abl complex translocation involving another chromosome (20, 33, 40, 46). Interestingly, the change from chronic phase CML to acute blast crisis is associated with numerous additional cytogenetic abnormalities, including trisomy 8, +19, isochrome 17, an additional second PH chromosome, and, at times, loss of the bcr/abl rearrangement (47). The exact mechanism by which abnormal tyrosine kinase activity leads to malignant transformation also remains a puzzle. Thus, the genetic basis of CML is more complicated than a single chromosomal translocation.

The development of transgenic mice has allowed us to observe the influence of various oncogenes in animal models. Transgenic mice allow the introduction of an oncogene or genetic sequence of interest into the fertilized egg or germ line cell of a mouse, which can result in the expression of this sequence in the adult animal (23, 73, 74). This allows the characterization of the effects of overexpression of specific genes. For example, Adams et al. demonstrated that overexpression of the c-myc oncogene induced lymphoid malignancies of a pre-B-cell type in transgenic mice (75, 76).

The past 5 years has brought significant improvement in our ability to study DNA-protein interactions that are important in regulating gene expression. For example, gel retardation studies have been extremely beneficial in establishing some of the protein-protein and protein-nucleic acid binding properties of many of these important regulatory molecules. The procedure requires mixing a protein with a radiolabeled DNA probe of interest followed by gel electrophoresis and autoradiography (25, 35). The demonstration of slower movement through the gel, or retardation, of the mixed product in reference to an isolated probe implies the formation of a bound, larger complex, and thus, affinity between the molecules.

The use of all of the above techniques has brought us closer to understanding the genetic basis of disease. Returning to APL, the absence of region A in RAR-α results in the loss of the regulatory component of a protein that binds to the responsive elements of a promoter in particular DNA sequences. This loss of a potential genetic inducer presumably plays a role in the blocking of granulocyte differentiation in this form of acute myeloid leukemia (43, 46, 67, 68). Rearrangement of the c-myc oncogene locus of chromosome 8, placing it under the influence of enhancers of immunoglobulin synthesis, is purported to play an important role in the development of Burkitt lymphoma (14–16). The rearrangement of the T-cell α-receptor (TaR) gene located at chromosome 14q11 is thought to play an important role in the pathogenesis of T-cell ALL where it is often found (15, 16). Mutations of the ras oncogenes, particularly at codon 12, 13, and 61, have been found by various investigators to occur at rates from 25–70% in AML and MDS. These particular codon locations are critical binding sites for GDP and GTP, and the resultant mutated proteins have been shown to contain reduced GTPase activity (15, 16, 22, 23, 74).

The pattern of the genetic abnormalities discovered in the various hematologic disorders provides some patterns of homogeneity, such as in CML and APL. However, the more striking characteristic is the heterogeneity in the variety and number of different genetic alterations that occur among the individual types of neoplasms. This picture and the data presented in this chapter provide strong evidence for the theory of a multistep oncogenic process required for the development of malignancy. In a rare event, a single genetic alteration may be solely responsible for malignant transformation. However, in general, just as the growth of a human being or animal requires numerous developmental changes, so does the transformation of a normal cell into a malignant cell. As further evidence, studies involving the cross-breeding of transgenic mice have now demonstrated the synergistic effect of more than one oncogene in the development of lymphomagenesis (73).

The Clinical Realm

The step-by-step molecular processes known to exist as part of the pathogenesis of CML have been identified in the 46-year-old patient described above. However, despite our improved understanding of the molecular pathogenesis of CML, the results of treatment have not improved dramatically. It is quite likely that the next decade will see corresponding advances in our ability to treat these diseases.

The development of PCR has greatly expanded our diagnostic capabilities. cDNA from the leukocytes of a patient with CML can be subjected to PCR for identification of the bcr/abl rearrangement. This technique has become important in the diagnosis of pH-negative CML, as well as in the evaluation of the efficacy of its therapy. Historically, standard chemotherapy offers prolongation of survival, but no potential for cure. More recently, with the development of allogenetic bone marrow transplantation, prolonged disease-free survival is obtainable in about 50% of patients <40 years old who are seen clinically with a chronic phase and have available HLA-matched donors (47). The use of PCR in the detection of minimal residual disease (MRD) in patients posttransplant is rapidly becoming an important diagnostic tool. PCR for the detection of rearranged T-cell receptor and immunoglobulin heavy chain genes is also gaining importance (21, 23).

Several hybridization techniques have also demonstrated efficacy for diagnosing genetic abnormalities. Tissue in situ hybridization has been useful in evaluating individual cells of prepared tissue sections. Radioactive cloned nucleic acid probes that are complementary to a specific mRNA of interest are placed on tissue sections under annealing conditions and then autoradiographed over time. As in chromosomal hybridization techniques, this process allows the clinician to detect specific RNA fragments with a direct comparison to the cellular morphology (23). Use of fluorescence in situ hybridization (FISH) analysis allows the identification of chromosomal abnormalities not only in metaphase nuclei, but in the interphase nuclei of single intact cells. Labeled probes surrounding a DNA region of interest are hybridized to intact cells and subsequently fluorescently marked for microscopic analysis. FISH analysis has been used for the detection of several genetic translocations: bcr/abl in CML patients with purported cytogenetic remission, the various translocations associated with Burkitt lymphoma, the translocation of the bcl-2 protooncogene with the heavy chain (J^H) locus seen in the t(14;18) abnormality of follicular lymphomas and lymphosarcoma cell leukemia, as well as in detection of particular chromosomal aberrancies in leukemic cells such as −7, +8, and +12 (46). This newer technique is not only quite sensitive, but also inherently simple, and it is hoped will make its way into the routine laboratory analysis of hematologic disorders with known chromosomal abnormalities.

Many of these genetic abnormalities have also been important as prognostic indicators. The finding of a Philadelphia chromosome or the bcr/abl rearrangement in patients with acute leukemia has a direct correlation with a poor response to therapy and shortened life expectancy (21, 33, 40, 47). In AML, the finding of either a t(8;21) or t(15;17) translocation has a more favorable prognosis, whereas abnormalities of chromosome 5 or 7 and trisomy 8 carry more unfavorable prognostic significance. Similarly, the finding of hyperdiploidy (>50 chromosomes) in ALL is associated with a more favorable prognosis, while the finding of hypodiploidy and tetraploidy carries a much poorer outcome. Other prognostically significant chromosomal changes have been described (21) (table 15.8). There have been numerous cytogenetic alterations found in patients with chronic lymphocytic leukemia, including trisomy 12, deletions of the long arm in chromosome 6, 11, and 13, and a 14 q+ chromosome. In general, patients with CLL who had a normal karyotype survived significantly longer than those with genetic alterations (21, 77). As mentioned, the development of acute phase or blast crisis of CML is often associated with other cytogenetic abnormalities. These acute leukemias along with those which develop from myelodysplastic syndrome (MDS), which similarly are usually accompanied by various cytogenetic changes, also carry a more dismal prognosis and respond poorly to therapy (21, 22, 78). Among the individual myelodysplastic syndromes, abnormal karyotypes also signify prognostic importance. MDS patients with a normal-appearing chromosome pattern or with a deletions of 5q ("5q-syndrome") have median survival >2 years. The presence of trisomy 8, a single chromosome 7, deletions of the long arm of chromosome 7, or complex genetic defects signify a much shorter survival (21, 78) (table 15.8). There have been several well-described translocations of particular genes associated with neoplastic disorders of B-lymphocytes (bcl-1, bcl-2, bcl-3) and T-lymphocytes (tcl-1, tcl-2, tcl-3, tcl-5).

Table 15.8. Prognostic Significance of Cytogenic Abnormalities in Acute Leukemia and Myelodysplastic Syndromes: Cytogenic Findings with Prognostic Significance*

Hematologic Diseases	Favorable	Unfavorable
AML	t(8;21)(q22.3)	Abnormalities of chromosome 5
	Abnormalities of 16q22	Abnormalities of chromosome 7
	t(15;17)(q22;q12-q21)	Trisomy 8
		Abnormalities of 11q23
		Deletion of 12p
		Trisomy 13
		Complex karyotypes
ALL	Hyperdiploidy (>50 chromosomes)	t(9;22)(q34;q11)
		t(4;11)(q21;q23)
		t(8;14)(q24;q32)
		t(1;19)(q23;p13)
		Near-tetraploidy
Myelodysplasia	Normal	−8
	del 5q	del 7q
		−7
		complex defects

*AML, Acute myeloid leukemia; ALL, Acute lymphoblastic leukemia.

The t(14;18) (q32;q21) translocation involving the bcl-2 gene located on chromosome 18 is often found in the more indolent follicular lymphomas. The bcl-1 gene is more commonly found in B-cell CLL. In the involved B-cell malignancies, the gene is rearranged with an immunoglobulin gene, and in the T-cell malignancies it is rearranged with the T-cell receptor gene located at 14q11. The prognostic implication of this finding is directly related to the disorders with which they are associated (14–16). In general, the higher the number of chromosomal abnormalities that are identified in a patient with a particular disorder, the poorer the overall survival will be.

These data lend support to the concept of the multihit hypothesis of neoplastic development. Concurrent with the advancement of the technical feasibility for the detection of genetic abnormalities, the frequency and the number of the associations of genetic changes with hematologic malignancies has greatly expanded. The techniques of molecular biology have thus given us a microscope into the genetic realm for diagnostic purposes and lent strong support to the idea of a clonal change becoming a part of the definition of a malignancy. Overall, these advancements, as well as developments in flow cytometry enable clinicians to better diagnose and counsel their patients with hematologic disorders.

Therapeutically, there have been a few advances at the molecular level that have led to improvements in clinical treatment. The use of all-trans retinoic acid in patients with APL has demonstrated >90% complete remission in several studies, albeit with small numbers of patients (43, 79–82). The initial interest in this therapy was promulgated by the molecular discoveries of the altered retinoic acid receptor associated with this disorder. Although this therapy is associated with minimal toxicity compared with high-dose chemotherapy, thus far it has not produced sustained responses. At this point, it appears that this therapy is an important component of combination therapy in patients with APL. More recently, a phase I trial involving the use of synthetic oligonucleotides complimentary to regions of the bcr/abl rearrangement in patients with the acute phase of CML has been initiated (83). Initial results are not available. As yet, there have been no dramatic developments borne from our understanding of the genetic pathophysiology of CML that can offer hope to patients with CML.

Summary

Leukemia and lymphoma are well-known malignant disorders of hematopoietic cells. Our knowledge of their clinical phenotypes and responses to various modalities of therapy is extensive. However, the genetic pathophysiology leading to their development is only now being uncovered as a result of major recent advances in molecular biology. This chapter has introduced and described many of the developments of molecular biology that have allowed scientists and researchers to uncover genetic alterations and their influences on hematologic and other disorders. The illustrated case of a patient with CML was quite helpful in this approach, enabling us to review the extensive amount of work already done on this disorder, as well as review the clinical ramifications that can be drawn and are currently in use. The understanding of the mechanics of these molecular techniques will help interpret future molecular and clinical investigative findings. The bridge between genes and clinical phenomena has now been erected, leading to new forefronts of clinical application. It stands ready to be crossed.

Acknowledgments
We wish to thank Andrew J. Carroll, Ph.D., for his contribution, and Barbara Wilson for her assistance.

REFERENCES

1. Dorland's illustrated medical dictionary. 27th ed. Philadelphia: WB Saunders 1988:261.
2. Lightman MA. Chronic myelogenous leukemia and related disorders. In: Williams WJ, Beutler E, Erslev AJ, Lichtman MA, eds. Hematology. 4th ed. New York:McGraw-Hill, 1990:202–223.
3. Nowell PC, Hungerford DA. A minute chromosome in human chronic granulocytic leukemia. Science 1960;132:1497.
4. de Klein A, van Kessel AG, Grosveld G, et al. A cellular oncogene is translocated to the Philadelphia chromosome in chronic myelocytic leukemia. Nature 1982;300:765–767.
5. Willman CL, Whittaker MH. The molecular biology of acute myeloid leukemia. Clin Lab Med 1990;10:769.
6. Fialkow PJ, Jacobson RJ, Papayannopoulou T. Chronic myelocytic leukemia: clonal origin in a stem cell common to the granulocyte erythrocyte platelet and monocyte/macrophage. Am J Med 1977;63;125.
7. Rous P. Transmission of a malignant new growth by means of a cell free infiltrate. JAMA 1911;56:198.
8. Baltimore D. RNA-dependent DNA polymerase in virions of TNA tumor viruses. Nature 1970;226:1209–1211.
9. Temin HM, Mizutani S. RNA-dependent DNA polymerase in Rous sarcoma virus. Nature 1970;226:1211–1213.
10. Poiesz BJ, Ruscetti FW, Gazdar AF, Bunn PA, Minna JD, Gallo RC. Detection and isolation of type C retrovirus particles from fresh and cultured lymphocytes of a patient with continuous T-cell lymphoma. Proc Natl Acad Sci USA 1980;77:7415–7419.
11. Norley SG, Kurth R. Retroviruses and malignant lymphoma. Blut 1989;58:221–227.
12. Miller DM, Blume S, Borst M, Gee J, Polansky D, Ray R, Rodu B, Shrestha K, Snyder R, Thomas S, Tran-Paterson R. Oncogenes malignant transformation and modern medicine. Am J Med Sci 1990;299:59–63.
13. Gutman A, Wasylyk B. Nuclear targets for transcription regulation by oncogenes. Trends Genet 1991;7:49.
14. Cline MJ. Oncogenes in hematologic neoplasia. Int J Cell Cloning 1989;7:213–222.
15. Butturini A, Sthivelman E, Canaani E, Gale RP. Oncogenes in human leukemias. Cancer Invest 1988;6:305–316.
16. Kluin PM, van Krieken JHHM. The molecular biology of B-cell lymphoma: clinico-pathologic implications. Hematology 1991;62:95–102.
17. Suzuki DT, Griffith AJF, Lewontin RC. An introduction to genetic analysis. San Francisco: WH Freeman, 1976.

18. Caspersson T, Gahrton G, Lindsten J, Zech L. Identification of the Philadelphia chromosome as a number 22 by quinacrine mustard fluorescence analysis. Exp Cell Res 1970;63: 238–240.

19. Rowley JD. A new consistent chromosomal abnormality in chronic myelogenous leukemia identified by quinacrine fluorescence and Giemsa staining. Nature 1973;243:290.

20. Cannistra SA. Chronic myelogenous leukemia as a model for the genetic basis of cancer. Hematol Oncol Clin N Am 1990; 4:337.

21. Baer MR, Bloomfield CA. Cytogenetics and oncogenes in leukemia. Curr Opin Oncol 1992;4:24–32.

22. Sheridan BL, Reis MD. Oncogene involvement in myelodysplasia and acute myeloid leukemia. Tumor Biol 1990;11: 44–58.

23. Kirsch IR. Molecular biology of the leukemias. Pediatr Clin N Am 1988;35:693.

24. Watson JD, Hopkins NH, Roberts JW. Molecular biology of the gene. 4th ed. Menlo Park, CA: Benjamin/Cummings, 1987.

25. Freifelder D. Molecular biology. 2nd ed. Boston: Jones and Bartlett, 1987.

26. Dean M, Vande Woude, GF. Principals of molecular cell biology of cancer: introduction to methods in molecular biology. In: DeVita VT, Hellman S, Rosenberg SA, eds. Cancer principles and practice of oncology. 3rd ed. Philadelphia: JB Lippincott, 1990:14–30.

27. Heisterkamp N, Groffen J, Stephenson JR. Chromosomal localization of human cellular homologues of two viral oncogenes. Nature 1982;299:747–749.

28. Dalla-Favera R, Gallo RC, Giallongo A, Croce CM. Chromosomal localization of the human homolog (c-sis) of the Simian sarcoma virus onc gene. Science 1982;218: 686–689.

29. Abelson HT, Rabstein LS. Lymphosarcoma: virus-induced thymic-independent disease in mice. Cancer Res 1970;30: 2213.

30. Konopka JB, Davis JL, Watanabe SM, et al. Only site-directed antibodies reactive with the highly conserved src-homologous region of the v-abl protein neutralize kinase activity. J Virol 1984;51:223.

31. Wang JYJ, Queen C, Baltimore D. Expression of an Abelson murine leukemia virus-encoded protein in *Escherichia coli* causes extensive phosphorylation of tyrosine residues. J Biol Chem 1982;257:13181.

32. Witte ON, Goff SP, Rosenberg N, et al. A transforming-defective mutant of Abelson murine leukemia virus lacks protein kinase activity. Proc Natl Acad Sci USA 1980; 77:4993.

33. Leibowitz D, Young KS. The molecular biology of CML: a review. Cancer Invest 1989;7:195–203.

34. Deuel TF, Huang JS, Huang SS, Stroobant P, Waterfield MD. Expression of a platelet-derived growth factor-like protein in simian sarcoma virus transformed cells. Science 1983;221:1348–1350.

35. Sambrook J, Fritsch EF, Maniatis T. Molecular cloning: a laboratory manual. 2nd ed. Cold Spring Harbor: Cold Spring Harbor Laboratory Press, 1989.

36. Southern EM. Detection of specific sequences among DNA fragments separated by gel electrophoresis. J Mol Biol 1975; 98:503.

37. Heisterkamp N, Groffen J, Stephenson NK. The human v-abl cellular homologue. J Mol Appl Genet 1983;12:57–68.

38. Heisterkamp N, Stephenson JR, Groffen J, Hansen PF. Localization of the c-abl oncogene adjacent to a translocation breakpoint in chronic myelocytic leukemia. Nature 1983; 306:239–242.

39. Leibowitz D, Schaefer-Rego K, Popenoe DW, et al. Variable breakpoints on the Philadelphia chromosome in chronic myelogenous leukemia. Blood 1985;66:243–245.

40. Epner DE, Koeffer HP. Molecular genetic advances in chronic myelogenous leukemia. Ann Intern Med 1990; 113:3.

41. Popenoe DW, Schaefer-Rego K, Mears JG, et al. Frequent and extensive deletion during the 9:22 translocation in CML. Blood 1986;68:1123–1128.

42. Heisterkamp N, Stam K, Groffen J, de Klein A, Grosveld G. Structural organization of the bcr gene and its role in the Ph translocation. Nature 1985;315:758–761.

43. Degos L. Retinoic acid in acute promyelocytic leukemia: a mode for differentiation therapy. Curr Opin Oncol 1992;2: 45–52.

44. Maxam AM, Gilbert W. A new method for sequencing DNA. Proc Natl Acad Sci USA 1977;74:560.

45. Sanger F, Nicklen S, Coulson AR. DNA sequencing with chain-terminating inhibitors. Proc Natl Acad Sci USA 1977; 74:5463.

46. Head DR, Downing JR. Pathology and immunology of leukemia. Curr Opin Oncol 1992;4:14–23.

47. Silver RT. Chronic myeloid leukemia. Curr Opin Oncol 1992;4:66–72.

48. Kantarjian HM, Kurzrock R, Talpaz M. Philadelphia chromosome-negative chronic myelogenous leukemia and chronic myelogenous leukemia. Hematol Oncol Clin N Am 1990;4:389.

49. Leibowitz D, Cubbon R, Bank A. Increased expression of a novel c-abl-related RNA in K562 cells. Blood 1985;65: 526–529.

50. Canaani E, Saltz D, Aghai E, Gale R. Altered transcription of an oncogene in chronic myeloid leukemia. Lancet 1984; 1:593.

51. Collins SJ, Kubonishi I, Miyoshi I, Groudine MT. Altered transcription of the c-abl oncogene in K562 and other chronic myelogenous leukemia cells. Science 1984;225: 72–75.

52. De The H, Chomienne C, Lanotte M, Degos L, Dejean A. The t(15;17) translocation of acute promyelocytic leukemia fuses the retinoic acid receptor alpha gene to a novel transcribed locus. Nature 1990;347:558–561.

53. Borrows T, Goddard AD, Sheer D, Solomon E. Molecular analysis of APL breakpoint cluster region on chromosome 17. Science 1990;249:1577–1580.

54. Longo L, Donti E, Mencarelli A, Avanzi G, Pegoraro L, Alimena G, Tabilio A, Venti G, Grignani F, Pelici PG. Mapping of chromosome 17 breakpoints in acute myeloid leukemia. Oncogene 1990;5:1557–1563.

55. Sefton BM, Hunter T, Cooper JA. Some lymphoid cell lines transformed by Abelson murine leukemia virus lack a major 36,000-dalton tyrosine protein kinase substrate. Mol Cell Biol 1983;3:56.

56. Konopka JB, Watanabe SM, Witte O. An alteration of the human c-abl protein in K562 leukemia cells unmasks associated tyrosine kinase activity. Cell 1984;37:1035.

57. Witte ON, Dasgupta A, Baltimore D. Abelson murine leukemia virus protein is phosphorylated in vitro to form phosphotyrosine. Nature 1980;283:826–831.

58. Pawson T. Non-catalytic domains of cytoplasmic protein-tyrosine kinases: regulatory elements in signal transduction. Oncogene 1988;3:491.

59. Prywes R, Foulkes JG, Baltimore D. The minimum transforming region of c-abl is the segment encoding protein-tyrosine kinase. J Virol 1985;54:114–122.

60. Konopka JB, Watanabe SM, Singer JW, et al. Cell lines and clinical isolates derived from Ph1-positive chronic myelogenous leukemia patients express c-abl proteins with a common structural alteration. Proc Natl Acad Sci USA 1985;82:1810–1816.

61. Ben-Neriah Y, Daley GQ, Mes-Masson AM, Witte ON, Baltimore D. The chronic myelogenous leukemia-specific P210 protein is the product of the bcr/abl hybrid gene. Science 1986;233:212.

62. Kloetzer W, Kurzrock R, Smith L, et al. The human cellular ABL gene product in the chronic myelogeous leukemia cell line K562 has an associated tyrosine kinase activity. Virology 1985;140:230–238.

63. Clark SC, McLaughlin J, Crist WM. Unique forms of the abl tyrosine kinase distinguish PH_1-positive CML from Ph1-positive ALL. Science 1987;235:85.

64. Davis RL, Konopka JB, Witte ON. Activation of the c-abl oncogene by viral transduction or chromosomal translocation generates altered c-abl proteins with similar in vitro kinase properties. Mol Cell Biol 1985;5:204.

65. Clark SS, McLaughlin J, Timmons M, et al. Expression of a distinctive BCR-ABL oncogene in Ph1-positive acute lymphocytic leukemia (ALL). Science 1988;239:775.

66. Kurzrock R, Shtalrid M, Romero R, et al. A novel c-abl protein product in Philadelphia-positive acute lymphoblastic leukemia. Nature 1987;325:631–635.

67. Chomienne C, Ballerini P, Balitrand N, Huang ME, Krawice I, Castaigne S, Fenaux P, Tiollasi P, Dejean A, Degos L, De The H. The retinoic acid receptor alpha gene is rearranged in retinoic acid sensitive promyelocytic leukemia. Leukemia 1990;4:802–807.

68. De The H, Lavau C, Marchio A, Chomienne C, Degos L, Dejean A. The PLM-RARα fusion mRNA generated by the t(15;17) translocation in acute promyelocytic leukemia encodes a functionally altered RAR. Cell 1991;66:675–684.

69. Kelliher MA, McLaughlin J, Witte ON, Rosenberg N. Induction of a chronic myelogenous leukemia-like syndrome in mice with v-abl and BCR/ABL. Proc Natl Acad Sci USA 1090;87:6649–6653.

70. Daley GQ, Van Etten RA, Baltimore D. Induction of chronic myelogenous leukemia in mice by the P210[bcr/abl]

71. Heisterkamp N, Jenster G, Ten Hoeve J, Zovich D, Pattengale PK, Groffen J. Acute leukemia in bcr/abl transgenic mice. Nature 1990;344:251–253.

72. Van Etten RA. Distinct effect of expression of the all-specific form of bcr/abl P190[bcr/abl] in murine bone marrow. Blood 1991;78:304.

73. Berns A, Breuer M, Verbeek S, van Lohuizen M. Transgenic mice as a means to study synergism between oncogenes. Int J Cancer 1989;4:22–25.

74. Adams JM, Harris AW, Pinkert CA, Corcoran LM, Alexander WS, Cory S, Palmiter RD, Brinster RL. The c-myc oncogene driven by immunoglobulin enhancers induces lymphoid malignancy in transgenic mice. Nature 1985;318:533–538.

75. Cory S, Adams JM. Transgenic mice and oncogenesis. Ann Rev Immunol 1988;6:25–48.

76. Greenberger JS. Ras mutations in human leukemia and related disorders. Int J Cell Cloning 1989;7:343–359.

77. Juliusson G, Gahrton G. Chromosome aberrations in B-cell chronic lymphocytic leukemia. Cancer Genet Cytogenet 1990;45:143–160.

78. List AF, Garewal HS, Sandberg AA. The myelodysplastic syndromes: biology and implications for management. J Clin Oncol 1990;8:1424–1441.

79. Huang ME, Ye YC, Chai JR, Lu JX, Zhoa L, Gu LJ, Wang ZY. Use of trans retinoic acid in the treatment of acute promyelocytic leukemia. Blood 1988;72:567–572.

80. Castaigne S, Chomienne C, Daniel MT, Ballerini P, Berger R, Fenaux P, Degos L. All trans retinoic acid as a differentiation therapy for acute promyelocytic leukemia. Blood 1990;76:1704–1709.

81. Degos L, Chomienne C, Daniel MT, Berger R, Dombret H, Fenaux P, Castaigne S. Treatment of first relapse in acute promyelocytic leukemia with all trans retinoic acid. Lancet 1990;336:1140–1141.

82. Warrel RM, Frankle SR, Miller WH, Scheinberg DA, Itri LM, Hittleman WN, Vyas R, Andreef M, Tafuri A, Jakuboswki A, Gabrilove J, Gordon MS, Dimitrovsky E. Differentiation therapy of acute promyelocytic leukemia with tretinoin (All trans retinoic acid). New Engl J Med 1991;324:1385–1393.

83. Reynolds T. First antisense drug trials planned in leukemia news. J Natl Cancer Inst 1992;84:288–290.

CHAPTER 16

Hodgkin Lymphoma

NICHOLAS DAINIAK, DAVID TUCK, WILLIAM T. PASTUSZAK

Hodgkin's paper 'On Some Morbid Appearances of the Absorbent Glands and Spleen' was read on January 10 and 24, 1832, before the Medical and Chirurgical Society and was published in its *Transactions*. Inasmuch as Hodgkin was not then a member of the society, his paper was read by the secretary, Robert Lee, M.D., F.R.S.
—Lee, *Transactions* (1832)

Introduction

Perhaps in no other disease has the integration of clinical acumen, histopathologic diagnosis, and (more recently) molecular biology tools been required to a greater extent for diagnosis and management than in Hodgkin lymphoma. Since approximately three-quarters of all patients with Hodgkin disease are curable in the 1990s, it is incumbent upon the physician to make the diagnosis quickly, assign the appropriate stage of disease, and select the most appropriate form of therapy. In this chapter, cases are selected that illustrate the many facets of a disease that has been recognized by physicians for over 150 years. The cases include early stage disease with good prognosis (case 1), advanced stage disease presenting with splenic involvement (case 2), and massive mediastinal disease of advanced stage that is refractory to traditional therapy (case 3).

Early Stage Disease

In nearly all instances, Hodgkin lymphoma arises in lymph nodes. Moreover, distinct from nodes involved with metastatic carcinoma (which are hard and fixed to underlying tissue), lymph nodes involved with lymphomas are often rubbery, firm, and matted together. In contrast to inflamed lymph nodes, nodes involved with lymphomas are nontender and of normal temperature. Hodgkin disease is believed to have a unifocal origin and to spread stepwise from one group of nodes to contiguous lymph node groups. The extent or stage of Hodgkin disease depends upon the number of lymph node regions and anatomical sites involved with disease. Recently, a new staging system, the Cotswolds staging classification (derived from an international meeting of lymphoma experts in the Cotswolds, United Kingdom), has been introduced that includes the use of computerized tomography (CT) as a staging tool (see table 16.1). Involvement of a single lymph node region or two or more regions on the same side of the diaphragm (stage I and II, respectively) is referred to as "early stage" disease. The following case illustrates a typical presentation of early stage Hodgkin disease.

Case 1

An 18-year-old Caucasian girl presented with a lump in the neck that was incidentally found by her mother while she dressed for a formal gathering. There was no history of fever, drenching night sweats, weight loss, or early satiety. Specifically, the patient denied recent sore throat, rash, weakness, malaise, or myalgias. Physical examination disclosed a rubbery mat of nontender right anterior cervical lymph nodes measuring 1×3 cm. There were no other enlarged lymph nodes in the neck or in the axillary, epitrochlear, inguinal, or popliteal areas. There was no splenomegaly by direct palpation of the patient in the supine or the right lateral decubitus positions, and dullness was not appreciated beneath the left upper quadrant. The physical examination was otherwise unremarkable.

Laboratory studies revealed a normal hematocrit of 41%, a normal platelet count of $260 \times 10^9/L$, and a normal white blood cell (WBC) count of $7 \times 10^9/L$. The WBC differential was unremarkable. Serum calcium and albumin levels, liver, and renal function tests were normal, while the erythrocyte sedimentation rate (ESR) was elevated at 35 mm/hr. A chest X-ray appeared normal and CT scan of the abdomen revealed no masses, enlarged lymph nodes, or splenomegaly. Bipedal lymphangiography revealed no abnormalities in lymph node size or architecture. Bilateral iliac crest bone marrow aspiration and biopsy specimens showed no evidence of disease.

The mat of lymph nodes was excised and on histology found to contain occasional Reed-Sternberg cells in a background pattern of dense interconnecting bands of sclerosing fibrous tissue (fig. 1A and B). Based upon the histopathologic diagnosis of Hodgkin disease, nodular sclerosing type, and the "negative" hematologic, biochemical, and radiologic workup, the patient was administered pneumococcal capsular polysaccharide vaccine and exploratory laparotomy with splenectomy performed. No evidence of intraabdominal disease was found. The patient was defined as having pathologic stage I-A disease, and radiation therapy was administered to

Table 16.1. The Cotswolds Staging Classification of Hodgkin Lymphoma*

Stage I. Involvement of single lymph node region or lymphoid structure (e.g., spleen, thymus, Waldeyer ring)

Stage II. Involvement of two or more lymph node regions on same side of the diaphragm (mediastinum is a single site, hilar lymph nodes are lateralized). Number of anatomical sites indicated by a suffix (e.g., II_3)

Stage III. Involvement of lymph node regions or structures on both sides of diaphragm

III_1. with or without splenic hilar, celiac, or portal nodes

III_2 with para-aortic, iliac, mesenteric nodes

Stage IV. Involvement of extranodal site(s) beyond the designated "E"

   A. Asymptomatic

   B. Symptomatic (fever, drenching, sweats, weight loss)

   X. Bulky disease

      $>\frac{1}{3}$ widening of mediastinum

      >10 cm maximum dimension of nodal mass

   E. Involvement of a single extranodal site, contiguous or proximal to known nodal site

  CS. Clinical stage

  PS. Pathologic stage

*Adapted from Lister and Crowther. Semin Oncol 1990;17:696, with the permission of the publisher.

the mantle area of the body, limiting the mediastinal dose to 3000 Gy.

Pathology

Despite its original description in 1832 (1), the etiology of Hodgkin disease and the nature of its characteristic cell, the Reed-Sternberg (RS) cell, remain controversial (2, 3). Although it has been argued that RS cells proliferate as part of an infectious or inflammatory process, recent cytogenetic and molecular genetic studies indicate their growth to be a clonal, neoplastic process (4, 5). RS cells are considered to be the neoplastic cells. However, RS cells are apparently "end-stage" cells (6, 7), while small, less obvious mononuclear cells may provide the proliferating clone (8).

Morphologically diagnostic RS cells have eosinophilic inclusion-like nucleoli in two or more nuclear lobes (fig. 1B). A binucleated, mirror-image "owl eye" appearance is the hallmark of the "classic" RS cell. Single and multinucleated variants of the RS cell generally have a nuclear halo due to chromatin condensed around the nuclear membrane. The cytoplasm is abundant with eosinophilicto-amphophilic staining.

The diagnosis of Hodgkin disease (HD) requires identification of diagnostic RS cells in an appropriate histopathologic background associated with a recognized subtype or variety (9). RS-like cells may appear in other disorders, including viral illnesses (10), non-Hodgkin lymphomas, benign lymphadenopathies, and tumors of epithelial and soft tissue origin (11). Because of the lack of distinguishing features, diagnostic confirmation by an experienced hematopathologist may be required. In particular, confusion may occur between the diagnosis of non-Hodgkin lymphomas and Hodgkin disease (11). Every case of suspected Hodgkin or non-Hodgkin lymphoma (NHL) should have fresh and/or frozen tissue reserved for possible performance of immunopathologic studies (flow cytometry or tissue immunopathology) and/or molecular genetic studies (DNA hybridization for clonal T or B cell gene rearrangements). Such studies may provide a definitive diagnosis in cases lacking distinguishing morphologic features (12–14).

The histopathologic classification of HD used today is based on the original proposal by Lukes et al. (15). This classification was modified at the Rye conference (16) when the original six categories were reduced to four categories. A relationship between survival, clinical stage, and histopathologic subtype is well documented (15). The four categories include: nodular sclerosis (NS), lymphocyte predominant (LP), mixed cellularity (MC), and lymphocyte depletion (LD) (17). The last three subtypes differ largely in the numbers of RS cells versus lymphocytes, with LP having the lowest frequency of RS cells and greatest number of small lymphocytes in the background, and LD having the reverse of these relative numbers. MC Hodgkin disease is intermediate and more commonly accompanied by a polymorphous background of cellular elements.

The cellular background of Hodgkin lymphoma is almost unique in neoplastic processes, leading to earlier considerations of an infectious or inflammatory nature. The bulk of lymphoid tissue is reactive and not neoplastic, since RS cells and variants comprise only 1–35% and may be as little as 0.03% of the total cells (18, 19). **LP Hodgkin disease** contains numerous small lymphocytes in the background. Occasional epithelioid histiocytes with abundant pale staining cytoplasm may be scattered about or in clusters, resulting in granuloma formation. The characteristic RS cell variant in LP Hodgkin disease is a large cell with a moderate amount of pale cytoplasm, a lobulated nucleus resembling popped popcorn, and a generally small nucleolus. These cells were termed L&H variants (lymphocytic and histiocytic) by Lukes and co-workers (15). Classic RS cells in LP are exceedingly rare and may require numerous paraffin block sections. **MC Hodgkin disease** has more readily apparent classic RS cells and a background of small lymphocytes, eosinophils, plasmacytes, epithelioid histiocytes that occasionally form granulomas, and fibrosis.

LD Hodgkin has bizarre, pleomorphic multinucleated RS cells in a background with diminished lymphocytes and increased fibrosis.

The **NS Hodgkin variety** constitutes 40–60% of cases (20, 21), and typically presents as a disease of supraclavicular lymph nodes and mediastinum in adolescent and young adult females. Our case illustrates typical NS Hodgkin lymphoma in a young girl. It appears to be separate from the other subtypes which are more interrelated

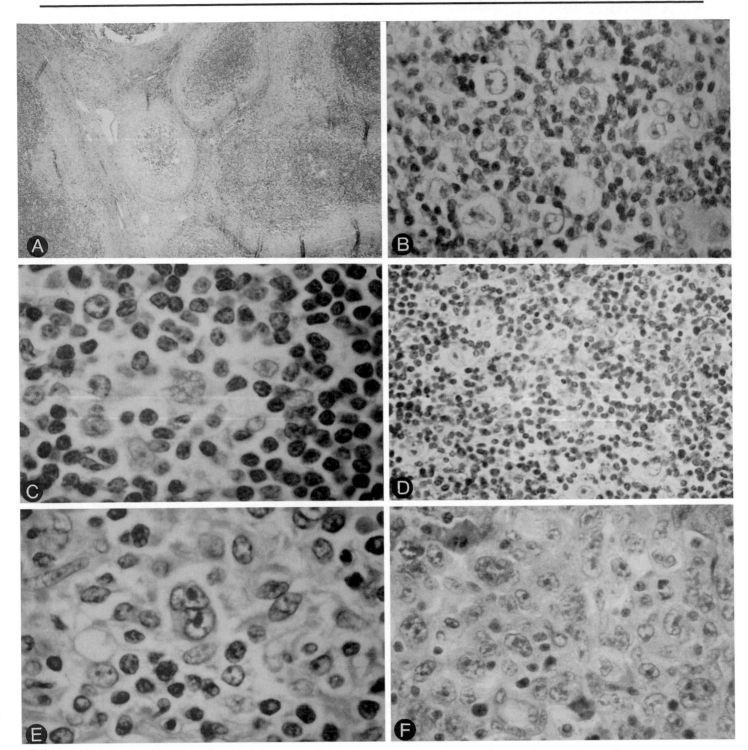

Figure 16.1. Photomicrographs of nodal tissue. Case 1. **A.** Low-power micrograph of nodular sclerosing Hodgkin disease; **B.** lacunar cells in nodular sclerosis; **C.** Popcorn LS cell variant.

Case 2. **D.** Mixed cellularity Hodgkin disease; **E.** Classic Reed-Sternberg cell in mixed cellularity Hodgkin disease. Case 3. **F.** Lymphocyte depletion Hodgkin disease.

and may undergo histologic progression to the LD variety. In NS Hodgkin disease, RS variants are found within nodules that are formed by deposition of dense interconnecting bands of birefringent, sclerosing fibrous tissue. Lacunar RS variants may be present which have abundant cytoplasm that has retracted during fixation, leaving large lacunar spaces around the nuclei. Lacunar cells have relatively small nucleoli in comparison to diagnostic RS cells.

Although lacunar cells may have many nuclear lobes, only an occasional lacunar cell has features of a diagnostic RS cell.

Sclerosis in NS Hodgkin disease is variable, and may present a problem for diagnosis and subclassification since early interfollicular disease with only lacunar cells may be diagnosed as reactive hyperplasia or possibly MC Hodgkin. This cellular phase of NS Hodgkin (9, 22) appears to be part of the spectrum of the disease, and may be due to sampling variability, or to degree of involvement within a lymph node. Progression to the sclerotic phase may be observed in simultaneous or subsequent biopsies (23). Recognition of the cellular phase of NS Hodgkin and potential confusion with other forms has lead to the requirement that the appropriate RS variant and background (lacunar cells and band-like sclerosis in NS Hodgkin) be identified (9).

Recently, RS cells have been found to be a source of lymphokines. Sclerosis in NS Hodgkin may be explained by induction of collagen synthesis by transforming growth factor-β that is secreted by RS cells (24). Other histologic subtypes may develop in response to lymphokine secretion by RS cells as well (25, 26), thereby explaining the unusual polymorphous cellular composition (i.e., necrosis, granulomas, and eosinophilia) that typifies the disease. Release of interleukin-5 (IL-5) from RS cells may stimulate eosinophil progenitor cell growth and contribute to generalized eosinophilia that is commonly found in Hodgkin lymphoma (27).

A potential diagnostic problem can be differentiating in NS Hodgkin from a syncytial variant of Hodgkin described by Strickler et al. (28). Cohesive sheets of lacunar cells may partially or totally replace nodal architecture and surround large necrotic foci, causing misdiagnoses such as carcinoma, melanoma, or large cell, non-Hodgkin lymphoma (28). Many cases of LD Hodgkin may actually be syncytial variants of NS Hodgkin. Immunopathology and examination of nodal tissue for rearrangement of immunoglobulin and T-cell receptor genes may be required for distinction from NHL.

Nodular sclerosis is distinct from other forms of Hodgkin disease not only with respect to its histologic appearance with lacunar cells and bands of sclerosis but also in the relative frequency of RS variants and lymphocytes. It has been proposed that NS Hodgkin be subcategorized (based on the numbers of RS cells) into lymphocyte predominant, mixed cellularity, and lymphocyte depletion subtypes (29). The last subtype is recognized as being clinically aggressive (29). It has been suggested that the presence of abundant RS cells may auger for a poor prognosis (30). NS Hodgkin has been also subclassified into grades I and II (based upon the appearance of LD areas in grade II disease) by the British National Lymphoma Investigation. Approximately 30% of cases fall into the grade II variety that is associated with a poor prognosis (30, 31).

NS Hodgkin has a predilection for the mediastinum, and generally presents as early stage disease with a good prognosis. **LP Hodgkin** generally presents as stage I disease in the neck or inguinal region, and is associated with a very good outcome as well. By contrast, advanced stage disease and poor prognosis are associated with LD Hodgkin, which often presents with abdominal and bone marrow involvement. MC Hodgkin has an intermediate prognosis, and may present with mediastinal or abdominal involvement.

Commentary

Hodgkin disease has a bimodal, age-specific incidence rate in the United States and, except for Japan, in other developed countries. One mode occurs at ages 15–35 years, while the other occurs above the age of 50 years. As exemplified in our young patient, the NS variety of Hodgkin disease has a disproportionate number of patients in the first modal peak. By contrast, Hodgkin disease in underdeveloped countries frequently occurs in children <10 years of age, where it often presents in the histologic varieties and in stages of more advanced disease (i.e., stage III and IV disease of the MC and LD varieties) (32–34). Reasons for these differences, including the lack of the "first peak" in Japan, are unexplained.

Case clustering and multiple cases in a single household have been described (35), suggesting a viral etiology. The Epstein-Barr virus (EBV) has been implicated in some cases and EBV genomes have been detected in DNA from up to 80% of tumor specimens (36, 37). Interestingly, EBV nucleic acids can be localized to RS cells and RS variants by in situ hybridization (38). Figure 16.2 shows strong EBV genome labeling of RS cells and variants in a patient with NS Hodgkin disease. Nevertheless, our patient illustrates the typical history of having had no preceding viral-like illness. Although chromosomal abnormalities of freshly isolated lymph node cells may be found in as many as one-half of the cases (39), specific cytogenetic abnormalities have not been associated with Hodgkin disease. It has been recently recognized that wood workers have an increased risk for developing Hodgkin disease. Accordingly, it is possible that Hodgkin disease represents a common pathologic response to a variety of environmental stimuli, including viruses (40).

Since our patient lacked symptoms of fever, drenching sweats, and weight loss, she is classified as having "A" disease. By combining normal plain chest radiography with this history and physical examination, nearly 90% of patients may be classified as having early stage disease (40). Adding bipedal lymphangiography will place approximately one-third of these patients into a higher stage. Today, most clinicians utilize CT scanning for staging as well, particularly to detect enlarged mediastinal and retroperitoneal lymph nodes (41). However, CT scanning of the thorax has limited utility, unless the plain chest radiograph is abnormal. Since lymphangiography detects not only size but also architecture (i.e., filling defects or "foamy" appearance of lymph nodes), many clinicians utilize the lymphangiogram (rather than the CT) as the most definitive test for disease, short of laparotomy (42, 43). Sensitivity of lymphangiography is approximately double that of CT scanning (85–98% vs 40–65% "true" positive results). In particular, lymphangiography is more sensitive than CT in detecting lower abdominal lymphadenopathy (44). In contrast to these radiologic procedures, gallium scanning is most useful in determining the presence or absence of residual mediastinal disease following the completion of therapy (45).

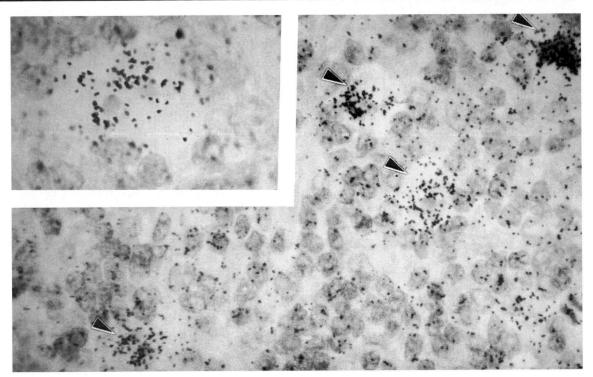

Figure 16.2 In situ hybridization for Epstein-Barre virus (EBV) nucleic acids in a patient with nodular sclerosing Hodgkin disease. Strong labeling of Reed-Sternberg variants and of a diagnostic RS cell (insert) is shown for formalin-fixed tissue embedded in paraffin and reacted with the Bam HI-W fragment of EBV DNA that had been radio-labeled with [^{35}S]-α-deoxycytidine triphosphate. Reproduced from Weiss et al. (N Engl J Med, 1989; 320:502), with the permission of the publisher.

The role of staging laparotomy has diminished over the last 10 years (46). This is due largely to acute surgical morbidity and the risk of serious infection (47). Overwhelming bacteremia due to encapsulated bacteria may occur following staging splenectomy, particularly in children. Since a normal antibody response to bacterial polysaccharides is observed in patients with pretreatment Hodgkin disease (48), administration of 14-valent pneumococcal vaccine is required prior to laparotomy. If radiation therapy is contemplated to treat early stage disease, it is incumbent upon the clinician to exclude stage III disease, which often requires chemotherapy. Furthermore, surgical staging accompanied by splenectomy may lessen the need for chemotherapy in early stage disease and permit smaller volumes of tissue to be irradiated. Therefore, in this patient, staging laparotomy was appropriate. It has been argued, nevertheless, that occasional very favorable presentations of early stage disease (i.e., clinical stage IA LP Hodgkin disease limited to the high neck) may be treated with radiotherapy without prior staging laparotomy (49, 50).

The liver is only rarely involved, when the spleen is not involved with disease. Patients with MC and LD Hodgkin have a higher likelihood of liver involvement. Approximately one-third of all patients with early stage disease will be placed into a higher stage after laparotomy (including one-half of patients with B symptoms and one-fourth of asymptomatic patients). Table 16.2 summarizes procedures that are recommended for staging Hodgkin disease.

Management of early stage disease varies, depending upon the risks and complications of therapy and the relative concerns of the patient. In the above case, radiation therapy administered to the mantle field (including the cervical, supraclavicular, axillary, infraclavicular, mediastinal, and pulmonary hilar lymph nodes) is considered standard therapy. The classic irradiation field for early stage subdiaphragmatic disease (that occurs in approximately 10% of patients with early stage disease) is the inverted-Y which includes paraaortic, splenic hilar, common and external iliac, and inguinal-femoral lymph nodes. Whereas extended-field radiotherapy that includes mantle and paraaortic fields is used routinely to treat supradiaphragmatic disease, the use of prophylactic subdiaphragmatic therapy to treat all patients with early stage disease is controversial.

Overall survival of approximately 90% and relapse-free survival of 75–80% after 10 years can be expected in patients such as the one described in case 1 (52, 53). At some university medical centers, paraaortic/splenic pedicle field radiotherapy may be also administered. However, it is unknown whether the addition of paraaortic field to mantle field therapy adds significantly to the long-term therapeutic outcome. It is important to remember that because recurrence rates may vary among different radiotherapy centers (for example, from 0–11% among patients with identical stage disease) (54), every clinician must know and

Table 16.2. Diagnostic Procedures for Staging Hodgkin Disease[*]

Radiologic procedures
    Plain chest radiography
    CT of thorax (unless chest film is normal)
    CT of abdomen and pelvis
    Bipedal lymphogiography
Hematologic procedures
    Complete blood count with differential WBC count
    ESR
    Bilateral bone marrow aspiration and biopsy
Biochemical procedures
    Liver function tests
    Serum albumin, lactate dehydrogenase, & calcium measurements
Procedures for use under special circumstances
    Laparotomy
    Ultrasound scanning
    MRI
    Gallium scanning
    Technetium bone scanning
    Liver-spleen scanning

[*]Adapted from Urba and Longo. N Engl J Med 1992;326:678, with permission of the publisher.
Abbreviations: CT, computerized tomography; ESR, erythrocyte sedimentation rate; MRI, magnetic resonance imaging; WBC, white blood cell.

understand the strengths and success rates of the local radiotherapy service.

While radiation therapy alone is the preferred treatment of stage IA disease, the risk for late second solid tumors must be recognized. Such tumors often occur in the second or third decade following therapy (55). There may be an even greater risk of second malignancy when radiation therapy is combined with chemotherapy (see Commentary, Advanced Stage Disease). Other potential complications of radiation therapy include skin reactions, hair loss in irradiated sites, dysphagia, dry cough, and nausea. Subclinical hypothyroidism may occur in one-third of patients receiving mantle irradiation and herpes zoster may occur in up to one-fifth of patients (51). For patients in whom reproductive potential is a major concern, the clinician must be aware that permanent azoospermia may complicate pelvic irradiation, unless the testes are shielded (56). Ovarian function in women over the age of 30 years can be affected from irradiation scattered from pelvic fields, although this is infrequently seen in younger women (57). Finally, mild radiation pneumonitis, chronic restrictive pulmonary fibrosis, and radiation carditis may occur in <5% of patients receiving mantle field therapy (51). The latter complications are related to dosage, rate, and volume of tissue irradiated (58).

Combined radiation therapy and chemotherapy has been used to treat early stage Hodgkin disease with results comparable to radiation alone (59). Recently, the combination of chemotherapy (using vinblastine, bleomycin, and methotrexate) together with radiation therapy has been used to treat patients with clinical stage IIB disease (60).

These patients are considered poor candidates for radiation therapy alone, since they have a high risk for both the presence of intrabdominal disease and relapse. Combined modality therapy has not been demonstrated to be superior to chemotherapy alone in stage IIB disease. Therefore, chemotherapy alone may be a good choice for some persons with clinical stage IIB disease (41).

Advanced Stage Disease

Involvement of Hodgkin disease in lymph node regions on either side of the diaphragm (stage III) and/or involvement of extranodal site(s) beyond that defined as "contiguous" (stage IV) is referred to as "advanced stage" Hodgkin lymphoma. As reviewed in table 16.1, the Cotswolds staging classification takes into account both tumor bulk (by adding the suffix X to patients having massive mediastinal disease or nodal masses >10 cm diameter), and location (upper vs lower lymphatics) of involved nodal sites within the abdomen. The following case illustrates several critical diagnostic and management issues in a patient with stage IIIA disease.

Case 2

A 25-year-old African-American man presented with left cervical and supraclavicular adenopathy of 2 months duration. According to the patient, the masses had waxed and waned during this interval. He denied recent weight loss, fever, drenching night sweats, pruritis, or alcohol-induced pain in the areas of adenopathy. On physical examination, firm, rubbery lymph nodes measuring 1–3 cm in size were palpable in the left anterior cervical chain, and in the left and right axillae. Abdominal examination revealed a spleen tip that was palpable 3 cm below the left costal margin. The remainder of the examination was unremarkable.

Laboratory studies revealed a hematocrit of 42%, platelets of 285×10^9/L, and WBC of 6×10^9/L with a normal differential. The ESR was elevated at 65 mm/hr. Uric acid and alkaline phosphatase levels were normal, while the lactate dehydrogenase was elevated at 620 U/L. Other tests of renal and liver function were normal, as were serum calcium and albumin levels.

The chest x-ray revealed an anterior mediastinal mass measuring slightly less than one-third of the diameter of the chest. A cervical lymph node biopsy was performed, a photomicrograph of which is shown in figure 1C. Microscopic review of the lymph node sections raised a differential diagnosis of mixed cellularity Hodgkin disease versus peripheral T-cell lymphoma.

Scattered RS-like cells were present in a background of small lymphocytes, eosinophils, plasma cells, histiocytes and areas of fibrosis. Immunopathologic analysis of the lymph node was requested (see Pathology section, this case 2).

CT scanning of the chest revealed mild bilateral hilar adenopathy in addition to the anterior mediastinal mass. Abdominal CT scanning revealed celiac lymph node en-

largement and splenomegaly with three identifiable splenic nodules. Bipedal lymphangiography revealed no abnormalities in the size or texture of the lower abdominal lymph nodes. Bilateral iliac crest bone marrow biopsies were completely normal.

The patient was defined as having clinical stage IIIA₁ Hodgkin lymphoma, mixed cellularity type. He was treated with six cycles of chemotherapy (doxorubicin, bleomycin, vinblastine, and dacarbazine), followed by involved field irradiation of the chest, and splenic pedicle.

Pathology

Histopathologic examination of the lymph node biopsy in this case was inconclusive in differentiating Hodgkin from non-Hodgkin lymphoma. Diagnostic RS cells were not apparent, while the polymorphous background of cellular elements with scattered atypical large mononuclear cells is a morphologic picture that is compatible with either entity, and may be a source of confusion with other lymphoid proliferations as well (10, 11, 61–63). Immunopathology and molecular genetics techniques may aid in the exclusion of morphologically overlapping entities.

A suspension of the lymph node cells was prepared and processed by flow cytometry. A predominant T cell population with a phenotype of CD2, CD3, CD4, CD5, CD7, and a small B-cell population expressing polyclonal immunoglobulin were evident by this analysis. Immunoperoxidase studies of nodal cells fixed in paraffin revealed the larger, mononuclear RS-like cells to have a phenotype of CD30+, CD15+, CD45−, L26−, and CD3 weak+. DNA hybridization and Southern blot analysis of nodal lymphocytes revealed no clonal T-cell receptor or B-cell (immunoglobulin) gene rearrangments in the Bam HI, Hind II, or Eco RI digestions, using probes to the constant region of the β-chain of the T-cell receptor complex (CTB) and the joining region of the immunoglobulin heavy chain (JH). Based on these studies, the diagnosis of Hodgkin disease was made.

Flow cytometry in this case revealed that the cells were predominantly T-cells with a phenotype of T helper cells without aberrant antigen expression (CD2, CD3, CD4, CD5, CD7). In addition, a small polyclonal B-cell population was also present. One should realize that RS cells are generally below the level of detection by flow cytometry. Moreover, there is no phenotype absolutely specific for RS cells (see Pathology section, case 1). Figure 16.3 shows the results of flow analysis of nodal cells from a patient with lymphoma. Typically, flow analysis is compatible with but not diagnostic of Hodgkin disease (63, 64). The absence of aberrant expression of T-cell antigens (loss of pan T-cell markers or an unusual phenotype for mature T-cells such as coexpression of CD4 and CD8) helps the histopathologist to exclude a T-cell lymphoproliferative disorder. Polyclonal expression of immunoglobulins mitigates against the diagnosis of a B-cell disorder, although a T-cell rich, B-cell neoplasm cannot be completely excluded.

Frozen section immunoperoxidase studies help to exclude the same NHL considerations that are discussed for

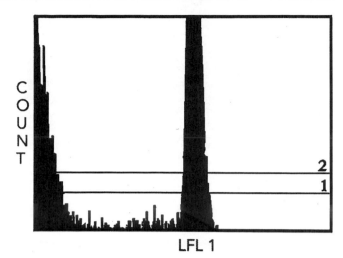

	MIN	MAX	PERCENT	MEAN
1	0.158	1023	62.0	6.164
2	0.302	1023	54.2	10.200

Figure 16.3. Typical flow analysis of nodal cells from a patient with mixed cellularity Hodgin lymphoma. The majority of lymphocytes are T helper cells on this CD4 histogram obtained using an EPICS profile analyzer.

flow cytometry but are of limited value in firmly establishing the diagnosis of HD. Again, due to their low frequency, RS cells are rarely identified in frozen tissue by this approach. The RS cell-associated lymphocyte activation marker, ki-l (CD30), and the granulocyte marker, Leu-M1 (CD15), can be readily identified in paraffin tissue. Thus, paraffin section immunopathology may provide valuable information regarding the phenotype of individual cells, and may be most helpful in establishing the diagnosis of HD when used in concert with analysis of fresh or frozen tissue. The paraffin tissue immunophenotype in the large cells in this case (CD30+, CD15+, CD45−, CD3) is compatible with HD but is not exclusive of a T-cell neoplasm.

A monoclonal antibody (designated CD30) has been developed to RS cell lines (65–67) that reacts with a 120-kd glycoprotein (Ki-l, Ber-H2, HRS-2, HcFi). However, this antibody reacts with activated lymphoid cells as well. Since CD30-positive cells also mark with other lymphocyte activation markers (HLA-Dr, CD25/IL-2, transferrin receptor), it is possible that RS cells represent a form of activated lymphocytes (68). It is unknown whether RS cell activation occurs prior to (i.e., a primary event) or following (i.e., a secondary event or epiphenomenon) the critical intracellular event that results in the transformation of a normal cell into a neoplastic cell. RS cells do not react with monoclonal antibodies to interdigitating reticulum cells, monocytes, or histocytes and, conversely, the latter cell types do not react with CD30 (69–72). Accordingly, suggestions that RS cells are of interdigitating reticulum cell origin or monocytic/histcytic origin appear to be unlikely (73, 74).

Kadin et al. (75) and Agnarsson and Kadin (76) demonstrated T-cell and/or B-cell antigens on the nodal lymphocytes from patients having nodular sclerosis (55%) and mixed cellularity (80%) Hodgkin disease. LP Hodgkin disease of the "nodular" subtype appears to be a B-cell disease, related to follicular centers (77, 78). It is also associated with progressive transformation of germinal centers in which secondary follicles become expanded by infiltration of the mantle zone with small lymphocytes (79–82). The "popcorn" RS variants in LPHD express B-cell antigens (83, 84) and sometimes express membrane or cytoplasmic monotypic immunoglobulin (85, 86). LP Hodgkin of the "diffuse" subtype may actually overlap with nodular LPHD since the use of CD20 (L26 in paraffin) and other B-cell markers reveals a diffuse rather than nodular distribution of cells (84, 85).

It has been speculated that LP Hodgkin is a B-cell disorder. This is supported by the immunophenotypic profile of LP Hodgkin, the relationship to germinal centers and progressive transformation of follicles and the association of LP Hodgkin with concurrent or subsequent B-cell non-Hodgkin lymphoma (86–89). Reports that bcl-2 can be identified in DNA amplified from nodal cells by the polymerase chain reaction and its association with t(14;18) in follicular lymphomas, have raised the possibility that Hodgkin disease is a follicular lymphoma variant (90, 91). However, cases of non-LP Hodgkin generally appear to be CD30+, CD15+, and CD45 (83), and by routine preparations do not express T- or B-cell surface antigens. Using more specialized techniques, one can variably demonstrate T-cell antigens (92–94), while B-cell antigens can be demonstrated in only 10% or less of non-LP Hodgkin

lymph node cells (92, 94). Therefore, it is possible that LP Hodgkin is a B-cell-related disorder, while non-LP Hodgkin is variably a T- cell or B-cell disorder.

In this case, the paraffin immunophenotype is compatible with HD. Additional testing for gene rearrangements may be used to confirm this diagnosis with greater certainty. T-cell and B-cell gene arrangements (TgR/BgR) characterize NHL. By contrast, routine DNA hybridization with Southern blot techniques fails to demonstrate diagnostic gene rearrangements in Hodgkin disease (12, 13). In this case, clonal TgR and BgR were absent, supporting the diagnosis of MC Hodgkin over a T-cell NHL.

Although the presence of immunoglobulin and T-cell receptor gene rearrangements has been suggested to support a lymphoid origin for RS cells (95–98), difficulty in obtaining and analyzing "pure" RS cell populations, and interference by "contaminating" lymphocytes make interpretation of these results difficult (95–96). Most HD cases do not show clonal gene rearrangements of the β-chain of the T-cell receptor complex. Faint bands may be visualized on Southern blots in <20% of HD cases (13, 19, 96–101). Therefore, while some information may be suggestive of a T- or B-cell nature for RS cells, a final conclusion remains to be established.

Commentary

As illustrated in this case, Hodgkin disease may occur in blacks as well as whites (approximately 10% of Hodgkin patients are African American). It frequently presents as disease in the chest (fig. 16.4). Whereas its frequency of in-

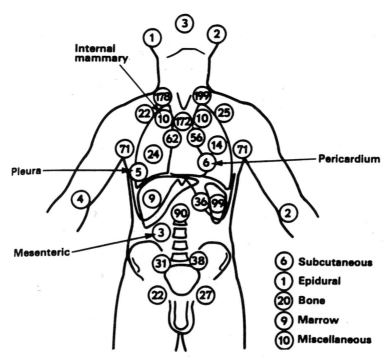

Figure 16.4. Anatomic sites of involvement of Hodgkin disease. Results of the cases of 285 unselected, consecutive patients from Stanford University who underwent routine laparotomy are shown. Reproduced from VT DeVita et al.

(Hodgkin's disease and the non-Hodgkin's lymphomas. In: Cancer: Principles and practice of oncology, Philadelphia: JB Lippincott, 1985, p. 1653) with the permission of the publisher.

volvement of epitrochlear and popliteal lymph nodes, the tonsil and Waldeyer ring are very low, involvement of the spleen is a common site of intra-abdominal disease (fig. 16.4). Often, disease below the diaphragm is unsuspected on physical examination. In this case, splenomegaly was detectable, suggesting that stage III disease was present. Interestingly, alcohol induced-pain in Hodgkin disease has been reported as an uncommon symptom that apparently coincides with heavy eosinophilic infiltration at the sites of lymphoma. If present, such pain may direct the clinician to a nodal site for biopsy.

The extent of mediastinal disease has been characterized by measuring the maximum single horizontal width of the mass on a standing PA chest radiograph, and dividing it by the maximum intrathoracic diameter. "Bulky" disease of the mediastinum is present when this ratio exceeds one-third. Patients with "bulky" mediastinal disease have a poor outcome when treated with single modality therapy (102). Staging laparotomy is rarely indicated because such patients should be treated with chemotherapy with or without radiotherapy, and surgery adds little to decision making. This patient did not have "bulky" mediastinal disease, but rather had splenic involvement at three apparently distinct sites with a disease of unfavorable histology (i.e., mixed cellularity type). In addition, both the lactate dehydrogenase level and ESR were elevated, suggesting that prognosis (i.e, complete remission, duration of remission, and overall survival) is poor (103, 104). Based upon these clinical manifestations, treatment with combined chemotherapy and radiotherapy is appropriate. As discussed below, the therapeutic option of chemotherapy alone may have been used as well in this case.

Recently, subdivision of stage III disease into stage III$_1$ and III$_2$ based upon the location of intraabdominal sites of disease has been introduced into the staging system (table 16.1). Some investigators have suggested that patients with presenting paraaortic, iliac, and/or mesenteric lymph node involvement have a poorer prognosis than those with splenic hilar, coeliac, and/or portal node involvement (105). However, this difference in response is observed in patients treated with radiation therapy but not with chemotherapy. Other investigators have found no significant difference in prognosis for stage IIIA$_1$ and stage IIIA$_2$ patients treated with total nodal radiation therapy (106). On the other hand, the number of splenic lesions does affect prognosis (106). The use of combined radiation and chemotherapy to treat stage IIIA Hodgkin disease (particularly those with unfavorable prognostic findings) has increased (107–109). This includes treatment of patients with stage III disease and extensive splenic involvement. Usually, chemotherapy is administered initially in order to reduce the overall mass of disease (in the above case, to shrink the mediastinal mass) and permit the use of more limited radiotherapy fields (and, therefore, less toxic amounts of irradiation). It is becoming clearer that combined modality therapy of patients with stage III disease is more effective than radiation therapy alone (110), al-

though no significant difference in response has been found in a prospective study of patients treated prospectively with combined modality therapy versus combination chemotherapy alone (111).

The most serious complication of curative therapy is the development of second malignancies, including acute nonlymphocytic leukemia, myelodysplastic syndrome, lymphoma and solid tumors such as melanoma, head and neck cancer, bone and soft tissue sarcomas, and cancer of the salivary glands (112–114). While the use of radiotherapy is associated with a low risk of leukemia (115, 116), administration of chemotherapy, primarily with alkylating agents (but not with nitrosoureas), is associated with a much higher risk of leukemia (117). It has been suggested that combined chemotherapy with doxorubicin, bleomycin, vinblastine, and decarbazine (ABVD) is less leukemogenic than combined chemotherapy with nitrogen mustard-, vincristine-, procarbazine-, and prednisone (MOPP)-like regimens (118). Risk of leukemia is higher in patients receiving chemotherapy for a longer duration, in patients receiving maintenance chemotherapy, in patients >40 years of age, and possibly in those who have undergone splenectomy (119–121). Since a fatal outcome frequently occurs when secondary malignancy develops, it is particularly frustrating to observe this complication in a patient who has been cured of Hodgkin disease.

Several chemotherapy regimens are effective in treatment of Hodgkin disease with overall complete remission rates of 81–97% (table 16.3). Administration of hematopoietic growth factors (e.g., granulocyte-macrophage colony-stimulating factor) may accelerate hematopoietic recovery following chemotherapy with MOPP (122), and its potential utility is under study as an agent that may permit the use of higher total doses where myelotoxicity is an issue. For most patients, six cycles of chemotherapy is sufficient to induce a complete remission. Usually, radiologic studies are performed after the fourth cycle of chemotherapy and again after the sixth cycle of therapy. Documentation of complete normalization or "no change" in radiographic abnormalities for 2 months during treatment is generally considered to be consistent with a complete response to therapy (even though tissue biopsy is not obtained). In approximately 15–20% of patients, more than six cycles of therapy are required to effect a complete therapeutic response. Treatment should be maintained until all of the radiologic studies have stabilized, after which two additional cycles of chemotherapy (i.e., "consolidation" treatment) are usually administered. *For the patient described here, administration of six cycles of chemotherapy, followed by radiation therapy, offers an excellent chance for complete remission. Recently, the use of two cycles of chemotherapy followed by radiation therapy was found to be as effective as more intensive treatment (123). There was no significant infertility and there was an approximately 1% actuarial incidence of acute leukemia at 15 years in patients with stage III$_1$ disease in this study (123).*

Table 16.3. Some Effective Chemotherapy Regimens for Treatment of Hodgkin Disease*

Drug Combination	Dose (mg/m²)	Route	Days Given	Complete Remission
MOPP[a]				84
Mechlorethamine (nitrogen mustard)	6	IV	1, 8	
Vincristine	1.4	IV	1, 8	
Procarbazine	100	PO	1–14	
Prednisone	40	PO	1–14	
ChlVPP[b]				85
Chlorambucil	6	PO	1–14	
Vinblastine	6	IV	1, 8	
Procarbazine	100	PO	1–14	
Prednisone	40	PO	1–14	
MVPP[c]				82
Mechlorethanime	6	IV	1, 8	
Vinblastine	6	IV	1, 8	
Procarbazine	100	PO	1–14	
Prednisone	40	PO	1–14	
ABVD[d]				81
Doxorubicin	25	IV	1, 15	
Bleomycin	10	IV	1, 15	
Vinblastine	6	IV	1, 15	
Dacarbazine	375	IV	1, 15	
MOPP/ABVD[e]				89
Alternating months of MOPP and ABVD				
MOPP/ABV hybrid[f]				97
Mechlorethamine	6	IV	1	
Vincristine	1.4 (max 2)	IV	1	
Procarbazine	100	PO	1–7	
Prednisone	40	PO	1–14	
Doxorubicin	35	IV	8	
Bleomycin	10	IV	8	
Vinblastine	6	IV	8	

*Abbreviations: IV, intravenous; PO, orally.
Regimens summarized from reference 103 (a), 124 (b), 125 (c), 126 (d), 127 (e) and 128 (f). Adapted from Urba and Longo. New Engl J Med 1992;326:678, with permission of the publisher.

Relapsed Hodgkin Disease

Approximately one-third of patients in complete remission from advanced stage Hodgkin disease will relapse at some time following completion of therapy. Of these patients, one-third will have a complete response to "salvage" therapy. Recently, aggressive, high-dose chemotherapy with autologous bone marrow transplantation has been performed in order to improve the results of salvage chemotherapy. The following case discusses these and other issues in a patient presenting with massive mediastinal involvement with Hodgkin disease who relapsed following successful combined modality therapy.

Case 3

A 32-year-old white man presented with bulky bilateral cervical and axillary lymphadenopathy. For several weeks he had experienced intermittent fevers of >101°F and drenching night sweats. He also reported a 15% weight loss in the previous 6 months. Recently, he had experienced a dry nonproductive cough, substernal discomfort, and easy fatiguability.

Physical examination revealed bilaterally enlarged cervical, supraclavicular, and axillary lymph nodes having a firm, rubbery consistency. His spleen was palpable 2 cm below the left costal margin. Chest x-ray revealed an anterior mediastinal mass greater than one-third the diameter of the chest (fig. 16.5).

Laboratory studies revealed a mild normochromic, normocytic anemia with a hematocrit of 35%. The serum iron and iron-binding capacity were mildly reduced. The WBC was 16×10^9/L with 10% eosinophils and lymphopenia. The alkaline phosphatase level was elevated at 200 U/L and the lactate dehydrogenase level was elevated at 1250 U/L. Renal function tests were unremarkable, while liver function tests revealed modestly elevated AST and ALT levels. Bilateral bone marrow biopsies revealed involvement with lymphoma.

A cervical lymph node biopsy was performed. Microscopic examination revealed sheets of pleomorphic, RS-like cells with occasional bizarre, multinucleated forms in the background of scattered lymphocytes and fibrosis. A differential diagnosis of lymphocyte depletion Hodgkin disease versus large cell, non-Hodgkin lym-

phoma was considered. Immunopathologic studies on frozen and paraffin-embedded tissue were performed. Frozen tissue immunoperoxidase studies revealed the pleomorphic large cells to have a phenotype that lacked B-cell antigens and surface immunoglobulin. The T-cell markers CD2 and CD4 were weakly expressed. Paraffin section immunopathology revealed the cells to be CD30+, CD15+, CD45−, L26−, CD3−, and staining for the epithelial membrane antigen (EMA) was negative. No clonal T- or B-cell gene rearrangements were detectable by analysis of DNA from lymphocytes, using molecular probes for T-cell receptor and immunoglobulin genes. Based on these findings, the diagnosis was made of Hodgkin disease, lymphocyte depletion type. The disease was determined to be pathological stage IVB.

Therapy was instituted with MOPP/ABVD hybrid chemotherapy (table 16.3), until a maximal tumor response occurred, as assessed by plain chest radiography and CT scanning after the fourth cycle of treatment. Two additional cycles of chemotherapy were administered as "consolidation" treatment, followed by extended field irradiation of the mediastinum. At this time, the ESR on two occasions was 25 and 40 mm/hr. Six months after completion of therapy, a repeat chest x-ray revealed widening of the mediastinum. A gallium scan demonstrated increased uptake over the mediastinum. Fine needle aspiration of the mediastinal mass revealed the presence of cells that were both morphologically and immunopathologically compatible with recurrent LD Hodgkin disease.

HLA typing of the patient and his 23-year-old sister revealed identity at the HLA-A, HLA-B, and HLA-Dr loci. In addition, no reaction among lymphocytes was observed in the mixed lymphocyte culture reaction. The patient was referred to a bone marrow transplantation center for evaluation for high-dose chemotherapy, followed by rescue with either allogeneic or autologous bone marrow stem cells.

Pathology

The histology in this case raises a differential diagnosis of LD Hodgkin disease versus large cell non-Hodgkin lymphoma. LD Hodgkin represents ≤5% of total HD cases, has a predilection for men, and usually presents as advanced stage disease (20, 21). Neiman and coworkers have suggested that the LD variant is a distinct clinicopathologic disorder of elderly men with an abdominal disease presentation; however, this has not been uniformly accepted by pathologists (129, 130). More recent studies employing immunopathologic and molecular genetic techniques indicate that both NS Hodgkin and large cell DHL have been misdiagnosed as LD Hodgkin (131, 132). Pathologic review of 39 cases originally diagnosed as LD Hodgkin and treated at the National Cancer Institute resulted in a changed diagnosis to NS Hodgkin (13 cases), other types of non-LP Hodgkin (7 cases), and NHL (10 cases) (131). Another review of 18 cases that were initially diagnosed as LD Hodgkin resulted in only 7 cases retain-

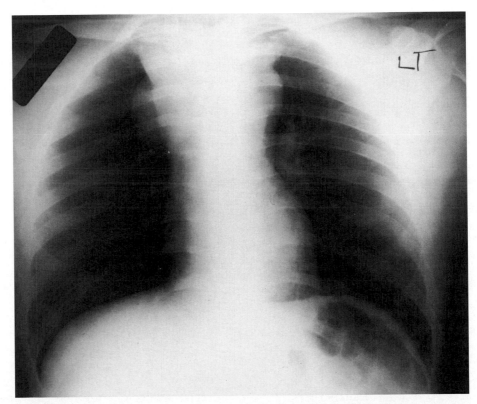

Figure 16.5. Plain chest radiograph showing mediastinal widening (case 3).

ing this diagnosis after histologic and immunopathologic evaluation review (132).

Morphologically, LD Hodgkin presents in either a diffuse fibrosis form with an acellular amorphous fibrosis that is distinct from birefringement NS fibrosis, or a reticular (i.e., sarcomatous) form with depleted lymphocytes and numerous pleomorphic and multinucleated RS cells. Paraffin immunopathology distinguishes LD Hodgkin from peripheral T-cell lymphomas (discussed in case 2), anaplastic large cell lymphomas (ki-1 positive) (68, 133–135), and other large cell lymphomas, especially those associated with sclerosis in the mediastinum (136, 138).

The leukocyte common antigen (CD45) is lacking from RS cells in most cases of HD (76, 138), except for LP Hodgkin (84, 139). LP Hodgkin can be confused with small cell NHL since both diseases typically have numerous small lymphocytes. However, it can be distinguished from small cell NHL by the expression of monotypic immunoglobulin on B-cells in NHL. CD30 (Ber-H2 in paraffin, Ki-1 in frozen tissue) and CD15 (Leu-M1) can be expressed in non-LPHD but not in the large cells in NHL.

The paraffin section immunophenotype expressed in this case (CD30+ CD15+ CD45+ L26− CD3−), is compatible with not only Hodgkin lymphoma but also with large cell NHL (LCNHL). In cases of LCNHL, in which CD45 may be absent and CD30 and CD15 are variably expressed, a T-cell neoplasm lacking CD3 and possibly Ki-1-positive lymphoma should also be considered. Interestingly, Ki-1-positive anaplastic large cell lymphoma (ALCL) (68, 132, 136, 137, 140–144) with variable T antigen expression (often CD4+) (135, 144) appears to be largely T-cell in nature. ALCL has an extranodal predilection and an age distribution similar to that of Hodgkin disease. However, infiltration of the subcapsular sinuses and the presence of sheets of tumor cells in ALCL distinguish this lymphoma from typical Hodgkin disease. Although ALCL

is positive for ki-1 (in common with HD), most ALCL cases are CD45+, CD15−, and epithelial membrane antigen (EMA)+ (142, 144–146). By contrast, EMA is not expressed on the surface of Hodgkin nodal cells. Thus, the paraffin immunopathology in this case (CD30+, CD15+, CD45-, L26−, CD3−, EMA−) favors the diagnosis of Hodgkin disease over that of NHL. Table 16.4 summarizes the recognition patterns for antibodies to these antigens in Hodgkin disease and NHL. Finally, negative molecular genetics studies reported in the case also favor of the diagnosis of Hodgkin disease over that of NHL.

Commentary

The therapeutic outcome of patients with mediastinal involvement with Hodgkin disease is directly related to the amount of disease present. Administration of chemotherapy alone has a high success rate for inducing complete remission. However, relapse rates of up to 50% can be expected (147). Relative to radiotherapy alone, combined modality treatment with chemotherapy and radiotherapy results in higher disease-free survival (148, 149) than does single-modality therapy. Today, most clinicians would recommend combined modality therapy for this patient. "Maintenance" chemotherapy administered following a complete response has not been shown to prolong remission (150) and is therefore not indicated in this case.

Persistent abnormalities of the mediastinum on plain chest radiography are present in up to 90% of the patients following treatment for mediastinal disease (151, 152). When abnormalities are stable, most clinicians administer an additional two cycles of chemotherapy without obtaining tissue by mediastinal biopsy. Therefore, treatment was appropriate in this case.

At 6 months following the completion of therapy, a suspicious chest x-ray was obtained that was pursued diagnostically with a gallium scan. In this setting, gallium scanning is very useful in detecting residual and/or recurrent disease (153). A clinical suspicion that recurrence will develop in this patient should have been raised by the unexplained elevated erythrocyte sedimentation rate obtained after therapy. Several patterns of such elevation have been found to correlate by multivariate analysis with recurrence of Hodgkin disease, including the pattern of oscillation between normal and elevated levels (154). Other patterns such as persistently elevated levels and levels that are high prior to therapy and normal after therapy are less commonly observed than oscillating values.

"Salvage" chemotherapy for patients who relapse following radiotherapy results in a 50–80% rate of complete remission (155). By contrast, remission rates vary for patients who have been treated previously with chemotherapy, depending on the nature of the initial response. Patients who have a prolonged initial response to chemotherapy (>12 months) have a >90% probability of achieving an additional complete remission with salvage chemotherapy (156). Patients whose initial complete remission

Table 16.4. Immunopathology of Hodgkin Disease and Some Non-Hodgkin Lymphomas (NHLs) using Parrafin Tissue Sections*

Disease	CD30	CD15	Marker CD45	L26	CD3
Hodgkin					
LP	+	−	+	+	−
Other	+	+	−	−	−
NHL					
B-cell	−	−	+	+	−
T-cell	−	−	+	−	+
ALCL	+	−	+	−	+/−

*These patterns are observed in the majority (but not all) cases. **LPHD**: lymphocyte predominant Hodgkin of the nodular form. Similar results are often present in diffuse Hodgkin disease. **Other**: nonlymphocyte predominant Hodgkin disease. **NHL**: non-Hodgkin lymphoma. **ALCL**: anaplastic large cell lymphoma. L26 is a CD20-related marker that is useful in analysis of tissue embedded in parrafin. CD3 is recognized by polyvalent antibody preparations that are currently available for parrafin use.

lasted <12 months have a <30% chance of obtaining a second complete remission (157). Recently, non-MOPP regimens have been used with increased popularity (158–160). A non-cross-resistant chemotherapy regimen that employs MOPP and ABVD as salvage chemotherapy has been reported to yield very high response rates (60%) and 5-year survivals (160). However, <10% 5-year survival rates were observed in subsequent studies (159, 161). Owing to patient selection, it is difficult to compare results of different salvage regimens. Nevertheless, it may be generalized that long-term, disease-free survival rarely occurs in patients who are truly resistant to MOPP, ABVD, or alternating MOPP and ABVD.

Recently, a new form of "salvage" chemotherapy has been introduced with very high doses of chemotherapy followed by "rescue" with hematopoietic stem cells. Steep dose-response curves have been demonstrated with many antineoplastic agents for Hodgkin disease, with a log-linear relation between tumor cell kill and dose over a certain range, followed by flattening of the curve in upper dose ranges (162). Myelosuppression is the major dose limiting toxicity of many agents, including cyclophosphamide, carmustine, etoposide, thiotepa, carboplatin, vinblastine, and melphelan. Therefore, combinations of these agents at close to the maximum tolerated doses are appropriate for use in bone marrow transplantation, if they have non-overlapping extramedullary toxicities.

To date, no prospective, controlled trials of allogeneic versus autologous bone marrow transplantation have been completed for relapsed Hodgkin disease. In a retrospective study, Applebaum et al. (163) compared the results of autologous, allogeneic, and syngeneic transplantation of patients with lymphomas. For those with Hodgkin disease, they found no significant difference in survival or relapse, using different marrow sources. Many patients with Hodgkin are unsuitable for allogeneic transplant regimens which commonly use total body irradiation, because they have already received prior mediastinal radiotherapy, or because no appropriate donor is available (for approximately 60% of potential transplant patients). Additionally, there is a high risk of opportunistic infections during the period of immune suppression that follows transplant (164), which may be exacerbated by pharmacologic immune suppression that is required after allogeneic transplantation. The immune sequelae of allogeneic transplant, including acute and chronic graft versus host disease, can be avoided by the use of autologous bone marrow rescue in patients who have no bone marrow involvement. For these reasons, allogenic transplantation is frequently preferable to autologous transplantation.

However, the patient discussed here presented with bone marrow involvement by Hodgkin lymphoma. A repeat bone marrow evaluation at the time of relapse is now indicated. If the marrow is uninvolved, cytogenetic studies of the marrow cells should be performed in order to exclude translocations that may indicate involvement with lymphoma and to evaluate for chromosomal abnormalities that are known to occur in myelodysplasia. The latter disease may result from prior chemotherapy and may presage transformation to acute leukemia (165).

Patients who have either morphologic or cytogenetic bone marrow involvement by Hodgkin disease and/or myelodysplasia and who are considered to be unsuitable for autologous bone marrow transplantation can be treated with peripheral blood stem cell transplantation. Hematopoietic stem cells and progenitors can be isolated by apheresis from peripheral blood, cryopreserved and reinfused following high-dose chemotherapy. Several studies have demonstrated the feasibility of reconstituting hematopoietic function, using peripheral blood stem cells after chemotherapy-induced marrow aplasia in patients with Hodgkin disease or other malignancies (166–168). If this patient had received irradiation of the pelvis, it would be difficult to harvest an adequate number of bone marrow mononuclear cells, and autologous peripheral blood transplantation would be an appropriate option. In the above patient, many transplant physicians would probably select autologous peripheral blood stem cell transplantation, holding allogeneic bone marrow in storage for subsequent transplantation for a future relapse. Nevertheless, as better regimens to prophylax for graft-versus-host disease and to treat posttransplantation infectious complications are developed, the role of allogenic transplantation in Hodgkin at earlier times during the course of the disease will undoubtedly increase.

Although results of prospective studies are unavailable to determine the optimal timing for transplant in relapsed Hodgkin disease, several investigators have suggested that patients transplanted early in the course of disease and with less disease will do better (169, 170). Jagannath et al. (170) studied prognostic factors in two patient groups. The "good" prognosis group had a performance status of 0 (no limitations), had failed (at most) two chemotherapy regimens, and were treated for disease that was sensitive to chemotherapy. The "poor" prognosis group consisted of all remaining patients who had performance status greater than 0 and/or who had failed more than two regimens and did not have chemotherapy-sensitive, relapsed disease. A study of 70 patients transplanted either early (36 patients receiving only one or two chemotherapy regimens and no bulky disease) or late (34 patients receiving three or more regimens, or bulky disease) showed that the group transplanted early had 65% complete responses and an early mortality of 6%. By contrast, the late group had a complete response rate of only 44% with 18% early deaths (169, 170).

Summary

The cases presented above have been selected to provide the reader with a feeling for the broad scope of issues that arise regarding the diagnosis, workup, and therapy of Hodgkin lymphoma. They provide a framework for discussing the natural history and clinical manifestations of the disease. Further cases could have been selected that reflect one or more of the unusual features of Hodgkin disease, such as complication with diffuse pulmonary infiltrates due to infection with the protozoan *Pneumocystis carinii*, development of Herpes zoster (shingles) which occurs in approximately 10% of treated Hodgkin disease patients, and 20% of treated patients who have undergone splenectomy, or presentation with acute cord compression due to vertebral body collapse or invasion of the epidural space from retroperitoneal lymph nodes. The serious student of this disease will be undoubtedly intrigued by patients whose clinical manifestations demand the highest clinical acumen and diagnostic precision. Because therapeutic outcomes are usually favorable, the student will be also rewarded by selecting appropriate successful therapy ranging from the administration of chemotherapy and radiotherapy to surgical exploration and extirpation.

REFERENCES

1. Hodgkin T. On some morbid appearances of the absorbent glands and spleen. Med-Chir Trans 1832;17:68.
2. Dorfman RF. The enigma of Hodgkin's disease: current concepts based on morphologic, clinical and immunologic observations. In: Hanaoka M, Kadin ME, Watanabe S, et al., eds. Lymphoma malignancy: immunology and cytogenetics. Philadelphia: Field & Wood, 1989.
3. Hsu S-M. The never-ending controversies in Hodgkin's disease. Blood 1990;75:1742.
4. Boecker WR, Hossfield DK, Gallmeier WM, et al. Clonal growth of Hodgkin cells. Nature 1975;258:235.
5. Weiss LM, Movahed LA, Warnke RA. Detection of Epstein-Barr viral genomes in Reed-Sternberg cells of Hodgkin's disease. N Engl J Med 1989;320:502.
6. Peckham MJ, Cooper EH. Proliferative characteristics of the various classes of cells in Hodgkin's disease. Cancer 1969;24:135.
7. Hsu SM, Zhao X, Chakroborty S, et al. Reed-Sternberg cells in Hodgkin's cell lines HDLM, L-428 and KM-H2 are not actively replicating and lack of bromodeoxyuridine uptake by multinuclear cells in culture. Blood 1988;71:1382.
8. Newcom SR, Kadin ME, Phillips C. L-428 Reed-Sternberg cells and mononuclear Hodgkin's cells arise from a single cloned mononuclear cell. Int J Cell Cloning 1988;6:417.
9. Lukes RJ. Criteria for involvement of lymph node, bone marrow, spleen, and liver in Hodgkin's disease. Cancer Res 1971;31:1755.
10. Lukes RJ, Tindle BH, Parker JW. Reed-Sternberg like cells in infectious mononucleosis. Lancet 1969;2:1003.
11. Strum SB, Rappaport H. Observation of cells resembling Reed-Sternberg cells in conditions other than Hodgkin's disease. Cancer 1970;26:176.
12. Pastuszak WT, Kosciol CM, Laird L. T and B cell gene rearrangements in lymphoma: correlation with immunophenotype. Mod Pathol 1991;4:81a.
13. Pastuszak WT, Kosciol CM, Rezuke WN. T and B cell gene rearrangements in Hodgkin's disease. Blood 1991;78:122a.
14. Miller TP, Byrne GE, Jones SE. Mistaken clinical and pathologic diagnoses of Hodgkin's disease: a Southwest Oncology Group Study. Cancer Treat Rep 1982;66:645.
15. Lukes RJ, Butler JJ, Hicks EB. Natural history of Hodgkin's disease as related to its pathologic picture. Cancer 1966; 19:317.
16. Lukes RJ, Craver LF, Hall TC, et al. Report of the nomenclature committee: Part 1. Cancer Res 1966;26:1311.
17. Banks PM. The pathology of Hodgkin's disease. Semin Oncol 1990;17:683.
18. Anatasi J, Variakojis D, Bauer KD. DNA content in Hodgkin's disease: a flow cytometric analysis with cytologic correlation. Am J Pathol 1987;128:573.
19. Cossman J, Sundeen J, Uppenkamp M, et al. Rearranging antigen-receptor genes in enriched Reed-Sternberg cell fractions of Hodgkin's disease. Hematol Oncol 1988; 6:205.
20. Berard CW, Thomas LB, Axtell LM, et al. The relationship of histopathological subtype to clinical stage of Hodgkin's disease at diagnosis. Cancer Res 1971;31:1776.
21. Colby VT, Hoppe RT, Warnke RA. Hodgkin's disease: a clinicopathologic study of 659 case. Cancer 1981;49:1848.
22. Kadin ME, Glatstein E, Dorfman RF. Clinicopathologic studies of 117 untreated patients subjected to laparotomy for the staging of Hodgkin's disease. Cancer 1991; 27:1277.
23. Strum SB, Rappaport H. Interrelations of the histologic types of Hodgkin's disease. Arch Pathol 1971;10:470.
24. Kadin ME, Agnarsson BA, Ellingsworth LR. Immunohistochemical evidence of a role for transforming growth factor-beta in the pathogenesis of nodular sclerosing Hodgkin's disease. Am J Pathol 1990;136:1209.
25. Kortman C, Burrichter H, Monner D, et al. Interleukin-1-like activity constitutively generated by Hodgkin derived cell lines: I, measurement in a human lymphocyte co-stimulator assay. Immunobiology 1984;166:318.
26. Burrichter H, Heit W, Schaadt M, et al. Production of colony stimulating factors by Hodgkin's disease cell lines. Int J Cancer 1984;166:318.
27. Samoszuk M, Nasen LI. Interleukin-5 mRNA detected in Reed-Sternberg cells of Hodgkin's disease with eosinophilia. Blood 1990;75:13.
28. Strickler JG, Michie SA, Warnke RA. The syncytial variant of nodular sclerosing Hodgkin's disease. Am J Surg Pathol 1986;10:470.
29. Bennett MH, MacLenna, Easterline MJ, et al. Analysis of histologic subtypes in Hodgkin's disease in relation to prognosis and survival. In: Quaglino D, Hayhoe FGJ, eds. The cytology of leukemias and lymphomas. New York: Raven Press, 1985;15:32.
30. Haybittle JL, Hayhoe FGJ, Easterling MJ, et al. Review of British National Lymphoma Investigation Studies of Hodgkin's disease and development of a prognostic index. Lancet 1985;1:967.
31. Wijhuizen TJ, Vrints LW, Jariam R, et al. Grades of nodular sclerosis (NSI-NSII) in Hodgkin's disease: are they of independent prognostic value? Cancer 1989;63:1150.
32. Cole S, MacMahon B, Aisenberg A. Mortality from Hodgkin's disease in the United States: evidence for the multiple etiology hypothesis. Lancet 1968;2:1371.
33. MacMahon B. Epidemiology of Hodgkin's disease. Cancer Res 1966;26:1189.
34. MacMahon B. Epidemiological evidence of the nature of Hodgkin's disease. Cancer 1957;10:1045.
35. Mueller N. An epidemiologist's view of the new molecular biology findings in Hodgkin's disease. Ann Oncol 1991; 2:23.
36. Mueller N, Evans A, Harris NL, et al. Hodgkin's disease and Epstein-Barr virus: altered antibody pattern before diagnosis. N Engl J Med 1989;320:689.

37. Pallesen G, Hamilton-Dutoit SJ, Rowe M, Young LS. Expression of Epstein-Barr virus latent gene products in tumor cells of Hodgkin's disease. Lancet 1991;337:320.

38. Weiss LM, Movahed LA, Warnke RA, et al. Detection of Epstein-Barr viral genomes in Reed-Sternberg cells of Hodgkin's disease. N Engl J Med 1989;320:502.

39. Tilly H, Bastard C, Delastre T, et al. Cytogenetic studies in untreated Hodgkin's disease. Blood 1991;77:1298.

40. Urba NJ, Longo DL. Hodgkin's disease (Review article). N Engl J Med 1992;326:678.

41. Armitage JO, Longo DL. Hodgkin's and non-Hodgkin's malignant lymphomas: management options. In: Hematology 1991 Education Program, American Society of Hematology, 1991:22–30.

42. Mansfield CM, Fabian C, Jones S, et al. Comparison of lymphangiography and computed tomography scanning in evaluating abdominal disease in stages III and IV Hodgkin's disease. Cancer 1990;66:2295.

43. Castellino RA, Hoppe RT, Blank N, et al. Computed tomography, lymphography and staging laparatomy: correlations in initial staging of Hodgkin's disease. AJR 1984;143:37–41.

44. Mansfield CM, Fabian C, Jones S, et al. Comparison of lymphangiography and computerized tomography scanning in evaluating abdominal disease in stages III and IV Hodgkin's disease. Cancer 1990;66:2295.

45. Hopper KD, Diehl LF, Lesar M, Barnes M, et al. Hodgkin's disease: clinical utility of CT in initial staging and treatment. Radiology 1988;169:17.

46. DeLaney TF, Glastein E. The role of the staging laparotomy in the management of Hodgkin's disease. In: DeVita VT, Hellman S, Rosenberg SA, eds. Cancer: principles and practice of oncology updates. Philadelphia: JB Lippincott, 1987:1–14.

47. Coker DD, Morris DM, Coleman JJ, et al. Infection among 210 patients with surgically staged Hodgkin's disease. Am J Med 1983;75:97.

48. Siber GR, Gorham C, Martin P, et al. Antibody response to pretreatment immunization and post-treatment boosting with bacterial polysaccharide vaccines in patients with Hodgkin's disease. Ann Intern Med 1986;104:467.

49. Russell KJ, Hoppe RT, Colby TV, et al. Lymphocyte predominant Hodgkin's disease: clinical presentation and results of treatment. Radiother Oncol 1984;1:197.

50. Sutcliffe SB, Gospodarowicz MK, Bergsagel DE, et al. Prognostic groups for management of localized Hodgkin's disease. J Clin Oncol 1985;3:393.

51. Hoppe RT. Radiation therapy in management of Hodgkin's disease. Semin Oncol 1990;17:704.

52. Carde P, Burger JMV, Henry-Amar M, et al. Clinical stages I and II Hodgkin's disease: a specifically tailored therapy according to prognostic factors. J Clin Oncol 1988;6:239.

53. Mauch P, Tarbell N, Weinstein H, et al. Stage IA and IIA supradiaphragmatic Hodgkin's disease: prognostic factors in surgically staged patients treated with mantle and para-arotic irradiation. J Clin Oncol 1988;6:1576.

54. DeVita VT, Jaffe ES, Hellman S. Hodgkin's disease and the non-Hodgkin's lymphomas. In: DeVita VT, Hellman S, Rosenberg SA, eds. Cancer: principles and practice of oncology. Philadelphia: JB Lippincott, 1985:1623–1709.

55. Tucker MA, Coleman CN, Cox RS, et al. Risk of second cancers after treatment for Hodgkin's disease. N Engl J Med 1988;318:76.

56. Pedrick TJ, Hoppe RT. Recovery of spermatogenesis following pelvic irradiation for Hodgkin's disease. Int J Radiat Oncol Bio Phys 1986;12:117.

57. Horning SJ, Hoppe RT, Kaplan HS, et al. Female reproductive potential after treatment for Hodgkin's disease. N Engl J Med 1981;304:1377.

58. Hellman S, Mauch P, Goodman AL, et al. The place of radiation therapy in the treatment of Hodgkin's disease. Cancer 1978;42(Suppl 2):971.

59. Longo DL, Glatstein E, Duffey PL et al. Radiation therapy versus combination chemotherapy in the treatment of early-stage Hodgkin's disease: seven year results of a prospective randomized trial. J Clin Oncol 1991;9:906.

60. Horning SJ, Hoppe RT, Hancock SL, et al. Vinblastine, bleomycin and methotrexate: an effective adjuvant in favorable Hodgkin's disease. J Clin Oncol 1988:1822.

61. Lukes RJ, Bulter JJ. The pathology and nomenclature of Hodgkin's disease. Cancer Res 1966;26:1063.

62. Waldron JA, Leech JH, Glick AD, et al. Malignant lymphoma of peripheral T-lymphocyte origin: immunologic, pathologic, and clinical features in six patients. Cancer 1977;40:1604.

63. Maggi E, Parronchi P, Macchia D, et al. High numbers of CD4+ T cells showing recognition of DR antigens in lymphoid organs involved by Hodgkin's disease. Blood 1988, 71:1503.

64. Poppema S, Bhan AK, Reinherz EL, et al. In situ immunologic characterization of cellular constituents in lymph nodes and spleens involved with Hodgkin's disease. Blood 1982;59:226.

65. Schwab U, Stein H, Gerdes J, et al. Production of a monoclonal antibody specific for Hodgkin's and Sternberg-Reed cells of Hodgkin's disease and a subset of normal lymphoid cells. Nature 1982;229:65.

66. Hecht TT, Longo DL, Cossman J, et al. Production and characterization of a monoclonal antibody that binds Reed-Sternberg cells. J Immunol 1985;134:4231.

67. Pfreudschuh M, Mommertz E, Meissner M, et al. Hodgkin's and Reed-Sternberg cell associated monoclonal antibodies HRS-1 and HRS-2 react with activated cells of lymphoid and monocytoid origin. Anticancer Res 1988; 8:217.

68. Stein H, Mason DY, Gerdes J, et al. The expression of the Hodgkin's disease associated antigen K-1 in reactive and neoplastic lymphoid tissue: evidence that Reed-Sternberg cells and histiocytic malignancies are derived from activated lymphoid cells. Blood 1985;66:848.

69. Dorreen MS, Habeshaw JA, Stansfield AG, et al. Characterization of Sternberg-Reed and related cells in Hodgkin's disease: an immunohistological study. Br J Cancer 1984; 49:465.

70. Jones DB, Gerdes J, Stein H, et al. An investigation of Ki-1 positive large cell lymphoma with antibodies reactive with tissue macrophages. Hematol Oncol 1986; 4:315.

71. Schwarrting R, Gerdes J, Ziegler A, et al. Immunoprecipitation of the interleukin-2 receptor from Hodgkin's disease-derived cell lines by monoclonal antibodies. Hematol Oncol 1987;5:57.

72. Stein H, Gerdes J, Ulrich S, et al. Evidence for the detection of the normal counterpart of the Hodgkin Sternberg-Reed cells. Hematol Oncol 1983;1:21.

73. Kadin M. Possible origin of the Reed-Sternberg cell from an interdigitating reticulum cell. Cancer Treat Rep 1982; 66:601.

74. Payne SV, Wright DH, Jones KJM, et al. Macrophage origin of Reed-Sternberg cells: an immunohistochemical study. J Clin Pathol 1982;35:159.

75. Kadin ME, Muramoto L, Said JW. Expression of T-cell antigens on Reed-Sternberg cells in a subset of patients with nodular sclerosing and mixed cellularity Hodgkin's disease. Am J Pathol 1988;130:345.

76. Agnarsson BA, Kadin ME. The immunophenotype of Reed-Sternberg cells: a study of 50 cases of Hodgkin's disease using fixed, frozen tissues. Cancer 1989;63:2083.

77. Timens W, Visser L, Poppema S. Nodular lymphocyte predominance type of Hodgkin's disease is a germinal center lymphoma. Lab Invest 1986;54:457.

78. Poppema S. The nature of the lymphocytes surrounding Reed-Sternberg cells in nodular lymphocyte predominance and in other types of Hodgkin's disease. Am J Pathol 1989; 135:351.

79. Poppema S, Kaiserling E, Lennert K. Nodular paragranulomas with lymphocyte predominance nodular type (nodular paragranuloma) and progressively transformed germinal centers: a cytohistological study. Histopathology 1979; 3:295.

80. Poppema S, Kaiserling E, Lennert K. Nodular paragranuloma and progressively transformed germinal centers. Virchows Arch [B] 1979;31:211.

81. Burns BF, Colby TV, Dorfman RF. Differential diagnostic features of nodular L&H Hodgkin's disease, including progressively transformed germinal centers. Am J Surg Pathol 1984;8:253.

82. Osborne BM, Bulter JJ. Clinical implications of progressive transformation of germinal centers. Am J Surg Pathol 1984; 8:725.

83. Pinkus GS, Said JW. Hodgkin's disease, lymphocyte predominance type, nodular: further evidence for a B cell derivation. L&H variants of Reed-Sternberg cells express L26, a pan B cell marker. Am J Pathol 1988;133:211.

84. Coles FB, Cartum RW, Pastuszak WT. Hodgkin's disease, lymphocyte-predominant type: immunoreactivity with B-cell antibodies. Mod Pathol 1988;1:274.

85. Schmid C, Sargent C, Isaacson PG. L and H cells of nodular lymphocyte predominant Hodgkin's disease show immunoglobulin light chain restriction. Am J Pathol 1992;139:1281.

86. Hansman M-L, Stein H, Fellbaum C, et al. Nodular paragranuloma can transform into high-grade malignant lymphoma of B type. Hum Pathol 1989;20:1169.

87. Miettinen M, Franssila KO, Saxen E. Hodgkin's disease, lymphocytic predominance type: increased risk for subsequent non-Hodgkin's lymphoma. Cancer 1983; 51:2293.

88. Rappaport H, Harris NL. Society for hematopathology symposium: controversies in Hodgkin's disease. Am J Surg Pathol 1987;11:148.

89. Sundeen JT, Cossman J, Jaffe ES. Lymphocyte predominant Hodgkin's disease nodular subtype with coexistent "large cell lymphoma": histological progression or composite malignancy? Am J Surg Pathol 1988;12:599.

90. Clearly M, Rosenberg SA. The bcl-2 gene, follicular lymphoma and Hodgkin's disease. J Natl Cancer Inst 1990; 82:808.

91. Stetler-Stevenson M, Crush-Stanton S, Cossman J. Involvement of the bcl-2 gene in Hodgkin's disease. J Natl Cancer Inst 1990;82:855, 858.

92. Falini B, Stein H, Pileri S, et al. Expression of lymphoid-associated antigens on Hodgkin's and Reed-Sternberg cells of Hodgkin's disease: an immunocytochemical study on lymph node cytospins using monoclonal antibodies. Histopathology 1987;11:1229.

93. Said JW, Sasson AF, Shintaku IP, et al. Absence of bcl-2 major breakpoint region and JH gene rearrangement in lymphocyte predominance Hodgkin's disease: results of Southern blot analysis and polymerase chain reactions. Am J Pathol 1991;138:261.

94. Louie DC, Kant JA, Brooks JJ. Absence of t(14:18) major and minor breakpoints and of bcl-2 protein overproduction in Reed-Sternberg cells of Hodgkin's disease. Am J Pathol 1992;138:1231.

95. Weiss LM, Strickler JG, Hu E, et al. Immunoglobulin gene rearrangements in Hodgkin's disease. Hum Pathol 1986; 17:1009.

96. Brinker MG, Poppema S, Buys CHCM, et al. Clonal immunoglobulin gene rearrangements in tissue involved by Hodgkin's disease. Blood 1987;70:186.

97. Sundeen J, Lipford E, Uppenkamp M, et al. Rearranged antigen receptor genes in Hodgkin's disease. Blood 1987; 70:96.

98. Griesser H, Feller AC, Mak T, et al. Clonal rearrangements of T cell receptor and immunoglobulin genes and immunophenotypic antigen expression in different subclasses of Hodgkin's disease. Int J Cancer 1987;40:157.

99. Knowles DM, Neri A, Pellici PG, et al. Immunoglobulin and T cell receptor beta chain gene rearrangement analysis of Hodgkin's disease: implications for lineage determination and differential diagnosis. Proc Natl Acad Sci USA 1986; 83:7942.

100. O'Connor NTJ, Crick JA, Gatter KC, et al. Cell lineage in Hodgkin's disease. Lancet 1987;2:158.

101. Griesser H, Mak T. Immunogenotyping in Hodgkin's disease. Hematol Oncol 1988;6:239.

102. Hoppe RT. The management of bulky mediastinal Hodgkin's disease: Hematology/Oncology Clinics of North America.

103. Longo DL, Young RC, Wesley M, et al. Twenty years of MOPP therapy for Hodgkin's disease. J Clin Oncol 1986; 4:1295.

104. Straus DJ, Gaynor JJ, Myers et al. Prognostic factors among 185 adults with newly diagnosed, advanced Hodgkin's disease treated with alternating potentially noncross-resistant chemotherapy and intermediate-dose radiation therapy. J Clin Oncol 1990;8:1173.

105. Stein RS, Golomb HM, Mauch P, et al. Anatomic substages of stage IIIA Hodgkin's disease: a collaborative study. Ann Intern Med 1980;92:159.

106. Hoppe RT, Cox RS, Rosenberg SA, et al. Prognostic factors in pathologic stage II Hodgkin's disease. Cancer Treat Rep 1982;66:743.

107. Glick JH. The treatment of stage IIIA Hodgkin's disease: what is the role of combined modality therapy? Int J Radiat Oncol Biol Phys 1978;4:781.

108. Prosnitz LR, Montalvo RL, Fischer DB. Treatment of stage IIIA Hodgkin's disease: is radiotherapy alone adequate? Int Radiat Oncol Biol Phys 1978;4:781.

109. Russell KJ, Donaldson SS, Cox RS, et al. Childhood Hodgkin's disease: patterns of relapse. J Clin Oncol 1984; 2:80.

110. Mauch P, Goffman T, Rosenthal DS, et al. Stage III Hodgkin's disease: improved survival with combined modality therapy as compared with radiation alone. J Clin Oncol 1985;3:1166.

111. Crowther D, Wagstaff J, Deakin D, et al. A randomized study comparing chemotherapy alone with chemotherapy followed by radiotherapy in patients with pathologically staged IIIA Hodgkin's disease. J Clin Oncol 1989; 2:892.

112. Tucker MA, Coleman CN, Cox RS, et al. Risk of second cancers after treatment for Hodgkin's disease. N Engl J Med 1988;318:76.

113. Blayney DW, Longo DL, Young RC, et al. Decreasing risk of leukemia with prolonged follow-up after chemotherapy for Hodgkin's disease. N Engl J Med 1988;316:710.

114. van Leeuwen FE, Somers R, Taal BG, et al. Increased risk of lung cancer, non-Hodgkin's lymphoma, and leukemia following Hodgkin's disease. J Clin Oncol 1989; 7:1046.

115. Lavey RS, Eby NL, Prosnitz LR. Impact on second malignancy of the combined use of radiation and chemotherapy for lymphomas. Cancer 1990;66:80.

116. Kaldor JM, Day WE, Clarke EA, et al. Leukemia following Hodgkin's disease. N Engl J Med 1990;022.7.

117. Devereaux S, Selassie TG, Vaughan-Hudson G, et al. Leukemia complicating treatment for Hodgkin's disease: the experience of the British National Lymphoma Investigation. Br Med J 1980;301:1077.

118. Valagussa P, Santoro A, Fossati-Bellani, et al. Absence of treatment-induced second neoplasms after ABVD in Hodgkin's disease. Blood 1982;59:488.

119. Pedersen-Bjergaard J, Specht L, Larsen SO, et al. Risk of therapy-related leukemia and preleukemia after Hodgkin's disease: relation to age, cumulative dose of alkylating agents, and time from chemotherapy. Lancet 1987; 2:83.

120. van Leeuwen FE, Somers R, Hart AAM. Splenectomy in Hodgkin's disease and secondary leukemias. Lancet 1987; 2:210.

121. van der Velden JW, van Putten WL, Guinee VF, et al. Subsequent development of acute non-lymphocytic leukemia in patients treated for Hodgkin's disease. Int J Cancer 1988; 42:252.

122. Hovgaard D, Nissen NI. Effect of recombinant human granulocyte-macrophage colony-stimulating factor in patients with Hodgkin's disease: a phase I/II study. J Clin Oncol 1992;10:390.

123. Henkelmann GC, Hagemeister FB, Fuller LM. Two cycles of MOPP and radiotherapy for stage III$_1$A and stage III$_1$B Hodgkin's disease. J Clin Oncol 6:1293.

124. Vose J, Armitage J, Weisenburger D, et al. MVPP an effective and well-tolerated alternative to MOPP therapy for Hodgkin's disease. Ann J Clin Oncol 1988;11:423.

125. Sutcliffe SB, Wrigley PFM, Peto J, et al. MVPP chemotherapy regimen for advanced Hodgkin's disease. Br Med J 1978;1:679.

126. Bonadonna G, Zucali R, Monfardini S, et al. Combination chemotherapy for Hodgkin's disease with adriamycin, bleomycin, vinblastiine, and imidazole carboximide versus MOPP. Cancer 1975;36:252.

127. Bonadonna G, Valagussa P, Santoro A. Alternating non-cross-resistant combination chemotherapy of MOPP in stage IV Hodgkin's disease. Ann Intern Med 1986;104:973.

128. Klimo P, Connors JM. An update on the Vancouver experience in the management of advanced Hodgkin's disease treated with the MOPP/ABV Hybrid program. Semin Hematol 1988;2:34.

129. Neiman RS, Rosen PJ, Lukes RJ. Lymphocyte-depletion Hodgkin's disease: a clinicopathology entity. N Engl J Med 1973;288:751.

130. Bearman KM, Pangalis GA, Rappaport HR. Hodgkin's lymphocyte depletion type: a clinicopathology study of 39 patients. Cancer 1978;41:293.

131. Kant JA, Hubbard SM, Longo DL, et al. The pathologic and clinical heterogeneity of lymphocyte depleted Hodgkin's disease. J Clin Oncol 1986;4:284.

132. Kinney MC, Greer JP, Collins RD. Assessment of lymphocyte depleted Hodgkin's disease, reticular variant (LDHD-R) by monoclonal antibodies (abstract). Lab Invest 1991; 64:75A.

133. Wolf BC, Gildchrist KW, Mann RB, Neiman RS. Evaluation of pathology review of malignant lymphomas and Hodgkin's disease in cooperative clinical trials. Cancer 1988; 62:1301.

134. Kadin ME, Sako D, Berliner N, et al. Childhood Ki-1 lymphoma presenting with skin lesions and peripheral lymphadenopathy. Blood 1986;68:1042,1049.

135. Agnarsson BA, Kadin ME. Ki-1 positive large cell lymphoma: a morphologic and immunologic study of 19 cases. Am J Surg Pathol 1988;12:264.

136. Addis BJ, Isaacson PG. Large cell lymphoma of mediastinum: a B cell tumour of probable thymic origin. Histopathology 1986;10:379.

137. Jacobson JO, Aisenberg AC, Lamarre L, et al. Mediastinal large cell lymphoma: an uncommon subset of adult lymphoma curable with combined modality therapy. Cancer 1988;62:1893.

138. Dorfman RF, Gatter KC, Pulford KAF, et al. An evaluation of the utility of anti-granulocyte and anti-leukocyte monoclonal antibodies in the diagnosis of Hodgkin's disease. Am J Pathol 1986;123:508.

139. Pinkus GS, Said JW. Hodgkin's disease, lymphocyte predominance type, nodular—a distinct entity? Unique staining profile for L&H variants of Reed-Sternberg cells defined by monoclonal antibodies to leukocyte common antigen, granulocyte-specific antigen, and B cell specific antigen. Am J Pathol 1985;118.

140. Kadin ME, Sposto R, Agnarsson BA, et al. Ki-1 antigen expression in childhood non-Hodgkin's lymphoma. Blood 1987;70:260a.

141. Bitter MA, Franklin WA, Larson RA, et al. Morphology in Ki-1 (CD30)-positive non-Hodgkin's lymphoma is correlated with clinical features and the presence of a unique chromosomal abnormality, t(2,5)(p23;q35). Am J Surg Pathol 1990;14:305.

142. Chott A, Kaserer K, Augustin I, et al. Ki-1 positive large cell lymphoma: a clinicopathologic study of 41 cases. Am J Surg Pathol 1990;14.

143. Kinney MC, Glick AD, Stein H, et al. Comparison of anaplastic large cell Ki-1 lymphomas and microvillous lymphomas in their immunologic and ultrastructural features. Am J Surg Pathol 1990;14:1047.

144. Kinney MC, Greer JP, Glick AD, et al. Anaplastic large cell Ki-1 malignant lymphomas: recognition, biological and clinical implications. Pathol Ann 1991;26:1.

145. Falini B, Pileri S, Stein H, et al. Variable expression of leukocyte-common (CD45) antigen in CD30 (Ki-1) positive anaplastic large cell lymphoma: implications for the differential diagnosis between lymphoid and nonlymphoid malignancies. Hum Pathol 1991;21:624.

146. Piris M, Brown DC, Gatter KC, et al. CD30 expression in non-Hodgkin's lymphoma. Histopathology 1990; 17:211.

147. Bonadonna G, Valagussa P, Santoro A. Prognosis of bulky Hodgkin's disease treated with chemotherapy alone or combined with radiotherapy. Cancer Surv 1985; 4:439.

148. Gomez GA, Panahon AM, Stutzman L, et al. Large mediastinal mass in Hodgkin's disease: results of two treatment modalities. Am J Clin Oncol 1984;7:65.

149. Crinkovich MJ, Hoppe RT, Rosenberg SA. Stage IIB Hodgkin's disease: the Stanford experience. J Clin Oncol 1986;4:472.

150. Longo DL, Young RC, DeVita VT Jr. Chemotherapy for Hodgkin's disease: the remaining challenges. Cancer Treat Rep 1982;66:925.

151. Jochelson M, Mauch P, Balikian J, et al. The significance of the residual mediastinal mass in treated Hodgkin's disease. J Clin Oncol 1985;3:637.

152. Radford JA, Cowan RA, Flanagan M, et al. The significance of residual mediastinal abnormality on the chest radiograph following treatment for Hodgkin's disease. J Clin Oncol 1988;6:940.

153. Hagemeister FB, Fesus SM, Lamki LM, et al. Role of the gallium scan in Hodgkin's disease. Cancer 1990;65:1090.

154. Henry-Amar M, Friedman S, Hayat M, et al. Erythrocyte sedimentation rate predicts early relapse and survival in early stage Hodgkin's disease. Ann Intern Med 1992; 114:361.

155. Buzaid AC, Lippman SM, Miller TP. Salvage therapy of advanced hodgkin's disease: critical appraisal of curative potential. Am J Med 1987;83:523.

156. Fisher RI, DeVita VT, Hubbard SM, et al. Prolonged disease-free survival in Hodgkin's disease with MOPP reinduction after first relapse. Ann Intern Med 1990;90:123.

157. Viviani S, Santoro A, Negretti E, et al. Hodgkin's disease: results in patients relapsing more than 12 months after first complete remission. Ann Oncol 1990;1:123.

158. Santoro A, Viviani S, Valagussa P, et al. CCNU, etoposide and prednimustine (CEP) in refractory Hodgkin's disease. Semin Oncol 1986;13:23.

159. Piga A, Ambrosetti A, Todeschini G, Cetto G. Doxorubicin, bleomycin, vinblastine, and dacarbazine (ABVD) salvage of mechlorethamine, vincristine, prednisone, and procarbazine (MOPP) resistant advanced Hodgkin's disease. Cancer Treat Rep 1984;68:947.

160. Tseng A Jr, Jacobs C, Coleman CN. Third-line chemotherapy for resistant Hodgkin's disease with lomustine, etoposide, and methotrexate. Cancer Treat Rep 1987; 71:475.

161. Harker WG, Kushlan P, Rosenberg SA. Combination chemotherapy for advanced Hodgkin's disease after failure of MOPP, ABVD, B-CAVe. Ann Intern Med 1984; 101:440.

162. Skipper HE. Dose response curves in animals. In: Some quantitative relationships that seem critical in cancer chemotherapy. Birmingham, AL: Southern Research Institute, 1984:39–68.

163. Applebaum FR, Sullivan KM, Thomas ED, et al. Allogeneic marrow transplantation in the treatment of MOPP-resistant Hodgkin's disease. J Clin Oncol 1985;3:1490.

164. Philips GL, Reece DE. Clinical studies of autologous bone marrow transplantation in Hodgkin's disease. Clin Haematol 1986;5:151.

165. Chao NJ, Auayporn PN, Gwynn DL, et al. Importance of bone marrow cytogenetic evaluation before autologous bone marrow transplantation for Hodgkin's disease. J Clin Oncol 1991;9:1575.

166. Kessinger A, Armitage JO, Smith DM. High-dose therapy and autologous peripheral blood stem cell transplantation for patients with lymphoma. Blood 1989;74:1260.

167. Korbling M, Holle R, Hass R, et al. Autologous blood stem cell transplantation in patients with advanced Hodgkin's disease and prior radiation to the pelvic site. J Clin Oncol 1990;8:978.

168. Hurd DD, Haake RJ, Lasky LC, et al. Treatment of refractory and relapsed Hodgkin's disease: intensive chemotherapy and autologous bone marrow or peripheral blood stem cell support. Med Pediatr Oncol 1990;18:447.

169. Longo DL. The use of chemotherapy in the treatment of Hodgkin's disease. Semin Oncol 1990;17:716.

170. Jagannath S, Armitage JO, Dicke KA, et al. Prognostic factors for response and survival after high-dose cyclophosphamide, carmustine, and etoposide with autologous bone marrow transplantation for relapsed Hodgkin's disease. J Clin Oncol 1989;7:179.

CHAPTER 17

Non-Hodgkin Lymphoma

M. A. RODRIGUEZ, F. C. CABANILLAS, A. B. DEISSEROTH

He found a definite pattern in the distribution, as most of the tumours were contained in a band which stretched across Africa, running between 10 degrees north and 10 degrees south of the Equator. The five million square miles within this band became known as the Lymphoma Belt.
—Dennis Burkitt, *British Journal of Surgery* (1958)

Case 1

The patient, a 25-year-old white woman presented to an emergency room for examination after an automobile accident. Routine physical examination and a chest x-ray were done. The chest x-ray demonstrated a 10-cm mediastinal mass (fig. 17.1). The patient denied any symptoms of fever, cough, or weight loss. There was no evidence of any further lymphadenopathy and no hepatosplenomegaly.

Resources

Differential Diagnoses

Differential diagnoses in a young woman with a mediastinal mass include Hodgkin disease, lymphoma, thymoma, thyroid carcinoma, or intrathoracic goiter. The management of each of these diseases is specific for each entity. Reaching the correct diagnosis is thus of paramount importance.

Background on Normal Lymphoid (B-Cell) Maturation and Malignant Arrest

Lymphoid malignancies are heterogenous, occurring at the different stages of lymphocyte differentiation. As expected, lymphomas can be derived from B- as well as T-lymphocytes. They express differentiation markers that correspond to the different stages of normal maturation (1–3). B-Cell lymphomas can be divided into two general categories of differentiation: the immature and the mature types. In order to better understand these disorders, we must first visualize the normal B-cell development conceptually (table 17.1, 17.2). The first step in B-cell differentiation occurs in the marrow and coincides of rearrangement of the heavy-chain gene (JH). The "pre-pre-B-cell," however, has not yet rearranged its light chain gene. TdT is present and CD10 (Calla) and CD19 antigens are prominently expressed on the cell surface. The malignancies that occur due to developmental arrest at this stage

are some acute lymphoblastic leukemias. As the lymphocyte continues to mature into a pre-B-cell, the light chain gene is rearranged, and TdT and CD10 expression is eventually lost, while CD20, CD22 (pan-B-antigens), and HLADR expression are gained.

At the next step of differentiation ("early B-cell"), the lymphocyte is still considered an immature cell. The characteristic pattern consists of both heavy and light chain rearrangement, no expression of TdT, variable CD10, and consistent expression of CD19, CD20, CD22, and HLADR. It is at this stage that surface immunoglobulin (SIg) is expressed for the first time in the form of IgM and light chains. Burkitt lymphoma and B-cell acute lymphoblastic leukemia are thought to be the malignant counterparts of the early B-lymphocyte.

The "mature resting B-cell," the next cell generated, is characterized by the simultaneous expression of SIgM and D, as well as CD19, CD20, CD22, and HLADR. Again, TdT and CD10 are no longer expressed at this stage. At this stage, as well as all subsequent stages of differentiation, the B-cell lymphomas can be considered mature B-cell neoplasms. Morphologically, the cells are small mature lymphocytes that circulate in the peripheral blood or reside in the mantle zones of the germinal follicles. The malignant counterpart is the B-cell chronic lymphocytic leukemia and the small lymphocytic lymphoma. A unique feature of this malignant B-cell disorder is the expression of CD5, which is otherwise primarily seen in T-lymphocytes (table 17.2).

Further B-cell differentiation proceeds in the germinal follicles. The mature B-cell enters the germinal center, where the cells already stimulated by antigen undergo morphologic changes. At this stage, the B-cell is known as follicular center cell and is characterized by heavy chain switching from IgM to IgG or IgA. This process of switching, however, does not alter the light chain type expression. All of the other pan-B antigens continue to be expressed at this stage. CD10 is variably expressed.

The most common lymphomas occur at the follicular center cell stage. The follicular lymphomas, as well as the diffuse large cell lymphomas, are the malignant counter-

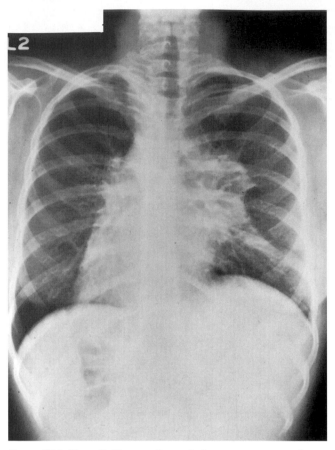

Figure 17.1 (Case 1) Chest radiograph demonstrating a mediastinal mass in asymptomatic 25-year-old woman.

parts of the different steps in the process of morphologic transformation that takes place within the germinal follicles as the cells respond to antigenic stimuli. The large noncleaved B-lymphocyte is the first step in the morphologic transformation process at the follicular center cell stage. This stage is followed by the large cleaved cell, which in turn is followed by the small cleaved cell. These are the basic cell types also seen in the follicular center cell lymphomas: large noncleaved, large cleaved, and small cleaved cell lymphomas. Most, but not all, of the follicular center cell lymphomas express SIg (either IgM, IgG, or IgA, as well as light chains) and the pan-B-antibodies, CD19, CD20, and CD22. Whenever SIg is not expressed, the lymphoma can still be identified as of B-cell lineage by the expression of the pan-B-antibodies.

The next step in the normal transformation process is the generation of an immunoblast that is characterized by the addition of cytoplasmic immunoglobulin (CIg). Surface immunoglobulin can be variably lost at this stage, as will definitely happen later as the cell continues to mature into a plasma cell. The immunoblastic lymphoma is the malignant equivalent of the normal immunoblast. It is histologically and clinically similar to the diffuse large cell lymphomas, except that cytologically it somewhat resembles a plasma cell. The last two steps in the process of maturation are the generation of the plasmacytoid lymphocyte and, finally, of the plasma cell. This step is thought to occur outside of the germinal follicle. At the plasma cell stage, there is loss of all the pan-B-antigens, as well as surface immunoglobulin, but CIg is prominently expressed as the cell typically manufactures

Table 17.1. Antigen Expression in B-Cell Differentiation

Normal	Heavy Chain Gene	Light Chain Gene	Tdt	CD10	CIg	SIg	CD19	CD20	CD22	CD21	CD5	HLA-DR	Neoplastic
Pre-pre-B-cell (B-cell precursor)	R	G	+	+	−	−	+	+/−	+/−	−	−	+/−	B-Cell ALL/LL
Pre-B-cell	R	+/−	+	+	+[a]	−	+	+/−	−	−	−	+	B-Cell ALL/LL
Early B-cell	R	R	−	+/−	−	+[a]	+	+	+	+/−	−	+	B-Cell ALL/LL Burkitt
Mature B-cell	R	R	−	−	−	+[b]	+	+	+	+/−	−	+	B-Cell CLL/SL
Follicle-center cell	R	R	−	+/−	−	+[c]	+	+	+	+/−	−	+/−	Follicular lymphoma
B-Immunoblast	R	R	−	−	+/−	+/−	+	+	+	−	−	+	Immunoblastic lymphoma
Plasmacytoid Lymphocyte	R	R	−	−	+	+	+/−	+/−	+/−	−	+/−	+	B-Cell/CLL plasmacytoid
Plasma cell	R	R	−	−	+[d]	−	−	−	−	−	−	+/−	Plasmacytoma/ myeloma

ALL, Acute lymphocytic leukemia; LL, Lymphocytic leukemia, CLL, Chronic lymocytic leukemia, R, Rearranged; G, Germline configuration, i.e., not rearranged.
[a]IgM.
[b]IgM/D.
[c]IgM, G, or A.
[d]IgG, M, or A.

Table 17.2. Antigen Expression in T-Cell Differentiation[a]

Normal Stage	T-cell Receptor Gene	CD45	TdT	CD10	HLA-DR	CD1	CD2	CD3	CD5	CD7	CD4	CD8	Neoplastic
Pre-pre-T-cell (T-cell precursor)	R	+	+	+/−	−	−	−	−	−	+	−	−	T-ALL
Cortical Thymocyte I	R	+	+	−	−	−	+	−	−	+	−	−	T-ALL/LL
Cortical Thymocyte II	R	+	+	−	+/−	+	+	−	+	+	+	+	T-ALL/LL
Thymocyte Stage III	R	+	+	−	+/−	+	+	+	+	+	+ or	+	T-LL
Peripheral T-Cell	R	+	−	−	+/−	−	+	+	+	+/−	+ or	+	T-CLL, Sezary/ Mycosis fungoides, Adult T-cell leukemia/ lymphoma, peripheral T-cell lymphoma

[a]ALL, Acute lymphocytic leukemia; CLL, Chronic lymphocytic leukemia; LL, Lymphocytic leukemia.

antibodies for secretion into the blood stream. The malignant equivalents of the plasma cell are multiple myeloma and plasmocytomas, while the equivalent of the plasmacytoid lymphocyte is the plasmacytoid small lymphocytic lymphoma that is also known as Waldenstrom macroglobulinemia when it is associated with an IgM monoclonal gammopathy. This malignant disorder, however, in contrast to the other small lymphocytic lymphomas, does not express CD5.

When a mature B-lymphocyte, which expresses either κ- or λ-light chains, becomes malignant, it will give rise to a monoclonal κ- or λ-population of lymphoma cells. All of the progeny that descend from this lymphoma cell will have essentially the same markers and the monoclonality of the population will be shown by its exclusive expression of either κ- or λ-light chains on its surface. In contrast, reactive benign B-cell proliferations will be polyclonal, because they are not derived from a single parent cell. Mature B-cell neoplasms, therefore, will express B-cell lineage antigens, such as CD19, CD20, and HLADR, but also will express frequently a clonal marker in the form of κ- or λ-light chains.

The Ki-1 antigen is an activation antigen which is expressed on a variety of cell types, such as Reed-Sternberg cells of Hodgkin disease and reactive immunoblasts. Ki-1 Positive large cell lymphomas usually are of T-cell origin, although they can be of null or B-cell type (4). They usually have a typical anaplastic morphologic appearance and they frequently involve the skin. Mediastinal involvement, seen in case 1, is not characteristic of those tumors.

Approximately 85% of diffuse large cell lymphomas (DLCL) will be of B-cell, and 15% of T-cell, origin after exhaustive testing. The null cell type is unusual in the DLCLs if all the necessary phenotyping and genotyping studies are done. In the absence of light chain expression, it is not possible to determine the monoclonality of this cell population by surface marker studies. The demonstration of a unique rearrangement of the immunoglobulin JH (heavy chain) gene in the cell population, however, confirms its monoclonal origin (5). Whenever a unique band for immunoglobulin gene rearrangement is detected (by the Southern blot technique), this indicates that at least 5% of the population of cells have exactly the same pattern of rearrangement, demonstrating that they arise from the same parent cell. This is the strong evidence for monoclonality. It normally precedes the expression on the cell surface of the immunoglobulin molecule. Consequently, in order to express the heavy or light chain molecule the cell must first rearrange its corresponding JH and light chain genes (6). As a normal B-lymphocyte differentiates, the first step that occurs at the level of the pre-pre-B-cell is the rearrangement of the JH gene. As the cell further progresses to the pre-B stage, the light chain gene also is rearranged. By the time it reaches the stage of a mature B-cell, both JH and light chain genes are always rearranged (Table 17.2B).

Case 1 (continued)

The patient was referred for a full evaluation that included radiographic and laboratory studies. The radiographic studies performed included a computerized tomographic (CT) scan of the abdomen and pelvis, as well as a CT scan of the thorax. The CT scan of the thorax revealed no evidence of parenchymal lesions, an anterior mediastinal mass, but no other lymphadenopathy. The patient's abdominal CT scan was negative for any evidence of adenopathy and showed no lesions in the liver or spleen. Laboratory studies indicated that the patient's serum lactic dehydrogenase (LDH) was elevated, but otherwise there were no other significant abnormalities. The serum B-2 microglobulin was normal. The patient was referred to the thoracic surgery department for a mediastinoscopy.

Pathology Findings

*The biopsy specimen contained evidence of fibrosis and a malignant lymphocyte proliferation consistent with either large noncleaved cell lymphoma or scyncitial variant of nodular sclerosis Hodgkin disease. Immunohistochemical markers revealed the following antigens: leucocyte common antigen (LCA) positive, LeuM-1 negative, CD19 and CD20 positive, and Ki-1 negative. κ- and λ-markers were negative. A Southern blot test revealed unique JH and K light chain gene rearrangements. Thus, the patient's diagnosis is consistent with a primary **mediastinal B-cell, large cell lymphoma** with sclerosis.*

This is a well-recognized entity that occurs with more frequency in young women (7). This contrasts with most of the other intermediate grade non-Hodgkin lymphomas that are more frequent in patients >50 years old and which occur predominantly in males. Histologically and clinically, these findings can also suggest Hodgkin disease, which, in young women, is often initially seen with a mediastinal mass (8). The diagnosis often needs to be clarified by immunohistochemical markers, which in this case demonstrated a pattern consistent with a non-Hodgkin lymphoma of B-cell differentiation. The LeuM 1 marker is expected to be positive in Hodgkin disease, Ki-1 is often positive, and the LCA marker is commonly negative (9). Conversely, in non-Hodgkin lymphoma, the LCA marker should be positive and LeuM-1 usually negative. Studies for specific differentiation of B-cell lineage such as molecular rearrangement of the immunoglobulin genes further identify the tumor within the category of B-cell non-Hodgkin lymphoma.

Classification and Epidemiology

The non-Hodgkin lymphomas are not only biologically heterogenous, they can also have a variety of histologic presentations, and in accordance with this variety of histologies, also manifest different clinical courses. A unified system of classification has been used in the United States and several countries under a convention called the International Working Formulation (10) (table 17.3).

The system divides lymphomas into three subgroups according to their clinical course. These are the *low-grade, intermediate grade,* and *high-grade lymphomas.* Within these subcategories of expected clinical behavior, there are several histologic subtypes. The large cell lymphomas fall

under an intermediate category, indicating that the expected survival for patients with this disease, when they are untreated or when they fail to respond to treatment, will be of the order of months. The working formulation, however, will likely be displaced in usage by a more recently proposed classification system (11) (table 17.2B).

The intermediate grade lymphomas constitute 30–40% of all the lymphomas seen in the United States and occur across a wide range of ages. Typically, however, they have

Table 17.2B. Lymphoma Classification

B-CELL NEOPLASMS
  I. PRECURSOR B-CELL NEOPLASMS: Precursor B-lymphoblastic leukemia/lymphoma
  II. PERIPHERAL B-CELL NEOPLASM
    1. B-cell chronic lymphocytic leukemia/polymphocytic leukemia/small lymphocytic lymphoma
    2. Lymphoplasmacytoid lymphoma/immunocytoma
    3. Mantel cell lymphoma
    4. Follicle center lymphoma, follicular provisional grades: 1-(small cell) 2-(mixed) 3-(large cell) provisional subtype: diffuse, predominantly small cell type
    5. Marginal zone B-cell lymphoma extranodal (MALT-type+/− monocytoid B cells) provisional subtype: Nodal (monocytoid B cells)
    6. Provisional entity: Splenic marginal zone lymphoma (+/− villous lymphocytes)
    7. Hairy cell leukemia
    8. Plasmacytoma/plasma cell myeloma
    9. Diffuse large B-cell lymphoma subtype: Primary mediastinal B-cell lymphoma
    10. Burkitt's lymphoma
    11. Provisional entity: High grade B-cell lymphoma, Burkitt-like
T-CELL AND PUTATIVE NK-CELL NEOPLASMS:
  I. Precursor T-cell neoplasm: precursor T-lymphoblastic lymphoma/leukemia
  II. Peripheral T-cell and NK-cell neoplasms:
    1. T-cell chronic lymphocytic leukemia/polymphocytic leukemia
    2. Large granular lymphocyte leukemia
       T-cell type
       NK-cell type
    3. Mycosis fungoides/Sezary syndrome
    4. Peripheral T-cell lymphomas, unspecified
    5. Angioimmunoblastic T-cell lymphoma
    6. Angiocentric lymphoma
    7. Intestinal T-cell lymphoma (+/− enteropathy associated)
    8. Adult T-cell leukemia/lymphoma
    9. Anaplastic large cell lymphoma, CD30+, T and Null-cell types
    10. Provisional entity: Anaplastic large cell lymphoma, Hodgkin-like
HODGKIN DISEASE:
  I. Lymphocyte predominance
  II. Nodular sclerosis
  III. Mixed cellularity
  IV. Lymphocyte depletion
  V. Provisional entity: Lymphocyte-rich classical HD

a median age of between 55 and 60 years. In general, these disorders are slightly more common in males, but for unknown reasons there is a strong female preponderance in the primary mediastinal large cell lymphomas and the age is usually also younger than for the rest of the large cell lymphomas. There are no specific etiologic factors known, although usually lymphomas appear to be more frequent in patients who live in areas where pesticides are used heavily, industries where organic chemicals are used (such as solvents in the dry cleaning industry, and petrochemical processing), postirradiation, and in immunosuppressed patients (12–15).

Staging and Prognosis

The currently accepted **staging** system for the non-Hodgkin lymphomas is the Ann Arbor staging system (16) (table 17.4). The system was originally devised for the staging of Hodgkin disease and it takes into consideration the anatomic distribution of disease. The non-Hodgkin lymphomas, however, do not spread b anatomic continuity, as the Hodgkin lymphomas more predictably do. This staging system is therefore not as clinically useful in predicting prognosis in non Hodgkin lymphoma. A number of investigators have attempted to arrive at more useful prognostic models (17–19). Several other factors that have been found to be of prognostic importance include: (a) the size of the tumor mass; (b) the level of the serum LDH; (c) the number of extranodal sites involved; (d) the patient's age; and (e) the patients serum β2-microglobulin level. By the Ann Arbor classification

Table 17.3. Working Formulation of Non-Hodgkin Lymphoma for Clinical Use

Low grade
  A. Malignant lymphoma, small lymphocytic, consistent with chronic lymphocytic leukemia, plasmacytoid
  B. Malignant lymphoma, follicular, predominantly small cleaved cell, diffuse areas of sclerosis
  C. Malignant lymphoma, follicular, mixed, small cleaved and large cell, diffuse areas of sclerosis

Intermediate grade
  D. Malignant lymphoma, follicular, predominantly large cell, diffuse areas of sclerosis
  E. Malignant lymphoma, diffuse small cleaved cell
  F. Malignant lymphoma, diffuse, mixed, small and large cell, sclerosis, epithelioid cell component
  G.[a] Malignant lymphoma, diffuse large cell, cleaved cell, non-cleaved cell, sclerosis

High grade
  H. Malignant lymphoma, large cell, immunoblastic, plasmacytoid, clear cell, polymorphous, epithelioid cell component
  I. Malignant lymphoma, lymphoblastic, convoluted cell, non-convoluted cell
  J. Malignant lymphoma, small non-cleaved cell, Burkitt follicular areas

[a]Most frequently seen histologic subtypes.

Table 17.4. Ann Arbor Staging Definitions

Stage I

I	Involvement of a single lymph node region (I) or a single extralymphatic organ or site (I_E)
II	Involvement of two or more lymph node regions on the same side of the diaphragm (II) or localized involvement of an extralymphatic organ or site (II_E)
III	Involvement of lymph node regions on both sides of the diaphragm (III) or localized involvement of an extralymphatic organ or site (III_E) or spleen (III_S) or both (III_{SE})
IV	Diffuse or disseminated involvement of one or more extralymphatic organs with or without associated lymph node involvement

[a]Asymptomatic
[b]Fever, sweats, loss of 10% of body weight

system, the patient described in case 1 has stage IA disease, and thus would have a very favorable prognosis category. By other tumor system classifications, however, the large size of the tumor in the mediastinum and the elevated level of the serum LDH would not place the patient in such a favorable category.

Treatment

The treatment of lymphomas depends on the histologic diagnosis, and therefore the initial step of diagnosis with appropriate histologic and immunohistochemical evaluation is critical. A laboratory that is able to do further studies, such as molecular analysis, can also be extremely helpful. In the case of the patient described in case 1, the most critical decision was the differentiation between Hodgkin and non-Hodgkin lymphomas, which might be treated quite differently.

Within the non-Hodgkin lymphomas the definition of the patient's illness as an intermediate grade is also important. The intermediate grade lymphomas can be curable with several currently available chemotherapeutic regimens (20–23). However, there is controversy as to which regimens are the most effective. What is undisputed is that all effective regimens for the management of these lymphomas should at least contain the drugs cyclophosphamide, doxorubicin, vincristine, and corticosteroids (24). Drugs that are also effective against these tumors and that have been added in various ways to different regimens include bleomycin, etoposide, methotrexate with or without leucovorin rescue, and arabinoside. Other drugs that are also effective against lymphomas and that are being explored for front-line regimens at this time include ifosfamide, novantrone, and cisplatin, the latter in synergy with arabinoside (25).

Case 2

The patient, a 65-year-old man, presented to his doctor for a routine physical examination. He had noted swollen lymph nodes in his neck waxing and waning for several years but was completely asymptomatic. On physical examination, the findings of note were multiple small lymph nodes ranging in size from 1–2 cm, palpable in cervical, axillary, and inguinal areas. The patient had no palpable splenomegaly.

Differential Diagnoses

In this patient with a history of small lymph nodes waxing and waning over a long period of time, a low-grade lymphoma is the most likely diagnosis. If the disease has been present for a long period of time, histologic transformation could have taken place. If a lymph node has exhibited recent rapid growth or if there is a lymph node that is clearly much larger than other adenopathy, this should be selected for a biopsy. Benign reactive adenopathy is unlikely because the adenopathy is diffuse, and an infectious etiology is also unlikely since there is a chronic or longstanding history of diffuse adenopathy without other systemic symptoms.

Background on Low-Grade B-Cell Lymphomas

Practically all of the follicular lymphomas, as well as 95% of the small lymphocytic lymphomas, are of mature B-cell derivation. These disorders express surface immunoglobulin with light chain restriction in a large proportion of the cases. As expected, both JH and light chain genes are usually rearranged. HLADR, CD19, and CD20 are uniformly positive in these disorders. CD10 is also expressed in the majority of the follicular low-grade lymphomas. The coexpression of pan-B antibodies such as CD19 and CD20, together with SIg and CD10, are typical of mature follicular center B-cells (see discussion of case 1). The most characteristic biologic finding in follicular low-grade lymphoma is the cytogenetic translocation t(14;18) (q32;q21) (26). Approximately 85% of these disorders will show this translocation by classic cytogenetics.

The site on chromosome 14 involved in this translocation is precisely the locus where the heavy chain immunoglobulin gene resides. The locus affected in chromosome 18 is the gene region called bcl-2 (27–29). This gene is usually rearranged in cases of follicular lymphoma, particularly if they show the t(14;18). Since this translocation juxtaposes the JH gene with the bcl-2 gene, it is assumed that this process takes place at the time that the B lymphocyte rearranges its JH genes.

The translocation (14;18) has been attributed to an error during the normal process of JH rearrangement, which instead of taking place within the JH gene in chromosome 14, mistakenly joins the JH region with another gene in another chromosome (in this instance with bcl-2 in chromosome 18). The fact that light chain rearrangement normally follows heavy chain rearrangement would imply that, if the t(14;18) translocation occurred at the pre-pre-B stage, then multiple light chain rearrangements would occur in a follicular lymphoma. The fact that only one light chain rearrangement is usually present suggests that t(14;18) translocation might actually occur at a later stage in maturation, following light chain rearrangement. However, it is also possible that the t(14;18) occurs early and that multiple clones with different light chain rearrangements also occur but do not necessarily impart a malignant phenotype to the cell. Perhaps other genetic changes are necessary for this cell with the t(14;18) translocation to become truly malignant. This hypothesis is supported by recent evidence that "benign" tonsils removed from children have been found to frequently contain several rearranged bcl-2 clones when examined by PCR technology (30). If this indeed is the case, then the bcl-2 gene rearrangement cannot be considered sufficient to produce a malignant cell.

The normal function of this gene is currently thought to be related to inhibition of programmed cell death ("apoptosis") (31). When bcl-2 is activated, as in the event of its juxtaposition with the JH gene, it would inhibit cell death, thus resulting in prolonged cell life without necessarily imparting a malignant potential to the cell. Again, this latter phenomenon most likely requires other genetic changes.

From the practical standpoint, the t(14;18) can be detected by molecular genetic studies using the Southern blot or polymerase chain reaction techniques (32). Probes are available for the most common bcl-2 breakpoints. Using these probes in conjunction with a JH probe, one can determine: (a) if there is a JH rearrangement that would indicate a monoclonal B-cell derivation; (b) if there is a bcl-2 rearrangement that would also indicate monoclonality as well as structural alteration of this gene; (c) if there is comigration of the JH and bcl-2 rearranged genes. The latter would indicate the probable juxtaposition of these two genes in the same DNA fragment, which would be an indication of the existence of a t(14;18). If such is identified, this would be acceptable evidence of the presence of this translocation, and cytogenetic studies would not be necessary to show it.

Case 2 (continued)

The patient had a chest x-ray as well as a CT scan of the abdomen and pelvis, a lymphangiogram, and bilateral bone marrow biopsies. The chest x-ray demonstrated no evidence of lymphadenopathy or other abnormalities. CT scan of the abdomen and pelvis showed some minimally enlarged lymph nodes throughout the paraortic and pelvic areas. The lymphangiogram showed diffusely enlarged lymph nodes with abnormal architecture in the pelvis and paraortic areas (fig. 17.2). Bone marrow biopsy showed that there were multiple paratrabecular

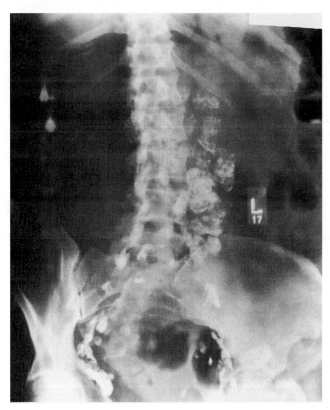

Figure 17.2. (Case 2) Lymphangiogram study showing enlarged and "foamy" appearance in pelvic and paraaortic nodes in a patient with follicular small cleaved cell lymphoma.

phomas (small and large cells). Histologically, the low-grade classification indicates a more differentiated morphologic appearance compared with the lymphomas of higher grade. The follicular lymphomas have retained the configuration of the normal germinal follicles, although normal lymphocytes are replaced by the aberrant malignant population (fig. 17.3). The follicular lymphomas are of B-cell origin, as their normal counterparts, i.e., the lymphocytes originating in the follicle, are B-cells. The small lymphocytic lymphomas arise in the cortex of the lymph nodes (outside of the germinal follicles), and although also predominantly of B-cell type, can also be of T-cell type. The small lymphocytic lymphomas, as opposed to the follicular lymphomas, do not have a cleaved appearance to the nucleus and, as expected, are diffuse in architecture because they don't arise from the germinal follicle. The phenomenon of histologic transformation occurs in at least 30% of low-grade lymphomas, with an average time from diagnosis to transformation of 5–7 years. In addition to a change in the histologic appearance of the cells, transformation also denotes a change in the biologic behavior of the tumor as supported by a rise in the S phase of the cells. It can be considered as dedifferentiation of the malignant cells.

foci of lymphocytic cells which appeared abnormal. The lymphocytic nodules constituted approximately 20% of the surface area of the cellular bone marrow. Other laboratory studies were done and these were within normal limits except for CBC with a hemoglobin level of 110 g/L and an elevated β2-microglobulin level of 4. The patient was referred to a surgeon for biopsy of a peripheral lymph node.

Pathology Findings

*On histologic examination the lymph node demonstrated a pattern of **follicular small cleaved cell lymphoma**, with immunohistochemical findings positive for monoclonal cell surface light chain restriction (κ), CD10, CD19, CD20, and HLADR expression. Flow cytometric analysis of the cells showed a low S phase, a normal DNA index, and normal RNA index. Southern blot revealed JH rearrangement as well as bcl-2 rearrangement. There was comigration of the rearranged genes.*

Diagnosis/Classification

The low-grade lymphomas in the working formulation consisted of the small lymphocytic lymphomas, follicular small cleaved cell lymphomas, and follicular mixed lym-

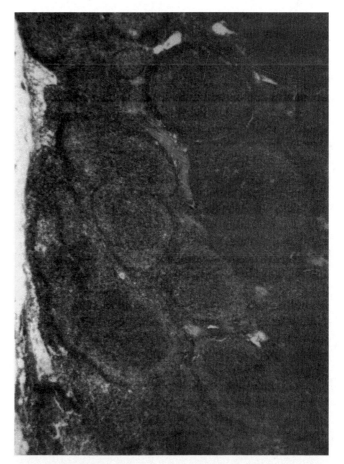

Figure 17.3. (Case 2) Histologic appearance of a follicular small cleaved cell lymphoma, where the underlying architecture of the previously normal follicles can still be appreciated.

Epidemiology

The low-grade lymphomas can occur at any age, but predominantly occur in older individuals. The median age is between 55 and 60 years of age (33). It is unusual for this process to occur in patients <30 years of age. Similarly to the intermediate grade lymphomas, there is no specific etiologic agent identified. Because the patients are frequently asymptomatic, occasionally they may remain undiagnosed until after they die of an unrelated illness. Most frequently, they are diagnosed when the disease is already disseminated. Overall, there is a slight predominance of females in this cell type compared with the large cell lymphomas.

Staging/Prognosis

The staging system used in the low-grade lymphomas is also the Ann Arbor system (16). Most patients at the time of diagnosis will have stage IV disease, predominantly with bone marrow involvement. A small subset of patients, however, will have limited disease, and it is important to define this subset of patients. A careful staging workup should therefore be done in all patients. The Ann Arbor system is helpful in defining a difference in overall survival as well as a pattern of disease- free survival between limited stage disease (I and II) versus extensive disease (III and IV). Within each of these stages, however, there are patients who manifest very aggressive disease. Attempts have been made, therefore, to define better prognostic indicators than the Ann Arbor system alone can. Factors that are known to bear significantly on the patient outcome include age, gender, tumor mass bulk, extent of bone marrow involvement, as well as the serum level of β2-microglobulin (34, 35).

Treatment

The treatment for the low-grade lymphomas is extremely controversial. There is no consensus as to which is the best approach for patients with stage IV presentations. These lymphomas are sensitive to a broad spectrum of chemotherapeutic agents, singly or in combinations. Irrespective of the treatment used, there has been a consistent trend for the median disease-free interval of these cases to fall between 1.5 and 3 years, and the survival also has consistently ranged from 5–9 years. The management options have ranged from "watch-and-wait," or observation without therapy until there is evidence of disease progression (enough to cause symptoms), to aggressive high-dose chemotherapy with bone marrow transplantation (36, 37). The reason for this controversy lies in the fact that in contrast to the large cell lymphomas, the stage IV low-grade lymphomas have not been shown to be curable with any of the current therapeutic approaches. This does not necessarily mean that they are fundamentally incurable. Whenever possible, these patients should be treated under

investigational protocols, aimed at developing such a curative approach. Recently, maintenance α-interferon has been shown to prolong the duration of complete responses of patients with stage IV low-grade lymphomas, after initial treatment with the combination regimen CHOP-Bleo (cyclophosphamide, doxorubicin, vincristine, prednisone, and bleomycin) (38). This observation is interesting in view of the frequent spontaneous remissions that occur in the low-grade lymphomas. This might indicate an important role for the host's immune mechanisms in controlling the growth of these tumor types. Whether α-interferon will result in a cured fraction of patients will have to await further followup since late relapses are very common in these cell types.

Because of the controversy of the "watch-and-wait" (W&W) approach, a randomized study was designed at the (U.S.) National Cancer Institute to compare this concept with an intensive approach, using a combination of drugs designated ProMACE-MOPP (prednisone, methotrexate, doxorubicin, cyclophosphamide, etoposide, nitrogen mustard, and procarbazine) plus total nodal radiation for patients with stage III–IV low-grade lymphomas (39). At a median followup of 50 months, 44% of the patients in the W&W arm have already required therapy, but only 43% of them have been able to obtain a complete response (CR); of the latter, only 71% remain in CR. The therapy used for the patients in the W&W arm at the time they progressed was the same used in the other arm of the study (ProMACE-MOPP and XRT). On the other hand, of the patients treated from the beginning on the ProMACE-MOPP arm, 78% have achieved CR and 86% of those remain in CR. According to the authors, the quality of life of the patients on the W&W arm who have required therapy has been poor in comparison to that of the ProMACE-MOPP-treated patients. Many of the former have needed almost continuous therapy, because, once treatment was required, their CR rate was low. So far, survival has not been different for the two arms of the study, but longer followup is necessary to determine whether aggressive therapy will affect this parameter.

Data on stage III low-grade lymphomas is very scarce, because most of the published series make no distinction between this stage and stage IV. Three series in the literature have indicated that the use of either radiation alone (total nodal) or radiation plus chemotherapy can result in 40–55% long-term (>5 years) disease-free survival (DSF) with an apparent plateau in the curve, suggesting the possibility that these patients might be cured (40–42). These data suggest that patients with stage III disease should receive particular attention, and that they should not be handled with the W&W approach or with minimal therapy.

Stage I–II presentations of low-grade lymphoma are also uncommon. Several studies, most of which are retrospective, have been published. Again, either radiation alone or with chemotherapy has yielded disease-free survivals beyond 5 years, ranging from 37–64%, with the best results associated with the combined modality management (43–47). A plateau in the DFS curve suggests again the likelihood of cure for these patients in the early stages.

Case 3

The patient, a 17-year-old male with a history of cough of approximately 2 weeks' duration, increasing shortness of breath, and facial swelling noted for 2 days prior to presentation to the emergency room. On physical examination, the notable findings were facial edema, prominence of the neck veins, and prominence of chest wall veins. The patient had rare wheezes on auscultation of the chest and his cardiac heart sounds were distant. There was no palpable lymphadenopathy or hepatosplenomegaly.

Differential Diagnosis

The presence of a large mediastinal mass and symptoms of superior vena cava compression are consistent with a rapidly growing tumor. The likely diagnosis in a male patient of this age group includes lymphoma, mediastinal germ cell tumor, or malignant thymoma. Hodgkin disease is a possibility, although it would be very unusual that it would present with superior vena cava syndrome. This clinical presentation indicates an urgency for diagnosis, and the priority is to obtain cytologic or histologic material for definitive diagnosis.

Background on T-Cell Lymphoid Differentiation

The T-cell lymphomas can be divided into mature and immature types in a way analogous to the B-cell lymphomas (see discussion of case 1) (3). The normal process of T-cell differentiation, however, proceeds in a different way. The first event is thought also to occur in the bone marrow and consists of rearrangement of the T-cell receptor gene (table 17.1B). Once their T-cell receptor genes rearrange, these lymphocytes migrate to the thymic cortex, where they have the morphologic appearance of lymphoblasts. They express TdT, CD45, CD2, and CD7 positivity. The third step in T-cell differentiation, which generates the cortical thymocyte II, involves the expression of CD1, CD3, as well as the simultaneous expression of CD4, and CD8 (helper and cytotoxic/suppressor T-cell markers). However, this cell is still not considered a mature helper or suppressor T-cell. It will have to lose the expression of both TdT and either CD4 or CD8, preserving only one of these latter two, before it can be considered a differentiated helper or suppressor cytotoxic T-cell. The next step is development of the thymocyte stage III, and consists of deletion of either CD4 or CD8, deletion of CD1, but preservation of TdT. As the cells proceed to lose their TdT positivity, they then leave the thymus to become mature "peripheral T-cells," in contrast to the immature "central or thymic" T-cells. The thymic T-cells,

which include all of the T-cells generated during the various different maturation steps inside the thymus, can become malignant at any of these points. Malignant transformation of any of these thymic cells would give rise to either a T-cell acute lymphoblastic leukemia or a T-cell lymphoblastic lymphoma (table 17.1B). Both of these would be considered as immature T-cell malignancies. Their cell surface markers would correspond to the level of differentiation at which the cell became malignant. Unlike B-cell lymphomas, the T-cell malignancies do not express any cell surface markers of clonality. In order to confirm monoclonal origin, it would be necessary to perform a Southern blot on tumor-derived DNA, using a probe for at least one of the genes coding for the T-cell receptor molecule. Similarly to the immunoglobulin molecule, the T-cell receptor (TCR) molecule is composed of separate chains that are coded by discontinuous genes. These genes are combined by rearrangement during the early differentiating stages of the T-cells. The T-cell receptor chains, designated T alpha (Tα), T beta (Tβ), T gamma (Tγ), and T delta (Tδ), are uniquely combined to generate antigenic determinant diversity. Thus, if a malignancy arises from a cell that manifests its own unique rearrangement, the clonal population of malignant cells will all share this same pattern of rearrangement. Again, as is the case for immunoglobulins, the detection of a unique band on a Southern blot analysis for one of the TCR chains indicates clonality in at least 5% of the cells in the sample tested (48, 49). T-Cell receptor gene rearrangement studies are usually not necessary in practice to confirm the existence of a lymphoblastic lymphoma because of its very distinct immature morphologic appearance (50). However, they could be important tests in the peripheral T-cell lymphomas, where the malignant T-cells appear mature, and are difficult to distinguish from reactive lymphocytes.

Case 3 (continued)

The patient was evaluated further with a chest x-ray that demonstrated a large mediastinal mass, small pleural effusions, and an enlarged cardiac silhouette. He was hospitalized and underwent additional workup. Laboratory studies showed a normal CBC, an elevated serum LDH, but otherwise normal chemistry profile. An echocardiogram demonstrated a moderate pericardial effusion, without compromise of cardiac function. Lateral decubitus films showed a free-flowing effusion in the right pleural space. A thoracentesis was performed.

Pathology Findings

The thoracentesis fluid demonstrated the following: protein in the fluid was elevated at 5 g/dl; glucose was decreased; LDH was elevated; and pH was 7.3. The cell count demonstrated a predominance of lymphocytes with convoluted nuclei that on cytologic spin appeared malignant. The immunohistochemical characteristics of these cells showed the following: TDT (+), CD 7 (+),

CD2 (+), CD 3 and CD 4 (−), CD 8 (−). Other markers analyzed included CD 10 (cALLa) (−) and CD 20 (B1) (−). Surface immunoglobulins were likewise negative. Gene rearrangement studies revealed a rearranged Tβ receptor gene with germ line (not rearranged) JH gene. Flow cytometry showed an S phase of 16%, with a DNA index of 1.5.

Diagnosis/Classification

In this case, the expression of CD2, CD3, CD7, and TdT with absence of CD4, CD8, CD3, and CD10 would correspond to the cortical thymocyte I level, the most immature type of all the thymocytes and thus consistent with a lymphoblastic lymphoma. The negative expression of CD20, a pan-B antigen, confirms its T-cell nature. The rearrangement of Tβ-receptor gene confirms its monoclonal derivation.

Patients with lymphoblastic lymphoma have a very different clinical presentation and behavior from those with peripheral T-cell lymphoma. The latter are malignancies of the mature T-cells and usually express either CD4 or CD8 (but not both) and are negative for TdT. Because they arise from immature T-cells originating from the thymus, lymphoblastic lymphomas will frequently present with a large anterior mediastinal mass that compresses the superior vena cava (as in case 3). This is very uncommon in the peripheral T-cell lymphomas, in which peripheral lymphadenopathy, splenic, and skin involvement are more common. This reflects the fact that the mature T-cell is a circulating blood cell. The frequent leukemic involvement of the bone marrow in lymphoblastic lymphoma (in which case it could be called "acute lymphoblastic leukemia" [ALL]) probably reflects the immature nature of the cell and its close proximity to the T-cell precursor, which originates from the bone marrow. In general, lymphoblastic lymphoma occurs in young patients with a median age in the second decade, while the peripheral T-cell lymphomas occur in an older patient population with median age in the sixth decade.

The lymphoblastic lymphomas are classified as high grade by the working formulation (10). The nucleic acid flow cytometry findings in this patient revealed an S phase of 16% and DNA index of 1.5. This high S phase is consonant with the high-grade nature of this lymphoma. Usually low-grade lymphomas have an S phase ranging from 1–5%, intermediate grade lymphomas from 6–14%, and high-grade >15%. The S phase reflects the percentage of all the cells undergoing DNA synthesis at a given point (51). The DNA index of 1.5 means that the malignant cells are hyperdiploid. Diploid cells have a DNA index of 1.0. Aneuploidy is characteristic of intermediate and high-grade lymphoma and reflects the abnormal genetic features of these malignancies.

Treatment

Lymphoblastic Lymphoma

Advances in the treatment of patients with lymphoblastic lymphoma are due in part to the recognition that this illness is very similar to ALL. The key elements to the success of the treatment schemas in ALL appear to be aggressive systemic chemotherapy consisting of induction, consolidation and possibly maintenance phases, and prophylactic chemotherapy to the central nervous system.

The largest published series of patients was from Memorial Sloan Kettering Hospital (52). The study described their experience over 15 years treating lymphoblastic lymphoma in the same protocols used for acute lymphoblastic leukemia. The distinctive components of their regimen design were aggressive induction, followed by aggressive consolidation, and a long maintenance phase with multiple drugs that lasted for 3 years. Patients received intrathecal methotrexate via an Ommaya reservoir, and radiotherapy was added to primary sites presenting with large masses. Fifty-one patients with lymphoblastic lymphoma were treated. There was no difference in the groups that presented with extensive bone marrow involvement, defined as >25% of bone marrow involvement by lymphoblastic cells, versus patients who did not have such a presentation. The complete remission in leukemic versus nonleukemic groups was 77% and 80%, respectively. There was no difference in the overall survival or disease-free survival at 5 years. Disease-free survival for these groups was 60% and 75%, respectively.

Several features that were identified in this study to designate a poor prognostic category included age >30 years, WBC >10 × 10⁹/L cells at presentation, and a prolonged time to accomplish remission (>4 weeks). Patients who did not accomplish complete remission during the induction phase had a median survival of only 9 months. Other investigators have described an elevated LDH level and the presence of central nervous system or bone marrow involvement as negative prognostic factors as well (53). For young patients in good performance status, allogenic bone marrow transplantation should be considered similarly to cases of acute lymphoblastic leukemia, either at first remission for those presenting with poor prognostic characteristics, or at second remission for those who relapse.

Case 4

The patient, a 20-year-old female, presented to her physician with a complaint of right lower quadrant pain, and a palpable right inguinal mass. She noted a small lump 3 days prior to her visit to the physician, but this lump had nearly doubled in size since she first noted it. She had not had any significant change in her body weight, had regular menses, and her only other complaint besides pain was constipation. Her physical examination results were significant for a right inguinal mass measuring 5 cm, and on pelvic examination had an ad-nexal mass in the right pelvis. She had active bowel sounds and guaiac- negative stool in the rectal vault.

Differential Diagnoses

In a young female, a right pelvic mass that is rapidly grow-ing could indicate a high-grade lymphoma, a germ cell tumor, sarcoma, or Wilms tumor. A definitive diagnosis is critical for appropriate management and must be done quickly given the rapid evolution of the patient's symptoms and findings.

Background on High-Grade B-Cell Lymphoma

The high-grade lymphomas of B-cell phenotype show im-mature markers as discussed in case 1. The classic example of this subset of malignancies is Burkitt lymphoma. The most characteristic finding in Burkitt lymphoma from the biologic standpoint is the presence of the T(8;14) trans-location (54). A small fraction of cases (approximately 10–20%) have either the variant translocations t(2;8) or t(8;22). The breakpoints in chromosomes 14, 2, and 22 contain the genes that code for JH, κ-, and λ-light chains, respectively. Lymphomas with the t(8;22) translocation have consistently been shown to be of the λ- light chain phenotype, while those with the t(2;8) translocation have proven to be of the κ-phenotype (55). Those with the t(8;14), where the breakpoint involves the JH in chromo-some 14, but do not specifically affect the light chain im-munoglobulin gene region, have shown roughly an equal distribution between κ- and λ-phenotypes.

Chromosome 8 is consistently involved in both the typi-cal as well as in the variant Burkitt lymphoma chromoso-mal translocations. The region consistently affected in chromosome 8 is band q24, which contains the C-myc oncogene (27). As a likely result of the juxtaposition of the C-myc oncogene with an immunoglobulin gene, activation of C-myc and deregulation of transcription occurs, leading to increased amounts of C-myc protein production. In the t(8;14) translocation, C-myc is always translocated from chromosome 8 to chromosome 14 and is frequently trun-cated, leading to a rearrangement of its DNA sequences, which can be detected by Southern blot analysis. The in-volvement of the C-myc oncogene is thought to be related to the high S phase that these tumors exhibit, since it ap-pears to play an important role in activating the entry of cells into reproductive cycle. This biologic observation is consistent with the very aggressive nature of this malignant neoplasm.

Case 4 (continued)

With a history of a rapidly growing mass, pain, and con-stipation, the primary concern was bowel obstruction due to mass. The patient was hospitalized for diagnostic

workup. A surgical consultation was obtained, and a biopsy of the right inguinal mass was done. Radi-ographic studies included the following: an obstructive bowel series, which showed dilated bowel loops, no de-finitive obstruction, or perforation; a CT scan of the ab-domen and pelvis which was positive for a large pelvic mass probably involving bowel, ovary, and uterus, dila-tion of the right ureter, inguinal and paraaortic adenopa-thy; chest x-ray is unremarkable. Laboratory studies were significant for elevated serum LDH and uric acid levels; creatinine and blood urea nitrogen (BUN) levels remained normal. HIV titers were negative. An upper gastrointestinal (GI) study with small bowel fol-lowthrough showed mass effect in the right lower quad-rant. Barium enema showed narrowing of the cecum.

Pathology Findings

*The biopsy specimen showed a monotonous diffuse malignant lymphoid proliferation of round cells, with basophilic staining of cytoplasm, cytoplasmic vacuoles, and a starry sky pattern typical of **Burkitt lymphoma** (fig. 17.4).*

Immunohistochemical stains CD19, CD20, CD22, and HLA-D12 were all positive. CD5 was negative. Surface

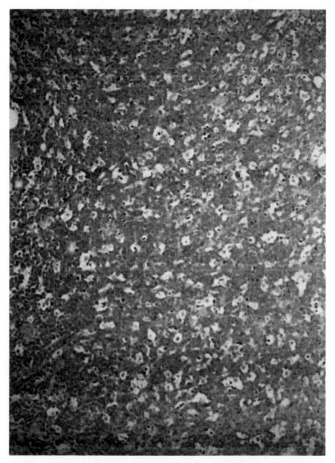

Figure 17.4. (Case 4) Histologic appearance of "starry sky" pat-tern in small non-cleaved cell lymphoma (Burkitt).

immunoglobulins were positive for IgM and κ. Cytogenetic studies revealed a t(8;14) (q14;q32). Flow cytometry showed an S phase of 30% with a DNA index of 1.2.

Diagnosis/Classification

The immunophenotype of this patient is typical of an early B-cell. Burkitt lymphomas are always of B-cell derivation and usually exhibit an immature phenotype (see discussion of case 1 and table 17.1). Frequently these disorders will be leukemic, a finding that is not surprising in view of the immature nature of the cells that have given origin to this lymphoma. It is a small noncleaved cell lymphoma classified as a high-grade malignancy by the working formulation, and the high S phase by flow cytometry is consistent with this classification (table 17.2). Histologically, not all small noncleaved cell lymphomas will show the "starry sky" pattern attributed to Burkitt lymphoma. There is no difference, however, between the clinical behavior of those that are designated "Burkitt" and those called non-Burkitt (56).

Staging

Although several staging systems have been used for Burkitt lymphoma, the classic staging system is that devised by Ziegler at the National Cancer Institute (57) (table 17.5). One study that compared the Ann Arbor system to Ziegler's system for prognostic significance found no major difference between them (58).

Epidemiology

In 1958 Burkitt first described the clinical entity that now bears his name (59, 60). He described a malignant disease that typically developed in the mandibular lymph nodes of children living in the areas of Africa in which malaria was endemic. After the original description of this lymphoma by Burkitt, the entity became recognized in multiple geographically diverse sites. The presentation of this illness outside of Africa has been termed nonendemic. Although the patients in Africa presented predominantly with adenopathies in the head and neck area, outside of Africa, and specifically in the United States, the adenopathy more commonly presents in the abdomen and other nodal sites outside of the head and neck area (57).

Table 17.5. Staging of Burkitt Lymphoma

Stage	Extent of Tumor
A	Single extraabdominal site
B	Multiple extraabdominal sites
C	Intraabdominal tumor
D	Intraabdominal tumor with involvement of ≥1 extraabdominal sites
AR	Stage C but with >90% of tumor surgically resected

Because of its peculiar geographic distribution in Africa, Burkitt had proposed that the illness could have a relationship with an unidentified infectious organism. A few years later, Epstein and his coworkers demonstrated the presence of a virus now known as the Epstein-Barr virus (EBV), in a cell line derived from a patient's lymphoma (61). EBV subsequently was found to be a B-cell tropic virus. Although this virus was hypothesized to be the underlying cause of Burkitt lymphoma, current molecular genetic studies actually have not conclusively demonstrated that the virus *causes* any specific genetic defect in the tumor cells.

More recent work has shown that patients who have malaria have underlying immune defects in their T-cell function (62). The co-incidence of malaria and Burkitt lymphoma could thus be explained on the basis of impaired T-cell immunity, leading to disregulated growth of EBV infected B-cells. EBV-related B-cell malignancies have been more recently described in patients who are immunosuppressed for various reasons, such as pharmacologically induced immunosuppression after renal or cardiac transplant, patients with inherited immune deficiency syndromes, and patients with AIDS from HIV infection (62–65).

Treatment

The chemotherapeutic agent cyclophosphamide has long been recognized as a active agent in the treatment of Burkitt lymphoma. Burkitt reported a series of cases with a possible cure in African children after one or two cycles of treatment with the drug (66). In the United States, patients with Burkitt lymphoma appeared to demonstrate overall a lower rate of cure with cyclophosphamide alone. Ziegler acknowledged that this difference was due principally to the more extensive presentation in the American cases. If survival was compared according to equivalent stages, results for both endemic African Burkitt lymphoma and nonendemic North American cases were similar (57).

The literature concerning the treatment of Burkitt lymphoma is largely focused on pediatric patients, since this disease is uncommon in adults. The National Cancer Institute (NCI) pioneered the treatment of Burkitt lymphoma by a multiagent chemotherapy program (55). In the original NCI protocol, 54 patients with Burkitt lymphoma were treated with a combination of cyclophosphamide, vincristine and methotrexate, with intrathecal methotrexate for prophylaxis against CNS recurrence, plus or minus prednisolone. The results demonstrated that in patients with stages designated A, B, and AR, the actuarial survival was 80% at 3 years, whereas for patients with stages C and D, the rate dropped to only 40%. For all patients combined, the overall survival rate was in the order of 50%.

Treatment strategies for adult patients have successively modified the original NCI strategy by addition of new chemotherapeutic agents and intensification of doses.

Stanford University Medical Center added doxorubicin and radiotherapy in a treatment program for adult patients (67). The characteristics that they recognized as indicators of poor prognosis in their patients included unresected tumor masses with bulk of >10 cm, pretreatment serum lactic dehydrogenase levels ≥500 IU/L (normal 200), or involvement of the CNS or bone marrow. Patients with these features had a projected disease free survival of 20% compared with 100% for patients who did not.

The largest published series of adult patients (44 cases) is from M. D. Anderson Cancer Center, in which an aggressive strategy of alternating chemotherapy regimens was used (58). The drugs etoposide, ifosfamide, arabinoside, and bleomycin were included, in addition to the drugs in the Stanford regimen. Results showed an excellent disease-free survival of 95% at 5 years for patients with Ziegler stages AR, A, B, or C. The series included 12 patients with HIV-positive serology. Patients with Ziegler stage D, however, still did poorly, with a disease-free survival rate of only 29%.

A recent study from Vanderbilt University selected patients with poor prognosis features, such as masses >10 cm, multiple extranodal sites, and poor performance status, for treatment with very dose-intensive drug combinations (68). The treatment required inpatient hospital management for all patients and had a treatment-related mortality of 10%. The results, however, were encouraging, given the selection of patient with poor prognosis. In 20 cases, the disease-free survival rate was 65%, with a calculated 5-year actuarial disease-free survival of 60%. Summarizing the observations from these studies, it is clear that there are subsets of patients with Burkitt disease who have extremely poor prognoses and in whom intensive treatment is appropriate. The cure fraction for patients who do not present with these features, however, is extremely good, with previously published combination chemotherapy regimens.

> For all the high-grade lymphomas, attention must be paid to the possibility of a tumor lysis syndrome, i.e., rapid tumor cell death resulting in hyperuricemia and thereby renal failure (69). In some patients, such as the patient in case 4, uric acid may already be elevated at presentation due to high cell turnover. It is recommended that patients be placed on Allopurinol prior to starting their first cycle of treatment and during that cycle of therapy. Electrolytes should be carefully observed at least twice daily, and hydration and urine alkalinization are recommended. If tumor lysis does occur, aggressive management of the renal failure with renal dialysis is indicated, since most patients do recover from the insult.

REFERENCES

1. Lukes RJ, Collins RD. Immunological characterization of human malignant lymphoma. Cancer 1974;34:1488–1503.
2. Foon KA, Todd RF. Immunologic classification of leukemia and lymphoma. Blood 1986;68:1–31.
3. Freedman AS, Nadler LM. Immunologic markers in non–Hodgkin's lymphoma. Hematol Oncol Clin N Am 1991; 5:871–889.
4. Agnarsson BA, Kadin ME. Ki-1 positive large cell lymphoma: a morphologic and immunologic study of 19 cases. Am J Surg Pathol 124:264–274.
5. Arnold A, Cossman J, Bakhshi A, et al. Immunoglobulin-gene rearrangements as unique clonal markers in human lymphoid neoplasms. N Engl J Med 1983;309: 1593–1599.
6. Korsmeyer SJ, Hieter PA, Ravetch JV, et al. Developmental hierarchy in immunoglobulin gene rearrangements in human leukemic pre-B cells. Proc Natl Acad Sci USA 1981; 78:7096–7100.
7. Levitt LJ, Ainsenberg AC, Harris NL, et al. Primary non-Hodgkin's lymphoma of the mediastinum. Cancer 1982;50: 2486–2492.
8. Kaplan HS. Hodgkin's disease. Cambridge, MA: Harvard University Press, 1972.
9. Hsu SM, Yang K, Jaffe ES. Phenotypic expression of Hodgkin's and Reed-Sternberg cells in Hodgkin's disease. Am J Pathol 1985;118:209–217.
10. The Non-Hodgkin's Lymphoma Pathologic Classification Project: National Cancer Institute sponsored study of classifications of non-Hodgkin's lymphomas: summary and description of a working formulation for clinical usage. Cancer 1982;49:2112–2135.
11. Harris NL, Jaffe ES, Stein H, et al. A revised European-American classification of lymphoid neoplasms: a proposal from the International Lymphoma Study Group. Blood 1994;84:1361–1392.
12. Ziegler JL, Beckstead JA, Volberding PA, et al. Non-Hodgkin's lymphoma in 90 homosexual men. N Engl J Med 1984;311:565–370.
13. Hardell L, Eriksson M, Lennet P, et. al. Malignant lymphoma and exposure to chemicals especially organic solvents chlorophenols and phenoxy acids: a case control study. Br J Cancer 1981;43:169–171.
14. Cantor KP. Farming and mortality from non-Hodgkin's lymphoma: a case control study. Int J Cancer 1982;29: 239–247.
15. Finch SC. Leukaemia and lymphoma in atomic bomb survivors. In: Boice JD, Fraumeni JF, eds. Radiation carcinogenesis: epidemiology and biological significance. New York: Raven Press, 1984;37–44.
16. Carbone P, Kaplan H, Musshoff K, et al. Report of the committee on Hodgkin's disease staging. Cancer Res 1971;31: 1860–1861.
17. Swan F, Velasquez WS, Tucker S, et al. A new serologic staging system for large cell lymphomas based on initial beta-2-microglobulin and lactate dehydrogenase levels. J Clin Oncol 1989;7(Suppl 10):1518–1527.
18. Coiffier B, Lepage E. Prognosis of aggressive lymphomas: a study of five prognostic models with patients included in the LNH-84 regimen. Blood 1989;74(2): 558–564.
19. Shipp MA, Harrington DP, Anderson JR, et al. A predictive model for aggressive NHL: the international non-Hodgkin's lymphoma prognostic factors project. N Engl J Med 1993; 329:987–994.
20. Miller TP, Dana BW, Weick JK, et al. Southwest Oncology Group clinical trials for intermediate- and high-grade non-Hodgkin's lymphomas. Semin Hematol 1988;25:17–22.

21. Klimo P, Connors JM. MACOP-B chemotherapy for the treatment of diffuse large-cell lymphoma. Ann Intern Med 1985;102:596–602.

22. Fisher RI, Longo DL, DeVita VT, et al. Long-term follow-up of ProMACE-CytaBOM in non-Hodgkin's lymphomas. Ann Oncol 1991;2(Suppl 1):33–35.

23. Boyd DB, Coleman M, Papish SW, et al. COPBLAM III: infusional combination chemotherapy for diffuse large cell lymphoma. J Clin Oncol 1988;6:425–433.

24. Fisher RI, Gaynor ER, Dahlberg S, et al. Comparison of a standard regimen (CHOP) with three intensive chemotherapy regimens for advanced non-Hodgkin's lymphoma. N Engl J Med 1993;328:1002–1006.

25. Cabanillas F, Rodriguez MA, Swan F. Recent trends in the management of lymphomas at M. D. Anderson Cancer Center. Semin Oncol 1990;17:28–33.

26. Bloomfield CD, Arthur DC, Frizzera G, et al. Non-random chromosome abnormalities in lymphoma. Cancer Res 1983;43:2975–2984.

27. Tsujimoto Y, Cossman J, Jaffe E, Croce CM. Involvement of the bcl-2 gene in human follicular lymphoma. Science 1985;228:1440–1443.

28. Rowley JD. Chromosome studies in the non-Hodgkin's lymphomas: the role of the 14;18 translocation. J Clin Oncol 1988;6:919–925.

29. Nowell PC, Croce CM. Chromosome translocation and oncogenes in human lymphoid tumors. Am J Clin Pathol 1990;94:229–237.

30. Limpins J, de Jong D, Voetdijk AMH, et al. Translocation t(14;18) in benign B lymphocytes. Blood 1990;76(Suppl 1):237a.

31. Hockenbery D, Nunez G, Milliman C, et al. Bcl-2 is an intermitochondrial membrane protein that blocks programmed cell death. Nature 1990;348:334–338.

32. Gulley ML, Dent GA, Ross DW. Classification and staging of lymphoma by molecular genetics. Cancer 1992;69(Suppl 6):1600–1606.

33. Jones SE, Fucks Z, Bull M, et al. Non-Hodgkin's lymphomas; IV, clinicopathologic correlation in 405 cases. Cancer 1973;31:806–823.

34. Romaguera JD, McLaughlin P, North L, et al. Multivariate analysis of prognostic factors in stage IV follicular low-grade lymphoma: a risk model. J Clin Oncol 1991;9:762–769.

35. Litam P, Swan F, Cabanillas F, et al. Prognostic value of serum ß2 microglobulin in low grade lymphoma. Ann Intern Med 1991;114:855–860.

36. Horning SJ, Rosenberg SA. The natural history of initially untreated low-grade non-Hodgkin's lymphomas. N Engl J Med 1984;311:1471–1475.

37. Lister TA. The management of follicular lymphoma. Ann Oncol 1991;2(Suppl 2):131–135.

38. McLaughlin P, Cabanillas F, Hagemeister F, et al. CHOP-Bleo plus α-interferon (IFN) in stage IV low grade lymphoma (abstract). Proc ASCO 1992;11:326.

39. Young RC, Longo LL, Glatstein E, et al. The treatment of indolent lymphomas: watchful waiting vs. aggressive combined modality treatment. Semin Hematol 1988;25(Suppl 2):11–16.

40. Cox JD, Komaki R, Kun LE, et al. Stage III nodular lymphoreticular tumors (non-Hodgkin's lymphoma): results of central lymphatic irradiation. Cancer 1981;47:2247–2252.

41. Paryani SB, Hoppe RT, Cox RS, et al. The role of radiation therapy in the management of stage III follicular lymphomas. J Clin Oncol 1984;2:841–848.

42. McLaughlin P, Fuller LM, Velasquez WS, et al. Stage III follicular lymphoma: durable remission with a combined chemotherapy-radiotherapy regimen. J Clin Oncol 1987;5:867–874.

43. Paryani SB, Hoppe RT, Cox RS, et al. Analysis of non-Hodgkin's lymphomas with nodular and favorable histologies stage I and II. Cancer 1983;52:2300–2307.

44. Gomez GA, Bercos M, Krishnamsetty RM. Treatment of early stages I and II nodular poorly differentiated lymphocytic lymphoma. Am J Clin Oncol 1986;90:40–44.

45. Lawrence TS, Urba WJ, Steinberg SM, et al. Retrospective analysis of stage I and II indolent lymphomas at the National Cancer Institute. Int J Radiat Oncol Biol Phys 1988;14:417–424.

46. Richards MA, Gregory WM, Hall PA, et al. Management of localized non-Hodgkin's lymphoma: the experience at St. Bartholomew's hospital 1972–1985. Hemat Oncol 1989;7:1–18.

47. McLaughlin P, Fuller L, Redman J, et al. Stage I-II low-grade lymphoma: a prospective trial of combination chemotherapy and radiotherapy. Ann Oncol 1991;2(Suppl 2):137–140.

48. Minden MD, Toyonaga B, Ha K, et al. Somatic rearrangement of T-cell antigen receptor gene in human T-cell malignancies. Proc Natl Acad Sci USA 1985;82:1224–1227.

49. Flug F, Pelicci PG, Bonettie F, Knowles DM, Dalla-Favera R. T-cell receptor gene rearrangements as markers of lineage and clonality in T-cell neoplasms. Proc Natl Acad Sci USA 1985;82:3460–3464.

50. Nathwani BN, Kim H, Rappaport H. Malignant lymphoma lymphoblastic. Cancer 1976;38:964–983.

51. Srigley J, Barlogie B, Butler JJ, et al. Heterogeneity of non-Hodgkin's lymphoma probed by nucleic acid cytometry. Blood 1985;65:1090–1096.

52. Slater DE, Mertlesman R, Koziner B, et al. Lymphoblastic lymphoma in adults. J Clin Oncol 1986;4:57–67.

53. Coleman CN, Picozzi VJ, Cox RS, et al. Treatment of lymphoblastic lymphoma in adults. J Clin Oncol 1986; 4:1628–1635.

54. Kodura PRK, Fillippa DA, Richardson ME, et al. Cytogenetic and histologic correlations in malignant lymphoma. Blood 1987;69:97–102.

55. Lenoir GM, Preud'homme JL, Berheim A, Berger R. Correlation between immunoglobulin light chain expression and variant translocations in Burkitt's lymphoma. Nature 1982;298:474–476.

56. Grogan MT, Warnke RA, Kaplan HS. A comparative study of Burkitt's and non-Burkitt's "undifferentiated" malignant lymphoma. Cancer 1982;49:1817–1828.

57. Ziegler JL. Treatment results of 54 American patients with Burkitt's lymphoma are similar to the African experience. N Engl J Med 1977;297:75–80.

58. Lopez TM, Hagemeister FB, McLaughlin P, Velasquez WS, et al. Small noncleaved cell lymphoma in adults: superior results for stages I-III disease. J Clin Oncol 1990;8:615–622.

59. Burkitt D. A sarcoma involving the jaws in African children. Br J Surg 1958;46:218–223.

60. Magrath IT. African Burkitt's lymphoma: history biology clinical features and treatment. Am J Pediatr Hematol Oncol 1991;13(2):222–46.

61. Epstein MA, Achong BG, Barr YM. Virus particles in cultured lymphoblasts from Burkitt's lymphoma. Lancet 1964;1:702–703.

62. Whittle HC, Brown J, Marsh K, Greenwood BM, et al. T-cell control of Epstein-Barr virus-infected B cells is lost during P. falciparum malaria. Nature 1984;312:449–50.

63. Hanto DW, Frizzera G, Purtillo DT, Sakamoto K, et al. Clinical spectrum of lymphoproliferative disorders in renal transplant recipients and evidence of the role of Epstein-Barr virus. Cancer Res 1981;41:4253–4261.

64. Saemundsen AK, Purtillo DT, Sakamoto K, Sullivan J, et al. Documentation of Epstein-Barr virus infection in immunodeficient patients with life-threatening lymphoproliferative diseases by Epstein-Barr virus complimentary RNA/DNA and viral DNA/DNA hybridization. Cancer Res 1981;41: 4237–4242.

65. Peterson JM, Tubbs RR, Savage RA, Calabrese LC, et al. Small non-cleaved B-cell Burkitt-like lymphoma chromosome t(8;14) translocation and Epstein-Barr virus nuclear-

associated antigen in a homosexual man with acquired immune deficiency syndrome. Am J Med 1985;78:141–148.

66. Burkitt D. Long term remissions following one- and two-dose chemotherapy for African lymphoma. Cancer 1967;20: 756–759.

67. Bernstein JI, Coleman NC, Strickler JG, et al. Combined modality therapy for adults with small non-cleaved cell lymphoma (Burkitt's and non-Burkitt's types). J Clin Oncol 1986; 4:847–858.

68. McMaster ML, Green JP, Greco FA, et al. Effective treatment of small non-cleaved cell lymphoma with high intensity brief-duration chemotherapy. J Clin Oncol 1991;9:941–946.

69. Codman EC, Lunberg WB, Bertino JR. Hyperphosphatemia and hypocalcemia accompanying rapid cell lysis in a patient with Burkitt's lymphoma and Burkitt cell leukemia. Am J Med 1977;62:282–290.

CHAPTER 18

Acute Lymphocytic Leukemia

SAMUEL GROSS, MD

"Lymphatic anaemia, Hodgkin's disease, pseudo-leukemia, anaemia lymphatica, adénie, malignant lymphoma, lymphadenoma, lympho-sarcoma, adenoid disease, lymphatic cachexia, desmoid carcinoma, diathèse lympho-gène, etc.

"A progressive non-leucocytic anaemia, depending on a wide-spread overgrowth of the lymphatic glands and sometimes of the spleen and other lymphatic tissues, together with the secondary development of heteroplastic lymphatic growths in various tissues of the body."
—Keating
Cyclopedia of the Diseases of Children, 1890

Introduction

The consistent feature of acute lymphocytic leukemia (ALL) is the clonal expansion and heterogeneous manifestation of normal-appearing precursors. The net effect is disordered cellular proliferation and asocial growth that leaves, in its wake, devastation, disorganization, and death.

Case 1

A 4-month-old, Asian-American female was seen by her physician because of a 2 week history of unexplained high fevers and scattered "black and blue" spots on her trunk and extremities. The remainder of her history, review of systems, and family history were noncontributory. Her parents were native-born Americans of Japanese-Filipino descent, and she had two full, older siblings, both males. The family lived in a middle-class neighborhood distant from toxic waste areas or high tension wires. Neither parent smoked nor worked with or stored volatile hydrocarbons; except for a visit by the paternal grandfather, who had chronic malaria, after the birth of this child, there was no history of malignant diseases or other untoward events in the family background.

The examination revealed a well developed and well nourished infant who was pale, ecchymotic, febrile (temperature, 39.5°C), and irritable. She had a protuberant abdomen with an enlarged liver and spleen. The remainder of her examination was unremarkable.

The clinical impression of a malignant process, probably leukemia, was supported by the following hematologic studies: Hgb, 90g/L; Hct, 28%; red blood cell count, 3.1 × 10^{12}/L; WBC, 30 × 10^9/L; platelet count, 25 × 10^9/L; and a 0.6% reticulocyte count. Her ANC was 0.3 × 10^9/L (10% mature granulocytes, 2% monocytes, 88% immature-appearing lymphocytes). The impression was verified by a marrow aspirate and biopsy that identified a cellular marrow, 80% of which was replaced mainly by 90% L1-appearing and 10% L2-appearing blasts (i.e., large round cells, most with scant cytoplasm, some with notched nuclei, and fewer yet with nucleoli).

Pertinent additional laboratory data included a normal urinalysis, elevated levels of LDH (800 IU/mL) and uric acid (15 mg/DL), normal prothrombin (PT), activated partial thromboplastin (aPTT) times, fibrinogen and antithrombin III levels. Electrolytes, particularly K+, P+, and Ca+, as well as renal and liver profiles, were normal, as were TORCH, EBV, and HIV titers. The patient's cerebrospinal fluid had 0.2 × 10^9 cells/L^3, consistent in appearance with those seen in the bone marrow. Chest films were normal. G-banding chromosome analyses revealed pseudodiploidy and an 11q23 rearrangement t(4;11)(q21;q23).

The morphologic diagnosis was L1 ALL, with disease involving the bone marrow, peripheral circulation, pia arachnoid, and probably the liver and the spleen as well.

In excess of 90% of marrow nucleated cell mass immunotyped HLA-DR+ and CD19+, 5% were CD34+/CD33+. The patient's cerebrospinal fluid cells also typed HLA-DR+ and CD19+. She did not type positive for CD10, and her DNA index was 1.2.

The diagnosis was infantile pre B-cell (CD19+) ALL with a t(4;11)(q21;23) translocation and very early myeloid markers.

The L1 designation, derived from the French-American-British (FAB) classification of the acute leukemias (1–3), is a morphologic type common to childhood ALL, which on univariant analysis, has favorable prognostic significance in all except infant ALL such as this case. CD19+ (CD10−) ALL is an early B lineage immunotype often in association with primitive myeloid markers (CD33+/34+). Moreover, patients with more than one clonal abnormality seemingly have an advanced stage of the disease.

The 11q23 rearrangement, as in this case and those involving chromosomes 11 and 19, is present both in ALL and ANLL and is particularly common in infants with poor prognostic features. The FAB classification and immunotyping features of ALL are detailed in Tables 18.1, 18.2, and 18.3.

Before the initiation of chemotherapy, the patient received 150 mg p.o. allopurinol q.d. (i.v. allopurinol would have been administered if there had been evidence of oral intolerance) and hydration with twice maintenance volume of alkalinized fluids i.v. to both decrease and solubilize, respectively, the urate load. Induction therapy consisting of vincristine, prednisone, daunomycin, and cytosine arabinoside (ARA-C) was initiated 24 hours later with a 33% dose reduction in Ara-C to accommodate upcoming CNS therapy and, accordingly, minimize the possibility of drug-induced central nervous system damage. Intrathecal medication included four weekly installations of methotrexate (MTX), ARA-C, and hydrocortisone (HC). At the end of 1 month, the patient's marrow aspirate and CNS examination, except for an occasional (drug-induced) macrophage in the CSF, seemed to be free of blast forms. She never developed problems with tumor lysis, e.g., elevated K+ and/or Ca+ levels, and her uric acid levels fell promptly after

Table 18.1. French-American-British Classification: ALL and ANLL

L1 ALL	Small, clumped chromatin Scant gray cytoplasm and rare nucleoli or vacuoles
L2 ALL	Large, fine chromatin, clefted nuclei, occasional nucleoli, abundant cytoplasm, ± vacuoles
L3 ALL	Large, fine chromatin with deep blue cytoplasm, many nucleoli, and numerous vacuoles
M1 Immature AML	Myeloblasts with rare or no granules
M2 Mature AML	Myeloblasts, 1+ granules
M3 Promyelocytic leukemia	Promyelocytes, 4+ granules
M4 Myelomonocytic leukemia	Myeloblasts, promyelocytes, promonoblasts, monoblasts
M5a Immature monoblastic leukemia	Large, poorly differentiated monoblasts
M5b Mature monoblastic leukemia	Differentiated monoblasts
M6 Erythroleukemia	Megaloblasts and myeloblasts
M7 Megakaryocytic leukemia	Megakaryoblasts

Table 18.2. ALL Subsets by Immunotypes

	Early Pre-B	Pre-B	Mature B	Early T	Mature T°
TdT (Nuclear)	+	+	−	+	+
HLA-DR	+	+	+	+/−	+/−
CD-19	+	+	+/−	−	−
CD-10	+	+/−	+/−	−	−
CD20	+/−	+	+	−	−
CD-24	+	+	+	−	−
CD-2	−	+	SIg	−	−
Cytoplasmic μ	−	+	−	−	−
CD-7	−	−	−	+	+
CD-2	−	−	−	+	+
CD-3	−	−	−	+/−	+/−
Cytoplasmic CD-3	−	−	−	+	−
CD-4	−	−	−	+	+
CD-8	−	−	−	+	+

°Small numbers of mature T cells do not mark for CD4 and CD-8

Table 18.3. ALL Subsets According to Age

Age in Years	Early Pre-B	Pre-B	B	T
<1.5	64 (50% cALLa)	26	4	6
2-10	68 (>90% cALLa)	18	1	13
10-15	58 (>85% cALLa)	18	1	23
>15 Adult	51°(50% cALLa)	?	4	22

°25% Null cell, mixed lineage AL in adults, 10% in children.

the administration of allopurinol and alkalinized fluids. If she had developed hypercalcemia or hyperkalemia, she would have received K+ exchange resins, a prednisone dosage boost, and replacement of alkalinization fluids by normal saline.

Her age, the markedly elevated tumor burden, including leukocytosis, and its unique karyotypic and immunocytologic features placed the patient in a high-risk category (4–6). She and her family were accordingly HLA tested in search of an allogeneic bone marrow transplant (alloBMT) donor. Neither of the siblings nor her parents was an acceptable match, and an unrelated donor search was initiated via the National Marrow Donor Program (NMDP).

While awaiting the results of the search, the patient received consolidation therapy consisting of a cyclophosphamide-etoposide combination alternating every 2–3 weeks with intermediate dose methotrexate-purinethol (6-mercaptopurine), along with a monthly schedule of intrathecal MTC and HC therapy. On the possibility that she might receive ARA-C in the BMT preparative regimen, it was removed from the intrathecal therapy regimen. She also received prophylactic trimethoprim sulfamethoxazole (TMP-SMX) three times each week for pneumocystis control.

The consolidation regimen was well tolerated, but within 5 months, primitive cells were once again present in the marrow. The CNS remained tumor free. A fully matched, unrelated donor (MUD) was identified at approximately the same time, and it was decided to attempt a pre-BMT reduction in tumor burden once again with prednisone, Ara-C, and l-asparaginase. After 4 weeks of therapy, the patient's marrow leukemic cell count fell to 3% and a decision was made to commence the BMT countdown with busulfan-cyclophosphamide rather than ARA-C and fractionated total body irradiation (FTBI), because of the risk of causing severe brain damage in a child whose neural development was not yet complete. Graft-versus-host disease (GVHD) prophylaxis was initiated with short-term i.v. MTX and continued with long-term i.v. cyclosporine (CSA). All of her viral studies were negative, and she received no additional prophylaxis other than cytomegalovirus (CMV)-blood product support.

As noted, the use of total body irradiation was believed to be ill advised because of the risk of damaging an incompletely developed neural system. Busulfan and cyclophosphamide (BuCy) are seemingly less neurotoxic than irradiation in infancy, but the real issues regarding BuCy concern (a) their therapeutic efficacy, and (b) the possibility of (an as yet ill-defined) long-term drug-induced toxicity.

The patient's BMT course was uneventful except for Grade 2 GVHD, which was readily responsive to high-dose prednisone. Evidence of engraftment was noted on day +16. On day +45, she was discharged on prednisone and CSA to the BMT ambulatory follow-up clinic. Six months later, blast-appearing cells were once again present in her circulation, and a repeat bone marrow aspiration showed virtual replacement by CD19+ cells.

This case highlights the fact that infant leukemia is a unique category in the pantheon of unfavorable prognostic features. In effect, this disease, which probably best fits the Greaves two-hit theory of intra-germ-line and extrauterine insults (7), is probably the poorest responder of all the leukemias, irrespective of best available therapy. It also raises concerns regarding the spectre of secondary malignancies attendant upon the use of etoposide in potentially susceptible individuals (8).

Thus, in establishing a table of unfavorable prognostic factors, one must include:

Age <1 year (infant ALL)
More than one clonal abnormality

Case 2

A 9-year-old Caucasian male was taken to his physician because of intermittent fevers, a chronic, nonproductive cough, and lethargy of approximately 3 weeks' duration. His U.S.-born parents of Dutch ancestry were distant cousins, and he had three living biologic siblings, of whom he was the eldest. One sibling with severe combined immunodeficiency disease died of an overwhelming fungal sepsis just before the initiation of a bone mar-

row allograft from his one-antigen-mismatched mother. There was no other pertinent history.

On physical examination, he was a chronically ill-appearing, febrile (38.9°C) male of stated age, without evidence of recent weight loss. He also had raspy, bronchial breathing.

Initial blood counts revealed the following: Hgb, 125 gm/L; Hct, 37%; RBC count, 4.1 × 10^{12}/L; WBC, 7 × 10^9/L; and platelets, 120 × 10^9/L. His differential included 35% granulocytes, 4% monocytes, 1% eosinophils, and 59% lymphocytes, none of which appeared to be atypical. Urinalysis was normal, as were renal chemistries, uric acid level, electrolytes, liver profile and serology, and clotting studies. The patient's LDH was elevated to 600 IU/mL. A chest film, obtained because of the bronchial findings, revealed an anterior mediastinal mass, inseparable from the thymus and without associated pulmonary infiltration.

The interpretation was anterior mediastinal mass, probably lymphoid in origin, with lymphoma, thymoma, and inflammatory mass to be ruled out.

Biopsy, if possible by mediastinoscopy, was contemplated, but it was proposed that a bone marrow assessment be carried out first on the possibility that the mass represented a T-cell lymphoma metastatic to the marrow. Such, apparently, was a reasonable assumption: his bone marrow was almost 60% replaced by primitive cells, not unlike those in case 1, but with 20% L2 type lymphoblasts in the L1/L2 mixture. As described in Table 18.1, the L2 cell, unlike the smaller, compact L1 cell, has a large cytoplasmic volume with occasional vacuoles and obvious nucleoli.

Flow cytometric analysis of the marrow population revealed a TdT+, CD5+, CD7+ positive clone and a DNA index of 1.3. The cerebrospinal fluid was entirely normal; and pending the outcome of the karyotype study, the impression was mature T-cell ALL, probably secondary to leukemic conversion of a mediastinal lymphoma.

He was considered to be in a good risk category because of age (between 2 and 10 years), white cell count (less than 25 × 10^9/L), and favorable DNA index (1.3). The only negative factor was the large extramarrow tumor burden, i.e., the thymic derived mass.

In general, two or more unfavorable features support a less favorable prognosis; in this regard, the suggestion that T-cell ALL is a poor prognostic feature is not borne out in children between 2 and 10 years of age, who present with low white cell counts.

Chromosomal studies revealed hyperdiploidy and a rare, prognostically insignificantly nonrandom, chromosomal translocation t(8:14)(p24;q11) that did not affect the prognosis. The patient did not have any of the unfavorable features often associated with T-cell ALL: hyperleukosis and the t(11;14)(p13;q11) abnormality.

Although difficult to prove, it is conceivable that many, if not all, of the cases of T-cell ALL begin as an extramedullary mass (usually in the mediastinum), despite the knowledge that thymic precursors probably migrate from the marrow to the mediastinal area to establish the anlage of the "mature" thymus gland. The premise for migration leading from a solid to a liquid phase malignancy, i.e., thymic lymphoma to marrow leukemia, gains support from the large number of patients, who present with partial marrow replacement and minimally reduced peripheral blood cell counts in the presence of a mediastinal mass, i.e., the early expression of a blatant marrow malignancy.

Initial therapy consisted of daily p.o. prednisone, weekly i.v. vincristine, and daily s.c. 1-asparaginase; the latter was a 9-day dose schedule commencing on day +2, along with a prophylactic TMP-SMX. The patient progressed well on this regimen until day +7, when he was noted to be disoriented and confused and had a dilated, sluggishly reacting right pupil. The clinical impression of a left cerebro-occipital "accident" was confirmed by a contrast-heightened CT scan, interpreted as a likely blood clot. The pretreatment PT and APTT increased threefold on day +4 of asparaginase therapy and then declined toward normal by day +7, at which time his previously normal antithrombin III level became undetectable. Impaired protein synthesis brought about by asparaginase is not restricted to leukemic lymphoblasts (9); but because of (a) its efficacy in ALL induction therapy and (b) its infrequent, albeit predictable toxicity, it is rarely if ever withheld. If the prescribed Escherichia coli derived 1-asparaginase had caused a hypersensitivity reaction, it would have been replaced either by an Erwinia or conjugated polyethylene glycol compound. However, in this circumstance, it was withheld altogether, and fresh frozen plasma was administered as an antithrombin III source. Shortly thereafter, his neurological deficit stabilized and then improved. One month later, he had no clinical residual and a repeat CT scan was unremarkable.

At the end of the third of three weekly doses of i.v. daunomycin, substituted for the 1-asparaginase, along with the remaining planned therapy, the patient's marrow was visibly free of disease. He then received an abbreviated (2-month) intensification course of intermediate dose MTX i.v. followed by daily p.o. 6-mercaptopurine and weekly s.c. MTX in a dose intensification schedule designed to maintain an ANC not less than 1×10^9/L and a platelet level above 75×10^9/L. Pneumocystis prophylaxis was continued. The three-dose course of triple intrathecal therapy as described in case 1, above, administered on consecutive weeks during induction, was continued on a monthly basis during the first year of maintenance, an approach based on data that established a heightened risk for the development of CNS disase after cessation of CNS prophylaxis before 1 year of total therapy (10). Commencing with year 2, spinal fluid examinations were performed every 3 months for diagnostic purposes only. At the end of 3 years of therapy, bone marrow, CSF, and testicular biopsy were free of disease, and therapy was discontinued. The patient remains disease-free 5 years after completion of therapy.

During the ensuing decade, the patient's chance of relapse will decline from approximately 5–7%, somewhat higher than that for females, to almost nil.

This case highlights the following: (*a*) patients between 2 and 10 years of age fall in a favorable risk factor category; (*b*) T-cell ALL, formerly believed to be a generally poor risk factor, is so usually in patients with elevations in WBC and in the presence of the t(11;14)(p13;q11) karyotype (not all karyotype abnormalities carry poor prognostic features); (*c*) failure to initiate CNS prophylaxis, or early cessation of CNS prophylaxis in the patient without evidence of CNS disease at onset, carries a 20% risk for late-occurring CNS relapse; and (*d*) L1 is commonly present in childhood ALL and, unlike the more common adult (L2) type, has favorable prognostic significance (11–14).

As the "unfavorable" prognostic features expand, additions would include:

Age >10 years
L2 Morphology
WBC >25 × 10^9/L
Specified T-cell ALL
Age <1 year (infant ALL)
More than one clonal abnormality

Case 3

A 5-year-old African-American female, the second of four biologic siblings (the youngest of whom had Down's syndrome), whose father and mother were a dentist and a schoolteacher, respectively, was taken to her family physician because of low-grade fever, anorexia of 2 weeks' duration, and lethargy. Three months previously, she had been evaluated by her physician because of complaints of diffuse bone pain of 1 month's duration.

When the patient was seen by her family physician and then by a rheumatologist, she had a slightly enlarged spleen and low normal white blood cell count and hemoglobin levels. A presumptive diagnosis of rheumatoid arthritis was made. Neither rheumatoid factor nor anti-DNA levels were positive. She had normal levels of complement and a slightly elevated ferritin level. The pain on ambulation and the splenic enlargement were verified, as were the borderline normal blood cell counts: Hgb, 110 g/L; Hct, 32.5%; RBC, 3.5 × 10^{12}/L; WBC, 3.0 × 10^9/L; reticulocytes, 0.1%; and platelets, 125 × 10^9/L. A stained peripheral blood film revealed 60% polymorphonuclear granulocytes, 5% mature monocytes, and 35% atypical/immature lymphocytes. The patient's erythrocytic sedimentation rate was 25 mm/hr. Long bone films revealed occasional distal metaphyseal disruptions. She received analgesics and was told to return in 1 month or longer if she felt better. However, after a brief pain-free interval, she worsened, and on her return, she was pale and had a palpable spleen and scattered ecchymoses. Her temperature was 39.5°C. A blood count revealed the following: Hgb, 80/dL; WBC, 100 × 10^9/L; platelets, 40 × 10^9/L; and a WBC differential of

80% L2 type blasts and 20% normal-appearing granulo-cytes. Review of the previous long bone films was rein-terpreted as consistent with leukemic disruptions of the metaphyses (15). Marrow aspirations were difficult to perform. Each tap was "dry." The only readily available marrow came from teased material from a biopsy speci-men that identified L2/L1 cells (80:20) that immuno-typed as TdT-, HLA-DR+ and CD10+/CD19+, consis-tent with pre-B ALL. Her cerebrospinal fluid was crystal clear and free of cells, and her DNA index was 1.3. Kary-otyping revealed pseudodiploidy and a t(9;22)(q34;q11) translocation, i.e., the Philadelphia (Ph) chromosome.

Diffuse bone pain, like unexplained fever and malaise, is a common presenting complaint in patients with acute leukemia. Of note is the fact that there are fairly distinct pediatric- and adult-related "pain involvement" areas. In adults, the pain usually originates in the sternum, ribs, and vertebral bodies, whereas in children, it is more commonly expressed in the long bones. In either situation, the pain is a consequence of densely packed marrow, the pressure of which, in turn, accounts for the bony irregularities in the distal metaphyses and the difficulty attendant upon aspira-tion of marrow.

With the exception of the patient's age and DNA index of 1.3, the tumor burden, predominance of L2 morphology, race, and the 9:22 translocation sup-ported a high-risk disease. The CD10+/CD19+ im-munotype, in this situation, did not influence the prog-nosis favorably.

Induction therapy consisted of vincristine, pred-nisone, l-asparaginase, and daunomycin; and because of the high risk of relapse, plans were set to HLA type the family. The eldest of the patient's three siblings was an identical, nonreactive match; at the completion of suc-cessful induction therapy, which included three courses of triple intrathecal therapy (MTC, ARA-C, HC), the BMT countdown began. Of note is the fact that poly-merase chain reaction (PCR) analysis of the patient's marrow at the completion of induction failed to reveal the presence of the Bcr/Abl oncogene.

The most revealing feature in this case is the pres-ence of a particular factor (i.e., the Ph chromosome, that impacts more unfavorably on prognosis. Other features, including black race, L2 subset, elevated WBC, and pseudodiploidy, were contributory but not predominant.

The t9;22 abnormality, which occurs in approximately 10% of all childhood and three times as often in adult ALL, involves the Bcr/Abl oncogenes typically seen in CML. A major distinction between the chromosomal features of CML blast crisis and ph+ ALL is the fre-quent presence of an added 8 chromosome or the emer-gence of a 17q chromosome in the former. In ALL, unlike the chronic phase of CML, successful induction of remission results in failure to detect the Bcr/Abl ab-normality.

As noted, the treatment of choice for Ph+ ALL in first remission is alloBMT.

Further additions to the list of unfavorable prognostic features include:

Black race
Pseudodiploidy (also hypodiploidy)
Specific karyotypic abnormalities
Age >10 years
L2 morphology
WBC >25 × 10⁹/L
Specified T-cell ALL
Age <1 year (infant ALL)
More than one clonal abnormality

Case 4

A 20-year-old male college student with type A Von Willebrand's disease went to the hospital infirmary be-cause of persistent fevers and lassitude of 1 month's du-ration. He had a recent history of a sore throat with en-larged, slightly tender cervical lymph nodes that went unattended. He was concerned about the possibility of infectious mononucleosis, or worse yet, that he was HIV positive. He did not recall receiving blood products for the treatment of his clotting disorder, neither was he an intravenous drug user nor was he sexually promiscuous. The patient was an excellent student on a full scholarship and the only child of working parents of Welsh descent; he was born and raised in a lower-middle-class area in the center of a major, river-based, inland industrial city.

On examination, the patient was deeply depressed, weary, and febrile (temperature, 38.6°C). He had a dif-fusely distributed, fine, macular rash on his trunk and extremities, a slightly injected posterior pharynx, and nontender, coalescing cervical, axillary, and epitrochlear lymph nodes along with a slightly enlarged, nontender spleen.

Laboratory studies revealed the following: Hgb, 100 g/L; Hct, 30%; RBC, 3.2 × 10¹²/L; WBC, 30.5 × 10⁹/L; platelets, 95 × 10⁹/L; and reticulocyte count, 1.5%. His absolute granulocyte count was 3.5 × 10⁹/L and, except for a rare eosinophil and 3% monocytes, the remainder of the smear consisted of two populations of lymphoid-appearing cells: a small number of irregularly shaped cells with gray-blue cytoplasm and occasional nonspecific granules and many slightly smaller cells with intense blue cytoplasm, clumped nuclear chromatin, readily apparent nucleoli, and numerous vacuoles. The mono-spot test was negative, as were the TORCH and HIV titers. The IgM (1:100) and IgG (1:250) Epstein-Barr virus titers were positive. Other studies included a total bilirubin of 1.5 mg% (direct bilirubin of 0.8 mg%), LDH of 3,000 IU/mL, mildly elevated liver enzymes, a weakly positive IgM direct Coombs' test, normal serum immunoglobulin levels, erythrocyte sedimentation rate of 35 mL/hr, and a throat culture of mixed bacterial growth including β-hemolytic streptococci. The possibil-ity of an infectious mononucleosis syndrome was consid-ered based on the following: (a) a blood film with a B-cell response (deep blue cytoplasm with occasional vacuoles *and nucleoli) to presumptively infected T cells (large, irregularly shaped lymphocytes with gray-blue cytoplasm, rare vacuoles, granules, and occasional nucleoli), (b) a questionable vasculitis or infiltration type rash, (c) positive (converting) EBV IgM-IgG titers suggestive of a relatively recent infection, and (d) a weakly positive (IgM) Coombs' test. However, the appearance of the B lymphocytes was of sufficient concern to warrant a bone marrow analysis, which revealed 65% replacement by L3 type cells with μ heavy chain surface Ig and which immunotyped CD20+, HLA-DR+, Tdt−. He had a hypodiploid karyotype with an 8;14 translocation [t(8;14)(p24;q32.3)] and a DNA index of 1.12.*

CSF examination revealed 0.15 × 10⁹ L3-type-appearing cells/L. The patient's urinalysis was normal; except for a borderline elevation in uric acid, his liver function tests, renal profile, and electrolytes were also normal. Repeat TORCH and hepatitis titres were unchanged, and his EBV titer was 1:1000 IgG, with barely detectable IgM.

The diagnosis was mature B-cell ALL (L3) with t8;14 translocation.

A triple-lumen intravenous catheter was inserted, and the patient was pretreated with allopurinol and alkalinization fluids. Systemic therapy consisted of high-dose cyclophosphamide, ARA-C, and MTX along with triple-drug intrathecal therapy, the latter every week for 6 weeks and then every 2 months for 12 months. Systemic therapy was administered every 3 weeks. At the end of 1 year, the patient was in complete hematological and clinical remission, and therapy was discontinued. Because patients with mature B-cell ALL and a low DNA index (historically) relapsed at a very high rate, both this patient and his parents were HLA typed. Even with this aggressive regimen, this "adult" patient had, at best, a 55% chance for longterm DFS leading to cure.

This case highlights a possible relationship between a viral agent (EBV) effecting a lymphoproliferative response and emphasizes the need to obtain comprehensive historical data in every newly diagnosed case of leukemia. It also emphasizes the necessity to provide aggressive systemic and CNS therapy to effectively treat a heretofore poorly responsive ALL subtype.

Completed additions to a table of unfavorable prognostic features would include:

DNA index <1.2
L3 morphology
Black race
Pseudodiploidy (also hypodiploidy)
Specific karyotypic abnormalities
Age >10 years
L2 morphology
WBC >25 × 10⁹/L
Specified T-cell ALL
Age <1 year (infant ALL)
More than one clonal abnormality

These cases, all U.S.-born patients (a 4-month-old female of Pacific-Asian descent, a 9-year-old male of French-Dutch descent, a 5-year-old female of African descent, and a 20-year-old "adult" male of Welsh descent) are prototypical in that they underscore the features that identify the biological underpinnings and the prognostic features of this complex group of disorders.

Incidence and Predilection

Age. The incidence of ALL in children who reside in the northern portion of the western hemisphere (data from the United States, Canada, and Western Europe, including the British Isles) through 15 years of age is 2.4/1000,000/annum. In adults, its incidence is approximately one-fourth that of children, or 0.7/100,000/annum. The peak incidence in children occurs between 2 and 5 years of age. In adults, there is no peak but rather a slow decline in incidence after 55 years of age. The ALL and ANLL incidences are mirror images in children and adults, i.e., ALL represents one-fourth of the adult acute leukemias, and the opposite is true in children 16–23 (fig. 18.1).

Race. The overall incidence among Caucasians is 2.9/100,000/annum, 1.37/100,000/annum among African-Americans; on the basis of extrapolations from Japanese data, the estimated incidence among Pacific-Asian Islanders is approximately two-thirds that of western hemisphere Caucasians. It is important to note that the demographics of acute leukemias in Western Asia and the easternmost parts of Europe differ significantly from the distribution of the acute leukemias in the western hemisphere (24, 25).

Sex. The ratio of male to female patients with ALL is slightly less than 1.25:1, primarily the result of a predominance of mature B- and T-cell subsets in males. This applies to all ages, except for infants in whom the sex ratio is essentially equivalent (26).

The demographics of age, race, and sex offer a number of unanswered questions. Why, for example, is ALL more common (a) in Caucasian Americans than in African-Americans and Pacific Asians, (b) why is it more common in males than in females, (c) why is it more common in children than in adults, and (d) what is the significance of age-, race-, and sex-related responses to therapy (27)?

Familial Relationships. The incidence of leukemia in siblings is approximately four times greater than it is in the general population; despite the extraordinarily rare report of mother-to-child transmission, there are no data to support a possibly vertical transmitted process. Among monozygotic twins, the incidence is much greater: approximately 30%, depending on both temporal and spatial relationships, viz., occurrence only in close association and rarely beyond 6–7 months of the initial diagnosis. Most occur within 3–4 months of each other. It is suggested that a likely explanation for the "nature" of the concordance is a shared genetic response to shared leukemogenic stimuli (28–30).

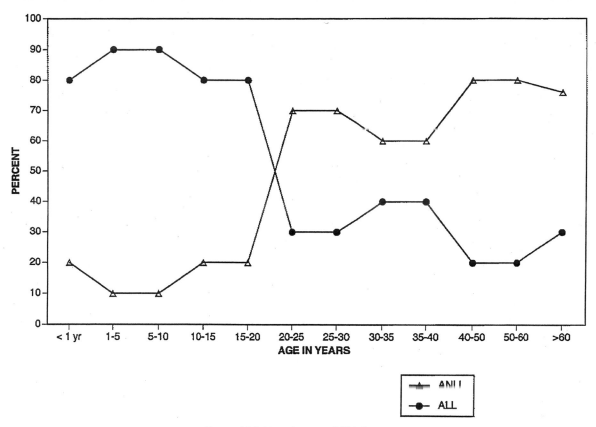

Figure 18.1 Distribution of ALL by age.

Genetic Disorders

Patients with **Down's syndrome** have a prepubescent frequency of leukemia, which is almost 70 times greater than that of the non-Down's syndrome population. After pubescence, it occurs at a rate no greater than that of the general population. With the exception of the rare examples of neonatal myelodysplastic-appearing disorders, most of the afflicted patients have risk factors otherwise concordant with all types of ALL. Unfortunately, these patients do not tolerate therapy well, and toxicity-induced dose modifications often result in poor outcome (31–33). There are no data to support a predilection for leukemia in siblings of individuals with Down's syndrome (case 3).

Patients with *ataxia telangiectasia* have an even greater chance of developing leukemia than do patients with Down's syndrome (and with no apparent age limit) (34, 35).

The risk of developing acute leukemia in patients with *Bloom's syndrome* is equivalent to that of ataxia telangiectasis (1:12), but there is a dropoff in the second decade as a consequence of losses directly attributable to the underlying disorder (36, 37).

Wiskott-Aldrich syndrome, like ataxia telangiectasia and Bloom's syndrome, is yet another example of an inherited immunologic disorder with a increased risk for the development of acute lymphocytic leukemia (38, 39). Although patients with a variety of immunological disorders

are at greater risk for the development of lymphopoietic malignancies, the risk does not apply to unaffected siblings (case 2).

In the **Fanconi syndrome,** the risk of developing acute (often monocytic or myelodysplastic) leukemia after a relentless pancytopenia, is much the same as it is in the immunological disorders noted above. However, there is a cutoff after late puberty, primarily because of the lethal consequences of prolonged aplasia (40).

In all of the above patients, there are nonrandom chromosomal abnormalities, but the molecular basis for induction of leukemic transformation is not at all clear. The relationship of T-cell ALL with **ataxia telangiectasia** (AT) may serve as a model of immune disorder-mediated chromosomal aberrations. In AT, translocations and breaks involving chromosome 7 and 14, which occur over time, apparently result in a clonal abnormality in the T-cell population, but the targeted gene has not been identified; the linkage with ALL and lymphomas, therefore, remains suspect (38). Even less certain is the process that occurs in other "inborn" immunologic disorders **(Bloom's Syndrome, Wiskott-Aldrich Syndrome, SCID).**

In the Fanconi syndrome, the characteristic karyotypic abnormality is widespread chromosomal breakage. The linkage between the pan-aplasia of Fanconi syndrome and leukemic transformation is unclear, notwithstanding the fact that chromosomal breaks have been identified in acute leukemia unassociated with the Fanconi syndrome and in normal siblings of FA patients (41, 42). Implicit in this and

Table 18.4. Common Chromosomal Changes in ALL

	Rearrangement	Features
A.	1;19 Translocation°	Occurs in two variations
	t(1;19)(q23;p13)	Usually present in L1 cALLa
		Commonly present in pre-B ALL, occasionally T cell All
B.	5;14 Translocation	Uncommon
	t(5;14)(q31;q32)	Chromosomal breaks occur at IL-3 sites on chromosomes 5 and 14
C.	8;14 Translocation°	
	t(8;14)(q24;q32)	
	t(2;8)(p12;q24)	L3, Mature B cell ALL
	t(8;22)(q24;q11)	
D.	4;11 Translocation°	Predominantly early pre-Ball ALL
	t(4;11)(q21;q23)	50% <1 year of age
		Associated with very high WBC count
		Lymphoblasts with myeloid markers
		L1 or L2 (T or B cell)
E.	9;22 Translocation°	Ph+ ALL and CML
	t(9;22)(q34;Q11)	Breakpoint in Bcr gene occurs 5′ to that observed in "Adult CML"
		L1 or L2 (T or B cell)
F.	Chromosome 9 short arm deletion°	
	9p22	Massive organomegaly
	dic(9;12)	Very high WBC counts
	(p11–13;p11–12)	
	dic(7;9)(p11–13;p11)	T-cell phenotype
		Inf$_{\beta-1}$ gene in deleted segment
G.	T-cell-specific abnormalities	
	Common:	Uncommon:
	t(1;14)(p32–34;q11)	Inv(14)(q11;q32)
	t(7;11)	
	(q34–36;p13–14)	t(14;14)(q11;q32)
	t(8;14)(q24;q11)	t(7;7)(p15;q11)
	t(11;14)(p13;q11)	t(7;14)(p15;q11)
		t(7;14)(p34–36;q11)
		t(7;19)(q34–36;p13)
		t(7;9)(q34–36;q34)
		t(7;9)(q34–36;q43)
	Summation:	44% of all abnormalities occur in adult/pediatric T cell ALL;
		70% occurs in non-T, non-B ALL;
		100% occur in mature B ALL

°Very high risk.

related instances is the fact that any sibling being HLA tested as a marrow donor should obviously be karyotyped as well.

It is increasingly apparent that genetic alterations, brought about by chromosomal deletions, translocations, or inversions, are often molecular hallmarks of events that either directly or indirectly influence leukemic transformation and, in the process, lend predictive value both to risk and response.

Cases 1, 3, and 4 are examples of poor prognosis genotypes involving abnormal ploidy or poor risk translocations. In case 2, the T-cell-related chromosomal ab-

normality was both uncommon and prognostically insignificant.

Table 18.4 lists the known chromosomal structural defects in ALL which, in combination with studies of chromosomal numbers have provided a wealth of information on the overall karyotypic abnormalities currently detectable in greater than 80% of all newly diagnosed cases of ALL (43).

Approximately two-thirds of the karyotypes are diploid or pseudodiploid; the remainder are hyperdiploid or hypodiploid. Pseudodiploidy is a poor prognosis feature, which occurs with high frequency in African-Americans, usually in association with elevated WBC numbers, L2 type, and chromosomal translocations. There is no selectivity between B- and T-cell ALL (44). Hypodiploidy is also a poor prognostic ploidy. Both pseudodiploidy and hypodiploidy are characteristic of mature B-cell ALL (L3, CD20+) (45–48). Conversely, hyperdiploid disorders have the fewest number of translocations and are frequently CD10+/CD19+. Patients with triploid or tetraploid numbers tend to be older, have L2 morphology, and like infant ALL, express early myeloid antigens (table 18.5). Among the structural abnormalities often associated with ALL, several deserve further commentary (table 18.4). The pH chromosome, t(9:22)(q34;q11), is uncommon, and like a child in case 3, often presents with leukocytosis and predominantly L2 morphology. The t(1;19)(q23;p13) translocation is the most frequently observed structural abnormality in childhood ALL and is commonly found in poor prognosis (pre-B) African-American patients with elevated WBC. The t(8;14)(p24;q32:3) is usually found in L3 type (B-cell) ALL, i.e., older patients with extramedullary disease (case 4). The t(4;11)(q21;q23) translocation (case 1) is typically present in poor prognosis infant ALL (elevated WBC, CD10−/CD19+, myeloid antigen), but it is also a prognostically poor finding in children >10 years of age. The t(11;14)(p13;q11) transformation is seen frequently in patients with T-cell ALL, most of whom are older and have leukocytes and mediastinal masses. The least frequent structural defect reported to date is the dic(9;12)(p11-p12;p12) abnormality, which has been found in low-risk patients. Whereas one may identify both food and poor prognosis karyotypes in children (<15 years of

Table 18.5. Chromosomal Numbers in ALL

	<15 years	>15 years
Pseudodiploid^1°	31.7	48.4
High hyperdiploid	23.1	12.5
Low hyperdiploid	11.7	7.8
Hypotriploid	7.0	4.7
Triploid/tetraploid	1.0	3.1
Haploid	0.4	0
Hypolipoid°	5.7	6.3
Diploid^2	19.4	17.2

^{1}46 chromosomes with rearrangements.
^{2}46 chromosomes.
°Poor prognosis.

age at diagnosis), adults tend to have predominantly poor prognosis structural defects, i.e., t(9;22), (t(4;11), and t(8;14) (49–53).

Case 1 was pseudodiploid and had well defined clonal abnormalities. Case 2 was hyperdiploid without identifiable karyotypic abnormality. Case 3 was pseudodiploid and had a t(9;22) abnormality, and Case 4 was pseudolipoid and had a t(8;11) karyotype. Based on ploidy and/or clonal abnormalities, Cases 1, 3, and 4 fell into the poor prognosis group.

Environmental Factors in the Etiology of AL

Viral and Parasitic Agents. As noted, the mechanism by which chromosomal changes are induced is unknown, but data derived from studies of cetain infectious agents support a causal, albeit usually indirect, relationship. Insight into the leukemia-initiation process is provided by the actions of the malarial parasite and the Ebstein-Barr virus (EBV) on the lymphoid system. Both agents include considerable proliferation-stimulating effects on lymphopoiesis, which may either enhance an existing proliferative defect or obscure existing chromosomal aberrations. The net effect may be a defect in lymphopoiesis, viz., lymphocytic leukemia (54).

The grandfather of the infant in case 1 was chronically infected with falciparium malaria, but this was presumably coincidental to the real but as yet unknown cause. The child was not infected, and there was no obvious invocable relationship between the grandfather's malaria and the child's leukemia. However, there may have been a more likely relationship in the case of the EBV-infected teenager who developed a mature B-cell ALL.

There is a body of evidence of EBV-induced (masked) chromosomal translocations that effect rearrangement of immunoglobulin genes in juxtaposition with an otherwise unobtrusive oncogene (e.g., c-myc), which together may trigger a B-cell malignancy (55–58). The biologic linkages responsible for this train of events are as yet unclear, and until such time as the mechanisms can be fully traced, a causal relationship (as in case 4) can only remain moot. However, the human T-cell leukemia group 1 virus (HTLV-1), which is endemic in certain parts of the Caribbean rim, Japan, southwest United States, and western Africa, is a "direct" viral inducer of a malignant T-cell response. It is transmitted in human (and animal) liquid matter, has a long latency period (which is why it is rarely if ever reported in children), is capable of immortalizing CD4+ cells in vitro, is initially IL-2 dependent before maturing into an IL-2 independent organism, and evokes a chromosomal response often seen in lymphopoietic malignancies, viz., the chromosomal 6q loss. It is also detectable in seronegative individuals by PCR (59–63).

Products of Combustion—Tobacco Smoke: *Case 4 did not smoke, but he was raised in an environment*
in which both parents and close relatives were heavy smokers.

Tobacco is both a carcinogen (for certain types of lung cancer) and a leukemogen for mostly myeloid malignancies. Its action is direct and the role of "secondhand smoke" is uncertain. No less uncertain is the role of tobacco during pregnancy as a late, or delayed, leukemogen. Ongoing epidemiologic studies will hopefully provide an answer to many of these questions (64–67).

Industrial Hydrocarbons—Benzene: The single most thoroughly evaluated industrial carcinogen is benzene, a known leukemogen that induces the occurrence of ANLL either via inhalation or direct skin contact. At issue is whether chronically low levels of benzene are as deleterious as short-term, intensive exposures (68–74). The role of benzene as an inducer of ALL is unknown.

Pesticides: Certain pesticides may also be leukemogenic, but the evidence is less certain than the data regarding benzene and tobacco. Most of the presumptive insecticide-based reports arose out of case studies of cigarette-smoking farmers who rode tractors powered by unleaded gasoline containing heavy benzene concentration (75, 76).

Nonionizing and Ionizing Irradiation: Whether high tension wires, e.g., nonionizing irradiation-induced magnetic field strength changes, are leukemogenic is a highly charged issue, which has generated considerable notoriety. The evidence is inconsistent. Application of data that support high risk in one site frequently fail to do so in other highly supsect areas (77–80).

Ionizing irradiation, on the other hand, is a well established leukemogenic process, which early on wreaked havoc with unsuspecting patients and physicians. Before the consequences of unprotected radiologic procedures were fully understood, the highest frequency of leukemia occurred among radiology physicians (81–85). Radiation fallout from atomic bombs during World War II affected a marked increase in both ALL and ANLL in direct proportion to the distance from the epicenter of the bomb blast. The changes were not vertically transmitted and, accordingly, did not persist beyond one generation (86–92).

On the basis of the preceding information, one may assume reasonably that certain genetic factors probably interact unfavorably with certain environmental factors, both as yet largely unknown, in the initiation of a leukemic event. Such, indeed, may be the predominant mechanism operative during the first 5 to 6 years of life, the critical time of both lymphoid upregulation and the peak period of childhood ALL (93–95).

Classification

Cytology. Before the efforts of a combined group of French, American, and British (FAB) investigators in 1976, there was little that was logical to the morphologic designation of the acute leukemias. The classification derived from the FAB group, with only few modifications, has stood the test of time both as a continuum for effective use of established histochemical techniques and as a foundation for subsequent immunophenotyping (1–3).

Neither FAB L1 nor L2 distinguishes immature B-cell leukemia from any of the T-cell leukemias, and on occasion, L2 even fails to distinguish ALL from ANLL M2 and M3 types. However, FAB L1 predicts a more favorable outcome than FAB L2 or L3. FAB L2 is commonly seen in the (poor prognosis) adult ALL patient. It is, in all likelihood, an independent prognostic factor, because L2 disease in young patients is also associated with poor outcome. Often, but not always, L2 is associated with elevated WBC counts. FAB L3 is unequivocal both in its appearance and its predictive value as a high-risk disorder irrespective of patient age, sex, or cell volume.

Histochemistry. The early introduction of vital dyes was designed to identify a variety of myeloid subsets and distinguish them from lymphoid malignancies. The FAB classification incorporated histochemical techniques into the body of contemporary knowledge and was heavily used until the advent of immunophenotyping (table 18.6).

Immunophenotyping. The most reliable method of identifying lineage, and to a somewhat lesser extent, offering predictive data, is via the use of immunophenotyping (96–102). Before its use, the conditions most commonly confused with acute leukemia were metastatic lymphoma, Ewing's sarcoma, stage D neuroblastoma, and to a somewhat lesser extent, infectious mononucleosis and aplastic anemia. Today, immunophenotype and karyotype analyses essentially preclude the likelihood of a mistaken diagnosis.

Additional refinements added to the earlier knowledge of predictive information. It is now apparent that there are distinct age-related differences in the frequency of the various B-cell and T-cell leukemias (fig. 18.1). Infants have the fewest (3%) and adults have the largest (20%) number of T-cell leukemias. T-cell disorders account for approximately 10% of ALL in children and adolescents. Both infants and adults experience approximately the same percentage of mature B-cell malignancies (4%), which is roughly four times the frequency of that in children and adolescents.

More than 90% of children and adolescents have cALLa disease (CD10+/CD19+), which is almost twice as common as it is in adults. Pre-B patients with CD10+/CD19+ phenotypes, except for those with at-tendant high-risk chromosomal abnormalities, carry a more favorable prognosis than patients with the CD10−/CD19+ phenotype.

Mixed lineage leukemia is easy to diagnose but difficult to categorize vis a vis predominant lineage. This unusual and prognostically unfavorable subset accounts for 10% of all acute leukemia groups, occurs most often in adults, and is treated with a patchwork of combination ALL and ANLL therapy. Because of its high-risk category, the treatment of preference is BMT. Approximately 25% of adults, as compared to 5% of children, have eithernontypeable (null-cell leukemia) and/or mixed-lineage leukemia (103, 104).

The features of mixed lineage AL are detailed in table 18.7.

Risk Factor Summation

As shown in Table 18.8, those factors that lead to high risk include age at diagnosis <2 and >10 years, white cell counts at diagnosis >25 × 10⁹/L, bulk disease, L2 morphology, specific chromosomal abnormalities, pseudodiploidy, hypodiploidy, lengthy induction time, B-cell and (conditional) T-cell disease; DNA indices <1.2, mixed lineage and null-cell leukemia, and African-American race. With rare exception, two or more adverse factors are sufficient to establish a high-risk category. B-cell ALL is designated as "high risk," because of the unique pre-

Table 18.7. Features of Mixed-Lineage Leukemia

α-Naphthyl butyrate positive
CD-41 positive
Cytoplasmic and surface Ig positive
Myeloperoxidase positve
Platelet peroxidase positive
T cell receptor positive
Ig hgb and chain rearranagements
Karyotype abnormalities
Auer rods
E-rosette formation

Table 18.6. Cytology and Histochemistry of the Acute Leukemias

Cytology	Histochemistry	Pre-B and T-Cell FAB L1, L2	B-Cell L3	Myeloid Series FAB M1–M7
ALL FAB L1-L3	Acid phosphatase	+/−	−	−
L1 = 90% Early Pre-B	Myeloperoxidase	−	−	−
Pre-B and T	Sudan black	−	−	+
	Chloroacetate esterase	+/−	+/−	+
L2 = 10-15% ALL L1, L2, L3	Non-specific esterase	−	−	+
	Platelet peroxidase	−	−	+M1–M4
L3 = >75% Mature B(L3)	TdT	+	−	+M4, M7
	Periodic acid schiff	+°	−	+M6

°Positive in Pre-B ALL.

Table 18.8. High Risk Factors in ALL

> *Very High Risk*
>   Leukocyte count >25 × 10⁹/L
>   Age <2, >10 years
>   M3 Day 14 bone marrow
>   B-cell L3 FAB morphology
>   DNA index <1.2
>   Specified chromosomal translocations
>   Pseudodiploidy, hypodiploidy
>   Mediastinal mass
> *High Risk*
>   L2 morphology
>   Specified T-cell ALL
>   Null-cell ALL
>   Mixed-lineage AL
>   CNS leukemia at diagnosis
>   Black race

sentation of the clonal translocation and its highly proliferative process. T-cell ALL is high risk only in association with translocations and/or elevated tumor volume.

Clinical Manifestations at Onset

There are no systems that escape the ravages of leukemic involvement. Like most malignant processes, it is asocial and respects no boundaries. Its major manifestation relates to hematopoietic failure, but leukemic cell invasion into sovereign sites accounts for the myriad of symptoms brought by this disorder.

Skin involvement, or petechial hemorrhages, are the result of a fragile vascular system brought about by insufficient numbers of platelets. Leukemic infiltration into dermal and epidermal layers also occurs, but for unexplained reasons, more commonly the result of myeloid infiltration (105).

Upper and lower gastrointestinal (GI) tract invasion, although relatively common, often goes unnoticed. Symptoms include pain and eructation. Pathologic examination reveals infiltration and bleeding (106).

Ocular involvement may result in local infiltration, hemorrhages, papilledema (see CNS), and loss of visual acuity. Iritis, hypopyon, and glaucoma may, on occasion, herald the disease (107).

Genitourinary tract abnormalities include renal enlargement with occasional development of hypertension. Less common are reports of priapism and involvement of the uterus, ovaries, and fallopian tubes. The most frequent involvement is testicular invasion (30% of males) (108–110).

Pulmonary disorders as presenting features are uncommon and usually restricted to bleeding diatheses. **Thymic** infiltration, however, is a major symptom contributor. Almost 10% of all patients present with mediastinal disease, often characterized by respiratory impairment (111, 112).

Cardiac involvement is also uncommon, but pericardial infiltration and tamponade may be presenting features on rare occasion (113).

Bone and joint pain is a frequent manifestation, and it is common for many patients who present in this manner to commence their journey through the hematology arena via the rheumatology clinic (114).

Table 18.9 is a compendium of the symptoms, signs, and hematologic data at presentation.

The CNS, along with the testes (and to a lesser extent the ovaries), are common extramedullary sites of disease activity, usually occult but occasionally reservoirs of resistant disease. Less than 5% of patients with overt CNS disease. The symptoms, however, are unequivocal. The disease begins in the pia arachnoid, extends into the surrounding blood vessels, and infiltrates solid tissues and ventricles. Symptoms range from focal neurologic defects to gross disturbances, usually the result of increases in intracranial pressure, and include vomiting, headache, nucchal rigidity, convulsions, papilledema, excessive appetite, weight gain, hirsutism, diabetes insipidus, lethargy, coma, and features of demyelination. In all cases, abnormal cells are identified in the cerebrospinal fluid (115–117). Signs and symptoms of CNS leukemias and the relative frequencies are presented in table 18.10.

Therapy

Until a definite form or group of therapies that uniformly effects cures is available, the single most effective approach to treatment will continue to be the use of well designed, peer-reviewed, protocol-driven chemotherapy regimens carried out by multi-institution participation. It is particularly noteworthy that in the United States at least 80% of all pediatric patients, as compared to only 3% of adults, are enrolled in protocol studies.

Treatment regimens are designed to address the fact that, at any given time, approximately 20% of the leukemic

Table 18.9. Presenting Symptoms, Signs, and Hematology in ALL

Symptoms	(%)	Signs	(%)	Hematology	(%)
Fever	(40)	Pallor	(30	Hct (%)	
Lethargy	(35)	Hepatomegaly	(25)	>31	(20)
Bone/ joint pain	(20)	Splenomegaly	(25)	22–30	(40)
Bleeding	(20)	Hepato- splenomegaly	(20)	<21	(40)
Anorexia	(10)	Bleeding	(15)	WBC (x10⁹/L)	
GI	(5)	Lymph adenopathy	(15)	>100	(10)
Neurological	(2)			25–100	(20)
				10–25	(25)
				1–10	(40)
				<1	(5)
				Platelets (10⁹/L)	
				>100	(25)
				50–100	(25)
				10–50	(30)
				<10	(20)

Table 18.10. Signs and Symptoms of CNS Leukemia

	Percentage
Headache	80
Papilledema	80
Vomiting	80
Lethargy	70
Irritability	60
Nystagmus	60
Paralysis	60
Vertigo	60
Autonomic dysfunction	40
Visual defects	40
Convulsions	40
Cushing syndrome	40
Slurred speech	40
Coma	20
Depression	20
Hirsutism	20
Hoarseness	20
Hydrocephaly	20
Diabetes insipidus	10
Weight gain	10

cells are in G_0[118] and that drug resistance along with occult disease is the basis for the occurrence of relapse. Accordingly, continuous, multi-agent, rotational therapy along with intensification and dose-escalation activities directed at active and potential sites of disease are the hallmarks of effective therapeutic intent. Drug combinations that include vincristine, prednisone, 1-asparaginase, and daunomycin have been successful in the induction of remission in 93% of childhood and in approximately 75% of adult ALL. The use of anthracyclines is designed primarily for use in high-tumor-burden patients as well as the adult ALL group. Cyclophosphamide probably contributes little to induction therapy and is best used for the consolidation or intensification phase. The best therapy for mixed lineage or null-cell disease is probably combination AML and ALL therapy (106–127).

Tables 18.11, 18.12, and 18.13 are summations of historical data regarding induction results, the types and activities of the therapeutic agents, and a guidepost for high-risk versus standard-risk therapy.

The use of intensification therapy is based on empirical observations that early aggressive therapy reduces the risk of emergence of drug resistance. It is common practice to introduce such regimens in all high-risk patients. Conversely, the need for intensification in otherwise good-risk individuals is overbalanced by excessive toxicity in the face of minimal, if any, gains in therapeutic efficacy. By combining more than one agent for induction, and by continuing induction into an intensification phase with additional "other" agents, usually paired as singlets or alternating doublets, markedly improved survival times have been recorded in the higher-risk patients. Examples of these combinations include daunomycin and cytosine arabinoside, cyclophosphamide, or etoposide; cyclophosphamide and etoposide or methotrexate; and etoposide and

methotrexate. Another efficacious approach in treating high-risk patients is the use of 1500 cGy irradiation to bulk disease (129–139). Although it is apparent that intensification has bought more remission-free time, there are no data as yet that support "the" single most effective regimen.

An equally germane issue centers around the durability of remission (140). Is it sustainable in high-risk patients? Only with carefully planned, concurrent, peer-reviewed studies that compare best available therapy, viz., alloBMT versus aggressive (nonmarrow ablative, cytokine-rescued) intensified therapy after successful induction of remission, will this issue be resolved (141).

Approximately 5% of all patients with ALL, usually those with white cell counts in excess of 50×10^9/L, present with overt CNS disease at diagnosis. For these patients, combination intrathecal chemotherapy consisting of methotrexate (15 mg/m²), hydrocortisone (15 mg/m²), and cytosine arabinoside (30 mg/m²), followed by 1800 cGy to the cranium and 3000 cGy to the spinal axis, is the treatment of choice in all but infant ALL. Maintenance intrathecal therapy essentially ensures a disease-free state. Prophylactic intrathecal therapy is essential for all patients in whom evidence of disease is lacking and should consist of a regimen designed to maintain a disease-free status with minimal toxicity, e.g., weekly during induction and every 2 months thereafter for 1 year. The three-drug therapeutic regimens of MTX, HC, and ARA-C, described above, are one example of an excellent prophylactic combination (142–150). Table 18.14 is an example of a successful dose drug regimen for us as CNS prophylaxis or therapy.

Table 18.11. Historical Induction Therapy Data in Children With ALL

	CR%
1970s:	
Prednisone and VCR are backbone of induction regimens.	
1. +L-asparaginase, +DNR	93
2. L-asparaginase +IT Med (1)	95
1980s:	
1. +L-asparaginase and DNR	96
+Cyclo and DNR	90
2. +ADR and MTX +IT Med (1)	96
3. +L-asp and VM-26 and ARA-C +IT Med (1)	88
1990s:	
1. +DNR and Cyclo and L-asp and ARA-C +IT Meds (2)	96
2. +DNR and L-asp and VM-26 and ARA-C +IT Meds (3)	96
Current BMT Remission Induction and 5-Year Survival Rates:	

	Induction	Survival
Children:	93%	75%
Adults:	82%	36%

The overall best induction results occurred in patients who had DNR/ADR and IT medications added to the prednisone/vincristine/L-asparaginase combination.

Best overall induction results in adults is 82% (range, 70–93%).

Table 18.12. ALL Chemotherapeutic Agents and Pertinent Properties

Chemotherapeutic Agents	Dose (m^2)/Administration	Activity	Resistance
Vincristine	1.5 mg (never >2) q.w. i.v.	Mitotic inhibitor Binds tubulin	MDR
Prednisone	40 mg q.d. p.o.[a]	Lympholysis	Loss of receptors
L-asparaginase	6000 IU i.m. q.o.d.[b]	↓ Protein synthesis	↑ Asparaginase synthase
Daunomycin	30–40 mg/i.v. q.d.[c]	Intercalation, DNA	MDR
Adriamycin	45–75 mg i.v. q.3w.	strand breaks; free radical formation	
Cyclophosphamide	250–2000 mg i.v./p.o. q.28d.	Cross-linkage	↑ DNA repair GT transferase
Methotrexate	7.5–30 mg i.v./p.o. q.w.[c]	↓ Folate metabolism	↑ Folate reductase ↓ Transport
6-Mercaptopurine	75–100 mg p.o. q.d.	↓ Purine synthesis	↑ Degradation
Etoposide (VP-16)	60–120 mg i.v. q.3w.	DNA strand breaks	MDR
Teneposide (VM-26)	70–180 mg i.v. q.d.[d]		
Cytosine arabinoside	3000 mg i.v.[e]	↓ DNA polymerase	↑ Deoxycytidine triphosphate ↓ Transport

[a]Usually given for 28 days during induction.
[b]10–14 doses.
[c]May be given as high-dose bolus.
[d]Usually as 3-day therapy every 3 wks.
[e]Usually high dose q12 × 6 schedule.

Table 18.13. General Chemotherapy Guidelines in ALL

	Standard Risk		High Risk
Systemic therapy induction	Prednisone	q.d. × 28x	Prednisone
	Vincristine	q.w. × 4	Vincristine
	L-asparaginase	q.o.d. × 10	
			L-asparaginase
		q.w. × 4	Daunomycin
CNS therapy	MTX		MTX
	HC	q.w. × 4	HC
	ARA-C		ARA-C
Systemic therapy	High-dose MTX	q3 w. × 4	
			Combination of ARA-C, VP-16;
Consolidation/maintenance	Standard dose 6Mp	q.d. × 2 mos	High-dose MTX–cyclophosphamide for 1 year
	Standard dose MTX	q.w.	then MTX and 6-MP q.d. x 9w. as
	Standard dose 6MP Total 3 years	q.d.	intrathecal therapy
CNS prophylaxis	MTX		MTX
	HC	q.60d. × 1 yr	HC
	ARA-C		ARA-C

For patients who experience a first relapse in an extramedullary site, reinduction therapy with radiation to the involved site is appropriate on the proviso that it has not been the subject of prior radiation therapy. Such therapy should also include a 2-year course of systemic therapy commencing with induction and following through with intensification and maintenance. The intent of this approach, after the relapse site has been presumptively "sterilized," is to prevent egress from the contaminated area. In addition, multiple relapses in a single extramedullary site are best treated in centers carrying out "investigative" research into such events. Unlike its use in first systemic relapse, alloBMT does not have a role in the treatment of

Table 18.14. Intrathecal Chemotherapy

Drugs[*]	Dose (mg/m^2)
Methotrexate	15
Hydrocortisone	15
Cytosine arabinoside	30

SCHEDULE:
Induction: q.wk × 4; Maintenance: q.8 wk.
1. One year in low-risk patients and to completion of systemic therapy in high-risk patients.
2. Includes cranio-spinal irradiation (1800 Gy) in patients with CNS disease at onset or relapse.

[*]Single agent (MTX) therapy may be as efficacious as triple therapy.

Table 18.15. Techniques for Detection of Residual Disease

Technique	Activity Site	Sensitivity
Light microscopy	Cytology	10^{-1}
Fluorescent in-situ hybridization	Chromosomes	10^{-2}
Cytogenetics	Chromosomes	10^{-2}
Fluorescent cell sorting	Antigens	10^{-3}
Gene rearrangement	DNA composition	10^{-3}
Polymerase chain reaction	DNA/RNA structures	10^{-5}
Clonogenic culture assays	In vitro assay	10^{-5}

first extramedullary relapse. Details of the use and timing of BMT are included in the chapters dedicated to auto- and alloBMT.

Failure to effect cure in any case of leukemia is related to considerable part to the failure of therapy to seek out minimal residual disease and/or overcome drug resistance. The latter may be the result of drug expulsion along specified internal channels or failure of therapy to gain access to cells in G_0 Means of overcoming either G_0 or the genetic control of calcium channel activity are part of ongoing investigative programs. No less important is the need to develop highly specific technologies to detect minimal residual disease. Table 18.15 is a summation of known detection modalities.

Iatrogenic Problems

Just as few systems escape the onslaught of the disease and/or its therapy, iatrogenic disturbances may leave permanent damage. Overdosing, or sometimes merely idiosyncratic responses, in addition to varying degrees of hematologic suppression, may lead to severe polyneuropathies (vincristine); acute or chronic cardiac degeneration (daunomycin, etc.); hemorrhagic cystitis/fibrosis or myocardial necrosis (cyclophosphamide); hepatitis (6 mercaptopurine/MTX); renal failure, pulmonary fibrosis, bone fractures (MTX); cerebritis (ARA-C); diabetes mellitus (corticosteroids); hypotensive shock (VP-16) and severe coagulopathies (1-asparaginase) (151–161). Secondary leukemias may also follow on the use of certain of the chemotherapeutic agents, including cyclophosphamide, cisplatin, melaphalan, doxorubicin, VP-16, and perhaps growth hormone (see Secondary Leukemias, Chapter 24) (164–166).

Supportive Therapy

Much of the success in effecting longterm survival leading to cure in ALL is the direct result of aggressive and intelligent use of supportive therapy, i.e., including anti-infective agents, nutrition, biologic response modifiers, and blood products. Guidelines for the use of any of the above approaches can only be addressed in general terms, but it is far safer to be aggressive and then back off when sufficient information permits a lessening of efforts than it is to attempt to catch up to a situation well out of control.

For example, a patient with unexplained fever and cardiovascular instability requires a thorough assessment of possible causes and aggressive use of empirical, broad-spectrum, anti-infective therapy. In effect, treatment of disease and/or therapy-related complications demands the same keen clinical sense that an understanding of the biologic features of the disease itself mandates. Other examples include the uses of parenteral nutrition and cytokine, i.e., biologic response modifier therapy. The former is an absolute necessity in any individual whose oral nutrition is inadequate to the needs of effective and aggressive treatment modalities. In the final analysis, responsible care includes a thorough appreciation of all disease-related phenomena, including an awareness of early changes or subliminal differences that may impede therapeutic efficacy. Cytokine therapy should not be withheld solely because of unsubstantiated concerns regarding the potential reintroduction of clones of malignant stem cells. However, cytokines should not be used without evidence to support their efficacy in shortening the intervals between therapy courses. Blood product support, and particularly the use of red cells and platelets, should be provided only when it is apparent that the decrements in red cells and platelets are associated with impending clinical impairment. The frequency of hepatitis and the chance of transmitting HIV or CMV to an immunosuppressed recipient, albeit uncommon, is nonetheless real. Whether there is a role for routine use of hyperimmune gammaglobulin is also highly suspect. It too, should be restricted to clearly proven approaches to therapy.

The Past and the Future

Forty years after the introduction of aminopterin (the first truly effective chemotherapeutic agent and the direct ancestor of methotrexate), the earlier feelings of hopelessness attendant upon the diagnosis of leukemia have been remarkably lessened. One can now predict outcome at the time of diagnosis with remarkable accuracy, and it is this knowledge that enables us to recognize how far we have come and how much further we must travel in pursuit of a 100% success goal. Improvements in the selection and use of chemotherapeutic agents, along with dramatic advances in the use of a variety of support systems, have further reduced the number of prognostic features to an understandable few. Nonetheless, drug resistance, residual disease, and toxicity-induced complications continue to be the most difficult obstacles to successful treatment in this group of disorders. In all likelihood, today's successes will be further enhanced in the years to come by the effective use of modulated stem cell transplantation along with gene targeting and, in selected cases, by the judicious use of vaccines.

REFERENCES

1. Bennett JM, et al. Proposals for the classification of the acute leukemias. Br J Haematol 1976;33:451.
2. Bennett JM, et al. Criteria for the diagnosis of acute leukemia of megakaryocytic lineage (M7). Ann Intern Med 1985;103:460.

3. Bennett JM, et al. The morphologic classification of acute lymphoblastic leukaemia: concordance among observers and clinical correlations. Br J Haematol 1981;47:553.

4. Spier CM, et al. Pre-B cell acute lymphoblastic leukemia in the newborn. Blood 1984;64:1064.

5. Crist W, et al. Clinical and biologic features predict a poor prognosis in acute lymphoid leukemias in infants. Blood 1986;67:135.

6. Reaman G, Zeltzer P, Bleyer WA, et al. Acute lymphoblastic leukemia in infants less than one year of age: a cumulative experience of the Children's Cancer Study Group. J Clin Oncol 1985;3:1513.

7. Greaves MF. The Sellafield childhood leukemia cluster: are germline mutations responsible? Leukemia 1990;4:391.

8. Ratain MJ, et al. Acute non-lymphocytic leukemia following etoposide and cisplatin combination chemotherapy for advanced non-small-cell carcinoma of the lung. Blood 1987;70:1412.

9. Homans AD, et al. Effect of 1-asparaginase administration on coagulation and platelet function in children with leukemia. J Clin Oncol 1987;5:811.

10. Pochedly C. Prevention of meningeal leukemia: review of 20 years of research and current recommendations. Hematol Oncol Clin North Am 1990;4:951.

11. Miller DR, et al. Prognostic implications of blast cell morphology in childhood acute lymphoblastic leukemia: a report from Children's Cancer Study Group. Cancer Treat Rep 1985;69:1211.

12. Kalwinsky DK, et al. Clinical relevance of lymphoblast biologic features in children with acute lymphoblastic leukemia. J Clin Oncol 1985;3:477.

13. Baccarani M, et al. Adolescent and adult acute lymphoblastic leukemia: prognostic features and outcome of therapy. A study of 293 patients. Blood 1982;60:677.

14. Leimert JT, et al. Prognostic influence of pretreatment characteristics in adult acute lymphoblastic leukemia. Blood 1980;56:510.

15. Thomas LB, et al. The skeletal lesions of acute leukemia. Cancer 1961;14:608.

16. McWhirter WR. The relationship of incidence of childhood lymphoblastic leukemia to social class. Br J Cancer 1982;46:640.

17. Greaves MF, et al. Collaborative group study of the epidemiology of acute lymphoblastic leukemia subtypes: background and first report. Leuk Res 1985;9:715.

18. Thiel E. Biological and clinical significance of immunological cell markers in leukemia. Rec Results Cancer Res 1984;93:102.

19. Kalwinsky DK, et al. Variation by race in presenting clinical and biologic features of childhood acute lymphoblastic leukemia: implications for treatment outcome. Leuk Res 1985;9:817.

20. Kasili EG. Leukemia and lymphoma in Keyna. Leuk Res 1985;9:747.

21. Kushawa MRS, et al. Leukemias and lymphomas at Luchnow India. Leuk Res 1985;9:799.

22. Stevens RG. Age and risk of acute leukemia. JNCI 1986;76:845.

23. Greaves MF. Speculations on the cause of childhood acute lymphoblastic leukemia. Leukemia 1988;2:210.

24. Kalwinsky DK, et al. Variation by race in presenting clinical and biologic features of childhood acute lymphoblastic leukemia: implications for treatment outcome. Med Pediatr Oncol 1975;1:143.

25. Pendergrass TW, et al. Prognosis of black children with acute lymphocytic leukemia. Med Pediatr Oncol 1975;1:143.

26. Miller DR, Leikin SL, Albo VC, Sather H, Hammond GD. Three versus five years of maintenance therapy are equivalent in childhood acute lymphoblastic leukemia: a report from the Children's Cancer Study Group. J Clin Oncol 1989;7:316.

27. Hoelzer D, Thiel E, Loffler H, et al. Prognostic factors in multicenter study for treatment of acute lymphoblastic leukemia in adults. Blood 1988;71:123.

28. Greene MH, et al. Lymphomas and leukemias in the relatives of patients with mycosis fungoides. Cancer 1982;49:737.

29. Miller RW. Persons with exceptionally high risk of leukemia. Cancer Res 1967;27:2420.

30. Pendergrass TW. Epidemiology of acute lymphoblastic leukemia. Semin Oncol 1985;9:661.

31. Levitt GA, et al. Prognosis of Down's syndrome with acute leukemia. Arch Dis Child 1990;65:212.

32. Peeters M, Poon A. Down's syndrome and leukemia: unusual clinical aspects and unexpected methotrexate sensitivity. Eur J Pediatr 1987;146:416.

33. Harnden DG. Inherited factors in leukemia. Leuk Res 1985;9:705.

34. Lerena JC, Mureru-Orlando M. Bloom's syndrome and ataxia telangiectasia. Semin Hematol 1991;28:95.

35. Filipovich AH, et al. The Immunodeficiency Cancer Registry. A research resource. Am J Pediatr Hematol Oncol 1987;9:183.

36. German J. Patterns of neoplasia associated with the chromosome-breakdage syndromes. In: German J, ed. Chromosome mutation and neoplasia. New York: Alan Liss, 1983.

37. Passarge E. Bloom's syndrome. In: German J, ed. Chromosome mutation and neoplasia. New York: Alan Liss, 1983.

38. Gatti RA, et al. Localization of an ataxia-telangiectasia gene to chromosome 11q22-23. Nature 1988;336:577.

39. Spector BD, et al. Genetically determined immunodeficiency diseases (GDID) and malignancy: report from the Immunodeficiency-Cancer Registry. Clin Immunol Immunopathol 1978:11:12.

40. Auerbach AD, et al. Acute myeloid leukemia as the first hematologic manifestation of Fanconi anemia. Am J Hematol 1982;12:289.

41. Garriga S, Crosby WH. The incidence of leukemia in families of patients with hypoplasia of the marrow. Blood 1959;14:1008.

42. Petersen-Bjergaard J, et al. Possible pathogenetic significance of specific chromosome abnormalities and activated protooncogenes in malignant diseases of man. Scand J Haematol 1986;36:127.

43. Secker-Walker LM. Prognostic and biological importance of chromosome findings in acute lymphoblastic leukemia. Cancer Genet Cytogenet 1990;49:1.

44. Pui C-H, Carroll AJ, Head D, et al. Near-triploidy and near-tetraploidy acute lymphoblastic leukemia of childhood. Blood 1990;76:590.

45. Pui C-H, Williams DL, Roberson PK, et al. Correlation of karyotype and immunophenotype in childhood acute lymphoblastic leukemia. J Clin Oncol 1988;6:56.

46. Look AT. The cytogenetics of childhood leukemia: clinical and biologic implications. Pediatr Clin North Am 1988;35:723.

47. Jackson JF, Pullen J. Patterson R, Land V, Borowitz M, Crist W. Favorable prognosis associated with hyperdiploidy in children with acute lymphocytic leukemia correlates with extra chromosome 6: a Pediatric Oncology Group study. Cancer 1990;66:1183.

48. Crist WM, Pui C-H. Clinical implications of cytogenetic and molecular analyses of pediatric acute lymphoblastic leukemia. Stem Cells 1993;11:81.

49. Crist W, Carroll A, Shuster J, et al. Philadelphia chromosome positive childhood lymphoblastic leukemia: clinical and cytogenetic characteristics and treatment outcome. Pediatric Oncology Group (POG) Study. Blood 1990; 76:489.

50. Pui D-H, Frankel LS, Carroll AJ, et al. Clinical characteristics and treatment outcome of childhood acute lymphoblastic leukemia with t(4;11)(q21;q23): a colloborative study of 40 cases. Blood 1991;77:440.

51. Ribeiro RC, Raimondi SC, Behm FG, et al. Clinical and biologic features of childhood T-cell leukemia with the t(11;14)(p13;q11) or t(11;14)(p15;q11). Blood 1991;78:466.

52. Huret JL, Heerema NA, Brizard A, et al. Two additional cases of tdic (9;12) in lymphocytic leukemia. Blood 1990; 76:1626.

53. Carroll AJ, Crist WM, Parmley RT, Roper M, Cooper MD, Finley WH. Pre-B cell leukemia associated with chromosome translocation 1:19. Blood 1984;63:721.

54. Facer CA, Playfair JKL. Malaria, Epstein-Barr virus and the genesis of lymphomas. Adv Cancer Res 1989;53:33.

55. List AF, et al. Lymphoproliferative diseases in immunocompromised hosts: the role of Epstein-Barr virus. J Clin Oncol 1987;5:1673.

56. Kieff E, Liebowitz D. Oncogenesis by herpes viruses. In: Weinberg RA, ed. Oncogenes and the molecular origins of cancer. Cold Spring Harbor: Cold Spring Harbor Laboratory Press, 1989.

57. Sullivan JL. Epstien-Barr virus and lymphoproliferative disorders. Semin Hematol 1988;25:269.

58. Cannon MJ, et al. Epstein-Barr virus induces aggressive lymphoproliferative disorders of human B cell origin in SCID/hu chimeric mice. J Clin Invest 1990;85:1333.

59. Blayney DW, et al. The human T-cell leukemia/lymphoma virus associated with American adult T-cell leukemia/lymphoma. Blood 1983;62:401.

60. Gallo RC. Human T-cell leukemia (lymphotropic) retroviruses and their causative role in T-cell malignancies and acquired immune deficiency syndrome. Cancer 1985; 55:2317.

61. Song-Staal F, Gallo RC. The family of human T-lymphotropic leukemia viruses: HTLV-1 as the cause of adult T cell leukemia and HTLV-III as the cause of acquired immunodeficiency syndrome. Blood 1985;65:253.

62. Bunn PA, et al. Clinical course of retrovirus-associated adult T-cell lymphoma in the United States. N Engl J Med 1983;309:257.

63. Kita K, et al. Epidemiologic and immunologic characteristics of acute lymphoblastic leukemia and adult T-cell leukemia in Japan. Leuk Res 1985;9:781.

64. Archimbaud E, et al. Influence of cigarette smoking on the presentation and course of chronic myelogenous leukemia. Cancer 1989;63:2060.

65. Garfinkel L, Bofetta P. Association between smoking and leukemia in two American Cancer Society prospective studies. Cancer 1990;65:2356.

66. Mills PK, et al. History of cigarette smoking and isk of leukemia and myeloma: results from the Adventist Health Study. JNCI 1990;82:1832.

67. Sandler DP. Epidemiology of acute myelogenous leukemia. Semin Oncol 1987;14:359.

68. Askoy M. Hematotoxicity and carcinogenicity of benzene. Environ Health Perspect 1989;82:193.

69. Askoy M. Chronic lymphoid leukemia and hairy cell leukemia due to chronic exposure to benzene: report of three cases. Br J Haematol 1987;66:209.

70. Askoy M. Benzene as a leukemogenic and carcinogenic agent. Am J Indust Med 1985;8:9.

71. Braier L. An hypothesis for the induction of leukemia by benzene. Arch Toxicol 1983; (Suppl 6):42.

72. Brett SM, et al. Review and update of leukemia risk potentially associated with occupational exposure to benzene. Environ Health Perspect 1989;82:267.

73. Berlin M. Low level benzene exposure in Sweden: effect on blood elements and body burden of benzene. Am J Indust Med 1985;7:365.

74. Austin H, et al. Benzene and leukemia. A review of the literature and a risk assessment. Am J Epidemiol 1988; 127:419.

75. Axelson O. Pesticides and cancer risks in agriculture. Med Oncol Tumor Pharmacother 1987;4:207.

76. Hoar SK, et al. Agricultural herbicide use and risk of lymphoma on self-tissue sarcoma. JAMA 1986;256:1141.

77. Coleman MP, et al. Leukemia and residence near electricity transmission equipment: a case-control study. Br J Cancer 1989;60:793.

78. Goodman R, Shirley-Henderson A. Exposure of cells to extremely low-frequency electromagnetic field: relationship to malignancy. Cancer Cells 1990;2:355.

79. Savitz DA, et al. Case-control study of childhood cancer and exposure to 60-Hz magnetic fields. Am J Epidemiol 1988; 128:21.

80. Severson RK, et al. Acute nonlymphocytic leukemia and residential exposure to power frequency magnetic fields. Am J Epidemiol 1988;128:10.

81. Cronkite EP. Is natural background or radiation from nuclear power plants leukemogenic? Prog Clin Biol Res 1990; 352:439.

82. Boice JD, et al. Radiation dose and leukemia risk in patients treated for cancer of the cervix. JNCI 1987;79:1295.

83. Bolvin J-F, et al. Leukemia after radiotherapy for first primary cancers of various anatomic sites. Am J Epidemiol 1986;123:993.

84. Curtis RE, et al. Leukemia risk following radiotherapy for breast cancer. J Clin Oncol 1989;7:21.

85. Evans JH. Leukemia and radiation. Nature 1990;345:16.

86. Kato H. Cancer mortality. In: Shigematsu I, Kagan A, eds. Cancer in atomic bomb survivors. Tokyo: Japan Scientific Societies Press, 1986.

87. Kellerer AM. Mathematical methods and models for radiation carcinogenesis studies. Leuk Res 1986;10:711.

88. Knox EG, et al. Cancer following nuclear weapons tests. Lancet 1983;1:815.

89. Land CE, et al. Childhood leukemia and fallout from the Nevada nuclear tests. Science 1984;223:139.

90. Maruyama T. Atomic bomb dosimetry for epidemiological studies of survivors in Hiroshima and Nagasaki. In: Shigematsu I, Kagan A, eds. Cancer in atomic bomb survivors. Tokyo: Japan Scientific Societies Press, 1986.

91. Matsuo T, et al. Reclassification of leukemia among A-bomb survivors in Nagasaki using French-American-British (FAB) classification for acute leukemia. Jpn J Clin Oncol 1988;18:91.

92. Archer VE. Association of nuclear fallout with leukemia in the United States. Arch Environ Health 1987;42:263.

93. Onions De, Jarrott O. Viral oncogenesis. Lessons from naturally occurring animal viruses. Cancer Surv 1987;6:161.

94. Wyke J. Principles of viral leukemogenesis. Semin Hematol 1986;23:189.

95. Hehlmann R, et al. Current understanding of virus etiology in leukemia. Rec Res Cancer Res 1984;93:1.

96. Crist WM, Grossi CE, Pullen DJ, Cooper MD. Immunologic markers in childhood acute lymphocytic leukemia. Semin Oncol 1985;12:105.

97. Jacobs AD, Gale RP. Recent advances in the biology and treatment of acute lymphoblastic leukemia in adults. N Engl J Med 1984;311:1219.

98. Pullen DJ, Boyett JM, Crist WM, et al. Pediatric Oncology Group utilization of immunologic markers in the designation of acute lymphocytic leukemia subgroups: influence on treatment response. Ann N Y Acad Sci 1984;428:26.

99. Vogler LB, Crist WM, Bockman De, Pearl ER, Lawton AR, Cooper MD. Pre-B-cell leukemia: a new phenotype of childhood lymphoblastic leukemia. N Engl J Med 1978; 298:872.

100. Crist W, Rivera G, Pullen J, Weinstein H. The leukemias of childhood. In: Rosenthal DS, Feinstein DI, Goodnight S, McArthus JR, eds. Hematology 1985. Education Program. New Orleans: American Society of Hematology, 1985;48.

101. Deleted in proof.

102. Sobol RE, Royston I, LeBien TW, et al. Adult acute lymphoblastic leukemia phenotypes defined by monoclonal antibodies. Blood 1985;65:730.

103. Mirro J, Zipf TF, Pui C-H, et al. Acute mixed lineage leukemia: clinicopathologic correlations and prognostic significance. Blood 1985;66:1115.

104. Mirro J, Kitchingman GR. The morphology, cytochemistry, molecular characteristics and clinical significance of acute mixed lineage leukemia. In: Scott S, ed. Leukaemia cytochemistry. Chichester, UK: Ellis Horwood, 1989;155.

105. Reed RJ, Cummings LE. Malignant reticulosis and related conditions of the skin. Cancer 1966;19:1231.

106. Prolla JC, Kirsner JB. The gastrointestinal lesions and complications of the leukemias. Ann Intern Med 1964; 61:1084.

107. Holbrook CT, Elsas FJ, Crist WM, Castleberry RP. Acute leukemia and hypopyon. J Pediatr 1978;93:626.

108. Givler RL. Involvement of the bladder in leukemia. J Urol 1971;105:667.

109. Wintrobe MM, Mitchell DM. Atypical manifestation of leukemia. G J Med 1940;9:67.

110. Hamlin JA, et al. Lymphomas of the testical. Cancer 1972; 29:1352.

111. Bodey GP, Powell RD Jr, Hersh EM, Yeterian A, Freireich EJ. Pulmonary complications of acute leukemia. Cancer 1966;19:781.

112. Gilmartin D. Leukemia involvement of the thymus in children. Br J Radiol 1963;36:211.

113. Jaffe N, Traggis DG, Tefft M. Acute leukemia presenting with pericardial tamponade. Pediatrics 1970;45:461.

114. Masera G, Carneli V, Ferrari M, Recchia M, Bellini F. Prognostic significance of radiological bone involvement in

115. Evans AE, Gilbert ES, Zandstra R. The increasing incidence of central nervous system leukemia in children. (Children's Cancer Study Group A). Cancer 1970; 26:404.

116. Hyman CB, et al. Central nervous system involvement by leukemia in children. Blood 1965;25:1.

117. Hagbin M, Zuelzer WW. A long-term study of cerebrospinal leukemia. J Pediatr 1965;67:23.

118. Hill BT, Baserga R. The cell cycle and its significance for cancer treatment. Cancer Treat Rev 1975;2:159.

119. Vaughn WP, Karp JE, Burke PJ. Two-cycle-timed sequential chemotherapy for adult acute nonlymphocytic leukemia. Blood 1984;64:975.

120. Bernard J, Boiron M, Weil M. Etude de la remission complete des leucemies aigues. Nouv Rev Fr Hematol 1962; 2:195.

121. Evans ZE, Farber S, Brunet S, Mariano PJ. Vincristine in the treatment of acute leukemia in children. Cancer 1963; 16:1302.

122. Selawry OS, Frei E III. Prolongation of remission in acute lymphocytic leukemia by alteration in dose schedule and route of administration of methotrexate. Clin Res 1964; 12:231.

123. Tan C, Tasaka H, Yu KP, et al. Daunomycin, an antitumor antibiotic in the treatment of neoplastic disease. Cancer 1967;20:333.

124. Oettgen HF, et al. Inhibition of leukemias in man by 1-asparaginase. Cancer Res 1967;27:2619.

125. Sackman MF, Pavlosky S, Penalver JA, et al. Evaluation of induction of remission, intensification, and central nervous system prophylactic treatment in acute lymphoblastic leukemia. Cancer 1974;34:418.

126. Pullen DJ, Sullivan MP, Falletta JM, et al. Modified LSA2-L2 treatment in 53 children with E-rosette-positive T-cell leukemia: results and prognostic factors—a Pediatric Oncology Group study. Blood 1982;60:1159.

127. Shaw MT, Raab SO. Adriamycin in combination chemotherapy of adult acute lymphoblastic leukemia: a Southwest Oncology Group study. Med Pediatr Oncol 1977;3:261.

128. Gottlieb AJ, Weinberg V, Ellison RR, et al. Efficacy of daunorubicin in the therapy of adult acute lymphocytic leukemia: a prospective randomized trial by Cancer and Leukemia Group B. Blood 1984;64:267.

129. Shinn LC, Cruz Jm, Powell BL, et al. A dose-intense cyclic treatment program for adult acute lymphoblastic leukemia (ALL) (abstract). Proc Am Soc Clin Oncol 1991; 10:224.

130. Riehm H, Gadner H, Henze G. The Berlin childhood acute lymphoblastic leukemia study, 1970–1976. Am J Pediatr Hematol Oncol 1980;2:299.

131. Riehm H, Feickert H-J, Lampert F. Acute lymphoblastic leukemia. In: Voute PA, Barrett A, Bloom J, eds. UICC cancer in children: clinical management. Berlin: Springer-Verlag, 1986;101.

132. Gaynon PS, Steinherz PG, Bleyer WA, et al. Intensive therapy for children with acute lymphoblastic leukaemia and unfavorable presenting features. Early conclusions of study CCG-106 by the Children's Cancer Study Group. Lancet 1988;1:921.

133. Clavell LA, Gelber RD, Cohen HJ, et al. Four-agent induction and intensive asparaginase therapy for treatment of

childhood acute lymphoblastic leukaemia. Arch Dis Child 1977;52:530.

childhood acute lymphoblastic leukemia. N Engl J Med 1986;315:657.

134. Krisham A, Paika D, Frei E III. Cytofluormetric studies on the action of podophyllotoxin and epidophyllotoxins (VM-26, VP-16-213) on the cell cycle traverse of human lymphoblasts. J Cell Biol 1975;66:521.

135. Ribera G, Dahl GV, Bowman WP, Avery TL, Wood A, Aur RJ. VM-26 and cytosine arabinoside combination chemotherapy for initial induction failures in childhood lymphocytic leukemia. Cancer 1980;46:1727.

136. Dahl GV, Rivera GK, Look AT, et al. Teniposide plus cytarabine improves outcome in childhood acute lymphoblastic leukemia presenting with a leukocyte count $\geq 100 \times 10^9/L$. J Clin Oncol 1987;5:1015.

137. Linker CA, Levitt LJ, O'Donnell M, et al. Improved results of treatment of adult acute lymphoblastic leukemia. Blood 1987;69:1242.

138. Pinkel D. Curing children of leukemia. Cancer 1987; 59:1683.

139. Shapiro E, Kinsella TJ, Makuch RW, et al. Effects of fractionated irradiation on endocrine aspects of testicular function. J Clin Oncol 1985;3:1232.

140. Land VJ, Berry DH, Herson J, et al. Long-term survival in childhood acute leukemia: "late" relapses. Med Pediatr Oncol 1979;7:19.

141. Herzig R, Bortin MM, Gluckman E, et al. Optimal timing of bone marrow transplantation in patients with high risk acute lymphoblastic leukemia. Lancet 1987;1:786.

142. van Eys J, Berry D, Crist WM, et al. Treatment intensity and outcome for children with acute lymphocytic leukemia of standard risk: a Pediatric Oncology Group study. Cancer 1989;63:466.

143. Aur RJ, Simone J, Hustu HO, et al. Central nervous system therapy and combination chemotherapy of childhood lymphocytic leukemia. Blood 1971;137:272.

144. Nesbit ME Jr, Sather HN, Robison LL, et al. Presymptomatic central nervous system therapy in previously untreated childhood acute lymphoblastic leukemia: comparison of 1800 rad and 2400 ad—a report for Children's Cancer Study Group. Lancet 1981;1:461.

145. Sullivan MP, Chen T, Cyment PG, et al. Equivalence of intrathecal chemotherapy and radiotherapy as central nervous system prophylaxis in children with acute lymphoblastic leukemia: a Pediatric Oncology Group study. Blood 1982;60:948.

146. Morra E, Lazzarino M, Brusamolino E, et al. Systemic high-dose cytosine arabinoside (HDARA-C) for treatment of central nervous system disease (CNS) in adult acute lymphoblastic leukemia (ALL) and non-Hodgkin's lymphoma (NHL). Proc Am Soc Clin Oncol 1986;5:161.

147. Winick N, Smith SD, Shuster J, Wharam MD, Buchanan GR, Rivera GK. Treatment of central nervous system relapse in children with acute lymphoblastic leukemia: a Pediatric Oncology Group study. J Clin Oncol 1993;11:271.

148. Rivera GK, Ochs J, Roberson PK, et al. Intensive salvage therapy for isolated initial CNS relapses in childhood ALL. Blood 1986;68:802.

149. Rivera GK, Mauer AM. Controversies in the management of childhood acute lymphoblastic leukemia: treatment intensification. CNS leukemia, and prognostic factors. Semin Hematol 1987;24:12.

150. Nesbit ME, Ribison LL, Ortega JA. Testicular relapse in childhood acute lymphoblastic leukemia: association with pretreatment patient characteristics and treatment. A report for Children's Cancer Study Group. Cancer 1980; 45:2009.

151. Shamberger RC, Weinstein HJ, Delorey MJ, Levey RH. The medical and surgical management of typhlitis in children with acute nonlymphocytic (myelogenous) leukemia. Cancer 1986;57:603.

152. Newberger PE, Cassady JR, Jaffe N. Esophagitis due to adriamycin and radiation therapy for childhood malignancy. Cancer 1978;42:417.

153. Nesbit M, Krivit W, Heyn R, Sharp H. Acute and chronic effects of methotrexate on hepatic, pulmonary, and skeletal systems. Cancer 1978;37:1048.

154. Coggins PR, Ravdin RG, Eisman SM. Clinical pharmacology and preliminary evaluation of cytoxan (cyclophosphamide). Cancer Chemother Rep 1959;3:9.

155. Warne GL, Fairley GF, Hobbs JB, et al. Cyclophosphamide-induced ovarian failure. N Engl J Med 1973; 289:1159.

156. Blum RH, Carter SK. Review of adriamycin, a new anti-cancer drug with significant clinical activity. Ann Intern Med 1974;80:249.

157. Ragab AH, Freich RS, Vietti TJ. Osteoporotic fractures secondary to methotrexate therapy of acute leukemia in remission. Cancer 1970;25:580.

158. Schriock EA, Schell MJ, Carter M, Hustu O, Ochs JJ. Abnormal growth patterns and adult short stature in 115 long-term survivors of childhood leukemia. J Clin Oncol 1991; 9:400.

159. Poplack DG, Brouwers P. Adverse sequelae of central nervous system therapy. Clin Oncol 1985;4:263.

160. Price RA, Jamieson PA. The central nervous system in childhood leukemia II. Subacute leukoencephalopathy. Cancer 1975;35:306.

161. Brouwers P, Riccardi R, Fedio R, Poplack DG. Long-term neuropsychological sequelae of childhood leukemia: correlations with CT brain scan abnormalities. J Pediatr 1985; 106:723.

162. Kelaghan J, Myers MH, Mulvihill JJ, et al. Educational achievement of long-term survivors of childhood and adolescent cancer. Med Pediatr Oncol 1988;16:320.

163. Ribiero RC, Pui C-H. The clinical and biological correlates of coagulopathy in children with acute leukemia. J Clin Oncol 1986;4:1212.

164. Chambers SK, et al. Development of leukemia after doxorubicin and cisplatin treatment for ovarian cancer. Cancer 1989;64:2459.

165. Greene MH, et al. Melphalan may be a more potent leukemogen than cyclophosphamide. Ann Intern Med 1986; 105:360.

166. Fisher DA, et al. Leukemia in patients treated with growth hormone. Lancet 1988;1:1159.

CHAPTER 19

Chronic Lymphocytic Leukemia

ROBERT K. STUART

A doctor who cannot take a good history and a patient who cannot give one are in danger of giving and receiving bad treatment.
—Anonymous

Chronic lymphocytic leukemia (CLL) is a neoplastic disease characterized by the accumulation—in the blood, bone marrow, and lymphatic organs—of morphologically mature but immunologically dysfunctional lymphocytes. In almost all cases, the abnormal lymphocyte population represents a clone of malignantly transformed B-cells.

Case 1

In 1982 a 62-year-old retired executive evaluated because of abnormal electrocardiogram (ECG) results during exercise was found to have severe coronary artery disease. Preparation for coronary artery bypass surgery included a complete blood count (CBC) that was normal except for a white blood cell (WBC) count of 12.3×10^9/L with 69% lymphocytes on differential cell count. After recuperation from surgery, the patient left the country for a 3-year period. Upon his return, he revealed that he had obtained old records of annual "executive physicals" required by his company. By chance, these had included CBCs and differential cell counts, and it was possible to document the onset of lymphocytosis in 1977 and the absence of significant progression since that time (table 19.1).

Commentary

The approach to the patient with lymphocytosis and normal physical findings begins with an examination of the peripheral blood film. Reactive lymphocytosis is usually easily distinguished from chronic lymphocytic leukemia (CLL) by the transient nature of the former versus the sustained lymphocytosis of CLL. In many cases of infectious lymphocytosis the large cell morphology of the lymphocytes and other clinical features allow distinction from CLL. In cases where there is doubt or where a rapid definitive diagnosis is desired, cell surface marker studies will distinguish the usually T-cell lineage and polyclonal nature of the reactive lymphocytosis from the monoclonal B-cell lymphocytosis of B-CLL. This will not resolve the question of the rare (2–5% of CLL) case of T-CLL, which may require more sophisticated studies.

Morphologically, CLL lymphocytes are usually typical small lymphocytes, although variable percentages of larger cells, including some with nucleoli, are seen, especially as the disease evolves. In the patient with significant lymphocytosis ($>30 \times 10^9$/L), marrow examination is not required to establish the diagnosis, especially with the demonstration of clonality of the blood lymphocyte population. However, marrow examination provides important prognostic information: diffuse lymphoid infiltration with massive replacement of normal marrow and fat correlates with advanced stage and poor survival (1); the other patterns of marrow involvement (interstitial, nodular, or mixed interstitial and nodular) are associated with lower stage and better survival. In patients without lymphadenopathy on physical examination, diagnostic imaging studies of thoracic, abdominal, and pelvic lymph nodes are not necessary; such information has not been incorporated into clinical staging systems. Imaging may be helpful in patients with suspected but nonpalpable splenomegaly or to investigate symptoms potentially attributable to visceral adenopathy.

Case 1 represents an increasingly common mode of presentation of CLL: a sustained absolute lymphocytosis discovered incidentally in an asymptomatic patient with no other clinical features of CLL. Such patients now represent at least 40% of newly diagnosed cases in France (2) and may be the majority of new cases in the United States.

The International Workshop on CLL (IWCLL) has suggested the minimum requirements for a diagnosis of CLL (table 19.2): the patient must demonstrate sustained blood lymphocytosis, which is defined as $>10 \times 10^9$/L; normal or near-normal lymphocyte morphology; and lymphocyte infiltration of the bone marrow. Mature-appearing lymphocytes must constitute $>30\%$ of nucleated cells in an aspirated specimen; marrow infiltration by mature lymphocytes on a biopsy specimen may be an acceptable alternative under some circumstances. In patients with sustained lymphocytosis in the $5–10 \times 10^9$/L range, the clonal nature of the lymphocytes should be demonstrated by cell marker studies before a diagnosis is made (3).

Table 19.1. Serial Complete Blood Count (CBC) Values: Case 1[a]

Date	White Blood Cells × 10⁹/L	% Lymphocytes	Total Lymphocytes × 10⁹/L
5/66	7.1	38	2.70
66–74	<similar values>		
9/75	6.7	33	2.21
8/76	7.9	34	2.69
9/77	**10.7**	**64**	**6.85**
9/78	8.5	**55**	**4.68**
9/79	**11.5**	**54**	**6.21**
1/81	**12.1**	**52**	**6.29**
1/82	**12.3**	**69**	**8.49**
5/85	**16.0**	**54**	**8.64**

[a]Abnormal values are given in **bold**.

Table 19.2. Diagnostic Features of B-Cell Chronic Lymphocytic Leukemia (CLL)[a]

Feature	Criteria
Sustained lymphocytosis	At least 5 × 10⁹/L, usually >10 × 10⁹/L
Characteristic morphology	Small mature lymphocytes, "smudge cells" (variants exist; see text.)
Bone marrow involvement	>30% of nucleated cells on aspirate
B-Cell CLL phenotype	CD 19 or 20, CD5, weak surface immunoglobulin (Ig), mouse erythrocyte receptor
Markers of clonality	κ/λ light chain restriction, clonal/ cytogenetic abnormalities, clonal Ig gene rearrangement, single Ig idiotype

[a]For diagnosis of B-cell CLL: A and B always required; in addition, if lymphocyte count is ≥10 × 10⁹/L, C, or D required if lymphocyte count is <10 × 10⁹/L, C, or D required. E is not required for diagnosis, but may be useful in some cases.
Source: International Workshop on Chronic Lymphocytic Leukemia (89).

The patient's evaluation in 1985 revealed no anemia, thrombocytopenia, lymphadenopathy, or hepatosplenomegaly; the WBC count was 16 × 10⁹/L with 54% lymphocytes. Reexamination of the peripheral blood film showed essentially normal lymphocyte morphology with occasional "smudge" cells (fig. 19.1). Flow cytometric analysis of the blood lymphocyte population showed weak surface immunoglobulin (sIg) positivity for coexpression of IgM and IgD heavy chains; monoclonal expression of λ-light chains; expression of CD5 (a "pan-T" antigen); and expression of the "pan-B" antigens CD19, CD20, and CD24. Iliac crest bone marrow aspiration and core biopsy revealed normal marrow elements and an interstitial pattern of infiltration with mature lymphocytes (fig. 19.2). The cardiology evaluation of the patient in case 1 confirmed his serious cardiac disease prognosis; however, he exhibited more concern about his "leukemia" than about his heart disease. The patient was reassured about his early stage, low-risk CLL and was followed-up without therapy.*

Case 1 illustrates a subset of low-stage CLL patients that has been termed "smoldering" CLL or "benign monoclonal B cell lymphocytosis" (4, 5). Originally identified as individuals having limited or no lymphadenopathy (Binet stage A—see below), a lymphocyte count <30 × 10⁹/L hemoglobin >13 g/dl, nondiffuse marrow infiltration, and a lymphocyte count doubling time of >12 months, such patients have a low probability of evolution to higher stages. Other groups have confirmed the utility of hemoglobin, lymphocyte count, lymphocyte doubling time, and marrow histology in identifying early-stage patients with low risk of disease progression and a survival rate that does not differ from age- and sex-matched normal individuals (6, 7). Cytogenetic studies of the CLL cells may also be prognostically helpful in that a normal karyotype is associated with a lower risk of progression.

As might be expected, some individuals with "smoldering" CLL (approximately 10%) will nevertheless progress to more advanced disease, and all current definitions have some degree of imprecision. Furthermore, it should be obvious that patients cannot be confidently identified as "smoldering" without some period of observation. The patient described above offered a splendid opportunity for retrospective observation of his clinical course (table 19.1). In practice, it is useful to obtain old records of any newly diagnosed early-stage patient to see if similar information exists that could assist in determining prognosis. As more individuals are diagnosed with early-stage CLL, as many as 50% of all newly diagnosed CLL patients may fall into the "smoldering" category. Most of these patients should be observed without treatment as long as they pursue an indolent course. In this situation, careful patient education is extremely important: the word "leukemia" is so emotionally charged with negative connotations that patients may have a distorted view of their illness and become unnecessarily psychologically burdened with anxiety.

CLL was probably included among the earliest recognized cases of leukemia in the years following the initial descriptions of what we now term "leukemia" by Bennett (8) and Virchow (9) in 1845. Virchow titled his report "Weisses Blut" (White blood), and later used the equivalent Greek term, *leukemia*. The associated hyperplasia of lymph nodes, spleen, and liver in many of the early cases led to speculation that these organs might be the source of the increase in WBCs, and the concept of leukemia as neoplasia gradually gained acceptance.

Virchow himself began to recognize the different types of white cells: most contained granules and irregular nuclei, but many had smooth round nuclei and lacked granules. He noted that the latter were increased in cases of leukemia that had particular enlargement of lymph nodes, whereas splenomegaly that was disproportionate to lymphadenopa-

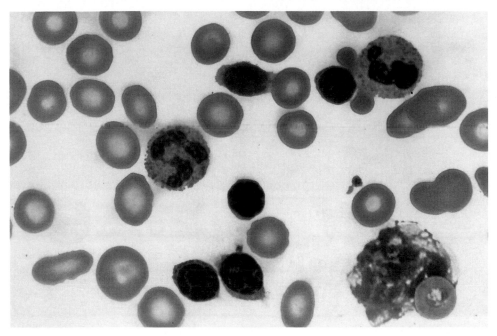

Fig. 19.1 Peripheral blood smear from a patient with early stage CLL. Note near normal lymphocyte morphology, "smudge" cells, and normal red cells, platelets, and neutrophil.

thy was usually associated with increased numbers of the granular white cells with irregular nuclei. He proposed to divide the leukemias into two types: "lymphatic" leukemia characterized by lymph node enlargement, and "splenic" leukemia characterized by splenomegaly, each with its own associated type of white cell in excess in the blood (10). Neumann (11) later noted that the marrow was at least equally involved in "splenic" leukemia, and later authorities began to use the terms "splenomedullary" leukemia, and finally "myeloid" (marrow-derived) leukemia. In 1889, Ebstein introduced the term "acute" leukemia (12) and the notion that leukemias could be classified (although only on clinical grounds at that time) into acute and chronic forms, with the former pursuing a rapidly fatal course and the latter often allowing more prolonged survival.

The introduction of Ehrlich's methods of staining blood cells (13) confirmed the different types of WBCs and their association with the different types of leukemia. Subsequent descriptions of the myeloblast and lymphoblast provided morphologic correlation with acute and chronic clinical courses, and allowed microscopic diagnosis of the acute and chronic leukemias.

The natural history of CLL as an entity was first described in 1924 by Minot and Isaacs (14), who also noted the age distribution and the effect of irradiation on the enlarged lymph nodes. Radiation therapy to lymph nodes and spleen emerged as the first effective palliative therapy, but its benefit in terms of survival was uncertain. The use of ^{32}P as systemic therapy for CLL was described in 1949 (15) but was largely abandoned with the development of glucocorticoids (16) and alkylating agents (17) in the 1950s. Currently, radiation therapy serves mainly as an adjunctive treatment modality.

A fundamental concept was supplied in 1967 by Dameshek (18) who described CLL as "an accumulative

disease of immunologically incompetent lymphocytes," one of the classic and most concise descriptions of a disease process in medical history. Galton had reached similar conclusions about the pathogenesis of CLL the previous year (19). In 1972, the monoclonal nature and predominant B-cell lineage of CLL was recognized by the demonstration of a restricted light chain immunoglobulin type on the surface of CLL lymphocytes (20). Although Boggs et al. had noted in the 1960s that survival in CLL inversely correlated with extent of disease at diagnosis (21), it was the introduction of staging systems by Rai et al. in 1975 (22) and by Binet et al. in 1981 (23) that allowed both more accurate prognostication and uniform patient entry into clinical trials. It is believed that ongoing studies of the molecular pathogenesis of CLL offer the best opportunity for understanding and controlling this common disease.

Epidemiology

Although rare in Asia, CLL is the most common type of leukemia overall in the Western world and is by far the most common type of leukemia in persons >50 years old (24). The median age of patients is about 60; the disease is sometimes found in young adults (<10% of patients are <40 years old), but essentially never in children (25). There is a 2:1 ratio of male to female patients that has never been explained.

CLL is clearly an acquired disorder, but its etiology is unknown. Although no evidence for inheritance has been found, there is an increased risk for lymphoid malignancies (26), some autoimmune disorders (26), and probably CLL itself (27, 28) among close relatives of patients with CLL. Some preliminary studies have identified links between CLL and residence in rural areas (29),

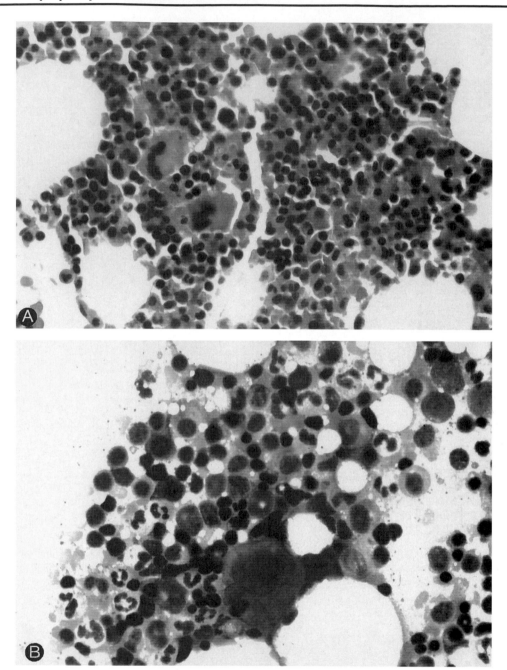

Fig. 19.2 Bone marrow preparations from a patient with early stage CLL. **A.** Biopsy showing interstitial infiltration of otherwise normal marrow by small lymphocytes. **B.** Aspirate smear with normal marrow elements and increased numbers of small mature lymphocytes.

farming (30, 31), and occupational exposure to rubber manufacturing (32, 33) and asbestos (34). Unlike the other forms of leukemia, there is no association between prior exposure to ionizing radiation and subsequent development of CLL.

Clinical Features

Symptoms

Many patients are asymptomatic at the time of diagnosis, especially if the diagnosis is made during routine screening. Symptoms, when present, are usually nonspecific.

While weakness, malaise, and fatigue are more typical symptoms of anemia, some patients may be initially seen clinically with anemia-induced angina. This type of presentation is not unusual given the age distribution of CLL and the prevalence of cardiovascular disease in such a population. Recurrent bacterial infections are common due to neutropenia and hypo-γ-globulinemia. An exaggerated response to insect bites is probably related to some overall dysfunction of the immune system. Any bleeding diathesis is usually due to thrombocytopenia. Constitutional symptoms typical of lymphoid malignancies, such as fever, chills, night sweats, and weight loss, can be present as well. Rapidly enlarging lymph nodes or compression of underlying structures can cause pain, directing attention to a specific area, and splenomegaly may produce abdominal discomfort and early satiety.

Physical Findings

The most common physical findings in CLL are lymphadenopathy and hepatosplenomegaly (22). Lymph nodes are typically firm, nontender, and movable; and, due to the indolent nature of the disease, lymphadenopathy can become massive before patients seek medical attention. The cervical, supraclavicular, axillary, and inguinal/femoral areas are most commonly involved, while involvement of Waldeyer ring is unusual. Secondary signs due to lymphadenopathy, such as extremity lymphedema, superior vena cava syndrome, dysphagia, bowel dysfunction, or jaundice are sufficiently rare to suggest another cause of lymphadenopathy. Similarly, symptoms or secondary signs due to spleen or liver enlargement are generally mild and compromise of organ function (other than splenic sequestration) is rare.

Laboratory Findings

The peripheral blood smear in typical B-cell CLL reveals lymphocytosis but normal morphology of the other cellular elements; indeed, the CLL cells themselves are usually identical to normal small lymphocytes (fig. 19.1). Larger cells with prominent nucleoli may be seen occasionally in any patient but are not conspicuous except in the variants described below. Disrupted leukocytes ("smudge cells") are commonly seen on the blood film, presumably because CLL cells are more vulnerable to mechanical shear forces in vitro. Granulocytes and monocytes are normal in appearance and absolute number, but may constitute only a few percent in a 100-cell differential cell count.

Red cell morphology is usually normal, even when anemia is present, unless severe autoimmune hemolytic anemia occurs with spherocyte formation and polychromatophilic macrocytes. Similarly, the platelets are normal unless immune thrombocytopenic purpura complicates the course of the disease, wherein platelets appear markedly reduced in number, and large platelets may be present.

The bone marrow always shows infiltration by the same lymphocytes as are present in the blood (fig. 19.2). Four patterns of marrow involvement are recognized on bone marrow biopsy and carry prognostic value (fig. 19.3). At diagnosis, approximately one-third of patients display an *interstitial* pattern of infiltration with preservation of normal marrow architecture; this is associated with early-stage disease and good prognosis. At the other end of the spectrum, about one-quarter of patients have very *diffuse* marrow involvement with virtual replacement of normal marrow elements by CLL cells. These patients have more advanced disease, often with marrow failure (anemia and thrombocytopenia) and a poor prog-

nosis. Intermediate patterns of marrow involvement are focal lymphoid nodules, called *nodular* involvement, seen in 10% of patients, and *mixed nodular-interstitial* involvement, seen in about 30%. In practice, distinction between *diffuse* and *nondiffuse* marrow involvement is most important.

Occasionally, a lymph node is biopsied in a CLL patient; the nodal architecture is replaced by sheets of small, well-differentiated lymphocytes, producing an appearance identical with what is termed "well-differentiated" lymphocytic lymphoma (fig. 19.4) when blood and marrow are not obviously involved. Infiltration of nonlymphoid tissues other than liver and prostate is rare except in extremely advanced disease, and involvement of organs such as the lung or the central nervous system (CNS) is sufficiently unusual that biopsy to rule out infection or other forms of neoplastic disease is warranted.

Lymphocyte Ontogeny

An elusive pluripotent stem cell gives rise to all the lymphoid and myeloid cells of the human lymphohematopoietic system. During fetal life B-lymphocytes develop in the liver, bone marrow, spleen, and lymph nodes, while the thymus provides the microenvironment necessary for the maturation of T-lymphocytes.

B-Cell Maturation

The earliest evidence for cellular commitment to the B-cell lineage is rearrangement of immunoglobulin heavy chain genes and expression of CD19 and Ia surface antigens (35, 36). Immunoglobulin heavy chain molecules, which appear in the cytoplasm during the pre-B-cell stage, ultimately will be found on the surface of mature B-cells (fig. 19.5).

A number of specific antigens that appear during B-cell maturation are not limited to B-cells. CD34, typically present on pre-B-cells, is an early hematopoietic progenitor cell antigen (37). A small group of normal differentiating B-cells from lymph nodes and spleen of 22–24-week-old fetuses also express the T-cell-associated antigen, CD5 (38). This antigen is paradoxically expressed strongly on the surface of B-cell CLL cells (39, 40). Exposure to antigens leads to activation of B-cells and expression of a number of new surface antigens, many of which are receptors for growth factors (e.g., CD71 [transferrin receptor] and CD25 [IL-2 receptor]) (41, 42). Following activation, various cytokines induce cellular proliferation and differentiation into mature immunoglobulin-secreting lymphocytes or plasma cells (43).

T-Cell Maturation

Certain lymphoid progenitors that migrate from bone marrow to thymus undergo maturation into mature T-lymphocytes (44). Analogous to the development of

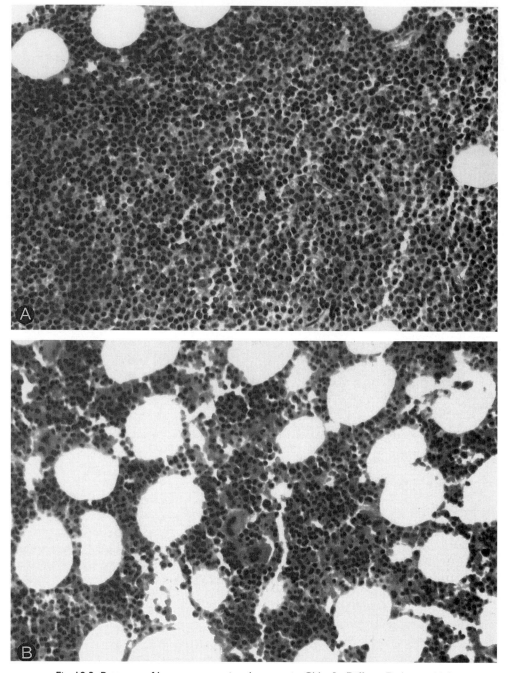

Fig. 19.3 Patterns of bone marrow involvement in CLL. **A.** Diffuse. **B.** Interstitial.

B-cells, a number of stage-specific surface antigens appear on T-cells (fig. 19.5) (45). The final stages of thymic-dependent maturation are characterized by the appearance of CD3 and the T-cell antigen receptor, both of which are necessary for recognition of foreign antigens in the context of major histocompatibility complex (MHC) gene products (46). Once the thymus-dependent maturation sequence is completed, T-cells are released into the circulation and two major subpopulations can be recognized, one defined by expression of CD4 (helper/ inducer phenotype) and the other by expression of CD8 (cytotoxic/suppressor phenotype).

Cell of Origin in CLL

Single cell mutation and ensuing clonal expansion is a well-documented and accepted pathophysiologic mechanism for most hematologic malignancies. The phenotype of the cell of origin of many lymphoid neoplasms can be correlated with a specific stage in the development of normal B-cells.

Although CLL cells morphologically resemble normal peripheral blood lymphocytes, major differences exist between the two. B-Cells in CLL have lower den-

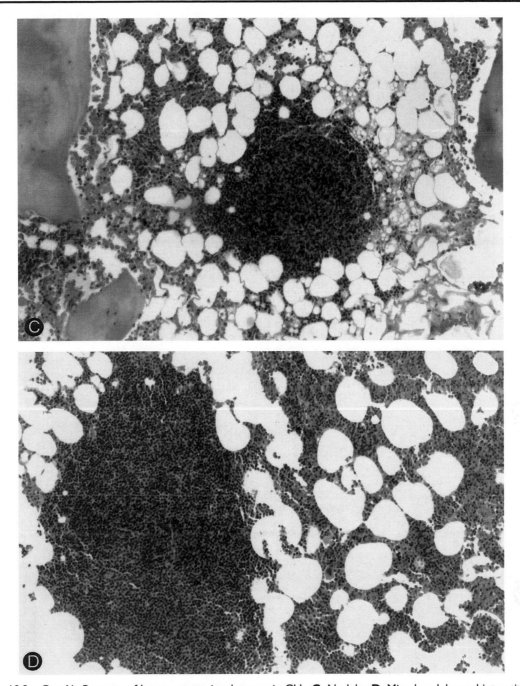

Fig. 19.3—Cont'd. Patterns of bone marrow involvement in CLL. **C.** Nodular **D.** Mixed nodular and interstitial.

sity of surface immunoglobulin and higher density of cytoplasmic immunoglobulin than normal lymphocytes of the corresponding stage of maturation (47). Malignant B-cells also express antigens such as the mouse red blood cell rosette receptor (MRBC-R) that are not present on normal lymphocytes (48). Another striking feature of the B-cell CLL phenotype is expression of CD5, an antigen present on normal T-cells past the stage III thymocyte and on only a small number of normal B-cells (49). CD5 has been shown to function as a receptor for another B-cell antigen, CD72,

which is expressed on pre-B and mature B-cells (50). On T-cells, CD5 stimulation leads to enhanced proliferation of T-cell antigen receptor-stimulated T-cells (51). Presence of the CD5 T-cell antigen on the surface of CLL B-cells could represent the aberrant nature of the differentiation of these malignant cells, or reflect expression of a B-cell antigen normally expressed on a small subset of activated B-cells (52). While the role of CD5 in B-CLL is not known, it is of interest to note that CD5-positive CLL cells are not (<1%) proliferating in vivo and require strong

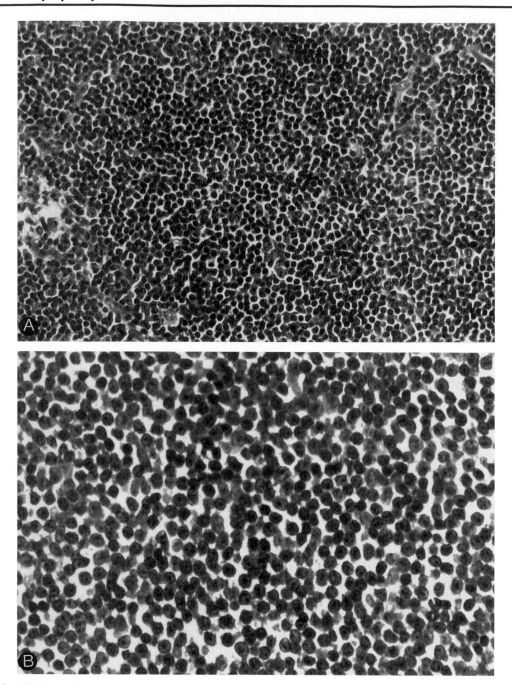

Fig. 19.4 Lymph node biopsy from a patient with CLL. **A.** Low-power view demonstrating diffuse nature of nodal hypercellularity. **B.** High-power view of uniform, small, mature lymphocytes.

mitogens to proliferate in vitro. Although it is generally accepted that the CLL B-cell phenotype correlates with an intermediate stage in development of normal B-cells, all of these differences suggest that B-CLL does not originate in normal peripheral blood lymphocytes.

A majority of the T-cells in T-CLL have mature T-helper cell phenotype, but unlike normal resting peripheral T-cells they also express CD25 (the interleukin-2 [IL-2] receptor) and proliferate in vitro in response to IL-2 (53), characteristics of activated T-cells.

Chromosomes and Oncogenes in CLL

Because CLL cells have a very low mitotic index, chromosome analysis of metaphase cells has been historically very difficult. However, if modern cytogenetic technology is employed, including the use of multiple B-cell mitogens (54), approximately 50% of patients with CLL will have detectable clonal chromosome abnormalities (55, 56). The single most common finding (in about 19% of patients) is trisomy 12. Although the genes of chromosome 12 that may be involved in CLL have not been identified, it appears that an extra copy of a gene or genes on the long arm

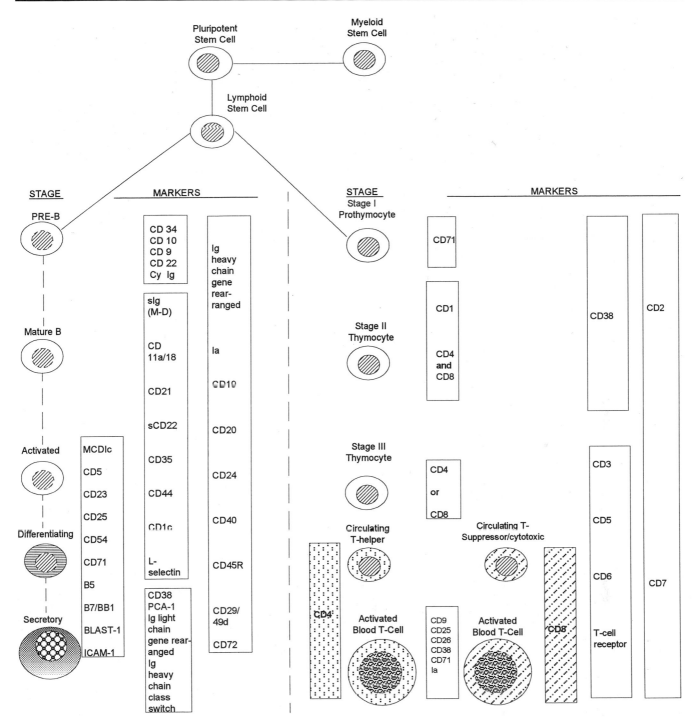

Fig. 19.5 Lymphocyte ontogeny. Adapted from Freedman AS, Nadler LM. Immunologic markers in B-cell chronic lymphocytic leukemia. In: Cheson BD, ed. Chronic lymphocytic leukemia: scientific advances and clinical developments. New York: Marcel Dekker, 1993:1–32 and Freedman AS. Immunobiology of Chronic Lymphocytic Leukemia (review). In: Canellos GP, ed. Chronic leukemias. Hematology/Oncology Clinics of North America. Philadelphia: WB Saunders, 1990:405–429.

of 12 is important because many of the infrequent structural abnormalities of chromosome 12 involve partial duplications, usually of regions q13-q22 (56). The second most common finding is structural deletions involving the 13q14 band (57), where the retinoblastoma tumor suppressor gene is located (58), suggesting a role for this antioncogene in CLL.

While activation of protooncogenes and chromosomal translocations are relatively rare in CLL, three, which are common in all types of B-cell neoplasms and not specific to B-CLL, have been studied in detail: t(11;14), t(14;18), and t(14;19). They all have in common juxtaposition of immunoglobulin heavy chain or light chain genes with protooncogenes bcl-1 (59), bcl-2 (60), and bcl-3 (61), respectively. The products of these genes appear to act as negative regulators of programmed cell death (apoptosis) and may help to give cells an abnormally long survival. What role these translocations play in the pathophysiology of CLL is not known, and their relevance is questioned by their rarity in CLL (<10% of patients studied) compared with their frequency in the follicular lymphomas (62).

Analogous to what has been found in other hematologic malignancies, the presence of clonal chromosome abnormalities adversely affects the prognosis in CLL (56, 63). Interestingly, unlike what is observed in chronic myelogenous leukemia or myelodysplastic syndrome, clonal evolution of chromosome abnormalities is rare in CLL and does not appear to have prognostic significance (64, 65).

Case 2

A 60-year-old plumber was initially seen with painful swelling of fingers, wrists, and knees, along with easy fatiguability and dyspnea on exertion. Physical examination showed tachycardia, bibasilar rales, and moderately active arthritis involving the wrists, knees, and metacarpophalangeal (MCP) joints of the hands. The spleen tip was palpable on deep inspiration. Laboratory evaluation revealed hemoglobin 81 g/L hematocrit 22%, reticulocytes 0.5%, platelets $56 \times 10^9/L$, and WBC $12.1 \times 10^9/L$ with 9% neutrophils, 21% lymphocytes, 2% monocytes, and 68% "atypical" lymphocytes. Examination of the blood smear showed a heterogeneous population of large lymphocytes with abundant cytoplasm and frequent scattered granules (fig. 19.6). The other blood cells were reduced in number but

morphologically normal. Bone marrow aspiration and biopsy revealed diffuse marrow infiltration by large lymphocytes similar to the circulating cells and a reduction in normal marrow elements. Flow cytometric cell surface marker analysis of the large lymphocyte population showed expression of CD3 and CD8 without expression of other T-cell, B-cell, or myeloid-specific antigens. Rheumatoid factor was detected at high titer in the serum.

This appearance was considered most compatible with the large granular lymphocytosis syndrome (see below). Prednisone 60 mg daily was begun with rapid resolution of his joint symptoms. With continued therapy, there was improvement in his anemia, neutropenia, and thrombocytopenia and in his marrow appearance; however, a small but significant number of cells with the morphologic and phenotypic characteristics of his original large granular lymphocytes persisted in both blood and marrow. Attempts to taper his prednisone dose <20 mg daily led to worsening of his arthritis and blood count abnormalities.

Commentary

Since the distinction between polyclonal reactive lymphocytosis (essentially always T-cell) and monoclonal B-cell lymphocytosis is easily made by cell surface marker studies (light chain ratio and CD3 expression), in practice, the more important differential diagnosis involves the other chronic lymphoproliferative disorders.

Case 2 illustrates a patient with lymphocytosis, anemia, thrombocytopenia, and splenomegaly, but who lacked the diagnostic morphologic and cell surface phenotypic features of CLL.

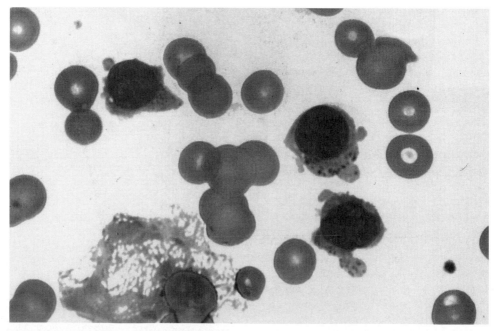

Fig. 19.6 Peripheral blood smear from a patient with large granular lymphocytosis syndrome. Note the abundant cytoplasm, frequent cytoplasmic granules, and cellular heterogeneity.

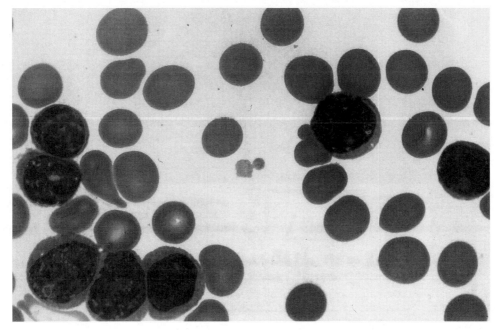

Fig. 19.7 Peripheral blood smear of a patient with prolymphocytic leukemia (PLL). The cells are large and show a prominent nucleolus.

CLL Variants—B-Cell

B-Cell Prolymphocytic Leukemia

Extreme lymphocytosis ($>100 \times 10^9$/L), splenomegaly, and minimal or absent lymphadenopathy are the hallmarks of prolymphocytic leukemia (PLL), a subacute form of lymphocytic leukemia poorly responsive to therapy with a median survival rate similar to advanced stage CLL (66). The diagnosis is based on lymphocyte morphology and confirmed by cell marker studies. The prolymphocyte, characterized by its large size, more abundant agranular cytoplasm, and prominent nucleolus, constitutes, by definition, at least 55%, and usually >70%, of the blood lymphocytes (fig. 19.7). In 80% of cases there is a B-cell marker phenotype that differs from CLL by strong expression of sIg, weak expression of CD5 and the mouse erythrocyte receptor, and positivity for the monoclonal antibody FMC7. A serum monoclonal immunoglobulin is present in a third of such cases.

CLL/PLL

Some patients present a morphologically mixed population of small lymphocytes and prolymphocytes. When the prolymphocytes represent ≤10%, the patients are usually considered to have CLL, although some prefer the designation CLL, mixed cell type. When there are ≥55% prolymphocytes, the patient is considered to have PLL. When prolymphocytes make up >10% but <55%, the term "CLL/PLL" is used (67, 68) (fig. 19.8). It is thought that CLL/PLL may represent "prolymphocytoid" transformation of CLL (69) rather than a distinct entity, but the point remains controversial. Currently, CLL/PLL describes both typical CLL that evolves into CLL/PLL as well as de novo presentation of CLL/PLL. In both situations, there are increasing tumor burdens, deficits of normal blood cells, relative resistance to treatment, and an aggressive clinical course.

Leukemic Phase of Non-Hodgkin Lymphoma

The follicular or diffuse small cleaved cell non-Hodgkin lymphomas (NHL) occasionally are seen with or develop circulating lymphoma cells, a situation termed "lymphosarcoma cell leukemia" in the past (70). With the associated lymphadenopathy and/or splenomegaly of the NHL, confusion with CLL is possible. Circulating NHL cells frequently are pleomorphic with nuclear clefting and/or nucleoli. Distinction from CLL is possible with cell marker studies: in contrast to CLL, NHL cells typically show strong sIg expression, weak mouse erythrocyte receptor positivity, CD5 negativity, and FMC7 positivity. In cases where cell morphology makes distinction from B-PLL difficult, lymph node biopsy may be useful to demonstrate the follicular or diffuse small cleaved cell NHL.

Splenic Lymphoma with Villous Lymphocytes

Splenic B-cell lymphomas with circulating villous lymphocytes (SLVL) may be confused with CLL with a massive spleen (71). The circulating lymphocytes in SLVL have short cytoplasmic villi and cell markers characteristic of NHL rather than CLL. Fever, sweats, weight loss, and pancytopenia except for moderate lymphocytosis (10–30

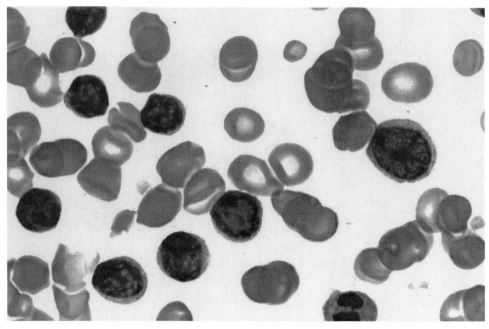

Fig. 19.8 Peripheral blood smear from a patient with CLL/PLL. There are two lymphocyte populations; small, mature-appearing lymphocytes and large prolymphocytes with prominent nucleoli.

$\times$ 10⁹/L) with plasmacytoid morphology, massive splenomegaly, lack of marrow infiltration, and small amounts serum of monoclonal protein are typical of SLVL. The disease frequently remits after splenectomy, like hairy cell leukemia with which it is frequently confused (72). However, in the SLVL spleen, the white pulp is primarily infiltrated, whereas the red pulp is principally infiltrated in hairy cell leukemia. Splenectomy usually results in prompt relief of constitutional symptoms and cytopenias in SLVL, whereas improvement after splenectomy occurs more slowly in hairy cell leukemia. Marrow aspiration and biopsy readily distinguishes the two entities.

Waldenström Macroglobulinemia

Patients with Waldenström macroglobulinemia (WM) may have circulating malignant lymphocytes, with typically "plasmacytoid" features: abundant basophilic cytoplasm and mature nuclei (73). Like CLL, WM occurs in older individuals and frequently involves lymph nodes and spleen. The IgM monoclonal paraprotein of WM and cell surface expression of CD38 and reactivity with PCA-1 (features of late B-cells and plasma cells) (fig. 19.5) help to distinguish it from CLL.

Hairy Cell Leukemia

Hairy cell leukemia (HCL) usually presents with cytopenias of normal blood elements, but some patients have leucocytosis with significant numbers of circulating malignant cells. When splenomegaly is present, such HCL cases may resemble CLL. The morphology of the circulating cells (abundant cytoplasm and cytoplasmic "hairy" projections),

tartrate-resistant acid phosphatase (TRAP) activity, and characteristic marrow biopsy histology help to distinguish HCL from CLL. In addition, cell marker studies in HCL typically disclose positivity for CD22, CD25, LeuM5, and HC2 results not seen in typical CLL (74). A variant form of HCL (HCL-V) has been described that shares some morphologic features with B-PLL (larger cells, nucleoli) and lacks some cell surface antigens of HCL (75). Its recognition may be important because, unlike HCL, it responds poorly to α-interferon and pentostatin. A rare T-cell variant of HCL (76), associated with HTLV-2 has been reported. It appears clinically identical to the more common "B-cell" HCL.

CLL Variants—T-Cell

T-CLL

Approximately 2–5% of patients with clinical features of CLL have lymphocytes that bear T-cell antigens other than CD5, such as CD2, CD3, CD7, and CD4 or CD8; these cases have been called T-CLL (77). Note that in T-cell lymphoproliferative disorders, clonality cannot be determined by cell surface markers, but is confirmed by rearrangement of the T-cell receptor genes (78) and/or clonal chromosome abnormalities (79). The term "T-CLL" historically has been applied to a heterogeneous group of patients with some features of CLL but with a mature T-cell phenotype on surface marker studies. Unfortunately, many published cases probably have been, in fact, other T-cell chronic lymphoproliferative disorders, such as T-γ-chronic lymphoproliferative disease (80) or T-cell prolymphocytic leukemia (81). This may account for the rather wide variability in clinical course reported, and makes description of "typical" T-CLL difficult.

Most cases of so-called T-CLL are of the helper (CD4) phenotype. The reported clinical characteristics are usually distinct from mycosis fungoides and Sezary syndrome (which also involve CD4 positive T-cells) and include younger age, marked lymphocytosis, lymphadenopathy, diffuse marrow infiltration, and frequent CNS involvement. As expected in patients with such characteristics, survival is poor. These features have led some authorities to suggest that all "T-CLL" cases are in fact one of the T-cell leukemia/lymphoma syndromes whose descriptions follow.

T-γ-Chronic Lymphoproliferative Disease

Also called large granular lymphocytosis syndrome, T-γ-CLL, or CD8-CLL, this condition results from a proliferation of large granular lymphocytes expressing CD2, CD3, and CD8, apparently derived from natural killer (NK) cells but lacking normal natural killer function (82, 83). The clinical syndrome is highly variable, but patients often have neutropenia, splenomegaly, and marrow infiltration. Rheumatoid arthritis or its seropositivity is frequent, and occasional patients have pure red cell aplasia. The clinical course is indolent in most patients, but a minority have a rapidly fatal outcome, often from complications of severe neutropenia. A variant syndrome has been described with CD8- negative, M1- and NKH1-positive lymphocytes displaying high levels of natural killer activity, but without clinical neutropenia or autoimmunity (84). Misdiagnosis of these conditions and treatment with aggressive acute lymphocytic leukemia therapy often results in fatal toxicity or lethal infections. Many patients are best managed symptomatically with corticosteroids and/or supportive care.

Cutaneous T-Cell Lymphoma

Mycosis fungoides and Sezary syndrome are cutaneous T-cell lymphomas with involvement of skin only in the former and systemic disease in the latter. Sezary syndrome may be confused with T-CLL with skin involvement (although most such latter cases probably represent T-PLL; see below): both have a CD4+ phenotype, and skin may be involved in T-CLL or T-PLL, while lymphadenopathy and splenomegaly may be present in Sezary syndrome. CD7 is usually expressed in T-CLL but not in Sezary syndrome; conversely, CD8 expression may occur in T-CLL or T-PLL but not in Sezary syndrome.

Adult T-Cell Leukemia/Lymphoma

Adult T-cell leukemia/lymphoma (ATLL) is an HTLV-1 associated aggressive disease with circulating lymphoid cells that may have a mature appearance, the only feature it shares with CLL. Skin lesions, lytic bone lesions, hypercal-

cemia, and a progressive clinical course distinguish it from CLL (85). Serologic evidence for infection with HTLV-1 also helps to identify patients with ATLL (86).

T-Cell Prolymphocytic Leukemia (PLL)

T cell PLL accounts for 20% of cases of PLL (see above), and although rare, in a recent review of 78 cases it was noted be the most common form of leukemia with a mature (postthymic) phenotype (81). Splenomegaly and hyperlymphocytosis ($> 100 \times 10^9$/L) are features shared with B-PLL, but lymphadenopathy occurs in half of cases and skin lesions in a quarter. Cell markers show a postthymic phenotype: TdT−, CD2+, CD3+, CD7+, with CD4+/CD8− in 65%, CD4+/CD8+ in 21%, and CD4−/CD8+ in 13% (81). Cytogenetic analysis in 30 cases showed only a single normal karyotype; consistent abnormalities of chromosome 14 with breakpoints at q11 (locus for the T-cell receptor α- and δ-chain genes) and q32 were observed in 76% of cases and trisomy 8 (including iso8q) occurred in 53%. The median survival was 7.5 months, and response to treatment was poor. A small cell variant was noted in 19%, with indistinct nucleoli by light microscopy always visible by electron microscopy (81). Similar cases have probably been misclassified as T-CLL in the past.

CLL—Staging

After a decade of increasing information linking prognosis in CLL with the clinical extent of disease at presentation, in 1975 Rai et al. (22) proposed a five-group staging system: *stage 0*—blood and marrow lymphocytosis only; *stage I*—lymphocytosis plus lymphadenopathy; *stage II*—lymphocytosis plus enlargement of spleen and/or liver, with or without lymphadenopathy; *stage III*—lymphocytosis plus anemia (hemoglobin <11 g/dl or hematocrit <33%), with or without lymphadenopathy or oganomegaly; *stage IV*—lymphocytosis plus thrombocytopenia (platelets $< 100 \times 10^9$/L), with or without the other features. In the original report, the median survival duration by stage was: 0—12.5 years; I—8.5 years; II—6.0 years; III—1.5 years; and IV—1.5 years. As noted by the authors, the five stages actually identified only three groups with substantially different survival probabilities. Subsequently, Rai (87) recommended a modification of the five-stage system that created three groups: low risk (original Rai et al. stage 0); intermediate risk (original stages I and II combined); and high risk (original stages III and IV combined). These groups originally constituted approximately 25%, 50%, and 25% of CLL patients, respectively. However, as noted above, more patients are being diagnosed in stage 0 currently than in the past. The modified Rai staging system still includes a large number of patients in the intermediate risk group, and there is a greater variability of survival in this group than would be desirable.

Table 19.3. Most Common Clinical Staging Systems for CLL

Modified RAI Stage	RAI Stage		Binet Stage	
Low risk	0 (>120)[a]	Lymphocytosis in blood and marrow	A (>102)	Lymphocytosis in blood and marrow; <3 areas of lymphoid involvement[b]
Intermediate risk	I (95)	Lymphocytosis + enlarged lymph nodes	B (61)	Lymphocytosis +3 or more areas of lymphoid involvement
	II (72)	Lymphocytosis + enlarged spleen and/or liver		
High risk	III (30)	Lymphocytosis + anemia (Hb <11 g/dL)	C (32)	Lymphocytosis + anemia (Hb <11 g/dL in men or <10 g/dL in women) or thrombocytopenia (platelets <100 × 10⁹/L)
	IV (30)	Lymphocytosis + thrombocytopenia (platelets <100 × 10⁹/L)		

[a]Figures in parentheses equal weighted median survival in months (89).
[b]Areas of lymphoid involvement: cervical, axillary, and inguinal lymph nodes (whether unilateral or bilateral); spleen and liver.

In 1981 Binet et al. (23) proposed a formal three-stage system, which has been popular in Europe. All CLL patients with anemia (hemoglobin <10 g/dl) and/or thrombocytopenia (platelets <100 × 10⁹/L) are assigned to stage C. All patients without anemia or thrombocytopenia are divided on the basis of lymphatic organ involvement with reference to five sites: cervical, axillary, or inguinal lymph nodes (each represents one site whether unilateral or bilateral), spleen, and liver. Stage A consists of two or fewer of these sites involved (clinically enlarged); stage B consists of three or more sites of involvement. In Binet's series, the survival of stage A patients was not different from the age- and sex-matched normal French population. The median survival for stage B patients was 7 years (comparable to modified Rai intermediate risk group) and for stage C patients, only 2 years (comparable to Rai high risk group). Table 19.3 summarizes the Rai and Binet staging systems.

The International Workshop on CLL (88) has recommended an integrated Rai-Binet system in which each Binet stage is further subdivided into the appropriate Rai stage, the later designation given as a Roman numeral in parentheses after the Binet letter designation. Although the International Workshop on CLL recently repeated its recommendation (89), there is little evidence that the integrated system is superior to either system used alone. In practice, most investigators use one or the other, with a preference for the Rai system in North America and for the Binet system in Europe.

While the available staging systems accurately identify the patients with poor prognoses (modified Rai high risk group and Binet stage C) with a median survival of ≤2 years, additional prognostic factors have been sought for the remaining patients (modified Rai low and intermediate risk groups and Binet stages A and B). Three factors appear to offer independent predictive ability for patients within a particular early or intermediate stage: the absolute blood lymphocyte count, the blood lymphocyte doubling time, and the histologic pattern of bone marrow involvement.

Two groups have reported patient series in which Rai stage I and II patients could be separated on the basis of their initial absolute blood lymphocyte count. Baccarini et al. (90) reported that patients with absolute lymphocyte counts above 50 × 10⁹/L had a more aggressive clinical course than similar stage patients with lymphocyte counts below this threshold. Rozman et al. (91) found that a lymphocyte count of 40 × 10⁹/L gave similar discrimination in their patients.

Galton's original publication on the pathogenesis of CLL included his observation that the individual patient's trend of increase in lymphocyte count over time predicted his or her clinical course (19). Later investigators (92, 93) confirmed the value of determining the blood lymphocyte doubling time (the actual or projected time required for an individual patient's blood lymphocyte count to double). Patients in low-risk and intermediate risk groups whose lymphocyte doubling time is >12 months tend to have an indolent course with projected median survival >12 years. Those with lymphocyte doubling times <12 months tend to have more rapid progression of disease and median survival of 5 years (94).

Finally, the histologic pattern of bone marrow involvement in CLL appears to have independent prognostic value for low- and intermediate risk patients (1, 95, 96). Patients with the diffuse pattern of bone marrow involvement—extensive replacement of both normal marrow elements and fat with malignant lymphocytes—have a more aggressive course than similar stage patients with one of the other three patterns: interstitial, nodular, or mixed.

Rai (25) has proposed use of the lymphocyte doubling time and bone marrow histologic pattern to identify subgroups of low-risk (stage 0 or A) and intermediate risk (stage I and II or B) patients. He proposes that when both prognostic factors are in agreement (doubling time >12 months and *nondiffuse* marrow pattern *or* doubling time <12 months and diffuse marrow pattern), then an indolent or aggressive course can be predicted with confidence. When the two prognostic factors are discrepant, i.e., one good prognostic factor and one poor one, then no inference can be drawn about clinical course beyond what is predicted by stage.

Case 3

A 74-year-old man was admitted with unstable angina. His physical examination was significant for bilateral cervical and axillary lymphadenopathy, a II/VI systolic flow murmur, and carotid and femoral bruits. Liver and spleen could not be palpated.

Laboratory data was significant for hemoglobin 50 g/L, hematocrit 14%, and absent reticulocytes. WBC count was 21.2 × 10⁹/L with 1% neutrophils, 99% lymphocytes, and many smudge cells seen on the smear. Platelet count was 265 × 10⁹/L. Direct Coombs test was positive for warm antibodies, but serum lactate dehydrogenase (LDH) and bilirubin levels were normal. On serum protein electrophoresis, a marked hypo-γ-globulinemia was present without monoclonal protein. Bone marrow aspiration and biopsy showed interstitial infiltration with small mature-appearing lymphocytes and a near absence of erythroid precursors. Flow cytometric analysis of cell surface markers showed a monoclonal population of lymphocytes in blood and bone marrow bearing low-density surface IgM, κ-light chains, CD19, CD20, and CD5, consistent with B-cell CLL.

Treatment with chlorambucil and prednisone led to gradual normalization of the hemoglobin and hematocrit values. The subsequent course was significant for recurrent bouts of Coombs- positive hemolytic anemia requiring retreatment with prednisone, which could not be tapered beyond an alternate day schedule. Hepatosplenomegaly developed, but over a period of 6 years of followup, the WBC remained in the range of 10—50 × 10⁹/L while platelets remained normal. His coronary artery disease was treated medically, but angina associated with hemolytic anemia necessitated intermittent blood transfusions and prednisone therapy. Pneumonia and urinary tract infections were managed with antibiotics. The patient finally succumbed to coronary artery disease without further progression of his CLL.

Commentary

Since CLL is a disease of lymphoid cells, it is not surprising that immune system function is abnormal in most patients. *Case 3 illustrates hypo-γ-globulinemia and autoimmune phenomena.*

Immunologic Complications

Hypo-γ-globulinemia

Hypo-γ-globulinemia, which eventually develops in the majority of patients with CLL, was present in case 3 from the time of diagnosis and probably contributed to recurrent infections later. Although the pathogenesis of hypo-γ-globulinemia has not been fully elucidated, it apparently reflects dysfunction of the residual normal (CD5 negative) B-cells in CLL patients (97). It is not clear whether this dysfunction is the result of simple replacement by the ma-

lignant clone or of inhibition by suppressor T-cells (98) or other lymphoid cells (99). Regardless of the mechanism, it is well established that patients with CLL do not respond with normal antibody production when challenged with certain antigens and often fail vaccinations. (It is of interest to note that the murine counterpart of human CD5-positive B-cells are also nonresponsive to foreign antigens). In addition to hypo-γ-globulinemia, about 5% of CLL patients are found to have a serum monoclonal immunoglobulin (usually IgM) of sufficient concentration to be apparent on conventional serum protein electrophoresis. However, with more sophisticated techniques such as agarose gel electrophoresis and immunofixation, small amounts of monoclonal immunoglobulin can be found in about 60% of patients, either in the serum or the urine (100).

Autoimmunity

Immune system dysfunction can also play a role in the bone marrow failure/hypoplasia syndromes in patients with CLL. Some patients such as the patient described in case 3 have isolated hypoproliferative anemia with near-zero reticulocyte counts and very few or no erythroid precursors in the bone marrow. This syndrome of pure red cell aplasia appears to be immunologically mediated via inhibition of erythroid precursor proliferation by suppressor T-cells (101, 102). Treatment with cyclosporine, in the absence of other CLL therapy, has reversed pure red cell aplasia in patients with CLL, although the experience is limited (103). Of course, it is important to distinguish this mechanism from anemia due to replacement of bone marrow with cells of the malignant B-cell clone, in which case treatment with cytotoxic therapy is appropriate. Other cellular immune system abnormalities reported in patients with CLL are diverse and contradictory (104–106). They include reversal of the T4:T8 ratio but increased absolute numbers of both T-cell subsets and of natural killer (NK) cells. The expansion of T-cells appears to be polyclonal, and they apparently are not a part of the malignant clone in B-cell CLL (107).

Autoimmune cytopenias are quite frequent in patients with CLL, and autoantibodies can be directed to all hemopoietic cells (108, 109). Interestingly, the autoantibodies are usually polyclonal and are not produced by the malignant CLL clone (110). Most common are anti-red cell IgG antibodies detected by the direct Coombs test, found in up to 35% of patients. Some patients (about 15%) will also have hemolytic anemia, but the balance are Coombs positive without hemolysis. Next in frequency are antiplatelet antibodies, usually detected as increased platelet-associated IgG, with only about 2% of patients exhibiting immune thrombocytopenia. Antineutrophil antibodies and immune neutropenia are rare in CLL. The patient described above (case 3) presented with a positive Coombs test but a clinical appearance of pure red cell aplasia. Later, repeated clinical episodes of Coombs-positive hemolytic anemia were noted.

The pathogenesis of autoimmune cytopenias in CLL is not fully understood. Because the murine equivalent of CD5-positive cells (Ly1 positive) are involved in autoimmune diseases (111), it is tempting to postulate a similar role for CD5-positive B-cells in patients with CLL as well. Increased numbers of CD5-positive B-cells that secrete rhematoid factor have been reported in patients with rheumatoid arthritis (112, 113), and there is some evidence of their direct role in autoimmunity in patients with CLL (114, 115). Alternatively, others have postulated that one of the consequences of hypo-γ-globulinemia is a lack of antiidiotypic antibodies that would normally antagonize CD5- positive autoimmune clones (116). This is a hypothesis that may resolve the association between CD5 expression and autoimmunity with evidence that CLL cells do not themselves produce the autoantibodies seen in CLL patients.

Other Complications

Infections

CLL patients are susceptible to a variety of infections, which contribute substantially to the morbidity and mortality of the disease. Significant immune impairment underlies the increased incidence of infection, including hypo-γ-globulinemia from B-cell dysfunction, altered T-cell immunity, and neutropenia. Due to the frequency of hypo-γ-globulinemia and neutropenia (in the chemotherapy era), bacterial infections are the most common (117), including both Gram-positive (hypo-γ-globulinemia) and Gram-negative (neutropenia) organisms. Patients are also susceptible to viral infections, especially due to human herpes viruses (*herpes simplex, varicella zoster*), and to a lesser extent cytomegalovirus and Epstein-Barr virus. Less commonly, fungal infections (usually in the setting of prolonged neutropenia and broad-spectrum antibacterial therapy) have been seen. Intravenous immunoglobulin (IVIg) infusions have been shown to decrease the incidence of bacterial infection in CLL patients with hypo-γ-globulinemia (118), although with no demonstrated effect on survival. Lack of cost effectiveness of prophylactic IVIg in CLL (119) restricts its prophylactic use (see below).

Recent experience with new agents, the nucleoside analogs fludarabine, cladribine, and pentostatin (see below), has confirmed an increased risk of opportunistic infections of a type not usually seen with alkylating agent therapy, such as *Pneumocystis carinii* pneumonia, listeriosis, and disseminated fungal infections.

Secondary Neoplasms

CLL patients have an increased incidence of solid tumors, especially lung and colorectal carcinoma, melanoma, and soft tissue sarcomas (120, 121). The secondary epithelial malignancies may be a function of CLL therapy, especially prolonged continuous chlorambucil (122). There is also a substantial increased risk of multiple myeloma (123), another B-cell–derived neoplasm, but the myeloma does not evolve from the malignant B-cell clone of the CLL (124, 125). Inexplicably, given the prolonged use of alkylating agents in CLL therapy, there appears to be no increased risk of secondary acute nonlymphocytic leukemia as is seen after such therapy for Hodgkin disease, ovarian cancer, and other primary neoplasms.

Evolution

Case 4

A 55-year-old electrician sought medical attention because of painful cervical lymphadenopathy. The patient recalled having "lumps in the neck" for a year, but stated that they had enlarged and become painful only over the previous 3 weeks. Physical examination was significant for generalized lymphadenopathy without hepatosplenomegaly. Hematocrit and hemoglobin were normal, WBC was 26.9 × 10⁹/L with 87% mature-appearing lymphocytes, 12% neutrophils, and 1% monocytes. Smudge cells were noted on the blood smear. Flow cytometry showed a monoclonal population of B lymphocytes bearing κ-light chain with μ- and δ-heavy chain surface immunoglobulin. A diagnosis of Rai stage II B-cell CLL was made, and because of symptoms, treatment with chlorambucil and prednisone was initiated, resulting in rapid resolution of pain and decrease in lymphadenopathy. However, the patient could not tolerate oral chlorambucil due to nausea, so he was treated with intravenous cyclophosphamide and vincristine plus oral prednisone (COP) intermittently and remained in a good partial remission. His course was complicated by recurrent respiratory infections and an episode of herpes zoster reactivation.

Three years after diagnosis, his cervical lymph nodes again increased in size, and treatment with COP was restarted for cosmetic reasons, but with little response. Fevers, chills, night sweats, and weight loss developed. No infectious cause for fever could be identified. The WBC increased to 150 × 10⁹/L and the lactate dehydrogenase (LDH) to 900 IU/dl. A chest x-ray showed widening of the mediastinum and hilar adenopathy. A CT scan of the abdomen showed a large pelvic mass. Biopsy of an axillary lymph node was compatible with CLL (fig. 19.9), but repeat biopsy of a submental node showed diffuse large cell lymphoma (fig. 19.9). The patient was then treated with combination chemotherapy, but after an initial response, the lymphoma progressed and he ultimately died of septic complications of further lymphoma therapy.

Commentary

Based on the original report by Richter (126), the term "Richter syndrome" is used for lymphomas developing in patients with CLL (127, 128). Richter used the term

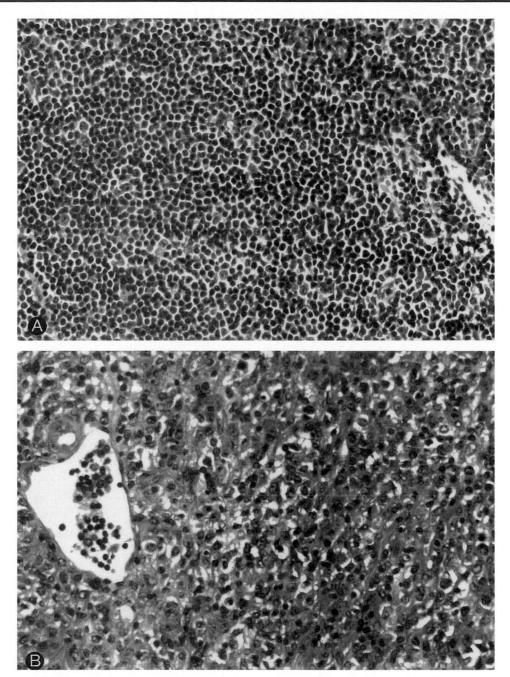

Fig. 19.9 Lymph node biopsies from a patient with Richter's syndrome. **A.** Diffuse small lymphocytic lymphoma, typical of CLL. **B.** Diffuse large cell lymphoma in a lymph node from another area.

"reticular cell sarcoma," but subsequently most of these lymphomas were classified as diffuse "histiocytic," or large cell, lymphomas. Controversy still exists about whether development of aggressive lymphoma represents true clonal evolution of otherwise indolent B-cell CLL. In some cases molecular and cell surface marker studies support the theory that the lymphoma cells derive from the same monoclonal population as the CLL (129–131); other reports reach the opposite conclusion (132).

The incidence of Richter transformation in CLL is 3–15% and the median interval between the diagnosis of CLL and development of lymphoma ranges between 24

and 49 months. Patients are usually in partial remissions when Richter syndrome develops, but in a few cases the lymphoma arises during clinical complete remission of CLL. There are no factors identified that can predict which patients are at risk to undergo this transformation. The most common symptoms are fever, increasing lymphadenopathy, weight loss, and abdominal pain. Laboratory data are generally nonspecific, but a rising LDH (as in case 4) is a marker of the increased proliferation of lymphoid cells associated with Richter syndrome.

Tissue is necessary for diagnosis, and an initial lymph node biopsy that shows only changes typical of CLL should not deter one from pursuing this diagnosis by biopsying another (preferably bulky) site in an appropriate clinical setting. Unfortunately, the prognosis after Richter transformation is extremely poor despite aggressive lymphoma treatment, and the median survival is only 4 months. Diagnosis of Richter syndrome is important for prognostic purposes and for considering these patients for novel therapeutic approaches, since their aggressive lymphoma is not controlled by CLL therapy and may not respond well to standard lymphoma therapy (see below).

Case 5

A 52-year-old man with a history of hypertension and a longstanding chronic seizure disorder was evaluated for weight loss, weakness, dizziness, and fatigue of 2 weeks' duration and the recent onset of headache. Massive nontender cervical, axillary, and inguinal-femoral lymphadenopathy and hepatosplenomegaly were noted. A CBC showed the following: hemoglobin 73 g/L, platelets 77×10^9/L, and WBC count 808×10^9/L with 2% neutrophils, 93% lymphocytes, and 5% prolymphocytes. Respiratory distress rapidly developed and the patient was transferred to a university medical center for further management. Upon arrival he was noted to be hypoxic despite application of oxygen by face mask. Physical findings were confirmed, and repeat CBC showed hemoglobin 37 g/L, platelets 58×10^8/L, and WBC count 887×10^9/L with peripheral blood findings similar to those already noted. Chest x-ray showed diffuse bilateral alveolar infiltrates.

Emergency management with hydroxyurea, packed red cell transfusion, and therapeutic leukapheresis improved the patient's respiratory function and chest x-ray appearance rapidly, although his WBC count was decreased only to 767×10^9/L. Bone marrow examination showed virtual replacement of normal elements by mature lymphocytes and occasional prolymphocytes with a diffuse pattern of infiltration on biopsy section. Cell surface markers were consistent with B-cell CLL: CD19, CD20, CD5, and weak sIg (IgM, IgD, and κ-light chains). Immunoglobulin profile revealed serum IgG and IgM levels within the normal range but undetectable IgA. He was considered to have Rai stage IV CLL, and he consented to treatment on a cooperative group clinical trial comparing chlorambucil plus prednisone with fludarabine monophosphate. He was randomized to and received fludarabine 25 mg/M² daily for 5 days, which was well tolerated. Nine days after the start of chemotherapy, he was discharged with a WBC count of 224×10^9/L.

Two additional 5-day fludarabine treatments were given in the outpatient setting at 4-week intervals, with little change in lymphadenopathy and WBC values ranging from $127-584 \times 10^9$/L. Shortly before his planned fourth treatment, he was admitted for signs and symptoms suggesting right lower lobe pneumonia. Admission blood examination showed hemoglobin 5 g/dl, platelets 68×10^9/L and WBC 301×10^9/L with 1% neutrophils, 84% lymphocytes, and 15% prolymphocytes. When a thorough evaluation failed to substantiate the suspected pneumonia, treatment with fludarabine was

resumed. On the 2nd day of therapy, he was noted to be tachypneic, lethargic, and poorly responsive; arterial blood gas analysis showed hypoxemia and acidosis. Fludarabine was subsequently withheld on suspicion of drug toxicity. However, a repeat WBC count was 536×10^9/L and examination of the blood film showed a predominance of prolymphocytes, increasing from 57->80% on subsequent differential cell counts. Two days later, with the patient's clinical condition rapidly deteriorating, therapeutic leukapheresis and CHOP (cyclophosphamide, doxorubicin, vincristine, and prednisone) chemotherapy were initiated. Despite these efforts, the patient rapidly succumbed to respiratory failure.

Commentary

Case 5 represents "prolymphocytoid transformation" of CLL (133) in a patient with an unusually short clinical course. Although this patient initially presented with advanced stage CLL, by the terminal illness his disease advanced to CLL/PLL (>10% but <55% prolymphocytes) and finally to PLL (>55% prolymphocytes). The features that predict prolymphocytoid transformation have not been described, and it remains a relatively rare (<10%) outcome in CLL. Even rarer, although reported (134, 135), is transformation to acute lymphocytic leukemia (ALL), which in some cases has been shown to represent clonal evolution of the original CLL population, as substantiated by cell marker studies (136).

It is interesting to note that in the patient described above signs and symptoms of leukostasis (obtundation, hypoxemia, acidosis) developed at a range of WBC (536×10^9/L) that had previously been tolerated without such symptoms. However, at the time of leukostasis, the predominant circulating cell had changed from a lymphocyte to a prolymphocyte. Presumably the larger prolymphocytes had different rheologic characteristics that produced more whole blood hyperviscosity at any given WBC count than the smaller CLL lymphocytes. This is not invariable, however. A patient with PLL managed by the authors tolerated a WBC count >1000 × 10⁹/L with only mild clinical leucostasis (somnolence).

Therapeutic measures in this patient were unsuccessful. Leukapheresis was only minimally effective in reducing the WBC count, both at presentation and at his terminal transformation. It may be that the large extravascular pool of malignant cells in a patient with massive lymphadenopathy and hepatosplenomegaly is readily mobilized to replace the cells removed from the vascular compartment during leukapheresis. The patient's initial response to fludarabine was encouraging, but after three cycles he still showed lymphadenopathy and organomegaly comparable to his appearance at presentation. It is also obvious that the prolymphocyte population was particularly resistant to fludarabine. Some PLL patients who are resistant to chlorambucil and prednisone respond to combination chemotherapy such as the CHOP regimen. Such responses are usually of short duration (a few months) and resistance to the combination then develops. Newer agents may be more promising in such cases.

Because in the majority of CLL patients progressive treatment-resistant disease eventually develops, it is important to determine the patient's position on important issues such as resuscitation and life support, preferably early in the course of the illness. Avoiding this type of discussion until the patient is in extremis may leave the physician with no clear directives at a time when they are needed.

Treatment

The single most important treatment principle in the management of most patients with CLL is this: *therapy is palliative*. With the possible exception of bone marrow transplantation, all current therapy in CLL is given with palliative rather than curative intent. In keeping with this principle, deciding who to treat (or perhaps who not to treat) is as important as deciding what therapy to use. Patient characteristics, such as age, comorbid disease, etc., are often as important as disease characteristics in the treatment decision.

Indications

Certain clinical situations require therapy, whereas others are appropriate for observation without treatment. After an initial bone marrow biopsy, low-risk and intermediate risk patients should be initially observed without therapy while serial blood counts are obtained at two 8-week intervals to determine the (extrapolated) lymphocyte doubling time. If chromosome analysis is available, it should be obtained before treatment.

Stage

Patients who are in low-risk stages should be observed without therapy until they progress to a higher stage or until a complication requiring treatment develops (see below). This recommendation includes patients in Rai stage O, Binet stage A, and some Rai stage I and II patients. The latter patients represent a heterogeneous group that requires further analysis before deciding whether to treat or not. One suggestion is to subdivide Rai I/II patients into Binet stage A and B, reserving treatment for Binet stage B patients (2). Another approach for Rai I/II patients is to look for non–stage-defining prognostic features, as noted above. Thus, a lymphocyte count $<40 \times 10^9$/L, a lymphocyte doubling time >12 months, and a nondiffuse pattern of marrow histologic involvement in an asymptomatic Rai I/II patient predicts an indolent course and allows observation off therapy with visits every 2–4 months for reevaluation. Similar stage patients with poor prognostic features (lymphocyte count $>40 \times 10^9$/L, lymphocyte doubling time <12 months, and diffuse marrow involvement) are likely to have rapidly progressive courses and should be treated with systemic therapy.

Two prospective, randomized cooperative group studies (122, 137) have shown no survival advantage for early treatment (chlorambucil) in low-risk patients such as those described above. In fact, in updated results (2) from one study (122), an excess of secondary epithelial malignancies and treatment refractoriness in patients who progressed on therapy resulted in *shorter* survival with chlorambucil than with no treatment. By contrast, it is generally agreed that Rai stage III and IV or Binet stage B and C patients should be treated (2, 3, 89), although even this has not been subjected to study by prospective, randomized trials.

Symptoms

Progressive, apparently disease-related symptoms such as fever, weight loss, night sweats, or disabling fatigue may respond to therapy, with improved quality of life. It is imperative to rule out other causes for such symptoms, especially infections, before attributing them to CLL. In early-stage CLL patients, such symptoms may be more likely due to infection, and therapy for CLL without specific treatment for the infection could aggravate the situation. Patients may also be symptomatic from lymphoid masses, such as bulky lymphadenopathy or splenomegaly. Such bulky disease may occasionally be painful, cause cosmetic problems, or compromise other tissues (ureteral or bowel obstruction, hypersplenic cytopenias, etc.). Local irradiation may be chosen over systemic therapy in some cases.

Immune Cytopenias

Coombs-positive autoimmune hemolytic anemia or immune thrombocytopenic purpura demand therapy. However, single-agent prednisone alone or with splenectomy may resolve the problem without need for further systemic therapy of CLL. Pure red cell aplasia often responds to cyclosporine (see below).

Hyperlymphocytosis

There is no generally accepted lymphocyte count per se that requires therapy in the absence of other criteria. However, the necessity to avoid the rare but severe and sometimes lethal complications of leukostasis (138) has led some authorities to recommend therapy for patients with lymphocyte counts $>150 \times 10^9$/L, especially when the rate of rise shows a short lymphocyte doubling time (25). Others may have a treatment threshold as high as 500×10^9/L in asymptomatic patients.

Transformation

Development of Richter syndrome or prolymphocytoid transformation in the patient without other indication for systemic therapy is rare, but these complications require immediate therapy.

Drug Therapy

Corticosteroids

Corticosteroids, usually prednisone, are frequently used in the management of CLL, either as a single agent in the therapy of immune cytopenias or in combination with chlorambucil or cyclophosphamide for systemic therapy of progressive or high-risk disease. For autoimmune hemolytic anemia or immune thrombocytopenic purpura, the usual prednisone dose is about 1 mg/kg daily in single or divided doses. Once maximum clinical response is obtained, the prednisone is slowly tapered to determine the minimum dose, if any, needed to sustain response. Patients who fail to respond to therapy or who require more than minimal prednisone doses chronically to maintain response should be considered for splenectomy. Intravenous immunoglobulin may be a useful adjunct in the short-term treatment of immune cytopenias in CLL (139).

Alkylating Agents

The most commonly used agent in the treatment of CLL is chlorambucil, which as a single agent is the standard treatment for low-risk and intermediate risk patients who warrant therapy. Chlorambucil is a well-tolerated, easily absorbed oral alkylating agent with few side effects other than dose-dependent bone marrow suppression. The two most common schedules of administration are essentially equal in efficacy and toxicity: daily low dose (0.07 mg/kg/day) or intermittent high dose (0.4–0.8 mg/kg every 3 or 4 weeks) (140). Dosing is adjusted on the basis of blood count monitoring to produce and maintain a WBC count in the range of $5–10 \times 10^9/L$ while avoiding bone marrow suppression. Approximately 60–80% of low-risk and intermediate risk patients will respond to this agent, almost all with partial responses (improvement in all disease manifestations) rather than complete responses (disappearance of all clinical signs of disease). Once a satisfactory response is attained, therapy is stopped and the patient observed for disease progression and reappearance of indications for treatment.

Cyclophosphamide is the alternate alkylating agent of choice in CLL. It has efficacy equivalent to chlorambucil but additional side effects of alopecia and hemorrhagic cystitis. It is only occasionally effective in patients who do not respond to chlorambucil. The usual oral dose is 1–3 mg/kg daily or 20 mg/kg every 2–3 weeks, either orally (4 mg/kg daily for 5 days) or as a single intravenous infusion. Blood counts are monitored as for chlorambucil to adjust doses. There is no advantage to the use of other alkylating agents in CLL.

Nucleoside Analogs

Several new agents are particularly promising in CLL patients who are resistant to alkylating agents. Approved by the U.S. Food and Drug Administration for alkylating agent–refractory CLL patients, fludarabine monophosphate is a fluorinated derivative of adenosine that is resistant to adenosine deaminase. In a study of previously treated CLL patients, an overall response rate of 57% was seen, evenly divided between clinical complete responses and partial responses (141). Even more exciting, in a small number of previously untreated CLL patients, fludarabine produced a 73% clinical complete response rate (including patients with residual lymphoid nodules in the marrow), better than any previous therapy (142). Trials are under way comparing fludarabine to CHOP (cyclosphamide, low-dose doxorubicin, vincristine, and prednisone) (143) in Europe and comparing fludarabine to chlorambucil and to the combination of fludarabine plus chlorambucil in North America. Fludarabine's toxicity at doses used in CLL (mainly marrow suppression and minor neurotoxicity) is mild, but its schedule of administration is inconvenient (25–30 mg/M² intravenously daily for 5 days, repeated monthly). With repeated cycles of therapy, profound depletion of circulating CD4-positive T-cells develops along with increased risk of opportunistic infections due to *P. carinii*, *Lysteria monocytogenes*, *Herpes zoster*, cytomegalovirus, and fungi (144), infections not typically seen in CLL patients treated with alkylating agents. Fludarabine also has activity against previously treated non-Hodgkin lymphoma, especially low-grade histologies (145) and Waldenstrüom macroglobulinemia (146).

A second new agent, cladribine (2'-chlorodeoxyadenosine or 2-CDA), another adenosine deaminase-resistant halogenated nucleoside derivative and potent inhibitor of ribonucleotide reductase, has activity in CLL similar to fludarabine. Response rates of 44–67% in previously treated CLL patients have been described (147–149). Toxicity is similar to that of fludarabine (myelosuppression, T-cell depletion, unusual infections), as is the approved route and schedule of administration (0.1 mg/kg daily for 7 days each month). An alternative dosing schedule (0.12 mg/kg by 2-hour infusion daily for 5 days each month) facilitates outpatient therapy (149). Early results in previously untreated CLL patients are also promising. Cladribine is also active in hairy cell leukemia (HCL), where a single 7-day course usually results in a durable complete remission (150), and in Waldenstrüom macroglobulinemia (151), and low-grade non-Hodgkin lymphoma (152).

Pentostatin (2-deoxycoformycin), a potent and long-acting adenosine deaminase inhibitor, produces responses in 25–30% of previously treated CLL patients with advanced disease (153, 154). The administration schedule (4 mg/M² every 2 weeks) is more convenient, but the response rate seems lower, especially in alkylating agent–resistant patients, and the toxicity profile at standard doses (prolonged T-cell suppression, infections, myelosuppression, gastrointestinal symptoms, and pruritus) may be worse than that of the other two agents. Neither cladribine nor pentostatin is currently approved for use in CLL in the United States, but both are licensed for the treatment of HCL.

Still to be determined is the extent of cross-resistance among these three agents. Despite an initial report of cladribine response in four of four CLL patients who had failed fludarabine therapy (155), it appears that cladribine is usually ineffective in truly fludarabine-refractory CLL patients (156).

These three nucleoside analogs are an intriguing group of new agents. All three would be expected to be active against proliferating cells based on their metabolism and in vitro activity, and in fact at high doses they have activity in acute leukemia (157). Why then is their major clinical activity observed in diseases (CLL, HCL, low-grade lymphomas) characterized by quiescent tumor cell populations? Although studies have indicated that cladribine may interfere with DNA repair in resting lymphocytes (158), and there is abundant evidence that cladribine and/or fludarabine induces apoptosis, or programmed cell death in normal lymphocytes (159, 160) and CLL cells (161, 162), our current understanding of the cytotoxic action of these agents in CLL is incomplete.

> The main question at present is whether these agents, especially fludarabine and cladribine, are superior to chlorambucil as initial therapy of CLL. This is being addressed in clinical trials, including an intergroup study nearing completion. A related question is whether the intent of therapy of CLL should be changed from palliative to curative, now that agents are available that induce clinical complete remissions in a substantial number of patients. Currently, the treatment-related toxicity of curative-intent approaches such as fludarabine/cladribine to complete remission followed by bone marrow transplantation (see below) prohibits widespread application to the majority of CLL patients. However, this approach should be studied in the small subset of young (<50-year-old) CLL patients.

Combination Regimens

For high-risk patients (e.g., Rai stage III and IV), the combination of chlorambucil and prednisone is regarded by some as the treatment of choice, although a prospective comparison of the combination to chlorambucil alone has not been reported. Chlorambucil is given on the intermittent schedule described above (0.4–0.8 mg/kg) along with prednisone 60–80 mg in divided doses daily for 5 days every 3–4 weeks. Some prefer to initially give prednisone at the above dose daily for 2 weeks, then at half dose daily for 2 weeks, before switching to the intermittent schedule. In high-risk patients, allopurinol to prevent urate nephropathy may be indicated when initiating therapy. In patients without significant toxicity, the chlorambucil dose may be escalated to produce the best response; therapy is then stopped to assess the durability of the response. Since treatment is palliative, there is no advantage in prolonged continuous therapy in responding patients.

A prospective trial comparing intermittent chlorambucil plus prednisone to no treatment in Binet stage A patients

has been under way for some time, but results have not been reported.

The three-drug combination of cyclophosphamide, vincristine, and prednisone, or COP (163), is also popular despite failure to demonstrate superiority over chlorambucil plus prednisone (164) or chlorambucil alone (165). Cyclophosphamide is given on the every 3-week intermittent schedule (300 mg/M^2 daily for 5 days) along with vincristine 1.4 mg/M^2 (maximum dose 2 mg) on day 1 and prednisone 40 mg/M^2 daily for 5 days. Other combinations (166, 167) show no advantage, except possibly the "CHOP" regimen—COP plus low-dose doxorubicin (25 mg/M^2 intravenously on day 1). One prospective randomized trial demonstrated a three-fold increase in survival (median 62 months vs 22 months) for Binet stage C patients treated with CHOP compared with COP (143). However, a subsequent trial found equivalent overall response to high-dose chlorambucil (15 mg daily until complete remission) and CHOP (168). In addition, other trials have shown median survivals similar to those reported for CHOP for high-risk CLL patients treated with chlorambucil plus prednisone or CVP (169). Another direct comparison between CHOP and chlorambucil plus prednisone in stage B and C patients has shown a higher response rate to CHOP on preliminary analysis, but survival data are not mature (170).

Radiation Therapy

Systemic radiation therapy, whether administered as ^{32}P, extracorporeal blood irradiation, or total body irradiation, is mainly of historical interest (2). However, local field radiation therapy remains useful in selected patients. Irradiation of bulky lymph nodes provides prompt palliation in most cases, and this approach may be especially appropriate in the management of symptomatic lymph node masses resistant to chemotherapy or in the patient with one or two areas of bulky disease but no other indications for systemic chemotherapy.

Splenic irradiation (171) usually results in rapid reduction in splenomegaly and may be associated with some systemic improvement. It is a temporary measure, but response may be maintained for as long as years in some cases. In patients who are poor operative candidates, it may be preferable to splenectomy. Although anemia and thrombocytopenia due to hypersplenism may improve after splenic irradiation, immune cytopenias generally are not relieved as they usually are after splenectomy. The main risk of splenic irradiation is myelosuppression due to incompletely understood mechanisms, sometimes referred to as the abscopal effect of (splenic) irradiation. Thrombocytopenia, particularly, is common after splenic irradiation, and may last for weeks.

Splenectomy

> Splenectomy is useful in the management of autoimmune hemolytic anemia and immune thrombocytopenic

purpura that have failed to respond to medical therapy (172, 173). The other main indication is bulky, painful, or otherwise symptomatic (e.g., early satiety) splenomegaly that is unresponsive to chemotherapy. Massive spleens present a surgical challenge and should be approached only by experienced surgeons. Pneumococcal vaccine is usually recommended before splenectomy, but CLL patients often do not respond to vaccination and should be managed after splenectomy with full asplenia precautions, including empiric antibiotics for fever.

Leukapheresis

Therapeutic leukapheresis (174) has a limited role in the treatment of CLL, being mainly useful for the adjunctive treatment of symptomatic hyperlymphocytosis (case 5). It is ineffective as a sole therapeutic maneuver because cells removed from the circulation are rapidly replaced by cells mobilized from other sites. Given in conjunction with chemotherapy, it may result in a more rapid reduction in lymphocyte count than chemotherapy alone.

Intravenous Immunoglobulin

The frequent occurrence of infection and hypo-γ-globulinemia in CLL patients has suggested the use of intravenous immunoglobulin for replacement therapy. A double-blind randomized study has demonstrated that intravenous immunoglobulin infusions (400 mg/kg every 3 weeks) can reduce the overall incidence of bacterial infections by 50% compared with placebo infusions (118). However, the incidence of *severe* bacterial infections or viral infections and the survival duration were equal in both groups. A subsequent study of the cost effectiveness of this approach in CLL has raised substantial doubts about its value as a general policy (119). There are individual patients who may benefit in a cost-effective way: these are patients with documented hypo-γ-globulinemia and recurrent infections without other predisposition (e.g., neutropenia) who otherwise have no indications for systemic chemotherapy of their CLL.

Bone Marrow Transplantation

Allogeneic bone marrow transplantation has been attempted in a small number of selected young patients with CLL, probably representing the first therapy in this disease to be administered with curative intent.

The European Group for Bone Marrow Transplantation reported 17 patients (mean age 40) allografted for advanced disease (175, 176), of whom 9 survived in continuous complete remission at a mean followup of 25 months. Two of the failures were due to relapse of CLL, and the remainder succumbed to transplant-related complications. While the eradication of the malignant CLL clone has still to be demonstrated with longer followup, these are en-

couraging results. Current patient selection practices among marrow transplant centers and the age distribution of CLL make it unlikely that this is a therapeutic option for more than a small fraction (5%?) of CLL patients.

Autologous bone marrow transplantation using bone marrow harvested in chemotherapy-induced complete remission is another approach under early investigation that may be applicable to a somewhat larger proportion of patients because of the lower treatment-related morbidity and mortality compared with allogeneic marrow transplantation (177). Because of the nature of CLL, long-term followup (5–10 years) and/or molecular confirmation of disease eradication (e.g., Ig gene rearrangement analysis using the polymerase chain reaction) will be necessary to evaluate the curability of CLL by this means.

Antibody/Immunotoxin Therapy

The relatively selective binding of antibodies and natural ligands to antigens and receptors on cell surfaces has led to the concept of targeted protein therapy of malignancies. This developing experimental field utilizes antibodies and natural ligands, either unmodified or coupled to plant toxins or high specific activity radionuclides, as cytotoxic agents in vivo. CLL is an appealing target for this approach because of expression of lineage-specific antigens (CD19,20) and disease-associated antigens (CD5). A relatively even more restrictive antigen, the common CLL antigen (cCLLa), is limited to CLL and HCL cells (178, 179).

Finally, CLL cells express surface immunoglobulin, usually IgM or IgM plus IgD (180), with variable regions containing antigenic determinants, called idiotypes, that can be common to variable regions of different Ig molecules (181). All these antigens represent potential targets for serotherapy (182).

Phase I clinical trials of an unmodified monoclonal antibody (designated T101) to CD5 demonstrated feasibility (although some schedules were associated with severe anaphylaxis), but efficacy was disappointing, limited to transient (1–3 days) decreases in circulating CLL cells without shrinkage of adenopathy or organomegaly (183–185). Preliminary trials of human-complement fixing antihuman lymphocyte rat monoclonal antibodies (the CAMPATH-1 family) produced more sustained and complete reduction in circulating lymphocytes (186), and these antibodies are currently under clinical study.

In an attempt to enhance the cytotoxicity of monoclonal antibodies, immunotoxins have been developed by conjugating monoclonal antibodies (or natural ligands) to toxins, such as saporin and pokeweed antiviral protein (187), *Pseudomonas* exotoxin, diphtheria toxin (188), and ricin (189).

The T101 antibody conjugated to ricin A-chain (190) has been as disappointing in early trials (191–193) as unmodified T101 antibody, due mainly to the transient nature of observed decreases in circulating CLL cells and lack of activity against lymph nodes. Subsequent studies showed little in vitro activity of this conjugate against CLL cells

(191), apparently because ricin A-chain conjugates have less cytotoxicity than intact ricin (A plus B chain) immunoconjugates. Currently of more interest is an immunotoxin called anti-B4-blocked ricin, in which intact ricin is conjugated to anti-B4 (a murine monoclonal antibody against CD19) and the native nonspecific ricin B-chain binding sites have been chemically blocked (194).

Another approach to immunotoxin therapy utilizes recombinant DNA technology to replace the receptor-binding portion of the diphtheria toxin gene with DNA sequences for human interleukin-2 (IL-2). The hybrid gene (expressed in *Escherichia coli*) results in a fusion protein, called DAB_{486} IL-2, which contains the binding domain of IL-2 (in place of the toxin B-chain binding domain) and the cytotoxic domain of diphtheria toxin (195). DAB_{486} IL-2 binds to and kills cells expressing the high-affinity IL-2 receptor (196); these include B-CLL and some lymphomas and activated but not resting T- and B-lymphocytes. Preliminary experience has included a substantial response in 1 of 4 CLL patients treated with DAB_{486} IL-2 (197), including reductions in marrow lymphocytosis, lymphadenopathy, and splenomegaly.

Although immunotoxin responses have been infrequent and incomplete, they are important because (a) all patients have been resistant to conventional therapies at the time of treatment, (b) dose schedules of immunotoxin therapies have only begun to be explored, and (c) theoretically these agents may have much greater efficacy in patients with low tumor burdens (perhaps as adjuvant therapy after drug-induced remission or following autologous bone marrow transplantation).

Summary

In summary, CLL is a largely indolent malignancy but one with a large number of immunologic complications. As with the lymphomas, much energy has been directed toward taxonomy and only latterly has the biology even begun to be explored, but no good molecular associations exist as for, e.g., CML. Historically, treatment has been conservative or palliative at the most, but newer pharmacologic initiatives point toward possibilities of cure.

REFERENCES

1. Rozman C, Montserrat JM, Rodriquez-Fernandez R, et al. Bone marrow histologic pattern—the best single prognostic parameter in chronic lymphocytic leukemia: a multivariate survival analysis of 329 cases. Blood 1984;64: 642–648.
2. Dighiero B, Philippe T, Chevret S, Fenaux P, Chastang C, Binet JL, and the French Cooperative Group on CLL. B-Cell chronic lymphocytic leukemia: present status and future directions. Blood 1991;78:1901–1914.
3. Cheson B, Bennett J, Rai K, et al. Guidelines for clinical protocols for chronic lymphocytic leukemia: recommendations of the NCI sponsored working group. Am J Hematol 1988;29:152–163.
4. Han T, Ozer H, Gavigan M, et al. Benign monoclonal B cell lymphocytosis. A benign variant of chronic lymphocytic leukemia: Clinical, immunologic, phenotypic and cytogenetic studies in 20 patients. Blood 1984;64:244–252.
5. Montserrat E, Virolas N, Reverter JC, Rozman C. Natural history of chronic lymphocytic leukemia: on the progression and prognosis of early clinical stages. Nouv Rev Fr Hematol 1988;30:359–361.
6. French Cooperative Group on Chronic Lymphocytic Leukemia: Natural history of stage A chronic lymphocytic leukemia untreated patients. Br J Haematol 1990;76: 45–57.
7. Binet JL, Catovsky D, Chasteng C, et al. Prognostic features of early chronic lymphocytic leukemia. Lancet 1989; 2:968–969.
8. Bennett JM. Two cases of disease and enlargement of the spleen in which death took place from the presence of purulent matter in the blood. Edinburgh Med Surg J 1845; 64:413–423.
9. Virchow R. Weisses Blut. Froriep's Notizen 1845;36: 151–156.
10. Virchow R. Die farblosen Blutökorperchen. In: Gesammelte Abhandlungen zur wissen-schaftlichen Medzin. Frankfurt: Meidinger, 1856:212–228.
11. Neumann E. Ein Fall von Leukümie mit Erkrankung des Knochenmarkes. Arch Heilk 1870;11:1–14.
12. Ebstein W. Ueber die acute Leukümie und Pseudoleukümie. Dtsch Arch Klin Med 1888–1889;44:343–356.
13. Ehrlich P. Farbenanalytische Untersuchungen zur Histologie und Klinik des Blutes. Berlin: Hirschwald, 1891.
14. Minot GP, Isaacs R. Lymphatic leukemia: age, incidence, duration and benefit derived from irradiation. Boston Med Surg J 1924;19:1–12.
15. Lawrence JH, Low-Beer BVA, Carpender JWJ. Chronic lymphatic leukemia: study of 100 patients with radioactive phosphorus. JAMA 1949;140:585–592.
16. Shaw RK, Boggs DR, Siberman HR, et al. A study of prednisone therapy in chronic lymphocytic leukemia. Blood 1961;17:182–190.
17. Galton DAG, Isreals LG, Nabarro JDN, et al. Clinical trials of p-(di-2-chloroethylamino)-phenybutyric acid (CD 1348) in malignant lymphoma. Br Med J 1955;2:1172–1180.
18. Dameshek W. Chronic lymphocytic leukemia—an accumulative disease of immunologically incompetent lymphocytes. Blood 1967;29:566–584.
19. Galton DAG. The pathogenesis of chronic lymphocytic leukemia. Can Med Assoc J 1966;94:1005–1010.
20. Preud'homme JL, Seligmann M. Surface-bound immunoglobulins as a cell marker in human lymphoproliferative diseases. Blood 1972;40:777–794.
21. Boggs R, Sofferman SA, Wintrobe MM, et al. Factors influencing the duration of survival of patients with chronic lymphocytic leukemia. Am J Med 1966;40:243–254.
22. Rai KR, Sawitsky A, Cronkite EP, et al. Clinical staging of chronic lymphocytic leukemia. Blood 1975;46:219–234.
23. Binet JL, Auquier A, Dighiero G, et al. A new prognostic classification of chronic lymphocytic leukemia derived from a multivariate survival analysis. Cancer 1981;48: 198–206.
24. Linet MS, Blattner WA. The epidemiology of chronic lymphocytic leukemia. In: Pollack A, Catovsky D, eds. Chronic lymphocytic leukemia. New York: Harwood Academic Publishers, 1988:11–32.

25. Rai KR. An outline of clinical management of chronic lymphocytic leukemia. In: Cheson BD, ed. Chronic lymphocytic leukemia: scientific advances and clinical developments. New York: Marcel Dekker, 1993:241–251.

26. Conley CL, Misiti J, Laster AJ. Genetic factors predisposing to chronic lymphocytic leukemia and to autoimmune disease. Medicine 1980;5:323–333.

27. Gunz FW. The epidemiology and genetics of the chronic leukemias. Clin Haematol 1977;6:3–20.

28. Heath CW Jr. The epidemiology of leukemia. In: Schottenfeld D, ed. Cancer epidemiology and prevention: current concepts. Springfield, IL: Charles C Thomas, 1975: 318–352.

29. Donham KJ, Berg JW, Savin RS. Epidemiologic relationship of the bovine population and human leukemia in Iowa. Am J Epidemiol 1980;112:80–92.

30. Blair A, White D. Leukemia cell types and agricultural practices in Nebraska. Arch Environ Health 1985;40: 211–214.

31. Burmeister LF, Van Lier SF, Isaacson P. Leukemia and farm practices in Iowa. Am J Epidemiol 1982;115: 720–728.

32. McMichael A, Andjelkovic D, Tyroler H. Cancer mortality among rubber workers: An epidemiologic study. Ann NY Acad Sci 1976;271:125–137.

33. Arp EW, Wolf PH, Checkoway H. Lymphocytic leukemia and exposures to benzene and other solvents in the rubber industry. J Occup Med 1983;25:598–602.

34. Kagan E, Jacobson RJ. Lymphoid and plasma cell malignancies: Asbestos-related disorders of long latency. Am J Clin Pathol 1983;80:14–20.

35. Korsemeyer JS, Arnold A, Bakshi A, et al. Immunoglobulin gene rearrangement and cell surface antigen expression in acute lymphocytic leukemias of T cell and B cell precursor origins. J Clin Invest 1983;71:301–313.

36. Nadler LM, Korsmeyer SJ, Anderson KC, et al. B cell origin of non-T cell acute lymphoblastic leukemia. J Clin Invest 1984;74:332–340.

37. Hurwitz CA, Loken MR, Graham ML, et al. Asynchronous antigen expression in B lineage acute lymphoblastic leukemia. Blood 1988;72:299–307.

38. Haynes BF, Eisenbarth GS, Fauci AS. Human lymphocyte antigens: Production of a monoclonal antibody that defines functional thymus derived lymphocyte subsets. Proc Natl Acad Sci USA 1979;76:5829–5833.

39. Boumsell L, Coppin H, Pham D, et al. An antigen shared by a human T cell subset and B cell chronic lymphocytic leukemic cells. J Exp Med 1980;152:229–234.

40. Martin PJ, Hansen JA, Siadak AW, et al. A new human T cell differentiation antigen: unexpected expression on chronic lymphocytic leukemia cells. Immunogenetics 1980; 11:429–439.

41. Neckers LM, Yenokida G, James SP. The role of the transferrin receptor in human B lymphocyte activation. J Immunol 1984;133:2437–2441.

42. Boyd AW, Fisher DC, Fox D, et al. Structural and functional characterization of IL-2 receptors on activated B cells. J Immunol 1985;134:2387–2392.

43. Kishimoto T. Factors affecting B cell growth and differentiation. Annu Rev Immunol 1985;3:133–155.

44. Moore MAS, Owen JT. Experimental studies on the development of the thymus. J Exp Med 1967;126:715–725.

45. Reinherz EL, Schlossman SF. The differentiation and function of human T lymphocytes: a review. Cell 1980;19: 821–827.

46. Acuto O, Reinherz EL. The human T-cell receptor: structure and function. N Engl J Med 1985;312:110–111.

47. Chen YH, Heller P. Lymphocyte surface immunoglobulin density and immunoglobulin secretion in vitro in chronic lymphocytic leukemia (CLL). Blood 1978;52:601–608.

48. Catovsky D, Cherchi M, Okos A, et al. Mouse red blood cell rosettes in B lymphoproliferative disorders. Br J Haematol 1976;33:173–177.

49. Kipps TJ, The CD 5 B cell (review). Adv Immunol 1989; 47:117–185.

50. Van de Velde H, von Hoegen I, Luo W, Parnes J, Thielemans K. The B cell surface protein CD72/Lyb-2 is the ligand for CD5, Nature 1991;351;662–665.

51. Ledbetter JA, Martin PJ, Spooner CE, Wofsy D, Tsu TT, Beatty PG, Gladstone P. Antibodies to Tp67 and Tp44 augment and sustain proliferative responses of activated T cell. J Immunol 1985;135:2331–2336.

52. Freedman AS, Freeman G, Whitman J, et al. Studies on in vitro activated CD5 1 B cells. Blood 1989;73:202–208.

53. Tsudo M, Uchiyama T, Umadome H, et al. Expression of interleukin-2 receptor on T cell chronic lymphocytic leukemia cells and their response to interleukin-2. Blood 1986;67:316–321.

54. Ueshima Y, Haren JM, Bird ML, Rowley JD. Culture conditions in chronic lymphocytic leukemia: relationship to karyotype. Leukemia 1989;3:192–194.

55. Juliusson G, Gahrton G. Chromosomal aberrations in B-cell chronic lymphocytic leukemia: pathogenetic and clinical implication. Cancer Genet Cytogenet 1990;5: 143–160.

56. Juliusson G, Gahrton G. Chromosome abnormalities in B-cell chronic lymphocytic leukemia. In: Cheson BD, ed. Chronic lymphocytic leukemia: scientific advances and clinical developments. New York: Marcel Dekker, 1993: 83–103.

57. Fitchett M, Griffiths MJ, Oscier DG, Johnson S, Seabright M. Chromosome abnormalities involving band 13q14 in hematologic malignancies. Cancer Genet Cytogenet 1987; 24:143–50.

58. Yunis JJ, Ramsay N. Retinoblastoma and subband deletion of chromosome 13. Am J Dis Child 1978;132:161–163.

59. Erikson J, Finan J, Tsujimoto Y, Nowell PC, Croce CM. The chromosome 14 breakpoint in neoplastic B cells with the t(11;14) translocation involves the immunoglobulin heavy chain locus. Proc Natl Acad Sci USA 1984;81: 4144–4148.

60. Adachi M, Cossman J, Longo D, Croce CM, Tsujimoto Y. Variant translocation of the bcl-2 gene to immunoglobulin lambda light chain gene in a chronic lymphocytic leukemia. Proc Natl Acad Sci USA 1989;86:2771–2774.

61. McKeithan T, Ohno H, Diaz M. Identification of a transcriptional unit adjacent to the breakpoint in the t(14:19) translocation of chronic lymphocyticleukemia. Genes Chromosomes Cancer 1990;1:247–255.

62. Weiss LM, Warnke RA, Sklar J, Cleary ML. Molecular analysis of the t(14:18) chromosomal translocation in malignant lymphomas. N Engl J Med 1987;317:1185–1189.

63. Juliusson G, Oscier D, Fitchett M, et al. Prognostic subgroups in B cell chronic lymphocytic leukemia defined by specific chromosomal abnormalities. N Engl J Med 1990; 323:720–724.

64. Nowell PC, Moreau L, Growney P, Besa E. Karyotypic stability in chronic B-cell leukemia. Cancer Genet Cytogenet 1988;33:155–160.

65. Oscier D, Fitchett M, Herbert T, Lambert R. Karyotypic evolution in B-cell chronic lymphocytic leukaemia. Genes Chromosomes Cancer 1991;3:16–20.

66. Galton DAG, Goldman JM, Wiltshaw E, Catovsky D, Henry K, Goldberg GJ. Prolymphocytic Leukemia. Br J Haematol 1974;27:7–23.

67. Bennett JM, Catovsky D, Daniel MT, Flandrin G, Galton D, Gralnick H, Sultan C. Proposals for the classification of chronic (mature) B and T lymphoid leukaemias. J Clin Pathol 1989;2:567–584.

68. Melo JV, Catovsky D, Gregory W, Galton D. The relationship between chronic lymphocytic leukemia and prolymphocytic leukemia: IV analysis of survival and prognostic features. Br J Haematol 1987;65:23–29.

69. Stark A, Limbert H, Robert B, Jones R, Scott C. Prolymphocytoid transformation of chronic lymphocytic leukemia: a clinical and immunological study of 22 cases. Leuk Res 1986;10:1225–1232.

70. Mintzer D, Hauptman SP. Lymphosarcoma cell leukemia and other non Hodgkin's lymphomas in leukemia phase. Am J Med 1983;75:110–120.

71. Melo JV, Hedge U, Parreira A, Thompson I, Lampert I, Catovsky D. Splenic B cell lymphoma with circulating villous lymphocytes: differential diagnosis of B cell leukemias with large spleens. J Clin Pathol 1987;40:642–651.

72. Neiman RS, Sullivan AL, Jaffe R. Malignant lymphoma simulating leukemic reticuloendotheliosis: a clinicopathologic study of ten cases. Cancer 1979;43:329–342.

73. Krajny M, Pauzanski W. Waldenström's macroglobulinemia: review of 45 cases. Can Med Assoc J 1976;114: 899–905.

74. Freedman AS, Nadler LM. Immunologic markers in B-cell chronic lymphocytic leukemia. In: Cheson BD, ed. Chronic lymphocytic leukemia: scientific advances and clinical developments. New York: Marcel Dekker, 1993:1–32.

75. Sainati L, Matutes E, Mulligan S, deOliveira MP, Rani S, Lampert IA, Catovsky D. A variant form of hairy cell leukemia resistant to α-interferon: clinical and phenotypic characteristics of 17 patients. Blood 1990;76:157–162.

76. Saxon A, Stevens RH, Golde TW. T–lymphocyte variant of hairy-cell leukemia. Ann Intern Med 1978;88:323–326.

77. Brouet JC, Flandrin G, Sasportes M, Preud'homme JL, Seligmann M. CLL of T-cell origin: immunological and clinical evaluation in 11 patients. Lancet 1975;2: 890–893.

78. Aisenberg AC, Krontiris TG, Mak TW, Wilkes BM. Rearrangement of the gene for the beta chain of the T-cell receptor in T-cell chronic lymphocytic leukemia and related disorders. N Engl J Med 1985;313:529–533.

79. Ueshima Y, Rowley JD, Variakojis D, Winter J, Gordon L. Cytogenetic studies in patients with chronic T cell leukemia/lymphoma. Blood 1984; 63:102–138.

80. Berliner N. T gamma lymphocytosis and T cell chronic leukemias. Hematol Oncol Clin N Am 1990;4:473–487.

81. Matutes E, Brito-Babapulle V, Swansbury J, et al. Clinical and laboratory features of 78 cases of T-prolymphocytic leukemia. Blood 1991;3269–3274.

82. Catovsky D, Matutes E. Leukemias of mature T cells: prolymphocytic and large granular lymphocytic leukemia. In: Knowles DM, ed. Neoplastic hematopathology. Baltimore: Williams & Wilkins, 1992:41–68.

83. Matutes E, Catovsky D. Mature T-cell leukemias and leukemia/lymphoma syndromes: review of our experience in 175 cases. Leuk Lymph 1991;4:81–91.

84. Chan WC, Link S, Mawle A, et al. Heterogeneity of large granular lymphocyte proliferations—delineation of two major subtypes with distinct origins, immunophenotypes, functional and clinical characteristics. Blood 1986;68: 1142–1153.

85. Blayney DW, Jaffe ES, Fisher RI, et al. The human T-cell leukemia/lymphoma virus, lymphoma, lytic bone lesions, and hypercalcemia. Ann Intern Med 1983;98:144–151.

86. Gallo RC, Kalyanaraman VS. Sarngadharan MG, et al. Association of human type C retrovirus with a subset of adult T-cell cancers. Cancer Res 1983;43:3892–3899.

87. Rai KR: A critical analysis of staging in CLL. In: Gale RP, Rai KR, eds. CLL recent progress and future direction. UCLA Symposia on Molecular and Cellular Biology. New York: Alan R. Liss, new series, 1987;59: 253–265.

88. International Workshop on CLL: Proposal for revised prognostic staging system. Br J Haematol 1981;48:365–367.

89. International Workshop on CLL. CLL: recommendations for diagnosis, staging and response criteria. Ann Intern Med; 1989:110;236–238.

90. Baccarani M, Cavo M, Gobbi M, Lauria F, Tura S. Staging of chronic lymphocytic leukemia. Blood 1982;59: 1191–1196.

91. Rozman C, Montserrat E, Feliu E, Granena A, Marin P, Nomdedeu B, Vives Corrons JL. Prognosis of chronic lymphocytic leukemia: a multivariate survival analysis of 150 cases. Blood 1982;59:1001–1005.

92. Montserrat E, Sanchez-Bisono J, Vinolas N, Rozman C. Lymphocyte doubling time in chronic lymphocytic leukemic leukemia: analysis of its prognostic significance. Br J Haematol 1986;62:567–575.

93. Vinolas N, Reverter JC, Urbano-Ispizua A, et al. Lymphocyte doubling time in chronic lymphocytic leukemia: an update of its prognostic significance. Blood Cells 1987;12: 457–470.

94. Lee JS, Dixon DO, Kantarjian HM, Keating MJ, Talpaz M. Prognosis of chronic lymphocytic leukemia: a multivariate regression analysis of 325 untreated patients. Blood 1987; 69:929–936.

95. Han T, Barcos M, Emrich L, et al. Bone marrow infiltration patterns and their prognostic significance in chronic lymphocytic leukemia: correlations with clinical, immunologic, phenotypic and cytogenetic data. J Clin Oncol 1984;6: 562–570.

96. Geisler C, Ralfkiaer E, Hansen MM, Hou-Jensen K, Larsen SO. The bone marrow histological pattern has independent prognostic value in chronic lymphocytic leukemia. Br J Haematol 1986;62:47–54.

97. Cone L, Uhr JW. Immunologic deficiency disorders associated with chronic lymphocytic leukemia and multiple myeloma. J Clin Invest 1964;43:2241–2248.

98. Fernandez LA, Macsween JM, Langley GR. Immunoglobulin secretory function of B cells from untreated patients with chronic lymphocytic leukemia and hypogammaglobulinemia: role of T cells. Blood 1983;62:767–774.

99. Kay NE, Perri RT. Evidence that large granular lymphocytes from B-CLL patients with hypogammaglobulinemia down-regulate B-cell immunoglobulin synthesis. Blood 1989;73:1016–1019.

100. Deegan MJ, Abraham JP, Sawdyk M, Van Slyck EJ. High incidence of monoclonal proteins in the serum and urine of chronic lymphocytic leukemia patients. Blood 1984;64: 1207–1211.

101. Mangan KF, Chikkappa G, Farley PC. T gamma cells suppress growth of erythroid colony-forming units in vitro in the pure red cell aplasia of B-cell chronic lymphocytic leukemia. J Clin Invest 1982;70:1148–1156.

102. Mangan KF, D'Alessandro L. Hypoplastic anemia in B-cell chronic lymphocytic leukemia: evolution of T cell-mediated suppression of erythropoiesis in early-stage and late-stage disease. Blood 1985;66:533–541.

103. Tura S, Finelli C, Bandini G, Cavo M, Gobbi M. Cyclosporin A in the treatment of CLL associated PRCA and bone marrow hypoplasia. Nouv Rev Fr Hematol 1988;30: 479–481.

104. Platsoucas CD, Galinski M, Kempin S, Reich L, Clarkson B, Good RA. Abnormal T lymphocyte subpopulations in patients with B cell chronic lymphocytic leukemia: An analysis by monoclonal antibodies. J Immunol 1982;129: 2305–2312.

105. Herrmann F, Lochner A, Philippen H, Jauer B, Ruhl H. Imbalance of T cell subpopulations in patients with chronic lymphocytic leukaemia of the B cell type. Clin Exp Immunol 1982;49:157–162.

106. Semenzato G, Pezzutto A, Foa R, Lauria F, Raimondi R. T lymphocytes in B-cell lymphocytic leukemia: Characterization by monoclonal antibodies and correlation with Fc receptors. Clin Immunol Immunopathol 1983;26:155–161.

107. Lucivero G, Prchal JT, Latwon AR, Antonaci S, Bonomo L. Abnormal T-cell functions in B cell chronic lymphocytic leukemia do not imply T-lymphocyte involvement in the leukemic process: report of a case with demonstrated "polyclonality" of T lymphocytes. J Clin Immunol 1983;3: 111–116.

108. Hamblin TJ, Oscier DJ, Young BJ. Autoimmunity in chronic lymphocytic leukemia. J Clin Pathol 1986;39: 713–716.

109 Foon KA, Rai KR, Gale RP. Chronic lymphocytic leukemia: new insights into biology and therapy. Ann Intern Med 1990;113:525–539.

110. Dighiero G. Hypogammaglobulinemia and disordered immunity in CLL. In: Cheson BD, ed. Chronic lymphocytic leukemia: scientific advances and clinical developments. New York: Marcel Dekker, 1993:167–180.

111. Hardy RR, Hayakawa K. Development and physiology of Ly-1 B and its human homolog, Leu-1 B. Immunol Rev 1986;93:53–79.

112. Hardy RR, Hayakawa K, Shimizu M, Yamasaki K, Kishimoto T. Rheumatoid factor secretion from human Leu-1+ B cells. Science 1987;236:81–83.

113. Casali P, Burastero SE, Nakamura M, Inghirami G, Notkins AL. Human lymphocytes making rheumatoid factor and antibody to ssDNA belong to the Leu-1+ B-cell subset. Science 1987;236:77–81.

114. Casali P, Notkins AL. CD5+ B lymphocytes, polyreactive antibodies and the human B-cell repertoire. Immunol Today 1989;10:364–368.

115. Sthoeger ZM, Wakai M, Tse DB, et al. Production of autoantibodies by CD5-expressing B lymphocytes from patients with chronic lymphocytic leukemia. J Exp Med 1989; 169:255–268.

116. Dighiero G. An attempt to explain disordered immunity and hypogammaglobulinemia in B-CLL. Nouv Rev Franc Hematol 1988;30:283–288.

117. Twomey JJ. Infections complicating multiple myeloma and chronic lymphocytic leukemia. Arch Intern Med 1973;132: 562–565.

118. Cooperative Group for the Study of Immunoglobulin in Chronic Lymphocytic Leukemia: Intravenous immunoglobulin for the prevention of infection in chronic lymphocytic leukemia: a randomized controlled trial. N Engl J Med 1988;319:902–907.

119. Weeks JC, Tierney MR, Weinstein MC. Cost effectiveness of prophylactic intravenous immune globulin in chronic lymphocytic leukemia. N Engl J Med 1991;325:81–86.

120. Quaglino D, Lusvarghi E, Piccinini L, diPrisco AU. The association between chronic lymphocytic leukaemia and a solid tumor: a survey study of 258 cases of chronic lymphocytic leukaemia covering an eleven year period. Haematologica 1976;61:456–469.

121. Pagnucco G, Castelli G, Brusamolino E. Risk of subsequent primary cancer in patients with chronic lymphocytic leukemia. In: Gale RP, Rai KR, eds. CLL recent progress and future direction. UCLA Symposia on Molecular and Cellular Biology. New York: Alan R. Liss, new series, 1987;59: 225–240.

122. French Cooperative Group on Chronic Lymphocytic Leukemia. Effects of chlorambucil and therapeutic decision in initial forms of chronic lymphocytic leukemia (stage A): results of a randomized clinical trial in 612 patients. Blood 1990;75:1414–1421.

123. Quaglino D, Paterlini P, De Pasquale A, Cretara G, Venturoni L. Association of chronic lymphocytic leukaemia and multiple myeloma: report of a case and review of the literature. Haematologica 1982;67:576–588.

124. Hoffman KD, Rudders RA. Multiple myeloma and chronic lymphocytic leukemia in a single individual: immunologic studies and review of the literature. Arch Intern Med 1977; 137:232–235.

125. Pedersen-Pjergaard J, Petersen HD, Thomsen M, Wiik A, Wolff-Jensen J. Chronic lymphocytic leukaemia with subsequent development of multiple myeloma: evidence of two B-lymphocyte clones and of myeloma-induced suppression of secretion of an M-component and of normal immunoglobulins. Scand J Haematol 1978;21:256–264.

126. Richter MN. Generalized reticular cell sarcoma of lymph nodes associated with lymphatic leukemia. Am J Pathol 1928;4:285–295.

127. Foucar K, Rydell RE. Richter's syndrome in chronic lymphocytic leukemia. Cancer 1980;46:118–134.

128. Harousseau JL, Flandrin G, Tricot G, Brovet JC, Seligmann M, Bernard J. Malignant lymphoma supervening in chronic lymphocytic leukemia and related disorders. Richter's syndrome: a study of 25 cases. Cancer 1981;48:1302–1308.

129. Bertoli LF, Kubagawa H, Borzillo GV, Mayumi M, Prchal JT, Kearney JF, Durant JR, Cooper MD. Analysis with antiidiotype antibody of a patient with chronic lymphocytic leukemia and a large cell lymphoma (Richter's syndrome). Blood 1987;70:45–50.

130. Delsol G, Laurent G, Kuhlein E, Familiades J, Rigal F, Pris J. Case reports: Richter's syndrome. Evidence for the clonal origin of the two proliferations. Am J Clin Pathol 1981; 76:308–315.

131. Michiels JJ, van Dongen JJ, Hagemeijer A, et al. Richter's syndrome with identical immunoglobulin gene arrangements in the chronic lymphocytic leukemia and the supervening non-Hodgkin lymphoma. Leukemia 1989;3:819–24.

132. McDonnell JM, Beschorner WE, Staal S, Spivak JL, Mann RB. Richter's syndrome with two different B-cell clones. Cancer 1986;58:2031–2037.

133. Enno A, Catovsky D, O'Brien M, Cherchi M, Kumaran TO, Galton DA. "Prolymphocytoid" transformation of chronic lymphocytic leukemia. Br J Haematol 1979;41:9–18.

134. Zarrabi MH, Grunwald HW, Rosner FL. Chronic lymphocytic leukemia terminating in acute leukemia. Arch Intern Med 1977;137:1059–1064.

135. Januszewicz E, Cooper IA, Pilkington G, Jose D. Blastic transformation of chronic lymphocytic leukemia. Am J Hematol 1983;15:399–402.

136. Frankel EP, Ligler FS, Graham MS, Hernandez JA, Kettman JR, Smith RG. Acute lymphocytic leukemic transformation of chronic lymphocytic leukemia: substantiation by flow cytometry. Am J Hematol 1981;10:391–398.

137. Shustik C, Mick R, Silver R, Sawitsky A, Rai K, Shapiro L. Treatment of early chronic lymphocytic leukemia: intermittent chlorambucil versus observation. Hematol Oncol 1988; 6:7–12.

138. Baer MR, Stein RS, Dessypris EN. Chronic lymphocytic leukemia with hyperleukocytosis: the hyperviscosity syndrome. Cancer 1985;56:2865–2869.

139. Besa EC. Use of intravenous immunoglobulin in chronic lymphocytic leukemia. Am J Med 1984;76:209–218.

140. Sawitsky A, Rai KR, Glidewell O, Silver RT. Comparison of daily versus intermittent chlorambucil and prednisone therapy in the treatment of patients with chronic lymphocytic leukemia. Blood 1977;50:1049–1059.

141. Keating MJ, Kantarjian M, Redman J, et al. Fludarabine: a new agent with major activity against chronic lymphocytic leukemia. Blood 1989;74:19–25.

142. Keating MJ. Fludarabine phosphate in the treatment of chronic lymphocytic leukemia. Semin Oncol 1990 17(Suppl 8):49–62.

143. French Cooperative Group on Chronic Lymphocytic Leukemia. Benefit of the CHOP regimen in advanced untreated CLL: results from a randomized clinical trial. Lancet 1986;1:1346–1349.

144. Kontoyianis DP, Anaissie EJ, Bodey GP. Infection in chronic lymphocytic leukemia: a reappraisal. In: Cheson BD, ed. Chronic lymphocytic leukemia: scientific advances and clinical developments. New York: Marcel Dekker, 1993:399–417.

145. Hochster HS, Kim KM, Green MD, et al. Activity of fludarabine in previously treated non-Hodgkin's low-grade lymphoma: results of an Eastern Cooperative Oncology Group study. J Clin Oncol 1992;10:28–32.

146. Kantarjian HM, Alexandian R, Koller CA, Kurzrock R, Keating MJ. Fludarabine therapy in macroglobulinemic lymphoma. Blood 1990;75:1928–1931.

147. Piro LD, Carrera CJ, Beutler E, Carson DA. Chorodeoxyadenosine: an effective new agent for the treatment of chronic lymmphocytic leukemia. Blood 1988;72:1069–1073.

148. Saven A, Carrera CJ, Carson DA, Beutler E, Piro LD. Phase II trial update of 2-chlorodeoxyadenosine treatment of advanced chronic lymphocytic leukemia (abstract). Proc Am Soc Clin Oncol 1990;9:212.

149. Juliusson G, Liliemark J. High complete remission rate from 2-chloro-2'-deoxyadenosine in previously treated patients with B-cell chronic lymphocytic leukemia: response predicted by rapid decrease of blood lymphocyte count. J Clin Oncol 1993;11:679–689.

150. Piro LD, Carrera CJ, Carson DA, Beutler E. Lasting remissions in hairy cell leukemia induced by a single infusion of 2-chlorodeoxyadenosine. N Engl J Med 1990;322:1117–1121.

151. Dimopoulos MA, Kantarjian H, Estey E, et al. Treatment of Waldenström macroglobulinemia with 2-chlorodeoxyadenosine. Ann Intern Med 1993;118:195–198.

152. Kay AC, Saven A, Carrera CJ, Carson DA, Thurston D, Beutler E, Piro LD. 2-Chlorodeoxyadenosine treatment of low–grade lymphomas. J Clin Oncol 1992;10:371–377.

153. Dillman RO, Mick R, McIntyre OR. Pentostatin in chronic lymphocytic leukemia: a phase II trial of cancer and leukemia group B. J Clin Oncol 1989;7:433–438.

154. Ho AD, Thaler J, Stryckmans P, et al. Pentostatin in resistant chronic lymphocytic leukemia: a phase II trial of the European organization for research and treatment of cancer (abstract). Proc Am Soc Clin Oncol 1990;9:206.

155. Juliusson G, Elmhorn-Rosenborg A, Liliemark J. Response to 2-chlorodeoxyadenosine in patients with B-cell chronic lymphocytic leukemia resistant to fludarabine. N Engl J Med 1992;327:1056–1061.

156. Saven A, Lemon RH, Piro LD. 2-Chlorodeoxyadenosine for patients with B-cell chronic lymphocytic leukemia resistant to fludarabine (letter). N Engl J Med 1993:328:812–813.

157. Plunkett W, Gandhi V. Cellular metabolism of nucleoside analogs in CLL: implications for drug development. In: Cheson BD, ed. Chronic lymphocytic leukemia: scientific advances and clinical developments. New York: Marcel Dekker, 1993:197–219.

158. Seto S, Carrera CH, Kubota M, Wasson DB, Carson DA. Mechanism of deoxyadenosine and 2-chlorodeoxyadenosine toxicity to nondividing human lymphocytes. J Clin Invest 1985;75:377–383.

159. Carson DA, Seto S, Wasson DB, Carrera CJ. DNA strand breaks, NAD metabolism, and programmed cell death. Exp Cell Res 1986;164:273–281.

160. Carson DA, Carrera CJ, Wasson DB, Yamanaka H. Programmed cell death and adenine deoxynucleotide metabolism in human lymphocytes. Adv Enzyme Reg 1987;27:395–404.

161. Robertson LE, Chubb S, Hittelman WN, Sandoval A, Plunkett. Programmed cell death (apoptosis) in chronic lymphocytic leukemia cells after fludarabine and chloroxeoxyadenosine. Blood 1991;78(Suppl 1):173a.

162. Carrera C, Piro LD, Saven A, Beutler E, Terai C, Carson DA. 2-Chlorodeoxyadenosine chemotherapy triggers programmed cell death in normal and malignant lymphocytes. Int J Purine Pyrimidine Res 1991;309·15–18.

163. Liepman M, Votaw ML. The treatment of chronic lymphocytic leukemia with COP chemotherapy. Cancer 1978;141:1664–1669.

164. Montserrat E, Alcala A, Parody R, et al. Treatment of chronic lymphocytic leukemia in advanced stages: a randomized trial comparing chlorambucil plus prednisone vs cyclophosphamide, vincristine and prednisone. Cancer 1985;56:2369–2375.

165. French Cooperative Group on Chronic Lymphocytic Leukemia. A randomized clinical trial of chlorambucil versus COP in stage B chronic lymphocytic leukemia. Blood 1990;75:1422–1425.

166. Kempin S, Lee BJ, Thaler HT, et al. Combination chemotherapy of advanced chronic lymphocytic leukemia: the M-2 protocol (vincristine BCNU, cyclophosphamide, melphalan and prednisone). Blood 1982;60:1110–1121.

167. Montserrat E, Alcala A, Alonso C, et al. A randomized trial comparing chlorambucil plus prednisone vs cyclophosphamide, melphalan and prednisone in the treatment of chronic lymphocytic leukemia stages B and C. Nouv Rev Fr Hematol 1988;30:429–432.

168. Jaksic B, Brugiatelli M, for IGCI (Vienna) CLL study group. High dose chlorambucil for the treatment of advanced B-chronic lymphocytic leukemia: results of two multicentric randomized trials (abstract). Blood 1990;76: 284a.

169. Bennett JM. The use of "CHOP" in the treatment of chronic lymphocytic leukemia (letter). Br J Haematol 1990; 74:546.

170. French Cooperative Group on CLL. Chlorambucil-prednisone vs CHOP polychimiotherapy in stage B chronic lymphocytic leukemia: results of a multicenter randomized clinical trial on 285 patients (abstract). Blood 1990;76:254a.

171. Roncadin M, Arcicasa M, Trovo MG, et al. Splenic irradiation in chronic lymphocytic leukemia: a 10-year experience at a single institution. Cancer 1987;60:2624–2628.

172. Thiruvengadam R, Piedmonte M, Barcos M, Han T, Henderson ES. Splenectomy in advanced chronic lymphocytic leukemia. Leukemia 1990;4:758–760.

173. Neal TF, Tefferi A, Witzig TE, Su J, Phyliky RL, Nagorney DM. Splenectomy in advanced chronic lymphocytic leukemia: a single institution experience with 50 patients. Am J Med 1992;93:435–440.

174. Marti GE, Folks T, Longo DL, Klein H. Therapeutic cytopheresis in chronic lymphocytic leukemia. J Clin Apheresis 1983;1:243–248.

175. Michallet M, Corronot B, Hollard D, et al. Allogeneic bone marrow transplantation in chronic lymphocytic leukemia: 17 cases. Report from the EB-MTC. Bone Marrow Transpl 1991;7:275–279.

176. Bandini G, Michallet M, Rosgi G, Tura S. Bone marrow transplantation for chronic lymphocytic leukemia. Bone Marrow Transpl 1991;7:251–253.

177. Stuart RK. Autologous bone marrow transplantation for leukemia. Semin Oncol 1993;20:40–54.

178. Faguet GB, Agee JR. Monoclonal antibodies against the chronic lymphatic leukemia antigen cCLLa: characterization and reactivity. Blood 1987;70:437–443.

179. Faguet GB, Agee JF. Immunophenotypic diagnosis of clinical and preclinical chronic lymphatic leukemia by using monoclonal antibodies against the cCLLa, a CLL-associated antigen. Blood 1988;72:679–684.

180. Freedman AS, Nadler LM. B cell development in chronic lymphocytic leukemia. Semin Hematol 1987;24:230–239.

181. Swisher EM, Shawler DL, Collins HA, et al. Expression of shared idiotypes in chronic lymphocytic leukemia and small lymphocytic lymphoma. Blood 1991;77:1977–1982.

182. Rabinowe SN, Grossbard ML, Nadler LM. Innovative treatment strategies for chronic lymphocytic leukemia: monoclonal antibodies. Immunoconjugates and bone marrow transplantation. In: Cheson BD, ed. Chronic lymphocytic leukemia: scientific advances and clinical developments. New York: Marcel Dekker, 1993:337–367.

183. Dillman RO, Shawler DL, Dillman JB, Royston I. Therapy of chronic lymphocytic leukemia and cutaneous T-cell lymphoma with T101 monoclonal antibody, J Clin Oncol 1984;2:881–891.

184. Foon KA, Schroff RW, Bunn PA, et al. Effects of monoclonal antibody therapy in patients with chronic lymphocytic leukemia. Blood 1984;64:1085–1093.

185. Dillman RO, Beauregard J, Shawler Dl, et al. Continuous infusion of T101 monoclonal antibody in chronic lymphocytic leukemia and cutaneous T–cell lymphoma. J Biol Resp Modif 1986;5:394–410.

186. Dyer MJS, Hale G, Hayhoe FGJ, Waldman H. Effects of CAMPATH-1 antibodies in vivo in patients with lymphoid malignancies: influence of antibody isotype. Blood 1989;73: 1431–1442.

187. Lambert JM, Blattler WA, McIntyre GD, Goldmacher VS, Scott CJ. Immunotoxins containing single-chain ribosome-inactivating proteins. Cancer Treatment Res 1988;37: 175–209.

188. Collier RJ. Effect of diphtheria toxin on protein synthesis: inactivation of one of the transfer factors. J Mol Biol 1967; 25:83–98.

189. Endo Y, Mitsui K, Motizuki M, Tsurugi K. The mechanism of action of ricin and related toxic lectins on eukaryotic ribosomes. J Biol Chem 1987;262:5908–5912.

190. Jansen FK, Blythman HE, Carriere D, et al. Immunotoxins: hybrid molecules combining high specificity and potent cytotoxicity. Immunol Rev 1982;62:185–216.

191. Hertler AA, Schlossman DM, Borowitz MJ, Blythman HE, Casellas, P, Frankel AE. An anti-CD5 immunotoxin for chronic lymphocytic leukemia: enhancement of cytotoxicity with human serum albumin-monensin. Int J Cancer 1989; 43:215–219.

192. Laurent G, Pris J, Farcet JP, et al. Effects of therapy with T101 ricin A-chain immunotoxin in two leukemia patients, Blood 1986;67:1680–1687.

193. Hertler AA, Schlossman DM, Borowitz MJ, et al. A phase I study of T101-ricin A chain immunotoxin in refractory chronic lymphocytic leukemia. J Biol Resp Modif 1988;7: 97–113.

194. Grossbard ML, Freedman AS, Ritz J, et al. Serotherapy of B-cell neoplasms with Anti-B4-blocked ricin: a phase I trial of daily bolus infusion. Blood 1992;79:576–585.

195. Williams DP, Parker P, Bacha P, et al. Diphtheria toxin receptor binding domain substitution with interleukin-2: genetic construction and properties of a diphtheria toxin-related interleukin-2 fusion protein. Protein Eng 1987;1: 493–498.

196. Bacha P, Williams DP, Waters C, Murphy JR, Strom TB. Interleukin-2 receptor cytotoxicity: Interleukin-2 receptor-mediated action of a diphtheria toxin-related interleukin-2 fusion protein. J Exp Med 1988;167: 612–622.

197. LeMaistre CF, Rosenblum MG, Ruben JS, et al. Therapeutic effects of genetically engineered toxin (DAB_{486}) IL-2 in patient with chronic lymphocytic leukemia. Lancet 1991; 337:1124–1125.

198. Freedman AS. Immunobiology of chronic lymphocytic leukemia (review). In: Canellos GP, ed. Chronic leukemias. Hemat Oncol Clin North Am. Philadelphia: WB Saunders, 1990:405–429.

CHAPTER 20

Plasma Cell Malignancies

ROGER HERZIG, GEETHA JOSEPH

So far as these investigations have gone, they appear to warrant the inference that . . . the cells seen in a cancer are only monstrosities of the normal cells.
—John Houston, Surgical Society of Ireland (1844)

Multiple Myeloma

Multiple myeloma is a B-cell malignancy characterized by abnormal proliferation of the end-stage or terminally differentiated B-cell (plasma cell). It accounts for 10% of hematologic malignancies and has an annual incidence of 3–5/100,000. The disease has been described in the literature for over 100 years. The median survival of untreated patients is 7–10 months (1). Chemotherapy with melphalan and prednisone, introduced in the late 1960s, increased the median survival to 30 months. Survival in multiple myeloma has changed little in the last 25 years despite advances in prognostic indices and the use of multiagent chemotherapy. New strategies including dose-intensive therapy with marrow support are being studied in an effort to prolong survival and achieve a cure in multiple myeloma.

Case 1

A 65-year-old woman presented to her family physician with complaints of weakness, shortness of breath, and low back pain. Physical examination revealed pallor, engorged retinal veins, fundal hemorrhages, and macroglossia. Signs of congestive heart failure were present with an S3 gallop, hepatomegaly, and peripheral edema. Percussion tenderness was elicited in the lumbar area. The following laboratory data were obtained: hemoglobin 84 g/L; hematocrit 30.1%; mean corpuscular volume (MCV) 98 fl; white blood cell (WBC) count 4×10^9/L; platelet count 133×10^9/L; blood urea nitrogen (BUN) 44 mg/dl; creatinine 2.2 mg/dl; calcium 11.8 mg/dl; albumin 3.0 g/dl; globulin 7.2 g/dl; uric acid 1.4 mg/dl; anion gap 4; erythrocyte sedimentation rate (ESR) 22 mm/hr.

Commentary

The immunoglobulins, or γ-globulins, which constitute the majority of the globulins, are produced by plasma cells in response to antigenic stimulation. Each plasma cell is committed to the production of a single epitope-specific antibody with either κ- or λ-light chains. Increased production of γ-globulins may be due to benign or neoplastic disorders. Benign causes of hyperglobulinemia include chronic antigenic stimulation of B-lymphocytes or immune dysregulation resulting in the production of polyclonal immunoglobulins. In contrast to monoclonal antibodies, polyclonal antibodies are heterogenous in terms of isotype, specificity, and light chain type. Monoclonal immunoglobulins (M proteins) are typified by the presence of only one light chain type and a specificity for the same epitope. The antigenic specificity of the M proteins is often not identifiable but is considered to be toward antigens to which the patient has been exposed in the past (2). The report of a patient who received horse serum as a child and developed myeloma 33 years later with M protein specificity against horse proteins corroborates this concept (3, 4). Some M proteins have been shown to react against viral and bacterial products. Others have been shown to be autoantibodies.

The uncontrolled production of a monoclonal immunoglobulin implies the neoplastic transformation of a single precursor cell. The malignant precursor cell in multiple myeloma was thought to be a pre-B lymphoid cell. However, the finding of myelomonocytic, erythroid, and megakaryocytic markers on precursor cells in multiple myeloma suggests that a more primitive stem cell may be involved (5, 6).

The role of cytokines, especially interleukin-5 (IL-5) and interleukin-6 (IL-6), as autocrine or paracrine growth factors in multiple myeloma is being investigated. Cultured human myeloma cells produce IL-6 and express receptors for IL-6 (7). In addition, antibodies to IL-6 inhibit the in vitro growth of myeloma cells (8). Interference with this autocrine pathway may be a therapeutic strategy in the future. In addition to IL-6 receptors, receptors for IL-5, α-interferon, vitamin D3, estrogen, progesterone, and glucocorticoids have also been demonstrated.

The interval from the neoplastic transformation of a single precursor cell to the overt manifestation of multiple myeloma has been difficult to determine but it appears to be several years. The doubling time of overt multiple myeloma based on doubling of M protein is roughly 6 months (9, 10). But doubling times invariably lengthen as tumor mass increases. The mass of plasma cells achieved before the disease is clinically detectable is approximately 1×10^{10} cells. It would take roughly 40 cell divisions or doublings. The malignant cell then would mature into a plasma cell and secrete M protein (fig. 20.1).

Initial estimates of the natural history of multiple myeloma from transformation of the precursor cell until clinically evident disease (1×10^{10}) projected a preclinical phase of 20–30 years. Based on the finding that myeloma cell growth is Gompertzian (logarithmic), newer estimates of the preclinical phase are 2–3 years. Once malignant transformation takes place, the plasma cell takes on neoplastic properties. It typically infiltrates organs such as the bone marrow, kidney, and bone, making this disease widespread or multifocal, and hence the terms "multiple myeloma" or "multiple bone marrow tumors." In a small proportion of patients, the plasma cell proliferation is focal and does not become diffuse: a solitary plasmacytoma. These tumors may also be associated with an M protein, and in the majority of patients, although adequately treated initially, overt multiple myeloma will eventually develop (11).

The clinical manifestations of multiple myeloma are related to the malignant behavior of the plasma cells as well as to the abnormalities produced by the monoclonal immunoglobulin.

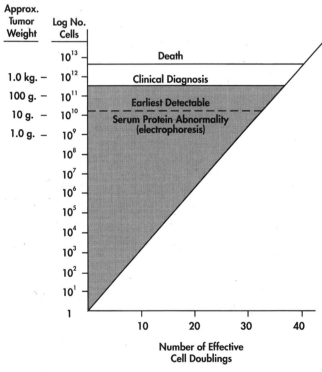

Figure 20.1. Relation of tumor weight and myeloma cell number to the number of effective cell doublings. Note that "effective cell doubling" is an idealized term, better expressed as tumor "doubling time," meaning in the number of times the tumor mass doubles. Tumor doubling time is not constant, as implied in this figure, but varies directly as a function of proliferative rate and indirectly in proportion to cell death rate. From Salmon SE. Immunoglobulin synthesis and tumor kinetics of multiple myeloma. Semin Hematol 1973; 10:135.

Plasma cell collections or tumors are called **plasmacytomas** and are found predominantly in the bone. Occasionally, extramedullary sites such as the upper respiratory tract, lung, testes, gut, and thyroid are involved (12). Involvement of the flat bones of the axial skeleton is most frequent. Bone involvement causes pain and often results in compression fractures of the vertebrae and pathologic **fractures** of the ribs and other long bones. Bone pain may be the first manifestation of multiple myeloma and is seen in over 70% of patients at presentation. The lesions in the bones are usually discrete and are seen as "punched-out" osteolytic lesions. This appearance is due to the secretion of **osteoclast activating factors** (OAF) by plasma cells, which stimulate osteoclasts around the plasmacytoma to resorb adjacent bone. Recently, OAFs have been identified as tumor necrosis factor (TNF) β- and interleukin 1-β (IL-1 B) (13). In some patients a diffuse osteoporosis is evident on radiography, but closer examination with microradiography or computerized tomographic (CT) scans detect trabecular destruction (14). The bone lesions of multiple myeloma are best viewed with plain X-rays or CT scans. Radionuclide scans are not reliable in the absence of osteoblastic activity. However, 2% of myelomas may be associated with osteosclerotic lesions. The most critical complication of bone involvement is the development of extradural **spinal cord compression** by plasmacytomas. This situation is a medical emergency requiring prompt diagnosis by myelography or magnetic resonance imaging (MRI), and treatment with steroids and radiation. Another sequela of bony involvement by multiple myeloma is hypercalcemia. **Hypercalcemia** is present in >30% of patients and is in large part mediated by OAFs which cause resorption of bone. In addition, renal dysfunction, hypoalbuminemia, and immobility contribute to the hypercalcemia. Some M proteins may bind calcium and protect against the effects of hypercalcemia (15).

More than 60% of patients present with **anemia** at diagnosis, and other cytopenias are also common. This myelophthisic appearance picture is often due to replacement of marrow by plasma cells, but can be associated with minimal marrow involvement. The presence of inappropriately low erythropoietin (Epo) levels and an appropriate response to Epo therapy raises the possibility that other factors are involved in the pathogenesis of the anemia (16). Later in the course of the disease, **cytopenias** are invariable and are usually related to progressive disease and therapy. A typical appearance of myelodysplasia can be seen after long-term alkylator therapy, which progresses to acute leukemia (usually myelomonocytic leukemia) in 2–6% of patients. Whether the leukemia is entirely due to therapy or part of the evolution of the disease from a pluripotent stem cell is not known. Reports of leukemia in untreated patients with multiple myeloma suggest that both hypotheses may contribute to leukemogenesis (17).

Rarely, patients present with numerous plasma cells (2×10^9/L) in the peripheral blood, i.e., **plasma cell leukemia**. These patients usually have IgE myeloma, but it can be a terminal event in other patients. The prognosis of plasma cell leukemia is poor either as the initial presentation or later in the course of the disease. The median survival of a patient with plasma cell leukemia is only 6–8 months (18).

The presence of a monoclonal M protein is seen in 99% of multiple myelomas, either in the serum or urine (19); 1% of cases are nonsecretory. The most common M protein is IgG (>60%), followed by IgA (20–25%), light chain only (10–15%), IgD (<1%), and IgE (very rare) (20). κ-Light chains are seen in >60% of cases. In 1–2% of cases, two monoclonal ("biclonal") M proteins are detected (21). Due to an inherent imbalance in immunoglobulin synthesis, there is usually an excess of light chains, which are filtered and catabolized in the kidney and detectable in urine.

The immunoglobulin profile at presentation shows markedly low levels of the other immunoglobulins in >90% of patients (22). In the murine model of myeloma, a secretion of plasmacytoma-induced macrophage substance (PIMS) appears to be responsible for this finding. PIMS suppresses B-cell function and therefore production of normal polyclonal immunoglobulins (23). An immunoglobulin-binding factor produced by T-cells has also been implicated in the pathogenesis of the decreased antibody production (24). The presence of decreased levels of normal immunoglobulins is only one of the reasons that patients with multiple myeloma have increased susceptibility to **infection**. Infection is one of the leading causes of death in patients with multiple myeloma. Infections with encapsulated Gram-positive and Gram-negative organisms, such as pneumococci and *Haemophilus influenzae* are common (25). Recently the spectrum of infections in these patients has changed to include more infections with Gram-negative bacilli. Neutrophil function has also been found to be defective in patients with multiple myeloma and may be related to abnormal chemotaxis and migration (26, 27). Cell-mediated immunity in multiple myeloma is usually normal.

The ability of certain subtypes of IgG (IgG3) and IgA to aggregate or polymerize gives rise to the syndrome of **hyperviscosity**. It is a relatively common occurrence in **Waldenstrom macroglobulinemia,** where the large, predominantly intravascular, monoclonal IgM molecules cause expansion of the intravascular compartment (28). In multiple myeloma, the smaller IgG proteins are found in the intravascular and extravascular spaces, and must therefore be present in extremely high levels to cause hyperviscosity. However, aggregates of IgG3 and IgA remain in the intravascular space and often lead to hyperviscosity. The viscosity of serum is usually compared with that of water. Normal serum viscosity is 1–1.8 (1.8 times more viscous than water). Symptoms of hyperviscosity rarely develop with a serum viscosity of <4. However, serum viscosity may underestimate whole blood viscosity because red cell mass contributes significantly to the latter (29). Measurement of whole blood viscosity at different levels of shear stress is the optimal method of determining whole blood viscosity; however, this test is not widely available, and needs to be standardized (30).

Besides the direct effects of hyperglobulinemia, the organ most commonly affected by myeloma is the kidney (50%). Myeloma affects the kidney in many ways: light chain toxicity, hypercalcemia, hyperuricemia, and amyloid deposition can all cause renal damage. The two main sites of damage in the kidney are the tubule and the glomerulus. The light chains in the plasma are filtered through the kidney and reabsorbed and catabolized in the tubules. Why some light chains and not others are nephrotoxic has not been elucidated, but more damage is associated with the λ-light chains. Certain physicochemical properties of the light chains such as their isoelectric points have been incriminated. Damage to tubular cells leads to the formation of protein casts. As many as 75% of patients have obstructive tubular casts with associated interstitial inflammation, leading to fibrosis and renal failure ("myeloma kidney") (31). Deposition of light chains in the tubular and interstitial space is common.

Acute **renal failure** in the setting of a monoclonal gammopathy strongly suggests the diagnosis of multiple myeloma. The etiology of the renal failure is multifactorial: dehydration, infection, hypercalcemia, and use of iodinated contrast material may all contribute. In >50% of cases, the renal failure is reversible, particularly when tubular cast formation is not extensive (32, 33). Glomerular lesions are due to deposition of κ-chains and develop gradually over the course of the disease.

The most damaging long-term effect of some paraproteins is the deposition of **amyloid**. Amyloid deposition is most often found in the kidney, heart, liver, spleen, skin, muscle, tongue, and gastrointestinal (GI) tract. Amyloid, associated with a paraprotein, is made up of free light chains. λ-Light chains are most likely to be involved (34). When the secretory mechanisms in the plasma cell are exceeded, the excess light chains collect within plasma cells as fibrillar inclusions ultrastructurally identical with amyloid. These are then released and further processed by macrophages to produce an amorphous material that stains with Congo red and exhibits apple green birefringence when viewed under the polarizing microscope (35). The ultrastructure of amyloid in multiple myeloma reveals a twisted β-pleated sheet configuration typical of all types of amyloid (36). Amyloid is insoluble, resistant to proteolysis, and often causes irreversible damage to vital organs, leading to death (37). The median survival of patients with multiple myeloma presenting with amyloidosis is 6–8 months.

Coagulation disturbances can be due to nonspecific interactions between the M protein and clotting factors and/or platelets. Diffuse mucocutaneous bleeding occurs commonly with hyperviscosity. The most common laboratory finding pertaining to coagulation in patients with multiple myeloma is a prolonged bleeding time due to coating of platelet surface receptors and a prolonged thrombin time (TT) due to interference with fibrin polymerization (38). Despite these abnormalities, clinically obvious bleeding is uncommon. In a few cases, the M protein has a specificity for von Willebrand factor or factor VIII, and causes an overt **bleeding diatheses** (39, 40).

Some of the M proteins are cold-insoluble and are termed "cryoglobulins." The presence of cryoglobulins gives rise to **Raynaud syndrome,** digital ischemia, and even gangrene (41).

Certain neurologic findings in multiple myeloma are caused neither by the M protein nor by the plasma cell. A typical "glove and stocking" distribution sensorimotor polyneuropathy may predate the onset of multiple myeloma by several years. A paraneoplastic multifocal leukoencephalopathy has also been described (42).

In certain patients a characteristic syndrome with the acronym **POEMS** has been described. This syndrome consists of the combination of **p**olyneuropathy, **o**rganomegaly, **e**ndocrinopathy (hypothyroidism, hypogonadism, and diabetes), an **M** protein, and **s**kin changes (hyperpigmentation) (43). These patients are more prone to solitary plasmacytomas and osteosclerotic bone lesions and these myelomas invariably produce λ-light chains. These findings usually disappear with treatment. Patients with the POEMS syndrome may not meet the criteria for the diagnosis of multiple myeloma.

Activities

*Based on the findings of hyperglobulinemia, anemia, azotemia, and bone pains, a serum and urine protein electrophoresis and bone marrow examination were ordered for the above-described patient. X-rays of her lumbosacral spine were also taken. The serum protein electrophoresis (SPEP) revealed a 6.9 g/dl monoclonal immunoglobulin, which was later characterized as IgG λ. Lumbar spine x-rays showed many lytic lesions in the vertebral bodies. The bone marrow aspiration and biopsy revealed 20% plasma cells. The combination of a monoclonal protein, along with evidence of abnormal plasma cell accumulation in the bone marrow and bones (lytic lesions), establishes the **diagnosis of multiple myeloma**.*

Due to the patchy nature of bone marrow involvement, more than one bone marrow aspiration may be required for diagnosis. More than 10% plasma cells in the aspirate is considered suggestive of multiple myeloma. In the event of negative bone marrow examination results, biopsy of a lytic lesion may confirm the diagnosis. The diagnosis is more difficult to make in nonsecretory myeloma because an M protein is not detectable. In the case discussed here, with a large amount of M protein, 20% marrow plasmacytosis and multiple lytic bone lesions, the diagnosis is straightforward.

Table 20.1 lists the major and minor criteria for the diagnosis of multiple myeloma and the various combinations required to fulfill the criteria for diagnosis (44).

The laboratory diagnosis of multiple myeloma involves the demonstration of the monoclonal immunoglobulin, which is seen as a sharp spike in the γ-globulin region on a densitometer tracing of the serum protein electrophoresis (see fig. 20.2). A serum M spike is found on serum protein electrophoresis in >85% of cases of multiple my-

Table 20.1. Diagnostic Criteria for Multiple Myeloma°

Major criteria
   I.   Plasmacytoma on tissue biopsy
   II. Bone marrow plasma cells >30%
   III. Monoclonal M spike on SPEP, IgG >3.5 g/dl, IgA >2g/dl, >1 g/dl light chains in 24 hr urine sample (without amyloid)
Minor criteria
   a. Bone marrow plasma cells 10–30%
   b. M spike but less than above
   c. Lytic bone lesions
   d. Normal IgM <50 mg, IgA <100 mg, IgG <600 mg/dl
To confirm diagnosis in symptomatic patients with progressive disease requires: 1 major + 1 minor or 3 minor criteria including a + b.
   1. I + b, I + c, I + d
   2. II + b, II + c, II + d
   3. III + a, III + c, III + d
   4. a + b + c, a + b + d

°Adapted from reference 44.

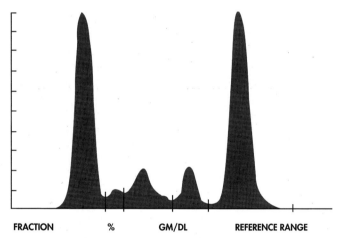

FRACTION	%	GM/DL	REFERENCE RANGE

Figure 20.2. Serum protein electrophoresis.

eloma. The remainder show hypoglobulinemia (light chain disease), a broad band, or normal serum protein electrophoresis. Light chain disease is detected by urine electrophoresis. The lower limit of detection of an M protein by serum protein electrophoresis is about 500 mg/dl (45). In addition, isolated heavy chains and aggregated IgA and IgG3 molecules are often seen as a broad band on serum protein electrophoresis migrating from the β- through the γ-region. Errors in interpretation of spikes in the α2- and β-regions may arise due to the formation of complexes between haptoglobin-hemoglobin in hemolytic anemias and large amounts of fibrinogen and transferrin. Confirmation of monoclonality is done by immunofixation or immunoelectrophoresis. Immunofixation and immunoelectrophoresis are much more sensitive than serum protein electrophoresis in identifying monoclonal heavy chains, small amounts of light chain, and aggregated molecules. Because of the rarity of IgD and IgE myelomas, immunoelectrophoresis is not routinely used to test for these myelomas. Bowing of the κ- or λ-arc on immunoelectrophoresis with negative results for IgG, IgA, and IgM should prompt screening for IgE and IgD. Sometimes the use of monospecific antibodies to heavy chains is needed to diagnose heavy chain disease. The urine should be tested for light chain excretion, which is common in multiple myeloma due to an imbalance with excess light chains. The presence of light chains excludes heavy chain disease. During therapy, the level of M protein must be followed in order to determine the efficacy of the treatment. Levels of M protein correlate well with response and dissociation between M protein levels, and disease progression is rare (22).

Performance of bone marrow aspiration and biopsy is a critical part of the diagnostic evaluation of multiple myeloma. Sternal aspiration is discouraged because of reports of fracture of the sternum during bone marrow aspiration (46). A level of 10% marrow plasmacytosis is suggestive of multiple myeloma. The specificity of this figure, however, is not high and therefore in the absence of an M protein other tissue evidence of plasma cell proliferation is required to confirm multiple myeloma. A level of >20% marrow plasmacytosis is very specific for multiple myeloma, especially if monoclonality can be proven. Immunohistochemical techniques to detect monoclonality are being widely used (47). Flow cytometric evaluation of bone marrow can also be done, although because these data are preliminary, they cannot currently be used in the diagnosis or prognosis of multiple myeloma. The erythrocyte sedimentation rate (ESR) is also often elevated due to the excess globulin. The serum β-2 microglobulin level is often elevated in multiple myeloma, and correlates with prognosis. Serum viscosity should be assayed only if indicated. Ancillary findings such as a narrow anion gap and pseudohyponatremia are related to the large amount of positively charged M protein.

Followup laboratory data while the patient is receiving therapy should include serum protein electrophoresis or 24-hour urine light chain quantitation and β-2 microglobulins done at 3–4 month intervals. While β-2 microglobulin levels are not routinely used to monitor response, rising levels may indicate relapse. β-2 Microglobulin levels are especially helpful in assessing response to therapy in patients with nonsecretory and light chain myelomas. Complete blood counts (CBCs) and blood chemistries should be monitored closely while the patient is receiving treatment. Chest x-rays and skeletal surveys should also be done.

Not all monoclonal proteins have pathologic significance. Certain clinical situations are associated with a transient finding of an M protein (e.g., recovery from infection or drug hypersensitivity) (48, 49). In a significant proportion of elderly individuals, a monoclonal immunoglobulin is often seen with no evidence of focal or diffuse malignant plasma cell activity. As many as 3% of people over the age of 70 and 15% over age 90 have an M protein of unknown significance (50). In the absence of malignant plasma cell behavior the term **"monoclonal**

gammopathy of undetermined significance" MGUS) is used. MGUS is diagnosed in as many as 67% of all patients with an M protein, and may be seen in association with cancers, leukemia, connective tissue disorders, and chronic inflammatory states (table 20.2). MGUS must be distinguished from smoldering and early stage multiple myeloma. This distinction is often difficult. The most compelling evidence for multiple myeloma is an increasing M protein on serial followup (table 20.3) (51). Some investigators have postulated that in MGUS there is a negative

Table 20.2. Disorders Associated with M Proteins°

Plasma cell proliferation	Multiple myeloma
	Solitary plasmacytoma
	Waldenstrom's macroglobulinemia
	Heavy chain disease
M protein induced	Primary amyloidosis
	Light chain deposition disease
	POEMS
	Papular mucinosis
	Systemic capillary leak syndrome
	Adult Fanconi syndrome
	Chronic cold agglutinin disease
Undetermined significance	MGUS
Chronic inflammation	Osteomyelitis, rheumatoid arthritis, TB, pyelonephritis, pyoderma
Immune dysregulation	Kaposi sarcoma, AIDS, old age
Malignancy	Bowel, breast cancer, leukemia
Lipodystrophies	Gaucher, xanthomatosis, familial hypercholesterolemia
Transient M protein	Viral infections, atypical pneumonias
	Post–valve replacement
	Associated with drug hypersensitivity (phenytoin, sulfa, penicillin)

°MGUS, monoclonal gammopathy of undetermined significance; TB, tuberculosis.

Table 20.3. Differences between MGUS and Myeloma Subsets°

	MGUS	SMM	MM
M protein	Yes	Yes	Yes
Level of M protein			
IgG <3.5 g, IgA <2 g, LC <1 g/day	90%	10%	10%
Stable M protein	Yes	No	No
Marrow plasmacytosis	<5%	10–20%	>10%
Anemia	No	No	Yes
Calcium	nl	nl	nl/high
Creatinine	nl	nl	nl/high
Labeling index	<1%	<1%	>1%
Normal immunoglobulins	nl	Low	Low

°MGUS, monoclonal gammopathy of undetermined significance; SMM, smoldering myeloma; MM, multiple myeloma, LC; light chains; nl, normal.

feedback system that controls the plasma cell proliferation. Removal of this inhibition leads to progression to multiple myeloma. The fact that there are reports of multiple monoclonal plasmacytomas arising in liver transplant patients who are taking the immunosuppressive agent cyclosporine as well as in patients with AIDS (suppressed T cell function) suggests that T cells may play a role in the control of plasma cell proliferation (52–54). Followup of a large cohort of patients with MGUS showed that in 10% of them multiple myeloma or a related disorder (amyloidosis, Waldenstrom macroglobulinemia) will develop (55). For this reason, M protein levels should be observed periodically in patients with MGUS.

Many different disorders are associated with a monoclonal protein and they are included in the differential diagnosis of multiple myeloma and MGUS. Chronic cold agglutinin disease is initially seen with intravascular hemolysis due to a monoclonal IgM cold agglutinin (56). Nearly 7% of low-grade lymphomas are associated with an M protein (usually IgM) (57). Waldenstrom macroglobulinemia is a plasmalymphocytic malignancy that has a clinical course similar to that of chronic lymphocytic leukemia (CLL) or an indolent lymphoma. It is associated with the production of an IgM M protein that causes symptoms of hyperviscosity in 70% of patients, variable lymph node enlargement, and hepatosplenomegaly (58). Unlike the case in multiple myeloma, however, no lytic bone lesions are seen. The presence of lytic bone lesions in addition to an monoclonal IgM is diagnostic of the very rare occurrence of an IgM myeloma.

Malignancies of the lung, breast, and colon may be associated with an M protein (59). Lytic bone lesions and 5–10% plasmacytosis suggestive of multiple myeloma may be present with metastatic cancer. In some situations, biopsy of a lytic lesion may be necessary to distinguish multiple myeloma from metastatic cancer. Primary amyloidosis may be initially seen with lytic lesions, making the distinction from multiple myeloma difficult (60). Biopsy of the lytic lesions, however, reveals amyloid and no plasma cell infiltrate. The association of an M protein and AIDS has also been reported. The incidence of an M protein in HIV-positive patients ranges from 2.5–4.6%, which is significantly higher than in age-matched controls (61). Light chain deposition disease is a rare condition characterized by the finding of predominantly κ-light chains in renal glomeruli. It may be confused with multiple myeloma. The monoclonal light chains in renal biopsies of patients with renal failure and proteinuria are not associated with evidence of plasma cell excess or with a serum or urine M spike. Bone marrow plasmacytosis and lytic lesions are absent, although anemia secondary to renal failure is common (62).

The finding of isolated heavy chains (α, γ, or μ) in the serum is suggestive of **heavy-chain disease.** Of these, α-heavy chain disease is the most common. It is usually seen in young people of Mediterranean descent. The clinical picture is dominated by fever, weight loss, and malabsorption (63). The α-heavy chain is detected in serum by serum protein electrophoresis in 50% of cases as a broad band. The M protein can be detected in the urine, saliva, and intestinal juice in many patients. In some instances, immunoperoxidase methods may have to be used to demonstrate the heavy chains in tissue sections (64). The two organs affected are the small bowel and the lung. α-Heavy chain disease may present with a mature plasma cell infiltrate, an atypical plasma cell infiltrate, or frank lymphoma. Most patients are treated with tetracycline but failure to respond to this requires institution of chemotherapy. γ-Heavy chain disease is a heterogeneous collection of disorders. Lymphadenopathy and hepatosplenomegaly are seen in 60% of patients. Interestingly, >30% of these patients have associated autoimmune diseases such as hemolytic anemia, Sjogren syndrome, lupus, or rheumatoid arthritis (64, 65). Some reports of γ-heavy chain disease are suggestive of MGUS, while others are associated with a transient γ-heavy chain associated with autoimmune illnesses. Some cases are typical of lymphomas, while others behave like multiple myeloma. Hypo-γ-globulinemia and bone marrow involvement are seen in 50–60% of patients. The age range varies from <20–>60 years of age. The course varies from benign to rapidly fatal. Treatment is based on the underlying condition. If definite evidence of malignancy is present chemotherapy is indicated. μ-Heavy chain disease is rare and usually associated with a CLL-like appearance.

Once the diagnosis of multiple myeloma is established, the tumor mass or stage must be determined. In 1975, Salmon and Durie established a staging system based on direct measurements of total myeloma mass (66). This system relies on the level of M protein, anemia, renal function, serum calcium, and the bony involvement detected on skeletal survey. The validity of this staging system with regard to prognosis has been established in prospective studies (67, 68). β-2 Microglobulin, which is the light chain of the human lymphocyte antigen (HLA) complex, has been found to be elevated in multiple myeloma (69). **β-2 Microglobulin** has proven to be an important prognostic variable in multiple myeloma and has been incorporated into a separate staging system (70). β-2 Microglobulin of >6 in the patient described above portends a poor prognosis. Accurate staging is especially important in younger patients as newer therapies such as bone marrow transplantation are available. It is important to distinguish between stage I multiple myeloma and "monoclonal gammopathy of undetermined significance," because the latter is much less likely to progress. "Smoldering myeloma" is a subset of stage I multiple myeloma characterized by a low labeling index (<1%) and an indolent course (table 20.3) (71). Anemia, hypercalcemia, renal failure, and a high IgG level put patients into the high tumor mass category (table 20.4).

Many prognostic factors have been studied in multiple myeloma (table 20.5). Some of these have the disadvan-

Table 20.4. Staging of Multiple Myeloma*

Low tumor mass (good 5 yr survival untreated, $<0.6 \times 10^{12}$
  plasma cells /m²) and all the following:
  Hemoglobin >100 g/l
  Serum calcium <12 mg/dl
  Serum IgG <5/dl, IgA <3 g/dl, ULC <4 g/d
  One or no lytic bone lesions
Intermediate tumor mass (may be indolent or progress rapidly,
  $0.6–1.2 \times 10^{12}$ plasma cells/m²) and all the following:
  Hemoglobin 8.5–100 g/L
  Serum calcium <12 mg/dl
  Serum IgG 5–7 g/dl, IgA 3–5 g/dl, ULC 4–12 g/d
  0–2 lytic bone lesions
High tumor mass (require therapy, $>1.2 \times 10^{12}$ plasma
  cells/m²) and any **ONE** of the following:
  Hemoglobin <8.5 g/L
  Serum calcium >12 mg/dl
  Serum IgG >7 g/dl, IgA >5 g/dl, ULC >12 g/d
  ≥3 lytic bone lesions
Subclassificaion
  A = Creatinine <2.0 mg/dl
  B = Creatinine >2.0 mg/dl

ULC, urinary light chains.
*Adapted from reference 66.

Table 20.5. Prognostic Variables in Multiple Myeloma*

Pretreatment variable	TM related	Resp	Surv	TTR
High tumor mass	Yes	Dec	Dec	Dec
High β-2 microglobulin	Yes	Dec	Dec	Dec
Low RNA index	No	Dec	?Dec	Dec
Low labeling index	No	ND	Inc	ND
DNA hypodiploidy	No	Dec	?Dec	ND
MDR expression	No	?Dec	ND	ND
High LDH	No	ND	Dec	Dec

*TM, tumor mass; Resp, response; Surv, survival; TTR, time to relapse; Dec, decrease; Inc, increase; ?Dec, suggested but not proven decrease; ND, no data.

tage of being subjective (Karnofsky performance, plasma cell morphology) (72, 73), some are subject to sampling error (marrow plasma cell percentage) (74), and some are technically difficult, not universally available, and therefore impractical for widespread use (labeling index, RNA index, ploidy) (75–77). The serum β-2 microglobulin and albumin levels are probably the most widely used and reliable prognosticators of survival (fig. 20.3) (70).

Because the reason for the heart failure in our patient was unclear, an electrocardiogram (ECG), echocardiogram, and serum viscosity were ordered. The ECG showed low voltage despite a large heart on chest x-ray. The echocardiogram excluded a pericardial effusion and revealed restricted wall motion of both ventricles. The relative serum viscosity was 11. Subtyping of the IgG showed it to be IgG3. The macroglossia was suggestive of amyloidosis. The large heart with low voltage on ECG and a restrictive defect by echocardiography was consistent with cardiac amyloidosis (78). The combination of cardiac amyloidosis and hyperviscosity was considered to be causing congestive heart failure.

The clinical features of hyperviscosity may be difficult to recognize and require a high index of suspicion to diagnose. Headaches, visual blurring, tinnitus, lethargy, heart failure, and confusion progressing to seizures and frank coma can be seen (79). Like cord compression, hyperviscosity is a medical emergency and treated with plasma exchange. Plasma exchange leads to rapid but temporary improvement until production of the abnormal protein can be halted by chemotherapy (80).

The patient improved dramatically after plasma exchange, although she remained anemic. Because red cells are important contributors to whole blood viscosity, the anemia was not treated with transfusions until removal of the M protein was accomplished.

Therapy with oral melphalan and prednisone was initiated, and the patient improved with a gradual decrease in her M protein to 3.1 g/dl. Six months later the M protein was increasing and salvage chemotherapy with high-dose dexamethasone was begun. A doxorubicin-based regimen was not given because of poor cardiac function. After 4 months of therapy, the patient experienced progressive heart failure and died from a complicating pneumonia.

The treatment of multiple myeloma has been disappointing. No therapy is indicated for stage I disease (71). All patients with stage III disease need treatment, as do most patients with stage II multiple myeloma. Despite response rates of 50%, very few cures or even complete responses are achieved with standard chemotherapy. The definition of response also varies from center to center and trial to trial. A 50% decrease in serum M protein or 90% decrease in urinary light chains, with resolution of hypercalcemia, anemia, and renal failure, is classified as complete response (81). Long-term survival after standard alkylator agent therapy has been reported anecdotally (82, 83). Newer therapies with myeloablative doses of melphalan with autologous marrow or peripheral stem cell support may result in "true CR" (disappearance of M protein by protein electrophoresis, <5% marrow plasma cells, and normalization of immune status) (84). Despite treatment, survival of patients with multiple myeloma is poor, and to date no cure exists for multiple myeloma unless allogeneic marrow transplant is done. Allogeneic marrow transplantation results in long-term survival in about 30% of patients (85). Unfortunately, allogeneic marrow transplantation is best suited for in patients <50 years of age with an HLA-identical sibling. About 5% of patients fall into this category (86). In addition, there is a 30% mortality associated with this form of therapy (87). Allogeneic marrow transplantation remains investigational and should be restricted to special centers. For the remaining patients, the choice of therapy is limited. Oral melphalan and prednisone are effective and well tolerated (provided myelosuppressive doses are used). Response rates of 50–60% have been reported. The response is gradual and reaches a plateau. The use of intravenous melphalan has been considered because of erratic oral absorption. The presence of an

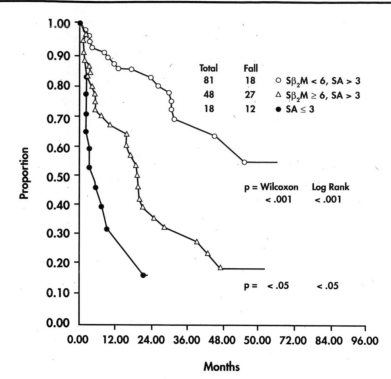

Figure 20.3. The Kaplan-Meier survival curves for patient with (1) a low Sβ₂M (<6 µg/ml) and a high serum albumin level (>3.0 g/dl), (2) a high Sβ₂M (≥6 µgt/ml) and a high serum albumin level (>3.0 g/dl), and (3) a low serum albumin level (<3 g/dl) are displayed. The differences between the curves are highly significant: 1 v 2, P < .001; 2 v 3, P < .05. The serum albumin values are missing for the 2 patients.

L-phenylalanine moiety in melphalan suggests that normal amino acid transport mechanisms are involved in absorption; this is hindered by the presence of food. Additionally, melphalan undergoes spontaneous hydrolysis at physiologic pH, which influences bioavailability. However, a randomized study comparing the use of oral to intravenous melphalan showed equal efficacy (88). The use of more intensive chemotherapy at the outset, such as vincristine, doxorubicin, dexamethasone, and the M2 protocol, has resulted in response rates similar to that of melphalan/prednisone (although time to response is shorter) but no difference in overall survival. Numerous randomized studies comparing melphalan/prednisone to other regimens have been reported and none show clear benefit over melphalan/prednisone (89–106). Meta-analysis of these studies shows a similar 2-year survival in patients treated with either melphalan/prednisone or combination chemotherapy (107). Some investigators have suggested that combination chemotherapy may be superior to melphalan/prednisone in patients with poor prognostic features. More recently, studies incorporating interferon with either melphalan/ prednisone or multiagent chemotherapy have reported high-response rates and prolongation in remission duration (108, 109). This strategy needs to be verified in randomized trials. The addition of an intravenous bisphosphonate (pamidronate) to standard therapy has shown significantly fewer skeletal events, less bone pain, and better quality of life in patients receiving pamidronate than standard therapy alone (109a).

Once maximal response has been obtained and remains stable, the benefits of continuing alkylator therapy are out-

weighed by the disadvantages, i.e., leukemogenesis (92). Randomized trials of maintenance therapy with melphalan/prednisone have not demonstrated prolongation of survival, although remission duration is prolonged (110). For this reason, chemotherapy is generally discontinued after a stable response is achieved, usually in 12 months. Mandelli et al. showed that in a randomized study, α-interferon significantly prolonged survival in patients who responded to treatment or had stable disease (111). A randomized trial by the Southwest Oncology Group, however, failed to confirm this (112). At the time of relapse (rising M protein) melphalan/prednisone may be reinstituted with a 50% chance of response, although the duration of this response is shorter than the first. However, if the relapse is within 6 months or no response is seen, the VAD (vincristine, doxorubicin, dexamethasone) regimen is most likely to be effective (40–50% response in melphalan/prednisone resistance) (113). This regimen has moderate toxicity and has 5–6% mortality, especially in older patients. Table 20.6 lists a number of different chemotherapy options.

Primary resistance to therapy, which occurs in 40% of patients, is defined as the failure to achieve >75% decrease in tumor synthetic rate, regression by >50% in serum M protein, and/or regression by >90% in light chain excretion despite myelosuppressive doses of melphalan/prednisone or other multiagent regimens. Secondary resistance is the failure to respond to myelosuppressive doses of a reinduction regimen after relapse from a previous remission. Therapy of primary resistance is difficult, although about 25% of patients will respond to high-dose steroids as a single agent (114, 115). The duration of primary resistance (stable disease) is of prognostic value, >12 months being worse possibly due to emergence of drug resistance (116). Secondary resistance usually responds fairly rapidly to the VAD regimen (40–50%), probably due to the higher number of dividing cells present in this situation (117).

One of the primary mechanisms of drug resistance in multiple myeloma is mediated via p-glycoprotein. The p-glycoprotein is a 170-kd glycoprotein responsible for the rapid efflux of certain chemotherapeutic agents from the target cell (plasma cell) (118). The drugs involved in this mechanism of resistance include anthracyclines, etoposide, and the vinca alkaloids (hence the term "multidrug resistance"). Resistance to the VAD regimen containing vincristine and doxorubicin is mediated via p-glycoprotein. Treatment with VAD-type regimens selects drug-resistant tumor cells, leading to relapse. Certain drugs are known to reverse the multidrug resistance

(MDR) phenotype, including calcium channel blockers (Verapamil), quinidine, dipyridamole, phenothiazines, and cyclosporine A (119). Verapamil in large doses has been shown to reverse MDR in patients resistance to the VAD regimen (120). Some of these agents are currently in clinical trials in a prophylactic setting to test whether expression of p-glycoprotein can be prevented. Resistance to alkylating agents (not p-glycoprotein mediated) can be overcome by dose escalation. Melphalan in doses of >90 mg/m^2 and total body irradiation (TBI) result in response rates of 60–80%. Despite these response rates and projected median survival times of 40–50 months, cure is rare and means of consolidating or maintaining these remissions need to be found.

Salvage chemotherapy is indicated when no response is seen with high-dose steroids in primary resistant disease, to an doxorubicin-based regimen in secondary resistance, or rapid relapse occurs following melphalan/ prednisone

Table 20.6. Commonly Used Chemotherapeutic Regimen in Multiple Myeloma Induction Therapy°

Regimen	Drug	Dose	Route	Days
M + P	Melphalan	9 mg/m2	Oral	1–4
	Prednisone	100–200 mg	Oral	1–4
		Repeat every 4–6 wk°		
M 2 protocol	Vincristine	0.03 mg/kg	IV	1
	Melphalan	0.25 mg/kg	IV	1–7
	Cyclophosphamide	10 mg/kg	IV	1
	BCNU	0.5 mg/kg	IV	1
	Prednisone	1 mg/kg	Oral	1–7
VAD protocol	Vincristine	0.4 mg/m^2	CIV	1–4
	Adriamycin	9 mg/m^2	CIV	1–4
	Dexamethasone	40 mg	Oral	1–4
				9 12
				17–20
	Bactrim	DS, bid	Oral	1–28
	Alternate cycles	Dexamethasone		1–4 only

°Document myelosuppression and escalate dose if no myelosuppression. IV, intravenous; bid, twice daily; CIV, continuous intravenous infusion.

Table 20.7. Salvage Chemotherapy°

Regimen	Drug	Dose	Route	Days
High-dose steroid	Dexamethasone	40 mg	Oral	1–4
				9–12
				17–20
VAD				
HDM	Melphalan	70–140 mg/m^2	IV	1
EDAP	Etoposide	100–200 mg/m^2	CIV	1–4
	Dexamethasone	40 mg	IV	1–5
	Ara-C	1 g/m^2	IV	5
	Cis-platinum	25 mg/m^2	CIV	1–4
HDM-TBI	Melphalan	140 mg/m^2	IV	1
	BI	170 cGy q12 h × 5		2–4
	BMT		IV	4/5
Thiotepa-TBI	Thiotepa	250-300 mg/m^2 q12 h x 3	IV	1-2
	TBI	170 cGy q12 h × 5		4–6
	BMT		IV	6/7

°TBI, total body radiation; CIV, continuous intravenous infusion, BMT, bone marrow rescue.
Adapted from reference 116. (See table 20.6).

(see table 20.7 for salvage regimens for refractory multiple myeloma). Response to salvage therapy is generally poor and the disease terminates in an acute phase analogous to the "blast crisis" in chronic myeloid leukemia.

> An important posttreatment prognostic factor is the β-2 microglobulin level. A high β-2 microglobulin level at relapse predicts poor response and survival, as do high lactate dehydrogenase (LDH) levels and hypodiploidy (121, 122).

Case 2

A 33-year-old black man was seen in the office with complaints of gradually worsening back pain which started after lifting a heavy object at home. The patient was evaluated and treated with analgesics. Three weeks later, the pain was no better and an x-ray of the painful area was taken. The x-ray showed a lytic lesion in the body of the T8 vertebra with a compression fracture. The following laboratory data was obtained: hemoglobin 1369/L; hematocrit 40.2%; WBC count 46 × 10⁹/L; platelet 244 × 10⁹/L; blood chemistry levels were found unremarkable on routine screening; urinalysis results were also unremarkable.

A radionuclide bone scan showed increased uptake at T8, but was otherwise normal. The chest x-ray appeared normal. A skeletal survey and a CT scan of the spine were also unremarkable except for the lesion at T8. The patient was scheduled for a biopsy of the involved vertebra. At surgery, the vertebral body was found to be necrotic. Microscopic examination of a wedge biopsy revealed sheets of atypical plasma cells. Immunohistochemical staining confirmed the monoclonality of the plasma cells, with only κ-light chains being detected. Bilateral iliac crest bone marrow biopsies were done and revealed no increase in plasma cells. A serum protein immunoelectrophoresis showed a small amount of IgG κ-M protein. The β-2 microglobulin was 3.1 ng/ml. Based on the findings, we made a diagnosis of solitary plasmacytoma of bone. The patient received primary radiotherapy to the affected area with 5000 cGy. Two months later, he was asymptomatic and the M spike had disappeared. The patient was followed up with serum protein electrophoresis and physical examination, but was lost to followup after 3 years. Five years after his original presentation, he experienced pain in his left leg while playing racquet ball that continued to worsen. An x-ray of the left femur revealed two lytic lesions in the neck of the femur. A skeletal survey revealed "punched out" lesions in the seventh and eighth ribs and the right humerus. The serum protein electrophoresis showed 5.3 gm/dl of an IgG κ-M protein. The hemoglobin was 8.1 g/dl and creatinine level was 1.6 mg/dl. Serum calcium was 10.8, albumen 2.9 g/dl, and LDH levels were normal. A bone marrow examination revealed >30% plasma cells, many of which were immature. The β-2 microglobulin was 6.4 ng/ml. Marrow specimens were analyzed for ploidy and cytogenetics. The marrow

plasma cells showed hyperdiploidy, and no chromosomal aberrations were noted.

Commentary

As demonstrated by the cases described above, multiple myeloma has a wide spectrum of clinical presentations, depending on localization of the disease, the extent or stage of disease (tumor burden), and whether or not the paraprotein causes clinical problems such as hyperviscosity or amyloidosis. Localized or limited disease includes solitary plasmacytoma of bone, solitary extramedullary plasmacytoma, and early stage I multiple myeloma with >10% marrow plasma cells, a small amount of M protein, and no other abnormalities. More advanced disease includes Salmon-Durie stages II and III and, at the extreme end of the spectrum, plasma cell leukemia, which has a very poor prognosis. Solitary plasmacytoma of bone is seen in 2–10% of patients with plasma cell malignancies. The most common sites of involvement are the spine and the pelvis, followed by the long bones. The presence of an M protein has been described in many cases. Persistence of the M protein after treatment of the solitary plasmacytoma suggests that the disease is more diffuse. Multiple myeloma ultimately develops in >50% of patients with solitary plasmacytoma of bone (123). Patients with extramedullary plasmacytomas seem to have a more indolent course and a lower incidence of progression to multiple myeloma (12). Like solitary plasmacytoma of bone, extramedullary plasmacytoma is usually treated by excision or radiation therapy. Patients are then observed closely for signs of more diffuse disease (124, 125).

Only 2% of patients with multiple myeloma are <40 years and 10–15% <50 years of age at presentation (126). Patients with extramedullary plasmacytoma or solitary bone plasmacytoma, however, may be younger, and patients as young as 3 years of age with plasmacytomas of lung have been reported (127). Despite multiple bone lesions, young patients often do not demonstrate bone marrow plasmacytosis and usually have a relatively indolent clinical course (128). It is not known why so few patients <40 years of age are affected by plasma cell malignancies.

Of interest is the observation that multiple myeloma can be seen in families (129). Reports of siblings, parent-child, and even husband and wife cases of multiple myeloma raise the possibility of a viral/infectious etiology for multiple myeloma. The finding of an HLA haplotype associated with multiple myeloma suggests a genetic predisposition to multiple myeloma.

The prognostic implications of DNA ploidy and cytogenetic abnormalities in multiple myeloma are being studied (130). Aneuploidy is seen in 80% and diploidy in 20%. Of the aneuploid cells, 10% are hypodiploid and the remaining 70% hyperdiploid. Hypodiploidy seems to be associated with light chain multiple myeloma, relative resistance to therapy, and an unfavorable outcome (131, 132). Chromosomal abnormalities in multiple myeloma have been difficult to study because of the low growth fraction, which makes chromosome analysis technically difficult. Consistent cytogenetic abnormalities are uncommon in multiple myeloma. In some studies only 20–35% of newly diagnosed patients and 40–50% of treated patients show abnormalities (despite aneuploidy in 80%). Cytogenetic abnormalities are more common in IgA multiple myeloma and relapsed multiple myeloma. Trisomy 3, 5, 9, and 15, and monosomy 13 and 16 are the most common chromosomal abnormalities. Translocation t(8;14) is associated with IgA multiple myeloma, although no specific prognostic significance is attached (133).

Case 3

A 38-year-old man with solitary plasmacytoma of bone was treated appropriately with local radiotherapy and followup. After 5 years he presented with findings of stage III A multiple myeloma with a β-2 microglobulin of >6 ng/ml, serum albumin of <3 g/dl, and stage III disease; his median survival is probably <12 months.

Various options for therapy exist. They include; (a) standard melphalan/prednisone or high-dose steroids in nonresponders; (b) rapid cytoreduction with VAD or VIMCP followed by allogeneic marrow transplantation; (c) high-dose therapy with stem cell/marrow support as initial therapy. Option (a), while reasonable in an older patient, offers no hope for cure in this 38-year-old patient with poor prognostic features. Melphalan/prednisone is thought to be superior to combination chemotherapy in patients with good prognostic factors. Option (b) offers potentially curative therapy; however, allogeneic marrow transplantation requires an HLA-identical donor or a mismatch with its associated problems. Also, despite a projected 28% 7-year overall survival with allografting, early mortality in 30% of patients makes this therapy a high-risk procedure (134). Given the poor prognostic features of the patient in case 2, option (b) may be justified. Although the data are preliminary, there is a trend toward better survival if allogeneic marrow transplantation is done early in the course of the disease. This prompts the initial use of VAD chemotherapy, which is associated with shorter time to response (135). The improved cure rate in allogeneic compared with autologous marrow support is possibly due to an immunologic graft-versus-myeloma effect, although only 9 of 162 patients are in continued complete response >4 years after allotransplant (132).

Option (c) may be preferable in patients <65 years of age or patients without HLA-identical siblings who respond to induction therapy. Autologous marrow or stem cell support is another option because there are no donor constraints precluding allogeneic marrow transplantation (table 20.8). Projected long-term survivals of >75% after dose-intensive therapy with stem cell support have been reported in patients responding to induction therapy (136). Results in refractory patients are disappointing (137). Delaying autologous transplantation until disease is far advanced or performance status is poor increases the treatment-related mortality from 5–10% to 30% (138). Advanced age (>65 years) is a relative contraindication to high-dose therapy with autologous stem cell support because of increased mortality. A cooperative trial of high-

dose melphalan (60–140 mg/m²), without marrow rescue, in previously untreated patients resulted in poor response rates (10%) and high mortality (29%), especially in older patients (>65 years) (139). McElwain et al. treated newly diagnosed patients with multiple myeloma with a VAD-type regimen followed by dose-intensive melphalan with or without autologous marrow support. Mortality was 10–15% and high complete response rates (50%) were seen; however, relapses were seen fairly early and median relapse-free survival was only 24 months (140). Recently, early high-dose therapy followed by autologous bone marrow transplant has shown improved survival compared with standard treatment. A randomized prospective study showed 5 year probability of overall survival to be 52% for high-dose versus 12% for standard therapy (140a). This data, combined with a 5% mortality from high-dose therapy, makes option (c) attractive. Prognostic factors may be helpful in selecting patients for high-dose therapy, since high pretreatment β-2 microglobulin, poor performance status, and refractory relapse are all associated with a poor outcome (136).

Trials of dose-intensive therapy with marrow rescue have demonstrated that the outcome is independent of the percentage of plasma cells in the reinfused marrow (141). This finding may be explained by the fact that the malignant precursor cell and not the plasma cell needs to be eliminated from the marrow. Thus, purging of marrow to remove plasma cells before reinfusion may not be important, and more effective cytoreduction prior to marrow rescue may improve results (142). Based on the finding that the malignant B-cell population is not able to grow in long-term cultures of bone marrow (unlike normal progenitors), a normalized source of autologous marrow could be obtained by long-term culture of the patient's marrow (143). The value of noncytotoxic maintenance therapy, e.g., interferon, after a dose-intensive approach is uncertain.

The use of newer agents to treat plasma cell neoplasms is being investigated. Anti-IL-6 antibodies have been used to treat a patient with plasma cell leukemia resistant to chemotherapy with some success (144). Radioisotopes with avidity for bone, such as samarium edegate trisodium monophosphate, are being considered in conjunction with chemotherapy to effect greater cytoreduction (145).

Various supportive measures are used in the management of patients with multiple myeloma. Radiation therapy is effective in the treatment of localized bone pain, cord compression, and imminent fractures (146). Myeloma is very radiosensitive, but care must be taken to avoid overuse of radiation to preserve marrow reserve. Hemi-body radiation to treat refractory multiple myeloma has been studied, although no randomized trials have been done to establish its efficacy compared with high-dose chemotherapy. However, hemi-body radiation has been shown to be inferior to chemotherapy for remission consolidation.

The effective use of recombinant Epo to treat the anemia of multiple myeloma has raised questions as to the eti-

Table 20.8. Is There a Dose Response in the Treatment of Myeloma?*

Treatment Modality	Percentage of CR	No. of Patients	Survival	Mortality (%)	Reference No.
Auto BMT	47	130	Median duration of relapse-free survival for the patients in C.R.: 28 mo	<5	163
Allo BMT	44	162	Relapse-free survival for the patients in C.R.: 34% at 6 yr	46	132
HDM w/o Auto BMT	32	63	Median duration of response: 18 mo	14	164
High-dose chemoradiotherapy + Auto PSCT	20	63	Median overall survival: 59 mo Median EFS 43 mo	11	165
1. Induction therapy 2. First HDM + Auto BMT 3. Second HDM + Auto BMT	1. 14 2. 27 3. 47	202	3 yr EFS survival: 60%	7	166 136
HDM + TBI + Auto BMT	22	100	28% 5 yr EFS	2	140a
VMCP/VBAP	5	100	10% 5 yr EFS		140a
MP VMCP VMCP/VBAP VBAP VBAD	6	243	Overall median survival: 27 mo Median survival for patients in C.R.: 42 mo Median survival for patients in P.R.: 42 mo		167

*Used with permission from Djulbegoric B, Begawoic S. Decision making in Oncology: evidence based on recommendation for management of malignant disorders Churchill/Livingstone, 1996 (in press).

ology of the anemia. Serum Epo levels are inappropriately low in some patients and therapy with Epo has improved the anemia in these cases (16). The level of anemia does not correlate with the M protein level or marrow plasma cell percentage. Lowering of the M protein with therapy also does not correlate with improvement of the anemia. No adverse effect on the disease was noted with doses of Epo of 150–250 u/kg subcutaneously three times a week.

Therapy of hypercalcemia is accomplished by saline hydration along with loop diuretics after euvolemia is achieved. The use of steroids is well-established and effective in the treatment of hypercalcemia in multiple myeloma (147). Suppression of OAFs by glucocorticoids in cell lines has also been demonstrated and is a likely explanation for this effect. Once chemotherapy is begun, the hypercalcemia is usually easy to control. The use of oral biphosphonates is effective for both control of bone pain and calcium levels. Although randomized trials have not shown any survival benefit from these agents (90, 148), a recent randomized trial using an intravenous bisphosphonate (pamidronate), has shown improvement in skeletal symptoms and quality of life compared with standard therapy alone (109a).

Hyperuricemia, which is common at presentation, should be controlled with allopurinol before chemotherapy is started. Uric acid nephropathy contributes to the renal failure seen with high tumor loads or rapidly progressing disease, but acute tumor lysis from therapy is uncommon.

Renal failure can be treated with hemodialysis concurrently with chemotherapy. Plasma exchange is beneficial in the treatment of renal failure in the presence of hyperviscosity. In 50% of cases, the renal failure is reversible. The prognosis for patients with irreversible renal failure is poor (149).

No data exists on the use of prophylactic antibiotics for patients with multiple myeloma. Early trials of intravenous immunoglobulin showed no benefit as prophylaxis against infection. More recent trials have shown promise, although further trials are necessary to prove this (150). The use of pneumococcal vaccines in multiple myeloma is controversial. Although in the majority of patients antibodies to the pneumococcal vaccine do not develop, the vaccine is so innocuous that it is reasonable to offer to patients (151).

Case 4

A 62-year-old man with adult-onset diabetes was seen with complaints of weakness and burning in his legs of 6 months' duration. He had noticed some weight loss and easy fatigability but denied having fevers or night sweats. Physical examination revealed slight pallor, but was otherwise unremarkable except for a palpable liver edge. There was a slight decrease in vibratory sense and light touch in the feet, but deep tendon reflexes were intact and no atrophy of the muscles was noted. Laboratory data showed: hemoglobin 115 g/L; hematocrit 34%; WBC count 38 × 10⁹/L; platelet 180 × 10⁹/L; creatinine 1.7 mg/dl; albumin 3.1 g/dl; cholesterol 334 mg/dl; γ-glutamyl transpeptidase (GGTP) 85 units (<50 normal); urinalysis; 2+ protein, 2+ glucose.

Serum protein electrophoresis showed a broad-based hyperglobulinemia. Based on the above findings, we considered the diagnosis of diabetic peripheral neuropathy and nephropathy. The hepatic enlargement was thought to be due to fatty liver. A chest x-ray showed borderline cardiomegaly, but was otherwise normal. The patient was counseled on dietary modification and his insulin dose was increased. One year later, he returned with leg weakness, left arm pain, and increasing pedal edema. Physical examination revealed a waxy complexion, moderate pallor, and mild periorbital ecchymoses. No lymphadenopathy was detected and the heart and lungs were normal. Abdominal examination revealed an enlarged liver and spleen. Laboratory data showed progressive anemia with a hemoglobin of 95 g/L, creatinine level of 2.0 mg/dl, and serum albumin of 2.4 g/dl. Prothrombin time (PT) was 17.4 seconds (control 11.6 seconds), PTT was 45.8 seconds (control 29.1 seconds) and fibrinogen was 315 mg/dl. Urinalysis showed 3+ proteinuria, quantitated at 6.4 g/24 hours. On chest x-ray, cardiomegaly had worsened and bilateral pleural effusions were seen. A lytic lesion was seen in the distal left humerus. Serum protein electrophoresis again showed a broad band in the β-γ-region. Serum and urine protein immunoelectrophoresis revealed 2.2 g/dl of IgG λ-M protein in the serum and free λ-light chains in urine along with albuminuria. A rectal biopsy showed amyloidosis. Aspiration of the lesion in the humerus showed amyloid with no evidence of plasmacytoma. Bone marrow aspiration and biopsy showed 8% atypical plasma cells. Therapy was begun with melphalan/prednisone but no significant improvement was noted. The patient died 6 months later.

Commentary

Amyloidosis is characterized by the finding of an amorphous eosinophilic material in tissue specimens. It has a very specific twisted β-pleated sheet structure determined by x-ray crystallography and infrared spectroscopy. It was described in 1853 by Virchow, who believed the material was a polysaccharide and hence used the term "amyloid," or starch-like. Amyloidosis is not one entity, but rather a variety of diseases resulting in the deposition of β-pleated sheet fibrils made up of different proteins by different pathogenic mechanisms (table 20.9) (37). This unique structure has not been found in any other mammalian tissues besides human ones. In addition, its unique structure makes it resistant to proteolysis and degradation, leading to the relentless deposition of inert amyloid fibrils and to death from vital organ dysfunction. In addition to the β-pleated protein, amyloid contains a glycoprotein, designated the p-component, which gives the characteristic periodic acid-Schiff (PAS) reaction. Amyloid deposition is also thought to be part of the natural aging process and more recently has been implicated in the pathogenesis of Alzheimer disease.

The incidence of amyloidosis is difficult to determine. The diagnosis is often missed because the symptoms are nonspecific. Primary or type I amyloidosis is a type of plasma cell dyscrasia, which manifests with multiorgan involvement due to deposition of amyloid fibrils made up of monoclonal light chains. Type I amyloidosis can be associated with multiple myeloma or arise de novo. In de novo amyloidosis, diffuse plasma cell infiltration of bone marrow or organs is not found, although as many as 10–20% atypical plasma cells have been reported in marrow samples. Primary amyloidosis without myeloma is similar to a light chain MGUS or smoldering light chain multiple myeloma, except that instead of being catabolized and excreted, light chains have a tendency to form a specific twisted β-pleated sheet of fibrils that is laid down in certain organs. No specific property of the light chain is known to predispose to the formation of amyloid (152). Primary amyloidosis is composed of λ-light chain in >70% of cases, but in association with multiple myeloma, κ- and λ-chains are more equally implicated. Biochemical evaluation of primary amyloid has revealed heavy chains and intact immunoglobulins on occasion (153). Amyloid deposition is seen in 10% of all patients with multiple myeloma but is more frequent (25%) in patients with light chain multiple myeloma. The association of amyloidosis with multiple myeloma decreases the median survival to 6–8 months. Amyloidosis without myeloma has a median survival of 15 months (154).

Amyloid is a chemically heterogenous compound not always made up of light chains. Numerous other proteins or molecules have been implicated in secondary or reactive

Table 20.9. Classification of Amyloidosis*

Clinical Disorder	Constituent Protein
Systemic Amyloidosis	
Immunocytic dyscrasia	Immunoglobulin
Plasma cell myeloma	light chain (AL)
Waldenstrom macroglobulinemia	
Heavy-chain disease	
γ-globulinemia	
lymphoid/immune malignacies	
Reactive	
Acute/chronic infection (TB, osteomyelitis, leprosy)	Serum AA protein (AA)
Chronic inflammation (rheumatoid arthritis)	AA
Hodgkin disease	AA
Nonlymphoid malignancy (renal & bladder cancer)	?
Heredofamilial	
Neuropathic	
Portuguese (type I)	Prealbumin (AFp)
Indians (type II)	?
Iowa (type III)	?
Finland (type IV)	?
Non-nueropathic	
Familial Mediterranean fever	AA
Ostertag cardiomyopathy	?
Localized Amyloidosis	
Immunocyte derived	
Respiratory tract, bladder, bone marrow	AL
Solitary plasmacytoma	AL
Light-chain deposition disease	AL
Cardiac (senile cardiomyopathy)	ASc
Cerebral placques	?
Cutaneous	?
Endocrine associated	
Medullary cancer of thyroid	Calcitonin (AE)
Insulinoma	Insulin (AE)
Glucagonoma	Glucagon
Gastrinoma	Gastrin
Hereditary	?
Corneal lattice dystrophy	?
Aging	

*Adapted from reference 37.

amyloidosis (37). In situations of chronic inflammation, e.g., osteomyelitis, the amyloid-forming substance has been identified as protein A; this type of amyloid is designated AA. Other compounds such as hormones (precalcitonin) and prealbumin have been implicated (table 20.9).

The clinical manifestations of amyloidosis are varied. Type I amyloid classically involves the skin, tongue, heart, gastrointestinal tract, muscle, carpal ligaments, and nerves. Periorbital bruising, or "raccoon eyes," is due to amyloid deposition in the skin and associated vascular fragility, or "pinch purpura," detected by the pinch or scratch test. Macroglossia can cause difficulty with deglutition and involvement of the esophagus and small bowel can cause dysphagia, diarrhea, and malabsorption. Cardiac involve-

ment leads to a restrictive cardiac defect and, finally, to congestive heart failure. These patients are prone to arrhythmias and are very sensitive to digitalis. Skeletal muscle involvement gives rise to muscle weakness, while carpal tunnel syndrome results from carpal ligament involvement. Neuropathies are common in amyloidosis with multiple myeloma and are difficult to treat. Occasionally, lytic bone lesions are seen in amyloidosis, and the distinction from multiple myeloma may be very difficult in this situation (61). These bone lesions consist of amyloid deposits and are not collections of plasma cells.

The prolongation of the prothrombin (PT) and partial thromboplastin time (PTT) is caused by an acquired deficiency of factor X (155). The production of factor X remains normal, but clearance is markedly increased. By radiolabeling factor X and using total body scans, the site of clearance of factor X was found to be the liver and the spleen. Levels of factor X varying from 2–50% of normal have been reported. Spontaneous bleeding is rare, but factor X levels of <10% may be initially seen with bleeding after trauma or surgery. The amyloid fibrils are thought to bind the factor, based on in vitro tests (156). Treatment of bleeding in this condition is difficult because of the rapid removal of transfused factor X by the liver and the spleen. Anecdotal responses to splenectomy have been reported.

Type II or reactive amyloidosis involves the liver, spleen, kidneys, and adrenals. Patients often present with hepatosplenomegaly and nephrotic-range proteinuria. There is a hereditary or familial form. A mixed type I and II pattern is seen in some cases. A fourth type is called "localized," or "organ-limited," amyloidosis and involves one organ only.

Activities

Diagnosis of amyloidosis requires a high index of suspicion due to the rarity of the disease. The presence of the nephrotic syndrome in an older person, associated with enlarged kidneys, is suggestive of amyloidosis, and is the most common presenting finding in amyloidosis. The incidence of amyloidosis is difficult to determine. The "gold standard" for the diagnosis is the demonstration of the typical apple-green birefringence under the polarizing microscope after Congo red staining (100% specific). The best diagnostic test is probably a rectal biopsy, although abdominal fat aspiration reportedly has equal sensitivity (80–90%) (157, 158).

Before a rectal biopsy can be interpreted as negative, adequate submucosal tissue (including arterioles) must be obtained. This requires technical expertise and carries a risk of bleeding. The abdominal fat aspiration is safe and sensitive in type I amyloidosis, but usually negative in localized forms of amyloid. It is not as sensitive as rectal biopsy in reactive amyloidosis. In localized forms of amyloidosis, specific organs may need to be biopsied. Despite reports of massive bleeding following liver biopsy in amyloidosis, biopsy of the liver and kidney can be safely done.

Distinguishing primary amyloid from secondary type in the laboratory is difficult. Once multiple myeloma has been excluded by clinical patterns of involvement, underlying conditions (e.g., rheumatoid arthritis or tuberculosis) or family history will help classify the amyloidosis. The finding of an M protein is not a prerequisite for the diagnosis of amyloidosis, but >90% of primary amyloidosis is associated with a light chain or complete M protein. Secondary amyloidosis, however, is associated with an M protein only 50% of the time (153).

The treatment of all types of amyloidosis is disappointing. Gertz et al. studied 153 patients with primary amyloidosis (without multiple myeloma), treating them with melphalan/prednisone. Only 27 (18%) responded to therapy; the median survival for the responders was 89 months compared with 15 for the nonresponders (159). A randomized trial of melphalan/prednisone versus colchicine showed a slight benefit for the former (160). Amyloidosis with multiple myeloma is treated like other types of multiple myeloma. Reactive amyloidosis is treated by controlling the underlying illness with antibiotics (osteomyelitis, tuberculosis), colectomy (inflammatory bowel disease), or immunosuppressive agents (rheumatoid arthritis) (161). Patients with familial types of amyloidosis (familial Mediterranean fever) are treated prophylactically with colchicine 1 mg/day to prevent amyloid deposition (162). More recently, colchicine has been reported to reverse nephrotic-range proteinuria in these patients (163).

REFERENCES

1. Osgood EE. The survival time of patients with plasmacytic myeloma. Cancer Chemother Rep 1960;9:1–10.
2. Merlini G, Farhangi M, Osserman EF. Monoclonal immunoglobulins with antibody activity in myeloma, macroglobulinemia and related plasma cell dyscrasias. Semin Oncol 1986;13:350–365.
3. Eichner ER. The plasma cell dyscrasias. Postgrad Med 1980;67:44–58.
4. Seligmann M, Sassy C, Chevalier A. A Human IgM myeloma protein with anti (alpha 2) macroglobulin antibody activity. J Immunol 1973;110:85–90.
5. Grogan TM, Durie BGM, Spier CM, Richter L, Vela E. Myelomonocytic antigen positive multiple myeloma. Blood 1989;73:763–769.
6. Akashi K, Harada M, Shibuya T, Fukagawa K, Kimura N, Sagawa K, Yoshikai Y, Teshima T, Kikuchi M, Niho Y. Simultaneous occurrence of myelomonocytic leukemia and multiple myeloma: involvement of common leukemic progenitors and their developmental abnormality of "lineage infidelity." J Cell Physiol 1991;148:446–456.
7. Klein B, Zhang X, Jourdan M, Content J, Houssiau F, Aarden L, Piechaczyk M, Bataille R. Paracrine rather than autocrine regulation of myeloma-cell growth and differentiation by interleukin-6. Blood 1989;73:517–526.
8. Kawano M, Hirano T, Matsuda T, Taga T, Horii H, Iwato K, Asaoku H, Tang B, Tanabe O, Tanaka H, Kuramoto A, Kishimoto T. Autocrine generation and requirement of BSF-2/IL-6 for human multiple myelomas. Nature 1988;332:83–85.
9. Salmon SE. Immunoglobulin synthesis and tumor kinetics of multiple myeloma. Semin Hematol 1973;10:135–147.
10. Laird AK. Dynamics of tumor growth: comparison of growth rates and extrapolation of growth curve to one cell. Br J Cancer 1965;19:278–283.
11. Knowling MA, Harwood AR, Bergsagel DE. Comparison of extramedullary plasmacytomas with solitary and multiple plasma cell tumors of bone. J Clin Oncol 1983;4:255–262.
12. Wiltshaw E. The natural history of extramedullary plasmacytoma and it's relation to solitary plasmacytoma of bone and myelomatosis. Medicine 1976;55:217–238.
13. Garrett IR, Durie BGM, Nedwin GE, Gillespie A, et al. Production of lymphotoxin, a bone resorbing cytokine, by cultured human myeloma cells. New Engl J Med 1987;317:526–532.
14. Kyle RA, Schreiman JS, McLeod RA, Beabout JW. Computed tomography in diagnosis and management of multiple myeloma and its variants. Arch Intern Med 1985;145:1451–1452.
15. Soria J, et al. Immunoglobulin bound calcium and ultrafiltrable serum in myeloma. Br J Hematol 1976;34:343–344.
16. Ludwig H, Fritz E, Kotzmann H, Hocker P, Gisslinger H, Barnas U. Erythropoietin treatment of anemia associated with multiple myeloma. N Engl J Med 1990;322:1693–1699.
17. Bergsagel DE. Chemotherapy of myeloma: drug combinations versus single agents, an overview, and comments on acute leukemia in myeloma. Hematol Oncol 1988;6:159–166.
18. Kyle RA, Maldonado JE, Bayrd ED. Plasma cell leukemia. Arch Intern Med 1974;133:813–818.
19. Osserman EF, Takatsuki K. Plasma cell myeloma: gamma globulin synthesis and structure. Medicine 1963;42:357–384.
20. Kyle RA. Multiple myeloma: review of 869 cases (subject review). Mayo Clin Proc 1975;50:31–40.
21. Kyle RA, Robinson RA, Katzmann JA. The clinical aspects of biclonal gammopathies: review of 57 cases. Am J Med 1981;71:999–1008.
22. Hobbs JR. Monitoring myelomatosis. Arch Intern Med 1975;135:125–130.
23. Jacobson DR, Zolla-Pazner S. Immunosuppression and infection in multiple myeloma. Semin Oncol 1986;13:282–290.
24. Lynch RG. Immunoglobulin-specific suppressor T cells. Adv Immunol 1987;40:135–149.
25. Savage DG, Lindenbaum J, Garrett TJ. Biphasic patterns of bacterial infection in multiple myeloma. Ann Intern Med 1982;96:47–50.
26. MacGregor RR, Negendank WG, Schreiber AD. Impaired granulocyte adherence in multiple myeloma: relationship to complement system, granulocyte delivery and infection. Blood 1978;51:591–599.
27. Penny R, Galton DAG. Studies on neutrophil function: II, pathological aspects. Br J Haematol 1966;12:633–645.
28. Somer T. Hyperviscosity syndrome in plasma cell dyscrasias. Duodecim 1977;93:586–603.
29. Phillips MJ, Harkness J. Annotation, plasma and whole blood viscosity. Br J Haematol 1976;34:347–352.
30. McGrath MA, Penny R. Paraproteinemia. Blood hyperviscosity and clinical manifestations. J Clin Invest 1976;58:1155–1162.

31. Hill GS, Morel-Maroger L, Mery JP, et al. Renal lesions in multiple myeloma: their relationship to associated protein abnormalities. Am J Kidney Dis 1983;2:423–438.

32. Alexanian R, Barlogie B, Dixon D. Renal failure in multiple myeloma. Arch Intern Med 1990;150:1693–1695.

33. Johnson WJ, Kyle RA, Pineda AA, O'Brien PC, Holley KE. Treatment of renal failure associated with multiple myeloma. Arch Intern Med 1990;150:863–869.

34. Stone MJ. Amyloidosis: a final common pathway for protein deposition in tissues. Blood 1990;75:531–545.

35. Nomura S, et al. Intracellular formation of amyloid fibrils in myeloma: cytochemical, immunochemical, and electronmicroscopic observations. Cancer 1984;54:303–307.

36. Glenner GG. Amyloid deposits and amyloidosis: the betafibrilloses. N Engl J Med 1980;302:1283–1292.

37. Glenner GG. Amyloid deposits and amyloidosis: The betafibrilloses. N Engl J Med 1980;302:1333–1343.

38. Goldsmith GH. Hemostatic disorders associated with neoplasia. In: Ratnoff OR, ed. Hemostatic Disorders. Philadelphia: WB Saunders, 1991;2:353–368.

39. Castaldi PA, Penny R. A macroglobulin with inhibitory activity against coagulation factor VIII. Blood 1970;35:370–376.

40. Zettervall O, Nilsson IM. Acquired von Willebrand's disease caused by a monoclonal antibody. Acta Med Scand 1978;204:521–528.

41. Gorevic PD, Kassab HJ, Lefo H, Kohn A, Meltzep W, Prose P, Franklin EC. Mixed cryoglobulinemia: clinical aspects and long-term follow-up of 40 patients. Am J Med 1980;69:287–308.

42. McCarthy J, Proctor SJ. Cerebral involvement in multiple myeloma: case report. J Clin Pathol 1978;31:259–264.

43. Bardwick PA, Zvaifler NJ, Gill GN, Newman D, Greenway GD, Resnick DL. Plasma cell dyscrasia with polyneuropathy, organomegaly, endocrinopathy, M protein, and skin changes: the POEMS Syndrome. Medicine 1980;59:311–322.

44. Durie BGM. Staging and kinetics of multiple myeloma. Semin Oncol 1986;13:300–309.

45. Reichert CM, Everett DF, Nadler PI, et al. High-resolution zone electrophoresis, combined with immunofixation, in the detection of an occult myeloma paraprotein. Clin Chem 1982;28:2312–2313.

46. Kyle RA. Diagnosis and management of multiple myeloma and related disorders. Progr Hematol 1986;14:257–282.

47. Davey FR, Elghetany T, Kurec AS. Immunophenotyping of hematologic neoplasms in paraffin-embedded tissue sections. Am J Clin Pathol 1990(suppl 1):S17–26.

48. Carpio JD, Espinoza LR, Lauter S, Osterland CK. Transient monoclonal proteins in drug hypersensitivity reactions. Am J Med 1979;66:1051–1056.

49. Young VH. Transient paraproteins. Proc R Soc Med 1969:62:778–780.

50. Waldenstrom JG. Benign monoclonal gammapathy. Acta Med Scan 1984;216:435–447.

51. Kyle RA. Multiple myeloma: an update on diagnosis and management. Acta Oncol 1990;29:1–15.

52. Schemankewitz E, Hammami A, Stahl R. Henderson JM. Check IJ. Multiple extramedullary plasmacytomas following orthotopic liver transplantation in a patient on cyclosporine therapy. Transplantation 1990;49:1019–1022.

53. Joseph UG, Barker RL, Yuan B, Martin A, Madeiros J, Peiper SC. Posttransplant plasma cell dyscrasias. Cancer 1994;74:1959-1964.

54. Karnad AB, Martin AW, Koh HK, Brauer MJ, Novich M, Wright J. Non-secretory multiple myeloma in a 26-year-old man with acquired Immunodeficiency syndrome, presenting with multiple extramedullary plasmacytomas and osteolytic bone disease. Am J Hematol 1989;32:305–310.

55. Kyle RA. Monoclonal gammopathy of undetermined significance: natural history in 241 cases. Am J Med 1978;64:814–826.

56. Evans RS, Baxter E, Gilliland BC. Chronic hemolytic anemia due to cold agglutinins: a 20-year history of benign gammopathy with response to chlorambucil. Blood 1973;42:463–470.

57. Alexanian R. Monoclonal gammopathy in lymphoma. Arch Intern Med 1975;135:62–66.

58. Mackenzie MR, Fudenberg HH. Macroglobulinemia: an analysis of forty patients. Blood 1972;39:874.

59. Migliore PJ, Alexanian R. Monoclonal gammopathy in human neoplasia. Cancer 1968;21:1127–1131.

60. Kramer MR, van Dijk JM, Hadas I, Hershko C. Destructive bone lesions in primary amyloidosis. Postgrad Med J 1986;62:1037–1041.

61. Crapper RM, Deam DR, Mackay IR. Paraproteinemias in homosexual men with HIV infection. Am J Clin Pathol 1988;88:348–351.

62. Randall RE, Williamson WC, Mullinar F, Tung MY, Shu WJS. Manifestations of systemic light chain deposition. Am J Med 1976;60:293–299.

63. Haghlighi P, Wolf PL. Alpha-heavy chain disease. Clin Lab Med 1986;6:477–487.

64. Fermand JP, Brouet JC, Danon F, Seligmann M. Gamma heavy chain "disease": heterogeneity of the clinicopathologic features: report of 16 cases and review of the literature. Medicine 1989;68:321–335.

65. Kyle RA, Greipp PR, Banks PM. The diverse picture of gamma heavy-chain disease: report of seven cases and review of literature. Mayo Clin Proc 1981;56:439–451.

66. Durie BGM, Salmon SE. A clinical staging system for multiple myeloma. Cancer 1975;36:842–854.

67. Bataille R, Durie BGM, Grenier J, Sany J. Prognostic factors and staging in multiple myeloma: a reappraisal. J Clin Oncol 1986;4:80–87.

68. Woodruff RK, Wadsworth J, Malpas JS, et al. Clinical staging in multiple myeloma. Br J Hematol 1979;42:199–205.

69. Bethea M, Forman DT. Beta 2-microglobulin: it's significance and clinical usefulness. Ann Clin Lab Sci 1990;20:163–168.

70. Bataille R, Durie BGM, Grenier J. Serum Beta₂ microglobulin and survival duration in multiple myeloma: a simple reliable marker for staging. Br J Haematol 1983;55:439–447.

71. Alexanian R, Barlogie B, Dixon D. Prognosis of asymptomatic multiple myeloma. Arch Intern Med 1988;148:1963–1965.

72. Sam Miguel JF, Sanchez J, Gonzales M. Prognostic factors and classification in multiple myeloma. Br J Cancer 1989;59:113–118.

73. Carter A, Hocherman I, Linn S, Cohen Y, Tatarsky I. Prognostic significance of plasma cell morphology in multiple myeloma. Cancer 1987;60:1060-1065.

74. Corrado C, Santarelli MT, Pavlovsky S, Pizzolato M, et al. Prognostic factors in multiple myeloma: definition of risk groups in 410 previously untreated patients. A Grupo Argention de Tratameiento de la Leucemia Aguda Study. J Clin Oncol 1989;7:1839–1844.

75. Durie BGM, Salmon SE, Moon TE. Pretreatment tumor mass, cell kinetics, prognosis in multiple myeloma. Blood 1980;55:364–372.

76. Barlogie B, Alexanian R, Gehan EA, Smallwood L, Smith T, Drewinko B. Marrow cytometry and prognosis in myeloma. J Clin Invest 1983;72:853–861.

77. Latreille J, Barlogie B, Johnston D, Drewinko B, Alexanian R. Ploidy and proliferative characteristics in monoclonal gammopathies. Blood 1982;59:43–51.

78. Buja LM, Khoi NB, Roberts WC. Clinically significant cardiac amyloidosis: clinicopathologic findings in 15 patients. Am J Cardiol 1970;26:394–405.

79. Pruzanski W, Watt JG. Serum viscosity and hyperviscosity syndrome in IgG multiple myeloma: report on 10 patients and a review of the literature. Ann Intern Med 1972;77:853–860.

80. Laesione NS, Nosanchuk JS, Oberman HA, et al. Therapeutic plasmapheresis in treatment of patients with Waldenstrom's macroglobulinemia. Transfusion 1968;8:174–178.

81. Chronic leukemia: Myeloma task force, NCI. Proposed guidelines for protocol studies: II, plasma cell myeloma. Cancer Chem Rep 1973;4:145–158.

82. Dutcher JP, Wiernik PH. Longterm survival of a patient with multiple mylenoma—a cure? Cancer 1984;53:3069–2072.

83. Kyle RA. Long-term survival in multiple myeloma. New Engl J Med 1983;308:314–316.

84. Richards F, Coleman M, Cooper MR, Ballard WP. Multiple myeloma: complete remission with high-dose melphalan. Cancer Chemother Invest 1985;3:15-21.

85. Selby PJ, MacElwain TJ, Nandi AC, et al. Multiple myeloma treated with high-dose intravenous melphalan. Br J Haematol 1987;66:55–62.

86. Alexanian R, Barlogie B. New treatment strategies for multiple myeloma. Am J Hematol 1990;35:194–198.

87. Gahrton G, Barlogie B. Bone marrow transplantation in multiple myeloma. Bone Marrow Transplantation 1991;7:71–79.

88. Osterborg A, Ahre A, Bjorkholm M, Bjoreman M, Brenning G, Gahrton G, et al. Oral versus intravenous melphalan and prednisone treatment in multiple myeloma stage II. Acta Oncol 1989:29:727–731.

89. Abramson N, Lurie P, Mietlowski WL, et al. Phase III study of intermittent carmustine (BCNU), cyclophosphamide, and prednisone versus intermittent melphalan and prednisone in myeloma. Cancer Treat Rep 1982;66:1273–1277.

90. Cohen HJ, Silberman HR, Tornyos K, et al. Comparison of two long-term chemotherapy regimens, with or without agents to modify skeletal repair, in multiple myeloma. Blood 1984;63:639–648.

91. Harley JB, Pajak TF, McIntyre OR, et al. Improved survival of increased-risk myeloma patients on combined triple-alkylating-agent therapy: a study of the CALGB. Blood 1979;54:31–41.

92. Bergasagel DE, Bailey AJ, Langley GR, et al. The chemotherapy of plasma-cell myeloma and the incidence of acute leukemia. N Engl J Med 1979;301:743–748.

93. Pavlovsky S, Corrado C, Santarelli MT, et at. An update of two randomized trials in previously treated multiple myeloma comparing melphalan and prednisone versus three- and five-drug combinations: an Argentine group for the treatment of acute leukemia study. J Clin Oncol 1988;6:769–775.

94. Alexanian R, Dreicer R. Chemotherapy for multiple myeloma. Cancer 1984;53:583–588.

95. Cooper MR, McIntyre OR, Propert KJ, et al. Single, sequential and multiple alkylating agent therapy for multiple myeloma: a CALGB study. J Clin Oncol 1986;4:1331–1339.

96. Salmon SE, Haut A, Bonnett JD, et al. Alternating combination chemotherapy and levamisole improves survival in multiple myeloma: a Southwest Oncology Group study. J Clin Oncol 1983:1;453–461.

97. Montalban C, Zapatero A, Blanco L, et al. Tratamiento del mieloma multiple en estadios II y III: estudio comparative del protocolo M-2 el de melfalan-prednisona. Sangre 1984;29:993–999.

98. Hansen OP, Clausen NAT, Drivsholm A, et al. Phase III study of intermittent 5-drug regime (VBCPM0 versus intermittent 3-drug regime (VMP) versus intermittent melphalan and prednisone (MP) in myelomatosis. Scand J Haematol 1985;35:518–524.

99. Palva IP, Ahrenberg P, Ala-Harja K, et al. Treatment of multiple myeloma with an intensive 5-drug combination or intermittent melphalan and prednisone: a randomized multicentre trial. Eur J Haematol 1987;38:50–54.

100. Osterborg A, Ahre A, Bjorkholm M, et al. Alternating combination chemotherapy (VMCP/VBAP) is not superior to melphalan/prednisone in the treatment of multiple myeloma patients state III-AA randomized study from MGS. Eur J Haematol 1989;43:54–62.

101. Kildahl-Andersen O, Bjark P, Bondevik A, et al. Multiple myeloma in central and northern Norway 1981–1982: a follow-up study of a randomized clinical trial of 5-drug combination therapy versus standard therapy. Eur J Haematol 1988;41:47–51.

102. Peest D, Deicher H, Coldewey R, et al. Induction and maintenance therapy in multiple myeloma: a multicenter trial of MP versus VCMP. Eur J Cancer Clin Onc 1988;24:1061–1067.

103. Jhorth M, Hellquist L, Holmberg E, et al. Initial treatment in multiple myeloma: no advantage of multidrug chemotherapy over melphalan-prednisone. Br J Haematol 1990;74:185–191.

104. Boccadoro M, Marmont F, Tribalto M, et al. Multiple myeloma: VMCP/VBAP alternating combination chemotherapy is not superior to melphalan and prednisolone even in high-risk patients. J Clin Oncol 1991;9:444–448.

105. Oken MM, Tslatis A, Abramson N, et al. Evaluation of intensive (VMCP/VBAP) vs. standard (MP) therapy for multiple myeloma (abstract). Proc Am Soc Clin Oncol 1987;6:203.

106. Gregory WM, Richards MA, Malpas JS. Combination chemotherapy versus melphalan and prednisone in the treatment of multiple myeloma: an overview of published trials. J Clin Oncol 1992;10:334–342.

107. Djulbegovic B, Blumenreich MS, Joseph UG, Hadley TJ. Melphalan prednisone vs combined chemotherapy in multiple myeloma: a meta-analysis (abstract). Proc Am Soc Hematol 1991;109.

108. Montuoro A, De Rosa L, De Blasio A, et al. Alpha 2a-interferon/melphalan/prednisone versus melphalan/prednisone in previously untreated patients with multiple myeloma. Br J Haematol 1990;76:365–368.

109. Oken MM, Kyle RA, Greipp PR, Kay NE, Tsiatis A, O'Connell MJ. Alternating cycles of VBMCP with interferon (rIFN-alpha 2) in the treatment of multiple myeloma (abstract). Proc Am Soc Clin Oncol 1988;7:868.

109a.Berenson JR, Lichtenstein A, Porter L, Dimopoulos MA, Gordoni R, Geoge S, et al. Efficacy of pamidronate in reducing skeletal events in patients with advanced multiple myeloma. N Engl J Med 1996;334:488–493.

110. Belch A, Shelley W, Bergsagel D, Wilson K, et al. A randomized trial of maintenance versus no maintenance melphalan and prednisone in responding multiple myeloma patients. Br J Cancer 1988;57:94–99.

111. Mandelli F, Avvisati G, Amadori S, Boccadoro M, Gernone A, Lauta V, Marmont F, et al. Maintenance treatment with recombinant interferon Alfa-2b in patients with multiple myeloma responding to conventional induction chemotherapy. New Engl J Med 1990;322:1430–1434.

112. Salmon SE, Crowley J. Impact of glucocorticoids and interferon on outcome in multiple myeloma (abstract). Proc Am Soc Clin Oncol 1992;11:1069.

113. Barlogie B, Smith L, Alexanian R. Effective treatment of advanced multiple myeloma refractory to alkylating agents. N Engl J Med 1984;310:1353–1356.

114. Alexanian R, Barlogie B, Dixon D. High-Dose glucocorticoid treatment of resistant myeloma. Ann Intern Med 1986;105:8–11.

115. Alexanian R, Yap BS, Bodey G. Prednisone pulse therapy for refractory myeloma. Blood 1983;62:572–577.

116. Barlogie B. Management of multiple myeloma. Blut 1990;60:1–7.

117. Alexanian R, Barlogie B, Ventura G. Chemotherapy for resistant and relapsing multiple myeloma. Eur J Haematol 1989;51:140–144.

118. Bellamy WT, Dalton WS, Dorr RT. The clinical relevance of multi-drug resistance. Cancer Invest 1990;8:547–562.

119. Beck WT. Modulators of p-glycoprotein-associated multidrug resistance. In: Ozols RF, ed. Molecular and clinical advances in anticancer drug resistance. Norvell, MA: Kluwer, 1991:151.

120. Dalton WS, Grogan TM, Meltzer PS, et al. Drug resistance in multiple myeloma and non-Hodgkin's lymphoma: detection of p-glycoprotein and potential circumvention by addition of verapamil to chemotherapy. J Clin Oncol 1987;7:415–424.

121. Garewal H, Durie BGM, Kyle RA, Finley P, Bower B, Serokman R. Serum Beta$_2$-Microblobulin in the initial staging and subsequent monitoring of monoclonal plasma cell disorders. J Clin Oncol 1984;2:51–57.

122. Barlogie B, Smallwood L, Smith T, Alexanian R. High serum levels of LDH identify a high-grade lymphoma-like myeloma. Ann Intern Med 1989;110:521–525.

123. Wasserman T. Diagnosis and management of plasmacytomas. Oncology 1987;1:37–41.

124. Corwin J, Lindberg R. Solitary plasmacytoma of bone vs. extramedullary plasmacytoma and their relationship to multiple myeloma. Cancer 1979;43:1007–1013.

125. Webb HE, Harrison EG, Masson JK. Solitary extramedullary myeloma (plasmacytoma) of the upper part of the respiratory tract and oropharynx. Cancer 1962;15:1142–1155.

126. Lazarus HM, Kellermeyer RW, Aikawa M, Herzig RH. Multiple Myeloma in young men: clinical course and electron microscopic studies of bone marrow plasma cells. Cancer 1980;46:1397–1400.

127. Hill LD, White Jr ML. Plasmacytoma of the lung. J Thor Surg 1952;**XX**:187–193.

128. Rapoport AP, Rowe JM. Plasma cell dyscrasia in a 15-year-old boy: case report and review of the literature. Am J Med 1990;89:816–818.

129. Hoenfeld Y, Shaklai M, Berliner S, Gallant LA, Pinkhas J. Familial multiple myeloma: a review of thirty-seven families. Postgraduate Med J 1982;58:12–16.

130. Latreille J, Barlogie B, Golde W, Johnston D, Drewinko B, Alexanian R. Cellular DNA content as a marker of human myeloma. Blood 1980;55:403–405.

131. Burn PA, Krasnow S, Makuch RW, Schlam M, Schechter G. Flow cytometric analysis of DNA content of bone marrow cells in patients with plasma cell myeloma: clinical implications. Blood 1982;59:528–535.

132. Gahrton G, Tura S, Ljungman P, Blade J, Brandt L, Cavo M, Facon T, et al. Prognostic factors in allogeneic bone marrow transplantation for multiple myeloma. J Clin Oncol 1995;13:1312–1322.

133. Gould J, Alexanian R, Goodacre A, et al. Plasma cell karyotype in multiple myeloma. Blood 1988;71:453–456.

134. Gahrton G, Tura S, Ljungman P, Belanger C, et al. Allogeneic bone marrow transplantation in multiple myeloma. N Engl J Med 1991;325:1267–1273.

135. Alexanian R, Barlogie B, Tucker S. VAD-based regimen as primary treatment for multiple myeloma. Am J Hematol 1990;33:86–89.

136. Anderson C. Who benefits from high dose therapy for multiple myeloma. J Clin Oncol 1995;13:1291–1296.

137. Fermand JP, Levy Y, Gerota J, et al. Treatment of aggressive multiple myeloma by high-dose chemotherapy and total body irradiation followed by blood stem cells autograft. Blood 1989;73:20–23.

138. Second International Workshop on Myeloma. Advances in biology and therapy of multiple myeloma. Cancer Res 1989;49:7172–7175.

139. Case DC, Coleman M, Gottlieb A, McCarroll K. Phase I-II trial of high-dose melphalan in previously untreated stage III multiple myeloma: Cancer and Leukemia Group B Study 8512. Cancer Invest 1992;10:11–17.

140. Gore ME, Viner C, Meldrum M, et al. Intensive treatment of multiple myeloma and criteria for complete remission. Lancet 1989; 2:879–882.

140a.Attal M, Harousseau JL, Stoppa AM, et al. High dose therapy in multiple myeloma: final analysis of a prospective randomized study of the "Intergroupe Francais du myeloma" (abstract). Blood 1995;86:124a.

141. Barlogie B, Epstein J, Selvanayagam P, Alexanian R. Plasma cell myeloma—new biological insights and advances in therapy. Blood 1989;73:865–879.

142. Shimazaki C, Wisniewski D, Scheinberg DA, et al. Elimination of myeloma cells from bone marrow by using monoclonal antibodies and magnetic immunobeads. Blood 1988; 72:1248–1254.

143. Visani G, Lemoli RM, Dinota A, et al. Evidence that long term bone marrow culture of patients with multiple myeloma favors normal hemopoietic proliferation. Transplantation 1990;48:1026–1031.

144. Klein B, Wijdenes J, Zhang XG, Jourdan M, et al. Murine Anti-interleukin 6 monoclonal antibody therapy for a patient with plasma cell leukemia. Blood 1991;78:1198–1204.

145. Appelbaum FR, Sandmaier B, Brown PA, Kaplan D, Ketring AR, et al. Myelosuppression and mechanism of recovery following administration of samarium EDTMP.

Antibody-immunoconjugates and radiopharmaceuticals. 1988:263–270.

146. Spiess JL, Adelstein DJ, Hines JD. Multiple myeloma presenting with spinal cord compression. Oncology 1988;45: 88–92.

147. Lazor MZ, Rosenberg LE. Mechanism of adrenal-steroid reversal of hypercalcemia in multiple myeloma. N Engl J Med 1964;270:749–755.

148. Paterson AD, Kanis JA, Cameron EC, et al. The use of dichloromethylene diphosphonate for the management of hypercalcemia in multiple myeloma. Br J Haematol 1983; 54:121–132.

149. Zucchelli P, Pasquali S, Cagnoli L, Ferrari G. Controlled plasma exchange trial in acute renal failure due to multiple myeloma. Kidney Int 1988;33:1175–1180.

150. Gordon DS, Hearn EB, Spira TJ, et al. Phase I study of intravenous gamma globulin in multiple myeloma. Am J Med 1984;76(suppl):111–116.

151. Schildt RA, Rubin RR, Schiffman G, et al. Polyvalent pneumococcal immunization of patients with plasma cell dyscrasias. Cancer 1981;48:1377–1380.

152. Solomon A, Weiss DT, Kattine AA. Nephrotoxic potential of Bence Jones proteins. N Engl J Med 1991;324: 1845–1851.

153. Isobe T, Osserman EF. Patterns of amyloidosis and their association with plasma-cell dyscrasia, monoclonal immunoglobulins and Bence-Jones proteins. N Engl J Med 1974; 290:473–477.

154. Kyle RA, Bayrd ED. Amyloidosis: review of 236 cases. Mayo Clin Proc 1975;54:271–299.

155. Furie B, Greene E, Furie BC. Syndrome of acquired factor X deficiency and systemic amyloidosis. N Engl J Med 1977; 297:81–85.

156. Furie B, Voo L, McAdam K, Furie BC. Mechanism of factor X deficiency in systemic amyloidosis. N Engl J Med 1981;304:827.

157. Duston MA, Skinner M, Shirahama T, Cohen AS. Diagnosis of amyloidosis by abdominal fat aspiration. Am J Med 1987;82:412–414.

158. Libbey CA, Skinner M, Cohen AS. Use of abdominal fat tissue aspirate in the diagnosis of systemic amyloidosis. Arch Intern Med 1983;143:1549–1552.

159. Gertz MA, Kyle RA, Greipp PR. Response rates and survival in primary systemic amyloidosis. Blood 1991;77: 257–262.

160. Kyle RA, Greipp PR, Garton JP, Gertz MA. Primary systemic amyloidosis: comparison of melphalan/prednisone versus colchicine. Am J Med 1985;79:708–716.

161. Gertz MA, Kyle RA. Secondary systemic amyloidosis: response and survival in 64 patients. Medicine 1991;70: 246–256.

162. Zemer D, Pras M, Sohar E, Modan M, Cabili S, Gafni J. Colchicine in the prevention and treatment of the amyloidosis of familial Mediterranean fever. N Engl J Med 1986; 314:1001–1005.

163. Baldini A, Guffanti BM, Cesana M, et al. Role of different hematologic variables in defining the risk of malignant transformation in monoclonal gammopathy. Blood 1996;87: 912–918.

164. Cunningham D, Paz-Ayres L, Gore ME, et al. High-dose melphalan for multiple myeloma: long-term follow-up data. J Clin Oncol 1994;12:765–768,

165. Fermand JP, Chevret S, Ravaud P, et al. High-dose chemoradiotherapy and autologous blood stem cell transplantation in multiple myeloma: result of a phase II trial involving 63 patients. Blood 1993;82:2005–2009.

166. Oken M. Standard treatment of multiple myeloma. Mayo Clin Proc 1994;69:781–786.

167. Blade J, Lopez-Guillermo A, Bosh F, et al. Impact of response to treatment on survival in multiple myeloma: results in a series of 243 patients. Br J Haematol 1994;88: 117–121.

EXERCISES AND TOOLS FOR LYMPHOCYTE AND PLASMA CELL DISORDERS AND GENETICS OF HEMATOPOIETIC MALIGNANCIES

Every member of the white cell series plays a role in immune surveillance but none is as diverse as the lymphocyte.

1. With the knowledge that lymphocyte diversity begins *in utero,* develop a schema that involves the relationships spawned by the knowledge of lymphocyte receptors on (a) cell types involved in the responses to injury and (b) the imposition of genetic controls in graft recognition.

2. Construct a paradigm that addresses the clinicopathological relationships between disease and the T, B, and NK lymphocyte subsets.

3. Taking into account the time sequences for the development of the various "hematopoietic" tissues, construct a clinicopathological paradigm between lymphocyte sources and subclasses for disorders involving the primary lymphoid organs (i.e., bone marrow and thymus) and the secondary organs (i.e., nodal tissues such as spleen, peripheral, tonsillar, gut, and peribronchial nodes).

4. Hematopoietic stem cells give rise to (a) myeloerythroid lineage and (b) lymphoid lineage cells, which help to sort out the underlying mechanisms in case studies of lymphoid malfunction. Markers common to both B and T lymphocytes (for example, CD-10) underscore the codependent nature of T and B lymphocyte development and the difficulty to determine the precise time of B-cell lineage irreversibility. In this context, explain how failure of stem cell maturation, i.e., the onset of stem cell leukemia, usually includes evidence of erythroid, myeloid, and lymphoid markers (antigens).

5. B, T, and NK cells respond to specific cytokines. Integrate the knowledge of these hematopoietic cell line inducers in terms of all lymphocyte disorders as well as the material presented in the chapters on bone marrow transplantation.

6. In reviewing B-cell development and related disorders, recall the distinction between antigen-dependent and antigen-independent activity and the fact that such activity crosses primary and secondary lymphoid tissue boundaries.

7. Note also that immunoglobulin diversity is typical of antigen-independent B lymphocytes. Only as these B-lineage cells mature do they show evidence of surface Ig. The cells show an immature expression until antigen stimulation awakens them to the antigen-dependent group of, initially, mature B-cells and, finally, plasma cells. Explain why development of B-cells from immature precursors requires a marrow-stromal cell contact.

8. The following information will help to develop constructs of T-cell related disorders. The T-cell micro environment is the thymus anlage, i.e., the third pharyngeal cleft. It is the earliest lymphocyte subset. T-cell precursors also arise in the sites of primitive marrow development and subsequently migrate to the thymus.

9. NK cells, the large granular lymphocytes, arise from the marrow and also possibly from the thymic tissue, but these lymphocytes destroy targets without prior processing and outside the confines of the major histocompatibility complex. That they preceded the appearance of immune memory containing cells and kill with antibody presentation supports the likelihood that they are the most primitive of all lymphocytes. Develop a theme that incorporates the stages of T-cell ontogeny with errors that may occur as a result of genetic or acquired influences.

10. With the use of tables of cytokine and cell receptor information construct and explain the nature of various lymphocyte-related disease entities such as acquired immune deficiency states, inherited disorders of T, B, or T and B lymphocytes ranging from nonfunctional to absence of activities. Also compare and contrast the same cytokine, cell receptor, and feedback mechanism scenario between combinations and interactions of lymphocyte and granulocyte-monocyte disorders, respectively. See material in Exercises and Tools for Biological Control Mechanisms.

11. Construct a mechanistic approach to the biology and therapy of acute and chronic lymphocytic leukemia and the plasma cell dyscrasias. Include an assessment of risk factors using a paradigm that includes genetics, environmental factors, principles of aging, cell kinetics, drug resistance, and pharmacokinetics.

12. With the information provided in the chapter on genetics, develop an expanded paradigm that uses genetic data involving all of the hematopoietic tissues in order to propose therapeutic modalities. For example, develop a construct that would target and repair the amino acid abnormality in sickle cell disease and then use that construct in a treatment vehicle. Con-

sider a transplantation effort in this regard, and include the factors that would enhance and inhibit this process. Include, in addition, the extent of success in the most favorable of all conditions. Apply this approach with appropriate modifications for all sorts of hematopoietic disorders.

13. See also Exercises and Tools for Myelocytes and Monocytes.

SECTION III APPENDIX

Appendix 1. Immunoglobulin Characteristics

	IgA	IgG	IgM	IgE	IgD
Molecular weight (KD)	150	150	950	190	185
Heavy chain	α	γ	μ	ϵ	λ
Light chain					κ, λ
Biological life (T$\frac{1}{2}$ days)	6	21	5	2	3
Percent distribution	15	80	<5	<1	<1

Myelocyte and Monocyte Disorders

CHAPTER 21

Quantitative and Qualitative Disorders of Granulocytes

YUVAL BRANDSTETTER, SAMUEL GROSS

> White blood cells (pus cells) migrate out through the walls of tiny blood vessels into inflamed tissues.
> —Cohnheim 1870

Nonmalignant neutrophil abnormalities fall into two major categories: quantitative disorders, that is, those that occur because of insufficient numbers, and qualitative disorders, that is, those that occur because of ineffective function. A less common group are those with combination defects. Neutrophil abnormalities are further subclassified as defects intrinsic or extrinsic to the bone marrow.

A quantitative defect, for example, neutropenia leading to impaired immune function, is defined as an absolute decrease in circulating neutrophils below the normal age, sex, and race-related absolute neutrophil count. Neutrophils include both polymorphonuclear leukocytes and band forms, the sum of which make up the absolute neutrophil count (ANC). Thus, a total leukocyte count of 6.0×10^9/L with 10% polymorphonuclear cells and 4% band forms has an ANC of 6.0×10^9/L $\times$ 14% (10% neutrophils and 4% bands) = 0.84×10^9/L. The lower limit a for normal ANC in Caucasians <1 year of age is 1.0×10^9/L. Beyond infancy, the generally accepted lowest norm is 1.5×10^9/L with somewhat lower levels for blacks and women. In all likelihood, the difference between infant and adult values is related to the size of the marrow pool. The reason for the race-related differences is not apparent (table 21.1)(1–4).

Qualitative neutrophil abnormalities cover the broad range of phagocytic function and encompass the complex processes and interactions of locomotion, ingestion, and killing.

Granulocyte Development

In order to appreciate the nature of these defects, it is appropriate to review granulocyte formation, production, function, and interaction. Committed granulocyte and monocyte precursors can be detected in the blood by week 5 in the embryo. By 16 weeks of development, mature neutrophils can be identified in human fetuses (in mature infants and even more so in premature infants, the granulocyte is functionally immature; its relatively rigid membrane impedes effective migration). In addition, granulocyte development lags behind red cell development. Conditions of high erythropoietin seen in the newborn may shift stem cells from myeloid to erythroid differentiation with resultant neutropenia. The combination of these factors probably contributes to the fact that the newborn infant is particularly sensitive to bacterial infections (5–12). This lag, or limited supply of reserve neutrophils, helps to account of the cytokine-responsive neutropenia frequently seen in bacterial infections in the neonate. In the adult, whose granulocyte reserve is considerably greater, neutrophilia is commonly seen following bacterial infections. Time sequences and cytokine relationships of granulopoiesis are noted in table 21.1. It takes around 7–9 days for a mature neutrophil to develop from a committed precursor. Another 3 days is used to fill the marrow reserve and a further 2 days to repopulate the peripheral circulation and the marginating pool. Newly formed granulocytes line the sinusoids of the bone marrow and form the mobilizable reserve. In the circulation they attach to the periphery of the vasculature and form the inducible vascular reserve. Fifty percent of the granulocytes at any given time occupy this vascular reserve. The granulocyte life span is difficult to assess, since all of the labeling techniques currently in use also influence the life span, but the consensus of information supports an approximately 24-hour life span from marrow release to cell death (table 21.2).

As maturation occurs, so do granules, locomotor apparati, and antigenic characteristics. Promyelocytes and myelocytes develop primary granules that are manufactured in the region of the Golgi apparatus. These primary granules, in common with those of basophils and eosinophils, in-

Table 21-1. Age, White Blood Cell Numbers and Distribution (mean $\times 10^9$)

Age in Years	Total WBC	Lymphocytes	Neutrophils	Monocytes	Eosinophils	Basophils
Full-term neonate	17.5	4.7	4.5	1.2	0.95	0.50
Infants (1–10)	12.0	6.6	4.7	0.65	0.47	0.30
Teenage (11–16)	9.6	4.5	5.6	0.63	0.45	0.45
Adults (16–45)	7.1	2.8	4.4	0.60	0.44	0.45

Table 21-2. Granulocyte Compartments and Production Times

Compartments and Volume	Identity
Mitotic group <2.1×10^9 cells/kg	Myeloblast, promyelocyte, myelocyte 140 hr
Maturation group 5.6×10^9 cells/kg	Metamyelocyte, band form, neutrophil 200 hrs
Circulating group 0.3×10^9 cells/kg	Neutrophil half life: 6.3hr
Marginating group 0.3×10^9 cells/kg	

Granulocyte Turnover Rate 1.6 cells/kg/24 hr

Table 21-3. Granulocyte Constituents: Golgi Apparatus and Organelles

Immature Granulocytes	Site
Primary Granules	Inner Golgi surface
Acid phosphatase	
α-Mannosidase	
Aryl sulfatase	
Basic proteins	
β-Glucuronidase	
Elastase	
5′ Nucleosidase	
Lysozyme	
N-acetyl-β-glucosaminidase	
Peroxidase	
Mature granulocytes	*Site*
Secondary (Specific) Granules	Outer Golgi surface
Alkaline phosphatase	
Aminopeptidase	
B_{12} binding protein	
Basic proteins	
Collaginase	
Lactoferrin	
Lysozyme	
Tertiary granules	Secretory organelles
gelatinase	

clude lysozymes, acid phosphatase, and peroxidase. Secondary granules develop principally at the level of the late myelocyte and include their contents alkaline phosphatase, myeloperoxidase, collagenase, lactoferrin, vitamin B_{12}-binding protein, and lysozyme. Specific granules, which account for the unique staining characteristics of basophils and esopinophils, develop alongside the primary and secondary granules and are followed by a tertiary crop of granules including gelatinase and related enzymes (13–21). The sum of all of these granules provides a mature cell with something like 150 enzymes (table 21.3).

Actin and tubulin, the filamentous structures that facilitate locomotion, are present in early granulocyte development but do not attain their full complement until maturity. It is important to emphasize the fact that, even in their primitive forms, these structures are present, which, in turn, permits egress outside the vascular system, as, for example, in leukemic infiltrates of the skin, central nervous system, testes, and other so-called sanctuary sites. The granulocyte surface architecture, in common with other cells, and particularly with other members of the leukocyte family, contains highly complex and well-integrated glycoprotein. Many of these structures provide recognition sites for specific monoclonal antibodies and surface receptors that include those for integrins and adhesion molecules as well as the Fc fragment of immunoglobulin (table 21.4) (22–25).

Quantitative Neutrophil Defects: Neutropenias

Case 1

A 2-year-old white boy was referred because of frequent skin infections. According to the parents, these began in early infancy as "boils" and kept recurring. Initially, these infections were infrequent, but after the first year they occurred almost monthly, lasted about 7–10 days and then cleared up, irrespective of the type of antibiotics administered. Recently, these infections involved more than the skin; they also included the middle ear, oropharynx, and tissues immediately surrounding an erupting premolar.

On examination, the child was well developed and nourished (40th percentile for weight and height), irritable and febrile, but not in acute distress. He had three 2 × 2-cm erythematous papules on his forearm and one on his right buttock. His vital signs were as follows: temperature 39°C, pulse 120 beats/min, respiration 25 breaths/min. Apart from the skin lesions, some minimally enlarged axillary and cervical nodes, and scarred tympanic membranes, the remainder of his examination was unrevealing. His upper airway and lower respiratory tract were normal as were his ophthalmologic exam results. He had no organomegaly and his cardiovascular, abdominal, genitourinary, locomotor, and neurologic systems were intact.

His laboratory studies were as follows: hemoglobin 114 g/L, hematocrit 34%, white blood cell (WBC) count

Table 21-4. The Granulocyte Membrane Selectin and
Integrin Families°

Integrin Family

p150,95 (CD-11c and CD-18) via their α_x- and β_2-integrins
bind to p150,95 counter receptors on endothelial cells
LFA-1 (CD-11a and CD-18) via their α_L- and β_2-integrins
bind to complementary ICAM-2 (CD-54) endothelial receptors
MAC-1 (CD-11b and CD-18) via their α_M- and β_2-integrin
bind to complementary ICAM-1 (CD-54) endothelial receptors
β_2 integrins, when activated, bind to opsonized bacteria

Selectin Family

LAM-1 attaches to its counter receptor on endothelial cells
ELAM-1 and GMP-140 counter receptors on granulocytes
interact with corresponding antigens on endothelial cells
GMP-140 is also present on platelets

°ICAM, intracellular adhesion molecule; ELAM, endothelial leukocyte
adhesion molecule; GMP, granule membrane protein; LAM, lectin adhesion molecule.

*5 × 10⁹/L with an ANC of 1 × 10⁹/L. The remaining cells
included 79% lymphocytes, 14% monocytes, 5%
eosinophils, and 1% basophils. His reticulocyte count
was 0.2% and his platelets numbered 150 × 10⁹/L. There
were no untoward appearing cellular elements on the peripheral smear. Urinalysis results were also normal.*

*The examiner believed that the neutropenia did not
represent a malignant process, but knowing that a monocytosis in concert with the history of frequent past infections suggested that granulocytes were about to appear,
she was concerned about the reticulocytopenia and the
low normal platelet count. A marrow aspirate and
biopsy revealed normal cellularity and a large number of
rapidly ripening granulocytes, that is, from promyelocytes to metamyelocytes with somewhat fewer band
forms and polymorphonuclear leukocytes. Both red cell
and platelet precursor activity was brisk.*

*Serum immunoglobulins and blood cultures drawn at
the initial contact were normal and unrevealing, respectively. A needle aspirate of one the papules grew out
Staphylococcus aureus, and appropriate antibiotic coverage was initiated.*

*According to familial history, the boy's mother's
brother had numerous bouts of skin infections during his
childhood that were severely disabling, and at age 10
years he died of an overwhelming "blood infection." The
subsequent arrival of the patient's prior medical records
added further revelations. On the few occasions when
blood counts were obtained at times of infections, his
white cell count was always low and marked by severe
neutropenia. Reticulocyte and platelet determinations
had not been carried out in the past.*

It appears that this may have been a case of **Cyclic
Neutropenia,** *and plans were made to follow the boy's
course over several months, during which time he did,
indeed, have cyclical production of granulocytes and*

*monocytes as well as marrow aspirates that showed ei-
ther no granulocytes and many monocytes or granulocytic recovery with few monocytes.*

The nature of this condition and the approach to therapy would best be served by assessing the nature of other
neutropenic conditions.

Intrinsic Quantitative Defects

Chronic Idiopathic Neutropenia proably represents a
group of disorders of varied clinical expression and inheritance that appear at or shortly after birth. This group
bears only marginal resemblance to the case in point.
The condition described in case 1 is milder, although
there is also an associated monocytosis at times of low
granulocyte levels. It is not a preleukemic stage, and in
some cases it disappears with age. It has no known associated immune system abnormalities. An autosomal pattern of inheritance has been described in Yemenite Jews
and in other scattered groups. The appearance of the
marrow varies within and among groups. In general,
there is a modest maturation arrest at almost any place
along the granulocytic series. Symptoms, which are rarely
serious, vary in accordance with the number of circulating neutrophils. Corticosteroids may have benefit in any
of the patients so afflicted, but with the exception of the
severe cases, the risks far outweigh the benefits. Individuals with severe symptoms should be evaluated for one
of the more severe neutropenic disorders and receive cytokine therapy whenever stem cell regulatory therapy appears to be indicated. Even in the chronic idiopathic
group, there are cases serious enough to benefit from cytokine therapy (26–29).

A neutropenic disorder of consanguinous marriage that
is common in the Amish population is **Cartilage Hair
Hypoplasia.** In addition to neutropenia, features common
to this disorder include fine hair, dwarfism, and, occasionally, defects in cellular immunity (30). For severely involved patients, the treatment of choice is allogenic bone
marrow transplantation (BMT). *Neither of the above examples relates to the nature of the process in case 1.*

Dyskeratosis Congenita is an X-linked inherited disease characterized by leukoplakia, hyperpigmentation, and
nail dystrophy. Serious infections are uncommon and related
immunologic abnormalities have not been described. Of the
approximately 50% of these patients who have modest neutropenia, half develop panhypoplasia leading to irreversible
aplasia, which is best treated by allogeneic BMT (31).

Myelokathexis is a lysosomal abnormality that leads to
impaired neutrophil production. It is characterized by distinctive granulocyte abnormalities consisting of cytoplasmic vacuoles and thin, filamentous nuclear lobar connec-
tions. Significant intraluminal neutrophil death is present
in an otherwise hyperplastic marrow. There is one report
of an associated hypo-γ-globulinemia with an effective response to rhG-CSF, but there are insufficient cases overall
upon which to identify an inheritance pattern (32).

Neutropenia with Immunoglobulin Defects is a disorder with abundant bone marrow precursors but little

postmyelocytic maturation and an associated type 1 dys-γ-globulinemia. Whether this is one disease or a complex of diseases is unclear because 30% of the patients with **X-Linked A-γ-globulinemia** experience neutropenia during the course of their illnesses. To confound matters, **Type 1 Dys-γ-globulinemia** may be associated with cyclic or persistent neutropenia. In the very serious forms, the only effective approach is allogenic bone BMT (33, 34).

None of the last three disorders is reminiscent of the findings in case 1.

Reticular Dysgenesis is an autosomal recessive disorder characterized by severe neutropenia and lymphopenia, arising from both thymus and marrow. The striking pathologic feature is the virtual absence of lymphoid follicles. Without BMT, it is rapidly fatal; the chances of living beyond 5 months are remote (35).

Its very nature clearly precludes it from consideration in the diagnosis of the case in question.

Shwachman Syndrome is an early onset, autosomal recessive disease involving many organs and characterized by dwarfism, metaphyseal chondrodysplasia, pancreatic insufficiency, neutropenia, and, to varying extent, diarrhea, weight loss, otitis media, eczema, and pneumonia. In all cases, there is a modest granulocytic hypoplasia; in approximately one fourth of the cases, bone marrow aplasia; and, on rare occasions, leukemic transformation. The neutropenia responds to the administration of rhG-CSF, and BMT has also been shown to be successful in otherwise uncontrollable patients in this group (36, 37).

The features of Shwachman syndrome do not fit the pattern of case 1.

Ineffective Granulopoiesis with resultant neutropenia is commonly seen in **nutritional disorders,** and specifically deficiencies of either/and **folic acid and vitamin B$_{12}$,** or both. **Starvation** and **alcoholism** and even **copper deficiency** may also cause neutropenia (38, 39).

Our patient was neither nutritionally deficient nor alcoholic.

The **Chediak-Higashi Syndrome (CH),** and its closely related disorder, **Specific Granulocyte Deficiency (SGD),** in addition to the associated anomalies in granule formation along with a predilection for leukemia, are characterized both by ineffective granulopoiesis and neutropenia (40). As shown in table 21.5, both of these disorders exhibit qualitative as well as quantitative abnormalities.

Neither CH nor SGD is consistent with the process that occurred in the propositus.

Isovaleric, propionic, and Methylmalonic Acid Hyperglycinemia, Type IB Glycogen Storage Disease, and Barth Syndrome are among a variety of metabolic disorders that lead to neutropenia. These disorders are inherited as autosomal recessive, and apart from correcting the underlying event, the only known effective therapy is the use of G-CSF (41–43).

There was no evidence in this patient to support a metabolic insult.

Extrinsic Quantitative Defects

Immune Neutropenia may present as **Isoimmune Neonatal Neutropenia** or a later occurring **Autoimmune Neutropenia.** In both instances marrow neu-

Table 21-5. Phagocyte Granule Defects: Chediak-Higashi and Specific Granule Deficiency Disease

Inheritance	Clinicopathologic Data	Therapy
Chediak-Higashi (CH) autosomal recessive	Misshapen, large granules (Also present in platelets, lymphocytes, melanocytes) Loss of cathepsin G, elastase Decreased platelet ADP and serotonin Impaired NK cell cytotoxicity Defective chemotaxis Impaired bacterial killing O$_2^-$ production normal Albinism Late-appearing lymphoproliferative disorders Death following infection	Trimethoprim-sulfamethoxazole or appropriate substitute Allogenic BMT is treatment of choice for severe disease
Specific Granule Deficiency (SGD) Autosomal recessive Acquired Neonates Burn patients	Bilobed nuclei often Loss of specific granules Absent B$_{12}$-binding protein, lactoferrin, cytochrome B alkaline phosphatase, gelatinase, CD-11/CD-18, FMPL receptors Abnormal chemotaxis Depressed bacterial killing O$_2^-$ production normal Patients rarely are mortally ill	Broad-spectrum antibiotics Allogeneic BMT is treatment of choice for severe disease

trophilic precursors are increased, and there is an associated monocytosis. The isoimmune abnormality is the result of the transfer of a maternally derived (IgG) antibody. The disease lasts from a few to as many as 12 weeks with serious infections attendant upon the degree of neutrophil depression. The majority of patients, however, recover without untoward sequelae. The neutropenia is the result of circulating neutrophil-specific agglutinating antibodies, identified by both direct and indirect immunofluorescent assays specific for subclasses of Ig. Among known underlying associations with autoimmune neutropenia are many of the connective tissue disorders, including Sjögren syndrome, Wegener granulomatosis, rheumatoid arthritis, systemic lupus erythematosus (SLE), chronic hepatitis, angioimmunoblastic lymphadenopathy, and Felty syndrome. It has been described following both autologous and allogenic BMT and after multiple whole blood transfusions. The underlying mechanisms are probably similar to those responsible for autoimmune anemias and thrombocytopenias. Only modest therapeutic success has been obtained with steroid administration. Other approaches include the use of intravenous γ-globulin (IVIG) and plasma exchange (44–58).

Vascular Trapping, most commonly in the spleen and often associated with neoplastic or infectious splenomegaly, is yet another known extrinsic cause of neutropenia.

Drug-Induced Neutropenia is typically idiosyncratic, the result either of marrow suppression and/or peripheral destruction; and for reasons that are unclear, occurs more commonly in women and in older persons. Included among the frequently incriminated agents are chloramphenicol, sulfonamides, antithyroid drugs, antipyretics, levamisole, phenylbutazone, phenothiazides, and various sedatives. A likely causative event is an adverse pharmacokinetic response, precipitated by host failure to detoxify any of the aforementioned agents. This process, in turn leads to an untoward immune response characterized by the development of a drug (innocent protein) complex or a hapten-like mechanism that directly targets neutrophils (59–64).

The commonest agranulocytic disorder in childhood is **Infection-Induced Neutropenia,** probably the result of ongoing viral replication in human endothelial cells, which, in turn, initiates an immune complex process, IgG plus C′, characterized by neutrophil adhesion to endothelium. The subsequent loss of circulating neutrophils, as in the CH syndrome, is an example of a combined defect. Parvovirus may directly effect a marrow shutdown leading to pancytopenia. The same applies to committed granulocyte precursors suppressed by bacteria and bacteria-like organisms, such as rickettsia, brucella, typhoid, paratyphoid, pasteurella, and tubercle bacilli, all via unknown mechanisms (65–68).

This group of disorders was not operative in case 1.

In reviewing all of the above, it is apparent that the patient had **Cyclic Neutropenia,** an autosomal recessive disorder of fairly consistent 21 day ANC peaks and troughs. Whether this disease is truly a cyclical neutropenia or more appropriately a cyclical hematocytopenia is worthy of consideration because of the knowledge that reticulocytes as well as platelets tend to follow the same sine wave typical of the granulocytes. Moreover, not all patients cycle every 21 days; some are intermittent, and not all disorders are manifest in the neonatal period. Some actually appear as late as the third decade.

The correlation between infection and low ANC is striking. Most of the infections are nosocomial, usually staphylococcal, invariably involving the skin, and are variable in intensity and duration in accordance with the severity and duration of the ANC depression. Although this disorder tends to be moderate in expression, on rare occasion the infection may be fulminant. Fatal outcome is rare today, but even in the recent past as many as 10% of cases experienced fatal outcome secondary to uncontrolled infections (69–71).

The precise nature of the underlying defect in cyclic neutropenia is not known; but it clearly involves inhibition at the stem cell level either by (poorly understood) fluctuations in thymidine phosphate, which, when elevated, inhibits ribonucleoside reductase and impedes cell production or fluctuations in differentiation factors. Knowledge of the pathogenetic mechanisms involving cyclical changes in cytokines (which control and/or direct hematopoietic stem cell production) has enhanced the efficacious use of combination antibiotics and rhG-CSF, thereby lessening the duration as well as the severity of the neutrophil nadir. Corticosteroids, androgenic steroids, epinephrine, lithium, and splenectomy or combinations of the above offer little of therapeutic value. There is also the occasional report of cyclic neutropenia in the presence of either a T- or B-cell abnormality, which may mandate more extensive biologic intervention, including the use of cytokines, antibiotics, infusions of γ-globulin and human recombinant γ-interferon (rhγIFn) (72–76).

Case 2

A 2-year-old white girl was referred to the infectious disease clinic to evaluate recurrent skin infections and a more recent respiratory illness characterized by cough and fever.

She was the product of a full-term, uncomplicated pregnancy and delivery. Both of her parents were well, and the mother received comprehensive prenatal medical attention. Shortly after delivery, the baby's umbilicus was noted to be erythematous and purulent. Streptococcus epidermidis was cultured from the wound, and long-term, broad-spectrum antibiotic usage was required in order to contain and ultimately eliminate its spread. Over the ensuing 2 years, the girl had numerous outbreaks of furuncles, purulent otitides, two severe respiratory infections, and two urinary tract infections. All responded, albeit very slowly, to the administration of broad-spectrum antibiotics. With rare exception, the infections were the result of S. aureus.

On examination, the girl was a thin, irritable, febrile child in the third percentile for length and weight. Her vital signs included a temperature of 39.8°C, with tachypnea and tachycardia. Her skin was replete with numerous healed scars, her tympanic membranes were sclerotic, and she had bilateral basilar rales with slight nasal flaring.

Her laboratory studies included a hemoglobin of 87 g/dL, WBC count of 13.8 × 10⁹/L with 73% lymhocytes, 19% monocytes, 3% eosinophiles, 1% basophils, and 4% myelocytes. She had a 1% reticulocyte count with hypochromic red cells and adequate numbers of platelets on smear. A bone marrow aspirate and biopsy carried out primarily to determine the reason for the lack of mature neutrophils revealed a granulocyte maturation arrest at the level of the promyelocyte/early myelocyte. Chest films supported the clinical impression of bilateral middle and lower interstitial pneumonitis.

The pathologic findings were clearly related to the clinical presentation, that is lack of circulating neutrophils because of maturation failure at the promyelocyte/myelocyte level leading to recurrent bacterial infections. The only unexplained factor was the underlying mechanism.

Case 2 has the features of Kostmann syndrome (KS). Had Case 1 presented in the same manner as this case, for more aggressive therapy would have been initiated.

Kostmann Syndrome is a (historically) lethal disorder characterized by failure of granulocytes to mature. Patients with this disease rarely have an ANC in excess of 2×10^9/L, despite the presence of adequate marrow precursors (77). Common presentations include fever, skin infections, perianal abscess formation, aphthous stomatitis, septicemia, meningitis, and peritonitis. The organisms most commonly involved in these complications include *Escherichia coli*, *S. aureus*, and *Pseudomonas aeruginosa*.

KS is characterized by a developmental defect occurring at the promyelocyte/early myelocyte level. Of note is the fact that Kostmann cells in culture do not suffer from a defect in phagocytosis (78–80). G-CSF added to granulocyte-monocyte marrow cultures obtained from patients with this syndrome affects normal granulocyte maturation, whereas the combination of IL-3 with GM-CSF enhances colony differentiation essentially into monocytes and eosinophiels. When stem cell factor (SCF) and G-CSF are added in culture, the results mimic those obtained with G-CSF and normal controls. The fact that G-CSF receptors on the surface of monocytes and neutrophils from KS patients are identical to those of normal controls points to a fundamental defect in G-CSF signal transduction, the result in most cases of an inherited defect in the intracytoplasmic signal transduction domain of the G-CSF receptor. Application of in vitro to in vivo studies supports the efficacy of

G-CSF over GM-CSF, with an acceptable therapeutic response in a daily dose range from 5–60 µg/kg. Prior to effective use of cytokine therapy, the treatment of choice was allogeneic BMT, which is now best reserved for those who respond poorly to cytokines. A major concern in patients with severe congenital neutropenia who respond well to recombinant G-CSF is the increased risk of the development of **Myelodysplasia** and/or **Acute Myelocytic Leukemia.** In a recent survey of 300 such patients, 11 were found to have either leukemia or preleukemic conditions; of these, 9 had a clonal deletion of chromosome 7, and 6 of the patients expressed the anomalous RAS protooncogene RNA. The malignant clones were not G-CSF dependent; it appears, therefore, that the abnormal myeloid progenitor is susceptible to malignant change in a manner similar to other progenitor diseases such as **Fanconi Anemia** and the **Shwachman-Diamond syndrome** (81–89).

Table 21.6 is a compendium of intrinsic and extrinsic quantitive defects of neutrophils.

Qualitative Inborn and Acquired Neutrophil Disorders

Defects in Chemotaxis and Phagocytosis

Case 3

A 9-year-old white boy, whose family lived in a small, rural mining community for many generations, was re-

Table 21-6. Extrinsic and Intrinsic Quantative Neutrophil Defects

Extrinsic
   Alcohol excess
   Drug induced
   Hypersplenism
   Infection
   Isoimmune and autoimmune neutropenia
   Nutritional deficiencies: folate, B_{12}, copper
   Radiation injury
   Vascular trapping

Intrinsic
   Barth syndrome
   Cartilage hair hypoplasia
   Chediak-Higashi syndrome
   Chronic idiopathic leukopenia
   Cyclic neutropenia
   Dyskeratosis congenita
   Glycogen storage disease, type 1B
   Hyperglycemia group
   Kostmann disease
   Leukemia
   Myelokathexis
   Neutropenia with B- or T-cell defects
   Reticular dysgenesis
   Shwachman syndrome

ferred for evaluation of repeated episodes of skin, oral, and gingival infections, often superficial, but sometimes penetrating (and on one occasion, systemic). His parents noted that, unlike their other three children (two males and one female), his umbilical cord dislodged slowly and was foul smelling and he needed extensive antibiotic usage. The only suggestive family information retelated to a maternal uncle who died in early childhood of an overwhelming infection, type unknown.

S. aureus, less frequently E. coli and P. aeruginosa, were the most commonly cultured skin infectious agents in this child. Numerous courses of antibiotics cleared up the infections but failed to effect any noticeable reduction in their frequency. Prophylactic antibiotics were not helpful. His physical examination revealed a chronically ill-appearing boy with normal vital signs. The only untoward physical findings included numerous healed skin infections as well as acute and chronic gingival disease. Initial laboratory data revealed a hemoglobin of 122 g/dL, a hematocrit of 37%, WBC count of $16 \times 10^9/L$ with 70% normal-appearing neutrophils and 12% band forms. Numerous cultures at multiple sites failed to reveal a consistent infective agent. A chest film appeared normal, and there was no indication to look for radio logic evidence of disease in any other site.

The elevated neutrophil count, along with a history of repeated infections, prompted a search for immune deficiency disorders, namely **Hypo-γ-globulinemia, A-γ-globulinemia, T-Cell Abnormalities, Hypocomplementemia,** or any of the functional granulocyte disorders, such as **Nuetrophil-Specific Granule Deficiencies (SGD)** or **Chediak-Higashi Syndrome** (90, 91).

*Serum γ-globulin levels were normal as were T- and B-cell subset and performance. SGD and CH syndrome were ruled out by the presence of normal-appearing granulocytes under light and ultramicroscopy, along with normal levels of neutrophil lactoferrin, vitamin B_{12}-binding protein, alkaline phosphatase, etc., and the absence of any of their respective clinical and/or hematologic stigmata. The possibility that this represented **Hyperimmunoglobulin E (Job Syndrome)** was quashed when IgE levels were shown to be normal.* In this disease, patients are highly susceptible to recurrent staphylococcal skin and lower respiratory tract infections, which often lead to chronic pruritic dermatitis and pneumatocele, respectively (92).

This patient did not have recurrent pneumonias, and serum complement levels, including C3, the protein precursor of C3b/C3bi that assists in phagocytic clearing of bacterial infections, were also normal (93).

The possibility that the child had the **Lazy Leukocyte Syndrome** is probably immaterial, because the disease likely represents a number of dysfunctional chemotactic disorders; and as more information accumulates on the molecular biology of neutrophils, this group may well be categorized according to defect specificity.

The next question concerned the possibility of an intrinsic defect in the ability of the leukocytes to interact with other leukocytes or with endothelial cells, that is the **Leukocyte Adhesion Deficiency Syndrome (LAD)**

(94). In this group of diseases, which are characterized by severe skin and gingival infections, granulocytes fail to accumulate at infectious sites irrespective of the numbers in the circulation. The process is readily demonstrable via the **Rebuck Skin Window,** or skin abrasion site (95).

This disorder occurs with different degrees of severity and involves a group of adhesion-promoting cell surface glycoproteins, known as β_2-integrins, the amount of which appears to correlate directly with the severity of the syndrome. A severe clinical phenotype is present when <0.5% of the β_2-integrins are present. Conversely, fewer symptoms are present when the adhesion-promoting glycoproteins are somewhere between 3% and 5% of normal.

The Rebuck skin window test, when carried out as prescribed (at 4 hours and again at 24 hours), failed to demonstrate the presence of neutrophils, thereby supporting the diagnosis of LAD. Of note also is the finding that the neutrophils in this patient failed to elicit oxidative bursts.

The leukocyte adhesion (LA) complex is best represented by the CD11b/CD18 glycoprotein, or the α-subunit of the β_2-integrin family (96). These integrins, which are present and active in the neonatal period along with certain of the immunoglobulins, interact in a cell/cell-cell/matrix fashion in order to maintain the adherence chemotaxis and phagocytic integrity of the granulocyte. The entire granulocyte adhesion complex is essential for interaction with endothelial cells, other neutrophils, and platelets, as well as a variety of adhesion molecules, cytokines (including IL-1), tumor necrosis factor (TNF), interferon-γ, lipopolysaccharides, and granulocyte membrane proteins.

The LA complex, which also involves certain of the clotting cascade factors (fibrinogen and factor X), is composed of a number of heterodimeric glycoproteins, each of which consists of an α-subunit linked to a β-subunit, the former variable and thus capable of conferring specificity (97–101). Adhesion, marginating, and aggregating proteins are not confined to these classes but also include LECAMS (leukocytic endothelial cell adhesion molecules) (102), ICAMS (intracellular adhesion molecules) (103), and laminin receptors (table 21.4) (104). Stimulation of neutrophils or other leukocytes in vitro increases the level of many such receptors, a situation which is presumably mirrored in vivo (96). Absence of these receptors leads to poor neutrophil-dependent defence because the first step in recruitment, i.e., adherence to local blood vessels, is ineffective.

A presumptive diagnosis is confirmed when the suspect neutrophils have neither surface adherence nor respond with oxidative bursts in the presence of serum-opsonized particles. In such individuals the membrane glycoprotein is missing or markedly reduced (99).

Of the four families of leukocyte integrins, the molecular defect in the child in case 3 involved the three members of the β_2-integrin family (CD18).

The subunits of leukocyte integrins bind directly to the cytoskeleton actin filaments using cytoskeleton-associated protein mediator attachments (105). Of note is the fact that macrophages, granulocytes, and natural killer (NK) cells express the β_2-integrins, whereas T- and B-lymphocytes express only (the internationally designated nomenclature) CD-11a/CD-18 antigen, also known as the leukocyte function related antigen (LFRJ-1) (106). In brief, the mechanism for **Leukocyte Adherence Deficiency** involves failure of mediation by integrins and selectins relative to the granulocyte attachment to endothelial and epithelial cells (107). The β_2-subunit integrins, which bind to their counterparts in endothelial cells, also include ICAM-1(CD54) and ICAM-2, members of immunoglobulin superfamily (ICAM is the intracellular adhesion molecule-1). The MAC-1 granulocyte component of the integrins is the receptor for C3bi opsonized microbes. Other factors that play a role in adherence of granulocytes to endothelium include three lectin proteins of the selectin family, (GMP-140, ELAM-1). LAM-1 (lectin adhesion molecule), ELAM-1 (endothelial leukocyte adhesion molecule), and GMP-140 (the 140-kd granulocyte membrane protein) (108–111).

Although the Rebuck window supports the diagnosis of LAD, it is limited solely to evaluating granulocyte migration. A more precise diagnosis requires the use of flow cytometry with monospecific antibodies directed against the surface expression of any of the β_2-integrin subunits (101). In the absence of flow cytometry, the diagnosis can be strongly suspected by the use of in vitro phagocytic assays designed to demonstrate adherence (97), chemotaxis (101), C3bi-mediated ingestion (108), and cytotoxicity (112).

Had the patient been younger and/or more severely infected, bone marrow transplantation would have been recommended as the treatment of choice. In view of the fact that this autosomal recessive disease belongs to a group of disorders caused by a number of potentially identifiable gene defects, the possibility exists that future therapy may incorporate gene replacement modalities (113).

The fact that this disease is not a **Neutrophil Actin Dysfunction (NAD)** disorder is in part because of the age of the patient (114). NAD is a very rare disorder involving a filamentous defect, which is present at infancy and results in early death. Impaired neutrophil actin impedes chemotaxis, as demonstrated by abnormal WBC polymerization when exposed to 0.6 M potassium chloride (115). Its unique features separate it from subsets of LAD. However, any newborn with severe limitation in phagocytic chemotaxis and ingestion, that is, the result of either LAD or NAD, should be prepared for allogenic BMT, which is the only currently viable therapeutic option.

A number of chemotactic disorders considered along with NAD include defects in the generation of chemotactic agents, namely **deficiencies of C1, C2, C3, and C4.** Deficiencies of C1, C2, and C4 are not associated with readily apparent problems, because the alternate complement pathway is still intact. Deficiency of C3 can be a problem, because it is the precursor of C3b and

C3bi, the complement opsonins that play a major role in oxidative bursts and chemotaxis. Patients with C3 deficiency require aggressive antibacterial therapy in combination with fresh (complement-rich) plasma in order to order to control routine infections from becoming fulminantly invasive.

Case 4

A 15-year-old, rural-dwelling white boy was examined by his physician following the sudden onset of high fever and chills. His past history included occasional eruptions of furuncles, which resolved slowly and only with prolonged antimicrobial therapy. As a toddler and on into his school years, he experienced frequent episodes of otitis media treated with prolonged courses of antibiotics and then subsequently with tympanostomy tubes. He was a shy child and spent much of his free time hiking through the valleys or splitting wood from fallen trees. His family history was unremarkable except for the death of a paternal aunt at 10 years of age following an acute infection of unknown etiology. His mother and father were well, and he had three normal sisters.

On examination, he appeared to be a well-nourished but chronically ill teenager with a fever (39.5°C), tachypnea, and tachycardia (without murmur). His skin revealed some scarring secondary to old furuncles. The only other significant findings were fine crepitant rales over the right lower lung field. A complete blood count revealed granulocytosis with a left shift (16 × 10⁹/L with an ANC of 12 × 10⁹/L). Platelet numbers as well as red cell and white cell morphology were normal. Chest films confirmed a right lower lobe consolidation. Blood and sputum cultures obtained prior to the onset of broad-spectrum antibacterial therapy and cultured on agar were unrevealing. His clinical course, as well as his chest films, worsened over the ensuing 2 days, whereupon a lung computerized tomography (CT) scan revealed a cystic-appearing mass with questionable early liquefaction. A change in antibiotic coverage was ineffective. Bronchoalveolar lavage carried out on day 4, failed to yield material from the distal bronchi, and skin tests for tuberculosis and Candida remained negative in the presence of appropriate controls. Reviews of the CT scan uncovered a small 3-mm opaque lesion in the upper right lobe of the liver that escaped observation at the initial evaluation and that when coupled with the cystic and suggestively granulomatous appearance of the lung lesion, supported the likely possibility of ineffective phagocytosis. On the following day, neutrophil and monocyte assays for glucose-6-phosphate dehydrogenase (G-6-PD), myeloperoxidase, glutathione peroxidase, glutathione reductase, and glutathione synthetase, as well as nitroblue tetrazolium (NBT) were performed.

The enzyme assays involve timed substrate-enzyme assays. In the NBT procedure, the oxidized form of nitroblue tetrazolium, a yellow soluble material that, when reduced by the release of superoxide electrons, crystallizes as deep purple-colored precipitates in cells undergoing respiratory burst activity.

There were neither pre- nor poststimulatory differences in the NBT tests, that is, no respiratory burst activity, which, in effect, supported the presumptive diagnosis of **Chronic Granulomatous Disease (CGD).**

An open right lung biopsy revealed a noncaseating granuloma that stained positive for budding yeast and mycelia on a trichrome/Gomori stain, and that cultured positive for Aspergillus fumigatus on Sabourraud media. Amphotericin and γ-interferon were added to the therapeutic regimen. Concern was expressed that the delay in initiating specific therapy would result in failure; but the patient improved dramatically, and after 5 weeks was discharged from the hospital with minimal pulmonary scarification and no evidence of the lesion in the liver.

When the boy's parents and three sisters were tested for NBT responsiveness, minimal levels were identified in both parents and in one of his three sisters; the other two sister's neutrophils had unequivocally normal activity. It was thus apparent that the autosomal recessive condition arose from two carrier parents, one of whom provided the gene for the single carrier sibling. It was also likely that the paternal aunt was a victim of this disorder either in its full-blown recessive expression or as a heterozygote with moderately impaired oxidative function.

The alacrity with which the infection responded once appropriate anti-infective therapy was initiated supports the therapeutic approach that includes antifungal agents, even in the absence of demonstrably involved sites when all appropriate cultures are organism-free in both known or suspected immunocompromised hosts. A review of the molecular biology and clinical relationships in this disorder will help the physician appreciate the nature of the process in this child, which was presumably initiated by fungal spores released during the process of cutting the limbs of dead wood infested with *Aspergillus*.

Chronic Granulomatous Disease occurs as either X-linked or autosomal recessive at a frequency of approximately 1:250,000 individuals with symptoms that range from mild to fulminant (116). The most vulnerable sites of infection are skin, gastrointestinal tract, respiratory passages, bones, and lymphatics. The commonest offending agents commencing with *Staphylococcus*, are *Aspergillus*, *Serratia*, *Salmonella*, and *Pseudomonas* (117–119). In known cases, failure to identify a bacterial organism in appropriate cultures strongly supports the likelihood that it is initiated by yeast or fungi. Not all microbial agents result in disease in CGD patients because of the inherent property of many organisms to undergo self-destruction following ingestion (120).

The granuloma formation in CGD represents an abortive attempt to defending against the lack of adequate granulocyte killing. In effect, a chronic cell/cell inflammatory reaction involving lymphocytes and macrophages produces the characteristic CGD granuloma, which slows a process that may otherwise be fulminant. In this patient, a slow "abscess" developed and remained asymptomatic until autolysis and

liquefaction caused pyrogen release. It is important to note that granuloma formation may also cause severe complications, including skip lesions throughout the entire gastrointestinal tract as well as the genitourinary system and, less commonly, the central nervous system (121, 122).

For reasons that are unclear, some of these patients, including carriers, develop a discoid, or even a blatant, form of SLE. The lupus appearance is virtually restricted to the X-linked carrier. The fact that the disease may begin in infancy, may be fulminant in some patients, may be relatively mild and only rarely express severe infections in yet others, or may not be apparent before the late teen or early adult years, supports its heterogenous nature (123, 124).

With the development of cell free systems capable of testing a variety of enzymatic activities, four different forms of CGD have been identified (125). In the normal individual the oxidative pathway follows a seemingly orderly fashion of reactions, beginning with the conversion of molecular oxygen to superoxide and thence to hydrogen peroxide, hypochlorous acid, and, finally, hydroxy radicals (126). With only little available mitochondria, normal phagocytes consume very small amounts of oxygen, with anaerobic glycolysis serving as the primary source of energy at rest. However, once "opsonized," infective agents are ingested, the energy burst shifts to an oxidative form of metabolism initiated by NADP oxidase, one of the heme-flavo enzymes (127). Table 21.7 outlines the nature of the oxidative burst process.

Phagocyte-initiated killing involves endogenously derived killing mechanisms, such as lysozymes, cathepsins, and lactoferrins, which do not have the capacity to destroy (the previously described) organisms that are unendowed with self-kill mechanisms (120), and which, therefore, require oxidative burst derivatives in order to complete the

Table 21-7. The Oxidative Burst Process

1. Initiation of **signal transduction (ST)** by foreign material
2. *ST initiates interaction of membrane (plasma) oxidases (gp91 and p22) with cytosol oxidases (p47 and p67) to form an active association in the presence of magnesium and GTP*
3. *Nascent O_2 formed by these reactions combines with NADPH to produce NADP and one molecule of H_2 which, in the presence of O_2, forms hydrogen peroxide (H_2O_2), hypochlorous acid (HOCl), and hydroxy radicals (OH −)*
4. The following enzymes play a major role in this process:
   - *NADPH oxidase converts NADPH to NADP, H_2 and nascent O_2*
   - *O_2 and H_2 are converted to H_2O_2 by superoxide dismutase*
   - *H_2O_2 is converted to HOCl by myeloperoxidase which simultaneously activates proteinase*
   - *H_2O_2 loses an electron and is converted to H_2O in the presence of GSH peroxidase and glutathione reductase*
   - *NADP gains an electron to form NADPH; and the cycle begins anew*

Oxidative burst does not occur in chronic granulomatous disease.

process of killing. There are six recognized oxidase subunits (126) (of which four are functionally essential [127]) designated by their biochemical and cellular origins. Because they are derived from phagocytes, they are identified by combining the first two letters of phagocyte and oxidase as *phox*, which is preceded by the molecular weights of their biochemical origins, that is, protein (P) or glycoprotein (GP). The various subunits are located in the plasma membrane (GP91-*phox* and P22-*phox*) or cytosol (P47-*phox* and P67-*phox*) (127). In addition, the cytosol of normal granulocytes contains several low molecular weight GTP-binding proteins within the ras p21 family—rac-1, rac-2, and rac-1A—that participate in the oxidative process along with the granulocyte membrane containing FAD component of oxidase, as illustrated in table 21.8 (128).

It is also important to note that, while oxidative metabolism is a potent killing mechanism, it is not without toxicity to surrounding tissues. Thus a series of supervening events are built into the entire process in order to maintain the integrity of the contiguous environment. In essence, antioxidant intervention is brought about both by endogenous and exogenous agents including enzymes such as superoxide dismutase, catalase, glutathione peroxidase, and nonenzymatic systems (e.g., α-tocopherol and ascorbic acid).

The underlying problem in this case involved ineffective NADPH oxidase as distinguished from other factors involved in the respiratory burst pathway, namely, myeloperoxidase, glutathione synthetase, glutathione reductase, glutathione peroxidase, and G-6-PD, all of which will be addressed subsequently (129–131).

Early on, it was difficult to determine why CGD occurred in various manifestations until two major processes were uncovered, namely that cytochrome b is not absent in all cases (132) (it is, in fact, present in the autosomal recessive form of CGD), and that both the membrane and cytosol participated in the catalytic process (133). In patients with normal levels of cytochrome b, the activity is found solely in the membranes, whereas patients who lack cytochrome b have solely cytosol activity. Cytochrome b consists of GP91-*phox* and P22-*phox* (134). P22-*phox* mutations apparently lead to the autosomal recessive form of the disorder, and mutations in GP91-*phox* lead to the

X-linked form of CGD. All known cases of CGD are seemingly attributable to abnormalities in the GP91-*phox*, P22-*phox*, P47-*phox*, or P67-*phox* (135, 136). Known mutations have been compiled (116).

Although further studies were not carried out in the propositus, it was assumed that he had a cytosolic CGD defect—in effect, an autosomal recessive disorder with its typically lesser severity.

An unusual mutation in GP91-*phox* gene merits particular attention. This X-linked CGD subtype includes the coinheritance of other X-linked diseases, for example, **Duchenne Muscular Dystrophy, Retinitis Pigmentosa,** and the **MacLeod Red Cell Disorder** (acanthocytic hemolytic anemia with low red blood cell antigen levels) (137).

The diagnosis of CGD is based on a combination of strong clinical evidence in association with a negative NBT test (138), with exceptions as noted. All studies should include family data, cytogenetics, measurements of respiratory burst activity, and flow cytometry (139, 140).

Once the diagnosis of CGD is made, prophylaxis and, when needed, aggressive therapy are mandated. Such activity includes administration of prophylactic trimethoprim sulfamethoxazole (TMZ), early use of parenteral antibiotics including antifungal drugs, surgical intervention as needed, and the use of recombinant human γ-interferon (γ-INf) (141). Granulocyte transfusions may have value if given daily and in sufficient quantities (which are virtually unattainable) (142). The best approach is attention to good hygiene, including appropriate, scheduled immunizations and dental care, careful attention to minor cuts and perianal cleanliness, as well as avoidance of constipation, abstinence from smoking cigarettes and marijuana, and avoidance of decaying plant material and mold ridden sites. Bone marrow transplantation is the treatment of choice for all patients with otherwise unmanageable disease (143).

Glucose 6-Phosphate Dehydrogenase (G-6-PD) Deficiency can cause a clinical picture similar to that seen in NADPH deficiency-induced CGD, because its absence results in diminished NADPH production and like its red cell counterpart, it is inherited as an X-linked recessive (144). G-6-PD assays should be carried out in patients presenting with recurrent infections similar to those identified in CGD. The treatment of neutrophil G-6-PD deficiency is essentially the same as that of CGD. That symptoms of neutrophil G-6-PD deficiency do not occur with the same frequency as those of red cell G-6-PD deficiency is based on the fact that severe depletion of neutrophil activity is required before the disease becomes manifest, which very likely accounts for the paucity of reported cases.

More common than CGD is **Myeloperoxidase (MPO) Deficiency** (145), with an incidence of 1:4,000 in its fully expressed form, and 1:2000 of the population in its partially expressed form. Unlike G-6-PD, it is inherited as an autosomal recessive, with the defect localized to the long arm of chromosome 17 (q22-q23) (146). MPO symptoms are generally mild because the respiratory burst in such in-

Table 21-8. The Biology of Chronic Granulomatous Disease

Source	M.W. Activity	Inheritance	Plasma	Cell Sol	NBT test
GP	91°*phox*	S	+		—
GP	91⁻ *phox*	S	+		✓
P	22° *phox*	A	+		—
P	22⁻ *phox*	S	+		—
P	47⁻ *phox*	A		+	—
P	67⁻ *phox*	A		+	—

GP, glycoprotein; P, protein; A, autosomal; S, somatic; (91, 22, 47, 67) MW, molecular weights (kd); *Phox*, phagocytic oxidase; °, normal protein concentration; —, decreased protein concentration.

dividuals tends to be more pronounced than it is in CGD, most likely the result of lesser impairment in production of hypochlorous acid (from chloride and hydrogen peroxide) and as a result a more stable NADPH oxidase system (147). Phagocytosis is unimpaired, but killing tends to be prolonged, particularly killing of *Candida* and *Aspergillus species;* but even in these latter instances, aggressive and prolonged therapy will bring about recovery (148).

Diseases resulting from the autosomal recessive inheritance of **Glutathione Peroxidase, Glutathione Synthetase,** and **Glutathione Reductase Deficiencies,** respectively, and from **Nutritional Selenium Deficiency,** are minimally severe and very rare. The gene for the reductase deficiency has been found at the p21.1 position of chromosome 8 (149). Patients with glutathione synthesis deficiency have elevated levels of 5-oxyproline (150), which produces an acidosis and a resultant mild neutropenia as well as hemolytic anemia (151). Vitamin E, selenium repletion, and riboflavin appear to be helpful in such individuals. In patients with glutathione peroxidase deficiency, concomitant CGD, heretofore undetected, may be the explanation for the symptoms (152, 153).

In order to engulf, ingest, and kill target organisms, neutrophils must be able to migrate to sites of inflammation. The cells migrate in the direction of a chemotactic gradient by the use of reciprocating gelling and dissolution mechanisms (Gelsolin), an ATP-consuming process (154). In this particular scenario, chemotaxis can be interrupted at multiple points, leading to increased susceptibility to infections caused by encapsulated organisms.

Case 5

A 22-year-old white woman was referred by the rheumatology group to the hematology division because of thrombocytopenia, anemia, and an incomplete heart block that did not require a pacemaker. She had earlier experienced fevers and episodes of small joint inflammation. Among the pertinent initial laboratory studies, she had an elevated erythrocyte sedimentation rate (ESR), both antinuclear and single-strand DNA antibodies, and anti-Smith antibodies, findings consistent with the diagnosis of SLE. Treatment consisted of the use of corticosteroids.

Her recent past history included the presence of staphylococcal skin infections that were slow to respond to antibiotics. At her last rheumatology outpatient visit, she appeared to be pale and had the following blood counts: hemoglobin 78 g/L, platelet count 80×10^9/L and WBC count 15×10^9/L without abnormal forms.

Physical examination revealed a pale young woman with moon-shaped facies and multiple skin ulcerations (some healing, others with minimal inflammation). Her interphalangeal joints were moderately inflamed, tender, and limited in range of motion. Her extremities were thin and her abdomen was protuberant.

Laboratory tests in the hematology clinic showed a WBC count of 13.5×10^9/L, with 45% neutrophils, 2% band forms, 42% lymphocytes 5%, monocytes, 4%

eosinophils, and numerous normoblasts (the corrected WBC was 8.5×10^9/L). In addition, her blood film revealed giant platelets and normal-appearing erythrocytes with polychromasia and a reticulocyte count of 6%. The neutrophils appeared to have normal granules and segmentation. Her indirect-reacting bilirubin was slightly elevated (4.0 mg/dL) along with a markedly decreased level of serum haptoglobin (10 mg/dL) and elevated amounts of serum "free" hemoglobin (15 mg/dL). Her bone marrow aspirate showed increased megakaryocytes and erythroid progenitors with normal myeloid numbers and maturation, which clearly ruled out the possibility of myelokathexis.

She had a minimal response to a Candida challenge. A Rebuck skin window showed very few granulocytes at 4 hours and a greater response at 24 hours. Buffy coat granulocytes exhibited both normal NBT test response and G-6-PD activity. There were no unusual immunophenotypes and T-cell cytotoxicity to allogeneic target cells was normal. Her nonalbino appearance and morphologically normal neutrophils ruled out the possibilities of CH syndrome or Pelger-Huet anomaly, respectively.

In order to test for disorders involved with ingestion and killing, washed neutrophils were incubated with Staphylococcus organisms and observed periodically: (a) ingestion was found to be rapid, (b) lysosome formation and degranulation progressed normally, and (c) organisms were readily digested. This test ruled out disorders of phagocytosis, for example, actin polymerization defects (155), granule content abnormalities, such as myeloperoxidase deficiency (144) and defensin deficiency (156). The experiment, when repeated with complement (C3bi)-coated polystyrene particles, showed normal engulfment, which, in turn, ruled out an LAD, for example, associated with deficiency of adherence glycoprotein CD11b/CD18. Immunophenotyping of neutrophils revealed normal levels of adhesion molecules, complement, and IgG-FC receptor (CD16) levels (157), although CD18b/CD11 levels were elevated during increased disease activity (158). When the test was repeated after stimulation with N-formylmethionineleucy-l-phenylalanine (NFMLP), a potent bacteria-derived stimulating factor, MAC-1 adhesion complex expression, was upregulated (as in normal neutrophils, thereby ruling out intracellular disorders of chemoattractant response). Because the Rebuck skin window demonstrated decreased chemotaxis in vivo, attention was turned to disorders of opsonization and chemotaxis.

Opsonins are proteins that attach to the target and allow the neutrophil to recognize and engulf it. Immunoglobulins of the G and A classes opsonize bacteria by presenting the FC domain to the phagocyte (159), which recognizes it via specific FC receptors. Other opsonins are complement fractions, especially C3bi. In the absence of immunoglobulins, or subclasses thereof, and in the absence of complement fractions, there is little opsonization.

Total IgG levels were elevated, but electrophoresis failed to uncover subclass deficiency. IgA levels were normal, which ruled out increased IgA-associated polymers with chemotactic inhibitory activity (160). Normal IgE activity ruled out a Job syndrome type of decreased chemotaxis, and levels of C3 and C5 were also normal.

The increased erythroid and megakaryocytic activity in the marrow, along with a positive direct Coombs test and antiplatelet antibody tests, supported intravascular destruction of red cells and platelets. The underlying condition, SLE, directed attention to the possibility of a chemotactic factor inactivator (CFI) (161), the presence of which was suspected because of the patient's nonresponse to the Candida antigen in the presence of normal T-cell activity.

One of the most potent chemotactic factors is the complement fraction, C5a. This chemoattractant becomes active in serum when coupled to a vitamin D-binding protein (162), and is rapidly converted in serum to C5arg by cleavage of arginine (163). Normal serum can generate the C5a fraction by exposure to zymosan particles (164) or *Candida* organisms. Inhibitors to C5a have been found both naturally and in association with various conditions such as leprosy and Hodgkin disease (165). Inhibitors to C5a are also found in normal human serum and synovial fluid (166) but are missing in serosal fluid from patients with familial polyserositis due to the action of a 55-kd protease (167). The absence of a chemotactic factor inhibitor (CFI) to C5a has been implicated in the increased levels of neutrophil migration into smokers' lungs (168). Nonsmokers' lungs have few, if any, neutrophils (169). CFI levels are depressed in bronchoalveolar lavage fluid of patients with adult respiratory distress syndrome (ARDS) (170), which suggests that C5a and its naturally occurring inhibitor(s) normally exist in a balanced state, thereby serving as a protective mechanism against untoward tissues invasion by phagocytes.

In this patient a CFI developed, which inhibited C5a-cochemotaxin activity, thereby abrogating chemotaxis and causing increased susceptibility to bacterial infections. In order to prove the presence and activity of the putative CFI, the Boyden chamber blind well method was employed (171).

The Boyden apparatus consists essentially of two chambers separated by a microfilter, typically of 3-μpore size. The bottom wells are filled with the chemoattractant, such as FMLP or zymosan-activated serum. Control samples consist of pooled serum or buffer. The top chamber is filled with the neutrophils (previously isolated from index and control blood by density centrifugation) and suspended in buffer. Following incubation, the filters are removed, stained with hematoxylin, and the trapped neutrophils are counted under the microscope. A chemotactic index (CI) is calculated wherein the numerator is the number of index (stimulated) counts, and the denominator is a random count without chemoattractant, as in buffer. The activity of a chemoattractant is expressed as the CI of attractant divided by CI of normal pooled serum. To test for the presence of CFI to C5a, index and control sera was

preconditioned by zymosan, (thereby generating C5a) and then inserted into the lower (blind well) chamber. Index and control neutrophils are inserted into the upper chamber. The presence of increased CFI is manifested by lower migration into the index filter.

The patient's serum demonstrated increased presence of CFI, affecting her own and control neutrophils, whereas her neutrophils, after isolation and washing, showed migratory function similar to those of controls. Once the CFI was proven to be present, its type remained to be determined.

The CFI, as described by Ayesh et al. (167) and Ward and Ozols (172), is a proteolytic inhibitor of C5a and IL-8. Yet another CFI has been described that exerts its action on the C5a cochemotaxin Gc-globulin (GcG) (173). To confirm these hypotheses, CFI, GcG, and C5a were purified by chromatographic methods, and specific antibodies raised against them. CFI, added to a chemotaxis assay with C5a, decreased the chemotactic index by 50%. Free GcG reversed this inhibition by binding to CFI. This binding was found to be specific for CFI in studies where radiolabeled CFI was incubated with GcG followed by exposure to anti-GcG antibodies covalently linked to Sephadex beads. The beads were centrifuged and CFI detected by scintillation counting. On the other hand, C5a serum depleted of GcG had a lower chemotactic index than GcG-replete serum. CFI added to GcG-depleted C5a-rich serum did not inhibit chemotaxis, but in the presence of GcG it did inhibit neutrophil migration.

An aliquot of the patient's serum was subjected to GcG depletion. The procedure did not increase chemotaxis. With the use of same methods, CFI depletion did not change the chemotactic inhibition displayed in the patient's serum. This ruled out the presence of a GcG-binding CFI. Recombinant IL-8 was used as a chemoattractant with the patient's serum and compared with purified C5a. The patient's serum showed CFI activity to C5a but not to IL-8, whereas control serum augmented chemotactic capacity in the presence of C5a and IL-8. It was thus apparent from this experiment that the patient's CFI was not a protease.

The presence of IgG antibodies to red cells and platelets supported the likelihood of an anti-C5a IgG antibody acting as a CFI. Goat antihuman C5a was coupled to Sepharose beads and incubated with both patient and control sera. The beads were centrifuged and resuspended, and radio-labeled rabbit anti-human FC was incubated with the beads. After centrifugation and washing, the beads were subjected to scitillation counting. The experiment showed that human IgG was attached to C5a in the patient's serum, whereas there was no such attachment in control serum. Finally, the patient's serum depleted of native C5a (and therefore specific anti-C5a antibody) and reconstituted with purified C5a was able to regain chemotactic capacity.

In conclusion, a patient with SLE developed multiple autoantibodies directed against red cells, platelets, and the chemotactic fraction of complement C5a, which, in turn, impeded neutrophil migration to sites of inflammation

Table 21.9. Inherited (I) and Acquired (A) Qualitative Neutrophil Defects

Adhesion

Drug- and disease-induced adhesion deficiencies (A)
Leukocyte actin deficiency (I)
Leukocyte adhesion deficiency (I)

Degranulation

Chediak-Higashi disease (I)
Specific granule deficiency disease (I)

Ingestion

Complement deficiency group: ↑ destruction, ↓ production (I)
Leukocyte adhesion deficiency (I)

Metabolism

Chronic granulomatous disease (I)
Disorders of glutathione metabolism (I)
Glucose-6-phosphate dehydrogenase deficiency (I)
Myeloperoxidase deficiency (I)
Selenium deficiency (A)

Motility

Prematurity (A)
89-kd protein deficiency (I)
Job (hyperimmunoglobulin E) syndrome (I)
Chemotactic factor inhibitor disease (A)

with resultant development of delayed hypersensitivity reactions.

Table 21.9 lists the inherited and acquired disorders of chemotaxis and phagocytosis.

Treatment modalities for this disorder include the use of intravenous IgG, plasmapheresis, and immunosuppressive drugs, any or all of which may provide moderate to complete symptomatic relief.

In this case, the disorder was still ongoing 2 years later but controlled with combination of all of the above.

Other acquired, albeit self-limiting, disorders of migration and phagocytosis are mostly iatrogenic and usually follow upon the use of myeloablative therapy for bone marrow transplantation. Such occurrences are discussed in the section on bone marrow transplantation.

Conclusion

When one considers the array of potentially adverse disease entities brought about by any one of a number of inherited disorders, it is to our everlasting good fortune that the vast biochemical complex within the confines of the granulocyte is so finely honed and surprisigly free of frequent and severe malfunctioning. It is also important to note, in this context, that many of the acquired qualitative and quantitative disorders are self-limited and/or readily controlled with appropriately utilized cytokine and/or anti-infective therapies.

REFERENCES

1. Orfanakis NG, et al. Normal blood leukocyte concentration values. Am J Clin Pathol 1970;54:647.
2. Shaper AG, Lewis P. Genetic neutropenia in people of African origin. Lancet 1971;2:1021.
3. Woodliff HJ, et al. Normal laboratory values for differential white cell counts established by normal and automated cytochemical methods (Hemalog DTM). Lancet 1972;2:875.
4. Xanthou M. Leucocyte blood picture in healthy full-term and premature babies during neonatal period. Arch Dis Child 1970;45:242.
5. Hasdahl H, Larsen JF. Hemopoiesis and blood vessels in human yolk sac: an electron microscopic study. Acta Anat (Basel) 1971;78:274.
6. Dommergues M, Aubeny E, Dumez Y, Durandy A, Coulombel L. Hematopoiesis in the human yolk sac: quantitation of erythroid and granulopoietic progenitors between 3.5 and 8 weeks of development. Bone Marrow Transplant 1992;(Suppl 1):23.
7. Mawas F, Weiner E, Ryan G, Sootholl PW, Rodeck CH. The expression of IgG Fc receptors on circulating leukocytes in the fetus and newborn. Transfus Med 1994;4(1):25.
8. Clapp DW, Baley JE, Gerson SL. Gestational age–dependent changes in circulating hematopoietic stem cells in newborn infants. J Lab Clin Med 1989;113(4):422.
9. Dos Santos C, Davidson D. Neutrophil chemotaxis to leukotriene B4 in vitro is decreased in the human neonate. Pediatr Res 1993;33:242.
10. Pharr PN, Hankins D, Hofbauer A, Lodish HF, Longmore GD. Expression of a constitutively active erythropoietic receptor in primary hematopoietic progenitors abrogates erythropoietic dependence and enhances erythroid colony-forming unit, erythroid burst-forming unit, and granulocyte/macrophage progenitor growth. Proc Natl Acad Sci USA 1993;90:938.
11. Ward CS, Westwood NB, Emmerson AJ, Pearson TC. The in vitro effect of high-dose recombinant human erythropoietin on granulocyte-macrophage colony production in premature infants using a defined serum deprived cell culture system. Br J Haematol 1992;81:467.
12. Mizuno S, Sasaki C, Kono H, Kojima S. Effect of recombinant human erythropoietic administration on peripheral blood neutrophil counts of premature infants. J Pediatr 1994;124:467.
13. Christensen RD, Rothstein G. Exhaustion of mature marrow neutrophils in neonates with sepsis. J Pediatr 1980;96:316.
14. Christensen RD, McFarlan JL, Taylor NL. Blood and bone marrow neutrophils during experimental group β streptococcal infection: quantification of the stem cell proliferation, storage and circulating pools. Pediatr Res 1982;16:549.
15. Gillan EF, Christensen RD, Suen Y et al. A randomized, placebo-controlled trial of recombinant human granulocyte colony-stimulating factor administration in newborn infants with presumed sepsis: significant induction of peripheral and bone marrow neutrophilia. Blood 1994;84:1427.
16. Warner HR, Athens JW. An analysis of granulocyte kinetics in blood and bone marrow. Ann NY Acad Sci 1964;113:523.

17. Athens JW, Haab OP, Raab SO. Leukokinetic studies. IV: the fetal blood, circulating and marginal pools, and the granulocyte turnover rate in normal subjects. J Clin Invest 1961;40:989.

18. Bainton DF, Ullyot JL, Farquhar MG. The development of neutrophilic polymorphonuclear leukocytes in human bone marrow: origin and content of azurophil and specific granules. J Exp Med 1979;134:907.

19. Weiss J, Victor M, Elsbach P. Role of charge and hydrophobic interactions in the action of the bactericidal/permeability-increasing protein of neutrophils on Gram-negative bacteria. J Clin Invest 1983;71:540.

20. Falloon J, Gallin JI. Neutrophil granules in health and disease. J Allergy Clin Immunol 1986;77:653.

21. Murphy G, Ward R, Hembry RM et al. Characterization of gelatinase from pig polymorphonuclear leucocytes: a metalloproteinase resembling tumour type IV collagenase. Biochem J 1989;258:463.

22. Packman CH, Lichtman MA. Activation of neutrophils: measurement of actin conformational changes by flow cytometry. Blood Cells 1990;16:193.

23. Junk LK. Association of aberrant F-actin formation with defective leukocyte chemotaxis and recurrent pyoderma. Clin Immunol Immunopathol 1991;61:41.

24. Krensky AM, Sanchez-Madrid F, Robbins E et al. The functional significance, distribution and structure of LFA-1, LFA-2, and LFA-3 cell surface antigens associated with CTL-target interactions. J Immunol 1983;131:611.

25. Mantovani B. Different roles of IgG and complement receptors in phagocytosis by polymorphonuclear leukocytes. J Immunol 1975:115:15.

26. Logue GL, Shastri KA, Laughlin M, Shimm DS, Ziolkowski LM, Iglehart JL. Idiopathic neutropenia: antineutrophil antibodies and clinical correlations. Am J Med 1991;90:211.

27. Weingarten MA, Pottick-Schwartz EA, Brauner A. The epidemiology of benign leukopenia in Yemenite Jews. Israel J Med Sci 1993;29:297.

28. Furukawa T, Takahashi M, Moriyama Y et al. Successful treatment of chronic idiopathic neutropenia using recombinant granulocyte colony-stimulating factor. Ann Hematol 1991;62:22.

29. Jakubowski AA, Souza L, et al. Effects of human granulocyte colony stimulating factor in a patient with idiopathic neutropenia. N Engl J Med 1989;320:38.

30. Makitie O, Rajantie J, Kaitila I. Anaemia and macrocytosis—unrecognized features in cartilage-hair hypoplasis. Acta Paediatr 1992;81:1026.

31. Putterman C, Safadi R, Zlotogora J, Banura R, Eldor A. Treatment of the hematological manifestations of dyskeratosis congenita. Ann Hematol 1993;66:209.

32. Bohinjec J. Myelokathexis: chronic neutropenia with hyperplastic bone marrow and hypersegmented neutrophils in two siblings. Blood 1981;42:191.

33. Kozlowski C, Evena DI. Neutropenia associated with X-linked agammaglobulinaemia. J Clin Pathol 1991;44:388.

34. Benkerrou M, Gougeon ML, Griscelli C, Fischer A. Hypogammaglobulimemia G and A with hypergammaglobulinemia M. Arch Fr Pediatr 1990;47:345.

35. Azcona C, Alzina V, Barona P, Sierrasesumaga L, Villa-Elizaga I. Use of recombinant human granulocyte-macrophage colony stimulating factor in an infant with reticular dysgenesis. Eur J Pediatr 1994;153:164.

36. Grill J, Bernaudin F, Lemerle S, Reinert P. Treatment of neutropenia in Shwachman's syndrome with granu-locyte growth factor (G-CSF). Arch Fr Pediatr 1993;50:331.

37. Barrios N, Kirkpatrick D, Regueira O et al. Bone marrow transplant in Shwachman Diamond syndrome. Br J Haematol 1991;79:337.

38. Beck WS, Ferry-Judith A. Case records of the Massachusetts General Hospital: weekly clinicopathological exercises: a 68-year-old man with recurrent fever and diarrhea after treatment for lymphoma. Case 51:1991. N Engl J Med 1991;325:1791.

39. Botash AS, Nasca J, Dubowy R, Weinberger HL, Oliphant M. Zinc-induced copper deficiency in an infant. Am J Dis Child 1992;146:709.

40. Zhao H, Boissy YL, Abdel-Malek Z et al. On the analysis of the pathophysiology of Chediak-Higashi syndrome: defects expressed by cultured melanocytes. Lab Invest 1994;71:25.

41. Hou JW, Wang TR. Isovaleric academia: report of one case. Acta Paediatr Sinica 1990;31:262.

42. Christodoulou J, McInnes RR, Jay V et al. Barth syndrome: clinical observations and genetic linkage studies. Am J Med Genet 1994;50:255.

43. Donadieu J, Bader-Meunier B, Bertrand Y et al. Recombinant human G-CSF (Lenograstim) for infectious complications in glycogen storage disease type Ib: report of 7 cases. Nouv Rev Fr Hematol 1994;35:529.

44. Huizinga TW, Kuijpers RW, Kleijer M et al. Maternal genomic neutrophil FcRIII deficiency leading to neonatal isoimmune neutropenia. Blood 1990;76:1927.

45. Shastro KA, Logue GL. Autoimmune neutropenia. Blood 1993 81:1984.

46. Neglia JP, Watterson J, Clay M et al. Autoimmune neutropenia of infancy and early childhood. Pediatr Hematol Oncol 1993;10:369.

47. Hartman KR. Anti-neutrophil antibodies of the immunoglobulin M class in autoimmune neutropenia. Am J Med Sci 1994;208:102.

48. Hartman KR, LaRussa VF, Rothwell SW et al. Antibodies to myeloid precursor cells in autoimmune neutropenia. Blood 1994;84:625.

49. Mascarin M, Ventura A. Anti-Rh(D) immunoglobulin for autoimmune neutropenia of infancy. Acta Paediatr 1993;82:142.

50. Ramakrishma R, Choudhuri K, Sturgess A, Manoharan A. Haematological manifestations of primary Sjögren's syndrome: a clinicopathological study. Q J Med 1992;82:547.

51. Keeling DM, Isenberg DA. Haematological manifestations of systemic lupus erythematosus. Blood Rev 1993;7:199.

52. Boxer LA, Yokoyama M, Wiebe RA. Autoimmune neutropenia associated with chronic active hepatitis. Am J Med 1972;52:229.

53. Carrington PA, Anderson H, Harris M et al. Autoimmune cytopenias in Castleman's disease. Am J Clin Pathol 1990;94:101.

54. Wandt H, Seifert M, Falge C, Gallmier WM. Long-term correction of neutropenia in Felty's syndrome with granulocyte colony-stimulating factor. Ann Hematol 1993;66:265.

55. Klump TR, Herman JH. Autoimmune neutropenia after bone marrow transplantation. Blood 1993;82:1035.

56. Klump TR, Herman JH, Macdonald JS et al. Autoimmune neutropenia following peripheral blood stem cell transplantation. Am J Hematol 1992;41:215.

57. Hisatomi K, Isomura T, Hirano A et al. Postoperative erythroderma after cardiac operations: the possible role of de-

pressed cell-mediated immunity. J Thorac Cardiovasc Surg 1992;194:648.

58. Calderwood S, Blanchette V, Doyle J et al. Idiopathic thrombocytopenia and neutropenia in childhood. Am J Pediatr Hematol Oncol 1994;16:95.

59. Stroncek DF. Drug-induced immune neutropenia. Transfus Med Rev 1993;7:268.

60. Durosinmi MA, Ajayi AA. A prospective study of chloramphenicol induced aplastic anaemia in Nigerians. Trop Geogr Med 1993;45:159.

61. Meyer-Gessner M, Benker G, Lederbogen S, Olbricht T, Reinwein D. Antithyroid drug-induced agranulocytosis: clinical experience with ten patients treated at one institution and review of the literature. J Endocrinol Invest 1994; 17:29.

62. Palcoux JB, Niaudet P, Goumy P. Side effects of levamisole in children with nephrosis. Pediatr Nephrol 1994; 8:263.

63. Strom BL, Carson JL, Schinnar R et al. Nonsteroidal antiinflammatory drugs and neutropenia. Arch Int Med 1993; 153:2119.

64. Moeller GH, Barver DL. Neutropenia in a patient receiving clozapine. Am J Psychiatry 1994;151:619.

65. Stark JM, van Egmond AW, Zimmerman JJ, Carabell SK, Tosi MF. Detection of enhanced neutrophil adhesion to parainfluenza-infected airway epithelial cells using a modified myeloperoxidase assay in a microtiter format. J Virol Methods 1992;40:225.

66. McClain K, Estrov Z, Chen H, Mahoney DH Jr. Chronic neutropenia of childhood: frequent association with parvovirus infection and correlations with bone marrow culture studies. Br J Haematol 1993;85:57.

67. Sporn LA, Lawrence SO, Silverman DJ, Marder VJ. E-selectin-dependent neutrophil adhesion to Rickettsia rickettsii-infected endothelial cells. Blood 1993;81:2406.

68. Etheredge EE, Spitzer JA. Chronic endotoxemia reversibly alters respiratory burst activity of circulating neutrophils. J Surg Res 1993;55:261.

69. Palmer SE, Dale DC, Livingston RJ, Wijsman EM, Stephens K. Autosomal dominant cycline hematopoiesis: exclusion of linkage to the major hematopoietic regulatory gene cluster on chromosome 5. Hum Genet 1994; 93(2):195.

70. Birgins HS, Karle H. Reversible adult-onset cyclic haematopoiesis with a cycle length of 100 days. Br J Haematol 1993; 83:181.

71. Dale DC, Bonilla MA, Davis MW et al. A randomized control phase III trial of recombinant human granulocyte conoly-stimulating factor (filgrastim) for treatment of severe chronic neutropenia. Blood 1993;81:2496.

72. Dinauer MC. Leukocyte function and nonmalignant leukocyte disorders. Curr Opin Pediatr 1993;5:80.

73. Yujiri T, Shinohara K, Kurimoto F. Fluctuations in serum cytokine levels in the patient with cyclic neutropenia. Am J Hematol 39:144.

74. Dale DC, Hammon WP. Cyclic neutropenia: a clinical review. Blood Rev 1988;2:1.

75. Ferrero D, Pregno P, Omeme P et al. Cyclic neutropenia and severe hypogammaglobulinemia in a patient with excess of CD-8-positive T lympocytes: response to G-CSF therapy. Haematology 1993;78:49.

76. Roilides E, Pizzo PA. Modulation of host defenses by cytokines: evolving adjuncts in prevention and treatment of serious infections in immunocompromised hosts. Clin Infect Dis 1992;15:508.

77. Kostmann RO. Infantile genetic agranulocytosis. Acta Paediatr 1956;105:1.

78. Kostmann, R. Infantile genetic agranulocytosis: a review with presentation of ten new cases. Acta Pediat Scand 1975;64:362.

79. Barak Y, Paran M, Levin S, Sachs L. In vitro induction of myeloid proliferation and maturation in infantile genetic agranulocytosis. Blood 1971;38:74.

80. Roseler J, Emmendorffer A, Elsner J et al. In vitro functions of neutrophils induced by treatment with rhG-CSF in severe congenital neutropenia. Eur J Haematol 1991; 46:112.

81. Welte K, Zeidler C, Reiter A et al. Differential effects of granulocyte-macrophage colony-stimulating factor and granulocyte colony-stimulating factor in children with severe congenital neutropenia. Blood 1990;75:1056.

82. Miyachi H, Nakamura Y, Shimizu H et al. Differential effects of IL-3, GM-CSF and G-CSF in an adult with congenital neutropenia. Int J Hematol 1992;56:113.

83. Hestdal K, Welte K, Lie SO et al. Severe congenital neutropenia: abnormal growth and differentiation of myeloid progenitors to granulocyte colony-stimulating factor (G-CSF) but normal response to G-CSF plus stem cell factor. Blood 1993;82:2991.

84. Guba SC, Sartor CA, Hutchinson R, Boxer LA, Emerson SG. Granulocyte colony-stimulating factor (G-CSF) production and G-CSF receptor structure in patients with congenital neutropenia. Blood 1994;83:1486.

85. Bernhardt TM, Burchardt ER, Welte K. Assessment of G-CSF and GM-CSF mRNA expression in peripheral blood mononuclear cells from patients with severe congenital neutropenia and in human myeloid leukemic cell lines. Exp Hematol 1993;21:163.

86. Elsner J, Roesler J, Emmendorffer A, Lohmann-Matthes ML, Welte K. Abnormal regulation in the signal transduction in neutrophils from patients with severe congenital neutropenia: relation of impaired mobilization of cytosolic free calcium to altered chemotaxis, superoxide anion generation and F-actin content. Exp Hematol 1993;21:38.

87. Welte K, Zeidler C, Reiter A, Riehm H. Effects of granulocyte colony-stimulating factor in children with severe neutropenia. Acta Haematol Pol 1994;25(suppl 1):155.

88. Rappeport JM, Parkman R, Newburger P. Camitta BM, Chusid MJ. Correction of infantile agranulocytosis (Kostmann's syndrome) by allogeneic bone marrow transplantation. Am J Med 1980;68:605.

89. Kalra R, Dale D, Freedman M et al. Monosomy 7 and activating RAS mutations accompany malignant transformation in patients with congenital neutropenia, with recombinant human granulocyte colony stimulating factor. Blood 1994 (suppl 1); (abs):313a.

90. Fernandez-Sola J, Monforte R, Ponz E et al. Persistent low C3 levels associated with meningococcal meningitis and membranoproliferative glomerulonephritis. Am J Nephrol 1990;110:426.

91. Sato A. Chediak and Higashi disease: probable identity of a new leukocytal abnormality: (Chediak) and congenital gigantism of peroxidase granules (Higashi). J Exp Med 1955; 61:201.

92. Jeppson JD, Jaffe HS, Hill HR. Use of recombinant human interferon gamma to enhance neutrophil chemotactic responses in Job syndrome (hyperimmunoglublinemia E) and recurrent infections. J Pediatr 1991;118:383.

93. Bilsland CA, Diamond MS, Springer TA. The leukocyte integrin p150,95 (CD11c/CD18) as a receptor for iC3b. Activation by a heterologous beta subunit and localization of a

ligand recognition site to the I domain. J Immunol 1994; 152:4582.

94. Arnaut MA. Structure and function of the leukocyte adhesion molecules CD11/CD18. Blood 1990;75:1037.

95. Rebuck JW, Crowley JH. A method of studying leukocyte functions in vivo. Ann NY Acad Sci 1955;59:757.

96. Detmers PA, Zhou D, Powell DE. Different signaling pathways for CD18-mediated adhesion and Fc-mediated phagocytosis. Response of neutrophils to LPS. J Immunol 1994;153:2137.

97. van Kessel KP, Park CT, Wright SD. A fluorescence microassay for the quantitation of integrin-mediated adhesion of neutrophil. J Immunol Methods 1994;172:25.

98. Au BT, Williams TJ, Collins PD. Zymosan-induced IL-8 release from human neutrophils involves activation via the CD11b/CD18 receptor and endogeneous platelet-activating factor as an autocrine modulator. J Immunol 1994;152:5411.

99. Lum H, Gibbs L, Lai L, Malik AB. CD18 integrin-dependent endothelial injury: effects of opsonized zymosan and phorbol ester activation. J Leukocyte Biol 1994;55:58.

100. Smith CW. Leukocyte-endothelial cell interactions. Semin Hemat 1993;30 (Suppl 4):45.

101. Bochsler PH, Neilsen NR, Slauson DO. Transendothelial migration of neonatal and adult bovine neutrophils in vitro. J Leukocyte Biol 1994;55:43.

102. Simon SI, Rochon YP, Lynam EB et al. Beta 2-integrin and l-selectin are obligatory receptors in neutrophil aggregation. Blood 1993;82:1097.

103. Altman LC, Ayars GH, Baker C, Luchtel DL. Cytokines and eosinophil-derived cationic proteins upregulate intercellular adhesion molecule-1 on human nasal epithelial cells. J Allergy Clin Immunol 1993;92:527–536.

104. Preciado-Patt L, Levartowsky D, Prass M et al. Inhibition of cell adhesion to glycoproteins of the extracellular matrix by peptides corresponding to serum amyloid A: toward understanding the physiological role of an enigmatic protein. Eur J Biochem 1994;223:35.

105. Pavalko FM, Otey CA. Role of adhesion molecules cytoplasmic domains in mediating intractions with the cytoskeleton. Proc Soc Exp Biol Med 1994;205:282.

106. Ginis I, Mentzer SJ, Faller DV. Oxygen tension regulates neutrophil adhesion to human endothelial cells via an LFA-1-dependent mechanism. J Cell Physiol 1993;157:569.

107. Erlandsen SL, Hasslen SR, Nelson RD. Detection and spatial distribution of the beta 2 integrin (Mac-1) and l-selectin (LECAM-1) adherence receptors on human neutrophils by high-resolution field emission SEM. J Histochem Cytochem 1993;41:327.

108. Scieszka JF, Maggiora LL, Wright SD, Cho MJ. Role of complements C3 and C5 in the phagocytosis of liposomes by human neutrophils. Pharmacol Res 1991;8:65.

109. Ohsaka A, Saionji K, Sato N et al. Granulocyte colony-stimulating factor down-regulates the surface expression of the human leukocyte adhesion molecule-1 on human neutrophils in vitro and in vivo. Brit J Haematol 1993; 84:574.

110. Hamburger SA, McEver RP. GMP-140 mediates adhesion of stimulated platelets to neutrophils. Blood 1990; 75:550.

111. Kansas GS, Muirhead MJ, Dailey MO. Expression of the CD11/18, leukocyte adhesion molecule 1 and CD44 adhesion molecules during normal myeloid and erythroid differentiation in humans. Blood 1990;76:2483.

112. Scollay R, Wilson A, D'Auico et al. Developmental status and reconstitution potential of subpopulation of immune phagocytes. Immunol Rev 1988;104:81.

113. LeDeist F, Blanche S, Keable H et al. Successful HLA nonidentical bone marrow transplantation in three patients with the leukocyte adhesion deficiency. Blood 1989; 74:512.

114. Roos D, Kuijpers TW, Mascart-Lemone F et al. A novel syndrome of severe neutrophil dysfunction:unresponsiveness confined to chemotaxin-induced functions. Blood 1993;81:2735.

115. Howard T, Li Y, Torres M, Guerrero A, Coates T. The 47-kD protein increased in neutrophil actin dysfunction with 47- and 89-kD protein abnormalities in lymphocyte specific protein. Blood 1994;83:231.

116. Roos A, De boer M, Kuribayashi F et al. Mutations in X-linked and autosomal recessive forms of chronic granulomatous disease. Blood 1996;87:1663.

117. Lacy DE, Spencer DA, Goldstein A, Weller PH, Darbyshire P. Chronic granulomatous disease presenting in childhood with pseudomonas cepacia septicaemia. J Infect 1993; 27:301.

118. Spencer DA, Darbyshire P. Resolution of hepatic abscess after interferon gamma in chronic granulomatous disease. Arch Dis Child 1994;70:856.

119. Spencer DA, John P, Ferryman SR, Weller PH, Darbyshire P. Successful treatment of invasive pulmonary aspergillosis in chronic granulomatous disease with orally administered itraconazole suspension. Am J Resp Crit Care Med 1994; 149:239.

120. Odell EW, Segal AW. Killing of pathogens associated with chronic granulomatous disease by the non-oxidative microbicidal mechanisms of human neutrophils. J Med Microbil 1991;34:129.

121. Smith FJ, Taves DH. Gastroduodenal involvement in chronic granulomatous disease of childhood. J Can Assoc Radiol 1992;43:215.

122. Dean AF, Janota I, Thrasher A, Robertson I, Mieli-Vergani G. Cerebral aspergilloma in a child with autosomal recessive chronic granulomatous disease. Arch Dis Child 1993; 68:412.

123. Yeaman GR, Froebel K, Galea G, Ormerod A, Urganiak SJ. Discoid lupus erythematosus in an X-linked cytochrome-positive carrier of chronic granulomatous disease. Br J Dermatol 1992;126:60.

124. Fischer A, Segal AW, Seger R, Weening RS. The management of chronic granulomatous disease. Eur J Pediatr 1993;152:896.

125. Gallin JI. Delineation of the phagocyte NADPH oxidase through studies of chronic granulomatous diseases of childhood. Int J Tissue React 1993;15:99.

126. Babior BM. The respiratory burst oxidase. Advances in enzymology and related areas of molecular biology: advances in enzymology of related areas of molecular biology. Biology 1992;65:49.

127. Dinauer MC. The respiratory burst oxidase and the molecular genetics of chronic granulomatous disease. Crit Rev Clin Lab Sci 1993;30:329.

128. El Benna J, Ruedi JM, Babior BM. Cytosolic guaninenucleotide binding protein Rac 2 operates in vivo as a compo-

nent of the neutrophil respiratory burst oxidase. J Biol Chem 1994;269:6729.

129. Quinn MT, Parkos CA, Walker L et al. Association of Ras related protein with cytochrome b of human neutrophils. Nature 1989;342:198.

130. Siflinger-Birnboim A, Malik AB. Neutrophil adhesion to endothelial cells impairs the effects of catalase and glutathione in preventing endothelial injury. J Cell Physiol 1993; 155:234.

131. Washko PW, Wang Y, Levine M. Ascorbic acid recycling in human neutrophils. J Biol Chem 1993;268:15531.

132. Rotrosen D, Yeung CL, Leto TL, Malect HL, Kwang CH. Cytochrome b558; the flavin binding component of the phagocyte NADPH oxidase. Science 1992;256:1459.

133. Heyworth PG, Curnutte JT, Nauseff WM. Neutrophil nicotineamide adenine dinucleotide phosphate oxidase assembly: translocation of p47 phox and p67 phox requires interaction between p47 phox and cytochrome b558. J Clin Invest 1991;87:352.

134. Parkos CA, Allan RA, Cochrane CG, Jesaitis AJ. Purified cytochrome b from human granulocyte plasma membrane is comprised of two polypeptides with relative molecular weights of 91,000 and 22,000. J Clin Invest 1987; 80:732.

135. Maly FE, Schuerer-Maly CC, Quilliam L et al. Restitution of superoxide generation in autosomal cytochrome-negative chronic granulomatous disease. J Exp Med 1993;178:2047.

136. Zhen L, King AA, Xiao Y et al. Gene targeting of X-chromosome-linked chronic granulomatous disease in human myeloid leukemia cell line and rescue by expression of recombinant gp91+.+phox−.− Proc Natl Acad Sci USA 1993; 90:9832.

137. Franke V, Ochs H, et al. Minor Xp21 chromosome deletion in a male associated with expression of Duchenne muscular dystrophy, chronic granulomatous disease, retinitis pigmentosa and McLeod syndrome. Am J Hum Genet 1985; 37:250.

138. Nathan DG, Baehner RL, Weaver DK. Failure of nitroblue tetrazolium reduction in the phagocytic vacuoles of leukocyts in chronic granulomatous disease. J Clin Invest 1969; 48:1895.

139. Kenney RT, Malech HL, Epstein ND, Roberts RL, Leto TL. Characterization of the p67+.+phox−.− gene, genomic organizational restriction fragment length polymorphism analysis for prenatal diagnosis in chronic granulomatous disease. Blood 1993;12:3739.

140. DeBoer M, Bolger BCJM, Sijmons RH et al. Prenatal diagnosis in a family with X-linked chronic granulomatous disease with the use of the polymerase chain reaction. Prenat Diagn 1992;12:773.

141. Curnutte, JT. Conventional versus interferon-gamma therapy in chronic granulomatous disease. J Infect Dis 1993; 1:S8.

142. Emmendorffer A, Logmann-Matthes ML, Roesler J. Kinetics of transfused neutrophils in peripheral blood and BAL fluid of a patient with variant X-linked chronic granulomatous disease. Eur J Haematol 1991;47:246.

143. Hobbs JR, Monteil M, McCluskey DR, Jurges E, el Tumi M. Chronic granulomatous disease 100% corrected by displacement bone marrow transplantation from a volunteer unrelated donor. Eur J Pediatr 1992;151:806.

144. Yeaman GR, Froebel K, Galea G, Ormerod A, Urbaniak SJ. Discoid lupus erythematosus in an X-linked cytochrome-positive carrier of chronic granulomatous disease. Br J Dermatol 126:60.

145. Kizaki M, Miller CW, Selsted ME, Koeffler HP. Myeloperoxidase (MPO) gene mutation in hereditary MPO deficiency. Blood 1994;82:1935.

146. Nauseef WM. Myeloperoxidase deficiency. Hematol Pathol 1990;4:165.

147. Chamulitrat W, Cohen MS, Masson RP. Free radical formation from organic hydroperoxides in isolated human polymorphonuclear neutrophils. Free Rad Biol Med 1991; 11:439.

148. Ludviksson BR, Thorarensen O, Gudnason T, Halldorsson S. Candida albicans meningitis in a child with myeloperoxidase deficiency. Pediatr Infect Dis J 1993;12:162.

149. McKusick VA. The human gene map. Clin Genet 1986; 29:545.

150. Jellum E, Kluge T, Boerassen HC. Pyroglutamic aciduria, a new inborn error of metabolism. Scand J Clin Lab Invest 1970;26:327.

151. Goebel KM, Goebel FD. Hemolytic anemia and pancytopenia in glutathione reductase deficiency: further experience with riboflavin. Acta Hematol 1972;47:292.

152. Bire JG, Corash L, Hubbard VS. Medical uses of vitamin E. N Engl J Med 1983;308:1063.

153. Cohen HJ, Chovaniec ME, Mistretta D, Baker SS. Selenium repletion and glutathione peroxidase-differential effects on plasma and red blood cell enzyme activity. Am J Clin Nutr 1985;41:735.

154. Wolach B, Baehner RL, Boxer LA. Review: clinical and laboratory approach to the management of neutrophil dysfunction. Israel J Med Sci 1982;18:897.

155. Roos D, Kuijpers TW, Mascart-Lemone F et al. A novel syndrome of severe neutrophil dysfunction: unresponsiveness confined to chemotaxin-induced functions. Blood 1993;81:2735.

156. Rice WG, et al. Defensin-rich dense granules in human neutrophils. Blood 1987;70:757.

157. Kew RR, Grimaldi Cm, Furie MB, Fleit HB. Human neutrophil gamma RIIIB and formyl peptide receptors are functionally linked during FMLP-induced chemotaxis. J Immunol 1992;149:989.

158. Molad Y, Buyon J, Anderson DC, Abramson SB, Cronstein BN. Intravascular neutrophil activation in systemic lupus erythematosus (SLE): dissociation between increased expression of CD11b/CD18 and diminished expression of l-selectin in neutrophil from patients with active SLE. Clin Immunol Immunopathol 1994;71:281.

159. Hostoffer RW, Krukovet I, Berger M. Increased Fc alfa R expression and IgA-mediated function on neutrophil induced by chemoattractants. J Immunol 1993; 150:4532.

160. Van Epps DE, Williams RC Jr. Suppression of leukocyte chemotaxis by human IgA myeloma components. J Exp Med 1976;144:1227.

161. Perez HD, Lipton M, Golstein M. A specific inhibitor of complement (C5) derived chemotactic activity in serum from patients with systemic lupus erythematosus. J Clin Invest 1978;62:29.

162. Perez HD, Kelly E, Chenoweth D, Elfman F. Identification of the C5a Des Arg cochemotaxin: homology with vitamin D-binding protein (group specific component globulin) J Clin Invest 1988;82:360.

163. Burgi B, Brunner T, Dahinden CA. The degradation product of anaphylatoxin C5a des arg retains basophil-activating properties. Eur J Immunol 1994;24:1583.

164. Kreutzer DL, O'Flaherty JD, Orr FW et al. Quantitative comparison of the various biological responses of neutrophils to different active and inactive chemotactic factors. Immunopharmacology 1979;1:39.

165. Ward PA, Berenberg JL. Defective regulation of inflammatory mediators in Hodgkin's disease: supernormal levels of chemotactic factor inactivator. N Engl J Med 1974;290:76.

166. Berenberg JL, Ward PA. Chemotactic factor inactivator in normal human serum. J Clin Invest 1973;58:129.

167. Ayesh SK, Azar Y, Babior BM, Matzner Y. Inactivation of interleukin-8 by the C5a inactivating protease from serosal fluid. Blood 1993;81:1424.

168. Robbins RA, Gossman GL, Nelson KG et al. Inactivation of chemotactic factor inhibitor by cigarette smoke: a potential mechanism of modulating neutrophil recruitment to the lung. Am Rev Resp Dis 1990;142:763.

169. Cooper JA Jr, Bridges TA, Kennedy JI Jr, Culbreth R. Alteration of cellular cytosolic calcium and chemotactic peptide binding by an inhibitor of neutrophil function. Am J Physiol 1994;267:71.

170. Robbins R, Maunder R, Gossman G et al. Functional loss of chemotactic factor inactivator in the adult respiratory distress syndrome. Am Rev Resp Dis 1990;141:1463.

171. Klempner MS, Noring R, Mier JW, Atkin MB. An acquired chemotactic defect in neutrophils from patients receiving interleukin-2 immunotherapy. N Engl J Med. 1990;322:959.

172. Ward FA, Ozols J. Characterization of the protease activity of the chemotactic factor inactivator. J Clin Invest 1976;58:123.

173. Robbins RA, Hamel FG. Chemotactic factor inactivator interaction with Gc-Globulin (vitamin-D binding protein): a mechanism of modulating the chemotatic activity of C5a. J Immunol 1990;144:2371.

CHAPTER 22

Monocytes, Macrophages, and Histiocytosis

MICHAEL J. JOYCE, PAUL A. PITEL

The disposal of microbes by phagocytes was not a simple affair. The microbes had to be "prepared" by some property of the blood before phagocytosis could take place. Wright gave the name "opsonic" to this property, from the Greek *opsono* meaning "I prepare victuals for."
—Almroth Wright, St. Mary's Medical School, London (1880)

In this chapter we will focus on the functions and disorders of the monocyte-macrophage system. This most primitive of cellular defense systems, formerly known as the reticuloendothelial system, includes the mononuclear cells of the bone marrow and circulating blood and free and fixed tissue macrophages. The monocyte-macrophage system is a central component of host immunity, participating in the processes of inflammation, antimicrobial killing, and cytokine secretion. The first part of the chapter will review monocyte-macrophage development, regulation, and functions in host immunity. The latter part of the chapter will be devoted to selected disorders of these cells.

Case 1

A 4-year-old African-American boy was brought to the emergency room with a 1-week history of fever as high as 39°C. The child had experienced decreased activity and appetite, weight loss, and night sweats. Physical examination revealed the following: bilateral shotty cervical lymphadenopathy, rales in both lung fields, and liver and spleen both palpable 2 cm below the costal margins. Laboratory studies included: hemoglobin 12.5 g/dl; white blood cell (WBC) count 11 × 10⁹/L; differential—50% neutrophils; 10% juvenile neutrophils; 20% monocytes; 20% lymphocytes; platelets 250 × 10⁹/L; electrolytes, normal; liver functions, normal. Chest x-ray revealed bilateral infiltrates (fig. 22.1). One month previously the child had been exposed to a relative with known tuberculosis. A first strength purified protein derivative (PPD) injected intradermally gave a 10-mm reaction after 48 hours. Culture of a gastric aspirate was positive for Mycobacterium tuberculi.

Commentary: The child's clinical presentation of fever, weight loss, and night sweats could be caused by a variety of systemic illnesses, including malignancies, infections, and collagen-vascular disorders. The presence of bilateral rales suggested the need for chest roentgenogram, with findings most compatible with an infectious process. The CBC and morphology were

within normal limits except for a monocytosis (normal <5%, or total monocyte count <0.5 × 10⁹/L). Further review of the child's medical history led to definitive intradermal skin testing and microbiologic culture results, establishing a diagnosis of pulmonary tuberculosis. A classic finding in active tuberculosis, monocytosis reflects the critical role of the monocyte-macrophage system in the immune system and the control and eradication of infectious organisms (1–4). From a conceptual viewpoint, this case raises at least three major issues. First, what is the etiology of the circulating and fixed cells of the monocyte-macrophage system? Second, what controls their number and location? Finally, what are their roles in the control of infections?

Monocyte Development and Regulation

The bone marrow is the chief, if not the only, source of monocytes and macrophages. Myelopoiesis begins with an extremely small number of marrow stem cells (probably <10⁶ cells) that undergo both self-renewal and differentiation to produce all subsequent hemic cells. Factors that influence the degree of self-renewal or the direction of differentiation include a variety of interleukins, colony-stimulating factors, and the local marrow hematopoietic microenvironment consistency of extracellular matrix proteins and other stromal elements. The daughter cells of the undifferentiated stem cells are capable of developing along any one of the hematopoietic lineages (fig. 22.2). Under the influence of microenvironmental and humoral factors, cells become further committed to specific cell lineages. The progenitor cell of the monocyte and granulocyte cell lines is the pluripotent colony-forming cell (CFC), which is capable of differentiation into the basophil, eosinophil, or granulocyte-macrophage lineage, depending upon the current mix of growth factors. Normally, most further differentiation is into the colony-

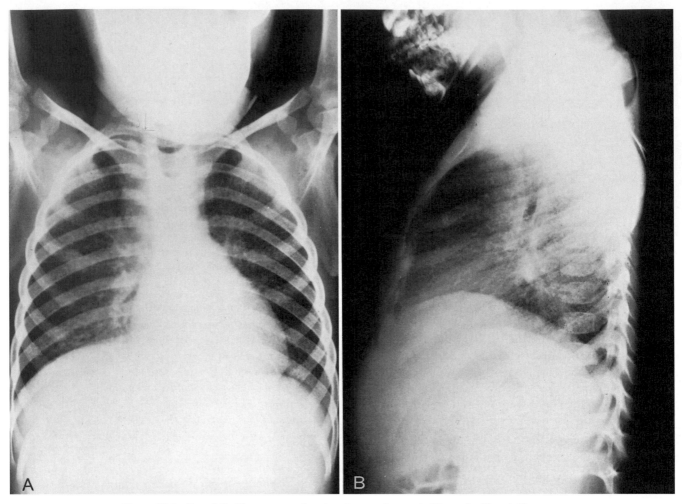

Figure 22.1. **A** and **B**. Chest x-ray of patient in case I reveals bilateral miliary infiltrates.

forming cells of the granulocyte-macrophage line—the CFC-GM (5–7).

These progenitor cells for the granulocyte-macrophage line were first identified in murine and then in human marrow lines. The CFC-GM has been detected in bone marrow, blood, spleen, and cord blood. Different colony assays for the progenitors of granulocytes, macrophages, eosinophils, basophils, and mast cells have been established (5).

Extensive research has focused on identifying and defining the roles played by a series of hemopoietic growth factors. These growth factors are proteins produced by a variety of cells, including T-cells, fibroblasts, endothelial cells, and monocyte-macrophages, and are categorized as erythropoietin, colony-stimulating factors, and interleukins. Among the better-defined factors are erythropoietin, interleukins (IL) 1–7, 9, and 11, and the colony-stimulating factors, granulocyte colony-stimulating factors, (G-CSF), granulocyte macrophage colony-stimulating factor (GM-CSF), and macrophage colony-stimulating factor (M-CSF). These factors are rarely lineage specific, usually influence several steps in hematopoiesis, and act in concert with multiple other factors (5, 8–10).

The terminal steps of monocyte-macrophage differential are under the control of IL-6, IL-3, GM-CSF, and M-CSF. Four cellular compartments of monocyte-macrophages are recognized: (a) the marrow mitotic compartment; (b) the marrow maturation-storage compartment; (c) the vascular (peripheral blood) compartment; and (d) the tissue compartment. Thus, during infections tissue macrophages engage the involving microorganisms and are stimulated to release cytokines such as IL-1, IL-6, and tumor necrosis factor (TNF) that activate T-cells and stromal cells to release further growth factors. These stimulate early marrow progenitor cells to divide and differentiate, myeloid cells are forced through the maturation pool, increased numbers of marrow storage cells are released, and circulating monocytes become capable of an enhanced respiratory burst (8, 11, 12).

Morphologically, the monoblast cannot be distinguished from the myeloblast by light microscopy. The promonocyte, which is 10–18 μm in diameter, is identifiable in blood and bone marrow. It has a well-developed Golgi apparatus and contains peroxidase-positive granules as well as nonspecific esterases. This cell is capable of endocytosis, but is poorly phagocytic. The monocyte has a diame-

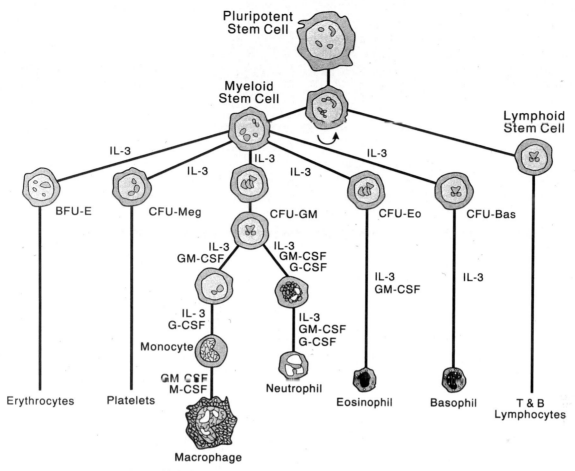

Figure 22.2. Hematopoiesis of monocytes from the pluripotent stem cell.

ter of 12–15 μm. The nucleus occupies half the cell, is eccentric in position, and is most often reniform in shape, but can be irregular or round. The cytoplasm is gray-blue with a variable number of faint azurophilic granules. As the monocyte matures into a macrophage, it increases in size until it is 25–50 μm in diameter. These cells have an eccentrically placed nucleus, with one or two distinct nuclei and finely dispersed nuclear chromatin. The cytoplasm shows fine granules and multiple azurophilic granules. The Golgi complex is well-defined as juxtapose clear zone. Concomitant with the maturation of the monocyte into a macrophage is an increase in the number of lysosomes and lysosomal enzymes. The diversity of lysosomal enzymes is appropriate for a cell whose functions include phagocytosis, microbial killing, catabolism, and removal of senescent blood cells (11, 13).

The monocyte-macrophage system differs in its kinetics from the granulocyte series. There is no substantial marrow storage pool, causing release into the peripheral blood several days earlier than marrow neutrophils. There is no significant peripheral blood marginated pool of monocytes, unlike that of neutrophils. The half-life of blood monocytes is 8 hours, after which the cells enter the tissues, where they differentiate into tissue macrophages (12, 14). Tissue macrophages are long-lived and remain in tissues for months performing the macrophage functions of

scavenging cellular debris and ingesting microorganisms.

The monocytes remain a numerically minor population in the peripheral blood. The average number of monocytes varies with the age of the patient and is greatest during the first 2 weeks of life, when the absolute monocyte count is more than 1000 cells/mm³. There is then a gradual decline in the monocyte count, which reaches a plateau of 400 cells/mm³ in adulthood. Monocytosis may be defined as an absolute monocyte count of >500 cells/mm³. After the newborn period, the differential count of monocyte is <5%. The number of fixed tissue macrophages is very difficult to estimate (12).

The cells of the tissue macrophage or histiocytic system can be further classified into two major subsets: antigen-processing or phagocytic cells and antigen-presenting or dendritic cells. Dendritic cells are essentially not phagocytic and act to present antigen to both T- and B-lymphocytes (15). Dendritic reticulum cells (DRCs) are found in lymph node follicles and present antigen to B-cells, while interdigitating reticulum cells (IRCs) and Langerhan cells (LC) present antigen to T-cells. LCs are found primarily in the skin and are rare in unstimulated lymph nodes but increase in certain reactive conditions. IRCs are prominent in the paracortex of lymph nodes.

All macrophages share many enzyme histochemical and immunophenotype characteristics. They have abundant lysosomal enzymes, including acid phosphatase and non-specific esterase. HLA-DR antigens and complement and Fc component of IgG receptors are present on cell surfaces. Thus, all are equipped for antigen recognition, and many have the capacity for phagocytosis and possible intracellular killing (8, 11).

Monocyte Function in Infection

Macrophages play important roles in the activation and effector phase of the immune response. Monocytes are antigen-presenting cells, capable of activating the humoral (B-cell) and cell-mediated (T-cell) responses. Macrophages can endocytose bacterial proteins, or soluble protein antigens, which become bound nonspecifically to surface molecules or to specific receptors on the macrophage surface. Once bound, the foreign protein is internalized by the process of phagocytosis or receptor-mediated endocytosis. The foreign antigen is then localized in intracellular membrane-bound vesicles known as endosomes, where it undergoes proteolysis and immunogenic peptides are formed. These peptides then bind to class II MHC molecules within the antigen-presenting cell. This process is thought to involve the fusion of endosomes with vesicles containing class II MHC molecules within the macrophage. Peptides that are not bound undergo further digestion. The complexes of peptides and class II molecules are then transported to and expressed

on the cell surface. This type of antigen processing is necessary for stimulation of helper T-cells to secrete a variety of cytokines, which magnifies the immune response (fig. 22.3). The binding of antigen-MHC related complexes to the T-cell receptor complex generates intracellular signals that result in the transcriptional activation of several genes that are quiescent in unactivated T-cells. T-cells proliferate due to the secretion of IL-2 and lymphotoxin. IL-2 simulates natural killer (NK) cells, T-lymphocytes, and B-lymphocytes. TNF and lymphotoxin activate neutrophils and endothelial cells. IL-5 activates eosinophils, while γ-interferon is a very potent activator of macrophages. Productions of IL-4 and IL-5 with IL-2 stimulates B-lymphocyte proliferation (8, 11, 16, 17).

Activated macrophages are functionally more efficient, and are the principal cells of cell-mediated immunity. γ-Interferon augments the process of phagocytosis and endocytosis and surface Fc receptors are increased, resulting in increased uptake of opsonized bacteria. The enzyme that generated the active oxygen species necessary for killing phagocytosed bacteria is also induced. Thus, one effect of macrophage activation is an increase in all processes involved in macrophage bacterial killing (8).

Activated macrophages stimulate acute inflammation through the secretion of inflammatory mediators, including platelet-activating factor, prostaglandins, leukotrienes, and tissue factor. TNF and IL-1 are secreted by activated macrophages, acutely augmenting the cell-mediated immunity response through their actions on T-cells, inflam-

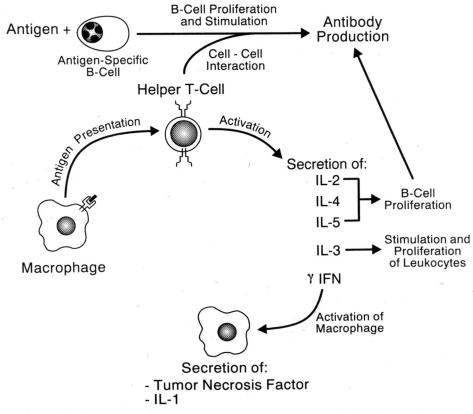

Figure 22.3. Interaction of the monocyte-macrophage system with T- and B-lymphocytes.

matory leukocytes, and endothelial cells (18, 19). The long-term effects of these cytokines is the stimulation of fibroblast and collagen formation. Platelet-derived growth factor and transforming growth factor β stimulate fibroblast proliferation and collagen production, respectively. In the setting of chronic antigenic stimulation, these secreted cytokines result in fibrosis. Thus, when elimination of the antigen is unsuccessful, fibrosis occurs (8).

Returning to consideration of case 1, the immune response to tuberculosis is the principal cause of tissue injury and disease. Intracellular bacteria such as mycobacteria are resistant to degradation and continue to replicate within the host cells. This resistance to phagocytic killing is the reason such bacteria cause chronic infections that are difficult to eradicate. The protein antigens of mycobacteria stimulate strong T-cell responses, resulting in macrophage production and activation. Muramyl dipeptide present in the cell walls of mycobacteria also directly activates macrophages. The chronic antigenic stimulation results in the formation of the granulomas, which are the hallmark of tuberculosis (8).

A granuloma is a compact, organized collection of macrophages. Initial T-cell activation results in the recruitment of polymorphonuclear leukocytes and mononuclear phagocytes. Resistant mycobacteria proliferate intracellularly and kill the phagocytic cells. With time, mononuclear cells predominate the inflammatory infiltrate and continued recruitment of monocytes occurs from the circulation. The mononuclear cells aggregate into loose sheets of cells and then into spherical aggregate. The monocytes assume an epithelioid appearance characterized by close packing of cells without interposed connective tissue. Hydrolytic enzymes released from living and dead macrophages and cytotoxic substances released from activated lymphocytes cause the necrosis termed "caseation," due to its appearance resembling crumbly cheese. This necrosis, which occurs 4 to 6 weeks after initial infection, causes local acidosis and hypoxia that inhibit the rapid proliferation of bacilli. After formation, a granuloma may follow one of several courses. If the number of bacilli continues decreasing, a fibrous capsule forms and the encapsulated granuloma become quiescent. After several years, the organisms may completely disappear. If the organisms are not eradicated, the granuloma may continue to enlarge and satellite granulomas form. The center of the caseous granuloma may liquify, permitting rapid extracellular growth and dissemination of disease (20).

Given the widespread roles of the monocyte in the immune system as well as the range of cytokines affecting monocyte production, it is not surprising that a variety of disorders are associated with monocytosis (table 22.1). Monocytosis is most typically associated with bacterial, protozoal, and rickettsial infections such as subacute bacterial endocarditis, tuberculosis, syphilis, Rocky Mountain spotted fever, and kala-azar (1, 21, 22). It may be prominent in malignant disorders such as acute myelomonocytic leukemia, chronic myelogenous leukemia, and a variety of

Table 22.1. Diseases associated with Monocytosis and Monocytopenia

Monocytosis
  Reactive monocytosis
    Infection
    Tuberculosis
    Syphilis
    Protozoal and rickettsial infection
    Tisteria
    Fever of unknown origin
    Collagen vascular disease
    Systemic lupus erythematosis
    Rheumatoid arthritis
    Myositis
    Chronic Inflammatory disorder
    Ulcertive cloitis
    Regional enteritis
    Sarcoidosis
    Chronic neutropenia
  Malignant disorders
    Leukemia
    Acute myelogenous leukemia
    Chronic myelogenous leukemia
    Acute lymphoblastic leukemia
    Hairy cell leukemia
    Lymphomas
    Hodgkin disease
    Non-Hodgkin lymphoma
    Preleukemia
    Malignant histiocytosis
  Miscellaneous
  Aplastic anemia
  Cyclic neutropenia
  Human Immunodeficiency virus infection (HIV)
  Glucocorticoid administration

Hodgkin and non-Hodgkin lymphomas. It is frequently noted in inflammatory and collagen-vascular diseases such as lupus erythematosus, sarcoidosis, rheumatoid arthritis, and myositis, as well as ulcerative colitis and Crohn disease (1, 22, 23). Monocytosis may be noted with some forms of neutropenia, such as cyclic neutropenia, and postsplenectomy. Patients whose marrow is recovering from myelosuppressive chemotherapy have peripheral monocytosis prior to the return of their neutrophils, reflecting their different marrow-release kinetics.

The evaluation of a patient with monocytosis should reflect this differential diagnosis. Appropriate studies should be obtained to complement the history and physical examination to focus on the broad categories of infectious, malignancy-associated, and inflammatory/collagen vascular diseases.

Although uncommon, monocytopenia may be noted in several diseases. It is characteristic of aplastic anemia as part of the global pancytopenia, in association with corticosteroid administration, in infections associated with endotoxemia, and in severe thermal injuries. The monocytopenia of these disorders may predispose individuals to serious infections (22, 24).

Primary Disorders of the Macrophage

In this section we will discuss primary disorders of the tissue macrophage, or histiocyte, system. Storage diseases, which secondarily involve this cell line, are discussed in chapter 23.

In 1987, the Histiocyte Society adopted a classification system for the childhood histiocytoses based on pathology (25). These diseases are grouped into three classes (table 22.2). Class I, or Langerhan cell histiocytosis, includes the diseases previously termed "histiocytosis X," and consists of those conditions in which the Langerhan cell is centrally involved. Class II histiocytoses, the largest group of disorders, are non-malignant conditions in which the predominant mononuclear cell is of the antigen-processing, or phagocytic, variety. This is in contrast with class I, for the LC is an antigen-presenting, or dendritic, cell. In class II disorders, the predominant cell involved is a normal mono-cyte/macrophage, functioning in an abnormal manner. Finally, class III disorders are the primary malignancies of the monocyte-macrophage system, including acute monocyte leukemia, malignant histiocytosis, and true histiocytic sarcoma (4, 26).

Case presentations and discussion will be grouped according to this pathophysiologic classification.

Class I Histiocytoses

Case 2

A 2-month-old white infant girl was brought to her pediatrician because of a "lump" on her head in the right temporal region. She appeared otherwise well, was the product of a normal pregnancy and delivery, and there was no history of trauma. Physical examination results were is unremarkable except for a 1½ × 2-cm raised area, apparently fixed to the skull in the area of the right temporal bone. Skull roentgenogram (fig. 22.4) demonstrated a bone lesion in the diploid space with erosion of the outer table of the temporal bone. CBC, serum blood chemistries, and metastatic bone survey were otherwise within normal limits. A biopsy of the lesion was performed.

Case 3

A 2-year-old white girl with a history of multiple ear infections since early infancy was brought to an otolaryngologist. She had normal speech pattern until 6 months previously, but her parents have since noted decreased hearing acuity and vocalization. Recently, she has begun to awaken during the night to drink liquids. Physical examination revealed an oily, seborrheic rash on her scalp and fluid accumulation in both auditory canals

Table 22.2. Classification of Histiocytosis Syndromes

Class	Diseases	Pathologic Features
Class I	Langerhans cell histiocytosis	Langerhans cells with cleaved nuclei and Birbeck granules
Class II	Infection-associated hemophagocytic syndrome Familial lymphohistiocytosis	Reactive macrophages with prominent erythrophagocytosis
Class III	Malignant histiocytosis Acute monocytic leukemia True histiocytic sarcoma	Neoplastic cellular proliferation of monocytes or macrophages

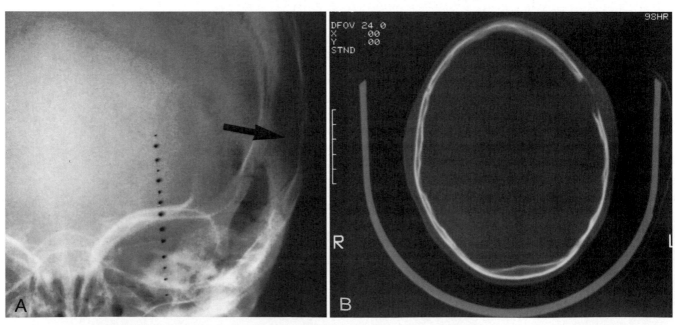

Figure 22.4. **A.** Lateral view of skull x-ray of patient described in case 2. **B.** CT scan of same patient revealing erosion of inner and outer tables of bone.

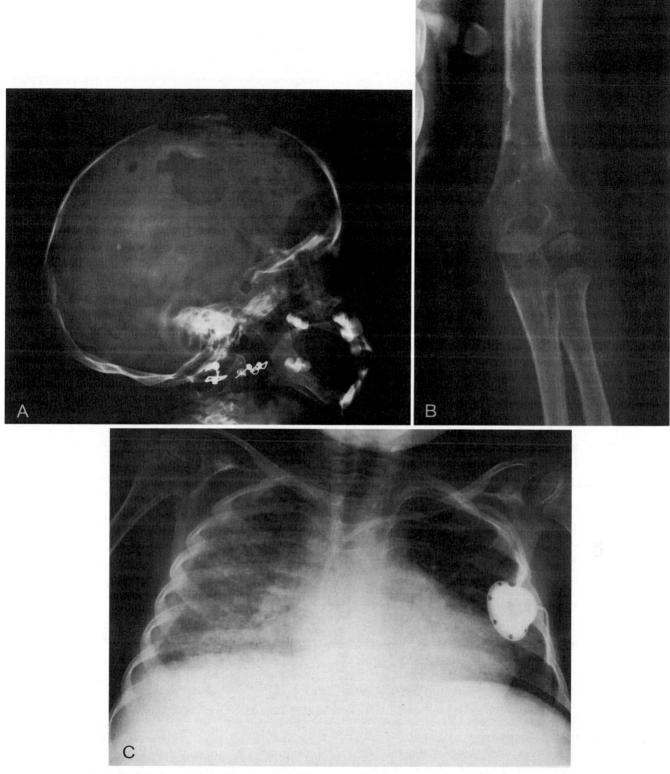

Figure 22.5. Radiologic findings of patient with multisystem described in case 3. **A.** Skull film reveals multiple lytic lesions. **B.** Humerus contains several lytic lesions. **C.** Chest x-ray demonstrates pulmonary involvement of Langerhan's cell histiocytosis.

precluding examination of the tympanic membranes. Roentgenograms of the mastoid bones revealed bilateral mastoiditis with marked osteopenia suggesting bone destruction. Computerized tomographic (CT) scan demonstrated destruction of the mastoid air cells and antrum and destruction of the temporal bones bilaterally. Skeletal survey revealed lytic lesions in the scapula and left second and third ribs (Fig. 22.5). Biopsy of the right mastoid bone was performed.

Case 4

A 1-year-old boy was referred by her pediatrician for evaluation and therapy. Over the past 2 months, the parents had noticed decreased appetite and activity, weight loss, increased thirst and urination, and, recently, jaundice. Physical examination revealed a jaundiced, ill-appearing child. A severe seborrheic dermatitis involved the scalp and external auditory canals. Both the liver and spleen were palpable 4 cm below the costal margins. Chest x-rays revealed prominent bilateral interstitial infiltrate, and skeletal survey demonstrated multiple lytic lesions in the skull and extremities (fig. 22.6). Liver chemistries were abnormal, with increased bilirubin, γ-glutamyl transpeptidase (GGT), and transaminase values. A skin biopsy of the involved scalp was performed.

Discussion: These three cases demonstrate much of the clinical spectrum of Langerhans cell histiocytosis. Case 2 represents the isolated lesion previously called unifocal eosinophilic granuloma of bone. Case 3 represents a variant of the condition previously referred to as Hand-Schuller-Christian disease, which has a classic triad of lytic skull lesions, diabetes insipidus, and exophthalmos. This triad rarely exists in a single patient, and a combination of dermatologic manifestations, skull lesions, and diabetes insipidus is most common. The disseminated form of the disease, previously called Letterer-Siwe disease, is most common in infants and young children and includes visceral involvement (4, 25, 26).

The differential diagnosis of the isolated bone lesion, is, of course, different from that of the disseminated disease. In case 2, infectious causes, such as osteomyelitis, benign bone tumors—including fibrosis dysplasia, neoplasm—including Ewing sarcoma, osteogenic sarcoma, and metastatic tumor, and, finally, Langerhans cell histiocytosis, need to be considered (27, 28). In the differential diagnosis of disseminated forms, the acute leukemias, metastatic tumors—including neuroblastoma, rhabdomyosarcoma, non-Hodgkin lymphoma, and Ewing sarcoma—and infectious causes, such as cytomegalovirus, must be considered. In nearly all instances, biopsy of an involved area will be necessary to establish a diagnosis (4, 26). Langerhans cell histiocytosis is a rare disease, occurring in 0.5/100,000 children to 1/3,300,000 children per year. Two-thirds of the cases occur prior to age 10 and 91% prior to age 30 (26). Langerhan cell histiocytosis has a variety of clini-

cal presentations. Lytic lesions of the bone are the hallmark of the disease, frequently cause pain and swelling, and may involve the skull, orbit, jaw, femur, rib, pelvis, vertebrae, scapula, humerus, or clavicle (27). Young children may be seen clinically with fever, chronic otitis media, or mastoiditis. Proptosis is usually seen in older children. Multiorgan involvement is associated with weight loss, fever, diabetes insipidus, lymphadenopathy, hepatosplenomegaly, anemia, and pancytopenia (4, 26, 29). The skin lesions of Langerhan cell histiocytosis resemble seborrheic dermatitis, but may be differentiated by skin biopsy. The gastrointestinal system, lung, and central nervous system may also be involved. Primary pulmonary histiocytosis, a disease of young adult males in which the lungs are the major site of involvement, is rare in children (31). It is of interest that it has been diagnosed in patients after treatment for Hodgkin disease (30).

Biopsy of the lesions demonstrates granulomas, which are commonly yellow-brown in color. The presence of LCs by light microscopy is the hallmark of these lesions. Macrophages, eosinophils, and lymphocytes are commonly noted within the bone lesions. Multinucleated giant cells and necrosis may be prominent. The presence of Birkeck granules, detected by electron microscopy, is the key diagnostic finding (fig. 22.7). These are racquet-shaped structures of variable length whose function is unknown. Immunohistochemistry studies will typically demonstrate the lesion to express S-100, CD1, CD11, CD14 (4, 25, 26, 32).

The etiology of Langerhans cell histiocytosis is unknown. It is clearly not a malignancy, and there is no evidence of clonal origin of the cells. It may reflect abnormal cytokine regulation of a normal antigen-processing cell, leading to their accumulation. Others have suggested that it is an autoimmune disease (4, 26, 32, 33).

Staging and Treatment of Langerhan Cell Histiocytosis

Since the spectrum and degree of involvement of various organ systems by Langerhans cell histiocytosis is extremely variable, it is important to characterize the degree of clinical involvement accurately and completely. A staging system for Langerhans cell histiocytosis, developed by Eugene Lahey, emphasized the number of organs involved and the age of the patient at the time of diagnosis (34, 35). More recently, the concept of organ dysfunction caused by histiocytic infiltration has been emphasized. Younger age of diagnosis and increased organ dysfunction remain the two most reliable prognostic factors of increased risk (28, 34, 35).

Once the diagnosis of Langerhans cell histiocytosis has been confirmed by biopsy, a complete diagnostic evaluation should be performed. The clinical history should focus on the occurrence of pain, irritability, loss of appetite, fever, polyuria, and polydypsia associated with diabetes insipidus

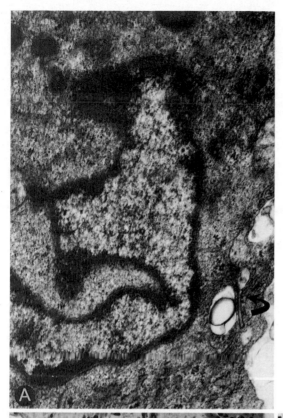

Figure 22.6. Pathology of Langerhan's cell histiocytosis **A.** Electron micrograph of pathologic Langerhans cell from case of LCH on bone in a 6-year-old girl. *Curved arrow* indicates a classical Langerhans cell granule in the cytoplasm of a histiocyte. ×18,000. **B.** Skin biopsy from an infant with disseminated LCH, including a maculopapular cutaneous eruption. Note the S-100 positive histiocyte in the papillary dermis with focal disruption of the epidermo-dermal basement membrane. S-100/PAP stain. ×200. **C.** Bone biopsy of an LCH lesion in a 6-year-old girl shows collections of large histiocytes and numerous eosinophils that form "abscesses" focally. H&E stain ×200.

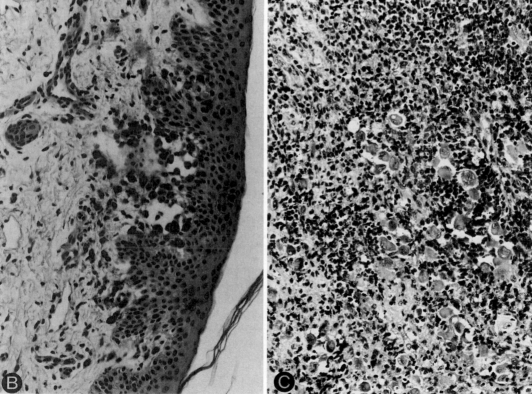

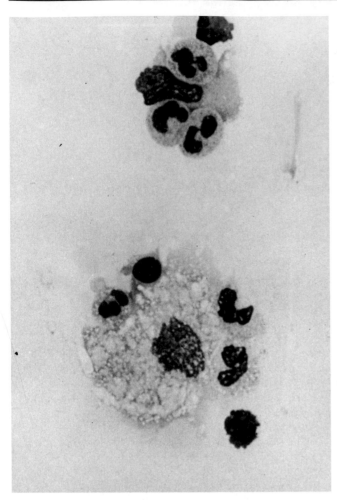

Figure 22.7. Bone marrow aspirate of patient in case 5 revealed hemophagocytosis.

Table 22.3. Mandatory Baseline Evaluations of All New LCH Patients[a]

Complete blood count
Liver function tests
Coagulation studies (PT, PTT, fibrinogin)
Quantitative immunoglobulins
Chest x-ray
Skeletal survey
Urine osmolality

[a]Any abnormal test should be followed monthly until results are normal for 6 months.
Unifocal LCH repeat skeletal survey once at 6 months.

and diarrhea. Physical examination should particularly note skin and scalp lesions, purpura, aural discharge, orbital abnormalities, hepatosplenomegaly, lymphadenopathy, oral lesions, ascites, and jaundice. A complete neurologic examination should be performed (4, 29, 33).

The laboratory and radiographic evaluation of a child with Langerhan cell histiocytosis should include a complete blood count (CBC), liver function tests, coagulation studies, chest roentgenogram, skeletal survey, and urine osmolarity after water deprivation test. Bone marrow aspiration should be performed in any patient with anemia,

leukopenia, or thrombocytopenia. Other laboratory and radiologic studies should be performed, depending on individual clinical symptoms or abnormal screening studies. Tables 22.3 and 22.4 outline initial diagnostic evaluation and the clinical indications for further evaluation (4, 26, 33, 36, 37, 38).

A complete review of the therapy of this disease is beyond the scope of this discussion. Isolated bone lesions may be treated with curettage and/or intralesional steroid injection (27, 39, 40). Multiple bone lesions or multisystem disease is usually treated with systemic therapy, lasting 6 months or longer. Steroids in different dosing regimens, vinblastine, and etoposide (VP-16 213) are the most commonly used agents (4, 26, 35, 41–45). Radiotherapy, typically involving doses in the 600–1000 cGY range, may be effective for controlling isolated lesions. Recently, a randomized international trial has been initiated to further study chemotherapeutic options.

Class II Histiocytosis

Case 5

A 3-year-old black girl was referred by her pediatrician for hematologic consultation. She had a 3-week history of persistent fever to 40.5°C associated with a papular rash of the face and trunk. Initial CBC demonstrated a hemoglobin of 98 g/L, WBC 9.1 × 10⁹/L with a differential of 71 neutrophils, 4 monocytes, 24 lymphocytes, and

Table 22.4. Clinical Indicators for Further Evaluation in Langerhans Cell Histiocytosis

Test	Clinical Indications
Bone marrow aspiration and biopsy	Anemia, thrombocytopenia, leukopenia
Pulmonary function tests	Abnormal chest x-ray
Lung biopsy or broncho alveolar lavage	Abnormal chest x-ray (chemotherapy patients only)
Small bowel imaging and biopsy	Chronic diarrhea, failure to thrive, malabsorption
Liver biopsy	Liver dysfunction
Imaging of brain (CT scan or MRI)	Hormonal, visual or neurologic abnormalities
Panorex	Oral lesions
Endocrine evaluation	Diabetes insipidus Growth failure Golartorrhea Delayed puberty Precocious puberty Abnormal CT or MRI Imaging of hypothalamus and pituitary
Otolaryngology	Aural discharge Hearing loss

[a]CT, computerized tomography; MRI, magnetic resonance imaging.

2 eosinophils, platelet count of 313 × 10⁹/L. Westergreen sedimentation rate was 92 mm/hr. After multiple studies for a fever of unknown origin, including a bone marrow aspiration, the child was discharged to home with a presumptive diagnosis of a collagen-vascular disease. She was readmitted to the hospital 5 days later with lethargy, dehydration, and fever to 41°C. At that time, she was pale, weak, poorly arousable, and clinically dehydrated. A CBC demonstrated hemoglobin of 45 g/L, WBC 4.5 × 10⁹/L, platelet count of 66 × 10⁹/L, and reticulocyte count of 0%.

Pertinent laboratory studies included a normal prothrombin time (PT) and partial thromboplastin time (PTT), ALT 1,531, lactate dehydrogenase 4,350, and creatine phsphokinase 64,000 international units. Direct and indirect antiglobulin tests were negative. Bone marrow aspiration was repeated and demonstrated marked hemaphagocytosis (fig. 22.7). Epstein-Barr virus serology was positive for recent infection.

Commentary: A persistent febrile illness of unclear etiology, which was carefully evaluated, developed in this 3-year-old girl. She was discharged to home with stable hematologic parameters after bone marrow aspiration demonstrated normal marrow morphology. A few days later, she was acutely ill, more febrile, and had markedly different hematologic and serum chemistry values. Bone marrow aspiration then demonstrated marked hemophagocytosis, with marrow macrophages engulfing and destroying hemic cells. This is a case of the unusual, and potentially fatal, disorder called **Infection Associated Hemophagocytic Syndrome (IAHS)**.

Patients with IAHS typically have fever, hematologic abnormalities involving one or more cell lines, liver function and coagulation abnormalities, and lymphadenopathy and hepatosplenomegaly. Bone marrow aspiration will typically demonstrate the presence of morphologically benign histiocytes, without cellular atypia, engaged in hemophagocytosis (fig.22.7). Lymph node and liver biopsy will demonstrate similar cellular abnormalities (4, 26, 46, 47). This condition has been seen in association with all human herpes viruses and a wide variety of fungal, bacterial, and protozoal infections (48–53). It has been reported in immunosuppressed individuals, including renal transplant patients taking immunosuppressants, and patients with the Chediak-Higeshi and X-linked lymphoproliferative syndromes.

The pathogenesis of IAHS is unknown, but probably reflects an abnormal immunologic response to the triggering infectious agents. Recent reports have focused on abnormal levels of T-cell-produced γ-interferon and other lymphokines, causing secondary macrophage stimulation and hemophagocytosis. Pediatric patients with IAHS have been demonstrated to have elevated γ-interferon, IL-6, G-CSF, and ferritin levels (54–57).

The hematologic abnormalities seen in these patients are multifactorial. Hemophagocytosis leads to direct hemic cell destruction, while bone marrow response is suppressed by cytokines inhibitory to hematopoiesis, including γ-interferon and IL-1.

The mortality rate with IAHS has been estimated to be as high as 30–40%. Immunosuppressants that can be discontinued should be. Underlying infections must be treated and aggressive supportive care instituted. Recently, intervenous γ-globulin has been reported to be effective in 3 patients, probably functioning through a combination of Fc-receptor blockage and down-regulation of cytokine production (58, 59).

Familial Hemophagocytic Lymphohistiocytosis (FHL), a clinically related disease, is an often fatal disorder affecting infants and very young children. More than 100 cases have been reported, nearly all occurring within the first 6 months of life. It is assumed to be a genetically transmitted disease, with consanguinities noted in several affected families (60).

The initial clinical symptom is usually fever, often accompanied by weight loss, vomiting, pallor, irritability, and often coma and seizures. Hepatosplenomegaly and lymphadenopathy are common. Laboratory findings, including hematologic and serum chemistry results, are similar to those in patients with IAHS. Bone marrow and/or lymph node biopsy demonstrates increased numbers of benign-appearing histiocytes with marked hemophagocytosis. The etiology remains obscure (61, 62).

FHL typically has a rapid and fatal course, with the average survival after diagnosis being only 6 weeks. Blood exchange transfusion has induced complete, but brief, remissions. Aggressive multiagent chemotherapy regimens based around etoposide (VP-16 213) have induced more prolonged remission (63). Allogeneic bone marrow transplant resulted in complete remission in 1 patient (64).

Class III Histiocytosis

Case 6

A 14-year-old white girl was brought to the emergency room with a 2-week history of intermittent fever, decreased activity, and weight loss. Over the past week, the parents had noted that she was more pale, had increased bruising, and recently had experienced bleeding of her gums with tooth brushing. Physical examination revealed a pale, ill-appearing adolescent with diffuse ecchymoses and petechiae. Gingival swelling was noted, along with moderate bilateral cervical lymphadenopathy. The liver and spleen were palpable 4 cm below the costal margins.

CBC revealed the following: hemoglobin 55 g/L, WBC 140 × 10⁹/L with 90% blasts and 10% lymphocytes, platelet count 15 × 10⁹/L.

Review of the peripheral smear revealed blasts consistent with French-American-British M5 monoblasts. Bone marrow aspiration and biopsy revealed a hypercellular marrow, with decreased megakaryocytes replaced with a monotonous population of monoblasts. Cytochemistries revealed the cells to be periodic acid Schiff (PAS) negative, myeloperoxidase negative, and nonspecific esterase positive in staining. Flow cytometry was consistent with acute monocytic leukemia, expressing CD11, CD14, and CD33.

Acute Monocytic Leukemia (AML)

Acute monocytic leukemia (M5 in the French-American British classification) is the classic malignancy of the mononuclear cell line and presents with symptoms related to marrow replacement. Anemia, thrombocytopenia with bleeding, and granulocytopenia with infection are common. Involvement of skin and mucous membranes is seen frequently. Gingival hyperplasia is noted in 10% of the cases of childhood AML. The diagnosis is confirmed by bone marrow aspiration with special stains and flow cytometry. Treatment of AML consists of intensive chemotherapy. HLA-identical matched sibling bone marrow transplantation and autologous purged bone marrow transplantation have been successful in treating this disease. Therapy of the acute leukemias is discussed in greater detail later (4, 26).

Malignant histiocytosis (MH) was first described in 1939 as histiocytic medullary reticulosis. Rappaport introduced the term "malignant histiocytosis" and characterized the disease as a malignant proliferation of cytologically neoplastic histiocytes within lymphoid organs (65). MH is a very aggressive disease that is often fatal and can be seen in all age groups. Clinical symptoms include fever, weight loss, malaise, sweating, and chest and abdominal pain. Lymphadenopathy may be localized or generalized and tender to palpation. Skin and pulmonary involvement are common. Laboratory features of MH include anemia, thrombocytopenia, and leukopenia. Elevations of lactate dehydrogenase, alkaline phosphatase, transaminase, and bilirubin are common (4, 26, 65–67). Abnormal mononuclear cells are visible in peripheral blood in rare cases.

The diagnosis of MH depends on an appropriate biopsy that reveals a malignant proliferation of histiocytes with distortion of the normal nodal architecture (65–67). There is cytologic atypia in all cases. Erythrophagocytosis may be present, but is not as prominent as in class II histiocytosis. Multinucleate cells are observed in two-thirds of cases and an occasional giant cell is seen. Lysozyme is a reliable marker in all cases of malignant histiocytosis (68, 69).

Recently, Nezelof et al. reviewed 20 cases of malignant histiocytosis and found the MH cell to react with acid phosphatase, α-naphthyl acetate esterase, antichymotrypsin, and antibodies directed against HLA-OR, CD25, CD30, CD68, and CD71. Cell lines derived from MH revealed a unique translocation involving the 5q35 breakpoint (70).

Malignant histiocytosis is an aggressive disease with death usually occurring within 6 months. Treatment of MH hasutilized multiagent anthrocycline-based chemotherapy.

True histiocytic lymphoma (THL) is a very rare disorder distinct from MH. THL involves the lymph nodes of the reticulocedothelial system, skin, and bones. Morphologic criteria for the identification of true histiocytic lymphoma are unsettled. Three microscopic features of typical cases are (a) cohesive type of growth, (b) monomorphic cellular components, and (c) cytologic resemblance to immunoblasts. The diagnostic requirement for THL includes negative immunologic studies for B-cell markers and positive histochemical studies of lysozyme and α-naphthylbutyrate esterase. Electron microscopy has a characteristic appearance in THL and is helpful in establishing the diagnosis (4, 67, 69). Lymph node biopsy shows effacement of the nodal architecture by a cohesive growth of large cells with large vesicular nuclei and abundant basophilic cytoplasm. Erythrophagocytosis is observed in most cases (69). Survival in THL is of short duration (often <6 months) and combination chemotherapy and radiotherapy have been utilized without any long-term success.

REFERENCES

1. Maldonado JE, Hanlon DG. Monocytosis: a current appraisal. Mayo Clin Proc 1965;40:248–259.
2. Hussey G, Chisholm T, Kibel M. Miliary tuberculosis in children: a review of 94 cases. Pediatr Infect Dis J 1991;10: 832–836.
3. Schuit KE. Miliary tuberculosis in children. Am J Dis Child 1979:583–585.
4. Snider DE, et al. Tuberculosis in children. Pediatr Infect Dis J 1988:271–278.
5. Metcalf D. Control of granulocytes and macrophages: molecular, cellular, and clinical aspects. Science 1991;254:529–533.
6. Demetri GD, Antman KHS. Granulocyte-macrophage colony-stimulating factor (GM-CSF): preclinical and clinical investigations. Semin Oncol 1992;19:362–385.
7. Young DA, Lowe LD, Clark SC. Comparison of the effects of IL-3, granulocyte-acrophase colony-stimulating factor in supporting monocyte differentiation in culture. J Immunol 1990;145:607–615.
8. Abbas AK, Lichtman AH, Pober JS. Cellular and molecular immunology. Philadelphia: WB Saunders, 1991.
9. Bajorin DG, Cheung NKV, Houghton AN. Macrophage colony-stimulating factor: biological effects and potential appliations for cancer therapy. Semin Hematol 1991;28 (suppl 2):42–48.
10. Cannistra SA, et al. Human granulocyute-macrophage colony stimulating factor induces expression of the tumor necrosis factor gene by the U937 cell line and by normal human monocytes. J Clin Invest 1987;79:1720–1728.
11. Groupman SE, Golde OW. Biochemistry and function of monocytes and macrophages in hematology. In: Williams W, Beutler E, Ersler A, Lichtman M, eds. Hematology. 4th ed. New York: McGraw-Hill, 1990.
12. Golde DW, Groopman JE. Cellular kinetics of monocytes and macrophages: production, distribution, and fate of

monocytes and macrophages in hematology. Hematology. 4th ed. In: Williams W, Beutler, E, Ersler A, Lichtman M, eds. New York: McGraw-Hill, 1990.

13. Douglas S, Hassan N. Morphology of monocytes and macrophages in hematology. In: Williams W, Beutler E, Ersler A, Lichtman M, eds. Hematology. 4th ed. New York: McGraw-Hill, 1990.

14. Curnutte J. Disorders of granulocyte function and granulopoiesis in hematology of infancy and childhood. 4th ed. Nathan D, Oski F, eds. Philadelphia: WB Saunders, 1993.

15. Ladisch S, Jaffe E. The histiocytoses in principles of pediatric oncology. 1st ed. In: Pizzo P, Poplack D, eds. Philadelphia: JB Lippincott, 1990.

16. Munk ME, Gatrill AJ, Kaufmann SHE. Target cell lysis and IL-2 secretion by y/o T lymphocytes after activation with bacteria. J Immunol 1990;145:1458–2439.

17. Ziegler-Heitbrock HW, et al.: Differential expression of cytokines in human blood monocyte subpopulations. Blood 1992;79:503–511.

18. Nathan CG, Murray HW, Cohn ZA. The macrophage as an effector cell. N Engl J Med 1980;303:622.

19. Nathan CF. Secretory products of macrophages. J Clin Invest 1987;79:319.

20. Kuhn C, Askin F. Lung and midiastinum. In: Kissane J, ed. Anderson's pathology. 9th ed. St. Louis: CV Mosby.

21. Stockman JA III, Ezekowitz A. Hematologic manifestations of systemic diseases: In: Nathan O, Oski F, eds. Hematology of infancy and childhood. 4th ed. Philadelphia: WB Saunders, 1993.

22. Lichtman MA. Monocyte and macrophage disorders: self-limited proliferative responses. Monocytosis and Monocytopenia. In: Williams W, Beutler E, Ersler A, Lichtman M, eds. Hematology. 4th ed. New York: McGraw Hill, 1990: 882–885.

23. Meas AS, Brineg J, Tiwell OP. Monocytes in inflammatory bowel disease; absolute monocyte counts. J Clin Pathol 1980; 33:917.

24. Twormey JJ, Douglass CC, Sharkey O Jr. The monocytopenia of aplastic anemia. Blood 1973;41:187.

25. The Writing Group of the Histiocyte Society. Histiocytosis syndromes in children. Lancet 1987;1:208–209.

26. Komp D, Lichtman M. Inflammatory and malignant histiocytosis. In: Williams W, Beutler E, Ersler A, Lichtman M, eds. Hematology. 4th ed. New York: McGraw Hill, 1990.

27. Greis PE, Hankin FM. Eosinophilic granuloma. Clin Orthop 1990;257:204–211.

28. Dimentberg RA, Brown KLB. Diagnostic evaluation of patients with histiocytosis X. J Pediatr Orthop 1990;10: 733–741.

29. Dunger DB, et al. The frequency and natural history of diabetes insipidus in children with Langerhans cell histiocytosis. New Engl J Med 1989;321:1157–1162.

30. Shanley DJ, Lerud KS. Luetkehans: development of pulmonary histiocytosis X after chemotherapy for Hodgkin disease. AJR 1990;155:741–742.

31. Nondahl SR, et al. A case report and literature review of "primary" pulmonary histiocytosis X of childhood. Med Pediatr Oncol 1986;14:57–62.

32. Favara BE. Langerhan's cell histiocytosis pathobiology and pathogenesis. Semin Oncol 1991;18:3–7.

33. Broadbent V, Gadner H, Komp DM, et al. Histiocytosis syndromes in children; II, approach to the clinical and labora-

tory evaluation of children with Langerhans cell histiocytosis. Med Pediatr Oncol 1989;17:492–495.

34. Lahey ME. Histiocytosis X-an analysis of prognostic factor. J Pediatr 1975;87:184–189.

35. Komp D. Concepts in staging and clinical studies for treatment of Langerhans' cell histiocytosis. Semin Oncol 1991;18: 18–23.

36. Gadner H. Langerhans cells histiocytosis: treatment protocol of the First International Study. Presented at the XXth Annual Meeting of the Histiocyte Society. April 1991.

37. Dunger OB, et al. The frequency and natural history of diabetes insipidus in children with Langerhans' cell histiocytosis. N Engl J Med 1989;321:1157–1162.

38. Chiumello G, et al. Magnetic resonance imaging in diabetes insipidus. Lancet 1989;1:901.

39. Greis PE, Hankin FM. Eosinophilic granuloma: the management of solitary lesions of bone. Clin Orthop 1990;257: 204–211.

40. Bollini GJM. Bone lesions in histiocytosis X. J Pediatr Orthop 1991;11:469–477.

41. Komp D, Broadbent V, Celi A. Therapeutic strategies for Langerhans' cell histiocytosis. J Pediatr 1991;119:274–295.

42. Raney RB. Chemotherapy for children with aggressive fibromatosis and Langerhans' cell histiocytosis. Clin Orthop 1991;262:58–63.

43. Stoll M, et al. Allogeneic bone marrow transplantation for Langerhans' cell histiocytosis. Cancer 1990;66:284–288.

44. Ringden O, et al. Allogeneic bone marrow transplanation in a patient with chemotherapy-resistant progressive histiocytosis X. Med Intell 1987;316:733–735.

45. Komp DM. Langerhan' cell histiocytosis. New Engl J Med 1987;316:747–748.

46. Risdall RJ, et al. Virus-associated hemophagocytic syndrome: a benign histiocytic proliferation distinct from malignant histiocytosis. Cancer 1979;44:993–1002.

47. Chen RL, et al. Fulminant childhood hemophagocytic syndrome mimicking histiocytic medullary reticulosis. An atypical form of Epstein-Barr virus infection. Am J Clin Pathol 1991;96:171–176.

48. Christensson B, et al. Fulminant course of infectious mononucleosis with virus-associated hemophagocytic syndrome. Scand J Infect Dis 1987;19:373–379.

49. Huang LN, et al. Human herpesvirus-6 associated with fatal haemophagocytic syndrome. Lancet 1990;30:60–61.

50. Lortholary A, et al. HIV-associated haemophagocytic syndrome. Lancet 1990;1128:171–176.

51. Ross CW, et al. Chronic active Epstein-Barr virus infection and virus-associated hemophagocytic syndrome. Arch Pathol Lab Med 1991; 115:470–474.

52. Risdall RJ, Brunning RD, Hernandez JI. Bacteria-associated hemophagocytic syndrome. Cancer, 1984;54: 2968–2972.

53. del Palacio A, et al. Disseminated neonatal trichosporosis associated with the hemophagocytic syndrome. Pediatr Infect Dis J 1990;9:520–522.

54. Daum GS, et al. Virus-associated hemophagocytic syndrome: identification of an immunoproliferative precursor lesion. Hum Pathol 1987;18:1071–1074.

55. Imashuklu S, Hibi S. Cytokines in haemophagocytic syndrome. Br J Haematol 1991;77:438–439.

56. Esumi N, et al. High serum ferritin level as a marker of malignant histiocytosis and virus-associated hemophagocytic syndrome. Cancer 1988;61:2071–2076.

57. Ishii E, et al. Prognosis of children with virus-associated hemophagocytic syndrome and malignant histiocytosis: correlation with levels of serum interleukin-1 and tumor necrosis factor. Acta Haematol 1991;85:93–99.

58. Goulder P, Seward D, Hatton C. Intravenous immunoglobulin in virus associated haemophagocytic syndrome. Arch Dis Child 1990;65:1275–1277.

59. Freeman B, et al. Intravenous gammaglobulin for the treatment of infection-associated hemophagocytic syndrome. J Pediatri 1993;123:479–481.

60. Janka GE. Familial hemophagocytic lymphohistiocytosis. Eur J Pediatr 1983;140:221–230, 1983.

61. Henter JL, et al. Hypercytokinemia in familial hemophagocytic lymphohistiocytosis. Blood 1991;78:2918–1922.

62. Miyashita T, Kawaguchi H, Mizutani S. Histiocytic medullary reticulosis, a lethal form of Epstein-Barr-virus-related disorder. Lancet 1991;337:986–987.

63. Fischer A, et al. Treatment of four patients with erythrophagocytic lymphohistiocytosis by a combination of epipodophyllotoxin, steroids, intrathecal methotrexate, and cranial irradiation. Pediatrics 1985;76:263–268.

64. Fischer A, et al. Allogeneic bone marrow transplanation for erythrophagocytic lymphohistiocytosis. J Pediatr 1986;108:267–269.

65. Warnke RA, Him H, Dorfman RF. Malignant histiocytosis (histiocytic medullary reticulosis). Cancer 1975;35:215–130.

66. Ben-Ezra J. Malignant histiocytosis X, a distinct clinicopathologic entity. Cancer 1991;68:1050–1060.

67. Burns BF, Evans WK. Tumours of the mononuclear phagocyte system: a review of clinical and pathological features. Am J Hematol 1982;13:171–184.

68. Shields JA, Shields CL. Clinical spectrum of histiocytic tumors of the orbit. Ophthalmol Otolaryngol 1990;42:931–937.

69. Nemes Z, Thomazy V. Diagnostic significance of histiocyte-related markers in malignant histiocytosis and true histiocytic lymphoma. Cancer 1988;62:1970–1980.

70. Nezelof C, Barbey S, Gogusev J, Terrier-Lancombe MJ. Malignant histiocytosis in childhood: a distinctive CD30-positive clinicopathological entity associated with a chromosomal translocation involving 5q35. Semin Diag Pathol 1992;9:75–89.

CHAPTER 23

Monocytes and Storage Diseases

JOEL M. RAPPEPORT

Enzyme deficiencies can be inborn and responsible for a variety of metabolic (and other) disorders.
—C. F. Cori and G. T. Cori, Nobel Laureates (1947)

As a medical student in 1882 Phillippe Charles Everett Gaucher noted unusual cells in a patient at postmortem examination. It was his considered opinion that the patient's abnormal cells were a new type of cancer (fig. 23.1).

Case 1

A 5-year-old boy, the product of an uncomplicated birth to unrelated parents of English-Irish background, was brought to an emergency room with marked swelling and pain in his left femur after having fallen from his bicycle. No abdominal trauma had been sustained. He had been in reasonably good health except that his mother had noted a slowly progressive decrease in appetite over the prior 6 months, a slightly swollen abdomen, and a tendency to increased bruisability and aches. He had had no fevers or recent viral infections. He had lived his entire life in central Connecticut, had not traveled to foreign countries or to the seaside, and had never received blood transfusions. He had two older, healthy siblings, and his mother was 14 weeks pregnant. The extended family history was negative for any disorders, including bone disease, anemias, bleeding diatheses, or unexplained early death.

On physical examination, marked swelling and tenderness were noted over the left lower femur. An extensive ecchymosis covered his left thigh. His abdominal examination revealed a nontender spleen palpable 6 cm below the left costal margin and a liver palpable 2 cm below the right costal margin. There was no lymphadenopathy or otherwise demonstrable masses. Results of neurologic examination were normal. The patient was in the 35th percentile for weight and head circumference, and in the 15th percentile for height. He was alert, attentive, and appropriately responsive.

X-Rays revealed a displaced fracture of the left midfemur and tapered appearances of the midshaft with widening of the distal femoral ends in both legs. A chest x-ray showed slight lordosis but no hilar adenopathy or anterior mediastinal mass. Additional bone films revealed mild cortical thinning of both proximal tibias and fibulas, with a suggestion of a few cystic lesions.

Laboratory examination revealed the following: hemoglobin 102 g/L, hematocrit 31%, mean corpuscular volume (MCV) 80 fL, platelet count $90 \times 10^9/L$, and white blood cell (WBC) count $3.6 \times 10^9/L$. The WBC differential revealed 60% polymorphonuclear leukocytes (PMNs), 2% bands, 29% lymphocytes, 8% monocytes, and 1% eosinophils. The smear revealed normochromic, normocytic red cells, with no abnormal white cells noted. A corrected reticulocyte count was 2.7%. Coagulation tests included a normal prothrombin time (PT) of 11.2 seconds (normal ≤13 seconds) and a prolonged partial thromboplastin time (PTT) of 51 seconds (normal ≤40 seconds). Bleeding time was 8 minutes (normal <13 minutes). Liver function tests included a total bilirubin of 2.0 mg/dL (normal <1.2), direct bilirubin 0.2 mg/dL (<0.2 normal), alanine transaminase (ALT), aspartate transaminase (AST), and alkaline phosphatase were normal for age. The blood urea nitrogen (BUN) and creatinine levels were also normal, as was the urinalysis. A nontartrate-inhibitable acid phosphatase was 6.2 U/L (normal 0–4.2 U/L). Mixing studies using normal plasma corrected the PTT and did not reveal evidence of an inhibitor. Further clotting studies revealed a deficiency of factor IX (15% of normal). Epstein-Barr virus (EBV) and antinuclear antibodies were negative, and urinary catecholamines were within normal limits.

The patient received 10 ml/kg of fresh frozen plasma, which corrected the PTT. He was then taken to the operating room where, under general anesthesia, a prosthesis was placed and the fracture reduced. Bone marrow aspirate performed at that time revealed numerous lipid-laden macrophages with a wrinkled tissue paper appearance. All hematopoietic elements with normal maturation were present, albeit in decreased numbers. Similar findings were noted in material taken from the tibia at the time of the reduction and repair of the fracture.

Subsequent evaluation over the next several weeks included a markedly elevated plasma glucocerebroside in

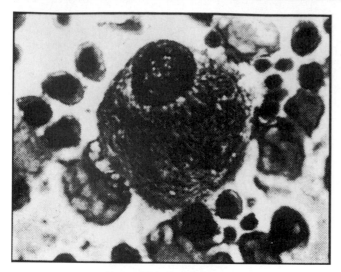

Figure 23.1. Gaucher cells.

the presence of a decreased leukocyte glucocerebrosidase level. Family studies utilizing functional enzymatic assays revealed that the patient's mother had a glucocerebrosidase level slightly below the lower limits of normal, while the father's level fell within the low normal range (1). One asymptomatic sibling had a glucocerebrosidase level slightly below normal, while the other sibling's level was normal.

Abdominal and chest computerized tomography (CT) scans verified the lack of lymphadenopathy, confirmed the marked splenomegaly and moderate hepatomegaly, and, additionally, noted the following: a number of both hypoechoic and hyperechoic splenic lesions, hyperechoic lesions, and surface lobulation of the liver. Magnetic resonance imaging (MRI) of the bones revealed low-intensity signals in the bone marrow. Technetium 99m sulfur colloid examination revealed expansion of hematopoiesis to peripheral bones with patchy areas lacking uptake. Imaging studies of the brain were normal.

This particular patient's sudden presentation with a pathologic fracture led to a rapid diagnosis of Gaucher disease, but with this disorder, the patient frequently may be initially seen with a more indolent progressive course. It is important to remember that Gaucher disease, despite being a genetic germline enzymatic defect, may appear clinically from infancy to as late as the seventh and eighth decade of life. Furthermore, the manifestations and progression of the disease are extraordinarily heterogeneous, even within families. Nevertheless, the single most common sign at presentation is splenomegaly, and this is clearly where the differential diagnosis begins.

Differential Diagnosis of Splenomegaly

The spleen may be palpable in as many as 30% of neonates and 10% of normal toddlers (2). However, in older individuals the spleen is usually enlarged 2–3 times normal before it is palpable at physical examination. As

noted in table 23.1, the differential diagnosis of splenomegaly is extensive. The degree of splenomegaly usually varies with the underlying disorder. Infectious causes, hemolytic anemias, and inflammatory disorders are usually associated with minimal-to-moderate splenic enlargement and may be difficult to palpate, while both extramedullary hematopoiesis and benign or malignant infiltrative disorders are associated with moderate-to-massive enlargement. The acuteness of the development of splenomegaly may also aid in establishing the diagnosis. An acute febrile illness associated with splenomegaly is suggestive of an infectious illness. On the other hand, splenomegaly in the presence of other signs or symptoms of chronic illness may suggest underlying hepatic disorders or benign or malignant infiltrative diseases including the myeloproliferative disorders. In some situations splenomegaly associated with chronic hemolytic erythroid disorders results from both increased splenic clearance of abnormal or antibody-coated cells and a secondary extramedullary hematopoiesis. The presence of lymphadenopathy is often important in establishing the correct diagnosis and may serve as an easily accessible source of tissue to establish diagnoses such as Hodgkin disease or other lymphomas. The relative frequency of various causes of splenomegaly will vary according to the patient's age. Myeloproliferative disorders are more frequent in the middle aged to elderly and less likely to occur in a 5-year-old child. Conversely, the splenomegaly of sickle cell disease (SCD) is limited to the young, with atrophy the hallmark of SCD in the adult (3). Patients with homozygous hemoglobin C or the heterozygous sickle cell hemoglobin C phenotype may have lifelong splenomegaly (4). Although the importance of the differential diagnosis often varies in accordance with age, it must be remembered that the diagnosis of Gaucher disease and other storage cell disorders as well, must be entertained in patients with painless splenomegaly from the very young to the aged.

The constellation of hepatosplenomegaly and skeletal disease is strongly suggestive of Gaucher disease at any age, and in combination with a neurodegenerative disorder, more likely to be the infantile or severely progressive

Table 23.1. Causes of Splenomegaly

Extramedullary hematopoiesis (compensatory and malignant)
Neoplastic infiltration
Nonneoplastic infiltration
Immune and Nonimmune hemolytic anemias
Passive congestion and abnormal splenic blood flow
Infections (bacterial, viral, protozoal, mycobacterial, fungal)
Inflammatory disorders and abnormal immunoregulation
Miscellaneous
   Sarcoidosis
   Hyperthyroidism
   Idiopathic splenomegaly
   Splenic cysts
   Trauma/Hemorrhage

type (5). It should be noted that other storage cell diseases and lipoidoses are often associated with hepatosplenomegaly (table 23.2). The bony pathology of Niemann-Pick, however, is usually limited to radiologic osteoporosis and widening of the medullary cavities (6). The pancytopenia that results from splenomegaly of all etiologies is due both to increased destruction of the cellular blood elements and to a hemodilution effect resulting from an increase in both the total blood volume and selective splenic pooling (7, 8).

Although the list of causes of an enlarged spleen is extensive, a carefully obtained family and travel history, as well as examination of the peripheral blood is extremely useful in establishing many of the diagnoses (9). Occasionally, multiple etiologies may result in a given patient's splenomegaly. Although any persistent splenomegaly must be evaluated, a small percentage of normal adolescents have a palpable spleen (10). The examination of the bone marrow adds significantly to the establishment of the diagnosis and, in the presence of lymphadenopathy, a lymph node biopsy may definitively identify the etiology of the splenomegaly. Ultimately, however, despite the use of sophisticated imaging techniques, morphologic diagnosis may be confirmed in some situations only by splenectomy with pathologic examination. The diagnosis of Gaucher disease is strongly suggested by bone marrow examination and confirmed by measurement of either leukocyte or fibroblast glucocerebrosidase enzymatic activity, plasma glucocerebroside levels, and molecular studies.

Pathology of Gaucher Disease

The Gaucher cell is a lipid-laden reticuloendothelial cell found wherever reticuloendothelial cells normally reside (11), i.e., in splenic histiocytes, hepatic Kupffer cells, and marrow macrophages and osteoclasts, respectively, as well as in lymph nodes, brain, and other sites (fig. 23.2). Gaucher cells are 20–100 μm in diameter with an eccentric nucleus and a "wrinkled tissue paper" cytoplasm. The appearance of the cell is usually distinctive enough to establish the diagnosis and to differentiate it from abnormal histiocytes seen in other muccopolysaccharidoses and lipoidoses (12). From a therapeutic point of view, it is important to note that these abnormal tissue histiocytes originate from the bone marrow monocyte-macrophage.

The morphologic presence of Gaucher cells in the bone marrow does not unequivocally establish the diagnosis of Gaucher disease, which is a specific genetic enzyme deficiency. "Pseudo-Gaucher" cells have been noted in the bone marrow of patients with chronic myelogenous leukemia, multiple myeloma, Hodgkin disease, AIDS, and hemoglobinopathies such as thalassemia (13–16). With excessive generation of glucocerebroside, a normal metabolic breakdown product resulting from rapid cellular turnover, the normal enzymatic machinery may be unable to cope with the large amount of substrate. This may result in excessive accumulation of glucocerebroside in reticuloendothelial cells and thus the formation of morphologic Gaucher-like cells. With treatment of the underlying diseases such as chronic myelogenous leukemia, the pseudo-Gaucher cells may markedly diminish or disappear. Conversely, it should be noted that multiple myeloma, acute leukemia, Hodgkin disease, and amyloidosis have been re-

Table 23.2. Classification of Storage Diseases

	Enzyme deficiency	Expression
Sphingolipidoses		
Gaucher disease	Cerebrocidase	Mild to fulminant
Niemann-Pick	Sphingomyelinase	Mild to fulminant
Farbers disease	Ceremidase	Fulminant
G$_{m1}$gangliosidosis	-galactosidase	Severe to fulminant
G$_{m2}$gangliosidosis	-hexosaminosidases	Severe to fulminant
Mucopolysaccharidases		
Hunter disease	Iduronate sulfatases	Severe
Sanfillipo disease		Mild to severe
Types A–D		Mild to severe
Murquois syndrome		
Types A and B	Galactosidase/sulfatase	Mild to severe
Morteaux-Lamy	Arylsulfatase	Severe
β-Glucuronidase deficiency	β-Glucuronidase	Mild to severe
Mucosulfatidosis	Arylsulfatases	Severe
Mucolipidoses		
Sialidoses	Neuraminidase	Mild to severe
Mucolipidoses II, III, IV	-phosphate transferase	Mild to fulminant
Others		
Fucosidosis	α-L-Fucosidosis	Mild to fulminant
α-Mannosidosis	α-Mannosidase	Mild
Aspartyl-glucosaminuria	β-Glucosidiminidase	Severe
Sialic acid storage disease	—	Mild to severe
Acid lipase deficiency (Wolman)	—	Fulminant
Cholesterol ester storage disease	—	Mild
Neuronal ceroid-lipofucsinosis		
Batten	—	Severe
Haltia-Santavuori	—	Fulminant
Jansky-Bielschlowsky	—	Severe to fulminant
Spielmeyer-Sjögren	—	Severe to fulminant
Kufs disease	—	Severe

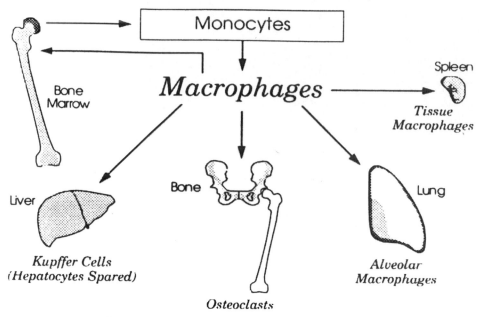

Figure 23.2. The pathophysiology of Gaucher disease.

ported in patients with underlying Gaucher disease, which might either be coincidental or result from an immunologic defect intrinsic to patients with Gaucher disease (17–20).

Clinical Manifestations of Gaucher Disease

Although the clinical expression of Gaucher disease may be extremely variable, three subtypes based on clinical signs and symptoms have been established, of which there are a number of excellent reviews (21–23) (table 23.3).

Type 1 nonneuronopathic Gaucher disease is the most frequent and accounts for >95% of cases. It is also the most varied in its clinical onset and progression and may be diagnosed in early childhood through to the seventh to eighth decade of life. This latter has been demonstrated in many Ashkenazi Jews, in whom life expectancy may be normal. On the other hand, type 1 Gaucher disease usually presents in childhood with progressively increasing splenomegaly, pancytopenia, and degeneration of the skeletal system. Less frequent occurrences are hepatic failure, pulmonary dysfunction, and involvement of the kidneys, heart, and lymph nodes. The clinical hallmark of type 1 Gaucher disease is its general lack of neurologic signs and symptoms, although Gaucher disease cells have been found in the perivascular region of the brain (24) (fig. 23.3).

The rarer type 2, or acute neuronopathic Gaucher disease, is uniformly fulminate in its presentation and course. The average age of onset is 3 months, and it is usually accompanied by rapid hepatosplenomegaly. Within a few months, usually at <1 year of age, neurologic manifestations develop with rapidly progressive deterioration and,

classically, cranial nerve nuclei and extrapyramidal tract involvement (fig. 23.4).

Trismus, oculomotor ataxia, strabismus, and spastic retroflexion of the head occur in the majority of affected patients. However, a wide variety of manifestations of neurologic deterioration are noted, including the development of seizures. Within a matter of months of the onset of the neurologic symptoms, death usually occurs from either aspiration pneumonia or apnea.

Type 3 Gaucher disease, or subacute neuronopathic Gaucher disease is clinically similar to type 1, and usually its diagnosis is established early in childhood. Like type 2 Gaucher disease, its course is accompanied by progressive neurologic deterioration, albeit less severe and less rapidly progressive. A few patients with type 3 Gaucher disease have been noted to have either localized neurologic lesions or nonspecific, diffuse, mild slowing on electroencephalogram (EEG). The phototypic type 3 Gaucher disease reported from Sweden is referred to as Norrbottnian Gaucher disease (25) (fig. 23.5).

The radiologic findings in the skeletal system in Gaucher disease vary from minimal to extensive. Approximately six different findings have been identified, and any combination of lesions may be present (26, 27). As the disease progresses, more extensive multiple processes are noted. The first and most frequent radiologic change results from intramedullary infiltration and cortical thinning. Lesions are most commonly noted in the femurs. Expansion of the distal diaphysis and metaphysis creates the radiologic appearance of an Erlenmeyer flask. These radiologic lesions can also be seen in patients with marked marrow hyperplasia, such as sickle cell anemia and thalassemia. The second finding is aseptic necrosis, often bilateral, and usually of the femoral heads. These lesions result from interruption of the blood flow by the expanding mass

Table 23.3. Demographics and Expression of Gaucher Disease

Disease Type	Onset	Duration	Organomegaly	Bone Defects	Neurologic Defects
Type 1 (95% of cases) (70% Ashkenazi Jews) 1/500–1/1000	Childhood to Adulthood	Generally normal	Mild to marked	Present	Rare, severe
Type 2 (all races) 1/100,000	Infants	1–2 yr	Mild	Rare	Severe
Type 3 (Swedish Norbottnian) 1/100,000	Juvenile	Teens to 4th decade of life	Mild	Present	Mild to severe

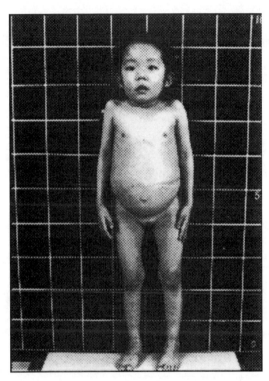

Figure 23.3. Gaucher disease, type 1.

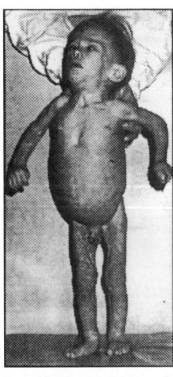

Figure 23.4. Gaucher disease, type 2.

of Gaucher cells. Less frequently aseptic necrosis is noted in the humeral heads and vertebral bodies. The third group of lesions is clinically associated with localized pain, swelling, and erythema, and appears on x-ray with periosteal swelling and new bone formation as well as rarefaction of the involved bone. These lesions are difficult to differentiate both radiologically and clinically from osteomyelitis. Radionuclear technetium 99 and gallium 67 scans may help in the differentiation, although it is important to note that true osteomyelitis may occur in the setting of Gaucher disease. The bony lesions often result in pathologic fractures. Finally, uncommonly expansive masses of Gaucher cells may result in isolated lytic lesions. Gaucher disease does not uniformly affect the skeletal system in a given patient (table 23.4). Sequential CT scans and MRI have been of value in determining both extent of disease and progression (28, 29). Of note is the fact that radiologic findings in other storage cell disorders are usually less marked.

Pathophysiology of Gaucher Disease

The pathophysiology of Gaucher disease is well understood (fig. 23.3). The disease is the result of excess accumulation, particularly in reticuloendothelial cells, of the metabolic breakdown product glucocerebroside (30). This intermediate product of catabolism is a glycolipid composed of ceramide and glucose. Ceramide is composed of the lipid sphingosine and variable length long-chain fatty acids. The majority of this material is derived from catabolism of cellular membranes. Under normal circumstances the membrane bound lysosomal enzyme glucocerebrosidase cleaves glucocerebroside into ceramide and glucose. A number of coenzymes, stimulators, and inhibitors of this glycoprotein have been identified in vitro (31, 32). The significance of these agents in clinical disease is uncertain, with the exception of a rarely reported saposin deficiency and its attendent disease state (33). Glucocerebrosidase is synthesized in ribosomes, and after translocation from the ribosome to

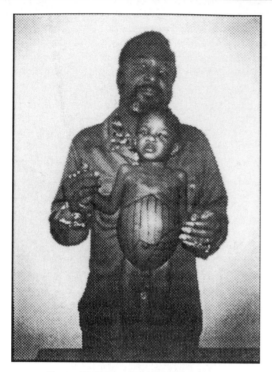

Figure 23.5. Gaucher disease, type 3.

Table 23.4. Bone Involvement in Gaucher Disease

Bone/Site	Manifestation
Femoral/shaft	Erlenmeyer flask/osteopenia
Femoral/head	Avascular necrosis/fracture
Humeral/shaft	Lytic lesions/osteopenia
Humeral/head	Avascular necrosis
Vertebral bodies/thoracic	Avascular necrosis/fracture
Pelvis	Avascular necrosis/fracture
Tibia-fibula/shaft	Lytic lesions/cortical erosion

[a]Ribs, mandible, maxilla, and other bones involved less frequently.

the endoplasmic reticulum and golgi apparatus, undergoes cleavage of a leader sequence and posttranslational glycosylation (34). The glycosylation process results in a number of cross-reactive species. The enzyme reaches lysosomes by as yet undefined mechanisms, where it hydrolyzes its substrate. In Gaucher disease both decreased enzyme protein and enzymatic activity have been detected (35). Most patients have normal synthetic processes with slightly diminished enzymatic activity, suggesting that the mutant enzymes are unstable in type 1 Gaucher disease and very unstable in types 2 and 3 (36). Other mutations have also been described, resulting in fusion proteins with a loss of functional activity or loss of activation sites. The molecular basis of these mutations will be described below.

Although this genetic enzyme deficiency is present in the germline and thus is abnormal in all cells, its major clinical manifestations result from an accumulation of the unmetabolized substrate in tissue macrophages. These

engorged cells are responsible for the splenomegaly, hepatomegaly, and bony disease. As yet unexplained is the frequently observed secondary hepatic fibrosis. Of greatest importance is the explanation for the absence of central nervous system (CNS) deterioration in type 1 disease and its devastating course in types 2 and 3 Gaucher disease. In all types of Gaucher disease cerebral perivascular Gaucher cells have been noted, but only in type 2 and less frequently in type 3 have parenchymal Gaucher cells been observed (37). The parenchymal cells are frequently surrounded by gliosis. Although plasma lipoprotein-bound glucocerebroside is markedly elevated in all types of Gaucher disease, elevated CNS levels are not found in type 1. In effect, the mechanism of the neurodegenerative disease is as yet unclear, but may result from a "toxic" effect of glucocerebroside on neuronal cells. Whether the difference in clinical syndromes results from differences in enzymatic levels or whether other contributory factors exist is also unknown.

Epidemiology of Gaucher Disease

Gaucher disease, the most common of all lysosomal storage disorders, is an autosomal recessive disease occurring in all populations. However, type 1 disease is seen most frequently in Ashkenazi Jews, and is the most common genetic disorder in this population. Since many of these patients may have benign and thus undiagnosed disease, the incidence may well be underestimated. In fact, utilizing a molecular probe of the most common defect to screen normal Jewish populations, the incidence of the disease appears to be as high as 1 in 850 births (38). Since the mutation used for screening only accounts for approximately 75% of the cases diagnosed in this population, the actual incidence of Gaucher disease is clearly higher. The other population with an increased incidence of Gaucher disease is a subgroup of Swedes with type 3 Norrbottnian disease. Most cases of Gaucher disease are type 1, and, given the rarity of types 2 and 3, no estimates of their incidence can be accurately made.

Molecular Biology of Gaucher Disease

Since 1985 the gene encoding for glucocerebrosidase has been fully cloned and the entire sequence of the gene has been described. The following is a brief description of current molecular knowledge of the gene. The glucocerebrosidase gene is localized on chromosome 1 in the q21 region, and is approximately 7.25 kb in length with 11 exons and 10 introns (39, 40). As is commonly seen with lysosomal enzymes, a hydrophobic leader sequence has been identified (41). An unusual aspect is that two functional-start codons have been localized. It is of importance that a pseudogene with a great deal of homology with the true gene has been located approximately 16 kb downstream from the functional gene (42). Although the pseudogene has an active promoter, there is no translation because of the loss of open reading frames, as well as absence of some exons and splice junctions. The identification of multiple polymorphic sites within the gene has aided in the clinical identification of mutations and in understanding the disease from an anthropomorphic point of view.

Within the glucocerebrosidase gene at least 30 mutations that result in clinical Gaucher disease have been identified. More than 2/3 of these mutations have been point mutations within exons (43). An additional upstream splice junction point mutation has been identified, as well as single mutations of nucleotide insertions and deletions. At least six unequal crossover events have resulted in recombinant events between the gene and pseudogene, resulting in a nonfunctional gene (44).

Population studies of patients with Gaucher disease have demonstrated a marked variation in the frequency of the mutations, with three mutations being very common, another nine uncommon, and the remainder usually occurring in single families. The frequencies are also variable within different ethnic groups. The single most common mutational allele, 1226G, is found in 75% of Ashkenazi Jews with Gaucher disease, while its frequency in non-Jewish patients is less (45). Whether the 1226G mutation's high frequency in the Jewish population represents positive selection is as yet unclear. The mutation 84GG represents an additional 13% of Jewish patients, and these two lesions plus the IVS2 + 1 and panethnic mutation 1448 account for 96% of the mutations found in Ashkenazi Jewish patients (46). In non-Jewish population studies, the two most frequent mutations are 1226G and 1448, while 20% of the mutations are comprised of the other rarer spontaneous mutations. Early studies suggest that the 3548 mutation may have a high frequency in Gaucher disease patients of Japanese descent (47). At present a substantive proportion of the non-Jewish mutations have yet to be characterized.

Description of the various molecular defects in the glucocerebrosidase gene has helped explain the clinical heterogeneity of Gaucher disease. In general, those patients homozygous for the 1226G mutation have mild nonneuronopathic disease, usually diagnosed in adulthood. Exceptions to this general rule have occasionally been noted in young children with early-onset severe disease who have the homozygous 1226G genotype. Conversely, this homozygous genotype has been noted in adults without any evidence of Gaucher disease. Ashkenazi Jews with this genotype tend to have milder disease than non-Jews with the same genotype (48). The explanation for this variability is currently unclear and possibly could be due to other associated genetic factors. Patients homozygous for the mutations 1448 and 84GG have severe neuronopathic disease in general. Patients with a heterozygous genotype, one allele of which is the mild 1226G mutation, tend to have a milder clinical course than those patients who are homozygous for the severe mutations (49). Thus, the age of onset of clinical disease in the patient with the 1226G/1448C genotype tends to be later than the homozygous 1448C patient, and has a slower clinical progression. Similar findings have been noted in the heterozygous 1226G/84GG genotype.

Although the description of the mutations in Gaucher disease have not fully explained any given patient's clinical course with certainty, these studies have been of immense help. Although not absolute, identification of the patient's genotype aids in prediction of the prognosis, and thus in therapeutic decisions to be entertained. Furthermore, these studies have led to an increased sophistication in genetic counseling, and have contributed to prenatal diagnosis. Molecular testing has allowed improved identification of the heterozygote carrier, particularly since functional enzymatic assays not infrequently overlap normal values. Cloning of the gene will lead to the ability to produce large amounts of purified enzyme for enzyme replacement at a lower cost than required for current purification of placentally derived enzyme. Finally description of the various mutations may ultimately lead to successful targeted gene transfer therapy.

Therapy of Gaucher Disease

Until relatively recently the only therapeutic modalities available for patients with Gaucher disease were supportive in nature. Experience with the orthopedic approach to fractures has suggested that, in general, a conservative course is preferable. When possible, immobilization will often result in fracture healing, while open surgical reduction may lead to subsequent osteomyelitis because of the underlying generalized bony disease. However, over time this conservative approach may lead to some chronic bony deformity. On the other hand, severe osteonecrosis of the femoral head may require arthroplasty or total hip replacement. Bony "crises" should be treated with analgesia and bedrest, with a constant watchful eye for true osteomyelitis.

The role of splenectomy has remained controversial for a number of decades. The removal of a massive spleen has resulted in immediate relief of a number of symptoms, including failure to thrive, early satiety, abdominal pain, and mechanical obstruction of the gastrointestinal tract (50). For those patients with high output cardiac failure and/or restrictive pulmonary disease, splenectomy may lead to immediate improvement. Furthermore, splenectomy will in most cases improve hematologic parameters, often correcting the pancytopenia. The older patient with benign disease manifesting only as splenomegaly and thrombocytopenia may only require a splenectomy. However, controversy remains over the long-term implications of splenectomy. Some data would suggest that by removing one of the major sources of glucocerebroside storage, an accelerated accumulation occurs in other organs, including both the liver and skeletal systems, and results in a more rapid clinical deterioration (51). Evaluation of other clinical series has not substantiated these findings. Nevertheless, this suggestion has led to attempted partial splenectomies, including splenectomies of 95% of the spleen (52). In such instances, more rapid progression of disease, as well as regrowth of the spleen have been noted. Whether there is an advantageous role for partial over total splenectomy is not yet clear.

Whether orthopedic surgical procedures or splenectomy are contemplated, or whether any other surgical procedure is considered in a patient with Gaucher disease, careful attention must be paid to potential hemorrhagic diathesis. Thrombocytopenia may lead to a prolonged bleeding time, and platelet transfusions in the presence of massive splenomegaly may lead to either no increment in the platelet count or a merely short-lived increase. Patients may have evidence of a bleeding diathesis that is greater than one would anticipate based on the platelet count alone. The increased PTT may result from a number of potential causes, including a variety of factor deficiencies, the most common being factor IX (53). Whether this represents decreased synthesis from liver dysfunction or a defect in the coagulation cascade has not been totally clarified. After careful evaluation, either fresh frozen plasma and/or platelet transfusions may be required for operative procedures.

In the mid-1970s attempts were made to infuse human placenta-derived glucocerebrosidase intravenously in a small number of patients. Infusion of relatively small quantities of enzyme was probably nonspecifically distributed to tissues, including hepatocytes, and thus no clinical beneficial effect was seen (54). In addition, only a small temporary biochemical effect was noted. It was recognized that since the major pathology of Gaucher disease resulted from the markedly increased mass of macrophages laden with cerebroside, the intact enzyme had to be delivered to macrophages. Early attempts to specifically target enzyme to macrophages included treatment with enzyme packaged in either liposomes or antibody-coated red cell ghosts (55, 56). These trials were also unsuccessful with minimal if any clinical improvement. These early failures were probably due both to limited enzyme and to failure deliver adequate enzyme to the macrophage. With the discovery of the mannose receptor on macrophages, it became possible to enhance biochemically specific targeting of enzyme to the macrophage (57). Limited deglycosylation of the oligosaccharide side chains of placental glucocerebrosidase was performed to expose mannose residues. Studies revealed that a 10-fold increase in modified enzyme was delivered to Kupffer cells in comparison with the unmodified native enzyme (58, 59).

A number of early clinical trials utilizing the modified enzyme have been reported (60–67). The results of treatment primarily in severely affected type 1 patients can be summarized as follows. Significant improvement in a number of clinical parameters has been noted, usually after a minimum of 3–4 months of treatment. Initially there has been reduction in both liver and spleen size, with an associated improvement in both anemia and often complete correction of thrombocytopenia. Skeletal improvement, albeit at a significantly slower rate, has also been observed. Patients have had improvement in the biochemical markers associated with their disease. In addition there has been improvement in growth and development in these children, as well as an improved sense of well-being.

Five major problems currently exist with this mode of treatment. The first is that the long-term effects of this lifelong therapy are unknown. Antibodies to the enzyme have developed in least 2 patients. Secondly, some of the effects associated with Gaucher disease may not be reversible. In at least 1 patient with associated cirrhosis, there has been no resolution of the cirrhosis. This observation is not totally unexpected given the results with bone marrow transplantation in both thalassemia and Gaucher disease, where, despite complete correction of the underlying disease, there has not always been an associated resolution of hepatic fibrosis. Therefore, treatment of patients with far-advanced disease may result in clinical improvement without resolution of secondary sequelae. The patient with variceal bleeding and cirrhosis may not be helped by this therapy. Thirdly, it is not clear at the current time whether exogenous enzyme administration will penetrate the CNS in patients with the neuronopathic forms of Gaucher disease. It is possible that circulating monocytes will ingest adequate enzyme with long-term stability to result in increased enzyme levels in the microglial cells of the brain. A second possibility is that decreased extracerebral glucocerebroside levels will ultimately decrease the substrate accumulation in the CNS. However, this therapy has not yet been tested sufficiently in patients with neuronopathic Gaucher. Fourthly, it is not yet clear as to the dose and frequency of enzyme administration. A number of protocols have been developed, all of which have had success over time, but the optimal dose and frequency have yet to be clearly determined. Finally, and perhaps one of the greatest problems at the current time, is the expense of therapy that may range *upward* from $250,000 per year depending on the dose and size of the patient. Given that this treatment is likely to be required for life, modified glucocerebrosidase may have the dubious claim of being the world's most expensive drug. This expense has had the following effects: (a) the drug's not being used frivolously, as in older, minimally symptomatic patients; (2) attempts being made to determine the minimal effective dose in appropriate patients; and (3) the production of a less expensive recombinant product is encouraged. Conversely, no appropriate candidates for this therapy should be denied treatment because of its expense.

The observation that tissue macrophages were of hematopoietic origin led to the belief that bone marrow transplantation might have a role in the treatment of Gaucher disease. In patients who received marrow grafts from opposite sex donors and were successfully engrafted, alveolar macrophages and hepatic Kupffer cells contained the cytogenetic markers of the donor (68, 69). Similarly, fixed tissue macrophages in the spleen, lymph nodes, tonsils, and peritoneum were also derived from hematopoietic cells. More controversial is the question of whether the microglial cell of the CNS is also derived from hematopoietic stem cells (70). Since the lipid-laden macrophage is the primary cause of the pathophysiology in nonneuronopathic Gaucher disease, it was logical to attempt to correct the macrophage disorder through marrow transplantation.

The first such patient with far-advanced disease after successful engraftment had rapid normalization of his peripheral blood enzyme levels (71). A more gradual decrease in his plasma glucocerebroside levels was noted, as was clearance of bone marrow Gaucher cells. However, the patient ultimately expired from the complications of his underlying cirrhosis. Approximately 17 reported and unreported patients have undergone allogeneic bone marrow grafting for Gaucher disease (71–73). One can conclude from this small and as yet early experience that when appropriate lymphohematopoietic ablative preparation is administered, stable long-term hematopoietic engraftment can be achieved. There is normalization of glucocerebrosidase activity in bone marrow–derived cells, with gradual disappearance of Gaucher disease cells from the marrow, spleen, and liver. There is also normalization of plasma and erythrocyte glucocerebroside levels. However, one must note with caution the persistence of hepatic fibrosis. Patients have enhanced growth, and there appears to be stabilization or partial normalization of skeletal lesions. Although most patients undergoing bone marrow transplantation for Gaucher disease have not had neurologic deficits, a few patients with the neuronopathic Norrbottnian type of Gaucher disease have been successfully transplanted (73). Some data would suggest a stabilization of oculomotor apraxia, but with a continued but attenuated slow decrease in intelligence testing. The long-term effects are clearly undefined, especially those of the CNS.

Currently, given the intrinsic risks of bone marrow transplantation, this therapy should be reserved for patients with aggressive life-threatening disease. The application of marrow grafting is limited by the identification of a histocompatible normal donor, although a heterozygous donor with a normal glucocerebrosidase gene and a single glucocerebrosidase mutation would be acceptable. The use of matched unrelated registry donors will increase the probability of identifying a histocompatible donor (74). The role of marrow grafting in neuronopathic forms of the disease is yet to be defined and must be approached cautiously. If this therapeutic option is to be undertaken, the

transplantation should be done prior to the development of irreversible nonhematopoietic organ damage, such as the development of hepatic cirrhosis. One might take the approach of initial temporary exogenous enzyme replacement in order to clinically stabilize the patient pending the identification of an appropriate bone marrow transplant donor. Bone marrow transplantation is likely to be less costly than lifelong exogenous enzyme replacement.

Future therapy might include gene therapy, with transvection of an expressible glucocerebrosidase gene into hematopoietic stem cells (75). This autologous transplant would provide a potential donor for all patients and would virtually eliminate the potentially life-threatening graft-versus-host reaction, a complication associated with allogeneic bone marrow transplantation. However, because the transvected hematopoietic stem cell would not be likely to have any growth advantage over the enzymatically defective cell, the patient would probably require lethal hematopoietic ablative preparation with its associated risks. Similarly, the role of this therapy in neuronopathic forms of the disease would need further definition.

Case 1

Discussion: *How, then, with the background information noted above, was this patient treated? His acute problem had been successfully treated surgically, and a presumptive diagnosis established. With the suggestion that the child probably had a genetic disorder, two basic paths were followed. The first was to confirm the diagnosis of Gaucher disease. A polymerase chain reaction–based Southern blot analysis revealed that the patient had both the 1226G point mutation and the 1448C lesion and thus was genotypically 1226G/1448C. Both parents were heterozygotes, with the boy's mother having the 1448C mutation in addition to a normal gene, and the father the 1226G lesion. The boy's clinically asymptomatic siblings were also tested, and the sibling with the normal enzymatic levels had a normal genotype. The other sibling was heterozygous, with the 1226G mutation being noted. Of major immediate concern to this family was the fact that the mother was pregnant. After full explanation of the disease and its course, the parents decided they would elect to terminate the pregnancy if the fetus were affected. A chorionic-villus biopsy showed a normal genotype. Amniotic fluid analyzed for enzymatic activity was also normal.*

It was pointed out to the parents that although the 1448C mutation was frequently associated with neuronopathic disease in the homozygous state, the genotype 1226G/1448C might not be associated with neurologic deterioration. An EEG, head CT scan, and MRI performed on the patient all were normal. In order to determine the potential long-term therapeutic options, the patient and his family were human lymphocyte antigen (HLA) typed. It should be noted that the major histocompatibility complex is encoded on the short arm of chromosome 6, and therefore is inherited independently from the Gaucher lesion, located on chromo-

some 1. Unfortunately, neither of the patient's siblings was HLA identical, with one of the siblings sharing one haplotype and the other having neither haplotype. However, HLA typing of the fetal amniotic fluid cells revealed HLA identity with the patient. Thus, the unborn child was a potential normal hemopoietic donor for the patient.

In effect the long-term therapeutic options available to this patient included the following: (a) symptomatic treatment, including the potential of performing a splenectomy, (b) exogenous enzyme replacement, (c) a bone marrow transplant, or (d) some combination of these options. The first option was not appealing to either the parents or the patient's physicians, since it was likely that given the age of presentation and degree of involvement, the patient would have a moderately rapid progression of his disease, leading initially to marked disability and ultimately death. Thus, although long-term followup of neither enzyme replacement nor marrow grafting was available at that time, a decision was made to follow either of these two courses. If a transplant were to be pursued, cord blood stem cells would be harvested at the time of the mother's anticipated delivery (76, 77). The parents were concerned about the possibility of nonengraftment because of inadequate umbilical cord stem cells and decided to delay the actual transplant until such time as the newborn would be capable of being a donor for a second transplant if necessary. Bone marrow harvests from donors as young as 5–7 months of age have been successfully performed. Therefore, the transplant would be delayed for approximately 1 year from the time of diagnosis. However, of concern was the fact that progression of the disease might lead to irreversible changes such as cirrhosis of the liver. The family's insurance company was approached about the possibility of reimbursement for exogenous enzyme replacement. Because the enzyme was to be used for only a limited period, the insurance company agreed to reimburse the family despite its exorbitant price.

The patient was thus begun on exogenous enzyme at a dose of 60 U/kg every other week. Treatment was not associated with any side effects. Approximately 6 months after the patient started treatment, his spleen had decreased by approximately 30% as measured by MRI. Similarly, the liver size decreased by 20%, and he had a marked improvement in appetite. The hematocrit increased to 35%, and the platelet count rose to 150 × 10^9/L. Plasma glucocerebroside levels decreased by 30%. No substantive changes were noted radiologically in the skeletal system. All improvements occurred during the course of enzyme therapy.

At the time of the mother's delivery, 120 ml of cord blood was harvested and cryopreserved. Approximately 1 year after diagnosis, the patient, who remained clinically stable on exogenous enzyme, underwent a bone marrow transplant. At the time of transplantation a significant number of Gaucher cells were evident in the bone marrow. Following preparation with busulfan in a total

dose of 16 mg/kg over 4 days and cyclophosphamide 1500 mg/M² daily for 4 days, the patient received 0.4 × 10⁸ cryopreserved umbilical cord–nucleated cells. Graft-versus-host disease (GVHD) prophylaxis was initiated with methotrexate and cyclosporin A. Engraftment was noted on day 18, and the patient was discharged from the hospital on day 35 without evidence of significant graft-versus-host disease or other regimen-related toxicity. Enzymatic assay of peripheral blood mononuclear cells at day 35 revealed normal enzyme activity. DNA analysis of the glucocerebrosidase enzyme confirmed complete engraftment. Continued improvement with further reduction of splenomegaly and hepatomegaly were noted, as was a continued gradual improvement in plasma glucocerebroside levels. Serial bone marrow studies revealed a slow but steady decrease in the number of Gaucher cells until 1 year posttransplant when they were no longer noted. Approximately 1 year posttransplantation there appeared to be stabilization or partial normalization of the skeletal lesions.

Conclusion

The presentation of splenomegaly in a young child may result from a variety of either inherited or acquired disorders. Full investigation is warranted in order to establish the correct diagnosis and initiate appropriate therapy. Associated signs and symptoms are often helpful in suggesting the diagnosis. Diagnostic approaches may include examination of pathologic material such as peripheral blood, bone marrow, lymph node, and, on occasion, the spleen itself. Given the possibility of a variety of infectious diseases, appropriate cultures and serologic tests may also be required. For inherited disorders, a variety of molecular probes may be employed in the evaluation and diagnosis. Currently, as demonstrated by this case, new therapeutic options may be available for the inherited disorders, and therefore a prompt and complete evaluation should be initiated.

REFERENCES

1. Furbish FS, Blair HE, Shiloach J, et al. Enzyme replacement therapy in Gaucher disease: large scale purification of glucocerebrosidase suitable for human administration. Proc Natl Acad Sci USA 1977;74:3560.
2. Mimouni F, Merlob P, Askhenazi S, et al. Palpable spleens in newborn term infants. Clin Pediatr 1985;24:197.
3. Pearson HA, Gallagher D, Chilcote R, et al. Developmental pattern of splenic dysfunction in sickle cell disorders. Pediatrics 1985;76:392.
4. Redetzki JE, Bickers JN, Samuels MS. Homozygous hemoglobin C disease: clinical review of fifteen patients. South Med J 1968;61:238.
5. Chang-Lo M, Yam LT. Gaucher disease. Am J Med Sci 1967;254:303.
6. Grunebaum M. The roentgenographic findings in the acute neuronopathic form of Niemann-Pick disease. Br J Radiol 1976;49:1018.
7. Crosby WH. Hypersplenism. Annu Rev Med 1963;14:349.

8. Zhang B, Lewis SM. Splenic hematocrit and the splenic plasma pool. Br J Haematol 1987;66:97.
9. Oclan LF, Tubergen DG. Splenomegaly in children: identifying the cause. Postgrad Med 1979;64:191.
10. McIntyre CR, Ebaugh FG. Palpable spleens in college freshmen. Ann Intern Med 1967;66:301.
11. Lee RE. The pathology of Gaucher disease. In: Desnick RJ, Gatt S, Grabowski GA, eds. Gaucher disease: a century of delineation and research. New York: Alan R. Liss, 1982:279.
12. Pick L. Uber die kipoidzellige splenohepatomegalie typus Niemann-Pick als stoffwechselerkrankung. Med Kin 1927;23:1483.
13. Scullin DC, Shelburne JD, Cohen JD. Pseudo-Gaucher cells in multiple myeloma. Am J Med 1979;67:347.
14. Lee RE, Ellis LD. The storage cells of chronic myelogenous leukemia. Lab Invest 1971;24:261.
15. Zaino EC, Rossi MB, Pham TD, et al. Gaucher cells in thalassaemia. Blood 1971;38:457.
16. Beutler E. Gaucher disease. Blood Reviews 1988;2:59.
17. Pinkhas J, Djaldetti M, Yaron M. Coincidence of multiple myeloma with Gaucher disease. Israel J Med Sci 1965;1:537.
18. Krause JR, Bures C, Lee RE. Acute leukemia and Gaucher disease. Scand J Haematol 1979;23:115.
19. Bruckstein AH, Karanas A, Dire JJ. Gaucher disease associated with Hodgkin's disease. Am J Med 1980;68:610.
20. Hanash SM, Rucknagel DL, Heidelberger KP, et al. Primary amyloidosis associated with Gaucher disease. Ann Intern Med 1978;89:639.
21. Buetler E. Gaucher disease (current concepts). N Engl J Med 1991;325:1353.
22. Barranger JA, Ginns EI. Glucosylceramide lipidoses: Gaucher disease. In: Scriver CR, Beaudet AL, Sly WS, Valle D, eds. The metabolic basis of inherited disease. 6th ed. New York: McGraw Hill, 1989:1677.
23. Martin BM, Sdransky E, Ginns EI. Gaucher disease: advances and challenges. Adv Pediatr 1989;36:277.
24. Nilsson O, Grabowski GA, Ludman MD, et al. Gycosphingolipid studies of visceral tissues and brain from type 1 Gaucher disease variants. Clin Genet 1985;27:443.
25. Dreborg S, Erikson A, Hagberg B: Gaucher disease—Norrbottnian type; I, general clinical description. Eur J Pediatr 1980;133:107.
26. Stowens DW, Teitelbaum SL, Kahn AJ, et al. Skeletal complications in Gaucher disease. Medicine 1985;64:310.
27. Pastakia B, Brower AC, Chang VH, et al. Skeletal manifestations of Gaucher disease. Semin Roentgenol 1986;21:264.
28. Rosenthal DI, Mayo-Smith W, Goodsitt MM, et al. Bone and bone marrow changes in Gaucher disease evaluation with quantitative CT. Radiology 1989;170:143.
29. Rosenthal DI Scott JA, Barranger J, et al. Evaluation of Gaucher disease using magnetic resonance imaging. J Bone Joint Surg 1986;68A:802.
30. Brady RO, Kanfer J, Shapiro D. The metabolism of glucocerebrosides: purification and properties of a glucocerebroside-cleaving enzyme from spleen tissue. J Biol Chem 1965;240:39.
31. Ho MW, O'Brien JS. Gaucher disease: Deficiency of "acid" B-glucosidase and reconstitution of enzyme activity in vitro. Proc Natl Acad Sci USA 1971;68:2810.
32. Dinur T, Osiecki KM, Legler G, et al. Human acid B-glucosidase. Isolation and amino acid sequence of a peptide containing the catalytic site. Proc Natl Acad Sci USA 1986;83:1660.
33. Christomanou H, Chabas A, Pampols T, Guardiola A. Activator protein deficient Gaucher disease: a second patient with the newly identified lipid storage disorder. Klin Wochenschr 1989;67:999.
34. Erickson AH, Ginns EI, Barranger JA. Biosynthesis of the lysosomal enzyme glucocerebrosidase. J Biol Chem 1985;260:14310.
35. Ginns EI, Brady RO, Pirruccello S, et al. Mutations of glucocerebrosidase: discrimination of neurologic and non-neurologic phenotypes of Gaucher disease. Proc Natl Acad Sci USA 1982;79:5607.
36. Jonsson LMV, Murray GJ, Sorrell S, et al. Biosynthesis and maturation of glucocerebrosidase in Gaucher fibroblasts. Eur J Biochem 1987;164:171.
37. Nilsson O, Svennerholm L. Accumulation of glucosylceramide and glucocylsphingosine (psychosine) in cerebrum and cerebellum in infantile and juvenile Gaucher disease. J Neurochem 1982;39:709.
38. Zimran A, Gelbart T, Westwood B, et al. High frequency of the Gaucher disease mutation at nucleotide 1226 among Ashkenazi Jews. Am J Hum Genet 1991;49:855.
39. Shafit-Zagardo B, Devine EA, Smith M, et al. Assignment of the gene for acid beta-glucosidase to human chromosome 1. Am J Hum Genet 1981;33:564.
40. Barneveld RA, Keljzei W, Tegelaers FPW, et al. Assignment of the gene coding for human-B-glucocerebrosidase to the region of q21-q31 of chromosome 1 using monoclonal antibodies. Hum Genet 1983;64:227.
41. Ginns EI, Choudary PV, Tsuji S, et al. Gene mapping and leader polypeptide sequence of human glucocerebrosidase: implications for Gaucher disease. Proc Natl Acad Sci USA 1985;82:7101.
42. Horowitz M, Wilder S, Horowitz Z, et al. The human glucocerebrosidase gene and pseudogene: structure and evolution. Genomics 1989;4:87.
43. Latham TE, Theophilus BDM, Grabowski GA, et al. Heterogeneity of mutations in the acid B-glucosidase gene of Gaucher disease patients. DNA Cell Biol 1991;10:15.
44. Beutler E. Gaucher disease: new molecular approaches to diagnosis and treatment. Science 1992;256:794.
45. Zimran A, Gelbart T, Beutler E. Linkage of the PvuII polymorphism with the common Jewish mutation for Gaucher disease. Am J Hum Genet 1990;46:902.
46. Beutler E, Gelbart T, Kuhl W, et al. Identification of the second common Jewish Gaucher disease mutation makes possible population-based screening for the heterozygous state. Proc Natl Acad Sci USA 1991;88:10544.
47. Kawame H, Eto Y. A new glucocerebrosidase gene missense mutation responsible for neuronopathic Gaucher disease in Japanese patients. Am J Hum Genet 1991;49:1378.
48. Zimran A, Sorge J, Gross E, et al. Prediction of severity of Gaucher disease by identification of mutations at DNA level. Lancet 1989;2:349.
49. Beutler E, Gelbart T, Kuhl W, et al. Mutations in Jewish patients with Gaucher disease. Blood 1992;79:1662.
50. Fleshner PR, Aufses AH, Grabowski GA, et al. A 27 year experience with splenectomy for Gaucher disease. Am J Surg 1991;161:69.
51. Ashkenazi A, Zaizov R, Matoth Y. Effect of splenectomy on destructive bone changes in children with chronic (type 1) Gaucher disease. Eur J Pediatr 1986;145:138.

52. Guzzetta PC, Ruley EJ, Merrick HF, et al. Elective subtotal splenectomy: indications and results in 33 patients. Ann Surg 1990;211:34.

53. Boklan BFK, Sawitsky A. Factor IX deficiency in Gaucher disease. Arch Intern Med 1976;136:489.

54. Brady RO, Pentchev, PG, Gal AE, et al. Replacement therapy for inherited enzyme deficiency: use of purified glucocerebrosidase in Gaucher disease. N Engl J Med 1974; 291:989.

55. Beutler E, Dale GL, Guinto E, et al. Enzyme replacement therapy in Gaucher disease: preliminary clinical trial of a new enzyme preparation. Proc Natl Acad Sci USA 1977;74:4620.

56. Blechetz PE, Crawley JCW, Braidman IP, et al. Treatment of Gaucher disease with liposome-entrapped glucocerebrosidase: B-glucosidase. Lancet 1977;2:1116.

57. Stahl PD, Rodman JS, Miller MJ, et al. Evidence for receptor-mediated binding of glycoproteins, glycoconjugates and lysosomal glycosidases by alveolar macrophages. Proc Natl Acad Sci USA 1978;75:1399.

58. Furbish FS, Steer CJ, Krett NL, et al. Uptake and distribution of placental glucocerebrosidase in rat hepatic cells and effects of sequential deglycosylation. Biochim Biophys Acta 1981;673:425.

59. Murry GJ. Lectin-specific targeting of lysosomal enzymes to reticuloendothelial cell. In: Green R, Widder KJ, eds. Drug and enzyme targeting; vol 149, methods in enzymology. San Diego: Academic Press, 1987:25.

60. Barton NW, Brady RO, Dambrosia JM, et al. Replacement therapy for inherited enzyme deficiency-macrophage-targeted glucocerebrosidase for Gaucher disease. N Engl J Med 1991;324:1464.

61. Beutler E, Kay AC, Saven A, et al. Enzyme replacement therapy for Gaucher disease. Blood 1991;78:1183.

62. Figueroa ML, Rosenbloom BE, Kay AC, et al. A less costly regimen of alglucerase to treat Gaucher disease. N Engl J Med 1992;327:1632.

63. Murray GJ, Howard KD, Richards SM, et al. Gaucher disease: lack of antibody response in 12 patients following repeated intravenous infusions of mannos terminal glucocerebrosidase. J Immunol Methods 1991;137:113.

64. Barton NW, Brady RO, Dambrosia JM, et al. Dose-dependent responses to macrophage-targeted glucocerebrosidase in a child with Gaucher disease. J Pediatr 1992;120:277.

65. Barton NW, Furbish FS, Murray GJ, et al. Therapeutic response to intravenous infusions of glucocerebrosidase in a patient with Gaucher disease. PNAS 1990;87:1913.

66. Fallet S, Grace ME, Sibille A, et al. Enzyme augmentation in moderate to life-threatening Gaucher disease. Pediatr Res 1992;31:496.

67. Barranger JA, Ohashi T, Hong CM, et al. Molecular pathology and therapy of Gaucher disease. Jpn J Inher Metabol Dis 1989;51:45.

68. Thomas ED, Ramberg RE, Sale GE, et al: Direct evidence for bone marrow origin of the alveolar macrophage in man. Science 1976;192:1016.

69. Gale RP, Sparkes RS, Golde EW. Bone marrow origin of hepatic macrophages (Kupffer cells) in humans. Science 1978;201:937.

70. Hoogerbrugge PM, Wagemaker G, VanBekkum DW Failure to demonstrate pluripotential hemopoietic stem cells in mouse brains. Proc Natl Acad Sc USA 1985; 82:4268.

71. Rappeport JM, Ginns EI. Bone marrow transplantation in severe Gaucher disease: slow turnover of storage cells following rapid correction of enzyme deficiency. N Engl J Med 1984;311:84.

72. Starer F, Sargent JD, Hobbs JR. Regression of the radiological changes of Gaucher disease following bone marrow transplantation. Br J Radiol 1987;60:1189.

73. Ringden O, Groth CG, Erkson A, et al. Long-term follow-up of the first successful bone marrow transplantation in Gaucher disease. Transplantation 1988;46:66.

74. Kernan NA, Barsch G, Ash RC, et al. Analysis of 462 transplantations from unrelated donors facilitated by the National Marrow Donor Program. N Engl J Med 1993;328:593.

75. Fink JK, Correll PH, Perry LK, et al. Correction of glucocerebrosidase deficiency after retroviral-mediated gene transfer into hematopoietic progenitor cells from patients with Gaucher disease. Proc Natl Acad Sci USA 1990;87:2334.

76. Gluckman E, Broxmeyer HE, Auerbach AD, et al. Hematopoietic reconstitution in a patient with Fanconi's anemia by means of umbilical-cord blood from an HLA-identical sibling. N Engl J Med 1989;321:1174.

77. Broxmeyer HE, Kurtzberg, J, Gluckman E, et al. Umbilical cord blood hematopoietic stem and repopulating cells in human clinical transplantation. Blood Cells 1991;17:330.

CHAPTER 24

Myelodysplastic Disorders

STUART ROATH AND SAMUEL GROSS

In treating a patient, let your first thought be to strengthen his natural vitality.
—Rhazes, Persian physician and philosopher (932)

The term "myelodysplastic disorders" covers a range of conditions that have in common ineffective hemopoiesis, of known or presumed clonal derivation, and that frequently terminate in acute nonlymphoid leukemia.

Case 1

S.K., a 77-year-old man, presented to his physician with symptoms of lethargy and dyspnea of 4 weeks' duration. Previously in good health, he had retired from ownership of a retail store 5 years previously. His past history included cigarette smoking for many years, but he had stopped 12 years earlier. He drank alcohol occasionally and had been diagnosed as having non–insulin dependent diabetes 5 years ago. This was controlled by weight reduction and diet. He had a history of hemorrhoids which had ben banded twice, 15 and 8 years previously. Physical examination revealed a well-nourished, fit looking man with obvious pallor and sallow complexion. The skin was clear, the sclera nonicteric, and no lymphadenopathy was found. There was a trace of ankle edema, and the dorsalis pedis pulses were absent on both sides. Examination of the cardiovascular system revealed a regular tachycardia of 110 beats/minute and a blood pressure of 190/105. The cardiac apex was felt 4 inches from the center, and a soft systolic blowing grade 2 murmur was heard in all areas. The lungs moved well and were normal with the exception of a few basal crepitations. The liver was felt 2 cm below the costal margin on inspiration; the spleen was not felt. Central nervous system (CNS) examination results were normal with nothing to indicate, for instance, subacute combined degeneration or peripheral neuropathy.

A presumptive diagnosis of anemia was made, and an automated blood screen showed the following: hemoglobin 85 g/L, white blood cell (WBC) count 3.2 (absolute neutrophil count [ANC]) 1.6×10^9/L, and platelets 98×10^9/L. Red blood cell (RBC) indices showed a mean corpuscular volume (MCV) of 99 fL, and an increased red cell distribution width (RDW). Examination of the peripheral blood film revealed anisocytosis with many macrocytes and an occasional nucleated RBC with small distorted nuclei and some cytoplasmic inclusions. The WBCs and platelets showed no gross morphologic abnormalities but the neutrophils were numerically low at 1.6×10^9/L. Urea, electrolytes, and liver function

test results were normal and his early morning urine showed 1+ positive for sugar but no heme products or bilirubin. Serum ferritin was at the upper limits of normal (330 μg/L), vitamin B_{12} was 900 pmol/L, and RBC folate 650 nmol/L, both in the high normal range. Serum immunoglobulin and albumin levels were normal.

The differential diagnosis included a secondary anemia, with cancer a possibility—a hematologic premalignancy or one of the myelodysplasias.

Bone marrow biopsy and aspirate were carried out showing hypercellularity with normal architecture. No tumor or granulomas were seen nor was there excess fibrosis or plasma cells. Blasts were <5%. Erythropoiesis was active but dysplastic showing nucleocytoplasmic asynchrony and so-called "megaloblastoid" features, the iron stain showing many sideroblasts, some with perinuclear rings of hemosiderin. (An iron stain done on a peripheral blood smear also showed siderocytes and some ringed normoblasts.) The marrow karyotype showed an extra number 8 chromosome in about 60% of the dividing cells, which on subsequent testing was found also in PHA-stimulated peripheral blood karyotyping.

A final diagnosis of myelodysplasia classified as Refractory Anemia with Ringed Sideroblasts (RARS) was made.

Other diagnoses considered initially among the **differential** were **Secondary, or Simple Chronic Anemia**. No systemic disease was found to account for this and pancytopenia, and the characteristic ringed sideroblasts are not found in this anemia.

The ineffective erythropoiesis and iron loading of **Megaloblastic Anemia** can be a feature of this disorder. The megaloblastic morphology is superficially confusing. Prior to the discovery of the relationship between vitamin B_{12}, folate, and hematopoiesis, it may have been difficult to identify the myelodysplasias. Older textbooks used the term **Achrestic Anemia** to describe what were probably megaloblastic and refractory anemias, but the normal levels of vitamin B_{12} and folate in this patient exclude a megaloblastic anemia.

Thalassemia is an iron-loading, ineffective erythropoietic disorder, which presents as a microcytic hypochromic anemia. Although hypochromia may also be a feature in the RBCs of patients with MDS, the clinical features of thalassemia and the presence of the globin chain synthesis abnormalities, including elevated levels of hemoglobin F and/or A_2, are distinctive. Modest elevations of hemoglobin F have been noted in myelodysplastic syndrome (MDS), especially in childhood MML.

Both primary, and especially secondary, **Acute Myeloblastic Leukemia (AML)**, especially AML of protracted onset, may be indistinguishable from MDS in some cases. French-American-British (FAB) classification M1 and M2 variants are those that develop in 25–50% of MDS cases and are presumably biologically related. **Preleukemia, or Smoldering, Leukemia** are older terms that probably included some cases of MDS.

Pyridoxine Responsive Anemia is another uncommon iron-loading anemia. Pyridoxine deficiency as such does not occur in man, but some persons with iron-loading anemias, including ringed sideroblast variants, respond to pharmacologic doses of pyridoxine. Familial cases have been reported and are usually X-linked (1).

Acquired Sideroblastic Anemia can also be associated with alcoholism, drugs such as isoniazid, copper deficiency, and lead poisoning. Defective heme synthesis associated with aminoeluvinic acid (ALA) metabolism or mitochondrial defects are probable causes.

The Myelodysplastic Syndrome

MDS was only recognized as a clinically coherent entity about 20 years ago, although refractory anemia and preleukemia had previously been described and their evolutionary relationship to AML recognized (2). It is still an underreported disorder in many countries and its frequency is uncertain. Joosten et al. (3) suggest an occurrence of 0.75/1,000/year in geriatric patients; where a special study has been made it may be >40/100,000/year in patients >70 years of age and twice that number in patients in their 80s (4) (fig. 24.1). Most larger reported studies suggest a mean age of onset of about 60–65 years. Because of referral patterns, tertiary treatment centers often deal with slightly younger patients, and many therapeutic trials in such centers deal with MDS patients much younger than this. The age and sex distribution and incidence presented in figures 24.1 and 24.2 represents a largely adult appearance, but the disease is seen at all ages, and reviewers have suggested an incidence of from 3–8% (5, 6) of pediatric hematologic malignancies. There appears to be only a slight predilection for males overall; but CMML is commoner in males and the 5q-abnormality is more common in females. Aul et al. (7) make the point that because of different ways of collecting data, and disease nomenclature, much of the epidemiology is difficult to assess comparatively. The FAB classification (8) of these diseases, shown in table 24.1, is totally morphologically based, has broad prognostic significance, but probably covers a number of disorders in which the morphology is a common end point rather than specifically related to any genetic or enzymatic background.

Clinical and Laboratory Features

As in this patient, the commonest presentation relates to symptoms of anemia, but 20% of patients with MDS are

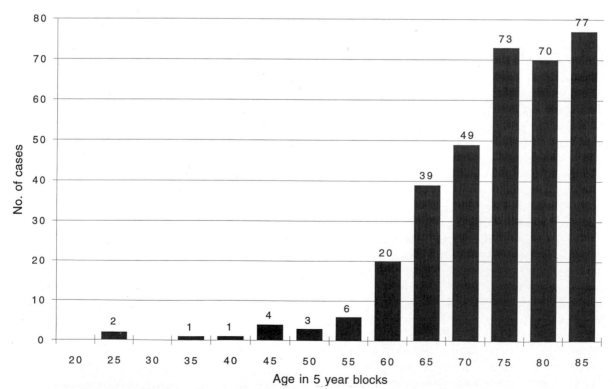

Figure 24.1. Age distribution of myelodysplasia cases diagnosed in Somerset, 1985–1993. (From Phillips M, Cull GM, Ewings M. Establishing the incidence of myelodysplasia syndrome. Br J Haematol 1994;88:186.)

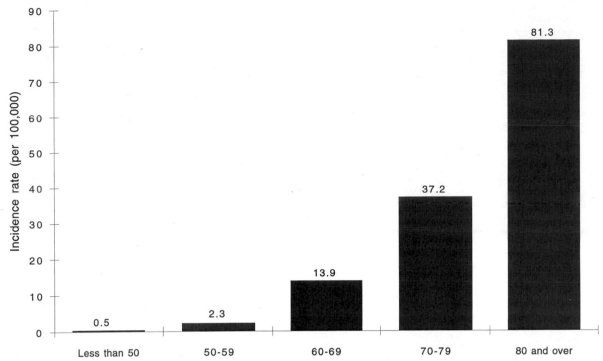

Figure 24.2. Age-specific incidence rates/100,000 of myelodysplasia diagnosed in Somerset, 1985–1993. (From Phillips M, Cull GM, Ewings M. Establishing the incidence of myelodysplasia syndrome. Br J Haematol 1994;88:186.)

Table 24.1. French-American-British (FAB) Classification*

Category	Abbreviation	Blood	Marrow
Refractory anemia	RA	Monocytes <1%	RS <15
		Blasts <1%	Blasts <5%
Refractory anemia with ringed sideroblasts	RARS or AISA	Monocytes <1%	RS >15%
		Blasts <1%	
Refractory anemia with excess blasts	RAEB	Blasts <5%	Blasts 5–20%
Refractory anemia with excess blasts in leukemic transformation	RAEBt	Blasts variable	Blasts >20%
Chronic myelomonocytic leukemia	CMML, or occasionally, CMMoL	Monocytes >1%	Blasts<5%
		Blasts <5%	

*RS, Ringed sideroblasts.

initially seen clinically with complaints due to thrombocytopenia or leukopenia (bleeding or infection). There is no predominant cluster of physical findings, except that in the CMML variant splenomegaly, skin lesions, and hepatomegaly are found more often, especially in the childhood form.

The anemia may be normocytic or macrocytic and the red cells strikingly abnormal in shape, appearance, and hemoglobinization. The MCV is rarely >110 fL and the RDW is increased. Hypochromia, inclusion bodies, and nucleated red cells may be seen in the peripheral blood smear. About 50% of patients have some degree of pancytopenia, and the neutrophils may show poor granularity and a Pelger-Huet-like defect in nuclear lobulation. Abnormalities in monocytes are not recognized except in the CMML.

Functional defects of no single nature are described in the MDS granulocytes. Adhesion, chemotactic abnormalities, and enzyme abnormalities have been reported (9, 10).

A relationship between these and complement receptors CR1 and CR3 and the FAB category has been suggested (11). Platelets may be reduced in 50% cases, but are morphologically normal. Platelet functional defects, including prolonged bleeding times and poor aggregation, have also been noted (12). Although lymphocytes do not show the overt morphologic changes seen in other blood cells, they are often numerically reduced, primarily due to decreases in CD-4 subsets. Similarly, natural killer (NK) cell numbers are reduced, but B-cells are more likely to be normal. Functional defects have also been described in these cells but their clinical significance is unclear (13). Polyclonal gammopathy occurs in about a third of MDS patients (14) and various autoimmune phenomena have been reported, but no consistent pattern of disorders emerges (13).

Bone marrow biopsy shows increased cellularity and variable gross morphologic features in about 90% of cases.

Table 24.2. French-American-British Classification (FAB) Type, Survival and ANNL Incidence[*]

FAB Type	Median Survival (mo)	Range	% ANNL	Range
RA	37	19–64	11	0–20
RARS	49	21–76	5	0–15
RAEB	9	7–15	23	11–50
RAEBt	6	5–12	48	11–75
CMML	22	8–60+	20	3–55
All patients	?	5–?	19	

[*]Modified from Deiss A. In: Lee GR et al., ed. Wintrobe's Clinical hematology, 9th ed. Philadelphia: Lea & Febiger, 1993:1956. RA. refractory anemia; RARS, refractory anemia with ringed sideroblasts; RAEB, refractory anemia with excess blasts; RAEBt, refractory anemia with excess blasts in leukemic transformation; CMML, chronic myelomonocytic leukemia.

Abnormal localization of immature cells (**ALIPs**) is rarely found **except in MDS and in some cases of AML,** and dysplastic small megakaryocytes may be prominent. Iron staining is usually heavy. Hypoplasia or fibrosis are seen in <10% of cases.

Marrow smears show the characteristic increase in normoblasts with misshapen or megaloblastoid nuclei lagging in development behind the cytoplasm and mitochondria contain iron-laden granules. Neutrophil abnormalities parallel these changes and include a preponderance of early precursors, as well as showing occasional Auer rods.

Attempts using multivariate analysis of the above clinical and laboratory findings to provide attribute "scores" for MDS have been undertaken. The FAB classification itself is of value in large populations, but the wide confidence limits in its prognostic values, as shown in the data collected by Ganser and Hoelzer (15), make it too crude to use as a basis for clinical trials (table 24.2). Like the FAB classification, these other guides are useful in generalizing about patient populations; but because different reports have dealt with noncomparable patient groups, their value is of interest mostly to taxonomists. They were reviewed by Mufti et al. (14). The purpose of classification and scores is to provide prognostic information and guidelines for treatment. At present it can be seen that **Refractory Anemia (RA)** and **Refractory Anemia with Ringed Sideroblasts (RARS)** have a better prognosis than the other forms, but CMML varies so much in its course that the prognosis is unpredictable. Childhood MDS is usually rapidly lethal if untreated. Cases of primary MDS in younger individuals appear to be more aggressive, but associated medical conditions and frailness in older populations can also contribute to poor survival (16).

Cytogenetics and Molecular Genetics

More precise classification has been sought by cellular and subcellular studies. MDS appears to be due to hemopoietic stem cell or pluripotential cell clonal defects. Glucose-6-phosphate dehydrogenase (G-6-PD) isoenzyme patterns, X-linked restriction fragment length polymorphism (RFLP), and the narrow pattern of karyotype abnormalities lend firm support to this hypothesis (17, 18).

Numerous studies have shown that 50–90% of patients with MDS have abnormal karyotypes (19, 20, 21). Although there is some overlap with the findings in acute myeloid leukemias (AMLs), the characteristic defects in MDS are deletions of whole or part of chromosomes. Mecucci and Van den Berghe describe 18 different p or q deletions (22). There are also some cases with trisomy 8 and a few with complex balanced translocations. More complex abnormalities tend to be found where frank leukemia is developing (table 24.3).

The 5q-syndrome, one of the most frequently found abnormalities in MDS (15–20% of cases), may correlate with the thrombocytosis seen in 10–20% of cases. It may also be associated with age, female sex, and a more prolonged indolent course and less frequent transformation to acute leukemia (23). In the syndrome, originally described by Van den Berghe et al. (24), the 5q- is associated with macrocytic anemia and thrombocytosis in elderly women, with a relatively good prognosis, but the abnormality is also found in other MDS patients without these features.

Loss of or deletion of part of chromosome 7 is frequently seen in childhood MDS and in secondary leukemias, and is typically associated with neutrophil functional defects and early leukemic transformation.

11q- is associated with sideroblastosis, especially the ringed form, but many cases with this finding do not demonstrate this particular karyotype.

Breakpoints in chromosomes 14 and 23 have been reported without specific association with MDS variants. *20q-* has been described in **Polycythemia Vera.** *Trisomy 8* is found in all forms of MDS, including a minority of CMML cases.

One form of MDS RA appears to be X-linked (Xq13 variant) (4), which is interesting in view of the benign X-linked sideroblastic anemias also reported (1). Followup studies on the earlier reported group were not reported but normal karyotypes were obtained at the time.

Survival may be related to karyotype only in that patients with normal cytogenetics survive longer than those with abnormalities; the VIth Workshop on Chromosomes in Leukemia showed that more abnormalities were found in the poorer FAB prognostic groups (25). However, others have shown poorer survival rates

Table 24.3. Percentage of Recognizable Cytogenetic Abnormalities

	MDS	Post-MDS	AML
t(8;21)	2	5	
t(15;17)		1	
Inv (10)	1	4	
+8	10	16	
−5/−7[°]	42	25	
Diploid	45	50	

[°]High risk factor for shortest survival with conventional therapy; −, loss of chromosome; +, additional chromosome.

with complex karyotypes or with monosomy 7 (26, 27). There may also be subgroups with nondeleted but abnormal karyotypes that are more difficult to identify, such as small balanced translocations that carry prognostic significance.

Despite the lack of an obvious common genetic background, the preceding chromosome abnormalities are of a nonrandom nature and support the clonal origin of MDS, which, unlike CML, may have many different regulatory mechanisms for hemopoietic growth and differentiation. Since all hemopoietic cells, including lymphocytes, may be involved, the commonest result is ineffective but hyperactive hemopoieses with as many as 70% of the marrow cells showing apoptosis in 90% of patients. The pace of development and takeover of the abnormal clone is slower than that observed in acute leukemia; and relatively stable "chimeras" of normal and MDS clones may coexist. The presence of a putative oncogene or the lack of a tumor suppressor gene would be noteworthy and has been sought (28).

The **RAS** family of oncogenes encode for 21-kd proteins involved in signal transduction from surface-generated signals to intracellular second messengers in the cell growth and differentiation process. They are found on chromosomes 1, 11, and 15 and are widely associated with the development of malignancy in many tissues. RAS mutations have been found in up to 25% of MDS patients and may signal preleukemic progression. One report (29) suggests a majority of CMML patients may have such a mutation. How the presence of such an oncogene is linked with the MDS process is unknown. RAS mutations have also been found in postchemotherapy or postradiotherapy patients without overt malignant hemopoieses. RAS oncogenes are located on chromosome 11, but there is no known relationship between MDS and the identification of a specific RAS mutation on no. 11. Most of the RAS mutations found in MDS (and leukemia) have been N type, rather than the K mutation found frequently in pancreatic and colon cancer. The presence of a RAS point mutation appears to be a bad prognostic finding and is associated with the development of AML (30). However, this may be a late development in MDS, and the mutation has been recorded as developing during the course of the disorder (31).

A possible explanation for its action may lie in the ability of this gene to control internalization of signals from hemopoietic growth factors, but a final link between its presence and MDS has not been made. The glutamyl transpeptidase (GTP) binding proteins controlled by this gene family indirectly control proliferation rates through intracellular GTP levels, but simple changes in cell proliferation do not account for the findings in MDS.

FMS protooncogenes may have a role in MDS development: the 5q- deletion may result in the loss of material on the 31 or 33 bands. This is an area rich in genes controlling or encrypted for control of many cytokines involved in hemopoiesis (IL-3, 4, 5, and 9, GM-CSF, or CSF-1, CD 14) (32). The FMS gene encodes for M-CSF receptor (the M-CSF gene is located on chromosome 1) and mutations of this gene at points 301 and 969 have been found in about 20% of MDS patients, more in the CMML variety but also in the others. Similar levels of mutations are found in AML. The connection between mutations or losses of FMS gene material and MDS is as yet unclear.

Tumor suppressor genes, such as the **p53** gene on chromosome 17, would be interesting candidates for involvement in MDS (33). Such gene mutations have been found at low frequency (approximately 5%) in this disease, sometimes with the rare 17p- chromosome abnormality or with the 5q/17p deletions. Recent investigations using PCR or single-strand conformational polymorphism sequencing (SSCP) and direct nucleotide sequencing cast doubt on a primary role for such mutations, which were found only in 4 of 26 cases of MDS. In effect, such mutations may have been terminal events (34). The tumor suppressor gene, EGR1, is located on 5q but has not yet been implicated in the evolution of MDS. An interferon-regulatory gene (IRFI) has been found on 5q31. In one study, this gene, which may have oncogene-antagonist activity, was found deleted in all 12 MDS patients (35).

The **DCC** gene **(Deleted in Colon Cancer)** is another tumor-suppression gene located on the long arm of chromosome 18. It encodes for a cell surface glycoprotein whose function is uncertain at present. However, it has been found to have absent or reduced expression in acute leukemia and MDS. Although absent in only 3 of 33 MDS cases, all became leukemic within 6 months; in others, when AML had already supervened, the gene expression was also absent (36). At present the significance of this and other findings in tumor suppression genes is not clear.

Hypermethylation of the Calcitonin gene has been reported in a majority of cases in another study, but correlation with the FAB classification was not obtained (37) and no other data were reported. Hutchison et al. (38) reported increases in a number of protooncogene RNAs in MDS but noted similar findings in nonmalignant perturbations of the bone marrow.

It could be argued for this and other deletions where oncogene or tumor suppressor genes are involved that if there is one normal chromosome, there should be no functional deficit except in the case of X-linked syndromes where the Lyon hypothesis can be applied. However, it is speculated that the corresponding gene on the apparently normal chromosome may be spatially or otherwise unbalanced, whereupon oncogene activation or masking of tumor suppressive genes may result.

Growth Factors or Receptors for these could be etiologically implicated. For instance, chromosome 5 deletions are one of the commonest defects in MDS. 5q33, or other sequences in this region, are responsible for G-CSF or GM-CSF receptors. No firm links between growth factor abnormalities and MDS variants are presently accepted (39). A few reports suggest that hemopoietic growth factor levels in vivo generally are low, suggesting that cyclic feedback mechanisms may be disturbed, pathologic autocrine growth stimulation has taken place, and opportunities for therapeutic intervention may exist. However, erythropoietin (Epo) levels are often normal or high in the initial stages of MDS despite the undoubted responses to this growth factor occasionally seen in vivo. Cytokines such as G-CF and GM-CSFs and Il-3 and 6 have been reported as being low (40), but these findings are not yet substantiated, and although, as with Epo, a clinical response can be observed sometimes with their in vivo use, they do not influence the course of the disease. There is even concern that the cytokines may accelerate the growth of the malignant clone.

There are further data relative to the biology of MDS, to cytokine production, and to their in vitro responses. In vitro growth of MDS bone marrow is variable and can be leukemic, normal, or mixed. The results of 20 different reported studies over a score of years (41) showed an inconsistent pattern of in vitro growth, but few of the reports could be compared. Although they often showed both poor differentiation and low growth, these were not always found, nor did they correlate well with clinical classification or FAB type. One notable finding may be significant— namely, three types of myeloblasts have been recognized, depending on morphology (42), and the types II and III, which are reputedly CD-34−, account for the increase in blasts in the advanced forms of MDS (43). This appears to be a critical difference between MDS and AML, where type I blasts are usually seen. A report on impaired CD-34+ cell responses in culture (44) would have to be interpreted carefully, since, if MDS blasts are CD-34−, then any work done with positive cells will be nonrepresentative. However, abnormal but variable responses were still seen. The gene responsible for the CD-34+ production is located on chromosome 1 and not known to be involved in MDS. This does not exclude the effect of another regulatory gene situated elsewhere, however.

Despite evidence compatible with disordered hemopoietic cell growth response in vitro and in vivo, no positive link between any single gene abnormality or product controlling hemopoietic cell development in vivo has been found in all MDS cases. More data are rapidly being assembled, however, which is likely to clarify the biologic basis for MDS and lead to better clinical approaches. Stephenson and her colleagues (45) have recently reviewed work in progress to this end. In all probability the biogenesis of MDS is a multistep pathway with many links that are presently unidentified (3).

Prognostic factors *relevant to this the patient described in case 1 would appear to be dependent on age, FAB type, and karyotype, although each is of limited value. Being elderly of itself carries an unfavorable prognosis. Childhood MDS has an entirely different outlook. The patient's RARS FAB category has a relatively good prognosis. His +8 karyotype carries an intermediate prognostic value. Therefore, his outlook appears to be* *average, and his management likely to be influenced more by his age than by the other factors.*

Management

The issues in management are fundamentally *supportive* therapy versus a more *aggressive* approach. The former would historically consist of blood transfusion, as clinically indicated. If this were protracted (some individuals could require as much as 100 units of packed cells), there may be a role for simultaneous iron chelation. Although hemosiderosis will occur eventually, it is rarely clinically damaging.

Cytokines can have a supportive role. The fact that this patient was able to accommodate to a single day's hospitalization for transfusion monthly does not warrant treatment with Epo, but this should be kept under review. The value of Epo in reducing the need for blood transfusion in this disorder is known and a recent meta analysis has reported the overall "significant response" rate in 205 patients studied to be 16% (46). Patients already being transfused and belonging to the RARS group responded least favorably. An unconfirmed preliminary report states that patients with the highest levels of endogenous Epo respond best (47). Occasional reports of increases in platelet counts are also recorded. Epo needs to be given by subcutaneous injection three times weekly, and its expense, inconvenience, and discomfort must be weighed against its possible benefit.

Additionally, if the neutrophil count should fall with resultant recurrent infections, the use of G-CSF or GM-CSF should be considered. As with Epo, this is occasionally of clinical value in these circumstances and can decrease disease morbidity successfully. The side effects, especially with GM-CSF, are also uncomfortable for some patients. An early report suggests that combinations of Epo and G-CSF might be better than Epo alone in supporting hemoglobin levels (48).

If our patient had been 52 rather than 72 years of age, he would have received measures aimed at cure, or at least remission, rather than support only.

The more aggressive options range from allogenic bone marrow transplantation to more aggressive chemotherapy programs, differentiating agents, and cytokines.

Bone Marrow Transplantation (BMT)

The use of bone marrow transplantation, is worth considering as a regimen for any form of MDS, as it is for chronic myelogenous leukemia (CML). MDS is lethal even when AML does not supervene. Many patients die of problems related to bone marrow failure, such as infections and bleeding, apart from the morbidity of the protracted "benign" course. A review of 260 transplanted patients (49) with a median age of about 33 years found disease-free survivals of 35–45% at various followup intervals. Indeed, the results for MDS appear to be better than those for secondary leukemia. If BMT is to be carried out, it should be done so as early as possible and preferably with matched donors (50). Only 10% of MDS patients qualify for this treatment (51), however, and the search for other therapy or improvements in the use of mismatched BMTs, needs to be continued. Numerous studies using mismatched transplants appear to be promising.

Conventional Antileukemic Therapy

Conventional antileukemic therapy has a remission rate approaching that for comparable cases of AML, but most of the older MDS patient population are unsuitable candidates for the most aggressive curative versions of this approach. However, patients in the age groups qualifying for aggressive AML chemotherapy can be similarly treated, and response rates of up to 55% have been reported (52). The different categories or cytogenetic groups are not noticeably different in outcome reports. Age is important in response and survival, and schemes of risk assessment (53) may give some guidance. Secondary MDS cases do worse than the primary ones (like AML). There is no one preferred regimen.

For the majority of MDS patients unsuitable for aggressive treatment, low-dose single-agent chemotherapy, especially with cytosine arabinoside, has been extensively used based on observations that, in vitro, it caused differentiation in HLA-60 cells. A few cases remitted, but many were worsened, and the approach has now been abandoned. No group of cases could be retrospectively identified as benefitting from this management, despite a number of variations in the mode of delivery. Older patients, especially, experienced considerable morbidity from the drug. Other single-agent therapy seems to have no benefit, although a recent brief report has shown promise with 5-azacytidine (54).

Differentiation Therapy

It was hoped that low-dose myelosuppressive therapy (see above) might prompt differentiation in MDS rather than suppression of a malignant hemopoietic clone, so that survival and quality of life would improve even in the absence of cure. In vitro data have supported this philosophy and led to the search for more suitable agents. The retinoic acids (both 13 cis and all trans) have been tried, including one controlled trial (55), with disappointing results to date. Vitamin D analogs are also capable of gene regulation and therefore are therapeutic candidates for disorders such as MDS, where gene regulation may be pathogenetically critical. As with other agents, the in vitro data were promising, especially in promoting macrophage differentiation. Their use in vivo has been limited by toxicity, and concentrations approaching those in vitro are unobtainable because of hypercalcemia and vitamin D toxicity. However, the search for less metabolically toxic analogs continues and vitamin D_3 derivatives may yet have a role to play in MDS. There has been a study of the potential differentiating agent hexamethylene bisacetamide (HMBA), which also promotes differentiation of HLA cells in vitro. To date (56), the response rate has been disappointing.

Another recent approach has involved the use of hemopoietic **Growth Factors,** not only for supporting ther-apy, but also to alter the course of the disease. Epo administration will reduce transfusion needs in some cases of indolent MDS, and both G-CSF and GM-CSF are effective in raising the white blood cell (WBC) levels. Both of these, as well as Il-3, were hoped to have some effect on the course of the disease. Currently there does not appear to be a marked survival advantage with any of these modalities.

Other biologic response–modifying agents include **Interferons,** especially γ-interferon. Anecdotal reports of response to interferons led to a number of small uncontrolled trials showing that both α- and γ-interferons produced rare remissions and some additional cases whose blood counts improved and transfusion requirements lessened. Overall, the results have had little impact on MDS management, and the side effects of the treatment discouraged its general application, especially in the less fit elderly. However, studies are still ongoing (57).

Weighing all the options in the patient in case 1, and discussing use of biologic response modifiers in particular, as well as more conventional therapy, we decided to treat him conservatively with periodic blood transfusion with monthly symptomatic evaluation and hematologic followup. After 1 year his transfusion needs were satisfied at 2 units of packed cells monthly, his platelets were adequate at $76 \times 10^9/L$, and his WBC averaged $3.2 \times 10^9/L$. Repeat bone marrow aspirate only showed <5% blasts in his marrow, along with unchanged karyotype and numbers of trisomy 8 cells.

Case 2

A 31-year-old woman was initially seen clinically with a 5- day history of severe menorrhagia. She had "always had heavy periods," but this was noticeably worse, and she had also noted some increased bruisability over the last month. A blood count showed her hemoglobin to be 83 g/L with an MCV of 105 fL. The WBC was $13.3 \times 10^9/L$ (absolute neutrophil count [ANC] 9.8, monos 1.6, lymphocytes $0.9 \times 10^9/L$), and platelets $30 \times 10^9/L$. Serum ferritin (70 μg/L), vitamin B_{12} 340 pmol/L, and red cell folate 285 nmol/L (all normal levels); lactic dehydrogenase (LDH) was 1008 U/L (normal − 530). Physical examination showed pallor and ecchymoses on the lower extremities; no enlargement of the spleen or liver was felt and no skin lesions were seen. Gynecologic examination revealed no pathologic findings other than confirming the excess vaginal blood loss. Because the cause for the anemia and thrombocytopenia was unknown, a bone marrow aspirate and biopsy were carried out, showing high cellularity but with reduced megakaryocytes, an appearance suggestive of an intrinsic marrow defect. Erythropoiesis was dysplastic, with distorted or megaloblastoid features and adequate storage iron found. Islands of such erythroblasts were seen. Immature monocytoid precursor cell were seen in clusters (ALIPs), and early granulocytes were increased. The megakaryocytes were small and lacked polyploidy of their nucleus. Blasts were increased at 8%; cytochemistry showed them to be of myeloid rather than mono-

cyte lineage. No Auer rods were seen. A karyotype of the blood and marrow showed poor metaphase yield but no abnormalities.

Differential Diagnosis: At presentation, the differential diagnosis would include most of the causes of thrombocytopenia. The anemia could be secondary, and the macrocytosis could be merely the appearance of reticulocytes associated with reticulocytosis. The leukocytosis was unhelpful. However, the abnormal marrow findings and normal hematinics levels suggested a diagnosis of MDS, refractory anemia with excess blasts (FAB classification RAEB).

Management: Initial management included treatment with platelet transfusions, followed by red cell infusions to stability. Prognostic factors were evaluated, and a management plan was then carried out.

This patient falls into the younger age group of patients who are sometimes said to do better, but that is because the group includes patients suitable for aggressive curative therapy. In most scoring or prognostic systems, the presence of anemia, thrombocytopenia, and >5% bone marrow blasts is linked to reduced survival. The presence of ALIPs is also considered unfavorable (58). The apparently normal karyotype of the patient could be considered a favorable prognostic factor, but the poor metaphase yield was suspicious and compatible with an abnormal clone. If a suitable FISH application had been available at the time of assessment, it might either have shown balanced translocation or located abnormal gene sequences.

Unlike the patient in case 1, the patient in case 2 could not be offered supportive treatment indefinitely because her thrombocytopenia was likely to be a problem. For 4 months while her therapeutic options were explored, however, her menorrhagia responded to danazol 600 mg daily and her hemoglobin was maintained with packed red cell transfusions. We noticed that her WBC was rising and blasts were now seen in the peripheral blood. She then re-presented for hyphema in the right eye. A repeat bone marrow aspirate showed 40% blasts, and her karyotype now showed a shortened q5 chromosome. A formal diagnosis of AML conversion was made and, in the absence of a suitable bone marrow donor, she was offered "conventional" AML therapy with cytosine arabinoside and mitoxantrone. Following two courses of this treatment, complicated by febrile neutropenia with unidentified pathogens, she swent into remission and received two more courses as consolidation. One more febrile episode occurred, which required antifungal treatment for resolution. Her progress was otherwise uneventful. She has been observed for 4 years without overt or cytogenetic relapse, but her platelet count has never risen above 150 × 10⁹/L.

Variants of MDS

There is relatively little difference clinically between cases classified as refractory anemia (RA) and those classified as refractory anemia with ringed sideroblasts (RARS). Refractory anemia with excess blasts (RAEB) and refractory anemia with excess blasts in leukemic transformation (RAEBt) are likely to be stages along the same disease progression pathway to acute leukemia. However the fifth category, CMML, deserves separate mention. CMML (sometimes termed CMMoL) resembles a myeloproliferative rather than a myelodysplastic disorder in many respects and is sometimes classified alongside pH-negative CML. CMML is *bcr* negative and thus clonally resembles only 1% of all CML cases in that respect. CMML may more closely resembles pH-negative juvenile CML. CMML is distinguished clinically by the more frequent presence of splenomegaly, hepatomegaly, and skin infiltrations with mononuclear cells. It has the same age and sex distribution in adults as MDS at large, but is characterized by the appearance of >1 × 10⁹/L monocytes in the peripheral blood as well as anemia with evidence of dyserythropoiesis and thrombocytopenia. Polyclonal increase in immunoglobulins is often reported, and there is a case report of an association with primary amyloidosis (59). The marrow shows an increase in monocytes, staining typically with nonspecific esterase, and is not reported as having a hypocellular variant as occurs in other cases of MDS or AML. Blast counts may be as high as 20%, but because monoblasts are always partly differentiated, this may not be as significant as in RAEB. Monosomy 7 is most often found, followed in turn by trisomy 8, 12p abnormalities, and in some blast transformations, 17q isochrome defects. 5q deletions are less frequent in CMML than in other categories of MDS (60, 61).

No specific oncogene or tumor suppressor gene abnormality has been consistently identified, and in all likelihood CMML is a heterogenous condition. Reported survivals range from 12–30 months median.

Secondary MDS should be included as a unique entity, because the pathogenesis appears better defined than the de novo cases so far described. All cases of secondary AML, whatever the underlying cause, probably go through a phase of MDS. However, not all cases at risk in who MDS or MDS-like changes develop are sure to develop AML in any specific period. The association between de novo acute leukemia with trilineage MDS, and the appearance of MDS as the remission phase of AML is well recognized (62) and fits the concept of a relationship between MDS and AML. The biogenesis of secondary MDS may be narrower than the primary forms. Secondary MDS appears in younger patients and has a worse prognosis than the primary form (63). Cytogenetic abnormalities are the rule (64), with monosomy 7 the most frequent, followed by deletions of 5q. Complex karyotype abnormalities are also found, and AML usually supervenes within months (65). The morphologic findings are the same in both secondary and primary MDS, but hypocellular and fibrotic bone marrow appearances are more common in the former.

Etiology of Secondary MDS

Treatment with alkylating agents, etoposide and radiotherapy, or other ionizing radiation and combinations of these have been implicated, as have chemicals causing AML such as benzene. The risk of leukemia developing after exposure to provocative therapy appears to peak at the 5–6 years of age. Dosage of alkylating agents may be critical (66), as may synergism between DNA intercalators and topoisomerase inhibitors in causing MDS or AML (67). Melphalan has been known to cause chromosome damage in those sites involved in leukemias (68), but not specifically MDS. However, benzene-associated leukemia often has a long prodromal period including MDS-like changes. The risk of MDS developing, as such, following benzene exposure seems not to be calculated, but for leukemia the risk is dose related; up to 10% overall for periods of surveillance for as long as 12 years (69). However, MDS changes in hemopoiesis may be transient and associated with the immediate posttreatment period of malignancies with drugs or radiation. Although better identification of genetic markers such as the bcr/abl oncogene in CML survivors has shown persistent subtle changes in long-term disease survivors apparently unaffected with the disease, few studies have been undertaken to look at hematologically normal patients given leukemogenic treatment years previously, but mutations in the RAS and FMS gene families have been noted (70, 71).

One may conclude that secondary MDS following certain chemical and/or ionizing radiation exposure follows a pattern similar to secondary AML. Other environmental factors, such as pesticides, are still under debate.

The prognosis for secondary MDS is poorer than for the primary form, and by the time of diagnosis the RAEB and RAEBt variants are usually found. The treatment of choice is allogenic BMT with limitations as noted; otherwise the treatment is the same as for AML in similar age groups.

AIDS and MDS

Numerous hematologic abnormalities are described with AIDS, including MDS (72, 73). Since AIDS rarely terminates as leukemia or has associated cytogenetic or genetic abnormalities such as those found with primary MDS, the significance of these findings is unclear. Although the anemia, leukopenia, and thrombocytopenia found in AIDS can be accompanied by hyperplastic bone marrow changes, these should be differentiated from those of typical MDS by the AIDS pattern of fat spaces separating hemic particles, along with frequent lymphoid or plasmacytoid aggregates (74). Ziduvodine (AZT) treatment of AIDS can cause marrow suppression and macrocytic RBCs, which complicate evaluation in some patients. The anemia and neutropenia seen in these subjects can sometimes be helped by Epo or GM-CFS, as in MDS.

MDS has also been recorded following *liver transplantation* (75), but the authors do not classify the 17 patients they reported other than to say that the changes were milder than in primary MDS; nor do they give details of immunosuppressive treatment or outcome, particularity secondary leukemia development.

Juvenile MDS is approached differently than the adult disorder and can be considered under more precise biologic categories rather than under the FAB classifications. Long dysplastic prodromal phases are uncommon, and rapidly evolving acute nonlymphoid leukemia is the expected termination in untreated cases.

Case 3

A 4-year-old white boy was initially seen because of a history of prolonged fever, marked enervation, and night sweats over a period of approximately 2 weeks. During that interval, and most notably in the 4 days prior to the first visit, he had lost his appetite completely. The remainder of his history, including immunization status, prior illnesses, family data, and systems review were noncontributory.

On physical examination, he was a chronically ill-appearing youngster in no acute distress. Vital signs included temperature 39.1°C, pulse 110 beats/minute, respirations 25 breaths/minute. His skin was clear and his mucous membranes were pale. Examination of his head and neck was unrevealing except for the presence of a few nonspecific anterior axillary nodes. His cardiovascular and pulmonary systems were intact and revealed only a grade 1 hemic murmur. Apart from a palpable spleen tip, there were no other untoward abdominal findings. Locomotion, except for the weakness, related in part to his underlying illness and to a lengthy stay in bed. Neurologic and genitourinary assessment were all normal.

His laboratory data were as follows: hemoglobin 97 g/L, hematocrit 28%, RBC count 280×10^{12}/L, reticulocyte count 0.5%, platelet count 150×10^9/L, and WBC count 4.1×10^9/L with 30% neutrophils, 5% metamyelocytes, 12% monocytes, 3% basophils, and 50% lymphocytes (5% of which were reactive appearing with prominent nuclear material and deep blue cytoplasm). A peripheral blood film revealed ovalocytes, poikilocytes, basophilic stippling, and Howell-Jolly bodies, as well as occasional hypersegmented neutrophils and bilobed neutrophils with vacuoles.

Additional data included a hemoglobin F of 7%, normal numbers of T- and B-lymphocytes (including a normal T4:T8 ratio) and normal electrolytes, renal function studies, and urinalysis.

The vitamin B_{12} and folate data returned with normal values following the results of the bone marrow analysis, carried out because the anemia, abnormal peripheral blood red cell and granulocyte morphology, and borderline neutrophil counts indicated that a hemopoietic disorder should be considered in the differential diagnosis. Marrow cellularity was normal, the boy's M:E ratio was 5:1, and there was evidence of megaloblastoid-appearing progenitors in all cell lines. The megakaryocytes often had double lobes, as did many of the erythroid precursors. There was distortion in the appearance of many of the granulocyte precursors, and there were slightly in excess of 3% blast forms of indeterminate lineage. Karyotyping revealed a monosomy 7 defect.

It was the impression of all those caring for the child that he had a monosomy 7 MDS, and exhaustive tests for

Epstein-Barr virus (EBV) or other infection were not identified. In such cases, so-called "conventional" chemotherapy has little to offer. Accordingly, arrangement was made to test for allogeneic transplantation. The child's only sibling was a perfect human lymphocytic antigen (HLA) match. Within 6 weeks of the diagnosis, a BMT was performed without untoward event after the graft was aggressively purged to prevent the appearance of graft-versus-host disease (GVHD). At 6 weeks post-BMT, the boy's marrow had recovered sufficiently to permit further karyotyping, which proved to be normal. His blood counts, including his platelets, were within normal range. Six months later, he returned to his local physician with fairly rapid onset of fever, pallor, ecchymoses, hepatosplenomegaly, and a laboratory study that revealed anemia, thrombocytopenia, and normal leukocyte numbers with 15% circulating blasts. The marrow had 60% blasts but no dyshemopoietic changes, and he again showed monosomy 7 on karyotyping. His blast numbers were reduced with high-dose cytosine arabinoside, and he was retransplanted with the same donor. The preparative regimen differed. The first time he received total body irradiation (TBI) and cytoxan; the second time he received busulfan and cytoxan without GVHD prophylaxis. Severe grade 3 GVHD developed, but the patient engrafted easily and stayed in remission for 2 years after a stormy GVHD-mediated course. His second relapse was marked by numerous infections, and after a brief remission on high-dose cytosine arabinoside, he succumbed to disseminated aspergillosis.

The constitutional symptoms and signs of splenomegaly, anemia, borderline WBC and platelet counts would have been compatible with many infections as well as with a hematologic malignancy. However, the peripheral blood RBC morphology was sufficient to warrant immediate bone marrow examination with karyotyping, which, in effect, led to the appropriate diagnosis. Occupancy of the marrow by leukemic blasts, nonhemic cells or hypoplasia/aplasia, would have been detected at this time. Had the bone marrow findings been nondiagnostic, a search for viral or other infections would have been undertaken. The establishment of the diagnosis of MDS calls for immediate assessment and a plan of management for curative therapy just as for an acute childhood leukemia.

Categories of Childhood MDS

The FAB classification is not usually applied to the childhood forms, but several well-defined biologic entities are described. The index case represents one of these.

Monosomy 7 is a preleukemic syndrome, found mostly but not exclusively in male children. It has been described both as a myeloproliferative and as a familial disorder, which suggests that it covers more than one variant (76, 77). Sometimes leukemia has already developed by the time of diagnosis and biphenotypic variants have also been described, suggesting that the genetic abnormality is related to control of the pluripotential stem cell. Non-

hemopoietic system abnormalities are rarely reported, but a defect of neutrophil chemotaxis has been found (78), as well as hypo-γ-globulinemia. As expected, these children have recurrent infections. The MDR-1 gene is located on the long arm of chromosome 7, and increased levels of its expression have been found in this syndrome (79). 1L-6 and Epo genes are also located on chromosome 7, as are protooncogenes ERB-B and MET (80). Possibly the effects of loss of different combinations of these genes and the function of those on the remaining chromosome 7, which may have previously masked mutant oncogenes, leads to the clinical variations in this syndrome. There is a description of 13 cases (5) with variable survival and clinical manifestations, and there are varying levels of, and responses to, Epo (81).

Several studies have shown siblings of children with chromosome 7 deletions to have similar abnormalities unrelated to DNA from a particular parent, which suggests the deletion itself may not be the only factor involved in the development of leukemia (82). There are probably familial and nonfamilial cases, but potential sibling bone marrow donors should be screened for occult defects of this kind. Also described is the "infantile monosomy 7 syndrome" (83). Prognosis and treatment are the same as for AML.

Other MDS variants seen in childhood include MDS associated with inherited or congenital disorders (table 24.4). With a few exceptions, the disorders are those associated with the development of AML also.

All of the first group are AML associated, and the MDS is assumed to be prodromal. However, trisomy 21 (Down syndrome) occasionally has been found to have transient abnormalities of hemopoiesis of an MDS-like nature (84). Some cases of monosomy 7 may be genuinely MDS, rather than AML, associated. There is another unexplained link between neurofibromatosis and juvenile CMML (JCMML) (85), wherein the karyotypic abnormality resides on chromosome 17 (an area rarely involved in blood disorders). No one pattern of biologic conditioning for MDS emerges, although the DNA repair disorders are obvious candidates for early tumor development. For example, there are reports of patients with Klinefelter syndrome and AML (86), which may add to the as yet undefined associations between germ line and X-chromosome abnormalities and AML/MDS.

Table 24.4. MDS Associated Disorders

Trisomy 21
Trisomy 8
Bloom syndrome
Shwachman syndrome
Fanconi anemia
Ataxia telangectasia
Diamond Blackfan syndrome
Neurofibromatosis
Monosomy 7 syndrome

JCMML appears to be confined mainly to boys <4 years of age with features much more florid than the adult variety hepatosplenomegaly, facial rash not unlike the butterfly rash of discoid lupus, adenopathy, and immunologic perturbations, including abnormal T-cells are reported. Save for the Ph+ chromosome and the bcr/abl abnormality, it resembles JCML. As in JCML, hemoglobin F levels are often as high as 10% (87, 88), but there are no identifiable gene defects and no characteristic karyotypic findings. The adult variety of CMML without these features can also be found in children.

Although less common in children, **secondary MDS** has been described after treatment of other malignancies. More cases are likely to arise in adolescents following greater success in the overall therapy of childhood neoplasia. Exposure to intrauterine or later X-radiation is a rare but accepted association with MDS, and parental exposure as a causative factor continues to be disputed (89, 90).

MDS in children is a more difficult disorder to diagnose and manage than the adult forms. As well as the congenital disorders directly linked to it, the congenital dyserythropoietic syndromes enter the differential diagnosis, and some infections, especially with EBV and cytomegalovirus (CMV), can cause ineffective hemopoiesis with thrombocytopenia, anemia, and the appearance of monocytoid cells in the peripheral blood films. Boundaries between myeloproliferative, dysplastic, and even aplastic diseases are blurred. At present, management is largely dependent on the needs of individual patients and the progress or stage of their disease. Vigorous supportive treatment, antileukemic chemotherapy, and BMT are established treatments. The results of aggressive chemotherapy are poorer than in the more common leukemias in this age group, and low-dose chemotherapy and differentiation or cytokine treatment is only occasionally effective, as with adults (91). BMT from a suitable donor is the best treatment at present and should be undertaken without delay when feasible. No prospect for gene therapy is seen until the nature of the genetic background is better understood.

Summary

Myelodysplasia is best regarded as a broadly based syndrome rather than a specific disorder, and probably contains a number of biologically different entities that have lack of control of hemopoietic cell development in common. Unlike CML, the genetic background in myelodysplasia is heterogenous and presumably reflects the complex and multifocal chromosomal loci that have input into the regulation of hemopoiesis. The association with congenital abnormalities and aging, radiation exposure, and cytotoxic therapy, with their respective array of DNA defects or repair faults corresponds with the concept of MDS as many disorders. The failure of a useful directed "standard" therapy to emerge is therefore not surprising; nor is the relative success of BMT that bypasses the pathologies responsible for the syndrome.

REFERENCES

1. Elves MW, Bourne MS, Israels MCG. Pyridoxine responsive anaemia determined by an X-linked gene. J Med Genet 1966;3:1.
2. Block M, Jacobsen L, Bethard WF. Preleukemic acute human leukemia. JAMA 1953;152:1018.
3. Joosten E, Pelemans W, Hiele M, et al. Prevalence and causes of anemia in a geriatric hospitalized population. Gerontology 1992;38:111.
4. Phillips M, Cull GM, Ewings M. Establishing the incidence of myelodysplasia syndrome. Br J Haematol 1994;88:186.
5. Hann IM. Myelodysplastic syndromes. Arch Dis Child 1992;67:962.
6. Hasle H, Jacobsen BB, Pederson NT. Myelodysplastic syndromes in childhood; a population based study of nine cases. Br J Haematol 1992;81:495.
7. Aul C, Gattermann N, Schneider W. Epidemiological and etiological aspects of myelodysplastic syndromes. Leuk Lymph 1995;16:247.
8. Bennett JM, Catovsky D, Daniel MT, et al. Proposals for the classification of the myelodysplastic syndromes. Br J Haematol 1982;51:189.
9. Ruutu P. Granulocyte function in myelodysplastic syndrome. Scand J Haematol 1986;36(suppl 45):66.
10. Ruutu P, Ruutu T, Vuopi I, et al. Defective chemotaxis in monosomy 7. Blood 1981;58:739.
11. Moretti S, Lanza F, Spisani S, et al. Neutrophils from patients with myelodysplastic syndromes: relationship between impairment of granular contents, complement receptors, functional activities and disease status. Leuk Lymph 1994;13:471.
12. Rasi V, Lintula R. Platelet function in the myelodysplastic syndromes. Scand J Haematol 1986;36(suppl45):7.
13. Hamblin TJ. Immunologic abnormalities in myelodysplastic syndromes. Hematol Oncol Clin N Am 1992;63:571.
14. Mufti GJ, Figes A, Hamblin TJ, et al. Immunological abnormalitires in myelodysplastic syndromes. 1. Serum immunoglobulins and autoantibodies. Br J Haematol 1986;63:1143.
15. Ganser A, Hoelzer D. Clinical course of myelodysplastic syndromes. Hematol Oncol Clin N Am 1993;6.3:612.
16. Mufti GJ. A guide to risk assessment in the myelodysplastic syndrome. Hematol Oncol Clin N Am 1992;6:587.
17. Taylor KM. Myelodysplasia. Curr Opin Oncol 1994;6:320.
18. Prchal JT, Trockmorton DW, Carroll AJ, et al. A common progenitor for myeloid and lymphoid cells. Nature 1978;274:590.
19. Janssen JWG, Buschle M, Layton M, et al. Clonal analysis of myelodysplastic syndromes: evidence of multipotent stem cell origin. Blood 1989;73:248.
20. Yunis JJ, Lobell M, Arnesen A, et al. Refined chromosome study helps define prognostic subgroups in most patients with primary myelodysplastic syndrome and acute myelodysplastic syndrome and acute myelogenous leukaemia. Br J Haematol 1988;68:189.
21. Chen Z, Morgan R, Berger CS, et al. Application of fluorescence in situ hybridization in hematological disorders. Cancer Genet Cytogenet 1992;63:62.
22. Mecucci C, Van den Berghe H. Cytogenetics. In: Koeffler HP, ed. Myelodysplastic syndromes. Hematol Oncol Clin N Am 1992;6:523.

23. Nimer SD, Golde DW. The 5q-abnormality Blood 1987;76: 1705.

24. Van den Berghe H, Vermaelen K, Cassiman JJ, David GG, et al. Distinct haematological disorder with deletion of long arm of N.5 chromosome. Nature 1974;251:437.

25. DeWald GW, Brecher M, Travis LB, et al. Twenty-six patients with hematologic disorders and X chromosome abnormalities: Frequent q13(X) abnormalities associated with pathologic ringed sideroblasts. Cancer Genet Cytogenet 1989;42:173.

26. Pierre RV, Catovsky D, Mufti GJ, et al. Clinical cytogenetic correlations in myelodysplasia (preleukemia). Cancer Genet Cytogenet 1989;40:149.

27. Musilova J, Michelova K. Chromosome study of 85 patients with myelodysplastic syndrome. Cancer Genet Cytogenet 1988;33:39.

28. Raymakers R, De Witte T, Joziasse J, et al. In vitro growth pattern and differentiation predict for progression of myelodysplastic syndromes to acute non lymphoblastic leukaemia. Br J Haematol 1991;78:35.

29. Bartram CR. Molecular genetics aspects of myelodysplastic syndromes. Hematol Oncol Clin N Am 1992;6:557.

30. Paquette RL, Landow EM, Pierre RV, et al. N Ras mutations are associated with poor prognosis and increased risk of leukemia in myelodysplastic syndrome. Blood 1992;82:590.

31. Van Kemp H, De Pijper C, Verlaan-de Vries M, et al. Longitudinal analysis of point mutations of n Ras proto oncogene in patients with myelodysplasia using archived blood smears. Blood 1992;79:1266.

32. Culligan DJ, Cachia P, Whittaker JA, et al. Clonal lymphocytes are detected in only some cases of MDS. Br J Haematol 1992;81:346.

33. Jonveaux P, Fenaux P, Quiquandon I, et al. Mutations in the p53 gene in myelodysplastic syndromes. Oncogene 1991;6: 2243.

34. Adamson DJA, Dawson AA, Bennett B, et al. p53 Mutations in the myelodysplastic syndromes. Br J Haematol 1995; 89:61.

35. Willman CL, Sever CE, Pallavicini MG, et al. Deletion of IRFI. Mapping to chromosome 5q31 in human leukemia and preleukemia myelodysplasia. Science 1993;259:968.

36. Miyake K, Inokuchi K, Nomura T. Expression of the DCC gene in human hematological malignancies. Leuk Lymph 1994;16:13.

37. Ihalinen J, Pakkala S, Savolainen ER, et al. Hypermethylation of the calcitonin gene in myelodysplastic syndromes. Leukemia 1993;7:263.

38. Hutchinson RM, Pringle JH, Knight SC. Oncogene expression in primary myelodysplasia: correlation with hematologic, karyotypic and clinical progression. J Clin Pathol 1992; 45:339.

39. Mittelman MM, Lessin LS. Oncogenes and growth factor genes in myelodysplasia. Hematol Pathol 1991;5:37.

40. Greenberg PL, et al. Production of granulocyte colony stimulating factor (G-CSF) by normal and myelodysplastic syndrome peripheral blood cells. Blood 1983;61:1035.

41. Richert-Boe KE, Bagby GC. In vitro hemopoiesis in myelodysplasia; liquid and soft gel culture studies. Hematol Oncol Clin N Am 1992;6:543.

42. Goasgyuen JE, Bennett JM, Cox C, et al. Prognostic implication and characterisation of the blast cell population in the myelodysplastic syndrome. Leuk Res 1991; 15:1159.

43. Oertel J, Huhn D. CD-34 immunophenotyping of blasts in myelodysplasia. Leuk Lymph 1994;15:65.

44. Sawada KI. Impaired proliferation and differentiation of myelodysplastic CD-34 cells. Leuk Lymph 1994;14:37.

45. Stephenson J, Mufti GJ, Yoshida Y. Myelodysplastic syndromes: from morphology to molecular biology; II, the molecular genetics of myelodysplasia. Int J Hematol 1993; 57:99.

46. Hellstrom-Lindberg E. Efficacy of erythropoietin in the myelodysplastic syndromes: a meta analysis of 205 patients in 33 studies. Br J Haematol 1995;89:67.

47. Rose EH, Rudnick SA, Abels RI, et al. Efficacy and safety of recombinant human erythropoietin (rHuEpo) in anemic patients with myelodysplastic syndrome. Proc Am Soc Clin Oncol 1991;10:306.

48. Negrin R, Stein R, Doherty K, et al. Granulocyte stimulating colony factor (G-CFSF) plus erythropoietin (Epo) for the maintenance treatment of the anemia of myelodysplastic syndromes. Exp Hematol 1994;22:703.

49. Loffler H, Schmitz N, Gassmann W. Intensive chemotherapy and bone marrow transplantation for myelodysplastic syndromes. Hematol Oncol Clin N Am 1992;6:619.

50. Uberti JP, Ratanatharathorn V, Karanes C, et al. Allogenic bone marrow transplantation in patients with myelodysplastic syndromes. Leuk Lymph 1994;14:379.

51. De Witte T, Gratwohl A. Bone marrow transplantation for myelodysplasia and secondary leukaemias. Br J Haematol 1993;84:361.

52. Trico G, Bogaerts MA. The role of aggressive chemotherapy in the treatment of myelodysplastic syndromes. Cancer 1989; 64:1812.

53. Hirst WRJ, Mufti GJ. Management of myelodysplastic syndromes. Br J Haematol 1993;84:191.

54. Silverman LR, Holland JF, Weinberg RS, et al. Effects of treatment with 5 azacytidine on *in vivo* and *in vitro* hemopoiesis in patients with myelodysplastic syndromes. Leukemia 1993;7(suppl 1):21.

55. Koeffler HP, Heitjan D, Mertelsmann R, et al. Randomized study of 3 cis retinoic acid v placebo in the myelodysplastic disorders. Blood 1988;71:703.

56. Andreeff M, Stone R, Michaeli J, et al. Hexamethylamine in myelodysplastic syndrome and acute myelogenous leukemia: a phase II clinical trial with a differentiating inducing agent. Blood 1992;80:2604.

57. Maiolo AT, Cortelezzi A, Calori R, et al. Recombinant alpha interferon as the first line therapy for high risk myelodysplastic syndromes. Leukaemia 1990;4:480.

58. Mangi MH, Mufti GJ. Abnormal localization of abnormal precursors (ALIPs) in the bone marrow myelodysplastic syndromes: current state of knowledge and future directions Leuk Res 1991;15:627.

59. Cohen AM, Mittelman M, Gal R, et al. Chronic myelomonocytic leukemia associated with primary amyloidosis. Leuk Lymph 1984;16:183.

60. Feneaux P, Jouet JP, Zandecki M, et Al. Chronic and subacute myelomonocytic leukaemia in the adult: a report of 60 cases with special reference to prognostic factors. Br J Haematol 1987;65:101.

61. Groupe Francaise de Cytogenetique Hematologique. Cytogenetics of chronic myelomonocytic leukemia. Cancer Genet Cytogenet 1986;21:11.

62. Tamura S, Kanamaru A. De novo acute myeloid leukemia with trilineage myelodysplasia (AML/TMDS) and myelodys-

plastic remission marrow (AML/MRM). Leuk Lymph 1995; 16:263.

63. Kantarjan HM, Estey EH, Keating M. Treatment of therapy related leukemia and myelodysplastic syndrome. Hematol Oncol Clin N Am 1993;7:81.

64. Berger R, Flandrin G. Chromosomal abnormalities in secondary acute myeloid leukaemia and the myelodysplastic syndromes. In: Galton DAG, Mufti JG, eds. The myelodysplastic syndromes. Edinburgh: Churchill Livingstone, 1992:129.

65. Heim S. Cytogenetic findings in primary and secondary MDS. Leuk Res 1992;16:43.

66. McIntyre OR, Pajak TF, Wiernik P, et al. Delayed acute leukemia in myeloma patients receiving pulsed vs continuous treatment. Blood 1981;58(suppl 1):167a.

67. Pederson-Bjergaard J, Philip P, Larsen SO, et al. Therapy related myelodysplasia and acute myeloid leukemia: cytogenetic characteristics of 115 consecutive cases and risk in seven cohorts of patients treated intensively for malignant disease in the Copenhagen area. Leukemia 1993;7:1975.

68. Jacobs A, Ridge SA, Carter G, et al. Fms and RAS mutations following cytotoxic therapy for lymphoma. Exp Hematol 1990;18:648.

69. Levine EG, Bloomfield CD. Leukemias and myelodysplastic syndromes secondary to drug radiation and environment exposure. Semin Oncol 1992;19:47.

70. Manuris Z, Prieur M, Dutrillax B, et al. The chemotherapeutic drug melphalan induces breakages of chromosome regions rearranged in secondary leukemia. Cancer Genet Cytogenet 1989;37:65.

71. Carter G, Hughes N, Warren N, et al. Ras mutations in preleukemia, patients following cytotoxic therapy and normal subjects. In: Spandidos DA, ed. The superfamily of RAS related genes. New York: Plenum, 1992:89.

72. Spivak JL, Bender BS, Quinn TC. Haematological abnormalities in the acquired immunodeficiency syndrome. Am J Med 1984;77:224.

73. Schneider DR, Picker LJ. Myelodysplasia in acquired immune deficiency syndrome. Am J Clin Pathol 1985;84:144.

74. Saba IH, Spiers ASD. Hematologic manifestations of acquired immune deficiency syndrome; Current understanding and management. Haematol Rev Comm 1994;9:51.

75. Clatch RJ, Krigman HR, Peters M, et al. Dysplastic hemopoiesis following orthoptic liver transplantation: comparison with similar changes in HIV infection and primary myelodysplasia. Br J Haematol 1994;88:685.

76. Carroll WL, Morgan R, Glader BE. Childhood bone marrow monosomy 7 syndrome: a familial disorder. J Pediatr 1985; 61:107.

77. Sieff CA, Chessels JM, Harvey BAM, et al. Monosomy 7 in childhood; a myeloproliferative disorder. Br J Haematol 1981;49:235.

78. Ruutu P, Ruutu T, Vuopi I, et al. Defective chemotaxis in monosomy 7. Nature 1977;265:164.

79. Holmes J, Jacobs A, Carter G, et al. Multidrug resistance in hemopoietic cell lines, myelodysplastic syndromes and acute leukemia. Br J Haematol 1989;72:44.

80. Culligan D, Jacobs A, Padua RA. The genetic basis for myelodysplasia. In: Brenner MV, Hoffbrand V, eds. Recent advances in haematology. Edinburgh: Churchill Livingstone, 1993:35.

81. Jacobs A, Culligan D, Bowen DT. Erythropoietin and the myelodysplastic syndromes. Contrib Nephrol 1991;88:266.

82. Shannon KM, Turban AG, Chang SSY, et al. Familial bone marrow monosomy 7. Evidence that the predisposing locus is not on the long arm of chromosome 7. J Clin Invest 1989; 84:984.

83. Chessels JM. Myelodysplasia. Bailliere's Clin Haematol 1991;4:459.

84. Gadner H. Myelodysplasia in childhood: In: Schwalz F, Mufti GJ, eds. Myelodysplastic syndromes. Berlin: Springer, 1992:31.

85. Kaneko Y, Maseki N, Sakurai M, et al. Chromosome pattern in juvenile chronic myelogenous leukemia, myelodysplastic syndrome and acute leukemia associated with neurofibromatosis. Leukemia 1989;3:36.

86. Mamunes K, Lapidus P, Roath S. Acute leukaemia and Klinefelter's syndrome. Lancet 1961;11:26.

87. Travis SF. Fetal erythropoiesis in juvenile chronic myelomonocytic leukemia. Blood 1983;62:602.

88. Weinberg RS, Leibowitz D, Weinblatt ME. Juvenile chronic myelogenous leukemia; the only example of truly fetal (not fetal like) erythropoiesis. Br J Haematol 1990;76:307.

89. Harvey EB, Boice JD, Honeyman M, et al. Prenatal X-ray exposure and childhood cancer in twins. N Engl J Med 1985; 312:541.

90. Longwengart RA, Peters JM, Cicioni C, et al. Childhood leukemia and parents' occupation and home exposures. J Natl Cancer Inst 1987;79:73.

91. Ganser A, Seipelt G, Lindemann A. Effects of human IL-3 in patients with myelodysplastic syndromes. Blood 1990; 73:31.

CHAPTER 25

Acute Myelocytic Leukemia

EDWARD D. BALL

> While there are several chronic diseases more destructive
> to life than cancer, none is more feared.
> —Charles H. Mayo, *Annals of Surgery* (1926)

Introduction

Acute myeloid leukemia (AML) is a form of leukemia arising within the myeloid lineage of bone marrow cells. This chapter will focus on the biology of AML, the consequences of the disease on the patient, and approaches to treatment.

Case 1

Menometorrhagia developed in a 17-year-old girl who had been in good health. While evaluating this problem, her gynecologist found her to have a prothrombin time (PT) of 14 seconds. The hematologist she was referred to for further workup found her PT to be 14.5 seconds (control 13.0 seconds), her partial thromboplastin time (PTT) to be 39 seconds (control 33.0 seconds), and the fibrinogen 143 mg/dl. Her white blood cell (WBC) count at that time was 2,400/μl, the platelet count was 189,000/μl, and the hemoglobin was 13.0 g/dl. Six days later her WBC was 1,100/μl with a differential of 16% neutrophils, 2% bands, 4% monocytes, 78% lymphocytes, and no abnormal cells. A bone marrow aspirate and biopsy showed a hypercellular marrow with replacement of normal architecture with immature myeloid cells. The marrow differential showed 63% myeloblasts containing Auer rods and 7% promyelocytes. Samples of bone marrow were sent for cytogenetic analysis and flow cytometry. The patient's serum fibrinogen was 109 mg/dl (0.01 I.U., normal range 0.2–0.4 I.U.), the D-dimer was 4 μg/ml (normal ≤0.5 μg/ml), and the lactic dehydrogenase (LDH) was 950 I.U. (normal range 275–650 I.U.). A diagnosis of AML accompanied by disseminated intravascular coagulation (DIC) was made.

Cytogenetic analysis showed an abnormal clone of bone marrow cells with the following karyotype: 47,XX, +8, t(15;17)(q22;11.2). Immunophenotyping of the leukemia cells showed them to be CD13+, CD33+, CD10 (CALLA)+, CD34+, and HLA-DR -. Cell-cycle analysis on the fluorescence-activated cell sorting (FACS) revealed that 95.5% of cells were in G_oG1, 3.8% in S, and 0.75% in G2/M of the cell cycle. After therapy with allopurinol and heparin was started, treatment with cytosine arabinoside (200 mg/m² for 7 days by continuous infusion) and daunorubicin (45 mg/m² intravenous bolus

days 1–3) was instituted. Her peripheral blood counts fell gradually over the next few days. When her granulocyte count was <500 cells/μl, a fever developed and she was placed on mezlocillin and tobramycin. She defervesced gradually but remained pancytopenic and required frequent red blood cell (RBC) and platelet transfusions. The dose of heparin was adjusted according to the levels of the D-dimer and fibrinogen.

A bone marrow aspirate obtained on the 14th day after chemotherapy was started revealed persistent leukemic blasts. Treatment with a second course of cytosine arabinoside (200 mg/m²) and daunorubicin (45 mg/m²) was begun, this time for 5 and 2 days, respectively. She continued to be pancytopenic following the second course of therapy.

Bone marrow aspirate and biopsy on the 28th day of therapy showed a hypoplastic marrow with no residual blasts. After another week of severe neutropenia, the neutrophil count began to increase gradually and all of her peripheral blood counts normalized within 7 weeks of the institution of chemotherapy.

Differential Diagnosis

The clinical presentation of an acute leukemia can be dramatic or subtle. Patients may present with very high peripheral blood blast counts and evidence of bleeding, bruising, fever, and petechiae. Alternatively, the peripheral blood counts may be normal or depressed and the patient may be seen with signs and symptoms of anemia. The patient in case 1 presented with early findings of disseminated intravascular coagulation with abnormal endometrial bleeding and slightly prolonged clotting times. Initially, although the WBC was somewhat decreased, her blood counts did not indicate leukemia. However, the WBC began to decrease relatively quickly as the marrow became crowded with blasts and promyelocytes. This case illustrates that "leukemia" is not really a blood disease as much as it is a bone marrow disease that eventually spills over into the peripheral blood as the marrow space becomes too crowded, or, in some cases, as other factors intrinsic to the leukemia cell produce changes in the blood, such as surface membrane changes that allow egress into the blood from the marrow sinusoids.

A bone marrow aspirate and biopsy are indicated to make a definitive diagnosis and to perform several helpful ancillary tests such as cytogenetic analysis, special stains on the blast cells, and immunophenotyping (all discussed below). The marrow aspirate allows careful examination of cellular morphology and the performance of special stains and immunologic studies on cell suspensions. The biopsy allows an assessment of the degree of marrow "cellularity." Typically, in leukemia, the marrow space is completely replaced with leukemia cells.

The first decision that must be made is whether a leukemic process is operative. "Benign" conditions, primarily infections, can mimic leukemia by causing the appearance of atypical lymphoblasts or a leukemoid reaction in the peripheral blood. Atypical lymphocytes are large vacuolated cells that can be seen in infectious mononucleosis and other mononucleosis syndromes such as cytomegalovirus (CMV) infection and toxoplasmosis. They are distinguished from malignant blasts by more pronounced clumping of nuclear chromatin, larger amounts of cytoplasm, and irregular nuclear borders. A leukemoid reaction is a leukocytosis that can occur in response to infection or stress. It is distinguishable from AML by the absence of blast forms in the blood and a relatively small percentage of blasts in the bone marrow.

Once leukemia is diagnosed, the clinician must determine whether it is lymphoblastic or myeloblastic. This determination is accomplished by examining the morphology of the blasts on Wright-Giemsa stained bone marrow aspi-

rates and by special histochemical stains that determine the presence of cytoplasmic enzymes characteristic of a particular lineage. Immunophenotyping and karyotyping give supportive, occasionally diagnostic, and always informative data.

Leukocyte Biology

Normal Hematopoiesis

Huge numbers of peripheral blood cells (a total of 6×10^9/kg/day of body weight comprised of 2.5×10^9 red cells, 2.5×10^9 platelets, and 1.0×10^9 granulocytes) are made each day by the normal bone marrow throughout life (1) (fig. 25.1). All of these cells arise from the self-renewing pluripo-tent stem cell in the bone marrow (2). The myeloidseries, defined as cells arising from a multipotential lineage-restricted hematopoietic progenitor cell, the colony-forming unit for granulocytes, erythrocytes, monocytes, and megakaryocytes (CFU-GEMM), originate from a pluripotent bone marrow stem cell (3). Studies in the mouse have shown that the pluripotent stem cell, the CFU-S (spleen), can be measured in vivo as a colony-forming cell in the spleens of lethally irradiated mice that were injected with bone marrow cells from the same species. In man, it has been possible to culture the multipotential CFU-GEMM progenitor cell in vitro (3) and a primitive "blast cell" colony (4), but not a true pluripotential stem

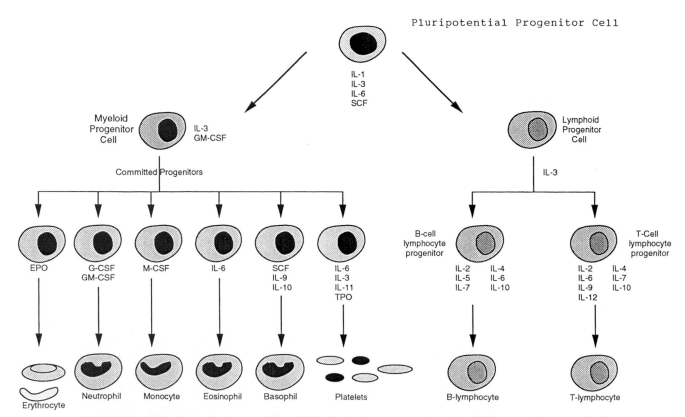

Figure 25.1 Generation of mature peripheral blood cellular elements from the pluripotential hematopoietic stem cell. This process is mediated by numerous cytokines acting at defined times and with lineage specificity as noted.

cell. Pluripotent stem cells exist in the bone marrow and the peripheral blood (including placental blood), as demonstrated by the success of both bone marrow and peripheral blood stem cell transplantation in fully reconstituting bone marrow function in patients treated with myeloablative therapy. Although the pluripotent stem cell must renew itself in order to maintain hematopoiesis for life, a portion of the daughter cells enter differentiation pathways forming intermediate progenitors capable of restricted differentiation into granulocyte/ monocyte (CFU-GM), erythrocyte (BFU-E), eosinophil (CFU-EOS), or megakaryocyte (CFU-MEG) colony formation. During this process, which takes place over a period of 7–14 days, the progenitor cells and their progeny become committed to one of eight final cellular blood elements with unique morphology, biochemistry, and function. This process of terminal differentiation into mature blood cells depends on the action of a family of colony-stimulating factors (M-CSF, GM-CSF, G-CSF, stem cell factor) and interleukins (IL-1, IL-3, and IL-6) (5). During this gradual process of cell differentation, expression of the cellular genome undergoes many changes, including altered protooncogene production, the loss and acquisition of cell surface antigens, and changes in morphology and function.

Leukemopoiesis

How Do Leukemia Cells Differ from Normal Cells?

Normally, hematopoietic cells are programmed for senescence. A neutrophil survives in the peripheral blood for about 8 hours, travels to sites of inflammation or injury, and dies in action as it extravasates the contents of its enzyme-containing granules. The primary cell kinetic problem in leukemia is that leukemia cells fail to differentiate and thus accumulate in the vascular space and, eventually, in the extravascular space. The cell cycle time and growth fraction of leukemia cells are actually lower than in normal myeloid precursors (6). Thus, the cells continue to divide instead of entering a final differentiation pathway and accumulate in the patient over a relatively short time of weeks to several months. When diagnosed with leukemia, a patient typically has approximately 10^{12} leukemia cells (a kilogram of cells) dispersed throughout the body.

Leukemia cells compete with normal stem cells and their progeny for space in the marrow and thus produce the cytopenias characteristic of the disease. Additional harmful effects of leukemia cells are generated from the release of a number of cytokines including interleukin-1 (7) and tumor necrosis factor (8), both of which could contribute to symptoms such as fever and fatigue. In addition, promyelocytic leukemia cells release thromboplastic substances that trigger the syndrome of disseminated intravascular coagulation, as seen in the patient described in case (see discussion as follows).

Effects of Leukemia on Normal Cells

Normal blood cell production is impaired in the patient with acute leukemia by at least two mechanisms. Examination of a bone marrow biopsy from a patient with AML demonstrates that the marrow space can be completely replaced with malignant cells, thus depriving normal hematopoietic elements of space in which to develop. A second mechanism, direct suppression by molecular means, is suggested by the presence of leukemia-inhibitory factors elaborated by leukemia cells that can inhibit normal hematopoiesis (9).

Growth Factors

Bone marrow progenitor cells respond to a family of cytokines called the hematopoietic growth factors (HGF) (table 25.1). The existence of such factors was suggested for years, but the recent and rapid progress in molecular genetics has revealed their individual identities and demonstrated the wide range of factors and activities. The best known factors are granulocyte-CSF (GM-CSF), monocyte-CSF, interleukin-3, erythropoietin (Epo), and stem cell factor (SCF). The genes for all of these molecules have been cloned using recombinant DNA technology and the proteins expressed in large quantities in bacteria or eukaryotic vectors allowing mass production and thus widespread use in vitro and in vivo. Numerous clinical trials have demonstrated that each of these factors used in vivo can increase WBC counts dramatically in patients having marrow failure states or undergoing myelosuppressive chemotherapy (10–12). These studies laid to rest many doubts about whether the growth factors would have any in vivo effects at all.

On the other hand, it is still unclear how important circulating growth factors are to normal hematopoiesis. It is possible, for example, that hematopoiesis is controlled by intrinsic processes and only minimally affected by the ex-

Table 25.1. **Hematopoietic Growth Factors**

| Molecule | Chromosomal | | Target Cells | |
	Molecular Weight (kd)	Location	Progenitor	Mature
G-CSF	18–22	17q11.2–21	CFU-G°	N
GM-CSF	14–35	5q23–31	CFU-GEMM, CFU-GM	N, Eos, M
M-CSF	70–90	5q33.1	CFU-M	M
IL-3	14–28	5q23–31	CFU-GEMM	Eos, M
EPO	34–39	7q11–22	CFU-E, CFU-Meg	None
Stem cell factor	28–35	4	CFU-blast	None

°G, granulocyte; GM, granulocyte-macrophage; M, macrophage; GEMM, granulocyte, erythrocyte, macrophage, megakaryocyte; E, erythrocyte; Meg, megakaryocyte; N, neutrophilic granulocyte; Eos, eosinophilic granulocyte.

ternal pressure of the endocrine actions of the hematopoietic growth factors. One model of hematopoiesis, the so-called "stochastic model," hypothesizes that stem cells make random "choices" to differentiate, mainly by turning off the genes necessary to fulfill certain differentiation pathways. In this model the growth factors are only permissive to the lineages they support. In addition to their actions as soluble systemically acting growth factors, the colony-stimulating factors may act locally in the bone marrow microenvironment either as cell membrane-bound factors on bone marrow stromal cells or in the extracellular matrix (13).

Leukemia cells both make and respond to the presence of the hematopoietic growth factors. AML cells variably express the receptors for all of the HGF (14). Detection of GM-CSF, G-CSF, and IL-3 receptors requires radiolabeled or fluorescent probes, because the density of these receptors on the cell surface is relatively low, from 0–1000 sites per cell in the case of G-CSF and GM-CSF (15–18). However, the M-CSF receptor is expressed in greater density and can be detected with monoclonal antibodies (19).

It is of interest that the M-CSF receptor has been shown to be a protein with tyrosine kinase activity encoded by a protooncogene, c-fms (20). This gene, normally located on the long arm of chromosome 5 in a region rich in other growth factor receptors and growth factors (M-CSF, GM-CSF, IL-3), is actively transcribed in about 70% of cases of AML as seen by Northern blotting and by studies with monoclonal antibodies directed to external epitopes of the cell surface protein (19). However, so far there is no compelling evidence that this protooncogene product plays any role in the pathogenesis of human AML. In cases of human AML, c-fms messenger RNA has not been found to be mutated or altered in any fashion and probably is expressed in a manner that mirrors the expression of the protein on normal myeloid cells (20).

Because AML cells bearing the appropriate receptors respond to the presence of the hematopoietic growth factors in vitro by proliferation, there has been little enthusiasm for the use of hematopoietic growth factors in vivo in AML to stimulate normal hematopoiesis following chemotherapy. It has been feared that the leukemic clone would proliferate. Interestingly, in several studies to date, this has not actually happened (12). In studies of patients with myelodysplasia treated with GM-CSF (21), G-CSF (22), and IL-3 (23), progression of the malignant clone into acute leukemia has occurred in only a few patients.

The leukemia cells from the patient described above were relatively quiescent, judging from the observation that only 4–5% of cells were cycling at the time of diagnosis. Some treatment strategies have taken advantage of the fact that the HGF will stimulate cell division in AML cells (24, 25). One strategy is to recruit cells into the cell cycle with the HGF and then institute therapy with cell-cycle-specific cytotoxic drugs such as cytosine arabinoside that will then kill a greater proportion of the leukemia cells.

The rationale for this approach is based on the knowledge that a proportion of leukemia cells will be resting in G_o and therefore be less susceptible to the cycle-active agents that are active in AML. This approach has been used successfully in patients with AML treated with GM-CSF prior to the use of S-phase specific cytotoxic drugs such as cytosine arabinoside (ARA-C).

Leukemia cells from some patients with AML secrete several cytokines including interleukin-1, tumor necrosis factor, GM-CSF, and M-CSF (26). This finding suggests that proliferation of the malignant clone in some cases of AML may operate by an autocrine and/or paracrine mechanism whereby the secreted factors have effects on their own growth or that of neighboring cells. Such mechanisms lend themselves to therapeutic interventions by blocking the feedback loop with antibodies, soluble receptors, or pharmacologic agents.

Etiology and Epidemiology

De Novo AML

As in case 1, the majority of patients in whom AML develops do not have an obvious environmental or genetic factor to blame for their misfortune. There are many known factors that predispose an individual to the development of AML and these lessons may be relevant to the cases where there is no known inciting event.

Rare in childhood, the incidence of AML steadily increases with age, thus accounting for 80% of the cases of acute leukemia in adults. The median age of onset of AML is 55 years. Overall, there are about 3 cases per year per 100,000 population and a slight male preponderance (27). There are several known occupational hazards, including exposure to benzene in the rubber industry (27, 28). It is has been known for some time that exposure to ionizing radiation is associated with excess risk of AML. Neonatal or congenital AML occurs in association with Down syndrome. These children display a transient elevation in WBC count at birth. In approximately a third of those who recover frank AML will develop, which, without therapy, is lethal. Until recently this subtype was considered to have a poor prognosis (29). More recent reports suggest that this group of patients is readily responsive to treatment (30).

Certain genetic conditions are associated with a higher incidence of AML (27). These include Bloom syndrome, Fanconi anemia, Down syndrome, and the Li-Fraumeni syndrome. Bloom syndrome and Fanconi anemia have in common the presence of DNA instability. The Li-Fraumeni syndrome is marked by the presence of a mutated recessive oncogene, the p53 gene on chromosome 17 (31). In addition to the higher incidence of AML, members of families with these syndromes have an excessive incidence of other cancers, primarily of the solid organ type such as sarcomas and breast carcinomas (31).

Secondary AML

Treatment-Related

AML occurs as a "secondary" neoplasm (see Chapter 27) in some patients treated for other malignancies such as ovarian carcinoma, multiple myeloma, Hodgkin disease, polycythemia vera, and acute lymphoblastic leukemia (32, 33). In fact, the incidence of AML following treatment of Hodgkin disease with combined modality therapy (chemotherapy and radiation therapy) is almost 5% (33). These secondary cases of AML are particularly difficult to treat because of considerable resistance to chemotherapy. It is believed that alkylating drugs such as cyclophosphamide, myleran, and nitrogen mustard are the inciting agents in these cases. A recent disconcerting observation is that patients treated for acute lymphoblastic leukemia with regimens containing epipodophyllotoxins (VP-16 or VM-26) have a 5% chance of secondary AML developing.

Myelodysplasia (MDS)

There is a group of marrow failure states associated with abnormal bone marrow morphology and maturation. These have been clustered together into a group of diseases called the "myelodysplastic syndromes." Patients with these disorders have a high propensity to AML's developing, at which time they have a very poor prognosis. The frequency of leukemia arising in patients with these disorders ranges from 10–75% (refractory anemia to refractory anemia excess blasts in transformation) (34). Cells from many of these patients have characteristic cytogenetic abnormalities, often involving whole or partial deletions of chromosomes 5 and 7.

Laboratory Features of AML

Morphology

The acute myeloid leukemias are classified according to the French-American-British (FAB) system (35) (fig. 25.2). Briefly, seven subtypes of AML are described by the FAB system according to the morphology and distribution of cell types in the bone marrow. M1 and M2 leukemias are generally myeloblastic in appearance. Promyelocytic leukemia cells, classified as M3, have abundant azurophilic granules and multiple Auer rods. A microgranular variant exists that is classified as M3V. The M4 subtype, myelomonocytic leukemia, displays both myeloblastic and monocytoid differentiation, whereas M5 cases are primarily monoblastic. Variants of the M2 and M4 subtypes that are characterized by a proliferation of abnormal eosinophils in addition to blast cells are referred to as M2 or M4 with eosinophilia (M2E or M4E). Likewise, M5 is subdivided into M5a and M5b, referring to the percentage of monoblasts (M5b having <80% monoblasts, M5a having more than 80% monoblasts). M6 refers to erythroleukemia wherein erythroblasts are abundant. M7 refers to megakaryoblastic leukemia.

This uncommon subtype of leukemia is difficult to diagnosis with conventional methods. Immunohistochemical staining with a platelet-specific monoclonal antibody and electron microscopy is helpful in making this diagnosis. The clinical course of M7 is variable. Some patients have hepatosplenomegaly and marrow fibrosis. Response to therapy, particularly in adults, is poor.

Auer rods, azurophilic rod-like structures in the cytosol, are found in about 33% of cases, primarily M3 and M5. These crystalline structures are important to identify because they are pathognomonic of AML (table 25.2).

Special Stains

A battery of histochemical stains are available to assist in the classification of cases into the myeloid lineage and the FAB subtypes (36). These include stains for the enzyme myeloperoxidase (MPO), which is commonly present in all of the FAB subtypes, excluding M5a and M7. The MPO stain is often used to differentiate AML from ALL, based on expression of MPO in at least 3% of blasts. Sudan black B, a fat-soluble substance that stains lipids in human cells, also commonly stains AML cells in a manner that correlates well with MPO staining.

In addition, a group of esterases can be detected by the addition of chromogenic substrates. A nonspecific esterase, detected with α-naphthyl acetate (ANA) or butyrate (ANB), is commonly present in FAB M4 or M5. The reaction is characteristically sensitive to NaF. A so-called "specific esterase" reacts with halogenated naphthol esters. Chloroacetate esterase (CAE) is commonly positive in FAB M1, M2, M3, M4E, and M6.

Cytogenetics

A large proportion of cases of AML have an abnormal karyotype (37) (table 25.3). However, in contrast to the situation in CML, where there is a consistent chromosomal abnormality (translocation of part of chromosomes 9 and 22), in AML there are a variety of less common abnormalities. If one examines the incidence of these abnormalities within the FAB subgroups, there are, however, some interesting associations in AML (see below). These associations raise the question of whether AML is really several different diseases, each with its own cell of origin or molecular basis.

About 50% of patients have abnormal karyotypes. The most common abnormalities are trisomy 8, monosomy 7 and 21, trisomy 21, and loss of the X or Y chromosome. The most common translocations are those of chromosomes 8 and 21 [t(8;21)], 15 and 17 [t(15;17)], and 9 and 11 [t(9;11)]. The patterns are often complex, with some patients having more than one detectable abnormality. Inversions of chromosome 16 (inv16) are associated with both myelomonocytic leukemia (FAB M4) and marrow eosinophilia, and have a somewhat better long-term survival (38). One of the most common translocation sites in pediatric AML (and infant AML) is chromosome 11q23.

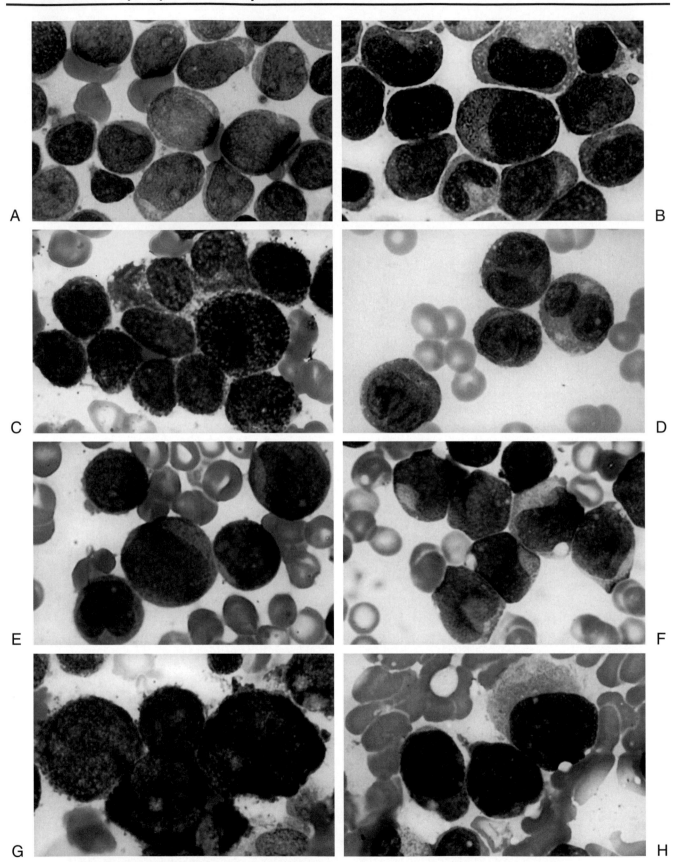

Figure 25.2 French-American-British (FAB) classification of acute nonlymphocytic leukemia. **(A)** AML FAB M1; **(B)** AML FAB M2; **(C)** AML FAB M3; **(D)** AML FAB M3v; **(E)** AML FAB M4; **(F)** AML FAB M5; **(G)** AML FAB M6; **(H)** AML FAB M7.

Table 25.2 Review of French-American-British Acute Leukemia Classification

Acute Lymphoblastic Leukemia

L1 Lymphoblast	Small cells, little or no cytoplasm and rare to no nucleoli	
L2 Lymphoblast	Larger cells than L1, abundant cytoplasm, irregular membranes, prominent nucleoli	
L3 Lymphoblast	Same size as L3, deeply basophilic cytoplasm, prominent nucleoli, and numerous cytoplasmic vacuoles	

Acute Non-Lymphoblastic Leukemia

M1	AML without maturation	Undifferentiated blasts	Rare myeloperoxidase (MY) and sudan black (SB)+ blasts
M2	AML with maturation	Early differentiation with promyelocytes	Frequent MY and SB+ blasts
M3	Promyelocytic leukemia	Hypergranulation	Frequent MY and SB+ blasts and Auer rods
M3V	Microgranular M3	Microgranules, folded nuclei	Same as M3
M4	Myelomonocytic leukemia	Monocyte and granulocyte components	MY and chloroacetate esterase (NASDA)+
M4Eo	Eosinophilic AML?	Many immature eosinophils	MY, NASDA, PAS+
M5a	Immature monocytic	>85% Monoblasts	MY+, fluoride inhibited NASDA
M5b	More mature monocytic	Promonocytes, monocytes	Same as M5a
M6	Erythroleukemia	Megaloblastic & dyspoietic	Ringed & PAS+ blasts
M7	Megakaryoblast leukemia	Polymorphonuclear blasts with blebs	NASDA & platelet peroxidase+

Myelodysplastic Syndromes

Cell Type	Peripheral Blood	Bone Marrow
Refractory Anemia (RA)	Reticulocytopenia, ovalocytes	Hyperplasia & dyspoiesis
RA with ringed sideroblasts	RA with basophilic stippling	Ringed sideroblasts
Chronic myelomonocytic leukemia	Mature cells, hypergranular polymorphonuclear cells	Increased monocytes and rbc's
RA with excess blasts (RAEB)	RA with multiple line dysplasia	Hyperplasia & dyspoiesis
RAEB	Increase in peripheral blasts	As above with Auer rods

This translocation is responsible for the creation of the MLL sequence that codes for a fusion protein (with intranuclear signalling abilities) related to the trithorax gene family of proteins that modulate the expression of DNA transcription factors. The association with pediatric leukemia before 6 months of age is so strong that it has been suggested that the translocation leading to transformation occurs in utero. The MLL sequence is present in multiple fusion proteins, depending on the chromosome with which the "promiscuous" 11q23 happens to couple. Each malignant clone has its own specific fusion MLL sequence, coding for a specific chimeric protein, which presumably is causal to the maturation arrest and malignant transformation (39).

Some abnormalities are associated with particular morphologies and FAB subclassifications. For example, as illustrated by case 1, almost all cases of M3 AML are associated with the translocation involving chromosomes 15 and 17, t(15;17)(q22;q11). Similarly, t(8;21) is common in FAB M2 and inv16 is common in M4E.

It is believed that the cytogenetic abnormalities may yield clues to the underlying pathology in AML by directing attention to the genes that may be affected by the chromosomal breaks. Thus, the recent discovery that cells from patients with M3 AML with t(15;17) have a characteristic breakpoint involving the α-subunit of the retinoic acid receptor (RAR) on chromosome 17 (40, 41) was received with great interest. This chromosomal lesion results in the fusion of a sequence on chromosome 15, termed "myl" (for "myeloid") with a rearranged RAR-α creating a fusion mRNA coding for a unique protein, analogous to the bcr/abl fusion protein in CML (42). Interestingly, cells with the t(15;17) respond in vivo and in vitro to pharmacologic doses of all transretinoic acid by undergoing terminal differentiation. Clinical remissions have been obtained in patients who failed to respond to con-

Table 25.3. Association of Specific Chromosome Aberrations with Morphology in Acute Myelocytic Leukemia (AML)*

	FAB Classification	Aberration
M1	AML without maturation	del(9)(q11q32), normal karyotype
M2	AML with maturation	t(8;21)(q22;q22), t(11;20)(p15;q11)
M3	Acute promyelocytic leukemia	t(15;17)(q22;q11), t(1;17)(p36;q11)
M4	Acute myelomonocytic leukemia	t(1;11)(q21;q23), del (11)(q23q24), t(11;17)(q23;q25)
M4Eo	AML with monocytic component and eosinophils	inv(16)(p13q22), t(16;16)(p13;q22), del(16)(q22)
M5	Acute monocytic leukemia	t(8;16)(p11;p13), t(6;11)(q27;q23), t(9;11)(p21;q23), t(10;11)(p11-15;q23-23), ins(10;11)(p11;q23q24)
M6	Erythroleukemia	i(21q), del(20)(q11q13), ring chromosomes
M7	Megakaryocytic leukemia	Too few cases studied to date

*Adapted from Machnicki and Bloomfield (45) with permission.
FAB, French-American-British.

ventional cytotoxic chemotherapy or who relapsed after such therapy (43, 44). The retinoic acid-induced remissions, however, are relatively short lived and require continuous treatment with transretinoic acid. Cytotoxic chemotherapy, either conventional dose or high-dose followed by bone marrow transplantation (BMT), is often required to consolidate the remission. The malignant cells apparently undergo differentiation under the influence of retinoic acid therapy, as seen by the presence of Auer rods in the maturing cells (43).

Protooncogenes and Antioncogenes (Table 25.4)

Myeloid leukemia cells express a number of protooncogene products, some in a manner correlating with FAB and with the state of proliferation and differentiation. It has been hypothesized that the various cytogenetic abnormalities seen in AML may affect the expression or structure of protooncogenes or other growth-modulating genes and thus contribute to the malignant phenotype. Except in the case of M3 AML discussed above where the RAR-α is rearranged, this is little direct evidence supporting this hypothesis to date.

The single most common abnormality found in AML cells is a group of point mutations in the ras gene family (46). Found in up to 25% of cases, these mutations affect either codons 12, 13, or 61 of the N-ras and K-ras gene.

Preliminary evidence suggests that these mutations are more common in patients with environmental exposure to toxins and that patients with the mutations actually have a better prognosis than their counterparts with normal ras gene structures (47).

A family of protooncogenes coding for proteins with tyrosine kinase activity is commonly expressed in AML cells. These include c-fms, c-fgr, c-scr, and hck. The expression of c-fms and c-fgr is partially linked to monocytoid differentiation and thus correlated with FAB M4 and M5 (48).

Many cases of AML have mutations in p53, an antioncogene, whose absence or functional debility may lead to excessive proliferation (49). However, this gene has been found to be altered in many malignancies and thus cannot be viewed as specific to the mechanism of leukemogenesis.

The genes coding for nuclear-binding proteins myc, fos, and jun, the so-called "early response genes," are expressed in proliferating cells, including AML cells. There is no evidence that they have been rearranged by the malignant process, although high levels of myc expression have been observed and correlated with aggressiveness of the disease (50).

Surface Antigens (Immunophenotyping)

Immunophenotyping can be useful in the diagnosis, subtyping, and prognostication in AML. Work in the field of tumor immunology suggested that AML cells expressed cell surface antigens specific to the malignant state, so-called "tumor-specific antigens." The advent of hybridoma technology stimulated the production of a large number of monoclonal antibodies that appeared to be specific to myeloid cells (51–54). However, these studies revealed that AML cells express the same repertoire of surface antigens as normal myeloid cells, rather than true tumor-specific surface antigens. The expression of surface antigens does correlate with the state of differentiation of the malignant clone, a fact that has been useful in studies of leukemia cell biology (51, 55). Workshops have been convened to organize the data from the large numbers of investigators working in this field of research. These workshops have defined leukocyte surface antigens into clusters of differentiation (CD) (56). Of particular relevance to

Table 25.4. Expression and Mutation of Protooncogenes in Acute Myelocytic Leukemia (AML)

Protooncogene	Type of Abnormality	Association with FAB* Subtype
_ras	Point mutation	All subtypes
p53	Point mutation, deletion	All subtypes
PML	Rearrangement	M3
AML1	Rearrangment	M2
fgr	High expression	M4, M5
fms	High expression	M4, M5
myc	High expression	All subtypes

*FAB, French-American-British.

myeloid cells are CD11b, CD13, CD14, CD15, CD16, CD32, CD33, CD34, and CD64, among others. Some of these molecules either have important functional activities such as adhesion proteins (CD11b) (57), receptors forendotoxin-binding protein (CD14) (58), or receptors for the Fc portion of immunoglobulin (CD16, CD32, and CD64) (59), or function as enzymes (CD13) (60). AML blasts commonly express one or more of the antigens in these CD groupings. The presence of the antigens on leukemia cells is easily determined by indirect immunofluorescence and flow cytometry. This technique, termed "immunophenotyping," is now commonly used for the diagnosis and classification of AML (61) (table 25.5).

The expression of surface antigens correlates with morphology and FAB subclass. For example, the expression of monocyte-associated antigens such as CD14 would be expected to correlate with FAB M4 and M5, the monomyelocytic and monocytic subtypes of AML. Typically, this has been found to be true. However, FAB M1-M3 cells are also commonly positive for CD14. Since CD14 is expressed on normal neutrophils, albeit in lower density and on myeloid precursors, it is not surprising to find CD14 on myelocytic leukemia cells. The CD34 antigen is expressed more commonly on FAB M1 and M2 cells. This is consistent with the view that CD34 is an early hematopoietic cell antigen that is not expressed on more differentiated cells. Both the type I and II Fcg receptors are expressed more commonly on FAB M4 and M5 cells, as expected in view of their higher expression on normal mononuclear phagocytes. Antigens expressed on both normal granulocytes and monocytes, such as CD13, are expressed on all subclasses of AML. One striking correlation is the absence of HLA-DR antigens on leukemia cells of FAB M3, as seen in case 1 above.

Case 2

A 48-year-old man was diagnosed with FAB M2 AML in January 1986. He was treated with cytosine arabinoside and daunorubicin and achieved a complete remission. He then received three additional treatments with the same regimen used to induce remission and was maintained for 1 year on subcutaneous cytosine arabinoside and oral 6-thioguanine. A bone marrow transplant was considered at this time. Peripheral blood leukocytes from the patient and his two siblings were submitted for histocompatibility antigen (HLA) testing. However, the patient and his siblings did not match at the HLA loci and, therefore, allogeneic bone marrow transplantation was not pursued.

In October 1988 he was found to be in relapse. He was treated with cytosine arabinoside (3 g/m² every 12 hours for a total of 12 doses) and achieved a second remission. The patient was referred to a transplantation center for an autologous bone marrow transplant. His marrow was harvested under general anesthesia and the cells then treated ex vivo with complement-fixing monoclonal antibodies directed to surface antigens expressed on his leukemia cells. The patient then was treated with cyclophosphamide (60 mg/kg given on each of 2 consecutive days) followed by total body irradiation (TBI) (1200 cGy in 6 fractions of 200 cGy twice daily for 3 days). His previously harvested marrow was infused through a central venous catheter. The patient experienced some nausea and vomiting, as well as oral mucositis. In addition, a thrombosis developed at the tip of his central venous catheter necessitating placement of a large bore catheter in the femoral vein. A thrombus developed around this catheter and began extending centrally. The patient was treated with heparin and then placed on coumadin. Unfortunately, a subdural hematoma developed several days later, which induced a grand mal seizure. A filter was placed in the inferior vena cava to prevent pulmonary embolism from the caval/femoral thrombosis and the patient was discharged from the hospital. He then experienced complete hematologic and physiologic recovery and is still in complete remission 3 years after his transplant.

Treatment

Remission Induction

Treatment is usually indicated immediately after a diagnosis of AML. Patients often are initially seen clinically with a fulminant illness that will lead to death from bleeding or infection within days without treatment. Occasionally the onset is more gradual, as shown in case 1. This gradual type of onset is more typical of treatment-related AML or AML evolving from a previous myelodysplastic syndrome.

The treatment of AML involves the use of cytotoxic chemotherapeutic agents and supportive care. The latter is important because of the profound effects of both the disease itself and the treatment on normal blood cells. The guiding principle of leukemia therapy is the selective killing of leukemia cells using cytotoxic chemotherapeutic

Table 25.5. Expression of Myeloid-associated Antigens on Acute Myelocytic Leukemia (AML) Cells

Antigen	Frequency in AML (%)*	FAB† Correlation	Reference No.
CD11b	56	M4, M5	55
CD13	57	M1–M6	55
CD14	77	M4, M5	55
CD15	91	M1–M6	55
CD16	26	M1–M6	62
CD32	67	M4, M5	62
CD33	71	M1–M6	55
CD34	45	M1, M2	63
CD64	58	M4, M5	62

*% of patients whose cells were positive for the respective antigen (positive usually defined as ≥20% of cells expressing the antigen in an individual patient).
†FAB, French-American-British.

agents. Leukemia cells are actively dividing while failing to differentiate. Thus, cell cycle–specific chemotherapy is relatively effective in killing these dividing cells while sparing normal hematopoietic stem cells. The mechanism of action of some antileukemia drugs, including cytosine arabinoside (ARA-C) and etoposide, involves initiation of a process called "programmed cell death," or "apoptosis." A characteristic of apoptosis is the finding of chromatin condensation followed by DNA fragmentation. This process is different from necrosis, where random and generalized destruction of cellular components occurs.

The standard of treatment at this time is the use of a 7-day continuous intravenous infusion of the S-phase specific antimetabolite ARA-C (100 mg/m²), along with an anthracycline antibiotic, usually daunorubicin (45 mg/m²), for 3 days. Continuous exposure of the blasts to cytosine arabinoside is efficacious, because most if not all of the blasts will eventually enter the S-phase of the cell cycle during the long infusion and thus increase the chances of eradicating the disease. This regimen will produce remissions in about 60–80% of patients. Remission is defined as a return to normal bone marrow cellularity and composition with <5% blasts and return of blood counts to normal. If no further therapy is given, >90% of patients will relapse. Therefore, a second phase of therapy is instituted. This phase has been called "consolidation," or "intensification," historical terms that are not very descriptive at the present time. There is a consensus that some form of postremission therapy is needed, but the exact drugs, dose, schedule, and duration of therapy are not presently known (64). Most physicians will treat with one or more intensive rounds of chemotherapy, often ara-C at 3 g/m² given 6 to 12 times every 12 hours (3 hours per infusion). Numerous studies of AML treatment with variations in the dose and schedule of postremission therapy have shown that about 20% of the total number of treated patients will achieve long-lasting remissions that are probably cures (65, 66). However, this means that improved therapy is needed for the majority of patients.

While less common in AML than in ALL, central nervous system (CNS) leukemia occurs in 5–10% of patients with AML and requires intrathecal treatment with either methotrexate or ARA-C as single agents, combined therapy with methotrexate and ARA-C, and, occasionally, the addition of cranial-spinal irradiation to refractory disease.

New Approaches to Therapy

New approaches to the treatment of leukemia involve the use of hematopoietic growth factors (HGF) to induce cells to proliferate and the use of differentiating agents to induce the malignant cells to overcome their block in differentiation.

There are two basic rationales for using the HGFs in the treatment of AML. HGFs recruit leukemia cells into active cell division in order to make them more susceptible to S-phase–specific drugs such as ARA-C (24, 25). HGFs also ameliorate the toxicity of chemotherapy against normal bone marrow cells when they are used after chemotherapy to stimulate hematopoiesis (11).

The rationale for the use of differentiation therapy arises from the observation that AML cells have the phenotype of normal myeloid cells that are arrested in an early stage of differentiation and that this block can be overcome by chemical agents, including certain vitamins such as 1,25 dihydroxyvitamin D₃ and retinoic acid. It has been shown that some mature myeloid cells in AML patients in remission are clonal by glucose-6-phosphate (G-6-PD) isoenzyme or restriction endonuclease fragment length polymorphism (RFLP) analysis, and that they are therefore probably derived from the malignant clone (67, 68). This observation suggests that the differentiation block can be overcome spontaneously.

More compelling support for the concept of differentiation therapy comes from studies of leukemia cell lines. For example, the HL-60 line, derived from a patient with promyelocytic leukemia, displays many of the features of AML cells from this subtype. Cells from this line can be induced to differentiate into either monocytoid or neutrophilic cells, depending on the differentiation agent used. One of the compounds that was found to have granulocytic differentiation-inducing activity was retinoic acid (69). This led investigators in France and China to use retinoic acid (RA) to treat patients with acute promyelocytic leukemia (APL) (70). All transretinoic acid (trans-RA) was found to be superior to cis-retinoic acid in vitro and in vivo in inducing differentiation of blast cells from patients. In fact, all trans-RA was capable of inducing remissions in patients with APL without the use of cytotoxic therapy (43, 70). It is believed that the mechanism of action of this therapy is pharmacologically induced differentiation of leukemic blasts. It is unclear whether this therapy will work in producing long-term remissions, since it has been observed that chronic therapy is necessary to maintain remission. It is of interest that the breakpoint in t(15;17) found in APL involves the gene of the α-isoform of the retinoic acid receptor generating a chimeric fusion messenger transcript comprised of the α-RAR and a sequence called "myl" (for myelocytic leukemia) analogous to the phenomenon in chronic myeloid leukemia involving bcr and the abl oncogene (4239) that also generates a fusion mRNA and protein.

Another type of differentiation therapy involves the use of a compound called "tiazofurin," an inhibitor of guanine nucleotide production that induces differentiation of HL60 cells (71) and has been reported to induce remissions in patients with AML (72).

The existence of AML-associated antigens, which could be targets for cytoreductive therapy, has been suggested by reports of antisera and of cytotoxic T cells reactive with leukemic blasts (73, 74). Although monoclonal antibodies to AML cells have not revealed any unique antigens, there are myeloid cell–associated antigens that are abundantly expressed on AML cells, including CD13, 14, 15, and 33 (61). It is possible to target these antigens with monoclonal antibodies coupled to toxin molecules (75, 76) (immunotoxins such as ricin) or to use the complement-activating property of antibodies (77).

There is evidence that natural killer (NK) cells may exert an antileukemia effect, especially after stimulation with interleukin-2 (IL-2) (78). The T-cell product, γ-interferon, also has been shown to have an antiproliferative effect on AML cells in vitro (79). Future studies may take advantage of these additional means of inhibiting AML cell proliferation.

Pharmacology of Antineoplastic Agents

Active agents for AML are shown in table 25.6. Notably, resistance to some of the agents most commonly used in the treatment of AML (the anthracyclines and etoposide) is mediated by a membrane protein termed multidrug resistance (MDR) protein-1. This protein, which acts as a drug efflux pump, can decrease the activity of the anthracyclines and the topoisomerase II inhibitors such as etoposide. Reversal of MDR-1 activity by agents such as calcium channel blockers has been attempted but without significant clinical benefit thus far. Several new agents that inhibit topoisomerase I or II, but are not targets for MDR-1-mediated resistance, include novobiocin (topo II) or camptothecin (topo I).

Complications of Therapy

Complications and adverse effects of chemotherapy are the rule in the treatment of AML. In many cases it is difficult to separate the effects of treatment from the disease itself, since myelosuppression results from both the inhibition of normal hematopoiesis and the effects of therapy.

Infection is common. The most common pathogens are bacteria. Invasive fungal infections caused by *Candida* species and *Aspergillus* are also common. Viral infection is not common, with the exception of cytomegalovirus (CMV) and the herpesviruses, because the therapy of AML is not generally toxic on a long-term basis to lymphocytes, and thus not immunosuppressive. However, the severe neutropenia induced by cytotoxic therapy puts patients at great risk for spontaneous bacterial infection arising from normal body flora (gastrointestinal and respiratory tracts). Both Gram-negative and Gram-positive organisms are causes of significant morbidity and mortality, requiring routine surveillance with cultures of blood, urine, and sputum and prompt institution of broad-spectrum antibiotics when the patient becomes febrile or a positive blood culture develops.

A second cause of toxicity following chemotherapy is the effect of the chemotherapeutic agents on other organs. For example, cytosine arabinoside can damage hepatocytes and lead to a mild hepatitis. Daunorubicin is cardiotoxic, especially after a cumulative dose of >550 mg/m².

Disseminated intravascular coagulation (DIC) is very common in patients with M3 AML, as illustrated by case 1 above. It is believed that thromboplastic substances are released from the granules of the leukemia cells. Some clinicians will use heparin prophylactically to reduce the consumptive coagulopathy (80). Others use replacement therapy (fresh frozen plasma and platelets) if indicated by the clinical situation (81). Thrombocytopenia caused by the disease and its therapy, independent of DIC, is a major problem in the management of patients with AML (discussed below).

Metabolic complications include hyperuricemia with its tendency to cause renal insufficiency, treated by the use of allopurinol to decrease urate formation and by alkalinization of the urine with sodium bicarbonate. Although theoretically possible, a tumor lysis syndrome during which the release of phosphorus, potassium, and uric acid from rapidly lysing cells leads to hypocalcemia and renal shutdown rarely occurs in AML.

Supportive Care

Because the leukemia patient is often neutropenic, infections with opportunistic organisms are common. If a leu-

Table 25.6.

Drug	Mechanism	Used in		
		Induction	Consolidation	Relapse
Cytosine arabinoside	Inhibits DNA synthesis	Yes	Yes	Yes
Anthracyclines	Inhibits DNA synthesis	Yes	Yes	Yes
Daunorubicin				
Mitoxantrone				
Idarubicin				
Etoposide (VP-16)	DNA strand breaks	No	Yes	Yes
Cyclophosphamide	Alkylator	No	Yes	Yes
AZQ (diaziquone)	Alklyator	No	Yes	Yes
m-amsa	DNA strand breaks	No	No	Yes
Carboplatinum	Alkylator	No	Yes	Yes
6-Thioguanine	Antimetabolite	Yes	Yes	No
1-Asparaginase	Depletes asparagine	No	Yes	Yes
2-Chlorodeoxyadenosine	Antimetabolite	No	Yes	Yes

kemia patient has a fever in association with a neutrophil count of <500/μl, institution of broad-spectrum antibiotic coverage adequate for Gram-negative and Gram-positive pathogens is indicated, usually employing an extended spectrum penicillin such as carbenicillin and an aminoglycoside, and often vancomycin because of the increased incidence of *Staphylococcus epidermidis* infection in immunosuppressed patients.

Both the disease process (replacement of normal marrow and suppression of normal hematopoiesis) and the therapy (myelotoxicity) commonly lead to a state of severe thrombocytopenia. Patients are prone to spontaneous bleeding from mucosal surfaces (gums, gastrointestinal tract) and internally, especially in the cranium, leading to subdural or intracerebral hemorrhage, often causing death. A common practice in AML therapy is to transfuse platelets when the platelet count is <20,000/ml of blood. Usually pooled concentrates of platelets are given first, followed by random donor platelets (if sensitization occurs to foreign HLA antigens), and finally HLA-matched platelets. Bleeding may be controlled via the use of antifibrinolytic agents such as ϵ-aminocaproic acid (AMICAR).

Alloimmunization to histocompatibility antigens (HLA) often occurs in multiply transfused patients, leading to poor responses to platelet transfusions due to rapid consumption of the antibody-coated platelets. The use of leukocyte filters during routine blood and platelet transfusion may decrease the rate of alloimmunization by removing a major source of HLA antigens (82). The use of intravenous immunoglobulin may play a role in decreasing the clearance of antibody-tagged platelets in alloimmunized patients (83).

Treatment at Relapse

The best treatment of the patient at relapse is not known. To some extent, treatment is dictated by the timing of the relapse in relation to the previous remission. For example, if a patient relapses more than a year after induction therapy, the same regimen used to induce remission may be used again. However, if the patient relapses sooner, it is considered unlikely that the same treatment will prove any better the second time around than it was at first. Numerous agents have activity in relapsed patients but there is no "gold standard" (table 25.5). Second remissions last a median time of 18 weeks, and only rarely do patients survive >1 year after the first relapse (84, 85). BMT at the time of first relapse may be the best option if a donor is available for an allogeneic transplant or if marrow has been harvested previously in order to perform an autologous BMT (86).

BMT with AML

For a number of the hematologic malignancies, including AML, BMT is often used as an attempt to prolong the interval of remission or even achieve a cure. BMT is effec-

tive largely because the high-dose chemotherapy employed exerts a cytotoxic effect on the malignant clone. However, there are other possible mechanisms, including a graft-versus-leukemia effect in allogeneic BMT mediated by alloreactive T-cells (87) and, in autologous BMT, a cytotoxic effect of NK cells on the malignant clone (88).

Allogeneic BMT is performed using an HLA-matched donor, often a sibling. Data from large pooled registries such as the International Bone Marrow Transplant Registry have shown that approximately 50% of patients transplanted in this manner will be cured. Performance of the BMT at relapse or in second remission results in a cure rate of about 25% (86). Earlier intervention probably is more effective because the leukemia cells are less drug resistant at that time. Other factors may contribute to the worse outcome in second remission including greater host susceptibility to infection and alloimmunization to platelet antigens, leading to more frequent bleeding episodes.

The biggest obstacle to allogeneic BMT is availability of suitable donors and the morbidity/mortality of graft-versus-host disease (GVHD). GVHD is more common and severe in older patients, particularly those >55 years of age. Thus, most centers will only perform HLA-matched sibling donor allogeneic transplants on patients <55 years of age. Organizations such as the National Marrow Donor Program are attempting to increase the pool of potential donors. This group maintains files on HLA-typing of large numbers of potential donors and aids in the "matching" of patients with suitable donors through a network of participating centers. It is too early to comment on the role that "matched unrelated donor" transplants may play in the approach to the patient with AML. However, there is a greater incidence of GVHD in this type of transplant with its attendant mortality (89). Thus, for the patient described in case 2, searching for a donor in the registry was not pursued because of the controversial nature of the role of unrelated donor allogeneic transplant in a patient who had a chance of already being cured from the initial chemotherapy.

One theoretical advantage that allogeneic transplantation has over autologous is the potential of a graft-versus-leukemia effect mediated by donor T-cells against the recipient's leukemia cells (87). This effect is seen most clearly in allogeneic BMTs for chronic myeloid leukemia when T-cell depletion is performed to abrogate GVHD, resulting in a very high relapse rate.

An alternative approach to the use of high-dose chemoradiotherapy and allogeneic BMT is the use of autologous BMT (ABMT) for patients who do not have an HLA-matched donor, such as the patient in case 2, or who are >45 years old, an age where allogeneic BMT has greater toxicity. This treatment option allows a wider use of BMT with AML and avoids the complication of GVHD and associated problems such as interstitial pneumonitis. Considerable activity in the use of ABMT has been reported over the past few years. Most centers in the United States have employed a purging technique, usually involving a cytotoxic drug such as 4-hydroperoxycyclophosphamide (4HC) or monoclonal antibodies directed to antigens expressed on leukemia cells in order to eradicate residual occult disease from the autologous marrow (90, 91). A recent analysis of data from a consortium of European centers has shown a benefit of purging with the chemical, mafosfamide (a cyclophosphamide congener), for patients transplanted within 6 months of attaining their first CR (92). In addition, the benefit of mafosfamide purging in second CR was shown in that study (92). Despite the optimism that investigators have for the use of purged marrows, no randomized studies comparing ABMT with and without marrow purging have been reported. However, since AML patients almost invariably relapse after achieving second or later standard chemotherapy-induced remissions, it seems clear that high-dose chemoradiation therapy and ABMT has been responsible for the long-term survivors in the BMT studies. Long-term disease-free remissions can be achieved in about 30% of patients in second and third remission at the time of ABMT, a similar outcome to that from allogeneic BMT used HLA-matched siblings. Lower relapse rates are seen following allogeneic BMT, but this is balanced by greater mortality from GVHD (87).

Although uncommon, late relapses occur after conventional chemotherapy and BMT (93). An interesting and unanswered question is how leukemia cells are triggered to proliferate again after relatively long periods of quiescence.

Prognostic Factors

Clinical Features

Since the outcome to treatment in AML is variable, it would be of value to determine, based on inherent features of the leukemia or of the patient, who might do better with therapy. Such a determination of prognosis could also contribute to progress in the evolution of therapy, because therapy could be tailored more appropriately to the patient. For example, patients with a very poor prognosis could be treated with more aggressive, or conceptually different, therapeutic modalities, in an effort to improve their outlook, while patients who do well with current therapeutic programs would not be subjected to unnecessarily experimental therapies.

Older patients do not do as well as younger patients. Patients >60 years of age have a lower complete remission rate than those younger (94). This is due in part to the fact that there are higher rates of death in these older patients during remission induction due to infection and other complications. In addition, the older population contains more patients with secondary leukemias arising from a previous myelodysplastic syndrome or from complications of treatment for a previous disease. These secondary leukemias have a worse outcome, apparently due to inherent features of the leukemia clone rendering it more resistant to chemotherapy.

Patients initially seen clinically with high blast cell counts (>100,000/μl) also have a worse prognosis, pre-

sumably related to the high proliferative potential of the leukemic clone and also due to early mortality from leukostasis, a process in which the malignant cells occlude capillaries in the lung and brain, leading to respiratory failure and obtundation.

Cytogenetics

Certain recurring cytogenetic findings have been shown to be associated with either better or worse prognosis in AML. Patients whose cells demonstrate translocations involving chromosomes 15 and 17 or 8 and 21 and inversions of chromosome 16 have a better prognosis than other patients (37). Conversely, those with deletions of chromosomes 5 or 7 do less well. It is not possible to know whether the cytogenetic lesion is a marker of biologic activity or directly associated with the behavior of the malignant clone.

Surface Markers

AML cells express a variety of cell surface markers indicative of cell lineage and state of differentiation. In the lymphoid malignancies, the expression of surface markers associated with lymphoid cells has been helpful in determining subsets, e.g., T-versus B-lineage, and this information has been useful clinically (95). At this time, it is less clear how surface marker determinations are helpful in AML. In general, AML blasts express antigens associated with the myeloid lineage. In one study patients whose cells reacted the My4 (CD14) or My7 (CD13) monoclonal antibodies had a poorer prognosis than those whose cells did not (96). It has also been found that patients whose cells expressed CD2 (OKT11 monoclonal antibody) had a better prognosis than the CD2- negative patients (97). This example of apparently mixed lineage leukemia is an exception to the usual observation that mixed-lineage leukemias behave more poorly than those displaying only myeloid antigens (98). It is important to note that prognostic markers may be dependent in part on the therapy used to treat the disease. Thus, as therapies evolve over time, the significance of a particular marker may decrease in importance.

Summary

What should be clear from the above discussion is that fundamental knowledge about the biology and treatment of AML is incomplete, although major advances have been made in recent years. A major factor impeding progress is the striking molecular and morphologic heterogeneity of the disease, leading one to surmise that AML is a family of diseases sharing some, but not all, phenotypic features, and possibly having different etiologies. Future progress will come from continued study of the molecular biology of the disease(s) and from therapy that is based on a better understanding of the fundamental properties of leukemia cells that differentiate them from normal bone marrow cells.

REFERENCES

1. Erslev A, Lichtman M. Structure and function of marrow. In: Williams WJ, Beutler E, Erslev AJ, Lichtman MA, eds. Hematology. 4th ed. New York: McGraw-Hill, 1990:37–47.

2. Till J, McCulloch E. A direct measurement of the radiation sensitivity of normal mouse bone marrow cells. Radiat Res 1961;14:213.

3. Fauser AA. Messner HA. Identification of megakaryocytes, macrophages, and eosinophils in colonies of human bone marrow containing neutrophilic granulocytes and erythroblasts. Blood 1979;53:1023.

4. Leary AG, Ogawa M, Strauss LC, Civin CI. Single cell origin of multilineage colonies in culture: Evidence that differentiation of multipotent progenitors and restriction of proliferative potential of monopotent progenitors are stochastic processes. J Clin Invest 1984;74:2193.

5. Groopman J, Molina J-M, Scadden D. Hematopoietic growth: biology and clinical applications. N Engl J Med 1989;321:1449–1459.

6. Henderson E. Acute leukemia: general considerations. In: Williams WJ, Beutler E, Erslev AJ, Lichtman MA, eds. Hematology. 4th ed. New York: McGraw-Hill, 1990: 236–250.

7. Bradbury D, Rogers S, Kozlowski R, Bowen G, Reilly I, Russell N. Interleukin-1 is one factor which regulates autocrine production of GM-CSF by the blast cells of acute myeloblastic leukemia. Br J Haemotol 1991;76:488–493.

8. Delwel R, Vanbuitenen C, Salem M, Oosterom R, Touw I, Lowenberg B. Hemopoietin-1 activity of interleukin-1 (IL-1) on acute myeloidl leukemia colony-forming cells (AML-CFU): in vitro IL-1 induces production of tumor necrosis factor-alpha which synergizes with IL-3 or granulocyte-macrophage colony-stimulating factor. Leukemia 1990;4: 557–560.

9. Metcalf D. The leukemia inhibitory factor (LIF). Int J Cell Clon 1991;9:95–108.

10. Nemunaitis J, Rabinowe S, Singer J, Bierman P, Vose J, Freedman A, Onetto N, Gillis S, Oette D, Gold M, Buckner D, Hansen J, Ritz J, Appelbaum F, Armitage J, Nadler L. Recombinant granulocyte-macrophage colony-stimulating factor after autologous bone marrow transplantation for lymphoid cancer. N Engl J Med 1991;324:1771–1778.

11. Gabrilove J, Kakubowski A, Scher H. Effect of granulocyte colony-stimulating factor on neutropenia and associated morbidity due to chemotherapy for transitional-cell carcinoma of the urothelium. N Engl J Med 1988;318:1414–1422.

12. Ohno R, Tomonaga M, Kobayashi T, Kanamaru A, Shirakawa S, Masaoka T, Omine M, Oh H, Nomura T, Sakai Y, Hirano M, Yokomaku S, Nakayama S, Yoshida Y, Miura A, Morishima Y, Dohy H, Niho Y, Hamajima N, Takaku, F. Effect of granulocyte colony-stimulating factor after intensive induction therapy in relapsed or refractory acute leukemia. N Engl J Med 1990;323:871–877.

13. Gordon M, Riley G, Watt S, Greaves M. Compartmentalization of a haematopoietic growth factor (GM-CSF) by glycoaminoglycans in the bone marrow microenvironment. Nature 1987;326:403–405.

14. Park L, Waldron P, Friend D, Sassenfeld H, Price V, Anderson D, Cosman D, Andrews R, Bernstein I, Urdal D. Interleukin-3, GM-CSF, and G-CSF receptor expression on cell lines and primary leukemia cells: receptor heterogeneity and relationship to growth factor responsiveness. Blood 1989; 74:56–65.

15. Budel L, Touw I, Delwel R, Clark S, Lowenberg, B. IL-3 and GM-CSF receptors on human acute myelocytic leukemia cells and relationship to the proliferative response. Blood 1989;74:565–571.

16. Budel L, Touw I, Delwel R. Lowenberg B. Granulocyte colony-stimulating factor receptors in human acute myelocytic leukemia. Blood 1989;74:2668–2673.

17. Begley C, Metcalf D, Nicola, N. Primary human myeloid leukemia cells: comparative responsiveness to proliferative stimulation by GM-CSF or G-CSF and membrane expression of CSF receptors. Leukemia 1987;1:1.

18. Begley C, Metcalf D, Nicola, N. Binding characteristics and proliferative action of purified granulocyte-colony stimulating factor (G-CSF) on normal and leukemic human promyelocytes. Exp Hematol 1988;16:71–79.

19. Ashmun R, Look A, Roberts W, Roussel M, Seremetics S, Ohtsuka M, Sherr C. Monoclonal antibodies to the human CSF-1 receptor (c-fms proto-oncogene product) detect epitopes on normal mononuclear phagocytes and on human myeloid leukemic blast cells. Blood 1989;72:827.

20. Sherr C. Colony-stimulating factor-1 receptor. Blood 1990; 75:1–12.

21. Vadhan-Raj S, Keating M, LeMaistre A, Hittelman W, McCredie K, Trujillo J, Broxmeyer H, Nenney C, Gutterman J. Effects of recombinant human granulocyte-macrophage colony-stimulating factor in patients with myelodysplastic syndromes. N Engl J Med 1987;317:1545–1552.

22. Negrin R, Haeuber D, Nagler A, Kobayashi Y, Sklar J, Donlon T, Vincent M, Greenberg P. Maintenance treatment of patients with myelodysplastic syndromes using recombinant human granulocyte-colony-stimulating factor. Blood 1990;76:36–43.

23. Ganser A, Seipelt G, Lindemann A, Ottmann O, Falk S, Klausmann M, Frisch J, Schulz G, Mertelsmann R, Hoelzer D. Effects of recombinant human interleukin-3 in patients with myelodysplastic syndromes. Blood 1990;76: 455–462.

24. Cannistra S, Groshek P, Griffin, J. GM-CSF enhances the cytotoxic effects of cytosine arabinoside in acute myeloblastic leukemia and in the myeloid blast crisis phase of chronic myeloid leukemia. Leukemia 1989;3:328–334.

25. Miyauchi J, Kelleher C, Wang C, Minkin S, McCullouch E. Growth factors influence the sensitivity of leukemic stem cells to cytosine arabinoside in culture. Blood 1989;73: 1272–1278.

26. Young D, Wagner K. Griffin, J. Constitutive expression of the GM-CSF gene in acute myeloblastic leukemia. J Clin Invest 1987;79:100–106.

27. Sandler D. Epidemiology of acute myelogenous leukemia. Semin Oncol 1987;14:359–364.

28. Rinsky R, Smith A, Hornung R, Filloon T, Young R, Okun A, Landrigan P. Benzene and leukemia: an epidemiologic risk assessment. N Engl J Med 1987;316:1044–1050.

29. Kojima S, Matsuyama T, Sato T, et al. Down's syndrome and acute leukemia in children: an analysis of phenotype by use of monoclonal antibodies and electron microscopic platelet peroxidase reaction. Blood 1990;76:2348.

30. Ravindranath Y, Abella E, Krischer JP, et al. Acute myeloyd leukemia (AML) in Down's syndrome is highly responsive to chemotherapy: experience of POG AML study 8498. Blood 1992;80:2210.

31. Malkin D, Li F, Strong L, Fraumeni J, Nelson C, Kim D, Kassel J, Gryka M, Bischoff F, Tainsky M, Friend, S. Germ

line p53 mutations in a familial syndrome of breast cancer sarcomas, and other neoplasms. Science 1990;250: 1233–1238.

32. Kaldor J, Day N, Clarke, A. Leukemia following Hodgkin's disease. N Engl J Med 1990;322:7–13.

33. Kaldor JM, Day NE, Pettersson F, Clarke EA, Pedersen D, Mehnert W, Bell J, Host H, Prior P, Karjalainen S, et al. Leukemia following chemotherapy for ovarian cancer. N Engl J Med 1990;322:1–6.

34. Mufti G, Stevens J, Oscier D, Hamblin T, Machin D. Myelodysplastic syndromes: a scoring system with prognostic significance. Br J Haematol 1985;59:425–433.

35. Bennett JM, Catovsky D, Daniel MT, Flandrin G, Galton DAG, Gralnick HR, Sultan C. Proposed revised criteria for the classification of acute myeloid leukemia: a report of the French-American-British (FAB) Cooperative Group. Ann Intern Med 1985;103:620–625.

36. Elghetany M, MacCallum J, Davey F. The use of cytochemical procedures in the diagnosis and management of acute and chronic myeloid leukemia. Clin Lab Med 1990;10: 707–720.

37. Bloomfield C, Chapelle DL. Chromosome abnormalities in acute nonlymphocytic leukemia: clinical and biologic significance. Semin Oncol 1987;14:372–383.

38. Arthur D, Bloomfield C. Partial deletion of the long arm of chromosome 16 and bone marrow eosinophilia in acute nonlymphocytic leukemia: a new association. Blood 1983;61: 994–998.

39. Kalwinsky DR, Raimondi SC, Schell MJ, et al. Prognoxtic importance of cytogenetic subgroups in de novo pediatric acute nonlymphocytic leukemia. J Clin Oncol 1990;8:75.

40. de The H, Chomeienne C, Lanotte M, Degos L, Dejean A. The t(15;17) translocation of acute promyelocytic leukaemia fuses the retinoic acid receptor a gene to a novel transcribed locus. Nature 1990;347:558–561.

41. Borrow J, Goddard A, Sheer D, Solomon, E. Molecular analysis of acute promyelocytic leukemia breakpoint cluster region on chromosome 17. Science 1990;249:1577–1580.

42. Stam K, Heisterkamp N, Grosveld G, de Klein A, Verma R, Coleman M, Dosik H, Groffen J. Evidence of a new chimeric bcr/abl mRNA in patients with chronic myelocytic leukemia and the Philadelphia chromosome. N Engl J Med 1985;313: 1429–1433.

43. Warrell R, Frankel S, Miller W, Scheinberg D, Itri L, Hittelman W, Vyas R, Andreeff M, Tafuri A, Jakubowski A, Gabrilove J, Gordon M, Dmitrovsky E. Differentiation therapy of acute promyelocytic leukemia with tretinoin (all-trans-retinoic acid). N Engl J Med 1991;324:1385–1393.

44. Castaigne S, Chomienne C, Daniel M, Ballerini P, Fenaux P, Degos L. All-trans retinoic acid as a differentiation therapy for acute promyelocytic leukemia; I, clinical results. Blood 1990;76:1704–1709.

45. Machnicki J, Bloomfield C. Chromosomal abnormalities in myelodysplastic syndromes and acute myeloid leukemia. In: Davey FR, ed. Clinics in laboratory medicine. Philadelphia: WB Saunders, 1990:755–768.

46. Bos J, Verlann-de Vries M, van der Eb A. Mutations in N-ras predominate in acute myeloid leukemia. Blood 1987;69: 1237–1241.

47. Taylor J, Sandler D, Bloomfield C, Shore D, Ball E, Neubauer A, McIntyre O, Liu E. ras oncogene activation and occupational exposure in AML. J Natl Cancer Inst 1991;84: 1626–1632.

48. Willman C, Stewart C, Longacre T, Head D, Habbersett R, Ziegler S, Perlmutter R. Expression of the c-fgr and hck protein-tyrosine kinases in acute myeloid leukemic blasts is associated with early commitment and differentiation events in the monocytic and granulocytic lineages. Blood 1991;77:726–734.

49. Slingerland J, Minden M, Benchimol S. Mutation of the p53 gene in human acute myelogenous leukemia. Blood 1991;77: 1500–1507.

50. Preisler H, Sato H, Yang P, Wilson M, Kaufman C, Watt R. Assessment of c-myc expression in individual leukemia cells. Leuk Res 1988;12:507–516.

51. Ball E, Fanger M. The expression of myeloid-specific antigens on myeloid leukemia cells: correlations with leukemia subclasses and implications for normal myeloid differentiation. Blood 1983;61:456–463.

52. Griffin JD, Lynch D, Sabbath K, Schlossman SF. A monoclonal antibody reactive with normal and leukemic human myeloid progenitor cells. Leuk Res 1984;4:521.

53. Andrews RG, Torok-Storb B, Bernstein ID. Myeloid-associated differentiation antigens on stem cells and their progeny identified by monoclonal antibodies. Blood 1983; 62:124–132.

54. Civin C, Strauss L, Brovall C, Fackler M, Schwartz J, Shaper J. Antigenic analysis of hematopoiesis: III, a hematopoietic progenitor cell surface antigen defined by a monoclonal antibody raised against KG-1a cells. J Immunol 1984;133:157–165.

55. Griffin JD, Mayer RJ, Weinstein HJ, Rosenthal DS, Coral FS, Beveridge RP, Schlossman SF. Surface marker analysis of acute myeloblastic leukemia: identification of differentiation-associated phenotypes. Blood 1983;62:557.

56. Knapp W, Dorken B, Reiber P, Schmidt RE, Stein H, von dem Borne AEGK. CD antigens. Blood 1989;74;1448.

57. Wright SD, Rao PE, Van Voorhis WC, Craigmyle, LS. Iida K, Talle MA, Westburg EF, Goldstein G, Silverstein SC. Identification of the C3bi receptor of human monocytes and macrophages by using monoclonal antibodies. Proc Natl Acad Sci USA 1983;80:5699.

58. Wright S, Ramos R, Tobias P, Ulevitch R, Mathison J. CD14 a receptor for complexes of lipopolysaccharide (LPS) and LPS binding protein. Science 1990;249:1431–1433.

59. Fanger M, Shen L, Graziano R, Guyre P. Cytotoxicity mediated by human Fc receptors for IgG. Immunol Today 1989; 10:92–99.

60. Look A, Ashmun R, Shapiro L, Peiper S. Human myeloid plasma membrane glycoprotein CD 13 (gp 150) is identical to aminopeptidase N. J Clin Invest 1989;83:1299.

61. Ball E. Immunophenotyping of acute myeloid leukemia cells. Clin Lab Med 1990;10:721–736.

62. Ball ED, McDermott J, Griffin JD, Davey FR, Davis R, Bloomfield CD. Expression of the three myeloid cell-associated immunoglobulin G Fc receptors defined by murine monoclonal antibodies on normal bone marrow and acute leukemia cells. Blood 1989;73:1951.

63. Borowitz MJ, Gockerman JP, Moore JO. Clinicopathologic and cytogenic features of CD34 (My 10)-positive acute nonlymphocytic leukemia. Am J Clin Pathol 1989;91:265.

64. Buchner T, Hiddemann W, Loffler G, Gassmann W, Maschmeyer G, Heit W, Hossfeld D, Weh H, Ludwig W, Thiel E, Nowrousian M, Aul C, Lengfelder E, Lathan B, Mainzer D, Urbanitz D, Emmerich B, Middelhoff G, Donhuijsen-Ant H, Hellriegel H, Heinecke A. Improved cure rate by very early intensification combined with prolonged maintenance chemotherapy in patients with acute myeloid leukemia: data

from the AML cooperative group. Semin Hematol 1991;28: 76–79.

65. Mayer R, Schiffer C, Peterson B, Budman D, Silver R, Rai K, Cornwell G, Ellison R, Maguire M, Berg D, Davis R, McIntyre O, Frei E. Intensive postremission therapy in adults with acute nonlymphocytic leukemia using various dose schedules of ara-C: a progress report from the CALGB. Semin Oncol 1987;14(suppl 1):25–31.

66. Champlin R, Gale R. Acute myelogenous leukemia: recent advances in therapy. Blood 1987;69:1551–1562.

67. Fearon ER, Burke PJ, Schiffer CA, Zehnbauer BA, Vogelstein B. Differentiation of leukemia cells to polymorphonuclear leukocytes in patients with acute nonlymphocytic leukemia. N Engl J Med 1986;315:15–24.

68. Fialkow P, Singer J, Adamson J, Berkow R, Friedman J, Jacobson R, Moohr J. Acute nonlymphocytic leukemia: expression in cells restricted to granulocytic and monocytic differentiation. N Engl J Med 1979;301:1–5.

69. Breitman TR, Selonick SE, Collins SJ. Induction of differentiation of the human promyelocytic leukemia cell line (HL-60) by retinoic acid. Proc Natl Acad Sci USA 1980;77:2936.

70. Degos L. All-trans-retinoic acid in the treatment of acute promyelocytic leukaemia. Presse Med 1990;19:1483–1484.

71. Goldstein B, Leary J, Farley B, Marquez V, Levy P, Rowley P. Induction of HL60 cell differentiation by tiazofurin and its analogues: characterization and efficacy. Blood 1991;78: 593–598.

72. Tricot G, Jayaram H, Lapis E, Natsumeda Y, Nichols C, Kneebone P, Heerema N, Weber G, Hoffman R. Biochemically directed therapy of leukemia with tiazofurin, a selective blocker of inosine 5′-phosphate dehydrogenase activity. Cancer Res 1989;49:3696.

73. Csako G, Binder R, Kales A, Neefe J. Cloning of human lymphocytes reactive with autologous leukemia cells. Cancer Res 1980;40:3218–3221.

74. Metzgar R, Mohanakumar T, Miller D. Antigens specific for human lymphocytic and myeloid leukemia cells: detection by nonhuman primate antiserums. Science 1972;178:986–988.

75. Roy D, Griffin J, Belvin M, Blattler W, Lanbert J, Ritz J. Anti-My9-blocked ricin: an immunotoxin for selective targeting of acute myeloid leukemia cells. Blood 1991;77: 2404–2412.

76. Myers D, Uckun F, Ball E, Vallera D. Immunotoxins for ex vivo marrow purging in autologous bone marrow transplantation for acute nonlymphocytic leukemia. Transplantation 1988;46:240–245.

77. Ball ED, Vredenburgh JJ, Mills LE, Cornwell GG, Schwarz L, Howell AL, Troy K. Autologous bone marrow transplantation for acute myeloid leukemia following in vitro treatment with neuraminidase and monoclonal antibodies. Bone Marrow Transplant 1990;6:277–280.

78. Oblakowski P, Bello-Fernander C, Reittie J, Heslop H, Galatowicz G, Veys P, Wilkes S, Prentice H, Hazlehurst G, Hoffbrand A, Brenner M. Possible mechanism of selective killing of myeloid leukemic blast cells by lymphokine-activated killer cells. Blood 1991;77:1996–2001.

79. Price G, Brenner M, Prentice H, Hoffbrand A, Newland, A Cytotoxic effects of tumour necrosis factor and gamma-interferon on acute myeloid leukemia blasts. Br J Haematol 1987;55:287.

80. Hoyle C, Swirsky D, Freedman L, Hayhoe F. Beneficial effect of heparin in the management of patients with APL. Br J Haematol 1988;68:283.

81. Goldberg MA, Ginsburg D, Mayer RJ, Stone RM, Maguire M, Rosenthal DS, Antin JH. Is heparin administration necessary during induction chemotherapy for patients with acute promyelocytic leukemia? Blood 1987;69:187–191.

82. Schiffer C. Prevention of alloimmunization against platelets. Blood 1991;77:1–4.

83. Sullivan K, Kopecky K, Jocom J, Fisher L, Buckner C, Meyers J, Counts G, Bowden R, Petersen F, Witherspoon R, Budinger M, Schwartz R, Appelbaum F, Clift R, Hansen J, Sanders J, Thomas E, Storb R. Immunomodulatory and antimicrobial efficacy of intravenous immunoglobulin in bone marrow transplantation. N Engl J Med 1990;323:705–712.

84. Keating M, Kantarjian H, Smith T, Estey E, Walters R, Andersson B, Beran M, McCredie K, Freireich, E. Response to salvage therapy and survival after relapse in acute myelogenous leukemia. J Clin Oncol 1989;7:1071–1080.

85. Arlin Z, Ahmed T, Mittelman A, Feldman E, Mehta R, Weinstein P, Rieber E, Sullivan P, Baskind P. A new regimen of amsacrine with high-dose cytarabine is safe and effective therapy for acute leukemia. J Clin Oncol 1987;5: 371–375.

86. Clift R, Buckner C, Thomas E, Kopecky K, Appelbaum F, Tallman M, Storb R, Sanders J, Sullivan K, Banaji M, Beatty P, Bensinger W, Cheever M, Deeg J, Doney K, Fefer A, Greenberg P, Hansen J, Hackman R, Hill R, Martin P, Meyers J, McGuffin R, Neiman P, Sale G, Shulman H, Singer J, Stewart P, Weiden P, Witherspoon R. Treatment of acute non-lymphoblastic leukemia by allogeneic marrow transplantation. Bone Marrow Transplant 1987;2: 243–258.

87. Sullivan K, Weiden P, Fefer A, Appelbaum F, Anasetti C, Buckner C, Clift R, Doney K, Fisher L, Martin P, Petersen F, Sanders J, Singer J, Stewart P, Witherspoon R, Hansen J, Thomas E, Storb R. Graft-versus-leukemia effect of allogeneic bone marrow transplantation in patients with acute nonlymphocytic leukemia. In: Gale RP, ed. UCLA Symposia on Molecular and Cellular Biology. New Series. New York: Wiley-Liss, 1990:391–402.

88. Reittie J, Gottlieb D, Heslop H, Leger O, Drexler H, Hazlehurst G, Hoffbrand A, Prentice H, Brenner M. Endogenously generated activated killer cells circulate after autologous and allogeneic marrow transplantation but not after chemotherapy. Blood 1989;73:1351–1358.

89. Beatty PG, Hansen JA, Thomas ED, et al. Marrow transplantation from HLA-matched unrelated donors for treatment of hematologic malignancies. Transplant 1991; 2:443.

90. Yeager A, Kaizer H, Santos G, Saral R, Colvin O, Stuart R, Braine H, Burke P, Ambinder R, Burns W, Fuller D, Davis J, Karp J, May W, Rowley S, Sensenbrenner L, Vogelsang G, Windgard J. Autologous bone marrow transplantation in patients with acute nonlymphocytic leukemia using ex-vivo marrow treatment with 4-hydroperoxycyclophosphamide. N Engl J Med 1986;315:141–147.

91. Ball E, Mills L, Cornwell G, Davis B, Coughlin C, Howell A, Stukel T, Dain B, McMillan R, Spruce W, Miller W, Thompson L. Autologous bone marrow transplantation for acute myeloid leukemia using monoclonal antibody-purged bone marrow. Blood 1990;75:1199–1206.

92. Gorin N, Aegerter P, Auvert B, Meloni G, Goldstone A, Burnett A, Carella A, Korbling M, Herve P, Maraninchi D, Lowenberg R, Verdonck L, de Planque M, Helbig W, Porcellini A, Rizzoli V, Alesandrino E, Franklin I, Reiffers J,

Colleselli P, Goldman J. Autologous bone marrow transplantation for acute myelocytic leukemia in first remission: a European survey of the role of marrow purging. Blood 1990;75:1606–1614.

93. Witherspoon R, Flournoy N, Thomas E. Recurrence of acute leukemia more than two years after allogeneic marrow grafting. Exp Hematol 1986;14:178.

94. Champlin R, Gajewski J, Golde D. Treatment of acute myelogenous leukemia in the elderly. Semin Oncol 1989; 16:51.

95. Vaickus L, Ball E, Foon K. Immune markers in hematologic malignancies [review]. Crit Rev Oncol Hematol 1991;11: 267–297.

96. Griffin J, Davis R, Nelson D, Davey F, Mayer R, Schiffer C, McIntyre O, Bloomfield C. Use of surface marker analysis to predict outcome of adult acute myeloblastic leukemia. Blood 1986;68:1232–1233.

97. Ball E, Davis R, Griffin J, Mayer R, Davey F, Arthur D, Wurster-Hill D, Noll W, Elghetany M, Allen S, Rai K, Lee E, Schiffer C, Bloomfield C. Prognostic value of lymphocyte surface markers in acute myeloid leukemia. Blood 1991;77: 2242–2250.

98. Mirro J, Zipf TF, Pui CH, Kitchingman G, Williams D, Melvin S, Murphy SB, Stass S. Acute mixed lineage leukemia: clinicopathologic correlations and prognostic significance. Blood 1985;66:1115–1123.

CHAPTER 26

Chronic Myelocytic Leukemias

DAVID A. MAYBEE, MD

"Leucocythaemia: a disease of haematopoiesis, characterized by a great and progressive increase in the number of white blood cells, and a diminution in the number of red blood cells, with hyperplasia of the spleen and bone marrow, and often of the lymphatic tissue."
—Keating
Cyclopedia of the Diseases of Children, 1890

The chronic myeloid leukemias are myeloproliferative disorders manifest by abnormal proliferation of a multipotent stem cell progenitor. Proliferation and differentiation of the affected stem cells in these disorders lead to multiple affected cell lines, thus earning the descriptive term "panmyelopathy" ("myelo" = marrow). Chronic myeloid leukemias are characterized clinically by excessive production of relatively differentiated cells, and in contrast to acute leukemias, they often are slowly progressive. However, within the spectrum of these diseases, there are instances of rapid clinical progression, sometimes culminating with findings resembling acute leukemia. These chronic leukemias account for more than 20% of all adult leukemias and for somewhat less than 5% of childhood leukemia. There are diverse and sometimes confusing presentations, as will be presented. Despite major advances in the understandings of the pathophysiology of these disorders, more effective treatment based on new insights has begun to emerge only recently. Adult and childhood forms (ACML and JCML) and their variants are described. Issues related to evaluation, pathophysiology, biology, and management will be discussed.

Adult Chronic Myelogenous Leukemia (ACML)

Also referred to as chronic myeloid leukemia (CML), chronic granulocytic leukemia (CGL), or chronic myelocytic leukemia, this is the most common of all leukemias and was the first leukemia to be recognized more than 150 yeas ago. The associated distinctive chromosome in CML cells, the Philadelphia chromosome, was identified in 1960 and was further described as a reciprocal translocation between chromosomes 9 and 22 by Rowley in 1973 (1). We will refer to Philadelphia chromosome positive (Ph+) chronic myelogenous leukemia as ACML (for "adult type") in this chapter.

The course of this illness is usually triphasic, with a slowly progressive chronic phase followed by a period of transformation (acceleration) and culminating in an acute and more primitive proliferation resembling an acute leukemia (blast crisis). As events unfold during the disease progression, specific therapeutic interventions can be undertaken. The following case is representative of some of the issues involved. It is divided into three parts, roughly pertaining to events occurring during these three phases of this disease.

ACML in an adult has been detailed in a case in Chapter 15, Cytogenetics. Because the issues are largely similar in adults and children with the adult form of the disease, we present a case of ACML in a child.

Case 1

A 4-year-old white male was in excellent health before a routine pediatric examination, at which time a CBC was drawn and showed marked elevation of the white count. The physical examination was unremarkable, except for spleen and liver edges 2 cm below the respective costal margins. On referral to the local hospital, the patient's white blood count was 88.8×10^9/L, with 41% polys, 15% bands, 6% metamyelocytes, 4% myelocytes, 17% lymphocytes, 6% monocytes, 7% eosinophils, 3% basophils, 1 NRBC, and no blasts. The hemoglobin was 11.7 gm/dL and the platelet count was 743×10^9/L. A myeloproliferative syndrome was suspected and a bone marrow biopsy was performed. This revealed marked hypercellularity, increased megakaryocytes, and a M/E ratio of approximately 10 to 1. The marrow cell differential showed 90% myeloid elements with 28% polys, 15% bands, 12% metamyelocytes, 23% myelocytes, 2% promyelocytes, and less than 1% blasts, with 5% eosinophils, 4% basophils, and 9% NRBC. Marrow megakaryocytes were morphologically normal and slightly increased. Marrow reticulin stain was negative. There were no dysplastic features (blood or marrow) in the myeloid or erythroid elements.

Further evaluation was undertaken. Liver enzymes and renal chemistries were normal, as were PT, PTT, and fibrinogen. Vitamin B12 was >2,000 pg/ml (normal, 140–750), leukocyte alkaline phosphatase (LAP) was 11 (normal score >32), and lactic acid dehydrogenase (LDH) was 560 u/L (normal, 28–186 u/L). Abdominal sonogram revealed the spleen to be three times normal volume. The peripheral blood karyotype was completely normal, but the bone marrow karyotype revealed 100% Ph+ cells. The diagnosis of ACML was made and the patient was started on alpha interferon therapy.

Clinical Findings

This childhood case and that of the 42-year-old man reviewed in Chapter 15 (Cytogenetics) demonstrate many of the characteristic presenting features of ACML. The median age at diagnosis is approximately 46 years (2, 3), but ACML is found from infancy to old age. There is a slight male predominance in adults and perhaps the opposite in children (4). The onset may be insidious, with up to one-quarter of all patients completely asymptomatic at the time of recognition of leukocytosis on CBC. Most commonly encountered symptoms at presentation are **malaise** and **fatigue, fever, weight loss, diaphoresis, sternal tenderness,** and **abdominal discomfort;** more than 80% of adults and more than 90% of children show moderate to massive **splenomegaly** and approximately one-third demonstrate **hepatomegaly** (4). Occasionally, patients will present with more striking symptoms, including **priapism** (5, 6), **hemorrhage** or **thrombosis** (less than 5%), severe **bone** and/or **joint pain, respiratory distress,** or **central nervous system signs** and **symptoms** including headache, visual disturbances, papilledema, sensory disturbances, stroke, ischemic digits, and cerebellar or cognitive disfunction (4, 7). In contrast to adult or childhood myeloproliferative disorders involving monocytes, ACML rarely presents with or subsequently develops skin rash or significant lymphadenopathy (8–10). Infection is seldom seen. If acute morbidity is experienced, it is usually caused by hyperleukocytosis or leukostasis (7).

Laboratory Findings

When presenting in what has been termed the "chronic" phase, most ACML patients will have **leukocytosis** with a mean WBC count in adults of over $200 \times 10^9/L$ (11) and with more than 80% of children having WBC greater than $100 \times 10^9/L$ (4, 7). The **peripheral blood morphology** is predominantly granulocytic and generally shows left-shifted myeloid maturation with large peaks in the number of myelocytes and neutrophils; less mature cells occur with decreasing frequency. However, it is not unusual to find that more than 30% of the peripheral blood myeloid cells are immature (from myelocytes to myeloblasts). The combination of myeloblasts and pro-myelocytes rarely exceeds 10%, and blasts in the peripheral blood rarely exceed 5%.

The peripheral smear often will show increased numbers of mature and immature basophils and eosinophils, and peculiar mixed granulated (eosinophilic/basophilic) leukocytes also are sometimes encountered (12). The absolute monocyte count may be slightly increased. Often, nucleated RBCs are seen. Morphologically, the myeloid elements in the peripheral blood appear normal (11). Dysplastic features have been recognized in ACML but are not a prominent feature.

Usually, there is a mild normochromic/normocytic **anemia** present, sometimes accompanied by a slight reticulocytosis. Anemia is more pronounced in children, with mean Hct of 25% in one series (13). Unless splenic sequestration is occurring, the **platelet count** usually will be high normal to markedly increased, especially in children, with more than 20% of children presenting with platelet counts in excess of $750 \times 10^9/L$. It is not unusual to see platelet counts in excess of $1000 \times 10^9/L$. Platelet morphology is normal.

When leukocytes are serially monitored in the peripheral blood of adults and children with ACML, they often will show a broad **oscillations** in a regular and predictable cycle, usually averaging an 8 to 10-week time span (2, 14, 15), with similar oscillations (not necessarily synchronous) in the platelet count.

The **bone marrow biopsy** and **aspirate** are invariably hypercellular and manifest granulocytic and sometimes megakaryocytic hyperplasia. Although the biopsy may show a slight increase in reticulin, significant marrow fibrosis is very unusual at presentation (2). The myeloid/erythroid ratio generally is greater than 10:1 and may be more than 50:1. As in the peripheral blood, marrow granulocytic elements are in all stages of maturation, including eosinophiles. Marrow basophilia may be extreme. The left shift in the granulocytic series is generally more pronounced than that in the peripheral blood, but blasts usually are less than 5%. Blasts are chloroacetate esterase and sudan black positive and do not stain cytochemically or immunologically for the monocyte lineage. Cell phenotyping is typical for the spread of differentiating granulocytes seen (mostly CD13 and 15 with a few CD33 and 34). An occasional finding, particularly in the marrow of adults with ACML, is the presence of lipid-laden histiocytes resembling Gaucher cells or sea-blue histiocytes (16). The significance of these cells is unknown. Red cell maturation is usually orderly and morphology is normal, and the RBC population lacks fetal characteristics (17, 18).

It should be stressed that not all patients with ACML are diagnosed in early chronic phase. Initial findings suggestive of a more advanced stage of the disease include increased blood/marrow basophilia, increased blood or marrow promyelocytes and/or myeloblasts, and evidence of increased marrow fibrosis (2). Occasionally, patients will present with an acute leukemia-like blood marrow/morphology called blast crisis, as will be discussed later.

Leukocyte alkaline phosphatase (LAP) activity invariably is decreased or absent in ACML at disease presentation at any age. Castro-Malaspina et al (4) found that 100% of children with ACML had LAP scores of less 40 (23% with 0 score) at presentation. More than 85% of adults present with low LAP levels (19). This can be helpful in distinguishing ACML from infectious and inflammatory states. It is quite common to find LAP scores returning toward normal (range, 32–130 in healthy adults) during clinical remission or in the face of concurrent inflammation or infection (19). The LAP scores also may increase as the disease accelerates.

Also invariably elevated in ACML are serum levels of vitamin B12, and the B12 binding protein, transcobalamin-I; serum B12 levels measured in the Castro-Malaspina series ranged from 1200 to 2500 pg/mL (4) (normal range, 200–900 pg/mL), and in adults, levels averaging 15 times normal have been reported (20). As with the LAP score, the serum B12 level also will return to normal when the leukemic mass is decreased by therapy. Decreased or negative LAP scores and elevated serum B12 levels are cardinal and reliable findings in ACML at presentation.

Serum and urine muramidase (lysozyme) levels are *not* increased in ACML. (21) Hyperuricemia and hyperuricacidurea are encountered commonly and occasionally may cause symptoms secondary to tissue and joint deposition or renal calculi, particularly in adults. Generally, there is no chemical evidence of hepatic or renal dysfunction. Lactic dehydrogenase (LDH) may be elevated. Serum immunoglobulins are usually normal.

The Philadelphia (Ph[1]) chromosome is found in 85–95% of all patients presenting with the classical ACML phenotype. Usually 90–100% of bone marrow cell metaphases will show the Ph chromosome at presentation and a lesser percentage in the peripheral blood cells. An additional 3–5% of Ph-negative patients will demonstrate the *bcr/abl* fusion gene by Southern blotting, PCR, or hybridization techniques, sometimes associated with more complex or subtler chromosomal rearrangements (22–26). However, there seems to be a "true" population of Ph-/*bcr/abl* patients, called "Philadelphia negative (Ph−) CML" (26), who appear to have a different clinical/laboratory profile.

The combination of the specific physical and laboratory phenotypic features and the cytogenetic abnormalitiy described above is pathognomonic for ACML. It generally is easy to arrive at the diagnosis quickly and to make a definitive plan concerning initial management, but some thought must be given to other disorders with overlapping presentations.

General Symptoms

Most symptoms encountered in ACML at presentation are the direct result of either mechanical changes induced by massive proliferation of the malignant cells or of the resultant hypermetabolic state. Hypermetabolism secondary to the malignant cell bulk can lead to weight loss, fever, fatigue, malaise, and diaphoresis. Such symptoms generally are less pronounced in the early chronic phase of ACML and may worsen as the disease progresses. This probably is due to increased turnover of more metabolically active cells.

Most other signs and symptoms can be attributed to massive cell volume. Extramedullary hematopoietic nodules (pseudochloromas) sometimes are found in organs, lymph nodes, or subcutaneous tissues (8). Bone pain and tenderness can be directly attributed to expansion of the bony medullary cavities and to periosteal and periarticular disease infiltration. Pain occasionally can become unbearable and prevent walking. Symptoms of this severity might invite a preliminary diagnosis of an arthropathy. Sometimes, sequestration of red cells or platelets due to *hypersplenism* becomes a significant complicating problem, as can the pain of splenic infarction. Occasionally, splenic pain from leukemic infiltration or cell sequestration can become so severe as to require urgent treatment. *Priapism* has been estimated to occur in 1–2% of adult men, especially in those with high blood leukocyte counts (6). It results from mechanical obstruction caused by leukemic cells with potential thrombosis of the corpora cavernosa, although it also may be caused by abdominal vein or nerve impingement. It is not the most common manifestation of hyperleukocytosis-induced leukostasis, Rowe and Lichtman (7) reviewed adult and pediatric leukostasis in ACML and reported signs and symptoms of leukostasis in 12% of adults and 60% children. Somewhat lower incidences have been found in children by others (2). Although priapism occurs in children as well as adults, the central nervous system, the retina, and the respiratory system are most frequently affected. Pulmonary leukostasis at all ages is usually manifested by tachypnea, dyspnea, and hypoxia but only rarely is severe enough to require emergency treatment.

The same authors also found a significant correlation between the incidence of leukostasis and high WBC as well as the percentage of blood granulocyte precursos. They noted an increased incidence of leukostasis in children compared to adults; children aso had higher counts at presentation than adults. There was a significant increased incidence of leukostasis in pediatric patients with white counts greater than $300 \times 10^9/L$; the average presenting white count was $294 \times 10^9/L$ in their 61 reported childhood cases. Finally, they noted an inverse correlation between height of the white count and the hemoglobin level. CNS leukostasis in their and other reported series almost invariably has been associated with a normal spinal fluid analysis.

The pathogenesis of this problem has been attributed to impaired blood flow in the microcriculation and possibly to the invasion of blood vessel walls (7, 27). Rowe and Lichtman's experience suggested that a leukocrit higher than 10% was required to make blood significantly more viscous than an equivalent volume of suspended red cells (7). Roath and Davenport (28) have reported that ACML leukocytes in whole blood demonstrate markedly increased viscosity at WBC levels corresponding to those found in AML patients, and Hild and Myers (29) found a direct correlation between the cytocrit (hematocrit plus leukocrit) and increased whole blood viscosity.

At present, it is uncertain if thrombocytosis complicates the leukostatic picture in ACML. Platelet counts in children also seem to average slightly higher than those in adults, with respective mean counts above 500×10^9/L and less than 450×10^9/L (2, 7). Only at very high platelet counts ($>1000 \times 10^9$/L) have increased thrombohemorrhagic complications been reported (30). Platelet function abnormalities are common in ACML, but the overall incidence of hemorrhage and thrombosis is low (30).

Hemorrhage, such as may be seen in the retina, may be caused by weakening of blood vessel walls secondary to leukocyte infiltration, changes in circulation or tissue oxygenation secondary to vaso-occlusion, or platelet abnormalities. However, it should be stressed that symptoms of hemorrhage are less prominent early in the course of ACML than they are in JCML.

Differential Diagnosis

The usual confusion in children is with JCML (see Table 26.2) or the Monosomy 7 syndrome (1). Contrary to ACML, these entities usually are associated with thrombocytopenia and significant anemia and seldom manifest extremely high white counts. Both are discussed later in this chapter and elsewhere.

Any cause of a **leukemoid reaction** or leukoerythroblastosis (31), including severe infection, metastatic cancer, congenital heart disease, or acute inflammatory states (such as Still's disease), might produce as high a white blood count, Particularly in young children, certain viral infections can elevate the WBC spectacularly. However, the peripheral blood leukocytes of a leukemoid reaction rarely contain blasts or promyelocytes nor does the white cell count attain levels reached in ACML, except in association with disseminated tuberculosis. Generally, a leukemoid reaction is accompanied by signs of an infection or an inflammatory state, and LAP scores are usually normal or elevated. Transient leukemoid reactions or myeloproliferative episodes are also common in Down's syndrome. Leukoerthyroblastosis must be considered, particularly if immature myeloid and erythroid elements are present (31).

Chronic neutrophilic leukemia (32) is much like a leukemoid reaction, with mostly mature neutrophils, no increase in basophils or eosinophils, only mild splenomegaly, and marrow myeloid hyperplasia. Organs are only moderately infiltrated with predominantly mature granulocytes. There are no cytogenetic abnormalities. This diagnosis is made by exclusion of causes of a leukemoid reaction and usually requires no treatment.

Chronic myelomonocytic leukemia (CMMoL), discussed later in this chapter and in Chapter 33 (MDS), is now classified as a myelodysplastic disorder. It lacks the Ph chromosome and is more easily confused with JCML than ACML.

In older adults, **myelofibrosis** may enter the differential diagnosis, especially if it is discovered when advanced. The gross splenomegaly and high WBC may mimic the findings of ACML, but anemia and thrombocytopenia are the rule. Similarly, some cases of **essential thrombocythemia** (33) or late stages of **polycythemia vera** might initially be considered in the differential.

Identification of the Philadelphia chromosome in the peripheral blood or bone marrow will discriminate between ACML and any of these conditions, but cases of Ph-negative ACML may need careful assessment.

Ph-Negative CML does not seem to be any different in the clinical and hematologic presentation, course, or response to treatment for Ph−, Bcr-abl+ ACML as compared to Ph+ ACML (22–25, 34). Although the mechanism for the juxtaposition of *abl* or *bcr* in these patients is unknown (22–26), essentially the same pathophysiology, clinical picture, and response to therapy results (34). *Internal rearrangements of the bcr gene also have been found in many* Ph−/bcr/abl− *patients presenting with the characteristic picture of ACML* (22–26). The 5–7% of CML patients who do not have either the standard 9:22 translocation, other rearrangements affecting the q34 and q11 regions of the 9 and 22 chromosomes, the *bcr-abl* oncogene, or internal rearrangements of bcr (23, 24, 26) may also share the clinical and hematologic features of ACML. However, such patients tend to be older, anemia is more prominent, and white blood counts are lower at presentation with elevated monocyte counts, low basophil counts, and dysgranulopoiesis (26, 35, 243). The course also differs from that of Ph+ CML; it is characterized by increasing organomegaly and leukocytosis, extramedullary infiltrates, and eventually bone marrow failure (35). Although blast transformation is less common (25–50%) (34), the prognosis is somewhat worse than in ACML, with rapid progression and shortened survival (23, 34, 35).

In the two cases presented here, and in Chapter 15, the diagnosis was confirmed by the typical karyotype as Ph+ CML (ACML).

Unusual Presentations

At least 10 cases of acquired **pure red cell aplasia** associated with ACML have been reported in adults (36). Such patients will present with the usual leukocytosis and a differential spanning the myeloid series, with platelet counts either normal or elevated, organomegaly, and either Philadelphia chromosome positivity or Ph-*bcr-abl* positivity. This is generally an acquired phenomenon in adults, with an autoimmune basis, but its relationship to ACML is uncertain. However, as the anemia does not always respond to erythropoietin, it is tempting to speculate that it is connected to the stem cell defect in ACML, which may include the erythroid cell compartment (37). Other unusual presentations of ACML have included **acne urticata** (38), isolated **optic nerve involvement** (39), isolated **thrombocytosis** (resembling essential thrombocythemia) (33), and isolated **eosinophilia** or **basophilia.**

Epidemiology

Most evidence suggests that ACML is caused by an acquired postzygotic leukemogenic change or changes in the stem cell, with subsequent gradual replacement of the stem cell compartment by the leukemic cells (15, 40). ACML shows no familial or hereditary pattern and lacks remarkable racial or sexual predilection. However, there have been rare reports of ACML occurring in identical twins (15, 41, 42). Consequently, researchers have sought both external and occult genetic factors, which could induce the malignant change. Although most patients have no evidence of an environmental factor that might be implicated, exposure to large doses of ionizing radiation seems to be the best known candidate at present.

Exposure to high-dose ionizing radiation has been studied extensively in survivors from Hiroshima and Nagasaki. The incidence of ACML occurring in the survivors was found to be markedly increased (43, 44). The intensity and duration of exposure seemed critical, correlating positively with earlier onset of ACML postexposure (43, 44) and with increased incidence at a younger age and favoring males (43–45). Holmberg has determined that the probability of a radiation-induced t(9;22) reciprocal translocation in exposed survivors at Hiroshima and Nagasaki is consistent with the observed incidence of affected individuals and thus could represent the primary leukemogenic event (46).

Although ACML has been reported in infants (47), to date there has been no association with intrauterine exposure to radiation at doses permissive of subsequent gestation (48). However, Holm et al (49) reported a significant increase in the incidence of ACML developing in a group of 35,000 patients who had received diagnostic doses of radioactive iodine. Also, there are many reports of ACML as a second malignancy, most recently described after I[131] therapy for thyroid cancer (50) and after extended-field radiation therapy for Hodgkin's disease (51).

The role of drugs and chemicals in the pathogenesis of ACML is uncertain. Older surveys of benzene-induced leukemia include occasional cases of ACML. A review by Aksoy (52) mentions several reports, but his own survey has none. Recent data on drug-associated leukemia (see Chapter 27) is focused on acute leukemia and MDS to the virtual complete exclusion of ACML.

It is interesting, in light of the above, that there is evidence that both maternal and paternal chromosomes are involved in the reciprocal T9,22 translocation. Recently, evaluation of 15 patients by Haas et al (53) demonstrated that the translocated chromosome 9 was of paternal origin and the translocated 22 was exclusively maternal, suggesting that an imprinting phenomenon may play a significant role in the acquired chromosomal rearrangement in ACML. It is reasonable to believe that there may be other molecular events occurring in association with predisposing genetic or environmental factors that have yet to be discovered (see Chapter 15).

Cellular Function

The malignant myeloid precursors in ACML leave the bone marrow microenvironment prematurely, and there is evidence that this may be due to defective adhesion to components of the stroma. This seems to be due largely to loss of expression in ACML cells of the anchoring molecule phosphatidyl inositol glycan (PIG) (54). Additionally, and unlike normal progenitors, 20–30% of ACML cells acquire adhesion receptors for laminin and collagens, perhaps explaining their ability to adhere to and penetrate subendothelial basement membranes in the bone marrow or in peripheral blood vessels (55). Defects in membrane sialylation also have been reported (56), which could contribute to defective adhesion. ACML granulocytes demonstrate other biochemical and functional defects, interfering with their chemotaxis (57) and ability to phagocytize and kill bacteria normally. Perhaps most significant is a defect in internalization of aggregated IGG, probably due to aberrations in phosphorylation of proteins (58).

These defects can only be partial, because ACML cells have been used successfully in the past to provide support for neutropenic patients or patients suffering from granulocyte dysfunction syndromes. They seem to have little significance in terms of presentation of the disease or its course; however, there is some continued loss of neutrophil function as the disease progresses, often despite normalizing of the LAP score and perhaps contributing to disease morbidity during acceleration.

The decrease in LAP activity consistently found in ACML patients has been attributed to the increase in circulating early myeloid forms in the chronic phase (59). This enzyme is a marker of terminally differentiated myelocytes (60). However, LAP is stimulated by G-CSF (60, 61), a monocyte-derived growth factor, suggesting that perhaps a relative decrease in monocyte mass, rather than defect in the LAP gene, might be the cause of LAP underproduction (61, 62). Lending support to the possible role of some extrinsic factor on LAP production is the finding that LAP activity may rise when ACML leukocytes are transfused into neutropenic hosts (although this may be simple selection for survival of LAP positive cells) (63, 64). The role of LAP in granulocyte function is unknown. There also is no known relevance of the increase in B12 and transcobalamin-I seen in CML. The increase in transcobalamin appears secondary to increased plasma concentration of the protein haptocorrin, which binds cobalamin. Normal granulocytes contain and release haptocorrin, and ACML cells make and release an increased amount of a specific haptocorrin (65). As increased transcobalamin is responsible for most of the increased binding of B12, and is in turn derived primarily from the markedly increased granulocyte pool, it is not surprising that B12 and transcobalamin levels rise and fall as the malignant white cell population fluctuates during treatment. Monitoring of LAP and B12/transcobalamin levels can be of value in assessing disease activity and response to treatment.

Pathogenesis

Chapter 15 has addressed the genetics of ACML, including the discovery of the Philadelphia chromosome and the translocated C-abl oncogene forming bcr-abl. This chromosomal marker is found in myeloid, megakaryocytic, erythroid, monocytic/macrophage, and B and T lymphocytic cell lineages (37, 66, 67), but not in fibroblasts (68) or other somatic tissues, supporting the contention that ACML originates from neoplastic transformation of a very early hematopoietic stem cell. Those tissues/cells showing the Ph chromosome always demonstrate just a single isoform of the G-6-PD enzyme, whereas those that do not will demonstrate both isoforms in women with ACML heterozygous for G-6-PD (69). Other evidence supports the clonal nature of ACML.

Does the Philadelphia chromosome and the bcr-abl molecular abnormality have functional significance in the pathology of ACML? A break or rearrangement of the 9q34 band at the site of c-abl has been proposed as the critical initiating step in the molecular events central to the pathogenesis of ACML (70). Bcr-abl messenger RNA was discovered in the mid-1980s. Subsequently, its product, a large protein named P210, was identified (by Western blotting) with a high level of tyrosine kinase activity. A major step in confirming a causal linkage between the Philadelphia chromosome, the synthesis of the p210 bcr/abl protein, and the initiation and progression of ACML was taken when bcr-abl cDNA was inserted into murine marrow cells infected with retroviruses, which when given to lethally irradiated mice, were found to induce a myeloproliferative syndrome consistent with the chronic phase of CML as well as the expression of P210 in the bone marrow of an adult animals (34, 71). This is not to say that bcr-abl gene products are solely responsible for oncogenesis, and additional events likely are necessary for ACML transformation into blast crisis. In fact, studies of G-6-PD heterozygotes with ACML have shown that some cells in their affected cell lines do not express the Ph chromosome, suggesting that abnormal proliferation of a clone might precede acquisition of the Ph chromosome (69, 72). Also, there are cases of the clinical and hematologic findings of ACML preceding the appearance of the Ph+ chromosome, and in other cases, persistence of those features during therapy despite disappearance of the Ph+ chromosome (73). Individuals "cured" of CML may also show persistent molecular abnormalities at the gene level. When this information is coupled with data presented earlier concerning the potential of ionizing radiation and

possibly other environmental factors to cause this postzygotic genetic event, the case is advanced for a multistep oncogenic process in the development of this clonal malignancy (72).

Growth Advantage of CML Clone

Why is it that ACML cells will expand to predominate in marrow, blood, and extramedullary sites? Studies of cell production in vitro and proliferative kinetics have suggested that the growth advantage results not from an increased *rate* of malignant cell proliferation but from *expansion of the pool* of committed granulocyte stem cells due to loss of sensitivity to regulatory molecules, changes in cellular adhesive interactions that might promote dissemination of cells, dysregulation of cytokine production, and possibly the production of substances that are inhibitory to normal hematopoietic stem cells.

Malignant precursor cells in children and adults with ACML do not divide more rapidly than normal precursors (74). Indeed, there is evidence that they divide more slowly (73). Derived CFU-GM and erythroid colonies require CSF and erythropoietin activity for growth (34), and colony formation appears normal in vitro. However, in ACML chronic phase, there is a marked expansion of the committed precursor pool, particularly CFU-GM. Marrow

Table 26.1 Clinical Differences Between JCML and ACML at Diagnosis

	JCML	ACML
Physical findings:		
Age (years)	usually <4	usually >4
Rash	present (usually facial)	absent
Hemorrhage	common	rare
Suppurative lymphadenopathy	common	rare
Infection (bacterial)	common	unusual
Hematologic findings:		
WBC >100 × 10⁹/L	<20%	>80%
Monocytosis in peripheral blood and bone marrow	prominent	rare
Platelets <100 × 10⁹/L	>70%	rare
NRBC	common	rare
Fetal hemoglobin	markedly increased	normal
Hb <120 g/L in absence of bleeding	>90%	<20%
Elevated immunoglobulins, autoantibodies	usual	rare
Cytogenetic findings	Ph chromosome negative	Ph chromosome positive
bcr/abl probe	negative	positive
Peripheral blood colony, growth assays	monocytic	granulocytic

suspensions from ACML patients in chronic phase produce several-fold the number of GM colonies produced by normal marrow, and ACML peripheral blood is even more productive of CFU relative to normal blood. These findings are at least partially attributable to changes in the signaling pathways for proliferative and maturational regulation of myeloid precursors. Implicated stimulatory cytokines include IL-1 and G-CSF, perhaps augmented by autocrine production by ACML cells (75). The altered tyrosine kinase activity of p210 *bcr/abl* has been implicated in this dysregulation (69), which among other things, results in one or more **additional cell divisions** during maturation (76) and a longer life for the progeny (69, 77). K562 cells expressing the *bcr/abl* fusion protein are resistant in vitro to the induction of apoptosis by various agents and conditions (77).

There are also abnormalities in feedback regulation of ACML myelopoiesis. At least three negative feedbacks ordinarily regulate myelopoiesis: *lactoferrin* (LF) is produced by mature leukocytes and acts to suppress granulopoiesis by decreasing monocyte/macrophage production of GM-CSF (78). *Prostaglandin E* (PG-E) and *acidic isoferritins* (AIF) are produced by monocytes and macrophages and seen to act on HLA-DR antigens on CFU-GM to inhibit growth under normal conditions. ACML granulocytes seem to have deficient LF production, and there is poor responsiveness of clonal monocytes and macrophages to LF. There also is decreased sensitivity of progenitor cells to PG-E and AIF. This suggests a fundamental defect in autocrine feedback mechanisms. Finally, ACML cells may release other factors suppressive to normal granulopoiesis but to which they are resistant (79). As yet, the contribution of these humoral inhibitory substances to disease pathogenesis is unclear, but at least some homeostatic control is retained, as witnessed by the persistence of cyclic oscillations in the blood leukocyte counts despite chemotherapy or interferon given at a constant dosage (41, 80).

The net result of these changes is massive overexpansion in the total granulocyte pool (81, 82), and an average ACML leukocyte half-life in the blood of up to 10 times that in normal persons (41, 73). Alterations in leukocyte adhesion molecules promote the early release of immature ACML cells from the marrow and their dissemination to extramedullary sites where they can continue to divide. As the chronic phase progresses, the increasingly immature cell population would have progressively more proliferative potential in these extramedullary locations, explaining the increasingly symptomatic course in accelerating ACML.

Management

Pretreatment Considerations

Table 26.2 details recommended studies to be accomplished before initiation of therapy for ACML. If the patient meets established criteria, HLA typing for alloBMT should be performed. This can also be done after initial cytoreduction. Fertility may be affected by some

Table 26.2 Pretreatment ACML and JCML Evaluations

Complete CBC and differential
Bone marrow aspirate *and* biopsy—for cytogenetics, in vitro colony assays, characterizations of cellular content, presence of fibrosis, cytochemical studies, and for flow cytometry
Peripheral blood karyotype and bone marrow karyotype—if possible with bcr-abl probes
Hemoglobin electrophoresis with *quantitative* A_2 and fetal hemoglobin
Blood leukocyte alkaline phosphatase determination
Serum B_{12}, muramidase (lysozyme)
Serum quantitative immunoelectrophoresis (consider serologies for autoantibodies)
Peripheral blood and bone marrow flow cytometry for cellular immunophenotyping
Peripheral or bone marrow blood in vitro clonogenic assays for CFC, with and without growth factor stimulation
Additionally consider:
Quantitative splenic sonography for volume, skin biopsy for histo-immunophenotyping
Peripheral blood RBC studies for I antigen, enzymes, and glycine/alanine ratio
HLA typing
Storage of semen

treatments, including busulfan and hydroxyurea, and αIFN and they may all be teratogenic. Cryopreservation of semen should be considered before initiation of specific therapy. The risks of teratogenesis and infertility should be discussed, and recommendations should be made for contraception if indicated.

Therapy for the Chronic Phase

After evaluation, the initial treatment goal for all cases of ACML, except those discovered incidentally, is to provide *symptomatic relief by debulking* the disease. Initial management problems mainly relate to side effects from cytoreductive therapy and to tissue/organ infiltration.

Hyperleukocytosis. Patients presenting with extremely high white counts may manifest signs and symptoms of leukostasis, particularly involving the brain, spleen, penis, lung, and retina (5, 7, 27). Consideration should be given to rapid cytoreduction in such patients by leukopheresis or exchange transfusion at the same time as cytotoxic chemotherapy is initiated (27, 83). *RBC transfusions, which increase blood viscosity, should be avoided during this period.* Initiation of high-dose single agent therapy, such as with hydroxyurea at 50–75 mg/kg/day i.v. (5, 83), is appropriate. However, there is the potential for cytotoxic drugs to precipitate symptoms of hyperviscosity due to loss of deformability of drug-injured ACML cells or from release of procoagulants (27). Use of interferons does not pose the same risk, but cytoreduction is more protracted with their use.

Central Nervous System (CNS) Symptoms. Secondary to leukostasis do not require directed therapy to the CNS, as they are responsive to leukopheresis and/or chemotherapy (7). Meningeal leukemia is virtually unknown in the chronic phase of ACML. Splenic infiltration, sequestration, or infarction can lead to massive and painful splenitis, sometimes necessitating emergency splenectomy or splenic irradiation. Priapism also can be persistent and painful: immediate intervention should include rest, analgesia, hydration, and local therapy such as ice packs or blood aspiration of the corpora cavernosa with simultaneous consideration for leukopheresis, irradiation, or high-dose single-agent therapy (6). Despite these measures, permanent penile flaccidity and impotence may result (6). Respiratory symptoms generally respond promptly to cytoreductive therapy (27).

Thrombocytosis. This rarely requires specific treatment because the infrequency of thrombotic or hemorrhagic complications (30). Generally, thrombocytosis responds to the treatment regimens used for leukocytosis, including αIFN (34). In refractory patients, anagrelide (84) has been effective; as a last resort, thiotepa (which is rapid acting) may be tried (34).

Metabolic. Cytolysis may lead to hyperuricemia, hyperkalemia, and hyperphosphatemia with hypocalcemia (27). These should be treated **prophylactically** with hydration, alkalinization of the blood and urine, and allopurinol. ACML in chronic phase tends to undergo massive and rapid cytolysis in response to chemotherapy, particularly hydroxyurea (85), but relatively few instances of severe metabolic disturbances have been documented.

Leukopheresis. Leukophresis is the preferred emergency treatment by some (27) and will give excellent temporary relief of symptoms while awaiting the effect of cytoreductive drugs. However, it does nothing to ameliorate the course of the disease (86).

Splenic Irradiation. Splenic irradiation will not only reduce splenomegaly but often lowers the peripheral white count, as well as decreasing the number of immature cells and even the mitotic index at sites distant from the spleen such as the bone marrow. This has been purported to result from interference with the release of cytokines from the splenic parenchyma into the circulation (87) or from the release of an inhibitor into the plasma (88). Before the availability of busulfan, this was the treatment of choice for chronic-phase CML. However, disease control was generally no longer than 6 months with no improvement in survival. Controlled trials comparing intermittent splenic irradiation with busulfan have demonstrated decreased control of leukocyte counts and worse survival for the irradiated patients (89, 90); thus, splenic irradiation should be considered only for relief of symptoms.

Splenectomy. Emergency splenectomy is occasionally warranted for pain relief, for hypersplenism, or to reduce the tumor burden pre-BMT. Despite reports of splenic origin of blast crises (91), several large, controlled trials have failed to demonstrate any benefit from splenectomy in prolonging chronic phase or survival (92). Thus, splenectomy should be considered only as "last stop" management for control of symptoms or for persistent splenomegaly despite optimal therapy, especially if associated with hypersplenism. There also seems to be no survival advantage conferred by splenectomy performed before or concomitant with alloBMT (92–94). Despite evidence of earlier hematopoietic recovery, splenectomy is associated with increased risk of GVHD. Additional morbidity from splenic irradiation or splenectomy includes the risk of overwhelming postsplenectomy sepsis and perhaps facilitation of extreme thrombocytosis.

Cytoreduction. Single-agent chemotherapy has been the standard for hematologic and clinical remission and symptomatic relief by lowering the white count and reducing the size of the liver and spleen. Single chemotherapeutic agents such as hydroxyurea will rarely achieve molecular remission, and it is rare for the bone marrow morphology or karyotype to normalize when the blood and organ involvement disappears. However, such treatment maximizes comfortable survival and allows arrangements to be made for more definitive and potentially curative therapy.

Hydroxyurea. Specific for the S phase of the cell cycle, hydroxyurea inhibits ribonucleoside diphosphate reductase. Control of the white count with hydroxyurea is somewhat less predictable than with busulfan, because it is short acting, so it is usually given daily at a starting dose of 10–20 mg/kg/day orally (83). However, it is easy to adjust the dose to the hematologic response and it seems effective in controlling and prolonging chronic phase CML (95, 96). Hydroxyurea has few side effects and lacks significant long-term consequences that might preclude subsequent BMT. It should be considered the starting agent of choice and is well suited to urgent cytoreduction, especially when given in doses up to 75 mg/kg/day.

Busulfan. Busulfan is an alkylating agent with a more protracted onset and prolonged duration of action; there will often be a lag of up to 2 weeks before the white count falls significantly after initiation of therapy. Splenomegaly disappears even more slowly, and clinical remission usually occurs within 4–6 weeks. The usual starting dose is 0.06 to 0.1 mg/kg/day p.o. (adult dose, 4 mg/day). The drug should be discontinued when the white cell count falls below 20×10^9/L as it will continue to fall for several weeks after the last dose. Overdose can result in severe and potentially irreversible marrow aplasia. Responsive patients may be maintained on a lower dose and intermittent therapy, as dictated by the white cell count (97). Because of the greater legacy effect from busulfan, the potential for other severe side effects, such as pulmonary or bone marrow fibrosis, and lack of survival advantage over hydroxyurea (97, 98), the latter is generally the preferred agent.

Multi-Agent Chemotherapy. Because single-agent therapy with busulfan and hydroxyurea rarely has resulted in prolonged reversion to marrow Ph-negative status in ACML (99, 100), there have been attempts to incorporate these drugs into multiple-drug regimens or to follow single-drug cytoreduction with multi-agent chemotherapy. Although cytogenetic remission has been achieved with such regimens, it almost invariably is of short duration and does not appear to lengthen the overall duration of the chronic phase or disease-free survival.

Intensive Therapy. Some reported successes, especially with busulfan, in inducing prolonged reversion to a Ph-negative status (99, 100) led to other attempts to use intensive multi-agent chemotherapy with or without splenectomy in chronic phase to ablate the Ph+ clone. Studies before 1985 have been reviewed by Clarkson (101). Although intensive combination chemotherapy regimens used to treat CML have achieved significant cytoreduction and even eliminated the Ph+ clone, none of these regimens have had much success in producing either a permanent disease-free survival state or a significantly improved survival.

A Change in Goals: Curative Treatment

Concomitant with the development of ACML treatment employing bone marrow transplantation and biologic response modifiers was a change in the treatment goals (34). Earlier therapy had been based on the belief that acquisition of the Ph chromosome was, in fact, a late phenomenon and that Ph-negative cells found in blood or marrow at any point in evaluation during or after treatment were still part of the clonal malignant process. Thus, in the early 1980s, there was no recognized therapeutic advantage in simply suppressing Ph+ cells. Several subsequent lines of investigation led to the realization that a normal stem cell pool would persist, even in the presence of massive proliferation of Ph+ cells, and that treatment strategies should try to take advantage of these residual normal stem cells and selectively target the Ph+ cells. Molecular evidence for this residual normal stem cell pool included findings of heterozygosity of certain markers of clonality and, more recently, evaluation for the hybrid bcr-abl mRNA in various subsets of ACML marrow precursors showing the persistence of normal clones (37, 72, 102, 103).

Implicit in this philosophy was the recognition that there was a direct relationship between the molecular events involving the Philadelphia chromosome and the onset and progression of the ACML. Recent work has suggested that there may be an early and a late myeloproliferative disorder induced in the murine CML model (discussed earlier) from bone marrow cells expressing P210 bcr-abl, with late onset murine CML undergoing a typical myeloid or lymphoid blast crisis and the early onset disease having a more gradual progression mimicking in the chronic phase of CML (104). Other researchers have demonstrated that normal, nonclonal Ph-negative cells would return in the human host with ACML after elimination of the disease (102). Thus, the cytogenetic events were necessary before any subsequent events that would lead to the natural progression of ACML through a biphasic or triphasic course. Accordingly, the goal of new therapies for ACML has been not only to eliminate the hematologic and bone marrow findings in ACML but also the cell clone with the Philadelphia chromosome or its molecular marker, bcr-abl. This is now considered synonymous with true remission of the disease (34). The use of cytokines (for which interferons are a paradigm), bone marrow transplantation, and other forms of cell manipulation is directed toward this goal.

Interferons

Those studied for therapeutic efficacy in ACML include alpha, beta, gamma, delta, and consensus interferon. Alpha interferon, by far, has been the most studied.

Alpha-Interferon

Many investigators have reported remarkable success in ACML disease control and cytoreduction with partially pure human leukocyte or recombinant alpha interferon (αIFN) as single-agent therapy (80, 105, 106) (recently reviewed by Kantarjian et al (34)). These studies report complete hematologic remissions (CHR) in 70–80%, and cytogenetic response in up to 60% of patients treated during chronic phase, with less than 35% Ph+ metaphases in as many as 40% of the cases and complete cytogenetic response (CCR) in 26% (34). To date, results seem to be similar in children (80, 107) and adults (34).

How does αIFN work? In vitro studies have suggested that αIFN selectively suppresses the proliferation of the malignant hematopoietic cells (108), although most were performed using extremely high IFN concentration (109). It has been demonstrated that αIFN will produce dose-dependent increase in adhesion of ACML cells in longterm culture, which can be inhibited by antibodies against integrins and other adhesion molecules. Thus, the mechanism might be one of reversing the pathologic adhesive changes previously discussed as possibly contributing to ACML cell growth advantage (110). There also may be an indirect affect on immune surveillance, particularly through NK or LAK cells (111). An earlier hypothesis that interferons induced 2'5' oligoadenylate synthetase (OAS) has been somewhat refuted by evidence that OAS titers do not seem to relate to clinical outcome with, or resistance to, IFN therapy. The dysregulation of cytokine production in ACML, including enhanced autocrine-production of IL-1, G-CSF, TNFα, and possibly IL-8, is also a likely target of αIFN therapy (75). There may be a dose-response relationship between αIFN and the suppression of Ph+ ACML clones, which is not yet fully explored.

Alpha IFN is usually given intramuscularly or subcutaneously, and a variety of different dosages have been employed successfully, ranging from 5 to 9 megaunits (Mμ) daily (105, 106) to three times per week in adults, to 30 Mμ/m²/day in children (80). Children seem to tolerate higher doses of interferon, but there is no proven dose-related efficacy in that age group as yet.

Interferon therapy is invariably associated with the onset of flu-like symptoms, including fever and chills, arthralgias and myalgias, malaise, and anorexia, or more intense gastrointestinal symptoms. Some of these constitutional symptoms might be exaggerated by the side effects of cytoreduction. Symptomatic relief can be obtained by administrating IFN at bedtime, pre-IFN acetaminophen (or other antipyretic/anti-inflammatory drug) dosing, and by starting IFN therapy at more tolerable doses, However, tachyphylaxis to "flu syndrome" invariably develops within a few weeks. *Later* and potentially dose-limiting side effects include persistent fatigue, depression, and other neurologic dysfunction, immune-mediated complications such as hemolytic anemia or thrombocytopenia, collagen-vascular diseases, and autoimmune nephritis and thyroid dysfunction (112). Life-threatening cardiac dysfunction also can occur. In general, most side effects can be controlled by dosage adjustment and do not require stopping therapy. In fact, withholding IFN therapy for more than a few days may exacerbate the flu-like symptoms (112, 113). Small doses of antidepressants at bedtime may help alleviate some of the more nonspecific symptoms (34). With proper dosage adjustment, αIFN can be used safely for long periods of time. In general, the younger the patient, the better tolerated the drug.

Response to αIFN is often sluggish, with median time to CHR in most studies of at least 6 weeks (80, 105, 106, 114). It is often associated with disconcerting oscillations in the white count, reminiscent of those seen during the natural course of ACML (82, 105, 106). Cytogenetic response is maximal by 20–24 months in most adults and children (34, 80 107). The effect of αIFN is apparently most effective in least bulky disease. This has led to attempts to combine αIFN with either debulking chemotherapeutic agent regimens (including hydroxyurea) or more chronically with intermittent or concomitant chemotherapeutic agents.

Longterm follow-up of AMCL patients (34) has revealed that most of those obtaining complete cytogenetic remission (CCR) will remain in CCR, even after discontinuation of interferon. Some have found that CCR is associated with improved survival (115–117), and response/survival with αIFN as compared to treatment with hydroxyurea is being studied prospectively (118). However, it has been estimated that 40% of ACML patients would have to attain CCR to produce even a 25% improvement in prognosis for this disease. Thus far, the experience with αIFN regimens suggests a median survival of 60–65 months, and 5-year survival of approximately 30% (34), clearly superior to that achieved with conventional chemotherapy. If subsequent results validate the positive impact on survival of αIFN, it may be advisable to recommend continuance of interferon therapy for all patients with ACML regardless of cytogenetic response to achieve the best survival benefit (34). Currently, only patients achieving a major or complete cytogenetic response should continue αIFN therapy—on the assumption that this is a group self selected on the basis of favorable response.

In αIFN-treated patients studied for complete or major cytogenetic remission, it has been shown by clonality analysis that granulocytes produced during the CCR are nonclonal (119). Clonogenic assays have not proven useful for pretesting for IFN sensitivity, but in vitro colony growth can reflect therapeutic efficacy if monitored over time (120). A method of preselecting patients likely to respond to IFN would be a therapeutic boon.

Other Interferons

Thus far, studies of other interferons in ACML have shown only moderate effectiveness, with a CHR of 20–30%. Interferon beta has been relatively ineffective; delta interferon and consensus interferon are still being studied. Combinations αIFN and γIFN have not proven any more effective than αIFN alone.

αIFN Combined with Other Agents

Combinations of αIFN with hydroxyurea, busulfan, intensive chemotherapy, and low-dose Ara-C have been explored. Most of these studies have been disappointing. The combination of low-dose Ara-C and αIFN administered in late chronic–phase ACML in at least one study has produced higher CHR rates (55%) as compared to those with αIFN alone (28%), as well as improvement in cytogenetic response rate and longer survival (121) Gilhot et al (122) also demonstrated a less striking but similarly positive effect on cytogenetic response when αIFN/hydroxyurea given for cytoreduction was followed by IFN/Ara C (45%) versus IFN alone (33%). Although results are mixed to date, this is an active area of investigation.

Bone Marrow Transplantation in Chronic Phase

Allogeneic BMT

Of all therapies for ACML, the best and longest disease-free survival rates have been achieved with alloBMT. At present, a matched or one-antigen-mismatched *related alloBMT* is most likely to provide cure in chronic-phase ACML. Younger patients do best. Data also suggest that alloBMT performed *early* has a better result than in late chronic phase (34, 123–125). The International BMT Registry (IBMTR) suggested a 5–10% difference in survival rates between those performed earlier versus later in

Table 26.3 Criteria Established by the International Bone Marrow Transplant Registry for Classifying the Phases of ACML

Chronic Phase
No significant symptoms (*after treatment*)
None of the features of accelerated phase or blastic phase
Accelerated Phase
WBC count difficult to control with conventional use of busulfan or hydroxyurea in terms of doses required or shortening of intervals between courses
Rapid doubling of WBC count (<5 days)
≥10% blasts in blood or urine
≥20% blasts plus promyelocytes in blood or marrow
≥20% basophils plus eosinophils in blood
Anemia or thrombocytopenia unresponsive to busulfan or hydroxyurea
Persistent thrombocytosis
Additional chromosome changes (evoling new clone)
Increasing splenomegaly
Development of chloromas or myelofibrosis
Blastic Phase
≥30% blasts plus promyleocytes in the blood or bone marrow

(Data from International Bone Marrow Transplant Registry, with permission.)

chronic phase (126). However, this seems to be secondary to an increased process-related mortality rate rather than due to leukemic relapse, suggesting that host factors such as organ toxicities from previous therapy, as well as recipient age, are at least partially resposible. It has been reported (123) that the duration of chronic phase and previous exposure to busulfan were independent prognostic factors for patient outcome. Criteria used by the IBMTR for classifying the phases of ACML are presented in Table 26.3. The European BMT Registry has discounted the importance of pre-BMT splenectomy, splenic irradiation, or prior interferon exposure on outcome (127, 128). Perhaps more significant is whether a T-cell-depleted or nondepleted alloBMT is performed. The decreased incidence of GVHD associated with T-cell-depleted BMTs has to be balanced against a higher incidence of leukemia relapse and of graft failure (126, 129).

AlloBMT performed in chronic phase was originally shown to produce a 40–64% disease-free survival (134, 124) compared to 25% or less when done after the disease

accelerates. Matched sibling alloBMT in chronic phase on patients younger than 20 years of age yields up to a 70% DFS (130). However, a 5-year disease-free survival rate of only 38% was found on review of long-term follow-up data from both the international and national registries, and a rather disconcerting tendency toward a pattern of late relapses was noted (127). Inclusion of T-cell-depleted BMT may have adversely affected survival in these patient cohorts. A variety of pre-BMT conditioning regimens seem to beeffective, allowing flexibility of choice in accommodat-ing such factors as organ toxicities from previous therapies (131).

AlloBMT using matched *unrelated donors* (MUD) predictably is associated with a higher incidence of graft failure and increased GVHD, both acute and chronic, but has yielded 2-year disease-free survival rates of over 35% when done in chronic phase (125), with better rates attained in younger and better matched patients. In children recently transplanted by the Minnesota Group, non-T-cell-depleted MUD AlloBMT yielded a 3-year DFS of 45%,

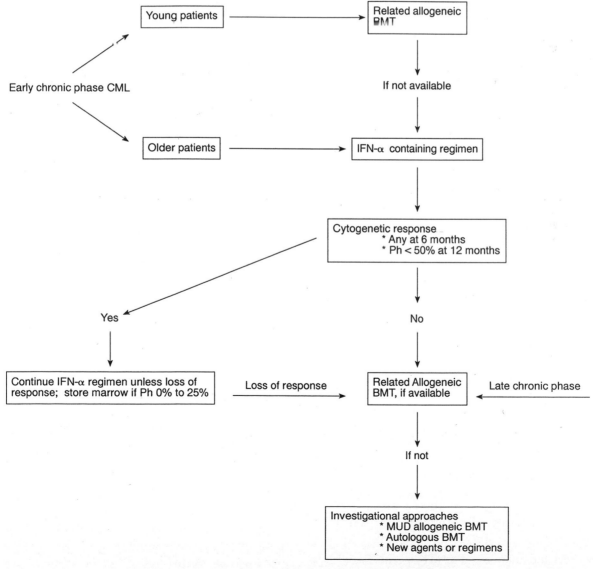

Figure 26.1. Proposed treatment approach for patients with ACML.

versus 78% for matched sibling donor BMTs (132). Thus, current data suggest that a MUD transplant would be indicated for patients either in late chronic phase or having other risk factors such as evidence of transformation.

Based on these findings and others, Kantarjian et al (34) have proposed an algorithm for therapeutic decision making for newly diagnosed patients with ACML (fig. 26.1). The algorithm takes into consideration opportunity for a matched allogeneic transplant, recipient age, and/or availability of a suitable donor, with the following considerations:

1. Any patient with ACML in acceleration or blast crisis or with a syngeneic donor should be offered alloBMT if suitable as a recipient (matched or one-antigen-mismatched related donor; recipient age less than 55 years, etc.)
2. Younger patients should be offered alloBMT in early chronic phase whenever possible (Consider age ≤40 as upper limit of "younger.") (109)
3. For patients not fitting categories 1 and 2, an initial trial of an αIFN-containing regimen should be undertaken. Those achieving a significant response would continue IFN unless the response is lose.
4. Patients who do not respond to αIFN as above should be offered a MUD alloBMT or other investigational treatments.
5. Patients who achieve a 6-month or longer CCR to αIFN should have autologous marrow storage. Freund and Huber (109) have proposed a more complicated but equally useful treatment strategy tree, including decision-making points according to timing and degree of response to IFN.

Finally, it should be noted that although αIFN therapy definitely is more effective during earlier stages of the disease, responses obtained to αIFN alone or with low-dose Ara-C in late chronic phase (121) suggest that a trial of αIFN may be indicated before BMT, even for those presenting with more advanced disease. In fact, secondary clonal phenomena evolving during acceleration will sometimes respond to αIFN dose escalation (133). αIFN can be effective when used repeatedly to suppress recurrent disease, has been used successfully to convert post-alloBMT relapses into chronic phase, and is being studied for continuous use in the post-alloBMT period in high-risk patients to prevent relapse (particularly in recipients of T-cell depleted marrow donors). Another promising therapeutic strategy under investigation for post-alloBMT relapses, and with potential for patients at high risk of relapse, is administration of donor lymphocytes. This therapy can be very toxic, but clearly demonstrates that allogeneic immune-competent cells can recognize and destroy the Ph+ clone.

Autologus Bone Marrow Transplantation (ABMT)

Most ACML patients will not have an HLA-matched related or unrelated donor for alloBMT or otherwise will be disqualified (over 55 years of age, etc). Use of stem cells harvested from patient blood or marrow obviates the need for a donor and generally is a less complicated procedure with a shorter hospital course than is required for allogeneic transplantation. ABMT has been attempted in ACML patients since the early 1980s. McGlave et al (134) recently analyzed results for 200 patients from eight hospitals so transplanted between 1984 and 1992. Almost three-quarters of the patients were in chronic phase at the time of ABMT; the median time diagnosis to transplant was 14.6 months. The rest were distributed equally between acceleration phase and blast crisis. Two-thirds of the patients received marrow and one-third received peripheral blood stem cells. Additional steps were taken ex vivo for some patients, including preinfusion cell culture (21) and incubation of the infusate with γ-IFN (23). Predictably, those in acceleration or blast crisis fared most poorly, although many achieved lengthy but transient responses (media 35+ months survival for ABMT patients in acceleration). At the time of publication, median survival for those in chronic phase had not been reached, with a plateau at approximately 60% at 43 months from ABMT and remaining stable for the next 4+ years. Patients younger than 40 years of age did better than older patients. As even older adults benefitted in this study, the use of ABMT may be worthwhile for ACML patients in their fifth or sixth decade of life. Normal or close-to-normal activity levels were achieved and maintained postABMT by most recipients. As most of the survivors had persistent or recurrent Ph+ positivity, it is a puzzle as to why the plateau in survival occurred and was so steadily maintained. These results are exciting but difficult to compare with alloBMT because of patient selection and lead-time bias as well as institutional variation in transplant methdology.

Many different strategies have been undertaken to improve response and survival for ABMT patients, including the following:

1. Aggressive preABMT preparative regimens such as busulfan/high-dose melphalan (135) or intensive chemotherapy plus IFN.
2. PostABMT immunomodulation including IFN and roquinimex (136).
3. Ex vivo purging of the stem cell infusate with mafosfamide (137), IFN, or by longterm marrow culture (138).
4. Ex vivo or in vivo stem cell collection using simple leukopheresis (139) or for exclusively benign progenitors using surface antigens (140).
5. Priming of patients preharvest with growth factors to obtain a better stem-cell yield (and hopefully shorten time to engraftment)

It has been shown that the autologous marrow or peripheral blood used to restore marrow function may contain Ph+ cells even after intensive therapy, but there is no evidence that a sufficient critical number of these cells must be present to contribute to relapse. Therefore, not only can the host fail but so can the infusate (141). In an attempt to develop a clinical model for prediction of outcome for autologous transplants, Butturini and Gale (142) analyzed relapse risk after T-cell-depleted alloBMTs (graft-versus-leukemia effect eliminated). Their data suggested that 50% of ACML patients in chronic phase and 10% in advanced phase might be cured by use of high-dose preABMT conditioning. This model did not try to account for any relapses that might occur from infusion of viable leukemia cells in the autograft infusate.

Other Considerations in Management
Pregnancy

As hydroxyurea and αIFN are teratogenic in some animal models, they should be avoided during the first two trimesters. Appropriate contraception should be practiced by a nonpregnant sexually active woman with ACML. Use of repeated leukopheresis has been recommended during the first and second trimesters for disease control (143).

Monitoring for Minimal Residual Disease

Once clinical disease disappears, it is common to still have persistent molecular evidence of the *bcr-abl fusion product*. In fact, for Philadelphia chromosome negative, *bcr*-positive patients, this is the only way to follow for cytogenetic improvement. Southern blot analysis can identify the presence of *bcr* but is more of value for screening. Polymerase chain reaction (PCR) or fluorescent in-situ hybridization (FISH) technology can be used to track cytogenetic response and/or progression in a more quantitative and sensitive way, as these techniques allow identification of residual disease up to the 10^{-5} cell level, whereas the discriminatory capability of standard chromosomal analysis is approximately 5% and Southern blot analysis approximately 1% (144).

Use of PCR to detect *bcr-abl* transcripts is important in two settings—for detection of minimal disease in patients attaining CCR, as with αIFN therapy and postBMT. Dhingra et al (144) were able to show that 15 of 18 patients achieving Ph negativity on IFN for a median of 22 months were positive for residual *bcr-abl* transcript by PCR analysis. Of the three still negative, a second amplification picked up the molecular marker in two. At present, the significance of these findings in prognosticating for long-term disease-free survival is unclear, but certainly late recurrences occur in ACML following any form of therapy, despite achieving CCR. The *bcr-abl* mRNA transcript has also been detected by PCR in most patients achieving CCR post-alloBMT (145). Here, the significance is even less clear, as the persistence of *bcr-abl* posttransplant is *not synonymous* with subsequent clinical relapse (34). However, one investigator (146) has adapted PCR for quantitative assessment of *bcr-abl* and demonstrated that increasing amounts of the mRNA have strong positive correlation with subsequent relapse. Another demonstrated that persistent *bcr/abl*/mRNA in patients with mixed T-cell chimerism post-alloBMT was highly predictive of relapse

(147). This suggested that T-cell chimerism might be a marker for the abrogation of graft-versus-leukemia activity, which has been considered pivotal for eradication of minimal residual disease post-alloBMT for ACML.

It is hard to use these data to suggest a plan for monitoring patients for residual disease, or for that matter, for decision making after detection of *bcr-abl*. Identification of the molecular marker clearly does not always herald reappearance of the Philadelphia chromosome. It seems reasonable to monitor for *bcr-abl* at perhaps 3-month intervals during or after treatment (including BMT) and to reserve decision making for intervention until such time as studies show that treatment of residual molecular disease is as important for prognosis as treatment of karyotypic or clinically evident disease.

Case 1

With treatment with αIFN, there was normalization of the peripheral blood white count by 14 days and the differential by day 29. By 90 days, the bone marrow aspirate had normalized, except for a slight increase in basophils. At that time, serum B12 was 1:330, LAP was 14, and the spleen was nonpalpable although still slightly enlarged by sonography. At that time, the marrow culture showed 16% Philadelphia chromosome metaphases.

The child was continued on αIFN and remained asymptomatic. However, at 6 months, the marrow Ph+ cells had increased to 43%. By 9 months, the bone marrow karyotype revealed 100% Ph+ cells as well as a second Philadelphia chromosome in more than one-third of them, and the splenic volume was slightly larger. Two months later, the white blood count began to increase with a shift toward more immature forms. The spleen became palpable, and the patient developed pain in his left foot. Marrow aspiration showed infiltration with Tdt-negative lymphoid cells (47%) that were considered reactive, not blasts. He was considered to be in accelerated phase and was taken off interferon. Shortly thereafter, he developed increasing pain in all extremities and was placed on hydroxyurea. Symptoms resolved, and he was referred for an allogeneic bone marrow transplant from a matched unrelated donor.

Disease Transformation

ACML chronic phase usually lasts 2–3 years, followed sometimes by a rapid onset of an acute blastic phase or, more commonly, by progression to an accelerated phase. As a patient might present well into the chronic phase, the interval until transformation may be short, as in our case, or it can last a decade. It can be difficult to distinguish loss of response to treatment from true acceleration (the latter has been difficult to define) (148). Criteria for all three phases, adopted by the Internationl Bone Marrow Transplant Registry are presented in Table 26.3. They seem to be appropriate for all ages and provide a framework for discussing disease progression, prognosis, and management.

The natural history of ACML chronic phase is characterized by continued proliferation of myeloid precursors. This may be associated with loss of sensitivity to or lack of response to initial therapy. Progressively increasing symptoms are secondary to increasing organomegaly (i.e., splenic pain, hypersplenism, abdominal discomfort), to infiltration of tissues with local proliferation (bone pain, arthralgia), to bulk disease and rapid cell turnover (fever, malaise, anorexia, weight loss), or to local massive proliferation (pseudochloromas). But at some point, the disease will undergo transition to a more aggressive and refractory phase in all patients. This natural history seems to be similar in children and adults.

More than 75% of ACML patients eventually will develop additional chromosomal aberrations if therapy does not lead to CCR (26–60% before blast crisis). These include duplication of the Ph chromosome, trisomy 8, and isochromosome 17 (73), which can occur even if the original clone is partially suppressed (as in our case). Secondary malignant clones distinguished by new karyotypic abnormalities can evolve in a step-wise fashion, perhaps because of relative growth advantage over the existing clone or clones. Approximately 50% are so affected (149). The presence at diagnosis of complex Ph rearrangements in chronic phase seems to have a delayed but significant impact on the disease progression or outcome (150).

During acceleration, new abnormal clones may evolve, the disease becomes refractory to therapy, a shift occurs more toward immature cells and an increasing rate of cell proliferation, and other changes in marrow and blood morphology and content occur. Clinical/laboratory response still may occur to other therapy, such as to hydroxyurea if used after interferon has begun to fail as in our case and, in fact, the second response may still be lengthy. If there is cytogenetic response to treatment initiated during chronic phase, disease progression often will be heralded by cytogenetic relapse before the clinical/cellular profile changes (as in our case). Further changes in the karyotype may precede other changes by up to 18 months and thus represent the first sign of acceleration.

Altmann (73) has estimated that 5% of patients undergo explicit evolution from chronic phase directly to **"blast crisis,"** 50% undergo a progressive but slower maturation defect producing the oncologic equivalent of an acute leukemia, and 45% undergo the gradual evolution of a more aggressive accelerated myeloproliferative state. Others cite somewhat different numbers for the incidence of blast crisis, depending on how they distinguish it from an acute leukemia (34, 73, 148, 149).

Prognostic Factors in Accelerated Phase

Bone marrow *myelofibrosis* has been considered by some (151, 152), but not all, (150, 153) to have adverse prognostic significance if recognized at diagnosis but otherwise is not a useful prognostic discriminant (150, 151, 154). Other features that have been associated with acceleration but are *not* of prognostic significance include

increasing drug dosage requirement, *marked* thrombocytosis (30), increased peripheral nucleated red cells, rising total WBC, rising LAP score (154), fever, bone pains, lymphadenopathy, splenomegaly, and skin involvement (148, 155). However, development of *thrombocytosis* during the chronic phase despite adequate control of the leukocyte count has been associated with disease acceleration and also a poor prognosis (30, 34). Recent multivariate analysis of these findings (34, 148) has found only the five criteria for acceleration listed in Table 26.4 to have additive independent prognostic significance (relative risk of death per day since development). Others have attempted to divide adult patients according to presenting features into risk groups with good, intermediate, or poor prognosis (equating respectively, to a 5-, 4-, or less than 3-year median survival) based on specific prognostic factors (153, 156). Kantarjian et al (34) have combined features at presentation with those significant for acceleration to create a staging system for therapeutic decision making (table 26.4). As yet, the impact of such prognostic discriminatory systems is not established. Pediatric ACML is less studied for prognostic factors, only peripheral blood and marrow blast counts are currently recognized as significant (4).

Pathogenesis

The events occurring in chronic phase that are responsible for the proliferative advantage and the progressive increase in tumor burden have been described as being caused by asynchronous and discordant maturation, increased cell longevity (delayed apoptosis), and additional cycles of division in later maturation compartments: these events contribute to the massive proliferation of ACML cells (69). What happens to cause the process to go through transformation? Although it has been suggested that the breakpoint

Table 26.4 Prognostic Staging System for ACML

Stage	No. of Characteristics	Characteristics for Poor Prognosis
1	0 or 1	Age ≥60 years
2	2	Spleen ≥10 cm below costal margin
		Blasts ≥3% in blood or ≥3% in bone marrow
3	≥3	Basophils ≥7% in blood or ≥3% in bone marrow
		Platelets ≥700 × 10⁹/L
4	*Any acceleration characteristic(s)*	**Accelerated-Phase Characteristics:**
		1. Cytogenetic clonal evolution
		2. Blasts ≥15% in blood
		3. Blasts and promyelocytes ≥30% in blood
		4. Basophils ≥20% in blood
		5. Platelets <100 × 10⁹/L

Modified with permission from Kantarjian HM, Deisseroth A, Jurzrock R, et al. Chronic myelogenous leukemia: a concise update. Blood 1993; 82(3):691–703.

location in the *bcr gene* is predictive of the duration of the ACML chronic disease phase, (157) no evidence has been found to show that a change in the species of *bcr-abl* fusion gene transcript leading to different mRNAs might be the cause of transformation. Activated RAS gene mutations have been found in only a few patients with late-stage ACML (157). More provocative is recent evidence linking the p53 gene to transformation; p53 is located on chromosome 17, and more than 20% of patients with late-stage ACML have abnormalities in that chromosome (158, 159). Although normal or even increased expression of p53 mRNA is found in most patients in blast crisis, deletions or rearrangements of the p53 gene do occur in up to 30% of all patients studied in transformed ACML.

Recently, researchers have noted a positive correlation between methylation of the calcitonin (CT) gene and the phase of ACML (157, 160). Abnormal DNA methylation, including the CT gene, has been noted previously in a variety of acute leukemias. Normal CT gene methylation is almost always seen in chronic phase of ACML, but hypermethylation has been identified in a high percentage of patients in acceleration, occurring on average as much as 6 months before clinical or laboratory signs of disease progression (160), and perhaps representing one manifestation of increasing genetic instability during disease progression (157).

Myelofibrosis

Investigators have found evidence of collagen overproduction in patients with ACML and of excessive platelet-derived growth factor secretion in ACML blasts (161). Recently, a case of fibrosis in lungs, spleen, and marrow was reported, associated with atypical megakaryocytic infiltration in the lungs (162). Although myelofibrosis occurs more commonly in patients with ACML after transformation, it should be cautioned that other causes for myelofibrosis may exist, especially from chemotherapy or interferon.

Drug Refractoriness

Why may transformation be characterized by drug refractoriness? Overexpression of *P-glycoprotein* (the MDR-1 gene product) has been implicated in ACML. In vitro, the ACML-derived cell line K562, when transfected with human MDR-1 cDNA, showed a several-fold increase in resistance to vinblastine and other chemotherapeutic agents (it tended to remain sensitive to cytosine arabinoside, 6-thioguanine, hydroxyurea, and methchlorethemine). These finginds could be reversed with cyclosporine, and there was increased responsiveness to differentiation with cytosine arabinoside. It would follow that drugs that differentiate rather than kill leukemic cells might be more effective with overexpression of P-glycoprotein, which seems to confirm what has been found clinically (163).

Monitoring

Monitoring for acceleration would include evaluation for and trending the criteria cited in Table 26.4. Extramedullary hematopoiesis, particularly in the liver and spleen, can be monitored for volumetric increases (164, 205). Additionally, it was observed recently that stainable marrow iron might be of value in monitoring disease. Patients with chronic-phase ACML usually have no stainable iron in the marrow but have normal serum iron, total iron-binding capacity, and serum ferritin levels. However, it has found by evaluation of sequential marrow aspirates that there is a switch from negative iron to positive iron coincident with the development of the accelerated stage or blast crisis (165). As yet, evaluation for stainable iron, for CT gene hypermethylation, or for changes in organ volume are not employed routinely for monitoring of disease escalation.

Case 1 (continued)

Our patient remained on hydroxyurea for 8 weeks. At pretransplant evaluation, he was still asymptomatic with normal CBC and differential. However, marrow aspirate revealed 90% blasts negative for peroxidase, sudan black, and esterase stains. Although PAS stain was negative, blasts had lymphoid morphology and were positive for Calla, Tdt, and CD19 and negative for myeloid, erythroid, megakaryocytic, and monocytic markers. Marrow karyotype was 100% positive for Ph chromosome. This was considered to represent **lymphoid blast crisis.** *He was placed on ALL induction therapy with vincristine, prednisone, L-asparaginase, and daunomycin and attained remission with 75% of marrow cells still Ph +. A MUD alloBMT was performed 6 weeks later (almost 1 year from diagnosis of ACML). Recovery was relatively uneventful with only mild GVHD and with reversion to complete Ph negativity. Evaluation for bcr-abl was not undertaken, and there was no therapy post-BMT. Six months later, he suffered a testicular/marrow relapse, 100% Ph + and pre-B-ALL by morphology markers and was placed on relapsed ALL chemotherapy. A year later, he experienced a second (CNS/marrow) relapse, also 100% Ph +, and died in blast crisis 3½ years after diagnosis.*

Blast Crisis

In approximately 5–25% of patients with ACML, a blast phase will develop without an intermediate accelerated phase in ACML (34, 73). The remaining 75% of patients have a more gradual transition through acceleration to either blast crisis or to a more differentiated myeloproliferative disorder, usually over 4–6 months, with increasing unresponsiveness to treatment. Ultimately, 39–80% will finally develop blas crisis by definition. The clinical picture is one of an acute leukemia, with 30% or more marrow blasts (see Table 26.3) and manifestations including anemia, thrombocytopenia and sometimes neutropenia (155). Blast crisis is strikingly associated with fever, diaphoresis, weight loss, and pleuritic or splenic pain. Generalized lymphadenopathy will occur occasionally, as will subcutaneous nodules. Basophilia sometimes may become extreme, leading to symptoms of excessive histamine release, including urticaria, pruritus, and even gastric ulceration (73). Leukostatic symptoms related to hyperleukocytosis are more commonly seen in blast crisis (2, 7), as is hemorrhage. Also, CNS leukemia may become overtly manifest with a positive CSF for blast cells. In more than 45% of lymphoid blast crisis patients, meningeal leukemia may develop (166), which may recur after initial control of blast crisis (2) despite appropriate neuroprophylaxis (166).

Blast crisis may involve proliferation of any of the bone marrow precursor lineages. The usual crisis is myeloblastic (60–70%). Myeloid crisis blasts have myeloid morphology and usually will display characteristic cytochemical and immunophenotypic staining. However, the myeloperoxidase stain is commonly negative and Auer rods are rarely seen. It is important to stress that other lineage-specific markers should be checked, particularly for the erythroid (glycophorin-A) (167) and megakaryocytic cell lineages and even monocytic phenotypes, as all of these have been reported. (168) The other one-third of blast crisis patients will have blasts with lymphoid morphology, cytochemistry, and immunophenotype, mostly related to early B-cell lineage. Rarely, T-lineage markers will be expressed (169, 170). Finally, it is not uncommon to find mixed lineage features in the cells of blast crisis.

Blast crisis is often associated with additional cytogenetic changes. These include multiple Ph chromosomes isochromosome 17q, or trisomy 8 or 19. Sometimes the karyotypic features and phenotype of blast crisis ACML will *match* those usually found in the corresponding *de novo (Ph negative)* acute leukemia subtype (171).

Evaluation

As therapy is usually tailored to the phenotype of the blast crisis, appropriate evaluation includes immunophenotyping and cytochemical staining of the blood or marrow. The patient and relatives also should be HLA-typed for alloBMT if this was not performed earlier.

Differential Diagnosis

For patients presenting in blast crisis without a preceding chronic phase, and especially if more classic features of ACML are not evident at presentation, **Ph+ acute leukemia** must be ruled out (73). The Philadelphia chromosome is found in up to 10% of childhood acute leukemias, almost one-third of adult acute lymphoid leukemias, and 2–3% of adult myeloid leukemias (172, 173). These are clinically similar to acute leukemias lacking the Ph chromosome and have few features other than prominent splenomegaly and basophilia to distinguish them from ACML blast crisis. Cytogenetic and molecular features are of value here; the specific karyotypic changes cited previously as heralding ACML blast crisis are not present; the novel p190 protein product of the *bcr-abl* fusion is seen in almost all children and half of all adults with Ph+ acute

leukemia and is not seen in PH+ ACML (which instead exhibits the 210kd protein) (174, 175). De novo Ph+ acute leukemia is responsive to conventional chemotherapy, as is ACML blast crisis. However, the Ph+ chromosome usually disappears with therapy, contrary to the more grudging disappearance of the ACML Ph chromosome. Both are rapidly fatal if untreated.

Treatment of Blast Crisis

The goal is to convert the disease back to a second chronic phase or to completely eliminate the Ph+ clone(s). At least two-thirds of *ACML lymphoblastic* crises will respond to standard ALL chemotherapy. Conventional neuroprophylaxis should be included in this therapy. Blast crisis involving *nonlymphoid* lineages generally responds poorly, with less than 25% reverting to chronic phase. Again, best results have been attained with conventional ANLL chemotherapy. Three-year leukemia-free survival after alloBMT from HLA-identical siblings for ACML patients in blast crisis is disappointing (15% in most series) (176, 177). IBMTR disease-free survival data for patients with ACML transplanted in acceleration phase and blast crisis are 35% and 12%, respectively (178). New post-BMT immunomodulatory therapies may improve the outcome for these high-risk patients.

The Treatment Outlook for ACML

Before the advent of new therapies, the median survival for adults with ACML was usually given as 3–4 years, with annual risk of death of 20–25% (156). Recently an analysis of survival of children (median age, 13 years; range, 2–19) with ACML showed a median survival of 4.1 years with annual risk of death of 20% (130). The major determinant is the length of the chronic phase, which historically is 2–3 years for all age groups. However, the overall prognosis has now improved, with a median survival at present of 60–65 months (34), attributed largely to earlier diagnosis, better supportive care, better therapeutic decision making in response to prognosis/risk considerations, and to better specific therapy (34, 179). New treatment strategies related to alloBMT and ABMT already have been presented. Other biologic response modifiers show promise. Interleukin-1 (IL-1) has a significant role in autocrine/paracrine pathways, particularly in acute leukemia and blast crisis, and IL-1 inhibitors (34) will suppress CML colony growth in vitro in a dose-dependent fashion. IL-4 suppresses CML colony growth in vitro. Retinoids and low-dose cytosine arabinoside can induce differentiation of ACML cells in vitro. Low-dose homoharringtonine has produced impressive hematologic and cytogenetic responses in late chronic-phase ACML and is being investigated in combination with αIFN (34). Finally, antisense oligonucleotides targeting the c-myb and c-kit proto-oncogenes have shown activity against the K562 CML cell line and ACML cells in blast crisis and may prove valuable as ex vivo or in vivo purging agents (180).

Juvenile Chronic Myelogenous Leukemia

Juvenile chronic myelogenous leukemia (JCML) typically differs from ACML in age of onset, associated respiratory and cutaneous manifestations, significant lymph node involvement, prominent thrombocytopenia with hemorrhage, markedly elevated fetal hemoglobin, monocytosis, evidence of immunodeficiency with frequent infections, absence of the Philadelphia chromosome or other specific cytogenetic marker, unique cell growth characteristics in vitro, and usually a rapidly progressive course. JCML represents less than 2% of all childhood leukemias and 30–40% of the chronic childhood leukemias in most published series of children younger than 18 years of age (9, 181, 183). It is more common in boys than girls. Before 4 years of age, it is much more common than ACML. JCML is difficult to define and treat.

Case 2

This 5-month-old black female was the product of an uncomplicated term delivery and had a negative family history and medical history. At routine 4-month well-baby check, splenomegaly was noted. CBC revealed an elevated white count, anemia, and thrombocytopenia. A bone marrow aspirate at the referring hospital was compatible with JCML. Laboratory evaluation additionally revealed persistence of fetal hemoglobin on electrophoresis and a negative sickle cell prep. The patient was referred for further evaluation.

Admission physical examination was unremarkable, except for shotty cervical, axillary, and inguina adenopathy, spleen palpable 6 cm below the left costal margin and liver palpable 3 cm below the right costal margin. CBC showed a WBC of 40×10^9/L with 32% segs, 9 bands, one metamyelocyte, 38 lymphs, 15 monos (AMC 6×10^9/L), three eosinophils, one basophil, and one nucleated red cell. Platelet count was 100×10^9/L. RBC morphology showed moderate aniso- and poikilocytosis and occasional ovalocytes and tear drops. The hemoglobin was 8.8 g/dL, with MCV of 74.7 fL and RDW of 15.4% (normal for age 11.5–14.5). Fetal hemoglobin was 10% (normal at 5 months is about 5%). LAP score was 80 (normal range, 13–130), serum B12 was 769 pg/mL (normal range, 140–750 pg/mL), and serum folate 31 Ng/mL (normal range, 2–14), with normal PT, PTT, and fibrinogen. Serum chemistries for renal and liver functions were normal. VDRL was negative as were serologies for CMV, HIV, rubella, EBV, syphilis, toxoplasma, and HSV. Serum IgG, IgA, and IgM were markedly elevated. Bone marrow aspirate revealed hypercellularity with slightly decreased megakaryocytes, monocytic and granulocytic hyperplasia, and slightly decreased erythropoiesis, with a M/E ratio of 7:1 (normal for age is 3:1) and elevated blasts at 5%. Bone marrow biopsy showed markedly increased cellularity without fibrosis. Karyotypes of bone marrow and peripheral blood showed no abnormalities. Peripheral blood flow cytometry demonstrated less than 1% progenitor cells (CD34 positive), 53% granulocytic, 19% mature monocytic, and approximately 23% cells of lymphoid origin. Bone marrow flow cytometry revealed 22% lymphoid lineage, 3% progenitor phenotype, 11% monocytic and 60% granulocyte lineage, and 4% erythroid lineage. Marrow assays for CFU-GEMM were performed and revealed greater than 1000 colonies per 10^5 plated cells (normal 10 per 10^5 plated), with or without added growth factors. Assays for CFU-GM, BFU-E, and other cell colonies were not performed.

***Assessment and Initial Management:** The laboratory and clinical pictures were believed to corroborate the diagnosis of **JCML**, and the patient was started on oral cis-retinoic acid (CRA), 100 mg per M², approximately2 weeks after admission. A search began for an HLA-compatible marrow donor. The patient tolerated the initial CRA dosage well with minimal side effects and decreasing symptoms and was discharged pending results of marrow donor search.*

Clinical Findings

This case illustrates many of the characteristics features of JCML. Newborns (183) and adolescents have been described, but more than 90% are diagnosed in the first 4 years of life (9, 182). Contrary to the early course of ACML, more than one-half of these children present with malaise, failure to thrive or weight loss, and fever or overt bacterial infection (10). Splenomegaly is a constant finding and is often massive. Significant hepatomegaly is seen in more than 30% of patients. Lymphadenopathy is common and can be striking. It usually is diffuse and nontender, but suppurative lesions can be seen (9, 10). Infections at presentation are mostly upper respiratory, but chronic bronchitis, reactive airway disease, and pneumonias, if not seen at diagnosis, invariably occur during the course of the illness. Bleeding, usually cutaneous and secondary to thrombocytopenia, is a presenting symptom in more than one-half of the cases and usually worsens as the disease progresses (9, 10, 182).

Cutaneous manifestations are seen in more than 40% of patients (9, 10, 182). Most typically, a maculopapular or eczematoid rash is seen on the face and trunk, varying from pale to deeply erythematous. Erythema nodosum-like lesions have been described. Additionally, xanthomas and cafe-au-lait spots are occasionally seen, with or without other stigmata of Von Recklinghausen's neurofibromatosis (10, 184). The cutaneous stigmata of JCML can antedate the onset of the hematologic picture by at least 12 months (185). Intensity of the rash commonly parallels disease activity.

Laboratory Findings

Peripheral blood findings in more than 80% of cases at presentation include WBC between 12 and 100×10^9/L (usually less than 50), with an absolute mononuclear count of $>5 \times 10^9$/L (normal for age is 0.4–0.6 AMC), and with significant numbers of immature granulocytes. Peripheral blood blasts (usually less than 5%) and nucleated RBCs are found in most cases. Platelet count is normal (in less than 20%) to severely decreased; platelets are functionally normal. Most patients are significantly anemic, and many demonstrate a decreased MCV with hypochromia, increased RDW, and decreased serum iron.

Fetal hemoglobin is markedly increased at diagnosis in more than 50% of cases (17, 18); this is a cardinal feature of JCML and levels above 25% are encountered frequently, with a mean of 38% (187, 189, 193). Serum and urinary muramidase often are markedly elevated. Serum B12 can be elevated, but not as consistently as in ACML (186). Similarly, the LAP score can be normal as in ACML (10, 182, 186). Most patients have markedly elevated serum immunoglobulins, and sometimes the presence of autoantibodies has been recorded (186, 187).

The **bone marrow aspirate,** as in our case, typically shows hypercellularity, normal to decreased megakaryocytes, myeloid hyperplasia with orderly maturation, notable increase in immature and differentiated monocytes, and generally greater than 5% blasts. Myelodysplastic changes are absent, and the usual M/E ratio is elevated at 5:1. Bone marrow and peripheral blood cytochemical stains and immunophenotyping will reveal primarily a granulocyte/monocyte cell population as in this case. **Marrow biopsy** corroborates the hypercellularity and very rarely demonstrates significant fibrosis.

None of the above features are truly pathognomonic, with the possible exception of the combination of markedly elevated fetal hemoglobin levels with thrombocytopenia. Best delineation of the diagnosis can be accomplished by combining these many features with cell surface antigen phenotyping, in vitro culture of peripheral blood or bone marrow, and cytogenetic analysis. The Philadelphia chromosome will not be found in JCML, and also in contrast to ACML, monocyte-macrophage colonies from these patients will proliferate in the absence of exogenous colony stimulating factors. *This latter phenomenon is indeed unique to JCML.*

Table 26.1 offers comparison of selected clinical, laboratory, and cytogenetic features of JCML at presentation with those of ACML. Refer to Table 26.2 for a suggested evaluation plan for childhood chronic leukemias.

Underlying Mechanisms

JCML is a rapidly progressing disease and usually comes to attention due to infections, failure to thrive, or hemorrhagic manifestations. Understanding the clinical course and pathogenic mechanisms is central to rationally approaching the diagnosis and management of JCML.

General Symptoms

Fever and malaise, bone pain, abdominal distention, failure to thrive, and weight loss are usually caused by organ and tissue neoplastic infiltration. The suppurative lymphadenopathy occasionally seen in JCML is probably also caused by infiltrating disease, which predisposes to bacterial infection. Splenomegaly can lead to hypersplenism, (182) with localized pain and worsening anemia and thrombocytopenia. Moderate to massive splenomegaly was found in more than 80% of a large case series retrospectively reviewed by Castro-Malespina et al (10).

Infections

The pathogenesis of the susceptibility to bacterial infections is unclear; diagnostic biopsy and postmortem evaluation of splenic, lymph node, liver, lung, and other tissues (10, 182, 186) has revealed extensive infiltration by mononuclear cells. Peribronchial and intra-alveolar infiltration by these functionally immature cells increasingly may predispose the patients to respiratory infections and may explain why they respond sluggishly to antibiotics and may improve with chemotherapy (182, 188). However, infection, particularly respiratory, was a major contributor to demise in early series (9, 10, 181).

Hemorrhage

No specific coagulation defect has been associated with the disease; bleeding seems to be almost entirely secondary to thrombocytopenia.

Fetal Erythropoiesis

The modest to marked elevation of fetal hemoglobin, noted in more than 60% of patients in most series, seems to be one of several manifestations of what has been described as "a reversion to fetal erythropoiesis." Fetal hemoglobin is uniformly distributed in the red cells (189), and the glycine to alanine ratio of hemoglobin F gamma chains has great similarity to that of newborn infants (190). Additionally, diminished expression of I antigen and a fetal profile of RBC glycolytic enzymes has been noted (190, 191), and most recently, the expression of the embryonic globins ϵ and ζ at the cell protein and mRNA level have been noted in cultured cells (unique for this leukemia) (192). These changes all become more prominent as the disease progresses. However, they seem to be expressed in a disordered fashion in the red cell precursors, suggesting that there is a failure in the coordination of gene expression rather than complete reversion to a fetal erythropoietic pattern (186). In addition, the changes do not interfere with the ability of JCML erythroid cells to reach functional and morphologic maturity. Nevertheless, fetal hemoglobin levels may be extraordinarily elevated, and if so, are strongly corroborative of the diagnosis of JCML. Quantitative fetal hemoglobin should be obtained at diagnosis and can be of value subsequently to monitor the course of the disease.

Integument

Integumental changes provoke some of the most intriguing diagnostic and biologic questions for this disease. The maculopapular/eczymatoid rash described in previous series (9, 182, 188, 189) is unresponsive to topical steroids, and on biopsy, a leukemic cellular infiltrate is seen in the dermal layer (185). Ng et al found that the neoplastic cells morphologically resembled monocytes, stained weakly for acid phosphatase and nonspecific esterase, and exhibited monocytic immunophenotypic markers. The cells also were positive for S-100 protein and thus shared features with dendritic cells as well as mononuclear phagocytes (194). The S-100 protein is a dimeric calcium-binding protein that was first identified in nervous tissue and later in many other tissues. In the lymphoreticular system, it can be found in Langerhans cells. It has also been found in T lymphocytes and T-cell lymphoma. The authors did not suggest that JCML is simply an atypical manifestation of disseminated histiocytosis-X, but they did propose that JCML may be derived from a stem cell common to dendritic cells and phagocytic histiocytes. Abnormally proliferating JCML colony-forming cells grown in vitro (184, 195, 196) have immunophenotypic features of monocytic-macrophage lineage. Shannon et al noted erythrophagocytosis, another feature common to histiocytic syndromes, in a patient with JCML with a cytogenetic marker in the involved monocytic cell line (184). It has been argued that JCML should be included in the working formulation as a major category in class III malignant histiocytic disorders (197).

The cutaneous manifestations of Von Recklinghausen's neurofibromatosis (VNF) also have an intriguing association with JCML. Many cases of simultaneous JCML and VNF have been documented (10, 198). Castro-Malaspina et al (10) noted that of their series of 38 patients, three had VNF and an additional five patients had xanthomas or cafe-au-lait spots. The monocyte-macrophage specific growth factor CSF-1 is recognized to stimulate production of CFU-GM in vitro. The cFMS proto-oncogene may encode for CSF-1. Cytogenetic and molecular evidence is accumulating implicating the NF1 oncogene in the regulation of production of monocyte/macrophage precursors. Whether NF-1 or cFMS will be linked to pathogenesis of JCML is speculative at this time (199).

Other Clinical/Laboratory Findings

Findings *not* helpful in initial differentiation of JCML from ACML include the following: degree of splenomegaly, immaturity of peripheral blood granulocytic series, LAP score, serum and urine lysozyme (muramidase), serum B12 and carrying proteins, other hepatic and renal chemistries (see table 26.1). **Serum and urine muramidase (lysozyme)** is elevated in least half of JCML cases (186), but not to the degree seen in adults with Philadelphia-chromosome-negative ACML. Elevated muramidase is probably secondary to increased turnover of granulocytes and monocytes. **LAP scores** are not useful in delineating the disease process, probably due to variability in degree of terminal differentiation of monocyte/granulo-

cytic precursors in JCML (60). **Serum vitamin B12** is elevated in most JCML patients, probably due to active granulocyte protein synthesis, as it is in ACML. The significance of the striking elevation of **serum IgG, IgA, and IgM** seen in 80% of children with JCML, along with frequent **light chain imbalance, polyclonality,** and the presence of **antinuclear and anti-IgG antibodies,** is unknown at this time (187).

Blood and Marrow In Vitro Cellular Assays

Numerous investigators have studied the precursor populations in blood and marrow from JCML patients (184, 186, 195, 196, 200, 201). Assays of CFU-C and CFU-GM have consistently shown two abnormalities: impaired growth of normal hematopoietic progenitors and excessive proliferation of exclusively monocyte-macrophage colonies even in the absence of added growth factors. Addition of appropriate growth factors did not always cause acceleration of colony growth. In liquid culture, this "autonomous" growth (73, 186, 195) would occur in the face of stromal layer depletion in the absence of added growth factor. The growing cells invariably were of monocyte-macrophage derivation (202). It could not be demonstrated that there was *increased GM-CSF production* in this disease either in vivo or in these culture systems. Most recently, Emmanuel et al demonstrated that the JCML erythroid nonadherent progenitors and granulocyte/macrophage populations were markedly hypersensitive to GM-CSF. They postulated that this hypersensitivity led to the selective proliferative advantage and clonal expansion in this disease (203).

Several investigators have also documented spontaneous erythroid colony growth in cells from selected patients, in the absence of added erythropoietin (192, 204). Cells derived from these colonies demonstrated the fetal characteristics (192) previously described. Blood and marrow assays for growth characteristics of CFU-GEMM have a major importance in defining this disease, and as in our case, play an important role in affirming the diagnosis.

Case 3

This 20-month-old female presented with fever, pallor, marked hepatosplenomegaly, and cardiomegaly with evidence of early congestive heart failure. No rash or adenopathy were noted. CBC showed the following. Hgb, 55 g/L; Hct, 15%, and platelets 77×10^9/L, with WBC 38×10^9/L, differential of 34 polys, four bands, three immature myeloid, thirty lymphocytes, 15 monocytes (AMC, 4.7×10^9/L), seven nucleated red cells, and four blasts. LAP was 113, vitamin B12 >2000 pg/mL, serum muramidase 16.6 μg/mL (NL, 3.0–12.8), and fetal hemoglobin 2.4% (normal for age is 2%). Bone marrow aspirate showed normal cellularity with M/E ratio of 8:1 (normal for age is 3.9:1), 1% monocytes and 1% blasts. Splenic sonography revealed splenic volume of 224 mL (normal for age 60) (205). Chromosome analysis showed monosomy 7. CFU-GEMM assays were not obtained.

The patient was diagnosed as JCML and transfused, with resolution of anemia and cardiac symptoms. She was started on high-dose recombinant α-IFN. Although leukocytosis resolved, thrombocytopenia persisted and worsened over the 3 months of IFN treatment, with increasing requirements for platelet and red cell transfusions. At 2 months of therapy, the patient developed massive splenomegaly, marked lymphadenopathy, and a raised, erythematous confluent facial rash that revealed infiltration with leukemic cells on biopsy. The patient died at home 4 months after diagnosis.

Cytogenetics

JCML always lacks the Philadelphia chromosome and rearrangements in the BCR region of chromosome 22 (206). Approximately 80% of patients have a normal karyotype, and the cytogenetic changes that have been identified are markedly heterogenous (10, 207). Monosomy 7, abnormalities of chromosome 8, and other C group chromosome changes are reported with JCML (208, 209). Abnormalities of chromosomes 7 and 8 have been seen in many other leukemias and myelodysplastic syndromes (MDS), and an association has been noted between acquired abnormalities of chromosome 8 and the Epstein-Barr virus (210). Such cytogenetic changes are invariably duplicated in cultured JCML CFC-GM (192, 195, 211, 212), and will persist in the affected cells (10, 200, 201, 207). These findings have led to the speculation that JCML is actually a group of disorders and not a homogeneous entity. Additionally, Symann reported two patients with JCML with monosomy 7 and spontaneous erythroid colony formation without added erythropoietin (204). There have even been cases of childhood Philadelphia-chromosome-positive CML that have some stigmata of JCML, including production of mainly CFU-GM in vitro from peripheral blood cells (213). The evidence of uniform clonality as cited for ACML does not link all JCML cases together, but at least some of the cases fitting the JCML phenotype are probably bonafide clonal diseases.

Evidence for association of JCML with a specific oncogene or with oncogene activation is scant. However, Miyauchi et al (214) recently found that 6 of 20 JCML patients had mutations of the N-ras gene, a finding similar to the incidence reported for AML and CMMoL, and seen only rarely in Ph+ CML. N-ras mutations seem to occur more commonly in AML subtypes involving monocytic lineage.

Differential Diagnosis of JCML

Mixed **leukemoid reactions** with both granulocytic and monocytic elements can be seen in children and can be confusing if associated with splenomegaly or thrombocytopenia. Clinical course, associated diseases states (i.e., collagen vascular disease, infection), and detailed evaluation should allow differentiation from JCML.

Monosomy 7 Syndrome

Numerous investigators have reported a childhood myeloproliferative or dysplastic syndrome similar to JCML. Purported differences from JCML include a younger age of onset (under 2 years), increased incidence in males (4:1

ratio), lack of cutaneous manifestations, higher incidence of infections, hypogammaglobulinemia, low or minimally elevated fetal hemoglobin, higher risk of a blast phase, and shorter survival time (10 months vs. 22 months for JCML) (204, 208, 209, 215). It has been suggested that the heightened susceptibility to infections is caused by association of defective chemotaxis with monosomy 7 (Chapter 21). *The Karyotypic abnormality* (monosomy 7) has been found in association with other myeloproliferative and myelodysplastic syndromes, as well as in the "classical" JCML phenotypes, as our case 3 portrays. Male sex and the associations with RAS and NFI mutations are common to both Monosomy 7 syndrome and JCML, suggesting common steps in pathogenesis.

Speculation that cytogenetically undetectable deletions or rearrangements in chromosome 7 exist in all patients with JCML, resulting in acquired hemizygosity of chromosome 7, has largely been put to rest by careful mapping of that chromosome (199), although very small deletions in chromosome 7, below the current level of detection, cannot completely be ruled out. A multistep model of JCML leukemogenesis has been proposed, based on known molecular and clinical data (199), and is included here in modified form (fig. 26.2)

Prolonged survival in JCML has been reported (10) and may represent one clinical extreme, whereas the short survival seen in patients with monosomy 7 may represent another. However, current knowledge does not allow the presence of monosomy 7 to alter the evaluation, monitoring or therapy undertaken for JCML, and the distinction between the "monosomy 7" myeloproliferative disorder and JCML remains unclear.

Persistent Epstein-Barr Virus (EBV)

An association has been recognized between JCML and EBV (209, 210, 216). Investigators have noted a condition that clinically was markedly similar to JCML but with increased anti-EBV antibody titers to VCA and EA present at diagnosis. Patient marrow and blood showed some spontaneous colony formation similar to true JCML but not exclusively of granulocyte/monocyte lineage. Evidence of chronic EBV infection has been associated with other chronic myeloproliferative and lymphoproliferative syndromes and with myelodysplasias and acute leukemias. Additionally, protracted EBV infection has been seen in at least one patient with both VNF and JCML (210). However, the serologic picture, cell culture characteristics, and spontaneous recovery should help differentiate this entity from JCML.

Infantile Cytomegalovirus Infection

Congenitally acquired CMV commonly presents with leukocytosis, anemia (often hemolytic), thrombocytopenia, and atypical lymphocytes and monocytoid cells. Organomegaly, sometimes respiratory symptoms and decreased marrow megakaryocytes, also are characteristic. These findings can make it hard to distinguish infantile CMV infection from JCML, but the two can be differentiated by (a) EM or histocytologic detection of typical CVM find-

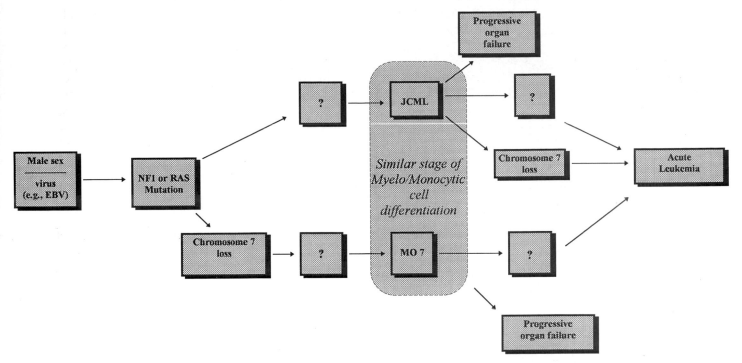

Figure 26.2. Multistep model for development of JCML and MO7. Question marks represent one or more additional events/occult genetic changes necessary to confer the proliferative growth advantages in both conditions and the subsequent changes involved in transformation to acute leukemia. (Modified with permission from Butcher M, Frenck R, Emperor J, et al. Molecular evidence that childhood monosomy 7 syndrome is distinct from juvenile chronic myelogenous leukemia and other childhood myeloproliferative disorders. Genes Chromosom Cancer 1995;12:50–57.)

ings, (b) direct demonstration of the virus or viral genome or seroconversion, and (c) marrow cell culture assays, as previously described, demonstrating the two characteristics JCML abnormalities of impaired growth of normal progenitors and excessive proliferation of CFU-GEMM and CFU-GM in the absence of exogenous growth factor (217). This approach could be adapted to differentiate JCML from any virus, producing a JCML-like clinical picture in early infancy.

Chronic Myelomonocytic Leukemia (CMMol or CMML)

An argument can be made that JCML is simply a childhood variant of adult CMMoL. Adult CMMoL is characterized by peripheral blood monocytosis (AMC $>1 \times 10^9$/L) with blasts, marrow proliferation of immature granulocytes and monocytes with partially differentiated monoblasts, thrombocytopenia and anemia, markedly elevated serum or urine lysozyme, hepatosplenomegaly and a chronic course with anemia, increasing lymphadenopathy and skin infiltrates, hyperimmunoglobulinemia, and infections (see Chapter 21) (218, 219, 220).

CMMoL represents 5–25% of reported series of MDS (218). It occurs primarily in adult men and has a poor prognsois with death either in chronic phase or after conversion to acute leukemia (20–40%) (220). Because of certain blood and marrow cellular characteristics, it has been classified as an atypical myelodysplastic syndrome (MDS) rather than a true myeloproliferative entity (47, 220, 221). CMMoL peripheral blood smears may display cells with monocytic morphologic and immunologic features but with peculiar unipolar ruffles and folds; these features are also described in leukemic monoblasts (218). Cytogenetic features, as in JCML, have been variable (223), and this disorder is always Ph chromosome and bcr negative (222).

Those reporting childhood cases of adult-type CMMoL (JCMMoL) have noted the clinical similarity to JCML but have made the distinction from JCML based on the usual only modest elevation of fetal Hb, a more chronic course, less prominent lymphadenopathy, and absence of skin rash (218, 219). Cultured cells from adult CMMoL and JCML are similar morphologically and by immunophenotyping, but cultured CMMol marrow appears to lack the exuberant and unique growth characteristics of JCML cells (218, 223). Cytogenetically, CMMoL and JCML have some striking similarities: a detailed analysis of cases having marker chromosomes has revealed presence of the marker in CFU-GM and CFU-E, but not T- or B-lymphocytic lineages (201). This suggested that abnormal clones in both CMMoL and JCML originate in a partially committed precursor common to granulocyte-macrophage and erythroid lineages (201). Castro-Malaspina et al (10) suggested that there might be several variants of childhood CMMoL, one of them following a much more indolent course and more accurately termed "chronic myelomonocytic leukemia," and another more closely resembling JCML. More than one-half of the 38 patients reviewed by these investigators diverged from the 37% displaying a more classic JCML disease progression, with one group of the divergent subjects (26%) manifesting a stable course (with one developing acute leukemia) and the other (37%) exhibiting disease regression from time of diagnosis but with persistent absolute monocytosis, worsening anemia, and, in the majority, thrombocytopenia. A high percentage of these patients died as a result of acute leukemia. Patients in the divergent group tended to be older, and six longterm survivors were off therapy for longer than 10 years.

Thus, it is unclear whether JCML and JCMMoL are indeed the same entity or are distinct within a spectrum of childhood MPS/MDS. Gadner and Haas (47) point out several factors leading to the confusion in classifying pediatric MDS and MPS. Most important is that dysplastic features, prominent in adult cases are much less pronounced in younger children. Secondly, EBV, CMV, and perhaps other viruses producing related syndromes may be associated with dysplastic hematopoiesis. Finally, the distinction between marrow failure and a proliferative state may be more subtle. They have proposed to classify both adult and juvenile JCMMoL as MPS and distinct from each other. In their proposal, JCML is JCMMoL and perhaps the former name should be completely dropped.

Chronic Monocytic Leukemia (CMoL)

CMoL has been reported to occur in children (224) but may represent a malignant histiocytic syndrome (225), a truly separate entity from JCML, or an unusual form of acute monocytic leukemia with a more benign course. It has an insidious course with pancytopenia and presence of increased numbers of mature monocytic cells and their precursors in the blood (224).

Familial Chronic Myelogenous Leukemia

A rare myeloproliferative syndrome exactly duplicating JCML has been described in infant siblings, involving at least three pairs (10, 226). It differs from classic JCML only in the long survival of one sibling from each of two sibships (183). Another large family group manifesting a Philadelphia chromosome negative myeloproliferative syndrome in children from multiple generations has been reported, with certain features suggestive of JCML (227). Some consider these entities to represent a distinct subgroup or division of childhood chronic myeloproliferative syndromes (182, 186).

Pathogeneis

JCML seems to be a clonal myeloproliferative disorder with a distinctive clinical and laboratory picture. There is little at this time to indicate a genetic predisposition, other than the cited cases of familial CML. It is tempting to postulate that a persistent EBV or other chronic infection might disrupt immune surveillance sufficiently to allow proliferation of a monocyte-macrophage-dominated malignant clone.

Cell culture and immunophenotyping have delineated biologic peculiarities of the disease that might explain selective proliferation of the malignant clone with its ultimate consequences of organ involvement and overwhelming body dysfunction (186, 195, 203, 228). Estrov et al (195) first demonstrated impaired growth of normal hematopoietic progenitors in cell culture and specific excessive proliferation of monocyte-macrophage colonies in the absence of added growth factors. It subsequently was demonstrated that this apparent "spontaneous" growth could be abolished if endogenous growth factor was eliminated, that the necessary factor was GM-CSF, and that in fact very small quantities of growth factor in vitro have an excessive stimulatory effect on the disregulated JCML cells (203, 228). Most recently, it has been determined that in vitro and in vivo GM-CSF production is not increased in this disease, that supernatants from the in vitro GM colonies will markedly inhibit normal cell growth, that the inhibitory cytokine is endogenously produced TNF-α, that TNF-α also has a JCML cell-growth-promoting effect, and that IL-1α augments these effects and may initiate them (186, 229, 230).

Thus, one can postulate that the JCML cells gain a selective proliferative advantage by two mechanisms: exquisite hypersensitivty to growth factors, which would allow continued proliferation in the face of a negative feedback signal, and the direct inhibition of normal colony development. With further proliferation of the disease, massive organ invasion occurs, setting the stage for decreased production of normal marrow elements, compromise of liver, lung, and other organs, eventual demise from tumor burden, and compromise of hematopoietic, respiratory, and other systems. Mechanisms potentiating acute leukemia in the end stages of the disease are totally unknown.

Theory

The multistep evolution of ACML (73) can be applied to the pathogeneiss of JCML. In this instance, the transforming event or events may be a preexisting cytogenetic abnormality such as monosomy 7 or molecular rearrangements on chromosome 7, an occult congenital genetic factor (related to male gender?), and/or an acquired transforming agent such as the EBV. In this instance, the nature of the transformation on a molecular level is unknown but could result in an N-ras or NFI mutation (fig. 26.2). This, in turn, could lead to the production of a clone of premalignant hematopoietic cells that have an aberrancy in signal transduction through IL-1 on GM-CSF. (214, 215)

As a part of the initial transformation event or as a subsequent development further in disease evolution, the clone aquires a growth advantage over normal stem cells, resulting in overproduction of more mature elements but with evidence of marked dysregulation (table 26-5). This growth advantage may be triggered by IL 1 and is largely due to excessive proliferative response to GM-CSF, and to a lesser degree, to inhibition of proliferation of normal marrow elements. The end result is production of a primarily monocyte-macrophage cell lineage and, in most instances, less conspicuously of erythroid and granulocytic components. The lymphoid lineage need not be involved, although the hyperimmunoglobulinemia seen in so many JCML cases

Table 26.5 JCML—Evidence for a Panmyelopathy
by Cell Lineage Involvement

Monocyte-macrophage—dominant cell lineage in vitro and in
 extramedullary sites
Myeloid—low LAP, recurrent infections despite marrow granulocyte hyperplasia
Erythroid—high fetal hemoglobin, other "fetal" red cell characteristics and peripheral blood shift toward immature cells
Platelet—thrombocytopenia, decreased marrow megakaryoctyes
Cytogenetic—chromosome markers (in occasional patients) appear in all cells

(187) and a recent report of a B-lineage lymphoid blast crisis (in a patient with JCML and a monosomy 7 marker in
both the original myelomonocytic marrow cells and in the
lymphoid cells) lend credence to the contention that JCML
is a "clonal disease of pluripotent stem-cell origin" (231).

Natural History

After the usual abrupt onset, with more than 50% of the patients manifesting symptoms at presentation, the course of
JCML is usually rapidly downhill, with death by 16 or fewer
months (9, 10, 182). Clinical parameters usualy directly reflect increasing organ involvement, as well as worsening
rash and thrombocytopenia, higher populations of monocyte-derived cells in the peripheral blood, increase in the
percentage of blasts, and a rising fetal hemoglobin in many
cases. Evidence of primitive erythropoiesis often increases
during the course of illness (191), and cytogenetic abnormalities also sometimes evolve. Generally, the terminal
stage of the disease is marked by severe anemia, overt
bleeding and/or overwhelming infection, and less commonly, development of acute leukemia. Because of the
small number of JCML patients and a more diverse clinical
picture, prognostic variables have not been studied by
many investigators. Castro-Malaspina et al, in their series of
38 patients, found that factors at presentation correlating
significantly with unfavorable prognosis included older age
(older than 2 years), hepatomegaly, bleeding, thrombocytopenia, and high blast counts in the peripheral blood.
Splenomegaly, fetal hemoglobin levels, total leukocyte
count, marrow blasts, as well as other parameters, had no
prognostic significance (10). They developed a discriminant function for prognostication from these data. However, considering the peculiar nature of their patient population with a cohort of long survivors and the high incidence
of terminal acute leukemia (which seems to be fairly unique
to their series), their system will need corroboration in further studies. In a recent report by the Italian National Registry for JCML, review of 22 evaluable cases suggested that
age younger than 1 year at presentation was the most significant favorable factor for probability of survival (232).
Others have suggested 6 months of age as the discriminant.

Immediate Management

It cannot be said that JCML is universally fatal without
treatment, as longterm survivors have been reported (10,
226). However, early rapid disease progression usually requires aggressive supportive care while definitive therapy
is being implemented. As death is almost always due to
bleeding or infection. Aggressive supportive care measures
should be implemented as clinically indicated, with
platelet and red cell transfusions as well as early institution
of antibiotic therapy for recognized infections. As bone
marrow transplantation continues to be the best option for
this disease, the early management plan should include tissue typing of siblings or other family members, and if indicated, the search for an unrelated matched bone marrow
donor. Also, marrow harvest and storage should be considered if the opportunity is permitted by response to initial
therapy. Splenectomy has been considered transiently effective for some patients, especially those with symptoms
of hypersplenism (10, 226), but is not warranted to control
the disease.

Acute Leukemia

If the percentage of blasts in the bone marrow is greater
than 30%, the disease should be considered acute leukemia. Patients who develop acute leukemia in JCML invariably show a myeloblastic cytochemical phenotype. In the
Castro-Malaspina series, none of the 11 acute leukemias
responded favorably to combination chemotherapy (10),
but others have noted response to such treatment (233).
Cases converting to acute leukemia should be considered
for aggressive combination chemotherapy or BMT.

Historical Therapeutic Strategies

Single chemotherapeutic agent therapy for JCML has
proven ineffective. **Splenectomy** and **splenic irradiation,** although sometimes effective in controlling massive
disease, have only transient benefit. Lilleyman et al (234).
described the use of sequential subcutaneous cytosine arabinoside and oral 6-mercaptopurine for JCML, and this
regimen has proven effective in the hands of others. However, most cases only will respond transiently. Subsequent
to the Castro-Malaspina review in 1984 (10), intensive
combination chemotherapy as employed for ANLL has
produced sustained remissions in a small series of patients
treated by Chan et al (233). However, 75% eventually relapsed; abnormal monocyte-macrophage cells had never
completely disappeared from the bone marrow during remission in the relapsed cases (200).

Biological Response Modifiers

There are case reports of responses to **cis-retinoic acid**
(CRA) and **alpha interferon.** Recombinant human
alpha interferon binds αIFN to JCML cells and causes
a sharp increase in certain intracellular metabolic
parameters that are related to interferon effect. Dose-
dependent growth inhibition of JCML colonies by αIFN
can be demonstrated in vitro (235), but clinical responses
to αIFN have been few and fleeting, and toxicity may be
unacceptable (232, 236–238). One case has been reported to date of response to combination therapy with
αIFN and hydroxyurea (239). **CRA** has been used more

extensively with significant although mostly brief responses. CRA is the geometric analog of vitamin A, a diterpine natural product, and induces the differentiation and maintenance of epithelial cell tissue and promote growth. It recently has been shown to abrogate spontaneous growth of JCML cultures in vitro and is presently being studied as single-agent therapy for JCML. However, aside from consideration for initial treatment of JCML patients with αIFN, combination chemotherapy, or CRA, the standard of care presently is allogeneic bone marrow transplantation.

Allogeneic Bone Marrow Transplantation

The first case report of a successful allogeneic bone marrow transplantation for JCML was published in 1979 (240). Recently, Sanders et al. (241) updated the Seattle experience with allogeneic transplantation in 14 children with JCML. Using a cyclophosphamide/TBI preparative regimen, unmodified allogeneic bone marrow was given to six patients from HLA-identical siblings and eight patients from one-haplotype-mismatched family members. Although five patients died of transplantation-related complications and three ultimately relapsed, six patients of this series remained alive from 6 months to more than 11 years post-transplantation; three of these had mismatched donors. Several have had chronic GVHD but maintain good quality of life. At present, evaluation for bone marrow transplantation would seem to be the top priority, hopefully to be accomplished while interval support with (242) or without chemotherapy or differentiating agents is initiated for disease control.

Summary

Chronic myeloid leukemias have provided unique insight into the biology of malignant disorders and demonstrated critically how genetic mechanisms, cell growth, and the process of disease are linked. ACML is currently the principal disorder in which rational biotherapy is being examined both at the cytokine and nucleotide levels. In this manner, it is the leader, as it was in the original discovery of a karyotypic abnormality associated with a specific malignancy.

REFERENCES

1. Rowley JD. A new consistant chromosomal abnormality in chronic myelogenous leukemia identified by quinine fluorescence and Giemsa staining. Nature 1973;243:290.
2. Canellos GP. Chronic granulocytic leukemia. Med Clin North Am 1976;60:1001–1018.
3. Li FP. The chronic leukemias: etiology and epidemiology. In: Wienik PH, Canellos GP, et al, eds. Neoplastic diseases of the blood. New York: Churchill Livingstone, 1985:7–14.
4. Castro-Malaspina H, Schaison G, Briere J, et al. Philadelphia chromosome-positive chronic myelocytic leukemia in children—survival and prognostic factors. Cancer 1983;52: 721–727.
5. Graw RG, Skeel RT, Carbone PP. Priapism in a child with chronic granulocytic leukemia. J Pediatr 1969;74:788–790.
6. Suri R, Goldman JM, Catovsky D, et al. Priapism complicating chronic granulocytic leukemia. Am J Hematol 1980;9: 295–299.
7. Rowe JM, Lichtman MA. Hyperleuekocytosis and leukostasis: common features of childhood chronic myelogenous leukemia. Blood 1984;63(5):1230–1234.
8. Barton JC, Conrad ME, Poon M. Pseudochloroma: extramedullary hematopoietic nodules in chronic myelogenous leukemia. Ann Intern Med 1979;91:735–738.
9. Hardisty RM, Speed DE, Till M. Granulocytic leukaemia in childhood. Br J Haematol 1964;10:551–566.
10. Castro-Malaspina H, Schaison G, Passe S, et al. Subacute and chronic myelomonocytic leukemia in children (juvenile CML): clinical and hematologic observations, and identification of prognostic factors. Cancer 1984;54: 675–686.
11. Spiers ASD, Bain BJ, Turner JE. The peripheral blood in chronic granulocytic leukaemia: study of 50 untreated Philadelphia-positive cases. Scand J Haematol 1977;18: 25–38.
12. Schmidt V, Mlynek ML, Leder LD. Electron microscopic characterization of mixed granulated (hybridoid) leucocytes of chronic myeloid leukemia. Br J Haematol 1988;68:175–180.
13. Homans HC, Young PC, Dickerman JD, et al. Adult-type CML in childhood: case report and review. Am J Pediatr Hematol Oncol 1984;6(2):220–224.
14. Vodopick H, Ropp EM, Edwards CL, et al. Spontaneous cyclic leukocytosis and thrombocytosis in chronic granulocytic leukemia. N Engl J Med 1972;286(6):285–290.
15. Goh K, Swisher SN, Herman EC. Chronic myelocytic leukemia and identical twins: additional evidence of the Philadelphia chromosome as postzygotic abnormality. Arch Intern Med 1967;20:214–219.
16. Dosik H, Rosner F, Sawitsky A. Acquired lipidosis: Gaucher-like cells and "blue cells" in chronic granulocytic leukemia. Semin Hematol 1972;9:309–316.
17. Sheridan BL, Weatherall DJ, Clegg JB, et al. The patterns of fetal haemoglobin production in leukaemia. Br J Haematol 1976;32:487–506.
18. Newman DR, Pierre RV, Linman JW. Studies on the diagnostic significance of hemoglobin F levels. Mayo Clin Proc 1973;48:199–202.
19. Rosner F, Schreiber ZR, Parise F. Leukocyte alkaline phosphatase: fluctuations with disease status in chronic granulocytic leukemia. Arch Intern Med 1972;130:892–894.
20. Beard MF, Pitney WR, Sanneman EH. Serum concentrations of vitamin B12 in patients suffering from leukemia. Blood 1954;9:789–794.
21. Perillie PE, Finch SC. Muramidase studies in Philadelphia chromosome-positive and chromosome-negative chronic granulocytic leukemia. N Engl J Med 1970;283(9):456–459.
22. Ganeson TS, Rassool F, Guo A-P, et al. Rearrangement of the BCR gene in Philadelphia chromosome-negative chronic myeloid leukemia. Blood 1986;68:957–960.
23. Kurzrock R, Blick MB, Talpaz M, et al. Rearrangement in the breakpoint cluster region and the clinical course in Philadelphia-negative chronic myelogenous leukemia. Ann Intern Med 1986;105:673–679.
24. Dreazen O, Klisak I, Rassool F, et al. Do oncogenes determine clinical features in chronic myeloid leukemia? Lancet 1987;1:1402–1405.
25. van der Plas DC, Hermans ABC, Soekarman D, et al. Cytogenetic and molecular analysis in Philadelphia negative CML. Blood 1989;73(4):1038–1044.

26. Wiederman LM, Karhi KK, Shivji M, et al. The correlation of breakpoint cluster region rearrangement and P210 Ph1/abl expression with morphological analysis of Ph-negative chronic myeloid leukemia and other myeloproliferative diseases. Blood 1988;71(2):349–355.

27. Lichtman MA, Rowe JM. Hyperleukocytic leukemias: rheological, clinical, and therapeutic considerations. Blood 1982;60(2):279–283.

28. Roath S, Davenport P. Leukocyte numbers and quality: their effect on viscosity. Clin Lab Haematol 1991;13:255–262.

29. Hild DH, Myers TJ. Hyperviscosity in chronic granulocytic leukemia. Cancer 1980;46:1418–1421.

30. Mason JE, DeVita VT, Canellos GR. Thrombocytosis in chronic granulocytic leukemia: incidence and clinical significance. Blood 1974;44(4):483–487.

31. Weick JK, Hagedorn AB, Linman JW. Leukoerythroblastosis: diagnostic and prognostic significance. Mayo Clin Proc 1974;49:110–113.

32. You W, Weisbrot IM. Chronic neutrophilic leukemia: report of two cases and review of the literatre. Am J Clin Pathol 1979;72:233–242.

33. Stoll DB, Peterson P, Exten R, et al. Clinical presentation and natural history of patient with essential thrombocythemia and the Philadelphia chromosome. Am Hematol 1988;27.77 83.

34. Kantarjian HM, Deisseroth A, Jurzrock R, et al. Chronic myelogenous leukemia: a concise update. Blood 1993;82(3):691–703.

35. Kurzrock R, Kantargian HM, Shtalrid M, et al. Philadelphia chromosome-negative chronic myelogenous leukemia without breakpoint cluster region rearrangement: a chronic myeloid leukemia with a distinct clinical course. Blood 1990;75(2):445–452.

36. Lion T, Gaiger A, Henn T, et al. Pure red cell aplasia in a case of Ph-negative Bcr/abl rearranged CML with t(12;14)(q23;p11). Cancer Genet Cytogenet 1991;56:189–195.

37. Fialkow PJ, Jacobson RJ, Papayannopoulou T. Chronic myelocytic leukemia: clonal origin in a stem cell common to the granulocyte, erythrocyte, platelet and monocyte/macrophage, Am J Med 1977;63:125–130.

38. Bryden J, Lucky PA, Duffy T. Acne urticata associated with chronic myelogenous leukemia. Cancer 1985;56:2083–2086.

39. Costagliola C, Rinaldi M, Coticelli L, et al. Case report: isolated optic nerve involvement in chronic myeloid leukemia. Leuk Res 1992;16(4):411–413.

40. Goldman JM, Lu D. New approaches in chroic granulocytic leukemia: origin, prognsois, and treatment. Semin Hematol 1982;19(4):241–256.

41. Stryckmanns PA. Current concepts in chronic myelogenous leukemia. Semin Hematol 1974;11(2):101–127.

42. Tokuhata GK, Neely CL, Williams DL. Chronic myelocytic leukemia in identical twins and a sibling. Blood 1968;31(2):216–225.

43. Miller RW: Leukemia and radiation. Pediatrics 1980;65(6):1160.

44. Bizzozero OJ Jr, Johnson KG, Ciocco A, et al. Radiation-related leukemias in Hiroshima and Nagasaki, 1946-1964. II. Observations on type-specific leukemia, survivorship, and clinical behavior. Ann Intern Med 1967;66(3):522–530.

45. Kanada N, Tanaka K. Cytogenetic studies of hematological disorders in atomic bomb survivors. In: Ishihara T, Saski MS, eds. Radiation-induced chromosome damage in man. New York: AR Liss, 1983:455–474.

46. Holmberg M. Is the primary event in radiation-induced chronic myelogenous leukemia the induction of the t(9;22) translocation Leuk Res 1992;16(4):331–336.

47. Gadner H, Haas OA: Experience in pediatric myelodysplastic syndromes. Hematol Oncol Clin North Am 1992;6(3):655–672.

48. Joblon S, Kato H. Childhood cancer in relation to prenatal exposure to atomic-bomb radiation. Lancet 1970;2:1000–1003.

49. Holm LE, Wiklung KE, Lundell GE, et al. Cancer risk in population examined with diagnostic doses of 131I. J Natl Cancer Inst 1989;81(4):302–306.

50. Walgraeve D, Verhoef G, Stul M, et al. Chronic myelogenous leukemia after treatment with 13I for thyroid carcinoma, report of a case and review of the literature. Cancer Genet Cytogenet 1991;55:217–224.

51. Bouabdallah K, Marit G, Reiffers J, et al. Hodgkin's disease and secondary Philadelphia chromosome-positive chronic myelogenous leukemia. Cancer Genet Cytogenet 1991;55:277–278.

52. Aksoy M. Benzene: leukemia and malignant lymphoma. In: Roath S, Wright J, eds. Topical Reviews in Haematology (no 2) Bristol: 1982;2:105.

53. Haas OA, Argyriou-Tirita A, Lion T. Parental origin of chromosomes involved in the translocation t(9;22). Nature 1992;359:414–416.

54. Gordon MY, Clark D, Goldman JM, et al. Deficiency of a phosphatidyl-anchored cell adhesion molecule in chronic myeloid leukemia. Nature (Lond.) 1984;328:342–344.

55. Verfaillie CM, McCarthy JB, McGlave PB. Mechanisms underlying abnormal trafficking of malignant progenitors in chronic myelogenous leukemia—decreased adhesion to stroma and fibronectin but increased adhesion to the basement membrane components laminin and collagen type IV. J Clin Invest 1992;90:1232–1241.

56. Baker MA, Taub RN, Welhton CH, et al. Aberrant sialylation of granulocyte membranes in chronic myelogenous leukemia. Blood 1984;63:1194–1197.

57. Anklesaria PN, Advani SH, Bhisey AN. Defective chemotaxis and adherence in granulocytes from chronic myeloid leukemia (CML) patients. Leuk Res 1985;9:641–648.

58. Desai H, Zingde S, Advani S, et al. Differential phosphorylation—cause for defective internalization of aggregated IgG by chronic myeloid leukemic granulocytes? Leuk Res 1992;16(3):235–245.

59. Pederson B. Functional and biochemical phenotype in relation to cellular age of differentiated neutrophils in chronic myeloid leukaemia. Br J Haematol 1982;51:339–344.

60. Rambaldi A, Terao M, Bettoni S, et al. Expression of leukocyte alkaline phosphatase gene in normal and leukemic cells: regulation of the transcript by granulocyte colony-stimulating factor. Blood 1990;76(12);2565–2571.

61. Chikkappa G, Wang GJ, Santella D, et al. Granulocyte colony-stimulating factor (G-CSF) induces synthesis of alkaline phosphatase in neutrophilic granulocytes of chronic myelogenous leukemia patients. Leuk Res 1988;12(6):491–498.

62. Sato N, Mizukami H, Tani K, et al. Regulation of mRNA levels of alkaline phosphatase gene in neutrophilic granulocytes by granulocyte colony-stimulating factor and retinoic acid. Eur J Haematol 1991;46:107–111.

63. Schiffer CA, Aisner J, Daly PE, et al. Increased leukocyte alkaline phosphatase activity following transfusion of leuko-

cytes from a patient with chronic myelogenous leukemia. Am J Med 1979;66:519–522.

64. Rustin GJS, Goldman JM, McCarthy D, et al. An extrinsic factor controls neutrophil alkaline phosphatase synthesis in chronic granulocytic leukemia. Br J Haematol 1980;45:381–387.

65. Gimsing P, Nex OE. The turnover of 57Co-labeled cyanocobalin bound to cobalamin binding proteins in patients with chronic myelogenous leukemia. J Lab Clin Med 1994;123(2):264–272.

66. Jonas D, Lubbert M, Kawasaki ES, et al. Clonal analysis of bcr-abl rearrangement in T lymphocytes from patients with chronic myelogenous leukemia. Blood 1992;79(4):1017–1023.

67. Fauser AA, Kanz L, Bross KJ, et al. T cells and probably B cells arise from the malignant clone in chronic myelogenous leukemia. J Clin Invest 1985;75:1080–1082.

68. Greenberg Br, Wilson FD, Woo L, et al. Cytogenetics of fibroblastic colonies in Ph-positive chronic myelogenous leukemia. Blood 1978;51(6):1039–1045.

69. Clarkson B, Strife A, Perez A, et al. Integration of molecular and biological abnormalities in quest for selective treatment of chronic myelogenous leukemia (CML). Leuk Lymphoma 1993;11(2):81–100.

70. Lewis JP. Evidence that 9pter→34::q34→qter is the initial DNA lesion converting benign to malignant hematopoiesis in chronic myelogenous leukemia (CML). Clin Research 1983;31(1):88A.

71. Daley GQ, Van Etten RA, Baltimore D. Induction of chronic myelogenous leukemia in mice by the P210bcr/abl gene of the Philadelphia chromosome. Science 1990;247:824–847.

72. Fialkow PJ, Martin PJ, Najfeld V, et al. Evidence for a multistep pathogenesis of chronic myelogenous leukemia. Blood 1981;58(1):158–163.

73. Altman AJ. Chronic leukemias of childhood. In: Pizzo P, Poplack D, eds. Principles and practice of pediatric oncology. 1993;2:501–518.

74. Chervenick PA, Boggs DR. Granulocyte kinetics in chronic myelocytic leukemia. Semin Hematol 1968;1(1):24.

75. Peschel C, Aman MJ, Rudolf G, et al. Regulation of the cytokine network by interferon: a potential mechanism of interferon in chronic myelogenous leukemia. Semin Hematol 1993;30(3)(Suppl 3):28–31.

76. Strife A, Clarkson B. Biology of chronic myelogenous leukemia: is discordant maturation the primary defect? Semin Hematol 1988;25(1):1–19.

77. McGahon A, Bissonnette R, Schmitt M, et al. BCR-ABL maintains resistance of chronic myelogenous leukemia cells to apoptotic cell death. Blood 1994;83(5):1179–1187.

78. Broxmeyer HE, Gentile P, Cooper S, et al. Functional activities of acidic isoferritins and lactoferrin in-vitro and in-vivo. Blood Cells 1984;10:397–426.

79. Olafsson T, Olsson T. Suppression of normal granulopoiesis in vitro by a leukemia-associated inhibitor (LAI) of acute and chronic leukemia. Blood 1980;55(6):975–982.

80. Maybee, D, Dubowy R, Krischer J, et al. High-dose interferon-alpha 2b(IFNα) treatment of Philadelphia chromosome positive (Ph+) chronic myelogenous leukemia (CML) in children. Proc ASCO 1995;14:A1043.

81. Galbraith PR, Abu-Zahra HT. Granulopoiesis in chronic granulocytic leukemia. Br J Haematol 1972;22:135–143.

82. Athens JW, Raab SO, Haab OP, et al. Leukokinetic studies X. Blood granulocytes kinetics in chronic myelocytic leukemia. J Clin Invest 1965;44(5):765–777.

83. Schwartz JH, Canellos GP. Hydroxyurea in the management of the hematologic complications of chronic granulocytic leukemia. Blood 1975;46(1):11–16.

84. Silverstein MN, Petitt RM, Solberg LA, et al. Anagrelide: a new drug for treating thrombocytosis. N Engl J Med 1988;318:1292–1294.

85. Allegretta GJ, Weisman SJ, Altman AJ. Oncologic emergencies I: metabolic and space-occupying consequences of cancer and cancer treatment. Pediatr Clin North Am 1985;32(3):601–611.

86. Hester JP, McCredie KB, Freirech EJ. Response to chronic leukapheresis procedures and survival of chronic myelogenous leukemia patients. Transfusion 1982;22:305–307.

87. Morris TCM, Vincent PC, Gunz FW, et al. Evidence following splenic radiotherapy for a highly dynamic traffic of CGU-GM between the spleen and other organs in chronic granulocytic leukemia. Leuk Res 1987;11(2):109–117.

88. Li JG. The leukocytopenic effect of focal splenic X-irradiation in leuekemic patients. Radiology 1963;80:471–476.

89. Report of the Medical Research Council's Working Party for Therapeutic Trails in Leukaemia. Chronic granulocytic leukemia: comparison of radiotherapy and busulfan therapy. Br Med J 1968;1:201–208.

90. Gratwohl A, Hermans J, Biezen AV, et al. Splenic irradiation prior to bone marrow transplantation in patients with CML in chronic phase. A prospective randomized study of the European group for bone marrow transplantation. Chronic Myeloid Leukemia, 2nd International Conference, Bologna, Italy, 1992:41.

91. Mitelman F, Brandt L, Nilsson PG. Cytogenetic evidence for splenic origin of nestic transformation in chronic myelogenous leukemia. Scand J Haematol 1974;13:87–92.

92. Italian Cooperative Group on Chronic Myeloid Leukemia. Results of a prospective study of early splenectomy in chronic myeloid leukemia. Cancer 1984;54:333–338.

93. Medical Research Council's Working Party for Therapeutic Trials in Leukemia. Randomized trial of splenectomy in Ph1-positive chronic granulocytic leukemia, including an analysis of prognostic factors. Br J Haematol 1983;54:415–430.

94. Gratwohl A, Goldman J, Gluckman E, et al. Effect of splenectomy before bone marrow transplantation on survival in chronic granulocytic leukemia. Lancet 1985;2:1290–1291.

95. Rushing D, Goldman A, Gibbs G, et al. Hydrozyurea versus busulfan in the treatment of chronic myelogenous leukemia. Am J Clin Oncol 1982;5:307–313.

96. Bolin RW, Robinson WA, Sutherland J, et al. Busulfan versus hydroxyurea in the long term therapy of chronic myelogenous leukemia. Cancer 1982;50:1683–1686.

97. Galton DAG. Chemotherapy of chronic myelocytic leukemia. Semin Hematol 1969;6(4):323–343.

98. Hehlmann R, Heimpel H, Kolb JH, et al. Randomized comparison of busulfan and hydroxyurea in chronic myelogenous leukemia: prolongation of survival by hydroxyurea. Blood 1993;82(2):398–407.

99. Brandt L, Mitelman F, Panani AS, et al. Extremely long duration of chronic myeloid leukemia with Ph1 negative cell Ph1 positive bone marrow cells. Scand J Haematol 1976;16:321–325.

100. Djaldetti M, Padeh B, Pinkas J, et al. Prolonged remission in chronic leukemia after one course of busulfan. Blood 1966;27:103–109.

101. Clarkson B. Editorial: chronic myelogenous leukemia: is aggressive treatment indicated? J Clin Oncol 1985;3(2):135–139.

102. Singer JW, Arlin Z, Najfeld V, et al. Restoration of nonclonal hematopoiesis in chronic myelogenous leukemia (CML) following a chemotherapy-induced loss of the Ph1 chromosome. Blood 1980;56(3):356–360.

103. Dube ID, Gupta CM, Kalousek DK, et al. Cytogenetic studies of early myeloid progenitor compartments in Ph positive chronic myeloid leukemia. I. Persistance of Ph1 negative committed progenitors that are suppressed from differentiating in vivo. Br J Haematol 1984;56:633–644.

104. Gishizky ML, Johnson-White J, Witte ON. Efficient transplantation of BCR-Abl induced chronic myelogenous leukemia-like syndrome in mice. Proc Natl Acad Sci USA 1993;90(8):3755–3759.

105. Talpaz M, Kantarjian HM, McCredie KB, et al: Clinical investigation of human alpha interferon in chronic myelogenous leukemia. Blood 1987;(5)69:1281–1288.

106. Talpaz M, Kantarjian HM, McCredit KB, et al. Interferon alpha produces sustained cytogenetic responses in chronic myelogenous leukemia Philadelphia chromosome-positive patients, Ann Intern Med 1991;114:532–538.

107. Dow LW, Raimondi SC, Culbert SJ, et al. Response to alpha-interferon in children with Philadelphia chromosome-positive chronic myelocytic leukemia. Cancer 1991;68:1678–1684.

108. Opalka B, Wandl U, Koppe J, et al. Molecular and in vitro stem cell analysis on patients (PTS) with chronic myelogenous leukemia (CML) under therapy with recombinant interferon α (IFN α-2B). Proc Am Assoc Cancer Res 1987;28:206(A818).

109. Freund M, Huber C. Interferon α has become a standard in the treatment of chronic myelogenous leukemia. Semin Hematol 1993;30(3):1–5.

110. Bhatia R, Wayner EA, McGlave PB, et al. Interferon α restores normal adhesion of chronic myelogenous leukemia hematopoietic progenitors to bone marrow stroma by correcting impaired β1 integrin receptor function. J Clin Invest 1994;94:384–391.

111. Meseri A, Delwail V, Brizard A, et al. Endogenous lymphokine activated killer cell activity and cytogenetic response in chronic myelogenous leukaemia treated with α-interferon. Br J Haematol 1993;83(2):218–222.

112. Quesada JR, Talpaz M, Rios A, et al. Clinical toxicity of interferons in cancer patients: A review. J Clin Oncol 1986;4(2):234–243.

113. Maybee D, Dubowy R, Pollock B, et al. Inadequacy of standard toxicity criteria in evaluation of complications of higher dose alpha interferon (αIFN) in children with Ph+ chronic myelogenous leukemia (CML). Proc ASPHO 1993;2:46.

114. Fernandez-Renada JM, LaVilla E, Odriozola J, et al. Interferon alpha 2 A in the treatment of chronic myelogenous leukemia in chronic phase. Results of the Spanish group. Leuk Lymph 1993;11(1):175–179.

115. Zuffa E, for the Italian Coopertive Study Group on Chronic Myeloid Leukemia. The Italian prospective study of interferon-alpha (Roferon-A) vs. chemotherapy—karyotypic response and survival at four years. Chronic Myeloid Leukemia, 2nd International Conference, Bologna, Italy, 1992:163.

116. Lazzarino M, Morra E, Merate S, et al. Evaluation of response to different therapies in chronic myelogenous leukemia according to risk assessment at diagnosis. Chronic Myeloid Leukemia, 2nd International Conference, Bologna, Italy, 1992:205.

117. Kloke O, Niederle N, Qiu JY, et al. Impact of interferon alpha-induced cytogenetic improvement on survival in chronic myelogenous leukaemia. Br J Haematol 1993;83(3):399–403.

118. Kluin-Nelemans JC, Louwagie A, Delannoy A, et al. CML treated by interferon α-2B vs. hydroxyurea alone: preliminary report of a large multicenter randomized trial. Blood 1992;80:358(A1423).

119. Claxton D, Deisseroth A, Talpaz M, et al. Polyclonal hematopoiesis in interferon-induced cytogenetic remissions of chronic myelogenous leukemia. Blood 1992;79(4):997–1002.

120. Wandl UB, Niederle N, Kranzhoff M, et al. Clonogenic assay is not predictive but reflects therapeutic efficacy of interferons in the treatment of chronic myelogenous leukemia. Int J Cell Cloning 1992;10(5):292–298.

121. Kantarjian HM, Keating MJ, Estey EH, et al. Treatment of advanced stages of Philadelphia chromosome-positive chronic myelogenous leukemia with interferon-α and low-dose cytarabine. J Clin Oncol 1992;10(5):772–778.

122. Guilhot F, Abgrall J-F, Harousseau J-L, et al. A multicentric randomised study of alpha 2b interferon (IFN) and hydroxyurea (HU) with or without cytosine-arabinoside (Ara-c) in previously untreated patients with Ph+ chronic myelogenous leukemia (CML): preliminary cytogenetic results. Leuk Lymph 1993;11(Suppl 1):181–183.

123. Goldman JM, McGlave P, Szydlo P, et al. Impact of disease duration and prior treatment on outcome of bone marrow transplants for chronic myelogenous leukemia. Blood 1992;80:(Abstr. Suppl. 1):170a.

124. Snyder DS, Negrin RS, O'Donnell MR, et al. Fractionated total-body irradiation and high-dose etoposide as a preparatory regimen for bone marrow transplantation for 94 patients with chronic myelogenous leukemia in chronic phase. Blood 1994;84(5):1672–1679.

125. McGlave P, Bartsch G, Anasetti C, et al. Unrelated donor marrow transplantation therapy for chronic myelogenous leukemia: initial experience of the National Marrow Donor Program. Blood 1993;81(2):543–550.

126. Advisory Committee of the International Bone Marrow Transplant Registry. Report from the International Bone Marrow Transplant Registry. Bone Marrow Transplant 1989;4:221–228.

127. Gratwhol A. Bone marrow transplantation for chronic myelogenous leukemia. The European Bone Marrow Transplantation experience in chronic myelogenous leukemia. Chronic Myeloid Leukemia, 2nd International Conference, Bologna, Italy, 1992.

128. Grotwhol A, Hermans J, Blezen AV, et al. Splenic irradiation before bone marrow transplantation for chronic myeloid leukemia: update of a prospective randomized study. Leuk Lymph 1993;11(1):227–231.

129. Butterini A, Gale RP. The role of T-cells in preventing relapse in chronic myelogenous leukemia. Bone Marrow Transplant 1987;2:351–354.

130. Marion T, Butturini A, Kantarjian H, et al. Survival of children with chronic myeloid leukemia. Am J Pediatr Heamtol Oncol 1992;14(3):229–232.

131. Santos GW. Busulfan and cyclophosphamide versus cyclophosphamide and total body irradiation for marrow transplantation in chronic myelogenous leukemia—a review. Leuk Lymph 1993;11(1):201–204.

132. Gamis AS, Haake R, McGlave P, et al. Unrelated-donor bone marrow transplantation for Philadelphia chromosome-positive chronic myelogous leukemia in children. J Clin Oncol 1993;11(5):834–838.

133. Claxton D, Kantarjian H, Kurzrock R, et al. Alpha interferon dose-dependent suppression of secondary clones in a patient with Philadelphia-positive chronic myelogenous leukemia. Acta Haematol 1990;83:149–151.

134. McGlave PB. De Fabritiis P, Deisseroth A, et al. Autologous transplants for chronic myelogenous leukaemia: results from eight transplant groups. Lancet 1994;343:1486–1488.

135. Reiffers J, Montastruc M, Marti G, et al. Autologous blood stem cell transplantation followed by recombinant alpha interferon as treatment for patients with high-risk chronic myelogenous leukemia: a report of 32 cases. Bone Marrow Transplant Unit, CHR Bordeaux, France. Leuk Lymph 1993;11(Suppl 1):297–299.

136. Rowe J, Ryan D, Diperiso J, et al. Autografting in chronic myelogenous leukemia followed by immunotherapy. Stem Cells 1993;11(Suppl 3):34–42.

137. Rizzoli V, Mangoni L, Almici C, et al. Autologous transplantation for chronic myelogenous leukemia with mafosfamide-treated marrow. Stem Cell 1993;11(Suppl. 3):25–30.

138. Gulati S, Lemoli R, Fraig M. Newer approaches in treating chronic myelogenous leukemia. Stem Cell 1993;11(Suppl 3):14–19.

139. Reiffers J, Trouette R, Marit G, et al. Autologus blood stem cell transplantation for chronic granulocytic leukaemia in transformation: a report of 47 cases. Br J Haematol 1991; 77:339–345.

140. Verfailie CM, Miller WJ, Boylan K, et al. Selection of benign primitive hematopoietic progenitors in chronic myelogenous leukemia on the basis of HLA-DR antigen expression. Blood 1992;79(4):1003–1010.

141. Deisseroth AB, Zu Z, Claxton D, et al. Genetic marking shows that Ph+ cells in autologous transplants of chronic myelogenous leukemia (CML) contribute to relapse after autologous bone marrow in CML. Blood 1994;83(10):3068–3076.

142. Butturini A, Gale RP. Clinical models of autotransplants in chronic myelogenous leukemia. Leuk Lymph 1993; 11(Suppl 1):255–257.

143. Fitzgerald D, Rowe JM, Heal J. Leukapheresis for control of chronic myelogenous leukemia during pregnancy. Am J Hematol 1986;22:213–218.

144. Dhingra K, Kurzrock R, Kantarjian H, et al. Minimal residual disease in interferon-treated chronic myelogenous leukemia: results and pitfalls of analysis based on polymerase chain reaction. Leukemia 1992;6(8):754–760.

145. Lee M, Khouri I, Champlin R, et al. Detection of minimal residual disease by polymerase chain reaction of bcr/abl transcripts in chronic myelogenous leukemia following allogeneic bone marrow transplantation. Br J Haematol 1992; 82(4):708–714.

146. Lion T, Henn T, Gaiger A, et al. Early detection of relapse after bone marrow transplantation in patients with chronic myelogenous leukaemia. Lancet 1993;341(8840):275–276.

147. Mackinnon S, Barnett L, Heller G, et al. Minimal residual disease is more common in patients who have mixed T-cell chimerism after bone marrow transplantation for chronic myelogenous leukemia. Blood 1994;83(11):3409–3416.

148. Kantarjian HM, Dixon D, Keating MJ, et al: Characteristics of accelerated disease in chronic myelogenous leukemia. Cancer 1988;61:1441–1446.

149. Ariad S, Seymour LK, McPhail AP, et al. Prognostic factors in chronic myeloid leukemia—importance of staging or disease biology. S Afr Med J 1992;81:299–303.

150. Gomez GA, Sokal JE, Walsh D. Prognostic features at diagnosis of chronic myelocytic leukemia. Cancer 1981;47:2470–2477.

151. Gralnick HR, Harbor J, Vogel C. Myelofibrosis in chronic granulocytic leukemia. Blood 1971;37(2):152–162.

152. Clough V, Geary CG, Hashmi K, et al. Myelofibrosis in chronic granulocytic leukemia. Br J Haematol 1979;42:515–526.

153. Tura S, Baccarani M, Corbelli G, and The Italian Cooperative Study Group on Chronic Myeloid Leukemia. Staging of chronic myeloid leukemia. Br J Haematol 1981;47:105–119.

154. Theologides A. Unfavorable signs in patients with chronic myelocytic leukemia. Ann Intern Med 1972;76:95–99.

155. Karanas A, Silver RT. Characteristics of the terminal phase of chronic granulocytic leukemia. Blood 1968;32(3):445–459.

156. Sokal JE, Cox EB, Baccarani M, et al. Prognostic discrimination in "good risk" chronic granulocytic leukemia. Blood 1984;63(4):789–799.

157. Nelkin BD, Przepiorka D, Burke PJ, et al. Abnormal methylation of the calcitonin gene marks progression of chronic myelogenous leukemia. Blood 1991;77(11):2431–2434.

158. Mashal R, Shtalrid M, Talpaz M, et al. Rearrangement and expression of p53 in the chronic phase and blast crisis of chronic myelogenous leukemia. Blood 1990;75(1):180–189.

159. Neubauer A, He M, Schmidt CA, et al. Genetic alterations in the p53 gene in the blast crisis of chronic myelogenous leukemia: analysis by polymerase chain reaction based techniques. Leukemia 1993;7(4):593–600.

160. Malinen T, Palotie A, Pakkala S, et al. Acceleration of chronic myeloid leukemia correlates with calcitonin gene hypermethylation. Blood 1991;77(11):2435–2440.

161. Kimura A, Nakata Y, Hyodo H, et al. Platelet-derived growth factor expression in accelerated and blastic phase of chronic myelogenous leukemia with myelofibrosis. Br J Haematol 1994;86(2):303–307.

162. Yamauchi K, Oda K, Shimamura K, et al. Pulmonary fibrosis with megakaryocytoid cell infiltration in accelerated phase of chronic myelogenous leukaemia. Br J Haematol 1993;84(2):329–331.

163. Hait WM, Choudhury S, Srimatkandada S, et al. Sensitivity of K562 human chronic myelogenous leukemia blast cells transfected with a human multidrug resistance cDNA to cytotoxic drugs and differentiating agents. J Clin Invest 1993; 91(5):2207–2215.

164. Baccarani M, Zaccaria A, Bagnara GP, et al. The relevance of extramedullary hemopoiesis to the staging of chronic myeloid leukemia. Boll Ist Sierotes Milan 1978;57(3):257–270.

165. Welborn JL, Lewis JP. Correlation of marrow iron patterns with disease status of chronic mydelogenous leukemia. Leuk Lymph 1993;10(6):469–475.

166. Saikia TK, Dhabhar B, Iyer RS, et al. High incidence of meningeal leukemia in lymphoid blast crisis of chronic myelogenous leukemia. Am J Hematol 1993;43(1):10–13.

167. Ekblom M, Borgstrom G, von Willebrand E, et al. Erythroid blast crisis in chronic myelogenous leukemia. Blood 1993;62(3):591–596.

168. Griffin JD, Todd RF III, Ritz J, et al. Differentiation patterns in the blastic phase of chronic myeloid leukemia. Blood 1983;61(1):85–91.

169. Griffin JD, Tantravahi R, Canelos GP. T-cell surface antigens in a patient with blast crisis of chronic myeloid leukemia. Blood 1983;61(4):640–644.

170. Bakhshi A, Minowada J, Arnold A, et al. Lymphoid blast crises of chronic myelogenous leukemia represent stages in the development of B-cell precursors. N Engl J Med 1983;309(14):826–831.

171. Bernstein R, Gale RP. Do chromosome abnormalities determine the type of acute leukemia that develops in CML? Leukemia 1990;4(1):65–68.

172. Priest Jr, Robison LI, McKenna RW, et al. Philadelphia chromosome positive childhood acute lymphoblastic leukemia. Blood 1980;56(1):15–22.

173. Kurzrock R, Shtalrid M, Kloetzer WS, et al. Expression of C-abl in Philadelphia-positive acute myelogenous leukemia. Blood 1987;70(5):1584–1588.

174. Kantarjian H, Talpaz M, Dhingra K, et al. Significance of the P210 versus P190 molecular abnormalities in adults with Philadelphia chromosome-positive acute leukemia. Blood 1991;78(9):2411–2418.

175. Heisterkamp, N, Jenkins R, Thibodeau S, et al. The bcr gene in Philadelphia chromosome positive acute lymphoblastic leukemia. Blood 1989;73(5):1307–1311.

176. Nathwani AC, Goldman JM. Management of chronic myeloid leukaemia in lymphoid blast transformation. Haematologica 1993;78:162–166.

177. Goldman JM, Apperley JF, Jones L, et al. Bone marrow transplantation for patients with chronic myeloid leukemia. N Engl J Med 1986;314(4):202–207.

178. Speck B, Bortin MM, Champlin R, et al. Allogeneic bone marrow transplantation for chronic myelogenous leukaemia. Lancet 1984;1:665–668.

179. Kantarjian HM, Keating MJ, Smith TL, et al. Proposal for a simple synthesis prognostic staging system in chronic myelogenous leukemia. Am J Med 1991;88:1–8.

180. Gerwirtz AM. Potential therapeutic applications of antisense oligodeoxynucleotides in the treatment of chronic myelogenous leukemia. Leuk Lymph 1993;11(Suppl 1):131–137.

181. Reisman LE, Trujillo JM. Chronic granulocytic leukemia of childhood: clinical and cytogenetic studies. J Pediatr 1963;62(5):710–722.

182. Smith KI, Johnson W. Classification of chronic myelocytic leukemia in children. Cancer 1974;34:670–679.

183. Clark RH, Taylor L, Wells R. Congenital juvenile chronic myelogenous leukemia: case report and review. Pediatrics 1984;73(3):324–326.

184. Shannon K, Nunez G, Dow LW, et al. Juvenile chronic myelogenous leukemia: surface antigen phenotyping by monoclonal antibodies and cytogenetic studies. Pediatrics 1986;77(3):330–335.

185. Heskel NS, White CR, Fryberger S, et al. Aleukemic leukemia cutis: juvenile chronic granulocytic leukemia presenting with figurative cutaneous lesions. J Am Acad Dermatol 1983;9(3):423–427.

186. Freedman MH, Estrov Z, Chan HSL. Juvenile chronic myelogenous leukemia. Am J Pediatr Hematol Oncol 1988;10(3):261–267.

187. Cannat A, Seligmann M. Immunological abnormalities in juvenile myelomonocytic leukaemia. Br Med J 1973;1:71–74.

188. Mays JA, Neerhout RC, Baby GC, et al. Juvenile chronic granulocytic leukemia: emphasis on cutaneous manifestations and underlying neurofibromatosis. Am J Dis Child 1980;134:654–658.

189. Weatherall DJ, Edwards JA, Donohoe WTA. Haemoglobin and red cell enzyme changes in juvenile myeloid leukaemia. Br Med J 1968;1:679–681.

190. Maurer HS, Vida LN, Honig GR. Similarities of the erythrocytes in juvenile chronic myelogenous leukemia to fetal erythrocytes. Blood 1972;39(6):778–784.

191. Travis SF. Fetal erythropoiesis in juvenile chronic myelocytic leukemia. Blood 1983;62(3):602–605.

192. Papayannopoulou T, Nakamoto B, Anagnou NP, et al. Expression of embryonic globins by erythroid cells in juvenile chronic myelocytic leukemia. Blood 1991;77(12):2569–2576.

193. Shapira Y, Polliack A, Cividalli G, et al. Juvenile myeloid leukemia with fetal erythropoiesis. Cancer 1972;30(2):353–357.

194. Ng CS, Lam TK, Chan JKC, et al. Juvenile chronic myeloid leukemia: a malignancy of S-100 protein positive histiocytes. Am J Clin Pathol 1988;90(5):575–582.

195. Estrov Z, Grunberger T, Chan HSL, et al. Juvenile chronic myelogenous leukemia: characteristics of the disease using cell cultures. Blood 1986;67(5):1382–1387.

196. Suda T, Miura Y, Mizoguchi H, et al. Characterization of hemopoietic precursor cells in juvenile-type chronic myelocytic leukemia. Leuk Res 1982;6(1):43–53.

197. Freedman MH, Estrov Z. Juvenile chronic myelogenous leukaemia and histiocytosis syndromes in children [letter]. Lancet 1987;1:754.

198. Clark RD, Hutter JJ Jr. Familial neurofibromatosis and juvenile chronic myelogenous leukemia. Hum Genet 1982;60:230–232.

199. Butcher M, Frenck R, Emperor J, et al. Molecular evidence that childhood monosomy 7 syndrome is distinct from juvenile chronic myelogenous leukemia and other childhood myeloproliferative disorders. Genes Chromosome Cancer 1995;12:50–57.

200. Estrov Z, Dubé ID, Chan HSL, et al. Residual juvenile chronic myelogenous leukemia cells detected in peripheral blood during clinical remission. Blood 1987;70(5):1466–1469.

201. Amenomori T, Tomonaga M, Yoshida Y, et al. Cytogenetic evidence for partially committed progenitor cell origin of chronic myelomonocytic leukaemia and juvenile chronic myelogenous leukaemia: both granulocyte-macrophage precursors and erythroid precursors carry identical marker chromosomes. Br J Hematol 1986;64(3):539–546.

202. Estrov Z, Zimmermann B, Grunberger T, et al. Characterizations of malignant peripheral blood cells of juvenile chronic myelogenous leukemia. Cancer Res 1986;46:6456–6461.

203. Emanuel PD, Bates LJ, Castleberry RP, et al. Selective hypersensitivity to granulocyte-macrophage colony stimulating factor by juvenile chronic myeloid leukemia hematopoietic progenitors. Blood 1991;77(5):925–929.

204. Symann M, de Montepellier C, Ninane J, et al. "Spontaneous" erythroid progenitor cells in the circulation and

monosomy 7 in juvenile chronic myelogenous leukemia. Cancer Genet Cytogenet 1982;6:183–185.

205. Dittrich M, Milde S, Dinkel E, et al. Sonographic biometry of liver and spleen size in childhood. Pediatr Radiol 1983; 13:206–211.

206. Nakamura H, Sadamori N, Ichimaru M, et al. Juvenile chornic myeloid leukemia: no rearrangement of the breakpoint cluster region. Cancer Genet Cytogenet 1988;36: 227–229.

207. Brodeur GM, Dow LW, Williams DL. Cytogenetic features of juvenile chronic chronic myelogenous leukemia. Blood 1979;53(5):812–819.

208. Ghione F, Meiucci C, Symonn M, et al. Cytogenetic investigations in childhood chronic myelocytic leukemia. Cancer Genet Cytogenet 1986;20:317–323.

209. Stollman B, Fonatsch CH, Havers W. Persistent Epstein-Barr Virus infection associated with monosomy 7 oschromosome 3 abnormality in childhood myeloproliferative disorders. Br J Haematol 1985;60:183–196.

210. Palmer CG, Provisor Al, Weaver DD, et al. Juvenile chronic granulocytic leukemia in a patient with trisomy 8, neurofibromatosis, and prolonged Epstein-Barr virus infection. J Pediatr 1983;102:888–892.

211. Inoue S, Ravindranath Y, Thompson RI, et al. Cytogenetics of juvenile type chronic granulocytic leukemia. Cancer 1977;39:2017–2024.

212. Inoue S, Shibata T, Ravinranath Y, et al. Clonal origin of erythroid cells in juvenile chronic myelogenous leukemia [letter]. Blood 1987;69:975–976.

213. Gay JC, Dessypris EN, Roloff JS et al. Juvenile features in adult-type chronic granulocytic leukemia. Am J Hematol 1984;16:99–102.

214. Miyauchi J, Asada M, Sasaki M, et al. Mutations of the N-*ras* gene in juvenile chronic myelogenous leukemia. Blood 1994;83(8):2248–2254.

215. Sieff CA, Chessells JM, Harvey BAM, et al. Monosomy 7 in childhood: a myeloproliferative disorder. Br J Haematol 1981;49:235–249.

216. Herrod HG, Dow LW, Sullivan JL. Persistent Epstein-Barr infection mimicking juvenile chronic myelogenous leukemia: immunologic and hematologic studies. Blood 1983; 61(6):1098–1104.

217. Kirby MA, Weitzman S, Freedman MH. Juvenile chronic myelogenous leukemia: differentiation from infantile cytomegalovirus infection. Am J Pediatr Hematol Oncol 1990; 12(3):292–296.

218. Thomas WJ, North RB, Poplack DG, et al. Chronic myelomonocytic leukemia in childhood. Am J Hematol 1981; 10:181–194.

219. Stockley RI, Eden OB. Chronic myelomonocytic leukaemia in infancy: a case report. Med Pediatr Oncol 1983;11:284–286.

220. Solal-Celigny P, Desaint B, Herrera A, et al. Chronic myelomonocytic leukemia according to FAB classification; analysis of 35 Cases. Blood 1984;63(3):634–638.

221. Kantarjian HM, Kurzrock R, Talpaz M. Philadelphia chromosome-negative chronic myelogenous leukemia and chronic myelomonocytic leukemia. Hematol Oncol Clin North Am 1990;4(2):389–404.

222. Martiat P, Michaux JL, Rodhain J, for the Groupe Francais de Cytogenetique Hematologipue. Philadelphia-negative (Ph−) chronic myeloid leukemia (CML): comparison with Ph+ CML and chronic myelomonocytic leukemia. Blood 1991;78(1):205–211.

223. Ohyashiki K, Ohyashiki J, Oshimura M, et al. Cytogenetic and *in vitro* culture studies on chronic myelomonocytic leukemia. Cancer 1984;54:2468–2474.

224. Pearson HA, Diamond LK. Chronic monocytic leukemia in childhood. J Pediatr 1958;53:259–270.

225. Orchard NP. Letterer-Siwe's syndrome: report of a case with unusual peripheral blood changes. Arch Dis Child 1950;25:151.

226. Holton CP, Johnson WW. Chronic myelocytic leukemia in infant siblings. Pediatr 1968;72:377–383.

227. Randall DL, Reiquam CW, Githens JH, et al. Familial myeloproliferative disease: a new syndrome closely simulating myelogenous leukemia in childhood. Am J Dis Child 1965;110:479–500.

228. Gaultieri RJ, Emanuel PD, Zuckerman KS, et al. Granulocyte-macrophage colony stimulating factor is an endogenous regulator of cell proliferation in juvenile chronic myelogenous leukemia. Blood 1989;74(7):2360–2367.

229. Freedman MH, Cohen A, Grunberger T, et al. Central role of tumour necrosis factor, GM-CSF, and interleukin 1 in the pathogenesis of juvenile chronic myelogenous leukaemia. Br J Haematol 1992;80:40–48.

230. Schirò R, Longoni D, Rossi V, et al. Suppression of juvenile chronic myelogenous leukemia colony growth by interleukin-1 receptor antagonist. Blood 1994;83(2):460–465.

231. Lau RC, Squire J, Brisson L, et al. Lymphoid blast crisis of B-lineage phenotype with monosomy 7 in a patient with juvenile chronic myelogenous leukemia (JCML). Leukemia 1994;8(5):903–908.

232. Arico M, Bossi G, Schiro R, et al. Juvenile chronic myelogenous leukemia: report of the Italian registry. Assoc Italiana di Ematologia Oncologia Pediatrica. Haematologica 1993;78(5):264–269.

233. Chan HS, Estrov Z, Weitzman SS, et al. The value of intensive combination chemotherapy for juvenile chronic myelogenous leukemia. J Clin Oncol 1987;5(12): 1960–1967.

234. Lilleyman JS, Harrison IF, Black JA. Treatment of juvenile chronic myeloid leukemia with sequential subcutaneous cytarabine and oral mercaptopurine. Blood 1977;49(4): 559–562.

235. Estrov Z, Lau AS, Williams BRG, et al. Recombinant human interferon alpha-2 and juvenile chronic myelogenous leukemia: cell receptor binding, enzymatic induction, and growth suppression *in vitro*. Exp Hematol 1987;15: 127–132.

236. Arico M, Nespoli L, Casselli D, Bonetti F, et al. Juvenile chronic myeloid leukemia and alpha-interferon. Eur J Pediatr 1989;148(4):379–380.

237. Hazani A, Barak Y, Berant M, et al. Congenital juvenile chronic myelogenous leukemia: therapeutic trial with interferon alpha-2. Med Pediatr Oncol 1993;21:73–76.

238. Maybee DA, Dubowy RL, Krischer J, et al. Unusual toxicity of high dose alpha interferon (αIFN) in the treatment of juvenile chronic myelogenous leukemia (JCML). Proc ASCO 1992;11:A950.

239. Suttorp M. Letter to the Editor: Interferon-alpha-2 (IFN) plus hydroxyurea for treatment of juvenile chronic myelogenous leukemia. Med Pediatr Oncol 1994;22: 358–359.

240. Sanders JE, Buckner CD, Stewart P, et al. Successful treatment of juvenile chronic granulocytic leukemia with marrow transplantation. Pediatrics 1979;63(1):44–46.

241. Sanders JE, Buckner CD, Thomas ED, et al. Allogeneic marrow transplantation for children with juvenile chronic myelogenous leukemia. Blood 1988;71(4):1144–1146.

242. Festa RS, Shende A, Lanzkowski P. Juvenile chronic myelocytic leukemia: experience with intensive combination chemotherapy. Med Pediatr Oncol 1990;18:311–316.

243. Shepherd PCA, Ganesan TS, Galton DAG. Haematological classification of the chronic myeloid leukemias. Baillierés Clin Haematol 1987;1(4):887–906.

CHAPTER 27

Secondary Leukemias and Lymphomas: Iatrogenic Hematologic Malignancies

STUART ROATH

When people's ill, they comes to I,
I physics, bleeds and sweats 'em;
Sometimes they live, sometimes they die.
What's that to I? I lets 'em.
—Lettsom, *On Himself*, 1815

The single most untoward complication of cancer chemotherapy in patients with seemingly long-term survivals has been the occurrence of second malignancies, including those of the hemopoietic system (1). Incriminated along with therapeutic irradiation (including isotopes) and prolonged immunosuppressive therapy are most of the commonly used antitumor drugs (Table 27.1). By far the most frequently encountered hematopoietic malignancy is acute myelogenous or myeloblastic leukemia (AML), but there are also reports of other acute leukemias, myelodysplasias, and non-Hodgkin's lymphoma.

Case 1

A 31-year-old male office worker presented with lassitude and dyspnea on exertion of gradual onset over approximately 3 months, unaccompanied by systemic symptoms such as fever, sweats, or weight loss. His history was significant in that 5 years previously, after investigation for night sweats, fever, weight loss, and cervical adenopathy, he had been diagnosed as having mixed cellularity Hodgkin disease stage IIIB, successfully treated with 6 courses of MOPP (nitrogen mustard, Oncovin, procarbazine, and prednisolone). No radiotherapy (RT) was administered. Follow-up, the last occasion being 6 months previously, had revealed no signs of recurrent disease or hematologic abnormality.

*Physical examination revealed a pale young man with no adenopathy or splenomegaly. His skin was free from petechiae or ecchymoses, and no retinal hemorrhages or infiltration were seen. The liver edge was just palpable, and he had a mild tachycardia at 94/minute. Chest x-ray showed no mediastinal or pulmonary disease nor significant cardiomegaly. His automated blood count showed an Hgb of 82 g/L; WBC, 1.9 × 10⁹/L (ANC 0.2 × 10⁹/L); and platelets, 55 × 10⁹/L. The film con-*firmed leukopenia and thrombocytopenia but also showed 25% of the mononuclear cells to be blast cells, subsequently identified by cytochemistry as moderately differentiated myeloblasts. The diagnosis of AML M_2 was confirmed by the bone marrow, which also showed a hypocellular picture with some fibrosis. Most cells were M2 myeloblasts with CD-13/CD-33 phenotype. Karyotyping showed a complex abnormality including partial deletion of #7 in most cells assessed.*

Differential Diagnosis. The causes of pancytopenia in an adult not acutely ill or on medication are limited. Hematologic neoplasms or other bone marrow infiltrating disorders, either malignant or granulomatous, would be considered first, followed by other causes of bone marrow failure such as de novo fibrosis and aplasia. Infection or autoimmune diseases may also cause pancytopenia, but they would be unlikely to demonstrate peripheral blood blast cells. The diagnosis was AML.

Assessment. In view of his previous history of Hodgkin's disease (HD) and the timing of the presentation, secondary AML associated with the treatment of his HD was strongly suspected. Because this usually has a poor prognosis, a search was immediately established for matched tissue typing among family and, if not available there, via the National Marrow Donor Registry, and remission induction treatment with idarubicin and cytosine arabinoside was begun.

Comment. Typically, secondary leukemia and myelodysplasia (MDS) present with fatigue or, somewhat less often (50%), fever. Bleeding manifestations tend to be found on examination rather than being presenting symptoms. Splenomegaly, gingivitis, and skin lesions are less common than in primary acute leukemia (AL). Ane-

Table 27.1. Known Leukemogenic Agents

Alkylating agents
  Busulfan
  Chlorambucil
  Cyclophosphamide
  Melphalan
  Nitrogen mustard (and derivatives)
  Nitrosoureas
    BCNU, CCNU
  Procarbazine
  Thiotepa
Topoisomerase inhibitors
  Etoposide (VP-16)
  Tenoposide (VM-26)
Platinum compounds
  Cisplatin
  Carboplatin

mia is usually found on laboratory investigation as is thrombocytopenia, but severe leukopenia or extreme leukocytosis is uncommon. Both the blood and marrow may show dysplastic changes in any lineage, and the percentage of blasts varies, as do bone marrow cellularity and fibrosis. Auer rods and cytochemistry showing differentiation are less marked than in primary AL. There are no specific CD phenotypes expected. Secondary leukemias and MDSs appear to be congruent in terms of presentation, biology, management, and prognosis.

Case 2

A 10-year-old Caucasian female was admitted to the hospital with a history of intermittent fever, pallor, and occasional petechiae of approximately 1 month's duration. Her past history, family history, and review of systems were unrevealing. On physical examination, the characteristic findings included fever and pallor, as noted, along with diffusely distributed petechiae and ecchymoses; cervical and axillary confluent adenopathy; and a slightly enlarged spleen. Blood counts were as follows: Hgb, 73 g/L; WBC, 25 × 10⁹/L; platelets, 40 × 10⁹/L; and a peripheral blood count revealed 30% blast forms that appeared to be predominantly L1 (25% L2). The presumptive diagnosis of acute lymphocytic leukemia was verified by bone marrow that was hypercellular and essentially replaced by HLA-DR-positive, TdT-negative, CD 10−, and CD 19+ lymphoblasts. Her cells were hypodiploid and showed a t(4,11) abnormality. Her cerebrospinal fluid was free of disease. She received an intermediate-risk regimen because of the modest increase in tumor burden, the CD 10− hypodiploid appearance, and her upper-limit age risk.

She underwent successful induction of remission with a combination of vincristine, prednisone, L-asparaginase, and daunomycin along with triple intrathecal (IT) therapy consisting of methotrexate hydrocortisone and cytosine arabinoside every 3 weeks. She also received intensification with intermediate-dose methotrexate

and cytosine arabinoside alternating with etoposide/cyclophosphamide. At the end of 6 months, therapy was changed to daily 6-mercaptopurine and weekly methotrexate. Monthly intrathecal therapy was discontinued at the end of the second year of therapy. All therapy was discontinued after 3 years; 6 months later she became febrile and pancytopenic. A blood film showed misshapen red cells as well as occasional primitive cells. She deteriorated rapidly and developed nucleated petechiae and purpura; her bone marrow revealed M₂ (CD 14+) myeloblasts. She again remitted on cytarabine and daunorubicin and received a bone marrow transplantation from an older sibling. Following this, she is in apparent hematologic remission.

Differential Diagnosis. In a child of this age, 3 years after the discontinuation of treatment for ALL, leukemic relapse still has to be considered. Additionally, there is an increased incidence of second tumors including clonally different acute leukemia or MDS. Acute viral illnesses and, even at this late stage, opportunistic infections with Pneumocystis or tuberculosis might occur. However, the appearance of blast cells in the peripheral blood pointed toward acute leukemia, which was confirmed as myeloid by the marrow analysis, cell phenotyping, and karyotyping.

In view of the previous history of Hodgkin disease in the patient in case 1 and ALL in the patient in case 2, respectively, and the timing of the presentation, therapy-induced secondary AML was diagnosed in both cases. Because of the poor prognosis typically seen in secondary AML, preparations were made for this patient as well to follow remission induction therapy with allogeneic bone marrow transplantation.

Comment: Causes of Secondary Leukemia. Although the relationship between ionizing radiation and leukemia development is well known, the risks of such a sequel are higher following the use of drugs (2), where chemotherapy-related leukemia or MDS are important complications of tumor treatment for long-term survivors. The relative risk calculated following RT alone in Hodgkin's disease is of the order of 10, while that for alkylating agents is 5–50 times as much again (2).

Drugs. Table 27.1 lists those drugs known to be leukemogenic. Most of those developed for the treatment of tumors, including leukemia itself, are incriminated in leukemogenesis: others, some also used to treat nonmalignant disease, have been said to occasionally cause leukemia or lymphoma. They and compounds such as benzene or pesticides are not considered under this heading.

Antitumor drugs in the anthracycline, antibiotic, and hormone categories, and agents such as the vinca alkaloids and asparaginase are less likely to be leukemogenic. Hydroxyurea and other antimetabolites or DNA precursor blockers are also relatively benign in this respect.

Although there is some crossover between mutagenicity and leukemogenesis, the mechanisms are dissimilar, and Table 27.1 is not an appropriate listing of mutagens.

The leukemias or lymphomas or related disorders secondary to therapy have certain characteristics of varying degrees of certainty, including:

1. An "incubation period" from 1–2 to 10 or more years
2. Leukemias are frequently myelogenous
3. MDS; for example, refractory anemia with excess blasts, transforming (RAEBt) precedes the above
4. Karyotypic abnormalities are nearly always present
5. The lymphomas resemble those occurring in AIDS patients
6. Drug/drug or drug/RT combinations are more leukemogenic than are single agents
7. Prognosis is often worse in therapy-induced leukemia than in the primary equivalent

Less certain relationships include:

8. The resulting second malignancy may be related to the type of therapy
9. Total drug dosage may be related to leukemogenesis
10. The mode of administration may be critical
11. Some underlying disorders may predispose to secondary leukemia or lymphoma

1. Incubation Period. Second neoplasms including leukemias and lymphomas may arise at any time following treatment or even during the later phases of therapy. However, the peak incidence is about 5 years, with a long tail of up to 20 years. The first of our patients fits well into this time span. Factors influencing the shape of the curve probably include (a) age (older adults have shorter intervals from the original therapy to the onset of leukemia than younger; children may also have short intervals as in our second case), (b) the type of treatment (e.g., etoposide may have a shorter period), and (c) intensity, which varies inversely with the latent period (3). The age-related curve of secondary AML incidence follows that of the primary disorder

2. All Types of AML Are Found Related to Therapy. M_1 and M_2 are the most frequent, but M_4 and M_5 occur in most cases of etoposide-related leukemias. There are a few reports of secondary ALL, but they are difficult to associate with any particular form of therapy and less well documented than AML. CML and CLL do not appear to occur as a result of drug or drug/radiation therapy, although accidental exposure to radiation is a cause of the former as well as both types of acute leukemia (4).

3. Most Cases of Secondary AML Are Preceded by MDS. If serial observations were carried out on all subjects at risk, this might be universally true. The MDS is usually RAEB or RAEBt at the time of presentation. However, dysplastic changes in hemopoiesis can be seen regularly following treatment with anticancer drugs and radiation, and these changes may persist for some time, so other factors (e.g., cytogenetics) need to be considered in confirming the diagnosis of secondary AML. Un-

like the primary form, the MDS seen is frequently associated with a hypocellular and/or fibrotic bone marrow (5), so biopsy is always necessary to confirm the pathology.

4. Virtually All Cases of Secondary, Therapy-Related Leukemia and Lymphoma Have Abnormal Karyotypes (6). The commonest changes, especially with alkylating agent–associated leukemia, are loss of material (i.e., either whole or partial deletions). As with primary MDS, chromosomes 5 and 7 are most frequently involved (about two-thirds of all cases) (7); less often, chromosomes 3, 12, 17, and 18. Chromosome 5 is known to be the location of a number of cytokine governors and growth factors, but how loss of material on the chromosome leads to leukemia is not known (discussed in the MDS section). Balanced translocations were not reported until the topoisomerase II–active drugs came into use. The high rate of DNA strand breakage due to these agents appears to give rise to rearrangements, especially in chromosomes 11(q23) or 21(q22) and, less often, 8, 9, 15, and 17.

It is difficult to construct a unified hypothesis for the molecular origins of the second malignancies following therapy. Although, like their primary counterparts, they are clonal, no single tumor suppressor gene, the most obvious candidate when chromosomal loss occurs, can be identified. Similarly, no single oncogene association such as a consistent fusion gene emerges from these abnormalities. The assumption must be made that at present, as with MDS and primary AL, there are multiple routes to the dysregulation of cell growth and development leading to secondary AL.

5. Lymphomas Resemble Those Occurring in AIDS Patients. The lymphomas reported following immunosuppressive therapy for kidney and heart transplantation are well studied, and a relationship between immunosuppression with azathioprine and especially cyclophosphamide, and infection with Epstein-Barr (EB) virus may facilitate the oncogenic potential of this virus (8). Its genomic material is found within the tumor DNA, which is otherwise of host origin except following bone marrow transplantation, when it is donor derived (9). Relatively few cases of secondary AL in the latter are seen; they are associated with graft-versus-host disease (GVHD) and its prophylaxis by T-cell reduction or by aggressive treatment. No one type of lymphoma is found, but B-cell disease is usually seen, and multiple monoclonal or polyclonal tumors can occur at the same time. Other B-cell malignancies, such as Burkitt's lymphoma and Kaposi's sarcoma, are suggested to have similar etiologies. Such malignancies occur not only in this situation but also in AIDS, where up to 20% of patients may develop non-Hodgkin's lymphoma and, less commonly, Burkitt's and Hodgkin's lymphomas. AML, ALL, myeloma, and polycythemia vera have also been reported in this situation (10). Other than AML, these are rarely reported following previous antitumor therapy. Secondary leukemias are much less common than lymphomas following immunosuppressive treatment for benign, usually autoimmune, states, but their incidence is greater than that in similar patients otherwise treated (11, 12).

6. Therapeutic Combinations Are More Leukemogenic Than Are Single Agents. Although single-agent chemotherapy can cause secondary hemopoietic malignancies, it is presumed that combination chemotherapy or, to a lesser extent, RT and chemotherapy may act synergistically in their provocation. The best-studied group of patients in whom different therapeutic modalities have been used is Hodgkin's disease; MOPP, given to the first patient, can be compared with ABVD (adriamycin, bleomycin, vinblastine, and dacarbazine). Within these groups, there are also RT-treated subgroups. The numbers studied are large enough, as are the long-term survivals, to give useful data. (Single-agent therapy against this disorder did not produce enough long-term survivals for study, so comparisons can not be made with patients so treated). However, animal experimental data have supported the concept that both of the MOPP alkylating agents (nitrogen mustard and procarbazine) are leukemogens when used alone. The incidence of AML in MOPP-treated HD in a typical study is given as 8.4%, compared with none for the ABVD group (both groups received RT). Secondary lymphomas and solid tumors were infrequent in either group (3.6% for the MOPP treated and 4.1% for the ABVD) (13). Some studies have shown much higher levels (14) and also noted increased rates in patients over 48 years of age. The risk with curative RT alone is said to be 1%. If chemotherapy added to RT has apparently worsened the outcome, this may only have been seen in some studies in which a special sequence of treatment has occurred (e.g., chemotherapy following failed RT) or in conditioning for bone marrow transplantation (BMT). In a study of 206 autologous BMT-treated patients with lymphoma, both HD and non-HD, 9 cases of MDS or AML were seen. All had received cyclophosphamide as part of their conditioning; half had received cyclophosphamide and VP-16, and all had total body irradiation (TBI) (15). Combination alkylating agent therapy or an alkylating agent/RT combination is most often used in BMT conditioning, and there is a reported 6- to 7-fold increase in second malignancies (16) following such management.

Although the incidence of secondary leukemia associated with BMT was once said to be "low" (17), this view has altered more recently, and an incidence of 6–18% at 5 years is reported from various sources if cases of MDS are included. Predisposing factors appear to include the total amount of pretransplant treatment and low platelet counts, but process-associated elements also need to be considered, such as graft manipulation and the timing of conditioning regimens. More data related to autologous BMT are beginning to emerge, and not surprisingly, the development of MDS or AML is becoming a serious hazard, as for example, posttreatment autologous BMT for certain cancers and lymphoma (15–17). Autografts should be screened for preleukemic and karyotypic abnormalities as well as gene rearrangement as technology becomes available. Such data may clarify the role of prior chemo-

therapy and process-induced changes in leukemogenesis (18).

Both etoposide (VP-16) and tenoposide (VM-26) are leukemogenic; the former may have been culpable in our second patient, but she also received an alkylating agent, cyclophosphamide, and an anthracycline, daunorubicin. It has been suggested recently that topoisomerase inhibitors are most leukemogenic when given with alkylating agents, platinum compounds, or anthracycline. Since DNA topoisomerase II is involved in DNA repair and DNA is damaged by these other agents, the operation gains credence. VP-16 and VM-26 are rarely given as single agents, so clinical proof of this synergism would be difficult to obtain (19).

7. Survival in Secondary Leukemias Is Usually Regarded As Poorer Than in Primary Leukemias. Rosenbloom (3) suggests 4–6 months, compared with a mean of 20 months in de novo AML patients. However, those patients suitable for BMT do not appear to be prognostically disadvantaged compared with primary AML. In addition, those with de novo type cytogenetic abnormalities such as t21/23 or t15/17 appear to have the same AML outcomes. The remainder, such as those with MDS-related AML, often respond poorly to treatment; those with deletions of 5 and 7 do badly, whether de novo or secondary. No special mode of therapy for the typical secondary leukemia has been suggested, so allogeneic BMT (alloBMT) appears to offer the only prospect for long-term survival or possible cure (20). Much lower remission rates and survivals appear to be obtained with combination chemotherapy, usually involving cytarabine; however, many patients are older and/or also have karyotypes generally regarded as unfavorable (1). Their prognoses parallel those of transformed MDS or CML patients.

8. Do Particular Treatments Result in Specific Tumors? Alkylator therapy seems to give rise to AML of any type but usually M0, M1, or M2. Deletions of chromosomes 5 and 7 are also strongly linked to this form of drug therapy. Topoisomerase II inhibitors usually give rise to myelomonocytic or monocytic leukemias, and immunosuppressants such as cyclosporine and azathioprine, to lymphoproliferative disorders. As it has become possible to more precisely identify genetic omissions, rearrangements, or substitutions, especially with secondary leukemias, so is it possible to increase our understanding of the putative mechanisms involved. Topoisomerase active drugs have been especially suitable for study because of their relatively narrow range of leukemia production and consistent cytogenetic abnormalities. Typically, the **11q23** abnormality is found in up to 85% of such secondary leukemias, which are clinically characterized by rapid onset, no prior diagnosis of MDS, AML with monocytoid (M4 or 5 FAB type) features and a response to treatment like that of de novo AMLs with the same karyotype. DNA analysis has shown breakdown clustering at the level of the 70-kDa mixed-lineage leukemia (MLL) proto-oncogene and revealed a narrow (8-kDa) cluster area suggesting a precisely located, induced lesion similar to that found in the primary form of the leukemia (21). The same group has also looked at secondary AMLs with the **t9:11** translocation, in which preliminary results have suggested a parallel lesion (22). This would suggest chromosome 11 as the source of the oncogene activity, probably in a fusion gene resulting from translocation. Other evidence also suggests the MLL genes as targets for this drug (23). HRX gene rearrangements have also been reported in secondary leukemias with this same karyotype involving fusion with material from a variety of other loci. The same HRX gene zinc finger fusion product has also been found in primary leukemia. MLL, HRX, and ALL-1 may all be the same gene, targeted by etoposide, whose expression is disturbed by the translocation. The gene product is either part of, or affects, neighboring transcriptional-rich areas of the chromosome. Related mechanisms may be operative in infant acute leukemia, in which MLL rearrangement was found in most patients studied with both the ALL and AML variants. However, secondary ALL has also now been reported following etoposide treatment with RT for Hodgkin's disease, as has acute promyelocytic leukemia (APML) with the expected 15:17 translocation. This suggests that other DNA alterations are also possible.

9. The Effect of Dose Variations. The effect of dose variations can best be found in the many studies on Hodgkin's disease, in which a relationship between incidence and rapidity of onset of the secondary leukemia and duration and amount of treatment can be determined (24, 25). Addition of RT in this group of patients appears to increase the rate of leukemia occurrence (26), and salvage chemotherapy doubles the AML percentage from 5 to 10% according to one report (27). A dose-response relationship has also been noted with ovarian cancer (28), polycythemia vera (29), and myeloma (30).

10. Modes of Drug Therapy Administration. The PRV Study Group report suggested a relationship between the frequency of chlorambucil administration and AML (29). Melphalan has been reported as less leukemogenic when given in pulsed treatment than when given continuously (31), though other studies have shed doubt on this finding. Few other relevant data are available.

11. Underlying Disorders. There may be different responses to leukemogenic drugs, depending on the underlying disorder. When there is already *disturbed immune responsiveness*, an increased incidence of spontaneous neoplasms is well known, as in CLL and congenital immune defects (32). The chapters on congenital disorders of neutrophil production and immune deficiency states describe some of these. The situation in CLL and other lymphoproliferative disorders, however, regarding secondary ALs is unclear with relation to the effects of therapy, because of the numerous but conflicting reports of coexistent neoplasms of other types, including MDS and AML, in untreated CL (33, 34). Probably the incidence of these is less than 1% (35). There are reports of CMML—an uncommon secondary leukemia—and M4,5 acute leukemias associated with myeloma. Survivors of this disease treated with alkylating agents were reported as having a 17.4% in-

cidence of AML 4 years later (36). Hodgkin's disease is also accompanied by variable cellular and humoral immune defects but, unlike polycythemia vera and CLL stage A, long survivals in untreated patients do not allow observation of any natural (therapy-unrelated) rate of second malignancies in this disease. In addition, when *hemopoietic* dysregulation is already disturbed, AML has an inherently increased appearance. In the case of congenital disorders, such as Schwachmann's syndrome and Blackfan-Diamond anemia, underlying disorders such as CML and aplastic anemia (37) and probably polycythemia vera (PV) to a lesser extent and paroxysmal nocturnal hemoglobinuria (PNH) in adults, have a high inherent incidence of terminal AML (38). This may be worsened by a "second hit" from a leukemogenic drug. A well-studied instance of the effect of alkylating agents in this situation is PV, in which the natural incidence of AML is ~1–2%, that following radiation via $_{32}$P is 6%, and following chlorambucil therapy, 11%, all within 6 years of beginning treatment (29). Additionally, since it has become possible to cure childhood ALL, cases of AML are now reported in survivors of that disorder (39), as happened in our second case. Presumably, there is an underlying trend to develop malignant disease, as evinced by the first childhood malignancy, capitalized on by the treatment originally given, producing the second tumor. Secondary leukemia follows brain tumors in frequency of occurrence in this group of individuals.

Germ cell tumors are also known to have an increased incidence of leukemia, especially following long-term survivors treated with platinum compounds and alkylating agents. Interestingly, some leukemias have been identified as of the same clonal origin as the original tumors and so may be derived from a common prehemopoietic stem cell (40). Again, no long-term *untreated* survivors are available to discover whether this is a naturally evolving phenomenon.

Breast (41), ovarian (42), GI, and lung are the main *cancers* with the most data available for analysis. The incidence of AML varies according to the structure of the study, and different agents such as cyclophosphamide, nitrosoureas, and busulfan have been involved. In summary, at 5 years, there appears to be a cumulative risk of about 5% with these agents, approaching 10% in 10 years. Fewer data exist for etoposide and platinum compounds at present, and the studies cited are apparently uninfluenced by RT, which is said not to be leukemogenic alone as an adjuvant following surgery for breast cancer, for example (43).

Autoimmune disorders treated with cyclophosphamide or azathioprine have been reported as developing both AML and lymphoma. The especially increased of the former is low, but the drugs appear to be active as leukemogens or coleukemogens, perhaps with factors related to the underlying disease (11, 12). Disorders such as psoriasis treated with methotrexate do not develop a notable increase in AML despite its known mutagenic effect. Absolutely normal individuals are not given known leukemogens, so the suspicion of a disease-related cofactor cannot be eliminated in the previous discussions.

Therapeutic Radiation. Despite the knowledge that large doses of ionizing radiation are leukemogenic, whether accidental (e.g., exposure to atomic explosion) or iatrogenic (e.g., with the use of thorotrast (44)), therapeutic radiation alone seemingly results in few cases of leukemia in many large series (24). It may be that the exposure of significant volumes of bone marrow, such as the pelvis or spinal column, accounts for the higher levels in some reports and an underlying genetically determined predisposition to leukemia in others (e.g., those with ankylosing spondylitis, in whom the incidence of leukemia is increased tenfold by radiation (45)). However, such genetic susceptibility may be more subtle; for example, the lack of a tumor suppressive gene may predispose to more than one neoplasm given a "second hit" from radiation. Most of the data for the effects of therapeutic radiation come from the treatment of Hodgkin's disease (46, 47), with contributions from the treatment of breast cancer, non-Hodgkin's lymphoma, and myeloma. Both these latter especially, often have gross immunosuppressive defects, which may also act as coleukemogens. Leukemia associated with RT alone is said to have a somewhat better prognosis than average for secondary AL and to be less frequently associated with chromosome 5 and 7 deletions (48). The evidence for diagnostic radiation as leukemogenic is inconclusive, and experimental data show that there is likely to be a threshold level for radiation dosage and effect. Probably no more than 1% of leukemia is so induced (49). In utero diagnostic radiation has been abandoned, as has the argument about its tumorigenic potential, and no increase in childhood leukemia has been noted in fetuses believed to be irradiated in association with atomic explosions or accidents (50).

Biologic Response Modifiers. Interferon has recently been reported to be associated with an unexpected incidence of second malignancies following its use in hairy cell leukemia (HCL) (51, 52). In one report, 13 of 69 and, in the second report, 6 of 199 individuals developed a variety of second cancers. Hematologic malignancies were seen; the natural incidence of such second tumors in HCL is unknown. However, powerfully active biologic-response modifiers have a clear potential for promoting or facilitating malignant cell growth, and their clinical use needs to be carefully documented in this respect.

Conclusion

In summary, secondary therapy-related leukemias are well recognized and make up to 10–15% of those seen in practice (53). They are usually AML and very likely preceded by MDS. The clonal nature of AML (and the secondary lymphomas) is established, but the presence of a common genetic defect is only indicated in the DNA topoisomerase–active drug-induced disease. Long-term moni-

toring of candidate populations, including serial examination of asymptomatic chemotherapy-treated individuals for possible oncogenes, is necessary to understand the nature of the problem and distinguish epiphenomena from the underlying etiology. Karyotypic analysis is useful in determining prognosis and the aggressiveness of management. BMT is the best treatment for suitable patients at present.

REFERENCES

1. Levine EG, Bloomfield CD. Leukemia and myelodysplastic syndromes secondary to drug, radiation, and environmental exposure. Semin Oncol 1992;19:47.
2. Pedersen-Bjergaard J. Therapy related myelodysplasia and acute leukemia. Leuk Lymphoma 1995;15(Suppl):11.
3. Rosenbloom R, Schreck R, Koeffler HP. Therapy related myelodysplastic syndromes. In: Koeffler PH, ed. Myelodysplastic syndromes. Hematol Oncol Clin North Am 1992; 6:707.
4. Moloney WC, Rosenthal D. Acute leukaemia in adults secondary to other disorders. In: Roath S, ed. Topical reviews in haematology. Bristol: Wright, 1980:138.
5. Bennett JM, Moloney WC, Greene MH, et al. Acute myeloid leukemias and other myelopathic disorders following treatment with alkylating agents. Hematol Pathol 1987;1:99.
6. Bloomfield CD. Chromosome abnormalities in secondary myelodysplastic syndromes. Scand J Haematol 1986; 36(Suppl 45):82.
7. Whang-peng J, Young RC, Lee EC, et al. Cytogenetic studies in patients with secondary leukemia/dysmyelopoietic syndrome after different treatment modalities. Blood 1988; 71:403.
8. Sullivan JL. Epstein-Barr virus and lymphoproliferative disorders. Semin Hematol 1988;25:269.
9. Fischer A, et al. Bone marrow transplantation for immunodeficiency and osteopetrosis. European survey 1968–85. Lancet 1986;2:1080.
10. Saba H. Hematological complications of AIDS. Haematol Rev Commun 1994;8:225.
11. Muller W, Brandis M. Acute leukemia after cytotoxic treatment for nonmalignant disease in childhood. A case report and review of the literature. Eur J Pediatr 1981;136:105.
12. Louie S, Schwartz RS. Immunodeficiency and the pathogenesis of lymphoma and leukemia. Semin Hematol 1978; 15:117.
13. Valagussa P, et al. Secondary acute leukemia and other malignancies following treatment for Hodgkin's disease. J Clin Oncol 1986;4:830.
14. Aisenberg AC. Acute nonlymphocytic leukemia after treatment with Hodgkin's disease. Am J Med 1983;75:449.
15. Miller JS, Arthur DC, Litz CE, et al. MDS after ABMT: an additional late complication of curative cancer therapy. Blood 1994;83:3780.
16. Deeg HJ, et al. Exp Haematol 1984;12:660.
17. Treleaven J, Smith C. Late effects of bone marrow transplantation. In: Treleaven J, Barrett J, eds. Bone marrow transplantation in clinical medicine. Edinburgh: Churchill Livingstone, 1992:345.
18. Ager S, Wimperis JZ, Tolliday B, et al. Autologous bone marrow transplantation for Hodgkin's disease—a five-year single center experience. Leuk Lymphoma 1994;13:263.
19. Pedersen-Bjergaard J, Philip P, Larsen SO, et al. Therapy related myelodysplasia and acute myeloid leukemia. Cytogenetic characteristics of 1125 consecutive cases and risk in

seven cohorts of patients treated intensively for malignant diseases in the Copenhagen series. Leukemia 1993;7:1975.

20. DeWitte T, Zwaan F, Hermans J, et al. Allogenic bone marrow transplantation for secondary leukemia and myelodysplastic syndrome. A survey by the leukemia working party of the European bone marrow transplantation group. Br J Haematol 1990;74:151.

21. Domer PH, Head DR, Raimondi SC. Breakpoint clustering in secondary acute non lymphocytic leukemia. Blood 1993; 82(Suppl 1):34.

22. Domer PH, Head DR, Renganathan N, et al. Molecular analysis of MLL/11q23 secondary acute leukemia translocation breakpoint. Blood 1994;84(Suppl 1):439.

23. Hilden JM, Kersey JH. The MLL(11q23) and AF-4 (4q21) genes disrupted in t(4;11) acute leukemia: molecular and clinical studies. Leuk Lymphoma 1994;14:189.

24. Pederson-Bjergaard J, Philip P. Incidence of acute non lymphocytic leukemia, preleukemia and the acute myeloproliferation syndrome after up to 10 years after treatment of Hodgkin's disease. N Engl J Med 1982;307:965.

25. Greene MH, et al. Evidence of a treatment dose response in acute nonlymphocytic leukemias which occurs after therapy of non-Hodgkin's lymphoma. Can Res 1983;43:1891.

26. Devereaux S, et al. Leukemia complicating treatment for Hodgkin's disease: the experience of the British National Lymphoma Investigation. Br Med J 1990;301:1077.

27. Bernstein ML, Vekemans MJ. Chromosomal changes in secondary leukemias of childhood and adults. Crit Rev Oncol Hematol 1986;23:5.

28. Greene M, Boice J, Greer B, et al. Acute nonlymphocytic leukemia after therapy with alkylating agents with for ovarian cancer. N Engl J Med 1982;307:1416.

29. Berk P, Goldberg J, Silverstein M. Increased incidence of acute leukemia in polycythemia vera associated with chlorambucil therapy. N Engl J Med 1981;304:441.

30. Gonzales F, Trujillo JM, Alexanian R. Acute leukemia in multiple myeloma. Ann Intern Med 1977;86:440.

31. McIntyre OR, Pajak TF, Wiemik P, et al. Delayed leukemia in myeloma patients receiving pulsed vs continuous treatment. Blood 1981;58(Suppl 1):70.

32. McPhedran P, Heath CW. Acute leukemia occurring during chronic lymphatic leukemia. Blood 1970;37:9.

33. Hamblin T. Immunologic abnormalities in myelodysplastic disorders. Hematol Oncol Clin North Am 1992;3:571.

34. Lawlor E, et al. Acute myeloid leukemia occurring in untreated chronic lymphatic leukaemia. Br J Haematol 1979; 54:277.

35. Bergsagel D, Bailey A, Langley G, et al. The chemotherapy of plasma cell myeloma and the incidence of acute leukemia. N Engl J Med 1979;30:743.

36. Foerster J. Chronic lymphocytic leukemia. In: Lee, et al., eds. Wintrobe's clinical hematology. Philadelphia: Lea & Febiger, 1993:2034.

37. Titchell A, Gratwahl A, Wursch A, et al. Acute hematological complications of severe aplastic anemia. Br J Haematol 1988; 69:413.

38. Nowell P, Bergman G, Besa E, et al. Progressive preleukemia with a chromosomally abnormal clone in a kindred with the Estren-Damashek variant of Fanconi's anemia. Blood 1984; 64:1135.

39. Pui CH, Behm FG, Raimondi SC, et al. Secondary AML in children with treated for acute lymphatic leukemia. N Engl J Med 1989;321:1356.

40. Vlasveld LT, Splintreer TAW, Hagemeier A, et al. Acute myeloid leukemia with + 11i(12p) shortly after treatment with of mediastinal germ cell tumor. Br J Haematol 1994; 88:196.

41. Rosner F, Carey W, Zarrati MH. Breast cancer and acute leukemia: a report of 24 cases and review of the literature. Cancer 1979;44:1470.

42. Resnor RR, Hoover R, Fraumeni F, et al. Acute leukemia after alkylating agent therapy of ovarian cancer. N Engl J Med 1977;297:177.

43. Curtis RE, et al. Leukemia not following radiotherapy for breast cancer. J Clin Oncol 1988;7:21.

44. Janower ML, Mieltinen OS, Flynn MJ. Effects of thorotrast exposure. Radiology 1972;103:13.

45. Court Brown WM, Doll R. Mortality from cancer and other causes after radiotherapy for ankylosing spondylitis. Br J Med 1965;4:1372.

46. Coltman C Jr. Treatment related leukemias. In: Bloomfield CD, ed. Adult leukemias. The Hague: Nijhof, 1982:62.

47. Koeffler HP, Rowley JD. Therapy related non-lymphocytic leukemias. In: Wiernik PH, et al., eds. Neoplastic diseases of the blood. New York: Churchill Livingstone, 1985:357

48. Pederson-Bejgaard J, Philip P, Larsen SO, et al. Chromosome aberrations and prognostic factors in therapy related myelodysplasia and acute nonlymphocytic leukemia. Blood 1990;76:1083.

49. Evans JS, Wennberg JF, McNeil BJ. The influence of diagnostic radiography on the incidence of breast cancer and leukemia. N Engl J Med 1986;315:810.

50. Ivanov EP, Tolochko GV, Shuvaeva LP, et al. Childhood leukemia in Gomel Vitebsk and Grodno Oblasts of Belarus prior to and after Chernobyl disaster. Haematol Rev Commun 1995, in press.

51. Kampmeier P, Spilkerge R, Diclistein R, et al. Increased incidence of second neoplasms in patients treated with interferon × 2d for hairy cell leukemia. Blood 1994; 83:2931.

52. Pawson R, Cakovsky D. Second malignancy in hairy cell leukemia. Possible effect of alpha interferon. Br J Haematol 1995;88(Supp 1):184.

53. Kantarjan HM, Keating ML. Therapy related leukemia and myelodysplastic syndromes. Semin Oncol 1987;14:435.

EXERCISES AND TOOLS FOR MYELOCYTIC AND MONOCYTIC DISORDERS

Inflammation is the reparative response to injury.

1. Recognize the clinical expressions of the acute and chronic phases of inflammation: *(a)* Rapid onset of neutrophilic accumulation and protein secretion. *(b)* Progressive monocytic infiltration along with vascular and fibroblastic proliferation.
2. Review the features of the granulocyte inflammation response cascade:
   a. Vascular permeability
   b. Margination
   c. Adhesion
   d. Migration
   e. Chemotaxis
   f. Degranulation
   g. Biodegradation
3. Recognize the diversity and assortment of messages that call in and direct phagocytes to sites of injury, including:
   a. Interleukins
   b. Interferons
   c. Lipopolysaccharides
   d. Tumor necrosis factors
   e. Cytokines
4. Review the dynamics of margination and adhesion integrins and their relationships with stimulation factors, immunoglobulins, and opsonins. With material from Biological Control Mechanisms construct an inflammatory response paradigm.
5. Construct clinical events based on molecular biological activities in disorders of
   a. Leukocyte actin and adhesion deficiencies
   b. Membrane disorders
   c. [Oxygen dependent] intracellular microbicidal activity
6. Recognize the unique differences between the response of phagocytes to acquired injuries and the disordered processes of inborn errors of metabolism.
7. Distinguish between the known initiators of the various acute myeloid (including monocytic and erythrocytic) leukemias (i.e., myeloproliferative states), myelodysplastic states, and chronic myelocytic leukemia with its lymphoid and/or myeloid crises. Develop a schema that accounts for the biological underpinnings of the "secondary" leukemias.
8. For the myeloid malignant states, development a paradigm that relates to the uncoupling of oncogene activities and the potential for the development of targeted therapy. Construct a tabulation that encompass cell cycling events with pharmacokinetics and the biological variables of resting cell and drug resistance.
9. Construct a paradigm for the relationship between the molecular biology and the clinical expression of risk factors among the various myeloid malignancies.
10. Review Exercises and Tools for Lymphocyte, Plasma Cell and Genetic Disorders.

SECTION IV APPENDIX

Appendix 1. Type and Frequency of Neutrophil Antigens

NA 1	Intermediate	40–60%
NA 2	Common	>85%
NB 1	Common	>95%
NB 2	Rare	<35%
NC 1	Common	75–95%
ND 1	Common	>95%
NE 1	Rare	<25%
HGA-3A	Rare	<25%
HGA-3B	Rare	<25%
HGA-3C	Rare	<25%
HGA-3D	Intermediate	50–60%
HGA-3D	Rare	<25%

Appendix 2. Histochemistry of Basophils, Mast Cells, and Eosinophils

	Basophils	*Mast Cells*	*Eosinophils*
Acid Phosphatase	+	−	
Alkaline Phosphatase	−	+	
Periodic Acid Schiff	3+	+	
Protease	−	+	
Peroxidase	+	−	+
Major Basic Protein	+	+	
Collagenase	+	+	
Eosinophil Cationic Protein			+
Eosinophil Neurotoxin			+
	Segmented Nucleus	Nonsegmented Nucleus	Segmented Nucleus
	Circulating Cells	Fixed Tissue Cells	Circulating Cells

SECTION 5

Hypocoagulable and Hypercoagulable State

CHAPTER 28

Immune Disorders of Platelets

KENNETH A. SCHWARTZ

The blood-plaques of Bizzozero, or haematoblasts of Hayem, are colorless, minute, homogenous or finely-granular, disk-like bodies, measuring from 1.5 to 3.5 micromillimeters, occurring isolated, or frequently agglomerated into the so-called Schultze's granule masses. Their origin and function are still subjects of much discussion but they are supposed to bear some part in the production of fibrin and the formation of clots. They are by most observers considered to be independent bodies; but in an elaborate paper recently published by Löwjts it is claimed that they are only the products of retrograde cells or of a precipitation from the plasma. There are probably 250,000 to 300,000 of them in the cubic millimetre of adult blood and decreased in the newborn.

What we now refer to as platelets.
—Keating, Cyclopedia of the Diseases of Children, 1890

Thrombocytopenia is the commonest acquired cause of bleeding. The causes are conveniently divided into immune- and nonimmune-based disorders. Those that are immunologically mediated involve destruction of formed platelets, and to a lesser extent, if the provoking antigen is carried on less mature cells, the megakaryocytes. Improvements in the technology of platelet antibody identification and the likelihood of a biologic process being identified in most cases have accordingly allowed the reallocation of the title **"ITP"** to **immune** rather than **idiopathic** thrombocytopenias. The remainder of the acquired thrombocytopenias (i.e., those of nonimmune origin) are discussed in the next chapter.

Case 1

Betty S., a 14-year-old caucasian girl, was brought to her physician by her mother. Betty appeared not to be in distress, although she looked pale. Since her severe nosebleed 4 days earlier, Betty has been listless, fatigued, and too weak to attend cheerleading and girls' basketball practice. Despite the use of pressure, ice, and a cotton pack, the nosebleed took 3 hours to stop. She noted a spontaneous bruise over her right arm. Her menstrual periods have occurred every 3–4 weeks over the past year, with moderately heavy flow (4–6 pads per day, 5–6 days). However, her most recent menses required a maximum of 10 pads per day. She reported no recent history of trauma or nose picking and no past history of bleeding from either dental procedures or incidental cuts. During the 6 weeks preceding her illness, she could not recall having had a cold or other type of viral illness. Her appetite remained good, with no significant weight change in the past year. She has no history of chronic medication intake and could not recall any exposure to chemicals or toxins. There was no family history of bleeding disorders.

Review of systems was significant for a single black stool 1 day before the physician visit. Her stool was brown on the day of the visit. She denied blood in her urine or sputum, as well as a past history of rash, joint pain or stiffness, or hair thinning.

Positive physical findings included pallor (most striking in the mucous membranes), a few petechial lesions on the outer surface of her right upper arm, ecchymotic areas on arms and legs (the largest is 5 cm in diameter), a funduscopic examination negative for bleeding, and pale mucous membranes.

Important laboratory findings included Hg 100 g/L (adult female normal, 120–160 g/L); Hct 30% (adult female normal, 37–47%); decreased platelets and occasional large polychromatophilic red cells on a blood film; and a platelet count of 15×10^9/L (normal, 150–400×10^9/L); a template bleeding time of 22 min (normal, 3–8 min); a prothrombin time of 13 sec (control, 12 sec); a partial thromboplastin time of 38 sec (control, 40 sec); fibrinogen 200 mg/dL (normal, 150–400 mg/dL); and a reticulocyte count of 7.2% (normal, 0.5–1.5%). Because of the low platelet count a bone marrow examination was carried out, which demonstrated increased numbers of megakaryocytes *but with otherwise normal appearing cells. Quantitative assay for autologous platelet-associated IgG (PAIgG) demonstrated 1500 molecules of IgG per platelet (normal <300).*

Discussion: *The patient's pale appearance coupled with her history of bruising, dark black bowel movement (bleeding into her bowel), and heavy menstruation suggests that she is bleeding from multiple sites. Her fatigue and weakness correlated with the recent decrease in hemoglobin, which was accompanied by a compensatory increase in red cell production, evidenced by the elevated uncorrected reticulocyte count of 7.2% (and the presence of increased numbers of polychromatophilic red cells observed on the blood film). smear. The recent onset of bruising and the petechiae and ecchymosis suggested that her bleeding was related to a problem with coagulation, which, in turn, was confirmed by the prolonged template bleeding time and the decreased platelet count. The increased number of platelet and red cell precursors indicated that the bleeding defect was peripheral and that red cell production was hastened in response to red cell losses. Abnormalities of the humoral coagulation factors were essentially ruled out by the normal prothrombin time, partial thromboplastin time, and fibrinogen value.*

In addition to confirming that her symptoms were secondary to a decrease in circulating platelets, the prolonged template bleeding time of 22 minutes was minimally shorter than the 26 minutes predicted from the formula in Figure 28.1. Thrombocytopenia secondary to marrow failure should produce prolongation of the template bleeding time that is close to this formula's prediction. Bleeding times that are longer than predicted suggest that the patient has either a hereditary or an acquired qualitative platelet disorder. Patients whose thrombocytopenia is secondary to increased platelet destruction with normal or increased compensatory platelet production may have a disproportionately shortened bleeding time. Hence comparisons of observed with predicted bleeding times help narrow the differential diagnosis of thrombocytopenia (1).

Discussion: *The pathophysiologic sequence leading to her illness supported the likelihood that Betty S. had immune thrombocytopenia.*

Because platelets are key components in the control of hemostasis, patients with thrombocytopenia usually present with evidence of bleeding (table 28.1). Most commonly, petechiae (fig. 28.1), red spots in the skin measuring millimeters in diameter and felt to represent capillary bleeding, are first seen in the dependent portion of the legs. Larger and darker petechiae occur with extremely low platelet counts and suggest that the hemostatic defect is especially severe. Bleeding can occur in almost every organ. As in this patient, skin bruising and gastrointestinal bleeding are common. A careful funduscopic examination seeking retinal hemorrhage as an index of intracranial bleeding is an especially important part of the physical examination.

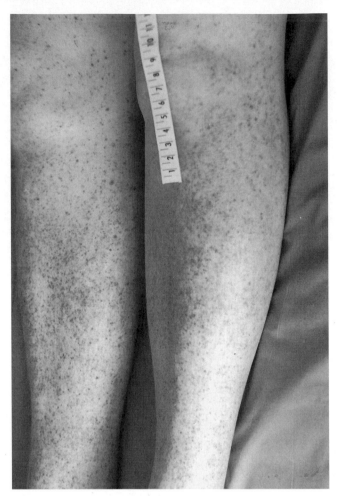

Figure 28.1 Petechia, anterior surface of legs in patient with thrombocytopenia secondary to quinidine.

Table 28.1. Signs and Symptoms of Thrombocytopenia

Signs	Symptoms
Petachia: skin and mucous membranes	"Red dots" on skin
Bruises	Black and blue marks in the skin
Internal bleeding	
Bowel	Vomiting blood or coffee-ground material or dark black or red stools
Urine	Blood in urine
Retinal hemorrhages	Central nervous system symptoms–like blurred abnormal vision
	Excess bleeding: gums after tooth extraction or brushing, muscle bleeds, menses, small cuts

Screening Tests for Suspected Coagulation Problems

Patients with untoward ecchymoses or black bowel movements will likely seek medical aid for these problems shortly after their onset. No less important, however, is screening asymptomatic patients for either hereditary or acquired coagulation defects. This is particularly important before surgery. The most sensitive screen is a careful history inquiring about prolonged bleeding following prior surgeries or accidental cuts or a family history of "easy bruising."

Routine performance of screening coagulation assays may lead to an erroneous conclusion. These assays lack the sensitivity to detect, for example, mild hemophilia and frequently are abnormally prolonged with mild coagulation abnormalities that do not produce clinical bleeding; hence, the best screen is a careful probing history (2).

General Considerations Concerning the Diagnosis of Idiopathic Thrombocytopenia

Idiopathic thrombocytopenic purpura (ITP) is an isolated hematopoietic event in a patient with normal or increased numbers of megakaryocytes and no other identifiable cause of the thrombocytopenia (3). The thrombocytopenia in the present case has neither clinical nor laboratory evidence of disseminated intravascular coagulation (DIC). The possibility of drug exposure, direct acting or immune mediated, as a cause of thrombocytopenia should be excluded (4). In addition, a history of a connective tissue abnormality such as systemic lupus erythematosus (SLE), rheumatoid arthritis, or hyperthyroidism should be investigated (5, 6). Malignancies, both lymphoid and solid tumors, along with severe nutritional deficiencies of folate or vitamin B_{12} must be ruled out (7). The multitude of factors leading to splenic trapping must be addressed. On rare occasions, primary bone marrow abnormalities including the acute leukemias or myelodysplastic syndromes will present with isolated thrombocytopenia. In patients with AIDS, the thrombocytopenia is likely to be immune mediated (8). Patients with none of the above most likely have the idiopathic variety of thrombocytopenia.

However, studies of PAIgG have demonstrated that 80–90% of such patients have detectable antiplatelet immunoglobulins (autoantibodies) against their own platelets (9). Since most ITP patients are felt to have immune-mediated thrombocytopenia, the "I" in ITP more likely refers to immune, rather than idiopathic, thrombocytopenic purpura.

Unlike that in adults, ITP in children has a different presentation, course, and therapeutic approach (10). Frequently, viral infections precede the onset of ITP in pediatric patients, while adults rarely have a history of a recent viral infection. The platelet count in children may improve spontaneously only to drop again after another viral infection (i.e., they may have a chronic relapsing course). The occurrence of spontaneous non-therapy-related recovery or multiple relapses is uncommon in adults.

General Clinical Considerations

Patients with DIC are usually extremely ill from an underlying disease and have clinical evidence of multiple active bleeding sites, including spontaneous blood loss from current and prior intravenous sites. If the clinician suspects DIC as a real possibility, then screening coagulation tests must include assays for fibrinogen and fibrin degradation products and analyses of prothrombin time and partial thromboplastin time (2). Drug exposure, including prescription medications and illegal drugs such as heroin, and a careful drinking history, including consumption of mixed drinks prepared with quinine water (tonic) should be sought (11). Connective tissue abnormalities can be evaluated with focused questions concerning arthritis and arthralgias, excessive hair loss, photophobia, pleuritis, and hematuria, as well as careful examination of the joints, hands, and skin and laboratory evaluation to include ANA and rheumatoid factor. The presence of malignancy should be assessed with a history of masses and/or weight loss and a physical examination that excludes significant adenopathy and enlargement of the liver and/or spleen. Neither hepatosplenomegaly nor each component is a feature of ITP. A bone marrow examination helps to exclude primary or metastatic marrow abnormalities, and as noted, the possibility of AIDS should be investigated (8). Pseudothrombocytopenia may be excluded by microscopic examination of a blood smear for platelet clumps. A normal platelet count obtained on citrate-anticoagulated blood helps to confirm the EDTA dependence of the platelet clumping, which thus accounts for the occasional observation of "pseudothrombocytopenia" (12, 13).

Distinction between Idiopathic and Immune Thrombocytopenic Purpura

Although sensitive micromethods are capable of detecting autologous antiplatelet immunoglobulins (14), there are no standards for uniform measurement of platelet antibodies. Comparisons of different methods show large variability in sensitivity, normal control values, and detection (9). Detection of antibodies in patient's sera or plasma does not differentiate between antibodies induced by a prior pregnancy or transfusion and a true autoantibody. In effect, autoantibodies can only be demonstrated if the patient's own platelets are tested. Because of the wide variability between the various methods, careful separation of antibody-positive from antibody-negative patients in terms of clinical course or response to treatment has not been described.

Pathogenic Mechanisms

Plasma collected from ITP patients usually contains a thrombocytopenic factor, and otherwise normal individuals may develop severe thrombocytopenia following transfusion with plasma from ITP patients (15) (fig. 28.2). Because

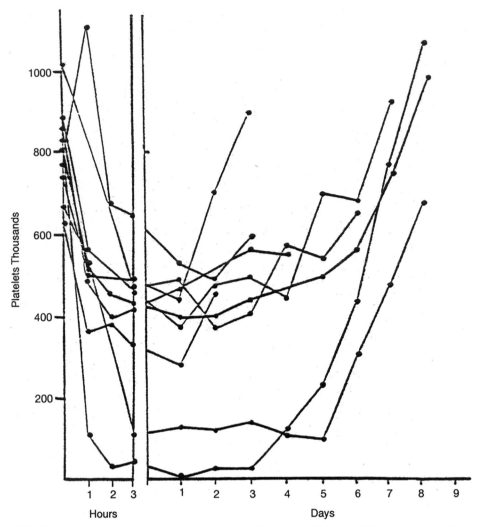

Figure 28.2 Throbocytopenia in eight normal volunteers following infusion of ITP plasma. (From Harrington WJ, Minnich V, Hollingsworth JW, Moore CV. Demonstration of thrombocytopenic factor in the blood of patients with thrombocytopenic purpura. J Lab Clin Med 1951;38:1.)

it is the immunoglobulin fraction from ITP patients' plasma that produces the thrombocytopenia and because radiolabeled platelet kinetic studies show markedly decreased platelet survival in ITP patients, (fig. 28.3), the pathogenic sequence is hypothesized to be antibody-mediated platelets destruction (16, 17). Antimegakaryocyte antibodies have also been demonstrated (18, 19). Platelet antibody assays can detect and quantitate platelet-associated immunoglobulins on the patient's own platelets (14).

Factors that are important in determining the patients' platelet counts include the rate of platelet destruction, which may be related to a number of different factors including (a) the number of immunoglobulin molecules attached to the platelet, (b) both the type of antibody (i.e., IgG, IgA, or IgM) and/or the subtype of immunoglobulin molecule (i.e., IgG subtype 1, 2, 3, or 4), and/or (c) the platelet attachment antigens (e.g., glycoprotein Ib, IIb-IIIa, the Fc receptor, or unidentified antigens) (20). In addition, the efficiency of the reticuloendothelial (R-E) system in removal of the immunoglobulin-coated platelet is important in determining how rapidly platelets are destroyed. Increased platelet production in the marrow, as

demonstrated with radiolabeled platelet turnover studies, is a moderately successful compensatory response (17). Hence, the level of the patients' thrombocytopenia can be approached by considering both the rate of immune-mediated platelet destruction and the compensatory increase in rate of platelet production.

Treatment Course (fig. 28.4): *Betty S. was initially treated with oral prednisone, 1 mg/kg/day, in three divided doses. Two weeks later, her platelet count had increased to 220 × 10⁹/L, and a 6-week prednisone dose-tapering schema was initiated. At the 10 mg/day dose, her platelet count fell to 20 × 10⁹/L. Two weeks after the prednisone was again increased to 50 mg/day, the platelet count leveled off at 180 × 10⁹/L. After a slow reduction in prednisone over the ensuing 4–6 weeks, there was another episode of severe thrombocytopenia, with a platelet count of 18 × 10⁹ on a daily dose of 15 mg of prednisone.*

Because of the unsuccessful weaning, it was decided to schedule her for splenectomy, which included increasing her prednisone dose back to 50 mg/day, with its resultant increase in platelet count to 190 × 10⁹/L. Three days af-

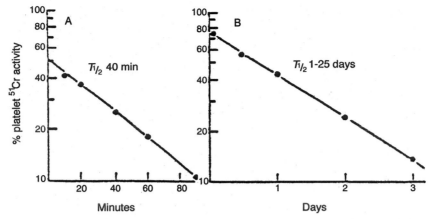

Figure 28.3 Decreased ^{51}CR labeled platelet survival in ITP patient. **A,** presplenectomy platelet survival measured in minutes with a platelet count of 6900/mm³. **B,** increased platelet count postspenectomy of 190,000/mm³ is relfected in the increased platelet survival of approximately 3 days. (From Harker L. Thrombokinetics in idopathic thrombocytopenic purpura. Br J Haematol 1970;19:95.

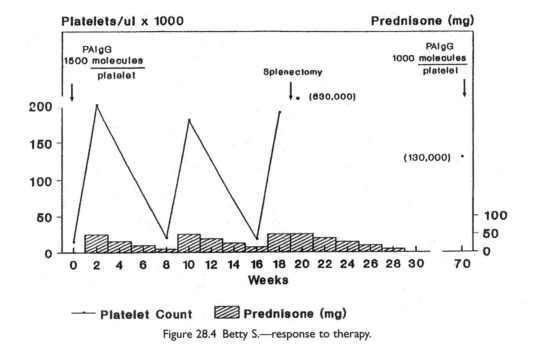

Figure 28.4 Betty S.—response to therapy.

ter her splenectomy, her platelet count maximized at a level of 630 × 10⁹/L. She was slowly weaned off prednisone, and 1 year postsplenectomy, her counts stabilized at a level of 130 × 10⁹/L. One year later, a consistent platelet count of 130 × 10⁹/L, coupled with a persistent autologous antiplatelet IgG elevation, supported a diagnosis of a compensated immune thrombocytopenic state, which paralleled the report by Harker (17) of a patient whose ⁵¹Cr platelet survival increased from just a few hours to several days (normal, 8–10 days).

Appropriate Therapy for ITP (Table 28.2)

Adult patients with ITP are initially treated with high-dose adrenocortical steroids. Generally, 1–2 mg/kg/day of pred-

nisone or its equivalent is started in patients whose platelet counts or clinical circumstances suggest that treatment is necessary (platelet count of 20 × 10⁹/L or less or bleeding at higher levels, 40–60 × 10⁹/L) and who do not have an absolute contraindication to steroids (21–23). Duration of steroid therapy varies according to the patient's clinical characteristics and response to the medication.

If the platelet count does not increase following a 3-month trial, splenectomy should be considered (21–23). Most patients will respond to steroids with a significant increase in platelet count, but only about 20% will the increase stabilize without therapy. Approximately 67% of patients will experience a stable increase in platelet count following splenectomy (24). Splenectomy serves two purposes: it removes one of the sites of an-

Table 28.2. Treatment of Adult ITP

Primary therapy
  Steroids (prednisone 1–2 mg/kg/day)
Secondary therapy
If no response or a satisfactory platelet count cannot be
  maintained without steroids and the patient can
  tolerate surgery, splenectomy
Tertiary therapy
If platelet count postsplenectomy greater than 50×10^9/L
  and patient hemostatically stable, off medication,
  consider no therapy.
If platelet count less than 50 and clinically appropriate,
  treatment with one of the medications listed may
  be considered.
  1. I.V. IgG 400 mg/kg d $\times$ 5 days or 1000 mg kg/day $\times$ 1 day
  2. I.V. vincristine, 2 mg/wk
  3. Oral alkylating agents cytoxan 50-150 mg/day or
     chlorambucil 2–6 mg/day
  4. Danazol 400–800 mg/day

tiplatelet antibody production as well as a formidable reticuloendothelial (sequestering) organ that removes antibody-coated platelets (25). Patients should be immunized presplenectomy with pneumococcal, *Haemophilus influenzae*, and meningococcal vaccines to decrease the risk of infection by opsonization-responsive encapsulated organisms because of the loss of major opsonization activity following splenectomy (26, 27). Although there is no indication to treat postsplenectomy patients with platelet counts above 100×10^9/L, there is still controversy about further therapy for patients with platelet counts below 50×10^9/L.

A variety of therapeutic options are available, depending on the patients' age and additional medical problems. Older patients may respond to orally administered alkylating agents, e.g., 50–150 mg per day of cyclophosphamide or 2–6 mg/day of chlorambucil (28). These medications function by destroying those cells capable of either antiplatelet antibody production and/or phagocytizing platelets. Because of the long-term carcinogenic potential of alkylating agents, they are relatively contraindicated in younger patients. Vincristine, at a dose of no more than 2 mg, or intravenous hyperimmune gamma globulin (IVIgG), at a dose of 400 mg/kg per day for 5 days or 1000 mg/kg as a single dose, can be used to increase platelet counts (29,30). In most patients, the increase in platelet count observed with either vincristine or IVIgG lasts for 5–7 days with the former and as many as 21 days with the latter. Nevertheless, these medications may be useful in supporting patients through acute bleeding thrombocytopenic episodes or as a means of increasing the platelet count prior to surgery such as splenectomy. IVIgG nonspecifically coats the platelets, thereby obscuring the presence of specific antiplatelet antibodies and rending them unseen to the phagocytic cells of the R-E system. Danazol, an synthetic attenuated androgen, has also shown some success in the treatment of ITP patients (31).

Plasmapheresis and pheresis performed by passing the patient's plasma over staphylococcal A protein columns (which nonspecifically bind certain of the platelet antibodies) also have nondurable efficacy in treating some otherwise refractory patients. However, evaluation of the stoichiometry of the binding of plasma IgG to the commercial staphylococcal A preparations suggests that only a small fraction of the total circulating IgG is removed by the staphylococcal A protein. Hence the mechanism of action cannot be simple removal of IgG antibody. Treatment of a single patient with a mouse monoclonal antibody against a low-affinity Fc gamma leukocyte receptor resulted in a dramatic increase in platelet counts of short duration (32). Infusion of anti-Rh (D) increased the platelet counts in Rh-positive ITP patients. In theory, the low level of hemolysis produced by the anti–red cell antibody may partially block phagocytic uptake of antibody-coated platelets (i.e., decrease the rate of platelet destruction). Anti-D appeared to be more effective in children than in adults and did not increase platelet counts in three splenectomized patients (33).

Idiopathic Thrombocytopenia Associated with the Human Immunosuppressive Virus (HIV)

Patients with HIV-ITP present with thrombocytopenia that is clinically indistinguishable from ITP (8). Marrow examinations demonstrate increased megakaryocytes in both disorders, and patients respond to similar therapy. Kinetic studies in HIV-ITP patients demonstrate shortened platelet survival, but additional data also suggest an abnormality in platelet production. Marked increases in platelet IgG, complement, and immune complexes are present. However, gel fractionation of some plasmas from HIV-ITP patients reveals antiplatelet IgG in the void volume, which contains immune complexes, but not in the 7S monomeric IgG fraction (34). Further evaluation suggests that some of the immune complexes contain antibody against HIV antigens that attaches to the platelet Fc receptor. Hence, current theory suggests that the thrombocytopenia may be immune complex–mediated increased platelet destruction and/or decreased platelet production.

Therapy in HIV-ITP is similar to that in ITP; patients are initially treated with steroids, prednisone 1 mg/kg/day or a comparable steroid equivalent. If a satisfactory increase in platelet count is not produced by steroids, then splenectomy should be considered. Of interest is the well-documented increase in platelet count following treatment with azidodeoxythymidine (AZT) (8). As in ITP, intravenous IgG is usually only transiently effective.

Isolated Thrombocytopenia in Infected Patients

Patients with both gram-negative and gram-positive sepsis, viral infections, and malaria may develop thrombocytopenia that is not related to increased consumption of clotting factors (i.e., there is no evidence for DIC) (35–37). Increased PAIgG has been reported in thrombocytopenic patients with either gram-negative or gram-positive sepsis.

Conversely, septic patients with normal platelet counts have not been reported as having increased antiplatelet IgG (38). Sera from patients with rubella or infections may have increased PAIgG that is not correlated with the patients' platelet counts (35). On the other hand, increased PAIgG was observed in 16 of 17 thrombocytopenic patients with malaria, the F(ab')$_2$ part of the IgG molecule bound to the malarial antigen present on the platelet surface (36). The significance of an increased PAIgG level in septic patients was questioned by a study that demonstrated increased PAIgG in thrombocytopenic and nonthrombocytopenic patients in both the acute and convalescent stages of their illness. Since these antiplatelet antibodies could only be demonstrated in EDTA anticoagulant, it was postulated that the antibodies might have been directed against cryptantigens exposed by EDTA (37).

Immune-Mediated Thrombocytopenia in Cancer Patients

ITP-like immune-mediated platelet destruction is associated with solid tumors, myelodysplasia, and lymphoproliferative malignancies including Hodgkin's disease, non-Hodgkin's lymphoma, and Waldenström's macroglobulinemia (7, 39–41). These patients have increased autologous antiplatelet antibodies, shortened platelet survival, and an increase in their platelet counts with therapy directed toward immune thrombocytopenia. Treatment may include steroids, splenectomy, and other "ITP" medications (7, 40). Specificity for platelet glycoprotein IIb or IIIa was demonstrated for an antibody from a Hodgkin's disease patient (42). Increased antiplatelet immunoglobulin may be detected in thrombocytopenic and nonthrombocytopenic cancer patients (40). If the patient has an antiplatelet antibody, immune-mediated thrombocytopenia should be suspected. However, confirmation of ITP in the cancer patient requires that the patient's platelet count is increased with "ITP" therapy such as steroids (fig. 28.5) and/or splenectomy.

Pregnancy-Associated Thrombocytopenia

If in later years Betty S. were to become pregnant, thrombocytopenia in the fetus would be a concern. Pregnancy-associated thrombocytopenia in the mother may be immune mediated or represent benign thrombocytopenia of unknown pathogenesis. Mothers whose ITP is associated with antiplatelet IgG antibodies may deliver a thrombocytopenic infant because of the ability of IgG to cross the placental barrier. During vaginal delivery, pressure on the head of a thrombocytopenic infant may lead to intracranial bleeding with the possible sequelae of mental retardation or death. In the main, this problem can be obviated by delivering the infant through cesarean section; hence the im-

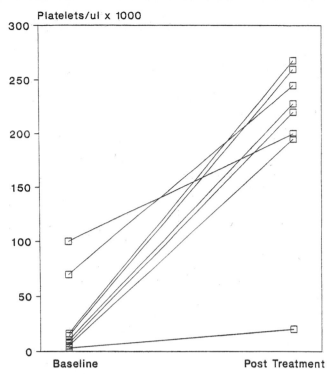

Figure 28.5 Immune thrombocytopenia associated with cancer: increased platelet count following treatment with steroids.

portance of separating immunemediated thrombocytopenia from the benign thrombocytopenia of pregnancy.

Benign Thrombocytopenia of Pregnancy

In general, patients with benign thrombocytopenia of pregnancy are found to be mildly thrombocytopenic during routine prenatal evaluations (43). Such patients do not have a history of easy bruising, excess bleeding, or bleeding with prior pregnancies or surgery. Petechia and ecchymotic areas are not present on physical examination. Bone marrows are normal, and evaluations for both autologous and plasma antiplatelet IgG are negative. These patients can be safely followed with serial platelet counts through pregnancy. If the platelet count remains above 100×10^9/L and there is no antecedent history of ITP or immune thrombocytopenia, then there is no contraindication to a normal vaginal delivery. A recent study of 162 pregnant patients with the presumptive diagnosis of ITP suggests that the lack of a diagnosis of ITP prior to the pregnancy coupled with the absence of an antiplatelet IgG in the patient's plasma indicates that the neonate is at minimum risk for thrombocytopenia (44). However, if the mother's platelet count is below 100×10^9/L, then caesarean delivery requires careful consideration (45).

ITP and Pregnancy

If Betty S., with known ITP and antiplatelet IgG on her platelets, were to become pregnant, she would most

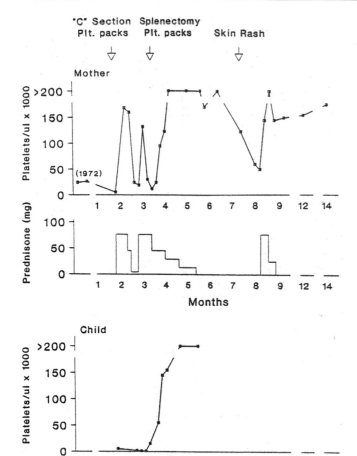

Figure 28.6 ITP pregnancy: treatment course for mother and child.

likely deliver a thrombocytopenic infant (fig. 28.6) (46). The concern about possible induction of intracranial bleeding during vaginal birth requires evaluation of both mother and infant.

If the mother has a history of ITP with a platelet count above 100×10^9/L and has not had a splenectomy, usually the infant's platelet count will be high enough to withstand a vaginal delivery. However, if the mother is currently taking steroids or her spleen has been removed, the clinical rule of "100,000" is no longer valid, and other criteria must be used to decide the appropriate route of delivery (45).

In an attempt to predict the fetus's platelet count, investigators have suggested that mothers with antiplatelet IgG in their plasma or on their platelets are at greater risk for delivering a thrombocytopenic infant and should have their infants delivered by cesarean section (47, 48). Unfortunately, this finding has not gained universal support (49, 50). When available, determinations of the fetus's platelet count in blood from either a scalp vein or the umbilical chord will help determine the appropriate delivery route. Both these procedures are associated with hazards and must be carried out by experienced physicians.

The route of delivery is a critical decision. Cesarean section with its associated problems must be balanced against the possibility of intracranial bleeding in a thrombocytic infant delivered vaginally. If the neonate's platelet count is unknown, most clinicians would recommend a cesarean section rather than risk the possibility that a thrombocytopenic baby might sustain brain injury in a vaginal delivery.

The mother's platelet count may be elevated with steroids. Karpatkin et al. reported significantly higher platelet counts in newborn infants of immune thrombocytopenic mothers treated with prednisone 10–20 mg/day than in those of untreated ITP mothers (51).

Neonatal Isoimmune Thrombocytopenia

Neonates may also develop immune-mediated thrombocytopenia secondary to a platelet antigen incompatibility between the mother and father. If the neonate inherits a platelet antigen from the father that the mother lacks, during the course of the pregnancy, the mother may produce an antiplatelet IgG antibody capable of crossing the placenta and producing thrombocytopenia in the fetus. Unlike mothers with ITP, mothers of infants with neonatal isoimmune thrombocytopenia are not thrombocytopenic and do not have a history of ITP (52). The immunology of this problem is analogous to Rh incompatibilities observed on red blood cells. First-born infants can be thrombocytopenic. Not all the infants from antigenically incompatible parents are thrombocytopenic. In a study by Blanchette et al., only 3 of 50 Pl^{A1}-negative mothers evaluated postpartum had anti-Pl^{A1} antibodies, and only 1 of the 3 delivered a thrombocytopenic infant (53). The authors estimated that only one of every 1000 pregnancies will develop alloimmunization to the Pl^{A1} antigen. Mothers with DR3, DRw52 HLA type are more likely to have this problem (54).

Usually the diagnosis of neonatal isoimmune thrombocytopenia is suspected because of either a previous pregnancy or a family history of neonatal thrombocytopenia that was unrelated to a concurrent infection or another perinatal illness. Platelet antibody studies require blood from both parents and the infant. The infant and the mother may have an antibody identified in their plasma that reacts with the father's platelets but not the mother's. If technically possible, antibody studies on the infant's own platelets should demonstrate increased platelet-associated IgG (52, 55). Laboratories with specific typing antibody should be able to demonstrate the specific antigen on the father's and infant's platelets and the lack of this antigen on the mother's. For example, the most common platelet antigen incompatibility is with the Pl^{A1} antigen (56). Appropriate studies would demonstrate that the father and infant carried the Pl^{A1} antigen and the mother did not. Although incompatibilities with the Pl^{A1} antigen are the most common, other platelet antigens may also produce neonatal isoimmune thrombocytopenia; these include Pl^{A2}, Br^a, Bak^a, Pen^a/yuk^b, Pen^b/yuk^a, Ko^a, and Pl^{E2} (57–62). Table 28.3 details expected platelet antibody results on blood

Table 28.3. Platelet Antibody Studies in Neonatal Thrombocytopenia

| | Mother's | | Father's | | | Baby's | | |
	(Auto)	Plasma	(Auto)	(Platelets with Maternal Plasma)	Plasma	(Auto)	(Platelets with Maternal Plasma)	Plasma
Neonatal isoimmune thrombocytopenia	−	+	−	+	−	+	+	+
Maternal ITP	+	±	−	±	−	±	+	±
Benign thrombocytopenia of pregnancy	−	−	na	na	na	na	na	nats

+ = Positive;
± = Postive or negative.
The key determinations are the mothers platelets and plasma. If autologous maternal platelet studies are positive, the mother has ITP. Conversely, if the mother is negative for autologous antibody, but has a plasma antiplatelet antibody that reacts with both the father's and baby's platelets, then the likely diagnosis is neonatal isoimmune thrombocytopenia, which can be confirmed with specific typing antiplatelet antibody demonstrating that the mother lacks an antigen present in both the father and the neonate. No maternal antibody should be demonstrated in benign thrombocytopenia of pregnancy. NA = not applicable.

and platelets from the neonate, mother, and father in neonatal isoimmune thrombocytopenia, ITP, and benign thrombocytopenia of pregnancy.

Counseling the family about outcomes of future pregnancies depends on whether the father was homozygous or heterozygous for the Pl^{A1} antigen. All of the infants from homozygous fathers will carry the Pl^{A1} antigen and will be at risk for thrombocytopenia, while only 50% of the infants from heterozygous fathers will be at risk. As an aid to genetic counseling, investigational platelet immunology laboratories may be able to differentiate homozygous from heterozygous Pl^{A1} positives.

Treatment

ANTE-natal therapy of the mother with IVIgG or with steroids may raise the neonate's platelet count enough to minimize or prevent intracranial hemorrhages (63). After birth, if the infant remains thrombocytopenic and requires platelet transfusion, the best source for antigen-negative platelets is the mother. Since maternal plasma contains the antiplatelet antibody, the mother's platelets should be washed before transfusion. If an antigen-negative nonfamily donor is selected for platelet donation, then a crossmatch using maternal plasma and donor platelets should be performed to be certain that the antiplatelet antibody produced by the mother and present in the infant will not react with the transfused platelets. This additional test is necessary because platelet antibody typing techniques and typing reagents are not standardized.

Drug-Induced Thrombocytopenia

Idiosyncratic drug-induced thrombocytopenia is suspected in patients with acute onset of petechia, ecchymoses, and/or overt hemorrhage or, less commonly, by presentation with asymptomatic thrombocytopenia detected with a screening platelet count. A careful medication history may reveal one or more drugs that may have caused the thrombocytopenia. Figure 28.7 shows the platelet count in a pa-

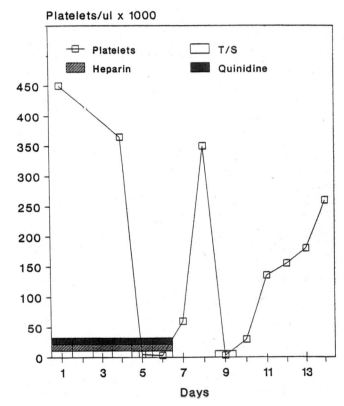

Figure 28.7 Recurrent thrombocytopenia caused by trimethoprim/sulfamethoxazole (T/S).

tient whose thrombocytopenia may have been related to three possible drugs: heparin, trimethoprim/sulfamethoxazole combination, and digoxin. Restarting the trimethoprim/sulfamethoxazole combination precipitated a recurrence of the patient's severe thrombocytopenia. Laboratory screening of the three possible drugs in a platelet antibody assay may have implicated the trimethoprim/sulfamethoxazole combination as a necessary cofactor for a positive result. Hence, the trimethoprim/sulfamethoxazole combination was the most likely medication to have caused the patient's thrombocytopenia, and the second thrombocytopenic episode could have been prevented. Certainly, recurrence of the patient's thrombocytopenia after repeat exposure to a suspected medication is excellent evidence that the patient's thrombocytopenia was caused by the drug.

Pathogenesis of Drug-Induced Thrombocytopenia

Drug-induced thrombocytopenia is an expected side effect of some of the cytotoxic anticancer drugs. These medications decrease platelet production through their toxic effects on megakaryocytes. Other toxins such as benzene and alcohol may also cause thrombocytopenia (64).

Idiosyncratic drug-associated thrombocytopenia occurs in a small percentage of patients. The thrombocytopenia may or may not be immune mediated and may involve direct interaction of the drug with a specific platelet receptor or the drug in conjunction with an antibody may attach to the platelet surface membrane (65). Interaction of drug and antibody may occur in the plasma, and then the complex may attach to the platelet, or the drug-antibody complex may form on the platelet surface. Some drug-induced thrombocytopenias require the presence of a drug, and some are non–drug dependent. Lerner et al. showed that drug-dependent immune thrombocytopenias require the Fc domain of the immunoglobulin molecule, suggesting that the drug and the antibody form an immune complex that is attached to the platelet via the Fc receptor. Conversely, drug-induced but non-drug-dependent antibodies can be demonstrated with just the $F(ab')_2$ fragments, suggesting that the antibody is binding to a specific platelet determinant (66). In addition, the drug may combine with a plasma protein, forming a haptenic complex that may interact with an antibody in the plasma or on the platelet. Eisner and Shaidi reported that an antibody to a metabolite of acetaminophen, but not the parent compound, was responsible for immune thrombocytopenia (67). Hence, antibody-mediated idiosyncratic drug thrombocytopenia may proceed via a variety of mechanisms that may or may not require the drug or a metabolite of the drug, a hapten, the platelet Fc receptor, or a specific platelet antigen.

Clinical Approach to Drug-Induced Thrombocytopenia

Causes of thrombocytopenia other than drugs should be investigated. Primary marrow pathology can be excluded with a bone marrow examination. The presence or absence of megakaryocytes will also be determined by studying marrow morphology. Testing for platelet antibodies in the presence and absence of each of the possible offending medications may help determine which drug, if any, caused the patient's thrombocytopenia (68). Stopping the medication that is suspected of causing the patient's thrombocytopenia and avoiding its future use is usually all

that is required to promptly restore the patient's platelet count to normal.

Quinidine

Quinidine commonly produces immune-mediated thrombocytopenia that is usually reversed a few days after the medication is stopped (69). Multiple antiplatelet antibodies directed against GPIb/IX and/or GPIIb/IIIa may be identified in the plasma from a single patient with quinidine-induced thrombocytopenia (70). In addition, both drug-dependent, Fc-mediated, and non-drug-dependent quinidine thrombocytopenias are reported (71).

Heparin

Heparin may induce thrombocytopenia in up to one-third of recipients (72). Most patients will develop a mild asymptomatic decrease in platelet count with no further clinical sequelae. A smaller proportion of affected patients on heparin will develop severe thrombocytopenia accompanied by thrombosis; these include venous thrombosis in the legs and pulmonary emboli, as well as arterial thrombi producing acute myocardial infarctions, strokes, and obstruction of limb arteries (73). Unfortunately, when the heparinized patient initially develops thrombocytopenia, determining whether the thrombocytopenia is benign and reversible, or progressive and associated with thrombosis, is not possible. Kelton et al. developed an assay based on platelet stimulation and release to determine retrospectively whether the patient's thrombocytopenia was heparin mediated (74).

Heparin-induced thrombocytopenia without symptoms of thrombosis may not be antibody mediated. However, severe heparin thrombocytopenia with thrombosis may be antibody mediated, with the antibody attaching to the platelet Fc receptor (72, 75).

Because the adverse effects of heparin thrombocytopenia with thrombosis may be severe and even fatal, deciding whether to stop or continue heparin is difficult. If heparin can be clearly implicated as the cause of the thrombocytopenia, then appropriate treatment is discontinuation of heparin and possible initiation of alternative anticoagulant therapy. Low-molecular-weight heparin is under investigation with the hope that the lower-molecular-weight polymer will have satisfactory anticoagulant properties without the side effects of thrombocytopenia and thrombosis. Heparinized patients with a mild decrease in platelet count must be followed with daily platelet counts and be observed carefully for recurrent thromboses. Asymptomatic benign mild decreases in platelet counts are common, but thrombocytopenia accompanied by thrombosis is frequently lethal. However, distinguishing benign decreases in platelet count from severe thrombocytopenia and thrombosis by clinical or laboratory criteria is currently not possible. Hence the difficulty.

Gold

Gold-induced thrombocytopenias may have a delayed onset as long as 18 months after the medication was stopped

(76, 77). Gold persists for a long time in tissues, which results in late induction of gold-initiated thrombocytopenia and lengthy persistence of symptoms (78). Antibody assays using plasma from gold-induced thrombocytopenic patients have demonstrated increased antiplatelet immunoglobulin (68, 79). Attempts to expedite the removal of gold with dimercaprol are inconclusively effective (75).

Vancomycin-Induced Thrombocytopenia

Vancomycin-induced thrombocytopenia may produce refractoriness to platelet transfusion in leukemia. Antiplatelet antibodies have been demonstrated against platelet glycoproteins IIb and/or IIIa. When the vancomycin is discontinued, refractoriness ceases (80).

Other Drugs

The list of drugs known to produce thrombocytopenia include, as noted, quinidine, quinine, heparin, cimetidine, and sulfa-containing medications. A literature review of drugs associated with idiosyncratic thrombocytopenia is presented in Table 28.4. Drugs with a plus sign were administered for a second time to the same patient and caused a recurrence of the patient's thrombocytopenia.

Patients may simultaneously take many drugs that could possibly cause thrombocytopenia. Where available, tests for platelet antibody with and without the possible offending drug may help to delineate the specific medication producing thrombocytopenia. Antibody that is dependent on the presence of a particular drug suggests that the drug produced the thrombocytopenia. If analysis for drug dependence in a platelet antibody assay is equivocal or not available, then the likelihood that a particular medication caused thrombocytopenia may be inferred from the number of case reports in the literature and the strength of the individual reports. Recurrence of thrombocytopenia in the same patient following repeat administration is strong evidence that the drug causes idiosyncratic thrombocytopenia.

Clinical decisions about stopping a particular drug should balance the importance of the medication for a particular patient's management against the probability that the drug produced the thrombocytopenia.

Posttransfusion Purpura

Approximately 5–10 days after a transfusion, patients may rarely develop what appears to be a transfusion-related thrombocytopenia. This occurs more frequently in multiparous women. Patients present with the usual signs of petechia, ecchymoses, and bleeding that accompany the acute onset of thrombocytopenia. Marrows show normal to increased numbers of megakaryocytes and are otherwise normal (81).

Patients usually have easily demonstrable antiplatelet antibodies in their plasma. However, the pathogenesis of immune-mediated destruction must reconcile the paradox that the antibody, most commonly anti-Pl^{A1},

has specificity for an antigen that is not present on the patient's platelets (i.e., patients with posttransfusion purpura and anti-Pl^{A1} antibody in their plasma are Pl^{A1} negative) (82). Similarly, patients who are negative for other platelet-specific antigens, Pl^{A2}, Bak^a, Bak^b, and Pen^a(Yuk^b), may have platelet antibodies in their plasma with specificity toward an antigen that is not present on their platelets (71).

The precise pathogenesis of this immune-mediated platelet destruction remains unknown. A popular hypothesis suggests that the prior transfusion stimulates the patient to produce an alloantibody directed against a foreign platelet antigen. How does this antibody produce thrombocytopenia when the specific platelet antigen it is directed against is not present on the patient's platelets? When Pl^{A1}-negative platelets are incubated with Pl^{A1}-positive plasma, the Pl^{A1} antigen will adhere to the Pl^{A1}-negative platelets (83). Hence, one theory suggests that the antigen is transfused into the patient, perhaps via platelet microparticles present in the Pl^{A1}-positive transfusion, and becomes attached to the patient's platelets (84). The transfused platelet antigen, now attached to the pretransfusion antigen-negative platelets, reacts with the antibody produced against the "foreign" transfused antigen, and the antigen-antibody reaction on the platelet surface leads to accelerated, immune-mediated, platelet destruction. It is also possible that the antiplatelet antibody binds to the antigen in the plasma, forming soluble antigen-antibody complexes that nonspecifically bind to the platelet via the platelets' Fc receptor.

Patients usually present with very low platelet counts, below 20×10^9/L. Currently accepted therapy includes steroids, 1 mg/kg prednisone or the steroid equivalent, and plasmapheresis. Removal of antibody by plasmapheresis may be effective through mechanisms that are not strictly based on antibody removal, as the decrease in antibody is much greater than would be expected by calculating the dilutional effect of removing plasma (85). Treating patients with intravenous IVIgG 400 mg/kg/day for 5 days has resulted in increased platelet counts in some patients (86). Most patients' platelet counts are back to normal within 3–4 weeks.

Platelet Transfusions (Table 28.5)

Platelet transfusions should be considered when the platelet count is below 50×10^9/L and the patient is actively bleeding. Depending on the pathogenesis of the thrombocytopenia, platelet transfusions may have variable efficacy. Platelet transfusions in patients with antibody-mediated thrombocytopenia may have very short platelet survivals, less than 24 hours. Unless a patient with antibody-mediated thrombocytopenia has life-threatening bleeding, platelet transfusions are not usually recommended. By comparison, platelet transfusions in patients with the same degree of thrombocytopenia that is secondary to decreased platelet production usually have platelet survivals of several days. Decreased platelet production in these patients may be secondary to aplastic ane-

Table 28.4. Idiosyncratic Thrombocytopenia Drugs

Drug	Positive in vivo Drug Rechallenge	Reference	Drug	Positive in vivo Drug Rechallenge	Reference
More than 50			**5 to 19** (cont'd)		
case reports			**case reports**		
Cimetidine		65, 68, 101	Penicillin		68, 116, 139, 140
Gold		41, 68, 76, 102	Pentosane polysulfate		141
Heparin	+	103-105 N	Phenylbutazone		123
Quinidine	+	65, 68, 106-111	Procainamide		111, 142, 143
Quinine	+	65, 68, 107-110, 112	Ranitidine		144, 145
Sulfonamides	+	68, 111, 113-115	Rifampin		146
20 to 50			Stibophen	+	65, 147
case reports			Sulindac		148
Acetylsalicylic acid		116	Vinyl chloride		123
Amrinone		117, 118	**Fewer than 5**		
Arsenical antileutics	+	65	**case reports**		
Heroin		119	Analgesics (nonsteroidal, antiinflammatory)		
Indomethacin		120	Antipyrine		123
Phthalazinol		121	Benoxaprofen		123
Sulfonamide derivatives			Diclofenac		149
Acetazolamide		68	Ibuprofen		150
Chlorpropamide		122	Meclofenamate	+	151
Chlorthalidone		111	Piroxicam		123
Clopamide		123	Sodium salicylate		123
Diazoxide	+	124	Tolmetin		123
Furosemide	+	125	Antimicrobials:		
Glibenclamide		123	Ampicillin		68, 111
Tolbutamide		126, 127	Apalcillin		123
Valproic acid		123	Carbenicillin		116
5 to 19			Cefotetan		143
case reports			Cephalexin		111
Acetmenophen		67, 128	Cephalothin	+	152
Actinomycin		129	Cefamandole		153
α Methyldopa	+	111, 130-132	Difluoromethy-lornithine		123
Bleomycin		123	Gentamicin		154
Chloroquinine		123	Isoniazid (INH)		123
Chlorothiazide	+	111	Methicillin	+	65, 155
Danazol	+	133	Mezlocillin		123
Digitoxin	+	65, 134	Moxalactam		123
Diphenylhydantoin		111, 113	Naxidixic acid	+	156
Fenoprofen		135	Nitrofurantoin		123
Hydrochlorothiazide		111	Norfloxacin		123
Insecticides: DDT, DDVP, others		136	Novodiocin	+	65
Noraminopyrine		116	Oxytetracycline		157
Oxyphenbutazone		123	P-aminosalicylate	+	138, 158
p-Aminosalicylate		137, 138			

mia, chemotherapeutic marrow toxicity, radiation therapy, or other causes of marrow failure. Hence, therapeutic platelet transfusions are recommended for actively bleeding thrombocytopenic patients, but prophylactic transfusions are usually reserved for patients whose thrombocytopenia is secondary to marrow failure and decreased platelet production (87–89).

Patients with marrow failure and platelet counts below 10×10^9/L probably should receive prophylactic random platelet transfusions. If the platelet count is below 5 ×

10^9/L, significantly increased amounts of blood can be demonstrated in the bowel (90). Although platelet count is an important determinant for platelet transfusion, clinical evaluation with special attention to the presence of fever, splenomegaly, and medications that inhibit platelet function should also be considered in evaluating patients for platelet transfusions (91).

Bleeding in patients with qualitative abnormalities may be controlled following platelet transfusion even if the platelet count is in the normal range. For example, during

Table 28.4. Idiosyncratic Thrombocytopenia Drugs

Drug	Positive in vivo Drug Rechallenge	Reference	Drug	Positive in vivo Drug Rechallenge	Reference
Fewer than 5 *(cont'd)*			**Fewer than 5** *(cont'd)*		
case reports			**case reports**		
Pentamidine		159	Cyclophosphamide		174
Streptomycin		123	Desferrioxamine		123
Sulfasalazine	+	160	Desipramine		175
Tobramycin		123	Diatrizoate	+	176
Trimethoprim		68, 161	Digitalis		123
Vancomycin		143, 162	Digoxin	+	65, 177
Sedatives, tranquilizers,			Diltiazem		123
anticonvulsants			Disulfiram		123
Allylisopropyl-		163	Eritinate		178
barbiturate			Flavone-8-acetic acid		179
Butabarbitone		123	Hydroxyquinoline		180
Carbamazepine		111	Iocetamic acid		181
Centalun		123	Iopanoic acid		182
Chlordiazepoxide		164	Isoniazid		65
Chlorpromazine		123	Isoretinoin	+	183
Clonazepam		165	Levamisole	+	65, 184, 185
Diazepam		113, 166	Levodopa		186
Fluphenazine		123	Lidocaine		123
Impramine		111	Mercurial diuretics		123
Meprobamate		111	Methylphenidate		187
Mianserin		123	Mexiletine		188
Paramethadione		5	Minoxidil	+	189
Phenyltoin		167	Morphine		190
Primidone		168	Nitroglycerin		123
Valproic acid		123	Nomifensine	+	65, 191
Miscellaneous:			Oxoprenolol		192, 193
Acetazolamide		163	Penicillamine		194
Allopurinal		123	Pentagastrin		195
Alprenolol	+	65	Pertussis vaccine		123
Aminoglutethimide		169	Prochlorperazine		196
Amiodarone	+	170	Propylthiouracil		123
Antazoline		37, 171	Sprironolactone		111
Captopril		123	Tetanus toxoid		197
Chenodeoxycholic acid		116	Thioguanine		111
Chlorpheniramine		172	Thiouracil		123
Clinoril		173	Ticlopidine		123
Clometacine		123	Tienilic acid		123
Clonazepam		65	Toluene diisocyanate		198
Co-trimoxazole		62, 161	Xylocaine	+	65

cardiac bypass surgery, platelet dysfunction may be induced by the bypass pump. Abnormal bleeding in these patients may be reversed with platelet transfusions regardless of the platelet concentration. Routine prophylactic platelet transfusions in nonbleeding cardiac bypass patients should be discouraged (92). Bleeding patients with other causes of dysfunctional platelets, such as myeloproliferative syndromes, leukemia, uremia, and certain drugs such as aspirin, antiinflammatory agents, and penicillin-based antibiotics, may benefit from platelet transfusions.

Usually adults are given random platelets collected from four or six donors (i.e., 4 or 6 units of random platelets). Pheresed platelets harvested from a single donor reduce the likelihood that the transfusion will transmit infection. In addition, exposure to fewer platelet donors decreases the number of antigens that the patients are exposed to and may delay the onset of immune reactions against platelets and possibly refractoriness, lack of increase in platelet count after transfusion of random platelets (93). Another strategy developed to reduce the incidence of refractoriness to platelet transfusions is the reduction of leukocytes in transfused platelets and red cells (94). Consensus about using platelets collected from multiple random donors or platelets pheresed from a single random donor, with or without removal of leukocytes, has not yet been reached; these questions are still under investigation.

Table 28.5. Indications for Platelet Transfusion

Bleeding patient
   Platelet count less than 50×10^9/L
   Qualitative platelet defect with prolonged template bleeding
      time—regardless of platelet count. Example: bleeding
      after cardiac bypass surgery.
Prophylactic platelet transfusion (non-bleeding patient)
   Thrombocytopenia secondary to marrow failure transfuse
      if platelet count less than 10 or less than 20×10^9/L
      depending on clinical assessment.

The efficacy of the platelet transfusion should be evaluated in terms of the effect on the patient's bleeding as well as the increase in platelet count, obtained 1 and 24 hours posttransfusion. Surgery on thrombocytopenic patients may proceed if platelet transfusions can raise the patients' platelet counts above 50×10^9/L for minor surgery and 100×10^9/L for major surgery.

Unfortunately platelet antigens that are important for platelet transfusions have not been delineated. Most patients receive platelets collected from random donors; when possible, the platelets are red cell antigens ABO and Rh compatible. Since the Rh antigen is not present on platelets, Rh-negative patients may receive platelets from Rh-positive donors without affecting the platelet transfusion (95). Small numbers of red cells are present in platelet concentrates and can result in immunization of Rh-negative recipients. Hence, Rh-negative women of childbearing age should not receive Rh-positive platelets.

Approximately two-thirds of all patients receiving serial platelet transfusions will develop antibodies against platelet antigens (96). A smaller percentage of patients with continued serial platelet transfusions will produce a strong enough antiplatelet immune response so that further platelet transfusions do not result in an increase in posttransfusion platelet counts. The transfused random platelets are probably being destroyed by an immune reaction, which may produce chills, fever, and other symptoms. Patients are said to be refractory to random platelet transfusion if after two sequential platelet transfusions there is no increase in their 1-hour posttransfusion platelet counts.

Platelet donors for refractory patients can be screened by two complementary techniques designed to select donors who are at least partially antigenically compatible. Since HLA A and B loci antigens are present on platelets, an HLA-compatible platelet donor can be chosen from an existing HLA donor computer program that stratifies perspective donors based on the degree of homology between the patient's and the perspective donor's HLA antigens (97). Platelet antibody assays may be used as a crossmatch, testing perspective donors' platelets with patient plasma; donors with negative crossmatches should be considered as possible platelet donors (98). Siblings are most likely to match for platelet antigens and should

be evaluated as possible platelet donors by testing for compatibility of their HLA type as well as reactivity of their platelets with the patient's plasma in a crossmatch assay. In an emergency, platelets from first-degree family members may be transfused while attempts to find HLA-compatible and/or crossmatch-negative donors are proceeding.

Patients such as those with acute leukemia who will probably require long-term serial platelet transfusions should have their HLA A and B loci typed when they are diagnosed. When possible, the patients' siblings should also be typed. If the patient becomes refractory to random donor platelets, a crossmatch using the patient's plasma and prospective family and community platelet donors can be used to select appropriate platelet donors. Monitoring platelet counts 1 and 24 hours after platelet transfusion will help determine which crossmatch-negative donors produce clinically beneficial increases in platelet counts. If necessary, a platelet donor may be pheresed daily without harmful effects to the donor.

Since intravenous IgG may decrease reticulendothelial uptake of antibody-coated platelets (30), IVIgG was evaluated as an adjuvant to platelet transfusions in refractory patients. Schiffer et al. found no benefit for IVIgG when used in conjunction with either random or partially HLA-matched platelets (99). However, Zeigler et al. documented improvement when IVIgG was used with platelets collected from the best HLA match available (100). Thus the use of IVIgG in refractory patients may depend on the degree of immune compatibility between donor and patient.

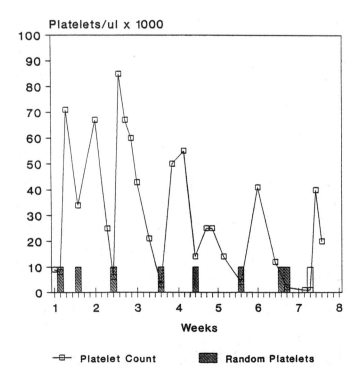

Figure 28.8 Increased platelet count following transfusion of HLA-matched platelets in patient refractory to random platelet transfusions.

Pheresis techniques are used to collect platelets from the donor whose platelets were selected for the refractory patient. If no increase in platelet counts is observed 1 hour after the transfusion, then another donor should be evaluated. Usually, either HLA-matched and or crossmatch-negative platelet donors provide platelets for transfusion that produce clinically satisfactory incremental increases in the refractory patients' platelet counts (fig. 28.8).

In conclusion, most acquired thrombocytopenias not due to marrow dysfunction will be of immune origin. The mechanisms for immune platelet destruction are generally similar to those for other blood cells, as are the underlying antigenic insults. An array of immunologic tests will aid in defining the pathology, and special cases such as children and pregnant mothers require sensitive assessment. Iatrogenic drug-based ITP is common and should always be considered. Treatment includes many immunoactive drugs and procedures, and splenectomy remains a worthwhile consideration in refractory cases.

REFERENCES

1. Harker LA, Slichteler SJ. The bleeding time as a screening test for evaluation of platelet function. N Engl J Med 1972; 287:155.
2. Thompson AR, Harker LA. Manual of hemostasis and thrombosis. Ed 3. Philadelphia: FA Davis, 1983.
3. McMillan R. Chronic idiopathic thrombocytopenic purpura. N Engl J Med 1981;304(19):1135.
4. Böttiger LE, Westerholm B. Drug-induced thrombocytopenia. Acta Med Scand 1972;191:541.
5. Karpatkin S, Strick N, Karpatkin M, Siskind. Cumulative experience in the detection of antiplatelet antibody in 234 patients with idiopathic thrombocytopenic purpura, systemic lupus erythematosus and other clinical disorders. Am J Med 1972;52:776.
6. Lamberg BA, Kivikangas V, Pelkonen R, Vuopio P. Thrombocytopenia and decreased life-span of thrombocytes in hyperthyroidism. Ann Clin Res 1971;98:98.
7. Schwartz KA, Slichter SJ, Harker LA. Immune-mediated platelet destruction and thrombocytopenia in patients with solid tumors. Br J Haematol 1982;51:17.
8. Karpatkin S. HIV-1 related thrombocytopenia. Hematol Oncol Clin North Am 1990;4:193.
9. Schwartz KA. Platelet antibody: review of detection methods. Am J Hematol 1988;29:106.
10. Bussel JB. Autoimmune thrombocytopenic purpura. Hematol Oncol Clin North Am 1990;4(1):179.
11. Reid DM, Shulman R. Drug purpura due to surreptitious quinidine intake. Ann Intern Med 1988;108:206.
12. Payne BA, Pierre RV. Pseudothrombocytopenia: a laboratory artifact with potentially serious consequences. Mayo Clin Proc 1984;59:123.
13. Pegels JG, Bruynes CE, Engelfriet CP, von dem Borne AEGK. Pseudothrombocytopenia: an immunologic study on platelet antibodies dependent on ethylene diamine tetra-acetate. Blood 1982;59:157.
14. Schwartz KA, Gauger JA, Davis JM. Precise quantitation of PAIgG: a new radiometric microtechnique. Am J Hematol 1990;33:167.
15. Harrington WJ, Minnich V, Hollingworth JW, Moore CV. Demonstration of thrombocytopenic factor in the blood of patients with thrombodytopenic purpura. J Lab Clin Med 1951;38:1.
16. Shulman NR, Weinrach RS, Libre EP, Andrews JA. The role of reticuloendothelial system in the pathogenesis of idiopathic thrombocytopenic purpura. Trans Assoc Am Physicians 1965;73:374.
17. Harker L. Thombokinetics in idiopathic thrombocytopenic purpura. Br J Haematol 1970;19:95.
18. Gernsheimer T, Stratton J, Ballem PJ, Slichter SJ. Mechanisms of response to treatment in autoimmune thrombocytopenic purpura. N Engl J Med 1989;320:974.
19. Hoffman R, Zakoen S, Yang HH, Bruno E, LoBuglio AF, et al. An antibody cytotoxic to megakaryocyte progenitor cells in a patient with immune thrombocytopenic purpura. N Engl J Med 1985;312:1170.
20. McMillan R, Tani P, Millard F, Berchtold P, Renshaw L, Woods VL. Platelet-associated and plasma anti-glycoprotein autoantibodies in chronic ITP. Blood 1987;70:1040.
21. Baldini M. Idiopathic thrombocytopenic purpura. N Engl J Med 1966;274:1245.
22. Burns TR, Saleem A. Idiopathic thrombocytopenic purpura. Am J Med 1983;75:1001.
23. Kelton JG, Gibbons S. Autoimmune platelet destruction: idiopathic thrombocytopenic purpura. Semin Thromb Hemost 1982;8:83.
24. Thompson RL, Moore RA, Hess CE, et al. Idiopathic thrombocytopenic purpura. Arch Intern Med 1972;130:730.
25. McMillan R, Longmire RL, Yelenosky R, Smith RS, Craddock CG. Immunoglobulin synthesis in virtro by splenic tissue in idiopathic thrombocytopenic purpura. N Engl J Med 1972;286:681.
26. Di Padova F, Durig M, Wadstrom J, Harder F. Role of spleen in immune response to polyvalent pneumococcal vaccine. Br Med J 1983;287:1829.
27. Giebink GS, Le CT, Schiffman G. Decline of serum antibody in splenectomized children after vaccination with pneumococcal capsular polysaccharides. J Pediatr 1984; 105:576.
28. Verlin M, Laros RK, Penner JA. Treatment of refractory thrombocytopenic purpura with cyclophosphamide. Am J Hematol 1976;1:97.
29. Ahn YS, Harrington WJ, Seelman RC, et al. Vincristine therapy of idiopathic and secondary thrombocytopenias. N Engl J Med 1974;291:376.
30. Fehr J, Hofmann V, Kappeler U. Transient reversal of thrombocytopenia in idiopathic thrombocytopenic purpura by high-dose intravenous gamma globulin. N Engl J Med 1982;306:1254.
31. Schreiber AD, Chien P, Tomaski A, et al. Effect of danazol in immune thrombocytopenic purpura. N Engl J Med 1987;316:503.
32. Clarkson SB, Bussel JB, Kimberly RP, et al. Treatment of refractory immune thrombocytopenic purpura with an anti Fc gamma receptor antibody. N Engl J Med 1986; 314:1236.
33. Bussel JB, Kimberley RP, Inman RD, et al. Intravenous gammaglobulin treatment of chronic idiopathic thrombocytopenic purpura. Blood 1983;62:480.
34. Walsh CM, Nardi MA, Karpatkin S. On the mechanism of thrombocytopenic purpura in sexually active homosexual men. N Engl J Med 1984;311:635.
35. Kahane S, Dvilansky A, Estok L, Nathan I, Zolotov Z, Sarov I. Detection of anti-platelet antibodies in patients with

idiopathic thrombocytopenic purpura (ITP) and in patients with rubella and herpes group viral infections. Clin Exp Immunol 1981;44:49.

36. Kelton JG, Keystone J, Moore J, Denomme G, Tozman E, et al. Immune-mediated thrombocytopenia of malaria. J Clin Invest 1983;71:832.

37. van der Lelie J, van der Plas-Van Dalen CM, von dem Borne AEGK: Platelet autoantibodies in septicaemia. Br J Haematol 1984;58:755.

38. Kelton JG, Neame PB, Gauldie J, Hirsh J. Elevated platelet-associated IgG in the thrombocytopenia of septicemia. N Engl J Med 1979;300:760.

39. Verdirame JD, Feagler JR, Commers JR. Multiple myeloma associated with immune thrombocytopenic purpura. Cancer 1985;56:1199.

40. Varticovski L, Pick AI, Schattner A, Shoenfeld Y. Antiplatelet and anti-DNA in Waldenström macroglobulinemia and ITP. Am J Hematol 1987;24:351.

41. Bellone JD, Kunicki TJ, Aster RH: Immune thrombocytopenia associated with carcinoma. Ann Intern Med 1983; 99:470.

42. Kubota T, Tanoue K, Murohashi I, Nara N, Yamamoto N, Yamazaki H, Aoki N. Autoantibody against platelet glycoprotein IIb/IIIa in a patient with non-Hodgkin's lymphoma. Thromb Res 1989;58:379.

43. Burrows RF, Kelton JG. Thrombocytopenia at delivery: a prospective survey of 6715 deliveries. Am J Obstet Gynecol 1990;162:731.

44. Samuels P, Bussel JB, Braitman LE, Tomaski A, Druzin ML, et al. Estimation of the risk of thrombocytopenia in the offspring of pregnant women with presumed immune thrombocytopenic purpura. N Engl J Med 1990;323:229.

45. Aster RH. Gestational thrombocytopenia: a plea for conservative management. N Engl J Med 1990;323:264.

46. Territo M, Finklestein J, Oh W, Hobel C, Kattlove H. Management of autoimmune thrombocytopenia in pregnancy and in the neonate. Obstet Gynecol 1973;41:579.

47. Cines DB, Dusak B, Tomaski A, Mennuti M, Schreiber AD. Immune thrombocytopenic purpura and pregnancy. N Engl J Med 1982;306:826.

48. Kelton JG, Inwood MJ, Barr RM, Effer SB, et al. The prenatal prediction of thrombocytopenia in infants of mothers with clinically diagnosed immune thrombocytopenia. Am J Obstet Gynecol 1982;144:449.

49. Piscitelli JT, Simel DL, Rosse WF. Does maternal platelet-associated or platelet-bindable IgG correlate with levels in umbilical cord blood or colostrum during normal pregnancy? Obstet Gynecol 1988;158:430.

50. Moutet A, Fromont P, Farcet JP, Rotten D, et al. Pregnancy in women with immune thrombocytopenic purpura. Arch Intern Med 1990;150:2141.

51. Karpatkin M, Porges RF, Karpatkin S. Platelet counts in infants or women with autoimmune thrombocytopenia. N Engl J Med 1981;305(16):936.

52. Kelton JG, Blanchette VS, Wilson WE, Powers P, Mohan Pai KR, Effer SB, Barr RD. Neonatal thrombocytopenia due to passive immunization. N Engl J Med 1980; 302:1401.

53. Blanchette VS, Chen L, Salomon de Friedberg Z, Hogan V, Trudel E, Decary F. Alloimmunization of the Pl^{A1} platelet antigen: results of a prospective study. Br J Haematol 1990;74:209.

54. Muller-Eckhardt G, Muller-Eckhardt C. Allioimmunization against the platelet specific Zwa antigen associated

with HLA-DRw52 and/or DRw6. Hum Immunol 1987; 18:181.

55. von dem Borne A, van Leeuwen E, von Riesz LE, van Boxtel CJ, Engelfriet P. Neonatal alloimmune thrombocytopenia: detection and characterization of the responsible antibodies by the platelet immunofluorescence test. Blood 1981; 57:649.

56. Mueller-Eckhardt C, Marks HJ, Baur MP, Mueller-Eckhardt G. Immunogenetic studies of platelet-specific antigen Pl^{A1}. Immunobiology 1982;160:375.

57. Mueller-Eckhardt C, Becker T, Weisheit M, Witz C, Santoso S. Neonatal alloimmune thrombocytopenia due to fetomaternal Zwb incompatibility. Vox Sang 1986;50:94.

58. von dem Borne AEGK, von Riesz E, Verheugt FWA, ten Cate JW, Koppe JG, Engelfriet CP, Nijenhuis LE. Bak^a new platelet-specific antigen involved in neonatal alloimmune thrombocytopenia. Vox Sang 1980;39:113.

59. Shibata Y, Matsuda I, Miyaji T, Ichibawa Y. Yuk^a, a new platelet antigen involved in two cases of neonatal alloimmune thrombocytopenia. Vox Sang 1986;50:177.

60. Kieffer N, Boizard B, Didry D, Wautier Jean-L, Nurden AT. Immunochemical characterization of the platelet-specific alloantigen Lek^a: a comparative study with the Pl^{A1} alloantigen. Blood 1984;64:1212.

61. Kiefel V, Santoso S, Katzmann B, et al. A new platelet specific alloantigen Bra. Report of 4 cases with neonatal alloimmune thrombocytopenia. Vox Sang 1988;54:101.

62. Barr AL, Whineray M. Case report. Immune thrombocytopenia induced by co-trimoxazole. Aust NZ J Med 1980; 10:54.

63. Bussell JB, Berkowitz RL, McFarland JG, Lynch L, Chitkara U. Antenatal treatment of neonatal alloimmune thrombocytopenia. N Engl J Med 1988;24:1374.

64. Deleted in proof.

65. Hackett T, Kelton JG, Powers P. Drug-induced platelet destruction. Semin Thromb Hemostas 1982;8:116.

66. Lerner W, Caruso R, Faig D, Karpatkin S. Drug-dependent and non-drug-dependent antiplatelet antibody in drug-induced immunologic thrombocytopenic purpura. Blood 1985;66:306.

67. Eisner EV, Shahidi NT. Immune thrombocytopenia due to a drug metabolite. N Engl J Med 1972;287:376.

68. Kelton JG, Meltzer D, Moore J, Giles AR, Wilson WE, et al. Drug-induced thrombocytopenia is associated with increased binding of IgG to platelets both in vivo and in vitro. Blood 1981;58:524.

69. Christie DJ, Diaz-Arauzo H, Cook JM. Antibody-mediated platelet destruction by quinine, quinidine, and their metabolities. J Lab Clin Med 1988;112:92.

70. Visentin GP, Newman PJ, Aster RH. Characteristics of quinine- and quinidine-induced antibodies specific for platelet glycoproteins IIb and IIIa. Blood 1991; 77:2668.

71. Taaning E, Killmann SA, Morling N, Ovesen H, Svejgaard A. Post-transfusion purpura (PTP) due to anti-Zw[+b] (−Pl[+A2]): the significance of IgG3 antibodies in PTP. Br J Haematol 1986;64:217.

72. Schwartz KA, Royer G, Kaufman DB, Penner JA. Complications of heparin administration in normal individuals. Am J Hematol 1985;19:355.

73. Warkentin TE, Kelton JG. Heparin and platelets. Hematol Oncol Clin North Am 1990;4:243.

74. Kelton JG, Sheridan D, Santos A, Smith J, et al. Heparin-induced thrombocytopenia: laboratory studies. Blood 1988; 72:925.

75. Coblyn JS, Weinblatt M, Holdsworth D, Glass D: gold-induced thrombocytopenia. Ann Intern Med 1981; 95:178.

76. Adachi JD, Bensen WG, Kassam Y, et al. Gold induced thrombocytopenia: 12 cases and a review of the literature. Semin Arthritis Rheum 1987;16:287.

77. Stafford BT, Crosby WH. Late onset of gold-induced thrombocytopenia. JAMA 1978;488:50.

78. Levin HA, McMillan R, Tavassoli M, Longmire RL, Yelenosky R, Sacks PV. Thrombocytopenia associated with gold therapy. Am J Med 1975;59:274.

79. von dem Borne AEGK, Pegels JG, van der Stadt RJ, van der Plas-van Dalen CM, Helmerhorst FM. Thrombocytopenia associated with gold therapy: a drug-induced autoimmune disease? Br J Haematol 1986;63:509.

80. Christie DJ, van Buren N, Lennon SS, Putnam JL. Vancomycin-dependent antibodies associated with thrombocytopenia and refractoriness to platelet transfusion in platelets with leukemia. Blood 1990;75:518.

81. Shulman NR, Aster RH, Leitner A, Hiller MC. Immunoreactions involving platelets. V. Post-transfusion purpura due to a complement fixing antibody against a genetically controlled platelet antigen. A proposed mechanism for thrombocytopenia and its relevance in "autoimmunity." J Clin Invest 1961;40:1597.

82. Abramson N, Eisenberg PD, Aster RH. Post-transfusion purpura: immunologic aspects and therapy. N Engl J Med 1974,29.1163.

83. Kickler TS, Ness PM, Herman JH, Bell WR. Studies on the pathophysiology of post-transfusion purpura. Blood 1986; 68:347.

84. Ehmann WC, Dancis A, Ferziger R, Karpatkin S. Post-transfusion purpura: conversion of PL^{A1}-negative platelets to the PL^{A1}-positive phenotype of stored plasma is not due to the presence of soluble PL^{A1} antigen. Proc Soc Exp Biol Med 1990;195:192.

85. Cimo PL, Aster RH. Post-transfusion purpura. Successful treatment by exchange transfusion. N Engl J Med 1972; 287:290.

86. Raniele DP, Opsahl JA, Kjellstrand CM. Should intravenous immunoglobulin G be first-line treatment for acute thrombotic thrombocytopenic purpura? Case report and review of the literature. Am J Kidney Dis 1991; 18:264.

87. Slichter SJ. Platelet transfusion therapy. Hematol Oncol Clin North Am 1990;4:291.

88. Murphy S. Guidelines for platelet transfusion. JAMA 1988; 259:2453.

89. Aster RH, Bartolucci A, Collins JA, Colton T, Gottlieb A, et al. Platelet transfusion therapy. JAMA 1987;257:1777.

90. Slichter SJ, Harker LA. Thrombocytopenia: mechanisms and management of defects in platelet production. Clin Haematol 1978;7:523.

91. Bishop JF, McGrath K, Wolf MM, Matthews JP, De Luise T, et al. Clinical factors influencing the efficacy of pooled platelet transfusions. Blood 1988;71:383.

92. Aster RH, Bartolucci AA, Collins JA, Colton T. Platelet transfusion therapy. Nat Inst Health 1986;6:1.

93. Sintnicolaas K, Sizoo W, Haije WG, Abels J, Vriesendorp HM, et al. Delayed alloimmunisation by random single donor platelet transfusions: a randomized study to compare single donor and multiple donor platelet transfusions in cancer patients with severe thrombocytopenia. Lancet 1981;750.

94. Sniecinski I, O'Donnell MR, Nowicki B, Hill LR. Prevention of refractoriness and HLA alloimmunization using filtered blood products. Blood 1988;71:1402.

95. Goldfinger D, McGinnis MH. Rh-incompatible platelet transfusions—risks and consequences of sensitizing immunosuppressed patients. N Engl J Med 1971; 284:942.

96. Howard JE, Perkins HA. The natural history of alloimmunization of platelets. Transfusion 1978;18:496.

97. Herzig RH, Herzig GP, Bull MI, Decter HP, Lohrmann FG, et al. Correction of poor platelet transfusion responses with leukocyte-poor HL-A matched platelet concentrates. Blood 1975;46:743.

98. Ware R, Reisner EG, Rosse WF. The use of radio-labeled and fluorescein-labeled antiglobulins in assays to predict platelet transfusion outcome. Blood 1984;63:1245.

99. Schiffer CA, Hogge DE, Aisner J, Dutcher JP, Lee EJ, Papenberg D. High-dose intravenous gammaglobulin in alloimmunized platelet transfusion recipients. Blood 1984; 64:937.

100. Zeigler ZR, Shadduck RK, Rosenfield CS, Mangan KF, Winkelstein A, et al. High-dose gamma globulin improves responses to single-donor platelets in patients refractory to platelet transfusion. Blood 1987;70:1433.

101. Glotzback RE: Cimetidine-induced thrombocytopenia. South Med J 1982;75:232.

102. Walker DJ, Saunders P, Griffiths ID. Gold induced thrombocytopenia. J Rheumatol 1986;13:225.

103. Cines DB, Kaywin P, Bina M. Heparin-associated thrombocytopenia. N Engl J Med 1980;303:788.

104. Lynch DM, Howe SE. Heparin-associated thrombocytopenia: antibody binding specificity to platelet antigens. Blood 1985;66:1176.

105. Sheridan D, Carter C, Kelton JG. A diagnostic test for heparin-induced thrombocytopenia. Blood 1986;67:27.

106. Shulman NR. Immunologic reactions to drugs. N Engl J Med 1972;287:408.

107. Christie DF, Mullen PC, Aster RH. Fab-mediated binding of drug-dependent antibodies to platelets in quinidine-and quinine-induced thrombocytopenia. J Clin Invest 1985; 75:310.

108. Smith ME, Reid DM, Jones CE, Jordan JV, Kautz CA, Shulman R. Binding of quinine- and quinidine-dependent drug antibodies to platelets is mediated by the Fab domain of the immunoglobulin G and is not Fc dependent. J Clin Invest 1987;79:912.

109. Kunicki TJ, Ruddell N, Nurden AT, et al. Further studies of the human platelet receptor for quinine- and quinidine-dependent antibodies. J Immunol 1981;126:398.

110. Berndt MC, Chong BH, Bull HA, Zola H, Castaldi PA. Molecular characterization of quinine/quinidine drug-dependent antibody platelet interaction using monoclonal antibodies. Blood 1985;66:1292.

111. Karpatkin M, Sisking GW, Karpatkin M. The platelet factor 3 immunoinjury technique reevaluated: development of a rapid test for antiplatelet antibody: detection in various clinical disorders, including immunologic drug-induced and neonatal thrombocytopenias. J Lab Clin Med 1977; 82:400.

112. Christie DJ, Mullen PC, Aster RH. Quinine- and quinidine-induced platelet antibodies can react with GPIIb/GPIIIa. Br J Haematol 1987;67:213.

113. Cimo PL, Pisciotta AV, Desai RG. Detection of drug-dependent antibodies by the ^{51}Cr platelet lysis test: docu-

mentation of immune thrombocytopenia induced by diphenylhydantoin, diazepam and sulfisoxazole. Am J Hematol 1977;2:65.

114. Hamilton HE, Sheets RF. Sulfisoxazole-induced thrombocytopenic purpura. JAMA 1978;239:2586.

115. Kiefel V, Santoso S, Schmidt S, et al. Metabolite-specific (IgG) and drug-specific antibodies (IgG, IgM) in two cases of trimethoprim-sulfamethoxazol-induced immune thrombocytopenia. Transfusion 1987;27:262.

116. Conti L, Fidani P, Chistolini A, et al. Detection of drug-dependent IgG antibodies with anti-platelet activity by the antiglobulin consumption assay. Haemostasis 1984; 14:480.

117. Ansell J, Tiarks C, McCue J, et al. Amrinone-induced thrombocytopenia. Arch Intern Med 1984;144:949.

118. Kinney EL, Ballard JO, Carlin B, Zelis R. Amrinone-mediated thrombocytopenia. Scand J Haematol 1983; 31:376.

119. Heer M, Von Felten A. Immune thrombocytopenia in narcotics addicts. Ann Intern Med 1985;103:645.

120. Camba L, Joyner MV. Acute thrombocytopenia following ingestion of indomethacin. Acta Haematol 1984; 71:350.

121. Koller RL, Blank NK. Strawberry pickers palsy. Arch Neurol 1980;37:320.

122. Morley A, Hirsch J. A case of thrombocytopenia associated with chlorpropamide therapy. Med J Aust 1964;2:988.

123. Williams WJ, Beutler E. Thrombocytopenia due to enhanced platelet destruction by immunologic mechanisms. In: Williams WJ, Butler E, eds. Hematology. 4th ed. New York: McGraw-Hill, 1990:1370.

124. Wales J, Wolff F. Hematologic side effects of diazoxide. Lancet 1967;1:53.

125. Duncan A, Moore SB, Barker P. Thrombocytopenia caused by furosemide-induced platelet antibody [Letter]. Lancet 1981; 1:1210.

126. Jost F. Blood dyscrasias associated with tolbutamide therapy. JAMA 1959;169:1468.

127. Balodimos MD, Camerine-Davalos RA, Marble A. Nine years' experience with tolbutamide in the treatment of diabetes mellitus. Metabolism 1966;15:957.

128. Shoenfeld Y, Shaidi NT, Livni E, et al. Thrombocytopenia from acetaminophen. N Engl J Med 1980;303:47.

129. Hodder FS, Kempert P, McCormack S, et al. Immune thrombocytopenia following actinomycin-D therapy. J Pediatr 1985;107:611.

130. Manohiharajah SM, Jenkins WJ, Roberts PD, Clark RC. Methyldopa and associated thrombocytopenia. Br Med J 1971;1:494.

131. Pai RG, Pai SM. Methyldopa-induced immune thrombocytopenia [Letter]. Am J Med 1988;85:123.

132. Benraad AH, Schoenaker AH. Thrombocytopenia after use of methyldopa. Lancet 1965;2:292.

133. Arrowsmith JB, Dreis M. Thrombocytopenia after treatment with danazol. N Engl J Med 1986;315:585.

134. Hess T, Riesen W, Scholtysik G, et al. Digitoxin intoxication with severe thrombocytopenia: reversal by digoxin-specific antibodies. Eur J Clin Invest 1983;13:159.

135. Katz MD, Wang P. Fenoprefen-associated thrombocytopenia. Ann Intern Med 1980;92:262.

136. Kulis JC. Chemically induced selective thrombocytopenic purpura. Arch Intern Med 1965;116:559.

137. Eisner EV, Kasper K. Immune thrombocytopenia due to a metabolite of para-aminosalicylic acid. Am J Med 1972; 53:790.

138. Feiging RD, Zarkowski HF, Shearer W, et al. Thrombocytopenia following administration of para-aminosalicylic acid. J Pediatr 1973;83:502.

139. Murphy MF, Riordan T, Minchinton R, et al. Demonstration of an immune-mediated mechanism of penicillin-induced neutropenia and thrombocytopenia. Br J Haematol 1983;55:155.

140. Salamon DJ, Nusbacher J, Stroupe T, et al. Red cell and platelet-bound IgG penicillin antibodies in a patient with thrombocytopenia. Transfusion 1984;24:395.

141. Follea G, Hamandijian I, Trzeciak MC, et al. Pentosane polysulphate associated thrombocytopenia. Thromb Res 1986; 42:413.

142. Meisner DJ, Carlson RJ, Gottieb AJ. Thrombocytopenia following sustained-released procainamide. Arch Intern Med 1985;145:700.

143. Christie DL, Lennon SS. Detection of drug-dependent platelet antibodies using immoblized staphylococcal protein A. Transfusion 1988;28:322.

144. Gibson PR, Pidcock ME. Immune-mediated thrombocytopenia associated with ranitidine therapy. Med J Aust 1986; 145:661.

145. Gafter U, Komolas L, Weinstein T, et al. Thrombocytopenia, eosinopnhilia and ranitidine. Ann Intern Med 1987; 106:477.

146. Blachman MA, Lowry RC, Pettit JE, Stradling P. Rifampicin-induced immune thrombocytopenia. Br Med J 1970;3:24.

147. Kahn HR, Brod RC. Thrombocytopenia due to stibophen. Arch Intern Med 1961;108:496.

148. Karachalios GN, Parigorakis JG. Thrombocytopenia and sulindac [Letter]. Ann Intern Med 1986;104:128.

149. Kramer MR, Levene C, Hershko C. Severe reversible autoimmune haemolytic anaemia and thrombocytopenia associated with diclofenac therapy. Scand J Haematol 1986; 36:118.

150. de al Coussaye JE, Mourad G, Canaud B, et al. Insuffisance renale aigne et thrombopenie a rechute par intolerance croisse a l'buprofene et an femoprotene. Presse Med 1983; 12:2764.

151. Schimizzi GF, Graehl PM, Michalski JP. Severe, reversible thrombocytopenia associated with meclofenamate. Arthritis Rheum 1982;25:359.

152. Gralnick HR, McGinniss M, Halterman R. Thrombocytopenia with sodium cephalothin therapy. Ann Intern Med 1972;77:401.

153. Lown J. Barr A. Immune thrombocytopenia induced by cephalosporins specific for thiomethyltetrazole side chain [Letter]. J Clin Path 1987;40:700.

154. Chen JH, Wiener L, Distenfeld A. Immunologic thrombocytopenia induced by gentamicin. NY State J Med 1980; 80:1134.

155. Schiffer CA, Weinstein HJ, Wiernik PH. Methicillin-associated thrombocytopenia [Letter]. Ann Intern Med 1967;85:338.

156. Meyboom RHB. Thrombocytopenia induced by nalidixic acid. Br Med J 1984;289:962.

157. Kounis NG. Oxytetracycline-induced thrombocytopenic purpura. JAMA 1975;231:734.

158. Wurzel HA, Mayock RL. Thrombocytopenia induced by sodium para-amino-salicylic acid. Report of a case. JAMA 1953;153:1094.

159. Levy MA, Senior RM, Sneider RE. Severe thrombocytopenic purpura complicating pentamidine therapy for pneumocystic carinii pneumonia. Cancer 1974;34:414.

160. Pena JM, Gonzalez JJ, Garciaal J, et al. Thrombocytopenia and sulfasalazine [Letter]. Ann Intern Med 1985; 102:277.

161. Claas FH, van der Meer JWM, Langerak J. Immunological effect of co-trimoxazole on platelets. Br Med J 1979; 2:898.

162. Walker RW, Heaton A. Thrombocytopenia due to vancomycin [Letter]. Lancet 1985;1:932.

163. Ackroyd JF. The immunological basis of purpura due to drug hypersensitivity. Proc R. Soc Med 1962;55:30.

164. Celada A, Herreros V, Rudolf H. Thrombocytopenic purpura during treatment with librax. Br Med J 1977;1:268.

165. Veall RM, Hogarth HC. Thrombocytopenia during treatment with clonazepam. Br Med J 1975;4:462.

166. Conti L, Gandolfo GM. Benzodiazepine-induced thrombocytopenia. Demonstration of drug-dependent platelet antibodies in two cases. Acta Haematol 1983;70:386.

167. Fincham RW, Hamilton HE, Schottelius DD. Late-onset thrombocytopenia with phenytoin therapy. Ann Neurol 1979;6:370.

168. Parker WA. Primidone thrombocytopenia. Ann Intern Med 1974;81:559.

169. Ragaz J, Buskard N, Manji M. Thrombocytopenia after combination therapy with aminoglutethimide and Tamoxifen: Which drug is to blame? Cancer 1984;68:1015.

170. Weinberger I, Rotenberg Z, Fuchs J, et al. Amiodarone-induced thrombocytopenia. Arch Intern Med 1987; 147:735.

171. Lanng-Nielsen J, Dahl R, Kissmeyer-Nielsen F. Immune thrombocytopenia due to antazoline. Allergy 1981; 36:517.

172. Eisner EV, LaBocki NL, Pinkney L. Chlorpheniramine dependent thrombocytopenia. JAMA 1975;231:735.

173. Stambaugh JE, Gordon RL, Geller R. Leukopenia and thrombocytopenia secondary to clinoril therapy. Lancet 1980;2:594.

174. Mueller-Eckhardt C, Kuenzlen E, Kiefel V, et al. Cyclophosphamide-induced immune thrombocytopenia in a patient with ovarian carcinoma successfully treated with intravenous gamma globulin. Blut 1983;46:165.

175. Rachmilewitz EA, Dawson RB, Rachmilewitz B. Serum antibodies against desipramine as a possible cause for thrombocytopenia. Blood 1968;32:524.

176. Lacy J, Bober-Sorcinelli KE, Farber KE. Acute thrombocytopenia induced by parenteral radiographic contrast medium. Am J Roentgenol 1986;146:1298.

177. Pirovino M, Ohnhaus EE, Vonfelte A. Digoxin-associated thrombocytopenia. Eur J Clin Pharmacol 1981;19:205.

178. Liang R. Thrombocytopenia associated with etretinate therapy. Acta Haematol 1988;79:112.

179. Davis HP, Newlands ES, Allain T, Hedge U. Immune thrombocytopenia caused by flavone-8-acetic acid [Letter]. Lancet 1988;1:412.

180. Khaleeli AA. Quinaband-induced thrombocytopenia purpura in a patient with myxoedema coma. Br Med J 1976; 2:562.

181. Insausti CLG, Lechin F, van der Dijs B. Severe thrombocytopenia following oral cholecystography with iocetamic acid. Am J Hematol 1983;14:285.

182. Hysell JK, Hysell JW, Gray JM. Thrombocytopenic purpura following iopanoic acid ingestion. JAMA 1977;237:361.

183. Johnson TM, Rapini RP. Isoretinoin-induced thrombocytopenia. J Am Acad Dermatol 1987;17:838.

184. El-Ghobari AF, Capella HA. Levamisole-induced thrombocytopenia. Br Med J 1977;555.

185. Andes WA. Thromboneutropenia and levamisole. South Med J 1982;75:895.

186. Wanamaker WM, Wanamaker SJ, Celesia GG, et al. Thrombocytopenia associated with long-term levodopa therapy. JAMA 1976;235:2217.

187. Grossman LK, Grossman NJ. Methylphenidate and idiopathic thrombocytopenic purpura—Is there an association? J Fam Pract 1985;20:302.

188. Fasola GP, Dosualdo F, Depangehe V, Barducci E. Thrombocytopenia and mexilitine. Ann Intern Med 1984; 100:162.

189. Peitzman SJ, Martin C. Thrombocytopenia and minoxidil. Ann Intern Med 1980;92:874.

190. Cimo PL, Hammond JJ, Moake JL. Morphine-induced immune thrombocytopenia. Arch Intern Med 1982; 142:832.

191. Green PJ, Nagrosea SM. Nomifensine and thrombocytopenia. Br Med J 1984;288:830.

192. Hare DL, Hicks BH. Thrombocytopenia due to oxprenolol [Letter]. Med J Aust 1979;2:259.

193. Dodds WN, Davidson RJL. Thrombocytopenia due to slow-release oxprenolol. Lancet 1978;2:683.

194. Harrison EE, Hickman JW. Hemolytic anemia and thrombocytopenia associated with penicillamine ingestion. South Med J 1975;68:113.

195. Arnved J, Shov PS, Winter K. Pentagastrin-induced thrombocytopenia [Letter]. Lancet 1985;2:1068.

196. MacFarland RB. Fatal drug reaction associated with prochlorperazine (Compazine): report of a case characterized by jaundice, thrombocytopenia, and agranulocytosis. Am J Clin Pathol 1963;40:284.

197. King HE, Cooper T. Thrombocytopenia: a clinical analysis of 500 cases. Postgrad Med 1962;31:532.

198. Jennings GH, Gower ND. Thrombocytopenic purpura in toluene diisocyante workers. Lancet 1963;1:406.

CHAPTER 29

Nonimmune Disorders of Platelets

PAULETTE MEHTA

If you prick us, do we not bleed?
—Shakespeare, 1596

Bleeding does not necessarily indicate that there is an underlying disorder. Many people have nosebleeds, but few of them have coagulation abnormalities. Therefore, the adequacy of response to bleeding is an important point. If adequate, diagnostic studies are not necessary; if not, they should be pursued.

Thus, the evaluation for platelet abnormalities is initially based on clinical judgment, which is largely formed during careful history taking. Does the patient bleed after brushing the teeth every day? (Some people think it's normal to bleed while brushing!) How many pads does she use during a menstrual period? How many bruises are "normal" for them?

Questions regarding family history need to be directed (Table 29.1). For example, were there prior stillbirths? Did anyone have splenectomy? Did family members ever require a blood transfusion? Who if anyone is on lifelong prophylactic antibiotics? Did any family members have a gallbladder removed?

Questions regarding drugs also must be direct. Many drugs—antibiotics, analgesics, antihistamines, antipruritics, antiemetics, antidepressants, and antiasthma medications—have profound effects upon platelets. Some patients forget about aspirin use, don't consider birth control pills medications, think that "Goodies" (one generic preparation of aspirin sold over the counter) are home remedies and not true medications, or discount other drugstore medications that may contain aspirin or other platelet inhibitors. Even foods like garlic, onion, mushrooms, and ginger, for example, may have potent platelet-inhibitory effects.

A Patient with a Platelet Aggregation

LW is a 4-year-old Caucasian girl who was admitted to the emergency room with an acute nosebleed. She had had frequent nosebleeds and ecchymoses in the past and had been previously evaluated by another physician who had suspected child abuse. This accusation had inhibited the family from seeking help for subsequent bleeding problems. This time, however, the bleeding could not be managed with ice and pressure alone. She was evaluated by the ENT service, where no

abnormalities were found, and she was then referred for evaluation of a bleeding disorder. She denied drug intake, recent viral infection, or change in diet. Review of history revealed that the bleeding manifestations were generalized; she often had mucosal bleeding and oozing from gums after brushing her teeth. Family history was significant in that other family members had similar problems; one family member had recurrent hemorrhages, and one infant had died of unknown cause in early life.

Bleeding time was more than 15 minutes (not repeated).

Laboratory studies showed a platelet count of 150 × 10⁹/L and a white blood cell count of 6 × 10⁹/L with 58% segmented cells, 38% lymphocytes, and 4% monocytes. Hemoglobin was 91 g/L, and hematocrit, 31%. The blood smear showed neither large, tiny, nor gray platelets. Platelet aggregation studied by optical density time measurement showed the following: epinephrine, 0%; ADP, 2 μM, 0%; ADP, 4 μM, 0%; ADP, 20 μM, 0%; ADP, 200 μM, 0%; thrombin, 0%; ristocetin, 0%; arachidonic acid, 0%; and collagen, 0% (fig. 29.1). With each of these reagents, the platelet aggregation pattern failed to show either a primary or a secondary wave. The aggregation pattern of the normal control subject was epinephrine, 80%; ADP, 2 μM, 80%; ADP, 4 μM, 100%; ADP, 20 μM, 100%; ADP, 200 μM, 100%; thrombin, 100%; ristocetin, 95%; arachidonic acid, 85%; and collagen, 85%. The control aggregation pattern showed an initial lag period, a primary wave, a slowing of the wave or plateau, and a final, rapid secondary wave.

Since LW had no aggregation response, one must search for other medical history, particularly intake of aspirin or aspirin-containing drugs, recent changes with diet, and recent infections. Changes in diet may be important to note, since ingesting onions, garlic, spices, fish, and other foods can cause decreased platelet aggregation (Table 29.2). The child's repeat platelet aggregation was unchanged; those of other family members were similar to those of control subjects. Counter immunoelectrophoresis was performed to evaluate platelet mem-

brane glycoprotein receptors, which showed that glycoprotein IIb/IIIa was missing.

LW continued to have recurrent nosebleeds, which were treated with platelet transfusions to which she developed antibodies and became refractory. She was begun on intranasal DDAVP (a synthetic derivative of vasopressin) at the time of nosebleeds, which helped decrease their severity, at least during the initial few hours of each day. We considered bone marrow transplantation, but no family members were compatible with the patient.

Discussion: This patient had a primary platelet aggregation defect that presented early in life. Her history

Table 29.1. Important Questions to Ask to Uncover a Bleeding Diathesis

1. Were bleeding episodes present since infancy? since childhood?
2. When did the first one begin?
3. How long do they last?
4. What makes them stop?
5. Was there excessive bleeding around the umbilical cord stump?
6. What happened at the time of circumcision? (if relevant)
7. Do you have gum bleeding after brushing your teeth?
8. Are multiple sites involved?
9. Is the bleeding spontaneous?
10. Is the bleeding slow and does it recur after a few days? (suggests deep bleeding as in factor deficiencies)
11. What happened during surgery or during accidents?
12. Are menstrual bleeding episodes excessive? (i.e., lasting more than 5–7 days, using more than 4–5 pads per day)?
13. Is a maternal uncle affected? (suggests factor VIII or IX deficiency)
14. Are the mother and a sister affected? (suggests platelet or vascular abnormality)
15. Did anyone in the family have transfusions, cholecystectomy, or splenectomy?

convinced us that she had a true bleeding disorder and not simply an exaggerated response to a bleeding stress. First, she had spontaneous generalized bleeding. Second, it was repeated over time. Moreover, the bleeding disorder was not related to thrombocytopenia, since her platelet count was normal. This was therefore a problem that needed to be investigated for a functional platelet or coagulation defect.

A history of having been accused of child abuse is common to parents of children with bleeding disorders. Child abuse always has to be considered in the differential diagnosis of ecchymoses, especially when there is no obvious laboratory abnormality. It can usually be ruled out, however, with careful history taking, with physical examination, by lack of other evidence of abuse, and by the generalized, spontaneous, and different types of bleeding. Overemphasis of this possibility can traumatize families who sincerely seek help and drive them away from medical facilities.

The first step in the laboratory evaluation of LW was a review of her blood count and smear (Table 29.3). The platelet count was normal, and the platelet morphology appeared normal. In the smear, we looked for clumps of platelets, which usually represents hyperactivity but can

Table 29.2. Foods and Spices Associated with Decreased Platelet Function

Ginger
Onions
Vitamin C
Vitamin E
Cumin
Turmeric
Garlic
Cloves
Alcohol
N-3 fatty acids
Chinese black tree fungus

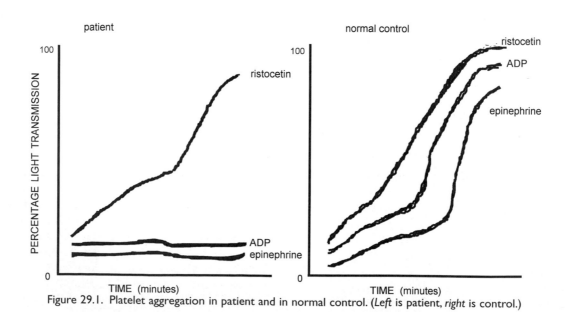

Figure 29.1. Platelet aggregation in patient and in normal control. (*Left* is patient, *right* is control.)

also indicate hypoactivity. For example, heparin induces a state in which platelets clump excessively and in which patients may develop arterial thrombosis and also have bleeding problems because of a relative thrombocytopenia at sites other than the thrombus. Disseminated intravascular coagulation (DIC) can cause a similar problem. Large platelets, which could indicate a compensated thrombolytic state, should be looked for.

When platelets are destroyed or consumed, as occurs in sequestration, thrombosis, or antibody-mediated destruction, the normal bone marrow responds with young, large, and optimally functional platelets. This is an important clue to diagnosis of thrombolytic state, since not all platelet-loss conditions cause thrombocytopenia; if the response from the bone marrow is sufficiently brisk, it may not occur or appear only intermittently. In LW, the platelets were not large, and it was therefore unlikely that she had a thrombolytic condition.

Large platelets can also suggest primary platelet dysfunction as in the Bernard-Soulier syndrome (Table 29.4). In this disease, platelets contain two to five times the normal amount of protein, and the bone marrow contains normal megakaryocytes. These patients lack glycoprotein Ib and therefore cannot bind von Willebrand's factor to the platelet membrane (Table 29.4, see below). The large platelets in this disorder are not associated with

a bone marrow thrombopoietic stress, rather they are related to a congenital abnormality (1).

Conversely, platelets can be extremely small; in particular, the platelets associated with Wiskott-Aldrich syndrome are tiny (1). Seeing such platelets should trigger a search for urticaria, allergic manifestations, and chronic infections by history. If these symptoms are identified, the possibility of Wiskott-Aldrich syndrome becomes real. (In LW, neither the history nor laboratory features suggested this possibility). The tiny platelets in this syndrome—like the huge ones in Bernard-Soulier syndrome—are related to congenital platelet abnormalities.

When platelets are very small or very large, electronic platelet counts become unreliable. Only platelets that fall within the normal platelet size range are counted on these machines; others will be counted as debris, if very small, or as red or white blood cells, if very large. These patients may therefore have spurious thrombocytopenia. Platelet morphology provides clues other than size. Certain conditions are associated with normal-sized, but abnormal-appearing platelets; in particular, patients with May-Hegglin disorder have bizarre platelets that appear folded over, hypersegmented, and granular and contain Dohle bodies. Patients with alpha storage pool disease also have abnormal-appearing platelets that appear gray and hypogranular.

In LW, the platelet morphology of the blood smear was normal. The sizing histogram obtainable on most modern automatic blood cell counters (PDW) is shown in Figure 29.2 and is similar to that of control subjects.

The original bleeding time was more than 15 minutes, which suggested a platelet or vascular abnormality. The bleeding time may be difficult to interpret, since it is variable (2–4). Many extraneous factors contribute to spuriously increased, decreased, or variable bleeding times (Tables 29.5 and 29.6). Also, many diseases cause prolonged bleeding time even though platelets are not involved in the disease or its complications (Table 29.5). In a recent critical review, Rodgers et al. evaluated 862 reports relating to 1321 studies and found that the bleeding time was not uniformly reliable in diagnosis, prognosis, or evaluation of therapy (3).

In this case, the history, normal blood smear, platelet count, and prolonged bleeding time convinced us that LW had a bleeding disorder. In addition, clinical history suggested a platelet or platelet–vessel wall abnormality rather than a coagulation defect, since the bleeding was superficial only; no joint or muscle bleeding had occurred, and bleeding did not recur after clot formation.

To pinpoint the diagnosis, *normal platelet physiology* is reviewed.

Normal Platelets: Under normal conditions, the platelet cytoplasm is surrounded by a membrane and an amorphous coat. In the cytoplasm, there are microtubular systems and

Table 29.3. Clues to Platelet Disorders on Blood Smear

Finding	Clue
1. Clumps of platelets	Spurious thrombocytopenia; platelet hyperactivity
2. Tiny platelets	Wiskott-Aldrich syndrome
3. Large platelets	Collagen vascular disease; excessive consumption; splenic trapping
4. Huge platelets	Bernard-Soulier syndrome
5. Gray platelets	Alpha storage pool disease
6. Granular and convoluted	May-Hegglin anomaly
7. Megakaryocyte fragments	Myeloproliferative disorders

Table 29.4. Features of Bernard-Soulier Disease

Mild-to-moderate bleeding disorder
Very large platelets
EM studies of platelets are normal
Platelet protein content is 2–5 times normal
Normal numbers of megakaryocytes
Normal platelet aggregation with ADP, collagen, epinephrine
Rate of aggregation is low in response to thrombin
No aggregation in presence of ristocetin or autologous plasma
Defective ristocetin-induced platelet aggregation is not corrected with normal plasma
No binding of platelets to radiolabeled vWF
Glycoprotein Ib is missing

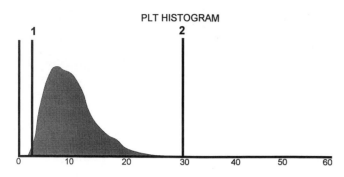

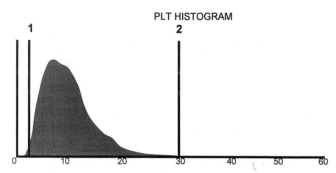

Figure 29.2. Platelet histogram in patient and in normal subject. *Top*, platelet histogram in this patient shows normal pattern of platelet size distribution. Microplatelets represent 13.9%, and macroplatelets 0.67%, of total population. *Bottom*, platelet histogram of normal subject is identical to that of patient.

Table 29.5. Conditions Associated with Abnormal Bleeding Time

Increased
    Increased cuff pressure
    Increased length or depth of cut
    Cut placement in antecubital fossa
    Changes in temperature
    Anxiety
    Younger age
    Female sex
    Pregnancy
    Anemia
    Thrombocytopenia
    Platelet functional defects
    vWD
    Some drugs
Decreased
    Previous bleeding test within 4 hours
    Cooling of skin
    Higher cholesterol diet
Variable effects
    Handedness
    Serum triglycerides
    Weight-to-height ratio
    Skinfold thickness
    Social class
    Direction of incision
    Ethnic group

Table 29.6. Diseases Associated with Prolonged Bleeding Time in Which Platelets Are Not Primarily Affected

Amyloidosis
Bartter's syndrome
Glycogen storage disease type 1
Congenital heart disease
Scoliosis
Collagen defects
    Osteogenesis imperfecta
    Ehlers-Danlos syndrome
Neurofibromatosis
Dysfibrinogenemia
Deficiencies of fibrinogen or factor V, VII, VIII, IX,
    X, XI, or XII
Factor VIII inhibitors
Vitamin K deficiency in newborn
Anemia
β-Thalassemia
Hepatic disease
Acute glomerulonephritis
Renal failure
Systemic lupus erythematosus
Hypothyroidism
Preeclampsia
Toxemia of pregnancy
Trisomy-21
Respiratory distress syndrome in the newborn

Table 29.7. Platelet Granules

Dense granules
    ATP
    ADP (storage pool)
    Calcium
    Pyrophosphate
    Serotonin
Alpha granules
    Platelet factor 4
    β-Thromboglobulin
    von Willebrand's factor
    Thrombospondin
    Fibronectin
    Factor V
    High-molecular-weight kininogen
    Platelet-derived growth factor (PDGF)

granules. The trilaminar membrane has many invaginated channels to the interior of the cell, allowing uptake of plasma-borne substances and extrusion of platelet contents. The dense tubular system in the cytoplasm is interspersed between the membrane invagination. Its function is not known. The microtubules are present at the circumference of the platelet and maintain its shape. The platelet membrane has at least 19 separate glycoprotein receptors. Some of these are related to ADP, thrombin, and collagen-induced aggregation; to sites of pore formation or membrane transport; and to cell-surface electrostatic charge. The amorphous coat surrounding the platelet membrane serves as a "sponge" to which fibrinogen and factors V, VIII, and XI attach (5).

Granules and Energy in the Platelets: Granules are present in the platelets; most numerous are α-granules and dense bodies (Table 29.7). Dense bodies contain ADP (storage pool), ATP, serotonin, and calcium. Another pool of ADP (metabolic pool) is freely available within the cytoplasm. Alpha granules contain platelet factor 4, β-thromboglobulin, thrombospondin, von Willebrand's factor, fibrinogen, factor V, kininogen, and platelet-derived growth factor (PDGF). The platelet also contains glycogen granules, RNA, and mitochondria. Energy is derived from ATP, most of which is generated from glucose metabolism through the Embden-Meyerhof glycolytic pathway, the rest from the Krebs cycle and the hexose monophosphate shunt. Energy is necessary for transport of protein in and out of the cell, for maintenance of shape, and for metabolism of proteins and fatty acids. Granules can be evaluated by election microscopy. Deficiency of dense or alpha granules results in platelet storage pool disease.

> **Platelet Function Tests Simulate In Vivo Activation:** Platelet function assays delineate step-by-step platelet physiology as shown in Figure 29.3. Under normal conditions, platelets flow through the vasculature without adhesion, sequestration, deposition, or alteration of function. Disruption of endothelium by chemical, toxic, trauma, infectious, or hemodynamic stress, however, results in adhesion of platelets, which is the initial step in hemostasis. Subsequent to adhesion, the platelet swells, spreads, and releases its granules (release reaction), which causes clumping of other platelets at the site of trauma, resulting in formation of a platelet plug. After the release reaction, only a few granules remain in the platelet.

Collagen in the subendothelium is a potent stimulus for attraction and deposition of (few) platelets at the damaged areas (adhesion). After a brief time lag, unbound platelets clump to the adherent platelets (aggregation). The most important mechanisms involved in the aggregation of platelets are (a) release of ADP; (b) activation of platelet phospholipase A_2 and C, which initiates the generation of cyclic endoperoxides PGG_2 and PGH_2 and subsequently thromboxane A_2, which per se induce aggregation and cause platelets to release their granule content; and (c) other mechanisms not involving ADP or endoperoxide-thromboxane pathway such as thrombin-induced aggregation. Platelet aggregation is accentuated by the synergistic actions of these mechanisms. Aggregation may be "primary," which is reversible and produced in vitro by low concentrations of aggregating agents, or "secondary," which is irreversible and is produced by high concentrations of aggregating agents and endogenous platelet secretions. The release reaction accounts for the irreversible secondary wave of aggregation in vivo; it requires that thromboxane A_2 be produced and secreted.

Platelet Function Requires Arachidonic Acid (AA) Metabolism: For platelet function, an entire metabolic pathway must be activated (Fig. 29.4). First, phospholipase A_2 or C must be activated and trigger the release of AA from the membrane phospholipids. AA is then available for oxidation as the first step in the formation of the prostaglandins, thromboxane, and prostacyclin via the cyclooxygenase pathway or to leukotrienes via the 5-lipoxygenase pathway or to other hydroperoxides (via 12- or 15-lipoxygenase), depending on the cell type, the enzymes present, and the stimulus. The metabolites are formed rapidly and are labile. In the platelet, cyclooxygenase converts arachidonic acid to endoperoxides G_2 and H_2. These are metabolized via thromboxane A_2 synthetase to thromboxane A_2, which is labile and rapidly hydrolyzed to thromboxane B_2, an inactive and stable product. This pathway will not proceed if phospholipase A_2 or C is missing, if cyclooxygenase is missing or inactivated (e.g., by indomethacin, aspirin, or some other nonsteroidal anti-inflammatory drugs), if thromboxane A_2 synthetase is missing or blocked, or if calcium mobilization does not occur normally.

> **Platelet Function Tests:** Tests that relate to platelet functions are listed in Table 29.8. Platelet adhesiveness can be studied in several different ways. A frequently used test involves passing the blood through a plastic tube filled with glass beads. The difference in platelet count between the affluent and effluent blood relates to the adhesion of platelets. However, during the procedure, platelets are lost in the glass-bead columns because of platelet-platelet aggregation occurring in layers over the initial glass-

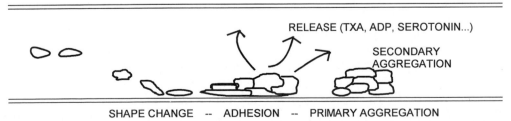

RELEASE (TXA, ADP, SEROTONIN...)

SECONDARY AGGREGATION

SHAPE CHANGE -- ADHESION -- PRIMARY AGGREGATION

Figure 29.3. Steps in platelet activation. Platelets circulate freely throughout circulation and become activated only at sites of endothelial disruption. Then, they change shape, adhere to subendothelium, and aggregate to each other. Primary aggregation triggers release reaction during which TXA_2, ADP, serotonin, and other vasoactive substances are secreted. This potentiates further platelet activation and results in secondary wave and irreversible platelet aggregation.

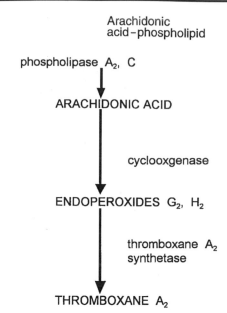

Figure 29.4. Arachidonic acid metabolism in platelets.

Table 29.8. Tests of Platelet Activity

In Vitro	*Ex Vivo*
Platelet adhesion	Platelet survival
Platelet aggregation	Plasma factor 4 level
Platelet release reaction	Plasma-thromboglobulin levels
Serotonin	Circulating platelet aggregates
ATP	Platelet prostaglandin generation

adherent platelet layer. This technique is difficult to standardize because several variables affect the results, and it is not considered specific for platelet adhesion.

Platelet adhesion to subendothelial surfaces can also be measured by direct morphometric techniques after perfusion of blood through chambers containing everted, deendothelialized strips of rabbit aorta. The attachment of platelets to surfaces can also be monitored by labeling platelets with a radioactive tag, such as indium-lll. The radiolabeled platelets can then be infused through a blood vessel obtained from a human or animal umbilical cord. Residual radioactivity can be measured and serves as an index of the attachment of platelets to the vessel wall.

Platelet aggregation is measured by direct microscopy and by light transmission methods (6). The latter are now the method of choice because subjective error is minimized. For either technique, platelet-rich plasma is obtained and an aggregation stimulant added to the platelet suspension. The amount of aggregation is evaluated by morphologic evidence of clumping of platelets on smear or by change in light transmission through the platelet-rich plasma. Light transmission is measured by means of a modified photometer that measures change in optical density as platelet-rich plasma becomes platelet-poorer as it

aggregates. (As the platelets clump and settle, the clear plasma allows more light to pass through.)

Although light transmission increases with aggregation, a temporary decrease occurs immediately after addition of the aggregating agent. This increase in density is due to the change of platelets from discoid to spherical shape and results in increased light scattering; this is referred to as "shape change." After shape change, the *primary wave* of aggregation takes place, resulting from platelets attaching to each other in suspension, either by a decrease in repulsive electrostatic charges or the stickiness of the external membrane surface of the platelets. Primary aggregation is reversible and activates the platelet to secrete and release granular contents including ADP, ATP, and serotonin, which then cause the *secondary wave* of platelet aggregation, which is irreversible. In some instances primary and secondary waves of aggregation might not be distinguishable. Fusion of the two waves occurs if reagent concentration is high or when certain reagents such as epinephrine are used. With collagen, aggregation may be delayed; this lag corresponds to the orientation of particulate material. Various parameters of platelet aggregation can be measured (but may be highly variable between laboratories). These include (*a*) the extent of primary wave aggregation, (*b*) the rate of primary wave aggregation, and (*c*) the extent of secondary wave aggregation.

Table 29.9 lists the commonly used platelet aggregation stimulating reagents (5). Various agents, their sites of action, and the type of aggregation pattern produced are mentioned. Use of various aggregation stimulating and inhibiting agents has allowed better understanding of the mechanism of platelet aggregation. *Platelet product release* can also be measured. Prior to the appearance of the secondary wave, platelets secrete and release constituents of their granules, including serotonin, ADP, ATP, platelet factor 4, β-thromboglobulin, fibrinogen, and other substances. The agents used to induce platelet product release are the same as the aggregating reagents. Secretion of metabolites from the various storage pools depends on the type of reagent used; for example, dense granules liberate ADP, serotonin, and calcium, alpha granules liberate acid hydrolyses, β-thromboglobulin, platelet factor 4 and fibrinogen.

Since secretory events do not occur simultaneously, measurement of one particular release product may not reflect the overall activity of platelets. Three criteria must be met to define platelet secretion: (*a*) the substance should be localized in the storage granules, (*b*) the extracellular increase should be balanced by intracellular decrease, and (*c*) secretion should be dependent on availability of metabolic ATP. The in vitro release reaction is commonly used to test for potential platelet hyperactivity and includes measurement of serotonin and ATP levels. The ex vivo release reaction is used to monitor actual release and is measured by plasma factor 4 and β-thromboglobulin levels.

Release of serotonin is triggered by many agents, such as thrombin, epinephrine, and collagen. This test is com-

Table 29.9. Platelet Aggregation Curves Induced by Various Aggregation-Stimulating Agents[a]

Agent	Lag Time	Shape Change	Primary Wave	Secondary Wave	Single Fused Wave	Dissaggregation
ADP—low conc.	0	+	+	0	0	+
ADP—med. conc.	0	+	+	+	0	0
ADP—high conc.	0	+	0	0	+	0
Collagen	+	+	0	0	+	0
Epinephrine—low conc.	0	±	+	+	0	0
Epinephrine—high conc.	0	±	+	+	±	0
Thrombin	±	+	0	0	+	0
Ristocetin	0	+	+	±	±	0
Serotonin	0	+	+	+	0	+
Cyclic endoperoxides	0	+	+	+	±	+

[a]Abbreviations: +, present; 0, absent; ± ,may be occasionally seen.

monly done by labeling platelets with ^{14}C, mixing labeled platelets with platelet-rich plasma, and adding release-inducing agent. The aggregated mixture is then centrifuged, and the supernatant counted in a scintillation counter. The percentage release of serotonin is then calculated. Serotonin release is a simple technique and has been used extensively to monitor release reactions. Simultaneous excretion of ATP and ADP and platelet aggregation can be measured by the Lumi-Aggregometer. Release of thromboxane A_2 (TXA_2) can be measured in platelet-rich plasma or in whole blood by radioimmunoassays of the stable metabolite (TXB_2).

Evaluation of Patient's Test Results: *There are several other tests of platelet activation that are useful for investigating "hyperactivity" or higher platelet turnover, rather than hypoactivity. These include platelet survival, platelet factor 4, β-thromboglobulin, and platelet prostaglandin production. However, these tests were not carried out in this patient because they measure platelet hyperactivity or increased destruction rather than hypoactivity. Since LW had problems with bleeding rather than with thrombosis or thrombolysis, platelet aggregation studies, electron microscopy, and receptor analysis were emphasized.*

Clinical experience dictates that the most common cause of deficient platelet aggregation is drug intake, in particular, aspirin and aspirin-containing drugs. However, LW's pattern of platelet aggregation did not resemble an aspirin-induced defect. In contrast to the pattern in LW, aspirin causes platelets to lose their responsiveness to epinephrine and ADP, but not to thrombin or ristocetin. Also, platelets from patients who have taken aspirin lose the secondary aggregation wave. In LW, the secondary wave is absent, but so is the primary wave. (In addition the history was negative for aspirin intake, even when the family was carefully questioned.)

Differential Diagnosis of the Abnormal Platelet Aggregation in This Patient: *In LW, it was necessary to search for a cause of primary and secondary wave platelet aggregation defects. (See Table 29.10 for a classification of platelet aggregation abnormalities.) Secondary wave platelet aggregation defects are much more common than primary defects and will be abnormal if*

Table 29.10. Classification of Platelet Function Abnormalities

I. Abnormal platelet adhesion (adhesion requires attachment of von Willebrand's factor to platelet glycoprotein Ib)
   A. von Willebrand's (vW) factor absent (vW disease)
   B. Platelet glycoprotein Ib missing (Bernard-Soulier disease)
   C. Barrier between von Willebrand's factor and the GPIb receptor (e.g., hypergammaglobulinemia)
II. Abnormal platelet aggregation
   A. Primary aggregation (the agonist must attach to its receptor)
      1. Selective defect: a particular receptor is missing
         α-Adrenergic receptor required for epinephrine-induced aggregation deficiency
         Thrombin deficiency
         ADP-receptor deficiency
         Endoperoxide/thromboxane A_2 receptor deficiency
      2. Generalized defect: platelet aggregation requires binding of agonists to receptors after attachment of fibrinogen to fibrinogen receptor
         A. Glycoprotein IIb/IIIA deficiency
         B. Several receptors absent
         C. Low fibrinogen (afibrinogenemia, hypofibrinogenemia)
         D. Glycoprotein IIb/IIIA receptor deficiency (Glanzmann's thrombasthenia)
   B. Secondary aggregation: (TXA_2 and ADP must be formed and released and granules must be present)
      1. TXA_2 or ADP not released (measure release reaction)
         A. Metabolic path may be interrupted
            1. Enzyme deficiency
               a. Cyclooxygenase
               b. Thromboxane A_2 synthetase
            2. Calcium mobilization defects
            3. Medication or drug that inhibits TXA_2 generation: aspirin, indomethacin, nonsteroidal antiinflammatories
            4. Storage pool deficiency (EM is diagnostic
               Alpha pool deficiency (gray platelet syndrome)
               Dense granule deficiency
               Combination of both

the necessary biochemicals are not generated and/or released during platelet activation. Thus, if the storage pools are deficient in substrates, then the products (i.e., ADP, histamine, serotonin, and others) necessary to drive the platelet to full activation will be deficient.

Alternatively, the secondary wave may fail to occur if the *enzymes* that drive the metabolic pathways are deficient. Under normal conditions, stimulation of the platelet membrane results in activation of phospholipase A_2 or C_2. This enzyme activation causes cleavage of arachidonic acid from the phospholipids on the platelet membrane. Once arachidonic acid is released into the cytoplasm, it is converted via cyclooxygenase to endoperoxides G_2 and H_2. These endoperoxides can then be metabolized to thromboxane A_2 via thromboxane A_2 synthetase. A deficiency of either of these two enzymes, cyclooxygenase or thromboxane A_2 synthetase, would prevent the formation of thromboxane A_2 and impair a secondary platelet aggregation response. Defective calcium mobilization, on which these steps depend, will similarly prevent the full expression of the secondary wave of platelet aggregation.

Other metabolic pathways and enzymes modulate this pathway. In particular, increases in cyclic AMP decrease platelet activity, while decreases in cyclic AMP promote it. Deficiencies of cyclooxygenase, of thromboxane A_2 and of calcium mobilization have all been described as congenital and familial syndromes (7–9).

In addition to congenital enzyme deficiencies, medication, drugs, and foods can also decrease platelet aggregation and result in secondary wave abnormalities (11) (Table 29.11). The most potent platelet-inhibitory drugs are aspirin and aspirin-containing medications that inhibit cyclooxygenase. Since cyclooxygenase cannot be synthesized in the platelet, the aspirin-induced platelet aggregation deficit persists for the entire life span of the platelet. Other medications that inhibit cyclooxygenase are indomethacin and sulfinpyrazone. Some medications actually increase platelet aggregation (Table 29.11).

In contrast to secondary wave aggregation defects, primary wave abnormalities are rare. In LW, the primary wave of platelet aggregation in response to both ADP and epinephrine was totally absent. This suggested that the receptors for ADP and epinephrine were not exposed. This happens only after fibrinogen binds to its receptor, glycoprotein IB. If fibrinogen is absent or if the glycoprotein lB receptor is missing, ADP- and epinephrine-induced platelet aggregation cannot occur.

The normal platelet aggregation in response to ristocetin ruled out von Willebrand's disease and Bernard-Soulier disease. In both of these diseases, ristocetin does not induce platelet aggregation, since ristocetin requires binding of von Willebrand's factor to its receptor, glycoprotein IIb/IIIa. If von Willebrand's factor or glycoprotein IIb/IIIa is missing, the patient will have a platelet adhesion deficiency, i.e., either von Willebrand's disease or Bernard-Soulier disease. Not all cases of von Willebrand's disease, however, are associated with abnormal ristocetin-

Table 29.11. Drugs Associated with Platelet Functional Abnormalities

A. Nonsteroidal antiinflammatory drugs
  1. Sulfinpyrazone
  2. Sulindac
  3. Indomethacin
  4. Aspirin
  5. Ibuprofen
  6. Diclofenac
B. β-lactam antibiotics
  1. Penicillins
    a. Carbenicilin, mezlocillin, piperacillin
    b. Ampicillin
    c. Penicillin G
  2. Cephalosporins
    a. Cephalothin
    b. Moxalactam
C. Cardiovascular drugs
  1. Dipyridamole
  2. Diltiazem
  3. Nifedipine
D. Anticoagulants
  1. Aminocaproic acid
  2. Heparin
E. Psychotropic drugs
  1. Imipramine
  2. Fluoxetine
  3. Amitriptyline
F. Anesthetics
  1. Cocaine
  2. Heroin
  3. Lidocaine
  4. Procaine
G. Chemotherapeutics
  1. Vincristine
  2. Asparaginase
  3. Daunorubicin
H. Antihistamines
  1. Diphenylhydramine
  2. Chlorpheniramine

induced platelet aggregation. In type IIb von Willebrand's disease, there is increased, not decreased, ristocetin-induced platelet aggregation.

Alternatively, deficient ristocetin-induced platelet aggregation (but normal platelet aggregation in response to other stimuli) could suggest Bernard-Soulier disease. This is an inherited platelet dysfunction associated with glycoprotein receptor IIb/IIIa deficiency, a lifelong bleeding diathesis, usually with mild thrombocytopenia and large platelets (Table 29.3). Thus, both von Willebrand's disease and Bernard-Soulier syndrome show decreased ristocetin-induced platelet aggregation but can be differentiated from each other by adding normal plasma. The defect in von Willebrand's disease will correct with normal plasma, since the missing von Willebrand's factor has now been added. The defect in Bernard-Soulier syndrome, however, will not do so, since the receptor to attach the

Table 29.12. Features of Glanzmann's Thrombasthenia

Bleeding disorder
Abnormal clot retraction
Mucocutaneous bleeding
Failure of platelets to aggregate in response to ADP, thrombin, collagen, or epinephrine
Platelets agglutinate in presence of ristocetin
Shape changes
Platelet degranulation
Platelets lack glycoprotein IIb/IIIa

von Willebrand's factor to the platelet membrane surface cannot be replaced by plasma.

In LW, Glanzmann's thrombasthenia was suspected in view of the normal platelet count and morphology, history of bleeding, and the decreased platelet aggregation induced by collagen, thrombin, and epinephrine but with normal platelet aggregation in response to ristocetin (Table 29.12).

To confirm the diagnosis of Glanzmann's thrombasthenia SDS-PAGE (sodium dodecyl sulfate–polyacrylamide gel electrophoresis) counterimmunoelectrophoresis was undertaken to determine that glycoprotein receptor IIb/IIIa was deficient and confirm the clinical suspicion of Glanzmann's thrombasthenia.

The platelet alloantigen PL A1, present in 97% of the normal population, is often absent in patients with Glanzmann's thrombasthenia (11). Most transfused platelets contain the antigen PL A1. Because patients with this disorder do not have this antigen, they are likely to produce antibodies against PL A1 following transfusions and are likely to become refractory to platelets very early in life. Therefore, they should be screened for this antigen, and if it is lacking, they should receive platelet transfusions from PL A1–negative individuals only.

More about the Receptor IIb/IIIa: Research on the nature of the receptor IIb/IIIa has led to surprising developments in antithrombotic therapy (12). Knowledge of the receptor biochemistry has led to synthesis of recombinant IIb/IIIa and to a monoclonal antibody against this receptor. This antibody has been tested in early animal and preclinical trials and appears promising in antithrombotic therapy (12). It may be an ideal agent, since it inhibits clot formation at the very first step, platelet activation and since it has no effects on other cell systems.

Had this been a sick child, the differential diagnosis would have been different; there are myriad reasons why platelets may function abnormally. Often the cause is multifactorial. Many of these factors have been sorted out; for example, various drugs, including antibiotics, antipyretics, antiemetics, and analgesics, impair platelet function (10) (Table 29.11). *Heparin,* even when used in very low doses as in flushing central catheters, is an often-overlooked agent that causes platelet dysfunction, thrombocytopenia, and sometimes arterial thrombosis (13). This he-

parin effect is independent of dose and may be related to the species origin of heparin. Thus, bovine heparin is more prone to alter platelets than is porcine heparin. The mechanism of heparin-induced platelet dysfunction is related to immune reactivity against heparin-platelet complexes in some cases and directly to altered arachidonic acid metabolism in others. The mere presence of an indwelling catheter can cause platelet injury. The catheter alters the platelet membrane surfaces as they travel through the thrombogenic, nonendothelialized surface of the catheter.

In *chronic renal disease,* decreased platelet adhesion, aggregation, platelet factor 3 release, and factor 4 release have been noted (14). The mechanisms of these impairments relate to the direct effects of unexcreted amino acids on platelets. Recently, Remuzzi et al. have also shown that nitric oxide production is increased in renal failure and that this is a potent platelet inhibitor (15). This could be another cause for platelet dysfunction.

Microangiopathies, associated with neoplasm, infection, and shock, can cause damage to red blood cells and to platelets, resulting in thrombocytopenia, anemia, and organ damage. If bone marrow compensation is adequate, patients may manifest platelet dysfunction without thrombocytopenia. Careful review of the blood film for red blood cell fragmentation and giant platelet size and simple laboratory evaluation of PT, PTT, fibrinogen, and fibrin split products should provide diagnostic information. Thrombotic thrombocytopenic purpura (TTP) and hemolytic uremia syndrome (HUS) are microangiopathies in which red cell fragmentation, thrombocytopenia, and organ dysfunction are present.

Treatment: *After the diagnosis of Glanzmann's thrombasthenia was established, LW was treated with platelet transfusions when bleeding occurred. She responded to platelet transfusions initially, but within 3 months became resistant to platelet transfusions and required single donor platelets from HLA-matched platelets. Refractoriness to platelets happens randomly in patients who are multiply transfused and is not necessarily related to the number of platelet transfusions. Patients with Glanzmann's thrombasthenia have a particularly high risk for developing refractoriness, as described above.*

LW was also started on desmopressin (DDAVP), a synthetic analog of vasopressin that has gained wide acceptance as a hemostatic agent. DDAVP is effective in many congenital and acquired platelet dysfunctional states as well as in other bleeding disorders. In some countries, DDAVP is even given to volunteer plasma donors to enhance factor VIII yield (16). (Agents that increase platelet function are listed in Table 29.13.)

Bone marrow transplantation can also be considered, and this may be the ideal treatment in view of the lifelong nature of Glanzmann's thrombasthenia, the severity of disease, and the rapid development of platelet refractoriness (17). Table 29.14 reviews treatment options.

Table 29.13. Agents That Increase Platelet Function

Prostanoids (e.g., thromboxane A_2)
Heparin
Cyclosporin
Ethanol
Saturated fatty acids
Cigarette smoke

Table 29.14. Methods of Treatment for Patients with Platelet Function Abnormalities

Local pressure
Ice
Packing
L-Desamino D-arginine vasopressin (DDAVP)
Estrogens
Platelet transfusions
Cryoprecipitate
Amicar (aminocaproic acid)
Bone marrow transplantation[a]

[a]May become treatment of choice as procedure becomes more refined.

Patient #2

JM is a 4-year-old Caucasian child who was well until he awoke one morning with widespread petechiae and ecchymoses. His physician examined him and performed laboratory tests. The platelet count was 60×10^9/L, and JM was referred for further evaluation. On admission, he was active, alert, and covered with numerous ecchymoses. He had not had any recent change in diet, medication intake, trauma, or viral infection, but he had had frequent episodes of upper respiratory infections in the past, each of which responded to antibiotics. He had not had episodes of severe infection such as meningitis or sepsis. Family history was negative for any blood dyscrasia, transfusion requirement, early deaths, splenectomy, or early cholecystectomy. The family denied any known child abuse. The natural parents lived together and did not smoke. The mother owned a cleaning company and maintained a stock of organic cleaners and paints and occasionally took JM to the area where they were used. The father worked in an office.

On physical examination, JM appeared well, alert, and active and had no evidence of heart disease, skeletal abnormality, organomegaly, or lymphadenopathy. He had many areas of petechiae and ecchymoses on face, arms, legs, back, and trunk.

A blood count showed a white blood cell count of 3×10^9/L, with 60% lymphocytes, 35% neutrophils, and 5% monocytes; Hb was 97 g/L; Hct, 27%; and platelet count, 60×10^9/L.

Review of the blood film showed neither large or giant platelets, nor unusual platelet morphology.

The platelet histograms were normal, with 13.9% small platelets and 0.67% large platelets, which was normal (Fig. 29.2). Folate and vitamin B_{12} levels were within normal ranges.

Viral studies showed an EBV titer of 1:640; HIV antibody was negative, as were CMV and TORCH titers.

A bone marrow examination showed normocellularity, with trilinear hematopoiesis and normal numbers of megakaryocytes. A platelet antibody screen was negative, antigranulocyte antibody studies were negative, and an extended antinuclear antibody panel was unremarkable. ESR was 36/mm/hour.

A presumptive diagnosis of post-EBV thrombocytopenia was made, and JM was seen weekly but not placed on treatment. Two months later, the platelet count decreased to 30×10^9/L, the neutrophil count to 10×10^9/L, and Hb to 50 g/L. He was treated with prednisone 2 mg/kg; the blood counts remained unchanged, but skin bleeding decreased.

A few months later, bone marrow aspiration was repeated. At this time, the marrow showed erythroid hyperplasia and normal trilinear bone marrow hematopoiesis. Chromosomal studies of the bone marrow were normal. JM continued with thrombocytopenia but remained asymptomatic and did not require therapy.

Discussion: Thrombocytopenia represents one of the more common childhood hematologic abnormalities. A review of the production, life span, and destruction of normal platelets will help to delineate which abnormality may be present in a given thrombocytopenic patient.

Normal Platelet Kinetics: The earliest committed precursor is the megakaryoblast, which is large, with basophilic cytoplasm and nonindented nucleus, and has up to 8N ploidy. Megakaryoblast granules contain demarcation membranes, alpha granules, and lysosomes, but no dense storage granules. These cells differentiate into promegakaryocytes, an intermediate form in which polyploidization stops. The nucleus is indented, and azurophilic granules are present. This cell differentiates into granular megakaryocytes with dense chromatin, an irregularly shaped nucleus, abundant cytoplasm, and alpha granules. The mature megakaryocyte begins to produce large amounts of platelet constituents including factor VIII R:Ag, actin, fibrinogen, platelet glycoproteins Ib, IIb/IIIa, platelet myosin, fibronectin, platelet factor 4, dense granules, and serotonin (18). Through a "fusion-fission" process, it develops demarcation membranes, which become margins for individual platelets that break away from the parent megakaryocyte.

Megakaryocyte maturation takes 4–5 days. Each megakaryocyte will release several thousand platelets, such that approximately 4×10^9/L will be made each day. In adults, most platelets are derived from bone marrow megakaryocytes, but pulmonary megakaryocytes will still contribute about 10% of total platelet production. Platelet production is regulated by colony-stimulating factors for megakaryocytes (CFU-mega), and thrombopoietin, a recently cloned hormone or biologic response modifier.

Once platelets are released from the bone marrow, two-thirds of them circulate and one-third reside in a splenic pool, exchanging freely with circulating platelets. The mechanisms of splenic platelet pooling is not completely understood, but apparently large numbers of platelets adhere to the surfaces of reticular cells and to the endothelial cells of the sinuses. Pooling is increased when the spleen is enlarged and may represent up to 80–90% of the total platelet mass. Platelets from the splenic pool are released into the circulation by epinephrine, stress, or infections.

Platelets *survive* in the circulation for 8–12 days, as measured by radiolabeling studies. Although they may aggregate in vivo in response to circulating ADP, serotonin, epinephrine, thrombin, or other agents, most such aggregates will dissociate. As the platelets age, their size, density, and functional capacity decreases. Large platelet size is therefore used as an index of age and function, although notable exceptions exist (19).

Most steps in platelet kinetics can be evaluated by in vitro or in vivo tests as shown in Table 29.15. An investigation into thrombocytopenia must attempt to determine if low counts are related to inadequate platelet production, accelerated destruction, or pooling. Platelet morphology is important. The blood film may provide evidence for a thrombolytic condition or congenital thrombocytopenia. Measurement of platelet-derived substances such as β-thromboglobulin and platelet factor 4 are helpful (20–21). These levels are increased in patients with shortened platelet life span or excessive consumption. Underproduction can be assessed by bone marrow examination for megakaryocyte number, ploidy, and morphology. If megakaryocytes are abundant, then thrombocytopenia is probably due to accelerated destruction; if sparse, thrombocytopenia is probably due to hypoplasia or aplasia.

Even if megakaryocytes are present in the bone marrow, platelet production will be ineffective if vitamin B_{12} or folate are deficient. In these cases, the megakaryocyte morphology may be megaloblastic.

Finally, evaluation of platelet survival can confirm shortened survival and increased destruction. A rough estimate of survival can be made from survival of transfused platelets into a thrombocytopenic person. When destruction is increased, an increase in count after platelet transfusion may be very small and transient. More accurate assessment can be made by radiolabeling platelets with radioactive isotopes of selenomethionine, indium, chromium, or disopropylfluorophosphate. After infusion of radiolabeled autologous platelets, the residual radioactivity in blood can be measured daily to provide in vivo platelet survival data. An advantage of indium-labeling is that the

area of platelet deposition can be detected by use of whole body scanners and a scintillation camera. This has allowed imaging of platelet thrombi in patients with increased platelet thrombus formation and, for example, platelet trapping in the spleen.

In confirming the etiology of the thrombocytopenia, a host of spurious thrombocytopenias must be ruled out. In some cases, platelets clump in EDTA-collected blood but not in citrate or heparin. In these patients, blood films from blood collected in EDTA show platelet clumping with low platelet numbers away from the clumps. This can be confirmed by a normal platelet count when blood is collected in sodium citrate rather than EDTA. Also, if the platelets are very large or very small, they may not be counted as platelets in an electronic counter. Large platelets may indicate Bernard-Soulier disease; patients with this disorder have decreased ristocetin-induced platelet aggregation and a lifelong predisposition to bleeding. In contrast, small platelets and megakaryocytes may indicate other thrombocytopenia with absent radius (TAR) syndrome, preleukemia, chronic myelogenous leukemia, and myelodysplastic syndrome.

While evaluating the blood smear, other clues may emerge. For example, fragmentation of red blood cells may suggest a microangiopathy such as thrombotic thrombocytopenic purpura (TTP), hemolytic uremic syndrome (HUS), or disseminated intravascular coagulation (DIC).

> Thrombocytopenia from a very early age always suggests a congenital disorder such as Wiskott-Aldrich disease, Epstein's syndrome, May-Hegglin abnormality, TAR syndrome, and other rare disorders (22–24). *Epstein's syndrome* is an inherited autosomal dominant disorder associated with renal defects, deafness, and thrombocytopenia. Patients with *May-Hegglin anomaly* also have mild thrombocytopenia. *TAR syndrome* is a rare and severe condition. Megakaryocytes are absent in the bone marrow. Skeletal abnormalities vary from absence of radii to more extensive phocomelia. (In contrast, in Fanconia's anemia, the thumb, but not the radius, is affected. Also, Fanconia's anemia almost always presents after 1 year of age and is associated with abnormalities of *all* blood cell lines.)

Megakaryocyte morphology can be evaluated by marrow aspirate smears, which also show size and maturation stage. Marrow biopsy is essential to evaluate megakaryocytic numbers. Flow cytometry measures megakaryocyte ploidy.

Most cases of amegakaryocytic thrombocytopenia are congenital. Some, however, are acquired. A review describes 30 adult cases of acquired amegakarycytic thrombocytopenia and suggests that it may be much more common than generally appreciated (25). Several pathogenetic mechanisms have been described, including absence of thrombopoietic activity in serum, presence of a humoral inhibitor to megakaryocyte colony-forming units or to granulocyte-macrophage colony-forming units; presence of a cytotoxic antibody against antigens on platelets and

Table 29.15. Investigation of Platelet Kinetics

Morphology of platelets
Platelet sizing
Detection of platelet-derived substances β-thrombin, platelet factor 4
Megakaryocyte number and mass
Platelet survival studies
Determination of sites of platelet deposition

megakaryocyte progenitor cells; T-cell suppression of CFU megakaryocytes; suppression of CFU-mega by adherent monocytes, possibly through a soluble factor elaborated by these cells, and an intrinsic defect at the level of CFU-mega. Spontaneous remissions occurred in 2 of the 30 reported cases; in others, immunosuppressive agents: methylprednisolone (2), cyclophosphamide (1), slow-infusion vinblastine (1), cyclosporine A (1), and antithymocyte globulin (2) seemingly induced remission. Vincristine pulse therapy was ineffective in six reported cases.

Thrombotic Thrombocytopenic Purpura (TTP) and Hemolytic Uremic Syndrome (HUS). Among the possible diagnoses of nonimmune thrombocytopenia are TTP and its related disorder, HUS. TTP is typically an adult disorder, about twice as common in females, often accompanied by a microangiopathic hemolytic process of moderate severity (60–100 g Hgb/L), modest thrombocytopenia ($10–50 \times 10^9$/L), and severe neurologic symptoms. HUS is more common in children, with an emphasis on renal rather than CNS findings. The etiology of TTP is unknown. Cases have been associated with autoimmune disorders (26), pregnancy (27), familial causes (28), bacterial (29), viral (e.g., HIV (30), HTLV-1 (31), rickettsial (32), and mycoplasma (33) infections as well as drugs (34) and toxins (35). It frequently follows gastrointestinal disorders, especially those resulting from Shigella (36, 37), Campylobacter (38), Yersinia (39), and HIV (40) infections and as a complication of chemotherapy (41), toxins (42), and bone marrow transplantation (43).

The clinical impression of TTP or HUS requires pathologic confirmation, which includes histologic evidence of sequential platelet aggregation in the microvasculature, followed by resolution of the thrombus so formed. Considerable data on the role of von Willebrand's factor multimers in TTP and HUS indicate that the largest of these are consumed in the initial platelet adhesion and aggregation but do not appear to be abnormal. However, the cause of the initial activation is unknown (44–45).

Disorders that have minimal similarities to TTP and HUS include systemic lupus erythematosus, Evan's syndrome (AIHA and ITP), and Henoch-Schönlein purpura. The course of TTP can be progressively fulminant or intermittent and on rare occasion may be self-limiting. HUS is usually an acute illness, with renal failure predominating. Improved renal care in HUS has led to good outcomes without specifically addressing correction of the pathology. In TTP, the use of splenectomy, corticosteroids, antiplatelet drugs, and anticoagulants has doubtful value. Both plasmapheresis and the administration of fresh plasma have been shown to correct the intravascular platelet-based clotting; and survival, which in its progressive form may be no more than a few months with less aggressive therapy, may be prolonged indefinitely with plasmapheresis and/or fresh plasma.

Many viral infections are associated with thrombocytopenia (Table 29.16), which may be acquired through blood transfusions, so a history of these must be sought in any patient presenting with thrombocytopenia, since HIV or other viral infection can cause, and even present with,

isolated thrombocytopenia (46). Increasing numbers of patients with HIV-related isolated thrombocytopenia are becoming recognized. The mechanisms of HIV-related thrombocytopenia are suppression of bone marrow by virus, immune-mediated destruction, opportunistic infections, and the effect of treatment of HIV with AZT (Table 29.17). All but the immune thrombocytopenias are often resistant to treatment.

A careful search for medications, both prescribed and illicit, must be made. Many medications cause nonimmune and immune thrombocytopenia, including amiodarone, penicillins, and cotrimoxazole.

Isolated thrombocytopenia is an uncommon presentation for leukemia. However, acute leukemia may present months to years after initial "preleukemia" signs such as thrombocytopenia, especially in older patients. "Preleukemia" is more easily determined if chromosome abnormalities are present.

An often overlooked cause of thrombocytopenia is type IIb von Willebrand's disease. In this disease, the patient has normal amounts of von Willebrand's factor but abnormal multimeric structures. Some of these patients have a bleeding diathesis, since the von Willebrand's factor does not function as a procoagulant. Nevertheless, the patients have increased, rather than decreased, platelet aggregation. Platelets therefore clump to each other; this results in a relative thrombocytopenia. These patients do not tolerate DDAVP (treatment of choice in other forms of von Willebrand's disease) and may develop more platelet clumping, thrombocytopenia, bleeding, and thrombostic episodes. von Willebrand's disease types should be distinguished before treating with DDAVP.

In JM, the platelets were normal-appearing and normal functioning. The megakaryocytes appeared normal and had normal ploidy and normal maturation.

Table 29.16. Common Viral Infections Associated with Thrombocytopenia

Measles
Rubella
Mumps
Herpes varicella zoster virus
Influenza A, B, or C
Hepatitis A, B, or C
Epstein-Barr virus
Cytomegalovirus
Parvovirus
HIV

Table 29.17. Causes of HIV-Related Thrombocytopenia

Decreased bone marrow production
Increased destruction
Splenic trapping
Treatment (e.g., AZT)
Other infection

There were no signs of platelet trapping or seques-tration. There were only two clues as to the possible cause of thrombocytopenia: (a) the prior EBV infection and (b) exposure to chemicals at the mother's work site, where cleaning and painting materials were stocked.

The protracted course of thrombocytopenia, the com-plete resolution of other apparent signs of the EBV in-fection, and the normal flow cytometry on bone marrow cells made it unlikely that the thrombocytopenia was due to a virus infection. The lack of ultrastructural damage to either platelets or megakaryocytes also made it un-likely that toxic injury was the cause of the protracted thrombocytopenia.

Thus JM remains with a diagnosis of chronic idio-pathic thrombocytopenia of nonimmune origin, without a recognizable cause for his thrombocytopenia. The un-derlying cause of thrombocytopenia may declare itself months to years after its presentation. These include leukemia, aplastic anemia, myelodysplasia, and some au-toimmune disorders. In these cases, the only approach to diagnosis and management is to wait and watch, repeat-ing relevant evaluations as necessary, until a diagnosis can be finalized, while withholding treatment.

In the newborn, the approach to diagnosis is different (Table 29.18). In the sick newborn, thrombocytopenia is often a secondary manifestation (e.g., of infection) that dis-appears as the primary illness improves. In the immunode-ficient infant, regardless of type, thrombocytopenia is com-mon, due either to an intercurrent infection or to an autoimmune process. In the well term infant, the most common cause of thrombocytopenia is passive neona-tal immune thrombocytopenia, but other conditions can also underlie neonatal thrombocytopenia. These include Kasabach-Merritt syndrome (hemangioma), TAR syn-drome, trisomies 13 and 18, familial thrombocytopenias, and cyanotic congenital heart disease. Cyanotic congenital heart disease can cause thrombocytopenia, either as an ar-tifact of collecting and measuring due to the high hemat-ocrit or due to low-grade platelet consumption. In the Kasabach-Merritt syndrome, consumption of platelets and or clotting factors occurs within the vascular system of hemangiomas. The hemangiomas may not be visible on physical examination because they are in the viscera or the central nervous system. Flow murmurs may be heard over these areas. Treatment of hemangiomas may include surgery, heparin, steroids, or radiation therapy.

In the ill, high-risk, newborn infant, thrombocytopenia has particular significance (47). The etiology is usually multifactorial and includes intrauterine infection and/or sepsis with or without DIC. In a study of thrombocy-topenia in 129 high-risk infants and 238 control infants, thrombocytopenia was more common in babies less than 37 weeks gestation and in sick babies than in healthy ones. Sixty percent of infants had no recognizable cause of thrombocytopenia. Features associated with thrombo-cytopenia included umbilical line placement, hyper-bilirubinemia, phototherapy, prematurity, respiratory dis-tress syndrome, respiratory assistance, low Apgar score, sepsis, meconium aspiration, and necrotizing enterocoli-tis. Thrombocytopenic babies had more complications, more hemorrhage, and greater mortality than nonthrom-bocytopenic babies. Platelet size was increased in two ba-bies with immune thrombocytopenia and in none of the others (48).

SUMMARY

These cases summarize approaches to the evaluation of platelet function and quantitative abnormalities. Platelet function and quantification abnormalities are common in children, with clinical manifestations that run the gamut from no symptoms to life-threatening hemorrhage. Care-ful history taking and physical examinations should provide the necessary clues for further evaluation, and targeted laboratory tests can almost always pinpoint the exact defect in platelet physiology that has caused the bleeding predis-position. Some treatment options (in particular, DDAVP) have reduced the need for platelet transfusion and blood products in selected situations, and some (e.g., bone mar-row transplantation) can effect cure. In adults, qualitative platelet defects are rare, and the nonimmune, like the im-mune, thrombocytopenias are usually associated with other primary disorders, especially those involving bone marrow.

Table 29.18. Thrombocytopenia in the Newborn

Well infant
  Neonatal immune thrombocytopenia
  Drug induced
  Maternal autoimmune disease (e.g., SLE)
    Neonatal autoimmune thrombocytopenia purpura
    Maternal alloimmune
    Maternal isoimmune
  Kasabach-Merritt syndrome (Hemangioma)
  Thrombocytopenia with absent radii (TAR syndrome)
  Trisomies 13, 18
  Familial
  Cyanotic congenital heart disease
Sick newborn
  Viral infections (TORCH)
  Sepsis
  Disseminated intravascular coagulation (DIC)
  Hypoxia
  Pulmonary hypertension
Older infant (1–12 months)
  Chronic thrombocytopenia (e.g., Wiskott-Aldrich syndrome)
  Hemolytic uremic syndrome
  Acute leukemia
  Aplastic anemia

REFERENCES

1. Rao AK. Congenital disorders of platelet function. Hematol Oncol Clin North Am 1990;4:65–86.
2. Diamond LK, Porter FS. The inadequacies of routine bleed-ing and clotting times. N Engl J Med 1958;259: 1025–1027.

3. Rodgers RP, Levin J. A critical reappraisal of the bleeding time. Semin Thromb Hemost 1990;16:1–20.

4. Lind SE. The bleeding time does not predict surgical bleeding. Blood 1991;77:2547–2552.

5. Mehta P, Mehta J. Evaluation of platelet function. In: Mehta J, Mehta P, eds. Platelets and prostaglandins in cardiovascular disease. New York: Futura Publishing, 1981: 37–53.

6. Born GVR. Aggregation of blood platelets by adenosine diphosphate and its reversal. Nature 1962;194:927–929.

7. Horellou MH, Lecompte T, Lecrubier C, et al. Familial and constitutional bleeding disorder due to platelet cyclooxygenase deficiency. Am J Hematol 1983;14:1–9.

8. Defryn G, Machin SJ, Carreras LO, et al. Familial bleeding tendency with partial platelet thromboxane synthetase deficiency: reorientation of cyclic endoperoxide metabolism. Br J Haematol 1981;49:29–41.

9. Hardisty RM, Machin SJ, Nokee TJC, et al. A new congenital defect of platelet secretion: impaired responsiveness of the platelets to cytoplasmic free calcium. Br J Haematol 1983;53:543–557.

10. George JN, Shattil SJ. The clinical importance of acquired abnormalities of platelet function. N Engl J Med 1991; 324:27–39.

11. McEver RP. The clinical significance of platelet membrane glycoproteins. Hematol Oncol Clin North Am 1990;4: 87–105.

12. Yasuda T, Gold HK, Fallon JT, et al. Monoclonal antibody against platelet glycoprotein (GP) IIB/IIIA receptor prevents coronary artery reocclusion after reperfusion with recombinant tissue-type plasminogen activator in dogs. J Clin Invest 1988;81:1284–1291.

13. Warkenti TE, Kelton JG. Heparin and platelets. Hematol Oncol Clin North Am 1990;4:243–264.

14. Carvalho AC. Acquired platelet dysfunction in patients with uremia. J Hematol Oncol Clin North Am 1990;4:129–143.

15. Remuzzi G, Perico N, Zoja C, Cornba D, Majcconi D, Vigano G. Role of endothelium-derived nitric oxide in the bleeding tendency of uremia. J Clin Invest 1990;86: 1768–1771.

16. DiMichele DM, Hathaway WE. Use of DDAVP in inherited and acquired platelet dysfunction. Am J Hematol 1990;33: 39–45.

17. Bellucci S, Devergie A, Gluckman E, et al. Complete correction of Glanzmann's thrombasthenia by allogeneic bone marrow transplantation. Br J Haematol 1985;59:635–641.

18. Han ZC, Bellucci S, Caen JP. Regulation of human megakaryocytopoiesis. Nouv Rev Fr Hematol 1990;32:395–396.

19. Karpatkin S. Heterogeneity of platelet function: correlation with platelet volume. Am J Med 1978;64:542–546.

20. Selgas R, Miranda B, Cuesta MV, et al. Measurement of the peritoneal platelet activity through the effluent betathromboglobulin levels in CAPD patients. Adv Perit Dial 1990; 6:26–30.

21. Jennings AM, Ford I, Murdoch S, Greaves M, Preston FE, Ward JD. The effects of diet and insulin therapy on coagulation factor VII, blood viscosity, and platelet release proteins in diabetic patients with secondary sulphonylurea failure. Diabetic Med 1991;8:346–353.

22. Najean Y, Lecompte T. Genetic thrombocytopenia with autosomal dominant transmission: a review of 54 cases. Nouv Rev Fr Haematol 1990;32:67–70.

23. Hedberg VA, Lipton JM. Thrombocytopenia with absent radii. A review of 100 cases. Am J Pediatr Hematol Oncol 1988;10:51–64.

24. Dowton SB, Beardsley D, Jamison D, et al. Studies of a familial platelet disorder. Blood 1985;65:557–563.

25. Manoharan A, Williams NT, Sparrow R. Acquired amegakaryocytic thrombocytopenia: report of a case and review of the literature. Q J Med 1989;70:243–252.

26. Ridolfi RL, Bell WR. Thrombotic thrombocytopenic purpura: report of 25 cases and review of the literature. Medicine 1961;60:413–428.

27. Upshaw JD Jr, Reidy TJ, Groshart K. Thrombotic thrombocytopenic purpura in pregnancy: response to plasma manipulations. South Med J 1985;78:677–680.

28. Waage A, Siegel J, Thorstensen K, Lamvik J. Thrombotic thrombocytopenic purpura in 2 siblings: defective platelet function and platelet factor deficiency occurring simultaneously. Scand J Haematol 1986;36:55–57.

29. Jaeschke R, Irvine EJ, Moore J, Kelton J. *Campylobacter jejuni* and thrombotic thrombocytopenic purpura. Can J Gastroenterol 1990;4:154–156.

30. Nair JMG, Bellevue R, Bertoni M, Dosik H. Thrombotic thrombocytopenic purpura in patients with the acquired immunodeficiency syndrome (AIDS)-related complex: a report of two cases. Ann Intern Med 1988;109:209–212.

31. Dixon AC, Kwock DW, Nakamura JM, et al. Thrombotic thrombocytopenic purpura and human T-lymphocyte virus, type 1 (HTLV-1) [Letter]. Ann Intern Med 1989;110:93–94.

32. Mettler NE. Isolation of a microtatobiote from patients with hemolytic-uremic syndrome and thrombotic thrombocytopenic purpura and from mites in the United States. N Engl J Med 1969;281:1023–1027.

33. Reynolds PM, Jackson JM, Brine JAS, Vivian AB. Thrombotic thrombocytopenic purpura: remission following splenectomy—report of a case and review of the literature. Am J Med 1976;61:439–447.

34. McShane PM, Bern MM, Schiff I. Thrombotic thrombocytopenic purpura associated with oral contraceptives: a case report. Am J Obstet Gynecol 1983;145:762–763.

35. Murgo AJ. Thrombotic microangiopathy in the cancer patient including those induced by chemotherapeutic agents. Semin Hematol 1987;24:161–177.

36. Raghupathy P, Date A, Shastry JCM, et al. Haemolytic-uraemic syndrome complicating *Shigella* dysentery in South Indian children. Br Med J 1978;1:1518–1521.

37. Baker NM, Mills AE, Rachman I, Thomas JEP. Haemolytic-uraemic syndrome in typhoid fever. Br Med J 1974;2:84–87.

38. Delans RJ, Biuso JD, Saba SR, Ramirez G. Hemolytic uremic syndrome after *Campylobacter*-induced diarrhea in an adult. Arch Intern Med 1984;144:1074–1076.

39. Davenport A, O'Connor B, Finn R. Acute renal failure following *Yersinia pseudotuberculosis* septicaemia. Postgrad Med J 1987;63:815–816.

40. Boccia RV, Gelmann EP, Baker CC, et al. A hemolytic-uremic syndrome with the acquired immunodeficiency syndrome [Letter]. Ann Intern Med 1984;101:716–717.

41. Kwaan HC. Miscellaneous secondary thrombotic microangiopathy. Semin Hematol 1987;24:141–147.

42. Van Buren D, Van Buren CT, Flechner SM, et al. De novo hemolytic uremic syndrome in renal transplant recipients immunosuppressed with cyclosporine. Surgery 1985;98: 54–62.

43. Craig JIO, Sheeman T, Bell K. The haemolytic uraemic syndrome and bone marrow transplantation. Br Med J 1987; 295:887.

44. Kelton JG, Moore J, Santos A, Sheridan D. Detection of a platelet agglutinating factor in thrombotic, thrombocytopenic purpura. Ann Intern Med 1984;101:589–593.

45. Murphy WG, Moore JC, Kelton JG. Calcium-dependent cysteine protease activity in the sera of patients with thrombotic thrombocytopenic purpura. Blood 1987;70: 683–1687.

46. Karpatkin S. HIV-1 related thrombocytopenia. Hematol Oncol Clin North Am 1990;4:115–138.

47. Bussel JB. Thrombocytopenia in newborns, infants and children. Pediatr Ann 1990;19:181–185.

48. Mehta P, Vasa R, Newman L, Karpatkin M. Thrombocytopenia in the high-risk infant. J Pediatr 1980;97:791–794.

CHAPTER 30

Disorders of Prothrombin Conversion

HIDEHIKO SAITO, JUNKI TAKAMATSU

In 1918 Fahraeus noted that red cell sedimentation rates varied in different disease states. These early observations were the anlage for the red cell estimated sedimentation rate, a test which more than 70 years later continues to be highly reliable and easily carried out.
—R. Fahraeus, Acta Med Scand, 1921

A 41-Year-Old Man

This patient was admitted to hospital because of numerous ecchymoses in the extremities and persistent gingival bleeding.

The patient had no history of bleeding problems during childhood. At the age of 21 years, he had an episode of massive gastrointestinal hemorrhage due to duodenal ulcer and underwent emergency gastrectomy with the transfusion of 2 L of blood. Several years later, the patient was found to have abnormal liver function tests. During the 6 months before admission he experienced the onset of increasing fatigability and weakness. Two weeks before entry he noticed ecchymoses and gum bleeding. He had ingested alcohol to excess in the past but had taken only small amounts during the several years preceding entry. The patient denied use of aspirin, other nonsteroidal antiinflammatory drugs, or warfarin. Family history was negative for bleeding disorders.

What Historical Aspects Are Important for the Patient with Hemorrhagic Diathesis?

The type of bleeding, the age at which hemorrhagic symptoms first appear, and how long the problem has been present are helpful when making the diagnosis. Ecchymoses are seen commonly with any kind of bleeding diathesis and do not give a clue to the diagnosis. Gum bleeding may occur with thrombocytopenia, coagulation factor deficiency, and uremia. In contrast, petechiae are almost always diagnostic of thrombocytopenia or vasculitis. Petechiae are usually prominent in areas of the body subjected to high venous pressures (e.g., legs) or to constriction by the external pressure of tight clothing. Spontaneous hemarthroses are usually associated with hemophilia. It is helpful to ask if the patient had any excessive bleeding during minor surgical procedures such as circumcision, tonsillectomy, and tooth extraction. The association of abnormal bleeding with past trauma should be

solicited. Questioning the patient regarding the need for previous blood transfusion is also important. In the female patient, a careful history about the degree and length of menstrual periods should be obtained. When bleeding begins during childhood, an inherited disorder is suggested; most of acquired disorders occur later in life. However, some inherited disorders such as mild hemophilia and hereditary hemorrhagic telangiectasia may have no bleeding symptoms until later in life. The incidence of acquired disorders is much higher than that of inherited disorders. Family history should be carefully evaluated for the presence of bleeding diathesis or consanguinity, but negative family history does not exclude a hereditary disorder; e.g., 30% of patients with hemophilia are sporadic (mutations).

Careful inquiry about medication must be made, because many drugs are known to cause bleeding complications. These include, among others, aspirin, warfarin, heparin, and tissue plasminogen activator (t-PA) (Table 30.1). Aspirin and aspirin-containing compounds are the most common cause of a hemostatic defect. The incidence of major hemorrhage in outpatients on long-term oral anticoagulant (warfarin) may be as high as 20% (1).

On physical examination, the conjunctivae were icteric and pale. Small amounts of blood were found in the gums. The head, neck, lungs, and heart were normal. Several vascular spiders were seen on the anterior chest wall. There were ascites and ankle edema, and many ecchymoses were noted over the abdomen and arms. The liver was not palpable, but the spleen tip was palpable.

Pertinent laboratory data showed the following results. The hematocrit was 38%, the white cell count was 1.8×10^9/L, and the platelet count was 87×10^9/L. The albumin was 26 g/L, the total bilirubin 4.0 mg/dL, serum aspartate aminotransferase 70 U (normal, 10–30), and cholinesterase was 0.25 (normal, more than 1). The prothrombin time (PT) was 16.5 sec, with a control

Table 30.1. Some Drugs That May
Cause Bleeding Complications

Site of Action	Drugs
Blood coagulation	Warfarin, heparin, ancroid, L-asparaginase
Platelet	Nonsteroidal antiinflammatory agents (aspirin, etc.), heparin, quinine, quinidine
Fibrinolysis	Streptokinase, urokinase, t-PA
Vascular wall	Adrenocorticosteroid

of 12.0 sec; the activated partial thromboplastin time (aPTT) was 75 sec (normal, 40–45). The administration of vitamin K 10 mg orally for 5 days did not improve the prolonged PT and aPTT. PT of a mixture of the patient's plasma and normal plasma was 12.5 sec. Hepatitis C virus antibody was positive.

This case illustrates a typical bleeding tendency accompanying liver damage.

What other bleeding symptoms might this patient have? Gastrointestinal bleeding from esophageal varices, duodenal ulcer, or gastric erosions is commonly seen in patients with liver cirrhosis. They may present with melena and/or hematemesis. Massive hemorrhage from ruptured esophageal varices may be life threatening. Epistaxis and bleeding from venipuncture sites may also occur.

Resources

Hemostatic Mechanisms

Normal hemostasis requires intact vessel wall, platelets, blood coagulation, and fibrinolysis (2). When a blood vessel is ruptured, three major mechanisms operate locally at the site of injury to control the bleeding and to limit blood loss: (*a*) vessel wall contraction, (*b*) platelet hemostatic plug formation, and (*c*) formation and maintenance of fibrin clots (blood clotting). All three mechanisms are essential for normal hemostasis, and they function in concert rather than at random. The rapid plugging of a hole in the vessel wall is achieved by a combination of vasoconstriction and platelet adhesion and aggregation. Platelets accumulate at the site of vascular damage and adhere to subendothelial or perivascular connective tissue that has become exposed to flowing blood. Platelets also adhere to each other and form a hemostatic plug. Further maintenance of hemostasis is achieved by the formation of a fibrin clot via blood coagulation. The clot, insoluble networks of fibrin, serve to solidify the platelet plug. Since the biology, biochemistry, and pathophysiology of platelets in hemostasis are discussed in other chapters, the following section focuses on the mechanisms of blood coagulation that are pertinent to the present case.

Blood Coagulation

Blood clotting is the end result of complex sequential reactions involving various trace plasma proteins called clotting factors (Fig. 30.1). All coagulation factors in human plasma have been isolated and characterized, and the genes encoding coagulation proteins have been cloned. We are now able to understand the detailed structure-function relations of these proteins at the molecular level (3). Most clotting factors (prothrombin, factors VII, IX, X, XI, XII) are zymogens of serine protease and are converted to their active forms by limited proteolysis; some factors (factors V and VIII and tissue factor) function as cofactors.

The blood coagulation cascade may be initiated by two separate pathways. Exposure of blood to injured tissue rapidly initiates blood clotting via the *extrinsic pathway* by the interaction of tissue factor (tissue thromboplastin) and factor VII. The prothrombin time screens the efficiency of this pathway. Contact of blood with a foreign surface also triggers blood coagulation via the *intrinsic pathway*. The partial thromboplastin time (PTT) and activated PTT (aPTT) are good monitors for this pathway. The extrinsic and intrinsic pathways share a common pathway after the activation of factor X. The concept of two pathways is of practical value, as the results of the prothrombin time and PTT or aPTT tests usually help to localize an abnormality in the coagulation scheme. However, the separation of two pathways is artificial, and whether the two pathways are sharply separable in vivo is not known. Furthermore, there is evidence to suggest that there are many links between them. For example, tissue factor and factor VII are known to activate not only factor X but also factor IX (4). Thus, the intrinsic and extrinsic pathways converge at *two* levels, factor X and factor IX. Since individuals with a deficiency of either factor XII, prekallikrein, or high-molecular-weight kininogen have no bleeding tendency (5), the in-

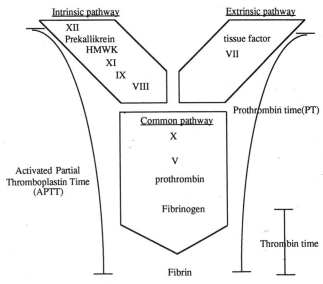

Figure 30.1. Scheme of blood coagulation and screening tests. HMWK, high-molecular-weight kininogen.

trinsic pathway seems not to be of great importance to in vivo hemostasis (3).

What Clotting Abnormality Do Prolonged Prothrombin Time and aPTT Suggest?

These test results suggest that there is either reduced activity of coagulation factors participating in the common pathway or a circulating anticoagulant. The two possibilities may be distinguished by aPTT or PTT of a mixture of the patient's plasma and normal plasma. If the addition of an equal volume of normal plasma corrects the abnormal clotting time, a circulating anticoagulant is not present. Deficiency of factors X, V, prothrombin, or fibrinogen is strongly suspected in the present case, since PT of a mixture of the patient's plasma and normal plasma was normal. Generally, deficiencies of multiple factors are present in an acquired disorder, whereas a deficiency of a single factor is usually due to an inherited disorder. If the PT or aPTT of a mixture of the patient's plasma and normal plasma is still prolonged, a circulating anticoagulant is present. *Circulating anticoagulants* are inhibitors of blood coagulation that interfere with various steps of the coagulation reactions. They include, among others, lupus anticoagulant, factor VIII inhibitor, and heparin. Lupus anticoagulant, which occurs in approximately 7% of patients with SLE (6), is an antibody against certain phospholipids and prolongs the phospholipid-dependent clotting tests such as aPTT and PT (7). Lupus anticoagulants appear to block the calcium-mediated binding of vitamin K–dependent coagulation factors to phospholipids. Most patients with lupus anticoagulant are rarely associated with a bleeding tendency. Paradoxically, some patients present with thrombosis (8), but the mechanism by which lupus anticoagulant induces thromboembolism is not fully known. Interestingly, lupus anticoagulant has been also reported in association with a history of recurrent abortions (9). The term **antiphospholipid syndrome** has recently been used to describe these patients with lupus anticoagulant (10).

What Additional Data May Be Helpful to Characterize the Patient's Coagulation Abnormality?

The failure of vitamin K administration to improve prolonged PT and aPTT is an important clue, since it excludes vitamin K deficiency. Clinical impression suggests that the coagulation abnormality is caused by the liver disease. The final diagnosis is established by specific assays of individual coagulation factors in the patient's plasma. The following results were obtained. The activities of prothrombin, factor V, and factor X were 60%, 50%, and 45%, respectively. Fibrinogen was 0.75 g/L. These results are due to decreased synthesis of fibrinogen, prothrombin, and factors V and X by the liver. In addition to these factors, the liver is the main site of synthesis of factors XIII, XII, XI, IX, VII, plasminogen, and naturally occurring anticoagulants such as antithrombin III, protein C, and protein S. Six of the coagulation fac-

tors produced by the liver (prothrombin; factors VII, IX, and X; and proteins C and S) are called vitamin K–dependent factors, since vitamin K (koagulation vitamin) is required for their production (11).

What Factors May Be Contributing to the Hemostatic Abnormalities in Liver Disease?

Since the liver plays a major role in maintaining normal hemostasis, it is not surprising to see multiple hemostatic defects in patients with liver disease (Table 30.2). More than one defect may be present in a single patient. The principal cause of bleeding in parenchymal hepatic disease, including liver cirrhosis, is decreased plasma levels of various clotting factors due to impaired protein synthesis. The present patient demonstrates not only low serum albumin and cholinesterase but also reduced levels of fibrinogen, prothrombin, and factors V and X. A qualitative abnormality of fibrinogen, dysfibrinogenemia, may also occur in liver disease (12).

The prothrombin time is a sensitive monitor for plasma levels of these clotting factors and has prognostic significance in patients with severe liver disease. A markedly prolonged prothrombin time suggests a poor prognosis in patients with cirrhosis (13). Antithrombin III and α_2-plasmin inhibitor, a major inhibitor of blood coagulation and fibrinolysis, are also produced by hepatocytes.

In addition to the role of the liver in the production of clotting factors and their inhibitors, the liver is believed to participate in the removal of activated clotting factors or plasminogen activators from the circulation (14). Impaired clearance of activated factors may predispose to disseminated intravascular coagulation (DIC) and enhanced fibrinolysis. Thus, patients with liver disease often show increased serum fibrinogen/fibrin degradation products (FDPs). FDPs interfere with the conversion of fibrinogen to fibrin and inhibit platelet aggregation, thereby contributing to disordered hemostasis. DIC and fibrinolysis also contribute to low titers of fibrinogen. A moderate degree of thrombocytopenia is commonly seen in patients with liver cirrhosis, as it is in this patient. Thrombocytopenia appears to be due to the splenic pooling of platelets by splenomegaly (15); another possible mechanism for thrombocytopenia is consumption coagulopathy. The combination of low platelet count, prolonged prothrombin time, low fibrinogen, and increased FDPs is a typical laboratory finding suggesting DIC (16). It is, therefore, difficult to make the diagnosis of DIC as such in the presence of severe liver disease.

Table 30.2. Hemostatic Abnormalities in Liver Disease

Decreased hepatic synthesis of coagulation factors
Decreased hepatic clearance of activated factors
DIC
Enhanced fibrinolysis
Thrombocytopenia

Vitamin K–Dependent Clotting Factors and the Role of Vitamin K in Their Biosynthesis

It has long been known that vitamin K is essential for the synthesis of certain clotting factors. How vitamin K functions in their production, however, was not clear until the discovery of a unique amino acid residue, γ-carboxyglutamic acid (γ-Gla), in prothrombin (17). Further studies demonstrated that γ-Gla is also present in factors VII, IX, X and proteins C and S (2). γ-Gla is critical for the function of vitamin K–dependent clotting factors by virtue of its ability to bind calcium ion and phospholipid (18). Table 30.3 lists six vitamin K–dependent factors that contain γ-Gla.

Prothrombin and factors VII, IX, and X are zymogens of serine protease and, upon activation, participate in the generation of thrombin. A more detailed discussion of prothrombin conversion is given below. Protein C is also a zymogen of serine protease and, together with protein S and thrombomodulin, participates in a major anticoagulant system that exerts a damping effect on the coagulation cascade (19). When excess thrombin is formed in circulating blood, it is bound to thrombomodulin, a thrombin receptor on endothelial surfaces. The thrombin-thrombomodulin complex then activates protein C. Activated protein C, a serine protease, selectively degrades factors Va and VIIIa by limited proteolysis. Activated protein C also stimulates fibrinolytic activity by inactivating plasminogen activator inhibitor 1 (PAI-1). Protein S is not a zymogen of serine protease but functions as a cofactor in these reactions.

The primary structures of prothrombin and factors VII, IX, and X are very similar (3). Ten to twelve γ-Gla residues are present at the NH2-terminal end of each protein, while the serine protease domain is present at the COOH-terminus. The serine protease domain is structurally related to trypsin and chymotrypsin. Recent studies have also shown that the genes encoding for vitamin K–dependent proteins share structural similarities (20). For example, the genes coding for factors VII, IX, and X and protein C all contain seven introns and eight exons, which occur in essentially the same positions throughout the amino acid sequence.

Biosynthesis of the vitamin K–dependent proteins occurs in the hepatocyte in two steps (Fig. 30.2). First, a polypeptide chain is produced on the ribosomes of the hepatocytes. Then a second carboxyl group is inserted into the gamma carbon of certain glutamic acid residues in the polypeptide chain by the action of a microsomal enzyme called carboxylase (21). It is interesting to know how this γ-carboxylation occurs only in the vitamin K–dependent proteins among the numerous polypeptide chains produced on the ribosomes. Recent studies showed that the propeptides of the vitamin K–dependent proteins contain the specific carboxylation-recognition site that is recognized by carboxylase (22). After carboxylation, the propeptide is cleaved, and mature proteins are secreted from the hepatocyte into the plasma. The reduced form of vitamin K is an essential cofactor for this posttranslational modification. In this process, vitamin K is metabolized to vitamin K epoxide but is regenerated to vitamin K by an enzyme, vitamin K epoxide reductase (21). When the supply of reduced vitamin K is limited, aberrant vitamin K–dependent factors without the normal complement of γ-Gla are produced. For example, abnormal prothrombin without γ-Gla is called PIVKA (proteins induced by vitamin K absence) (23), and it has markedly decreased coagulant properties.

Vitamin K is provided to man by two sources: dietary intake of green leafy vegetables and production by intestinal bacterial flora. The absorption of vitamin K, a fat-soluble vitamin, requires bile salts in the small intestine. Vitamin K deficiency may occur in several conditions (Table 30.4). It is most often seen in patients with malabsorption of fat (e.g., obstructive jaundice, malabsorption syndrome). Prolonged administration of oral antibiotics may also produce vitamin K deficiency in patients with poor dietary intake, since antibiotics suppress intestinal bacteria. Certain β-lactam antibiotics such as cefamandole and moxalactam that possess the methylthiotetrazole side group have been reported to cause hypoprothrombinemia by interfering with hepatic vitamin K metabolism (24). In the newborn who has marginal vitamin K levels, poor dietary intake and insufficient colonization of the intestinal flora may lead to frank vitamin K deficiency, hemorrhagic disease of the newborn. Breast-fed infants are more susceptible to this disorder, because human milk is poorer in vitamin K than cows' milk (25). This disease can be readily prevented by parenteral injection of vitamin K to the infant at delivery.

The most commonly used oral anticoagulant, warfarin, appears to exert its inhibitory effect by acting at two separate sites in the vitamin K cycle (Fig. 30.2). Warfarin inhibits the activity of both vitamin K reductase and vita-

Table 30.3. Some Properties of Vitamin K–Dependent Coagulation Factors

Factor	Molecular Weight	Plasma Concentration	Number of γ-Gla	In Vivo Half-Life (hr) ($T^{1/2}$)	Function
Prothrombin	72,000	100–150 mg/L	10	60	Zymogen of serine protease
VII	45,000	0.4–0.7 mg/L	10	6	Zymogen of serine protease
IX	55,000	30–50 mg/L	12	20–24	Zymogen of serine protease
X	67,000	50–100 mg/L	12	24–48	Zymogen of serine protease
Protein C	62,000	20–30 mg/L	11	6	Zymogen of serine protease
Protein S	69,000	3–5 mg/L	10	24–48	Cofactor of activated protein C

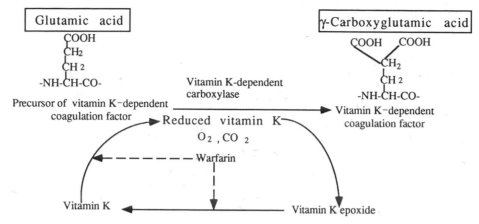

Figure 30.2. Role of vitamin K in the biosynthesis of vitamin K–dependent coagulation factors. *Broken lines* indicate the sites of the action of warfarin.

min K epoxide reductase, thereby blocking the recycling of vitamin K in the hepatocyte and limiting the action of the carboxylase (21). Warfarin thus depletes vitamin K and reduces synthesis of normally functioning vitamin K–dependent clotting factors. The plasma level of the various vitamin K–dependent factors after initiation of warfarin depends on the half-lives of these proteins (Table 30.3). The half-life of factor VII in the circulation is short (6 hr), and its concentration is the first to decrease during warfarin therapy. Since prothrombin has a long half-life (60 hr), at least 3 days of therapy are needed before all the vitamin K–dependent factors reach their lowest levels in plasma. A large number of drugs are known to interfere with the action of warfarin (26). Since patients are usually on warfarin for at least several months, the knowledge of the drug interaction is important for the management of patients on oral anticoagulants. Table 30.5 lists some commonly prescribed drugs that modulate the action of warfarin. Special caution should be taken when any drug is added to or removed from the regimen of a patient stabilized on warfarin.

Prothrombin Conversion

Prothrombin is a 72-kDa single-chain glycoprotein that is converted to its enzymatic form, thrombin, during blood coagulation. The activation of prothrombin to thrombin is mediated by activated factor X (Xa). Xa splits two peptide bonds in the prothrombin molecule and releases thrombin. Although Xa alone is able to activate prothrombin, the reaction is very slow. The rate of activation by Xa is accelerated about 300,000-fold by the presence of factor Va, phospholipids, and calcium ions compared with the rate by Xa alone (11).

The mechanism of this tremendous amplification may be considered as follows (Fig. 30.3). Both factor Xa and prothrombin bind to phospholipid surfaces (e.g., cell surface membrane) via their γ-Gla residues and calcium ions. Factor V, when activated to Va by a trace amount of thrombin, also binds to phospholipids and prothrombin. The common property of binding to phospholipids pro-

Table 30.4. Causes of Vitamin K Deficiency

Poor dietary intake
Malabsorption of fat
Malnourished patients on broad-spectrum antibiotics
Certain antibiotics (e.g., cephalosporins)
Hemorrhagic disease of the newborn
Oral anticoagulant (warfarin)

Table 30.5. Drugs That Alter the Anticoagulant Effect of Warfarin

Drugs that potentiate warfarin action	Drugs that inhibit warfarin action
Allopurinol	Alcohol
Aspirin	Barbiturates
Cimetidine	Carbamazepine
Clofibrate	Cholestyramine
Danazol	Glutethimide
Disulfiram	Griseofulvin
Isoniazid	Nafcillin
Ketoconazole	Rifampin
Metronidazole	
Omeprazole	
Phenylbutazone	
Quinidine	
Sulfinpyrazone	
Sulfamethoxazole-trimethoprim	
Tricyclic antidepressants	
Thyroxine	

vides a mechanism for bringing together prothrombin, factor Va, factor Xa, and calcium ions, which normally circulate separately, into a highly organized complex. Formation of this multimolecular complex (the prothrombinase complex) on the phospholipid surface brings molecules of prothrombin (a substrate) and factor Xa (an enzyme) into close proximity and increases their chance of interacting. It is the presence of γ-Gla that allows the generation of the enzymatically efficient prothrombinase complex. When factor Xa is associated with phospholipid and factor V, it is protected from inhibition by antithrom-

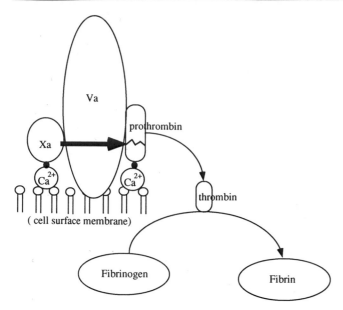

Figure 30.3. Conversion of prothrombin to thrombin. Formation of the prothrombinase complex on cell surface membrane is shown. *Dark circle* indicates γ-Gla.

bin III (27). Evidence suggests that a prothrombinase complex for the activation of prothrombin can form on the surface of stimulated platelets, endothelial cells, or white blood cells (28). It is likely that such a process localizes the generation of thrombin to the site of vascular injury under in vivo conditions.

Factor V, a large plasma protein (330 kDa), has no enzymatic activity of its own and participates as a cofactor in the activation of prothrombin by Xa. Amino acid sequence analysis and cDNA cloning revealed that factor V is structurally similar to factor VIII, another cofactor in blood coagulation (29). The liver is the main site of the production of factor V, and the titer of this clotting factor is reduced in parenchymal hepatic disease. How factor V accelerates the prothrombin conversion is not fully understood, but upon activation to Va, factor V has been suggested to affect prothrombin activation in three ways: a conformational change in the prothrombin molecule, an increase in the binding of Xa to the phospholipid surface, and promotion of the assembly of the enzyme-substrate complex.

Activities

This case represents typical hemostatic defects associated with parenchymal hepatic disease. The history and physical examination suggested that the patient has liver disease. Screening hemostatic tests showed prolonged prothrombin time and aPTT, indicating a common pathway deficiency. The patient could have vitamin K deficiency, but the prolonged prothrombin time was not corrected by administration of vitamin K. Thus, the most likely diagnosis is a bleeding tendency caused by severe underlying liver disease. It is usually not necessary to measure the

activity of individual clotting factors participating in a common pathway. In the present case, however, further studies demonstrated that the levels of fibrinogen, prothrombin, and factors V and X are decreased, which is consistent with reduced synthesis of these clotting factors by the liver. Enhanced fibrinolysis and DIC may also contribute to low titers of fibrinogen and factor V. As noted above, in addition to reduced levels of certain coagulation factors, thrombocytopenia due to splenic pooling is a risk factor for a bleeding tendency in liver cirrhosis. As mentioned above, hemostatic abnormalities in parenchymal hepatic disease are complex and multifactorial.

Assessment of the Bleeding Risk Prior to Surgery or Liver Biopsy

It is not uncommon to have patients with liver disease undergo liver biopsy. Screening hemostatic tests including platelet count, prothrombin time, aPTT, and fibrinogen provide useful information concerning the risk of hemorrhage. If the prothrombin time of the patient is more than 1.5 times that of the normal control, the risk of bleeding is high (30). Vitamin K (10 mg p.o. for 5 days) should be given, and the prothrombin time rechecked. If the ratio is not improved, liver biopsy is contraindicated. Thrombocytopenia (fewer than 80×10^9/L) is also a contraindication to biopsy (31). When surgical procedures are urgent, prophylactic transfusions of fresh frozen plasma and platelet concentrates are required.

Management of Hemostatic Abnormalities in Liver Disease

Not all patients with parenchymal hepatic disease require treatment of their bleeding symptoms. When the bleeding tendency seems to be life threatening or when surgery or liver biopsy is necessary, correction of hemostatic defects is indicated. First, intravenous administration of vitamin K 10 mg should be started, and the prothrombin time checked 24 hours later. As mentioned above, however, improvement after a dose of vitamin K is often insufficient. Thus, the mainstay of treatment is replacement therapy. The transfusion of fresh frozen plasma (FFP) provides the vitamin K–dependent factors, fibrinogen, and factor V that are deficient in such patients. The infusion of 20 mL/kg of FFP usually leads to partial correction of the hemostatic defects. Repeated transfusions may be necessary; improvement is transient because of the short half-life of factor VII. A limitation of replacement therapy with FFP is hypervolemia. Infusion of *prothrombin complex concentrates* that contain large amounts of the vitamin K–dependent clotting factors is not recommended in patients with liver disease, because untoward thrombotic complications have been associated with their use (32). It appears that some activated clotting factors in prothrombin complex concentrates cause

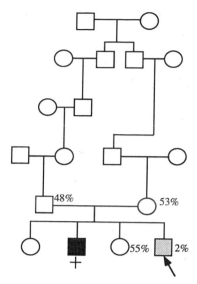

Figure 30.4. Family with hereditary factor VII deficiency. Factor VII activity of the proband, his sister, and parents is shown. *Arrow*, proband; +, died.

hypercoagulable states in such patients because of impaired clearance of activated factors by the liver. Acquired antithrombin III deficiency associated with liver cirrhosis may also contribute to the development of hypercoagulable states. When significant thrombocytopenia is present, platelet transfusion is indicated.

A 10-Year-Old Boy

This patient was referred because of recurrent episodes of nosebleeds and anemia.

The patient had no bleeding symptoms until the age of 1.5 years, when he first experienced severe epistaxis. Nosebleeds occurred once or twice a month without significant trauma and usually persisted for several days. Epistaxis apparently occurred from both nostrils. His mother reported that he bruised easily after minor trauma. He was seen by an otorhinolaryngolo-gist, who found no local lesion in the nose. Anemia (Hb, 6.5 g/dL) was discovered, and the patient was referred to the hematology service. No history of exposure to drugs was obtained. The family history is significant in that the patient's grandparents were cousins (Fig. 30.4). The patient's elder brother was said to have died of intracranial hemorrhage at the age of 10 years. Other close relatives including the parents are well, with no history of a bleeding tendency.

On physical examination the conjunctivae and mucous membranes were pale but not icteric. No lymphadenopathy was found. The head, neck, chest, and abdomen were normal. There was no ecchymosis, petechia, joint deformity, or edema.

The hematocrit was 22.4%; the white cell count was 4.5×10^9/L with a normal differential. The mean corpuscular volume (MCV) was 72 fL, and the mean corpuscular hemoglobin concentration (MCHC), 29%.

The platelet count was 224×10^9/L. The prothrombin time was 28.5 seconds, with a control of 11.0 seconds; the aPTT was 53.0 seconds (control, 54.6). Fibrinogen was 2.56 g/L. The bleeding time was normal. Liver function tests were within normal range.

What Hemostatic Abnormality Does This Patient Have? What Additional Tests Are Required to Pinpoint the Patient's Defect?

Epistaxis is commonly seen in children and does not always suggest a bleeding tendency. The frequency of epistaxis in this boy may not be abnormal, but his long-lasting nosebleeds and the absence of a local lesion appear to indicate a hemostatic abnormality. Microcytic and hypochromic anemia is probably caused by iron deficiency secondary to blood loss and illustrates the severe nature of the epistaxis. A congenital or inherited disorder is suspected, since the symptom began in infancy. The screening hemostatic tests revealed a normal platelet count and normal bleeding time, excluding the possibility of platelet disorders. The patient has markedly prolonged PT in the presence of normal aPTT (Fig. 30.1). Table 30.6 illustrates the differential diagnosis of coagulation abnormalities with PT, aPTT, and thrombin time. This patient most likely has factor VII deficiency. Another possibility might be the presence of an inhibitor against factor VII. The PT of a 1:1 mixture of the patient's plasma and normal plasma was 11.5 seconds, excluding the latter.

The activity of factor VII was found to be 2% of that in normal plasma. The activities of other vitamin K–dependent clotting factors, including prothrombin and factor X, were within normal range. The immunoreactive factor VII (factor VII antigen) was 5%. The factor VII activity of the patient's father and mother was 48% and 53%, respectively. Since the normal range of factor VII activity is 70–120%, these data are consistent with this patient having a homozygous factor VII deficiency and the parents being heterozygotes (Fig. 30.4).

Table 30.6. Differential Diagnosis of Coagulation Abnormalities with Screening Tests

Prothrombin Time	APTT	Thrombin Time	Deficiency States
Normal	Normal	Normal	Normal, XIII
Prolonged	Normal	Normal	VII
Prolonged	Prolonged	Normal	X, V, prothrombin
Prolonged	Prolonged	Prolonged	A(hypo)fibrinogenemia
Normal	Prolonged	Normal	Prekallikrein[a], HMWK[a,b], XII[a], XI, IX, VIII

[a]High-molecular-weight kininogen.
[b]No bleeding symptoms.

Resources

Factor VII and Its Role in Hemostasis

Factor VII, a 45-kDa glycoprotein, is a unique coagulation factor in that it participates exclusively in the extrinsic pathway (Fig. 30.1). Factor VII is produced by the liver in the presence of vitamin K and contains 10 residues of γ-Gla as described above. Since the plasma concentration of this factor is very low (0.4–0.7 mg/L), the isolation and characterization of factor VII from human plasma has been difficult. The complete structure of factor VII has been elucidated from cloned cDNA, and the gene has been localized to chromosome 13 (33, 34).

When vessel walls are ruptured and blood is exposed to subendothelial tissues, factor VII forms a complex with tissue factor (tissue thromboplastin) expressed on certain cell surfaces (35). γ-Gla plays an important role in the calcium-dependent binding of factor VII to the phospholipid portion of tissue factor. The factor VII–tissue factor complex may have weak activity to trigger the extrinsic pathway by activating factors X and IX. Factors Xa and IXa, in turn, catalyze the conversion of factor VII to its two-chain form, VIIa. The factor VIIa–tissue factor complex has 100-fold more coagulant activity than the factor VII–tissue factor complex, thereby accelerating the activation of factors X and IX. The reciprocal activation of factor VII by factors Xa and IXa appears to be critical for the explosive generation of thrombin. There is some evidence that factor VII bound to tissue factor has to be activated to VIIa before it can trigger blood coagulation (36), but the enzyme responsible for the initial activation of factor VII is not known. Anyway, factor VII appears to play a central role in in vivo hemostasis.

Recent studies showed that human plasma contains a specific inhibitor of the extrinsic pathway, called extrinsic pathway inhibitor (EPI) or tissue factor pathway inhibitor (TFPI). This is a plasma protein (38 kDa) that is synthesized by vascular endothelial cells as well as by hepatocytes. TFPI blocks the activity of the factor VIIa–tissue factor complex and, thereby, turns off blood coagulation initiated by factor VII (36). The mechanism by which TFPI functions as an inhibitor is complex and is not completely elucidated. The activity of TFPI is dependent on factor Xa, and it has been postulated that a TFPI–factor Xa–factor VIIa–tissue factor complex is formed with resultant loss of the activity of the factor VIIa–tissue factor complex. TFPI is present in human plasma at a concentration of approximately 0.1 mg/L, and its concentration is decreased in patients with DIC (37).

Tissue Factor (Tissue Thromboplastin)

Tissue factor is a transmembrane protein (44 kDa) that is present constitutively in the surface membrane of nonvascular cells such as fibroblasts and pericytes (38). Tissue factor is anatomically sequestered from the blood in the normal state. Prominent tissue factor expression is found in organ capsules, epidermis, cerebral cortex, and renal glomeruli. Under physiologic conditions, vascular endothelium and circulating blood cells do not express tissue factor, thereby contributing to the maintenance of blood fluidity. However, upon stimulation by endotoxin or interleukin-1, these cells may be induced to produce and express tissue factor. The fact that deep skeletal muscle and joints contain undetectable to low tissue factor levels is consistent with the well-known clinical observation that bleeding into deep muscles and joints is common in patients with hemophilia (factor VIII or IX deficiency) (39). The structure of tissue factor has been deduced from cloned cDNA; it is a single-chain polypeptide with 263 amino acid residues and consists of cytoplasmic, transmembrane, and extracellular domains (40–43). The extracellular domain is the factor VII receptor.

Hereditary Factor VII Deficiency

A rare disorder of blood coagulation, hereditary factor VII deficiency is inherited in an autosomal recessive manner (44). Homozygous patients usually have less than 5% factor VII activity and present with epistaxis, gum bleeding, hematuria, gastrointestinal bleeding, excessive hemorrhage after dental extraction, and menorrhagia. Hemarthrosis may also occur. The clinical presentation is variable, and there appears to be little relationship between factor VII activity and bleeding symptoms (45). Heterozygous patients have factor VII activity of 40–60% of normal and are asymptomatic.

Hereditary factor VII deficiency is a heterogeneous disorder, and a number of variants have been detected by various functional and immunologic assays (46). In most patients, the plasma levels of immunoreactive factor VII (factor VII antigen) are much higher than those of factor VII activity, suggesting the presence of an abnormal nonfunctional molecule. Such cases are called cross-reacting material–positive (CRM+) variants, since the plasma contains nonfunctional material that cross-reacts with a specific antibody against factor VII. In contrast, the plasma levels of factor VII antigen are reduced in parallel with those of factor VII activity in some patients; they are CRM− variants. Another type of variant is identified when factor VII activity is measured with a panel of tissue factor (thromboplastin) from various species and tissues. For example, factor VII Padua is a unique variant in which factor VII activity as measured with rabbit brain or lung thromboplastin is decreased, but the activity is almost normal using other thromboplastins (47). The molecular basis of these variants is not known. A recent study identified a point mutation in the factor VII gene resulting in an amino acid substitution in the catalytic domain of factor VII (48). Elucidation of the structural defects in abnormal nonfunctional factor VII should be useful in our understanding of the structure-function relationship of this coagulation factor.

Activities

This patient represents a homozygous factor VII deficiency. Early onset of a bleeding tendency is typical for a congenital or hereditary disorder. A markedly prolonged PT with a normal aPTT suggested factor VII deficiency, which was confirmed by the determination of factor VII activity. Family study showed that the patient's parents have reduced activity. These findings are consistent with an autosomal recessive pattern of inheritance. Although a number of variants of factor VII deficiency have been identified as described above, their clinical presentations are similar, and it is usually not necessary to perform detailed studies for the identification of variants.

Fresh-frozen plasma or prothrombin complex concentrates can be used to treat severe bleeding. A factor VII level of 10–20% of normal is sufficient for hemostasis and can be achieved by giving 5–15 mL of plasma per kg of body weight. Since the half-life of factor VII is very short (4–6 hr), replacement therapy should be given three times a day. If the patient is undergoing major surgery, factor VII concentrate is a treatment of choice.

REFERENCES

1. Landefeld CS, Goldman L. Major bleeding in outpatients treated with warfarin: incidence and prediction by factors known at the start of outpatient therapy. Am J Med 1989; 87:144.
2. Saito H. Normal hemostatic mechanisms. In: Ratnoff OD, Forbes CD, eds. Disorders of hemostasis. 2nd ed. Philadelphia, WB Saunders, 1991;18–47.
3. Furie B, Furie BC. Molecular and cellular biology of blood coagulation. N Engl J Med 1992;326:800.
4. Osterud B, Rapaport SI. Activation of factor IX by the reaction product of tissue factor and factor VII: additional pathway for initiating blood coagulation. Proc Natl Acad Sci USA 1977;74:5260.
5. Saito H. The contact factors in health and disease. Semin Thromb Hemost 1987;13:36.
6. Petri M, et al. The frequency of lupus anticoagulant in systemic lupus erythematosus. A study of sixty consecutive patients by activated partial thromboplastin time, Russell viper venom time, and anticardiolipin antibody level. Ann Intern Med 1987;106:524.
7. Pengo V, Thiagarajan P, Shapiro SS, Heine MJ. Immunological specificity and mechanism of action of IgG lupus anticoagulants. Blood 1987;70:69.
8. Bowie EJW, et al. Thrombosis in systemic lupus erythematosus despite circulating anticoagulants. J Clin Invest 1963; 62:416.
9. Lubbe WF, et al. Lupus anticoagulant in pregnancy. Br J Obstet Gynaecol 1984;91:357.
10. Harris EN, Asherson RA, Hughes GRV. Antiphospholipid antibodies—autoantibodies with a difference. Annu Rev Med 1988;39:261.
11. Mann KG, et al. Surface-dependent reactions of the vitamin K–dependent enzyme complexes. Blood 1990;76:1.
12. Martinez J, Palascak JE, Kwasniak D. Abnormal sialic acid content of the dysfibrinogenemia associated with liver disease. J Clin Invest 1978;61:535.
13. Tygstrup N. The prognostic value of laboratory tests in liver disease. Scand J Gastroenterol 1973;8(Suppl 19):47.
14. Deykin D, et al. Hepatic removal of activated factor X by the perfused rabbit liver. Am J Physiol 1968;214:414.
15. Harker LA. The kinetics of platelet production and destruction in man. Clin Hematol 1977;6:671.
16. Bick RL. Disseminated intravascular coagulation and related syndromes: etiology, pathophysiology, diagnosis, and management. Am J Hematol 1978;5:265.
17. Stenflo J, et al. Vitamin K–dependent modifications of glutamic acid residues in prothrombin. Proc Natl Acad Sci USA 1974;71:2730.
18. Esmon CT, Suttie JW, Jackson CM. The functional significance of vitamin K action: difference in phospholipid binding between normal and abnormal prothrombin. J Biol Chem 1975;250:4095.
19. Esmon CT. The roles of protein C and thrombomodulin in the regulation of blood coagulation. J Biol Chem 1989; 264:4743.
20. Furie B, Furie BC. The molecular basis of blood coagulation. Cell 1988;53:505.
21. Suttie JW. Vitamin K–dependent carboxylase. Annu Rev Biochem 1985;54:459.
22. Furie B, Furie BC. Molecular basis of vitamin K–dependent γ-carboxylation. Blood 1990;75:1753.
23. Hemker HC, Veltkamp JJ, Loeliger EA. Kinetic aspects of the interaction of blood clotting enzymes. III. Demonstration of an inhibitor of prothrombin conversion in vitamin K deficiency. Thromb Diath Haemorrh 1968;19:346.
24. Lipsky JJ. Mechanism of the inhibition of the γ-carboxylation of glutamic acid by N-methylthiotetrazole-containing antibiotics. Proc Natl Acad Sci USA 1984;81:2893.
25. von Kries R, Shearer MJ, Gobel U. Vitamin K in infancy. Eur J Pediatr 1988;147:106.
26. Hirsh J. Oral anticoagulant drugs. N Engl J Med 1991; 324:1865.
27. Teitel JM, Resenberg RD. Protection of factor Xa from neutralization by the heparin-antithrombin complex. J Clin Invest 1983;71:1383.
28. Tracy PB, Rohrback MS, Mann KG. Functional prothrombinase complex assembly on isolated monocytes and lymphocytes. J Biol Chem 1983;258:7264.
29. Kane WH, Davie EW. Blood coagulation factors V and VIII: structural and functional similarities and their relationship to hemorrhagic and thrombotic disorders. Blood 1988;71:539.
30. Chopra S, Griffin PH. Laboratory tests and diagnostic procedures in evaluation of liver disease. Am J Med 1985; 79:221.
31. Burroughs AK, McCormick PA, Sprengers D. Assessment of bleeding risk in chronic liver disease. Fibrinolysis 1988; 2(Suppl 3):56.
32. Cederbaum A, Blatt P, Roberts H. Intravascular coagulation with use of human prothrombin complex concentrates. Ann Intern Med 1976;84:683.
33. Hagen FS, et al. Characterization of a cDNA coding for human factor VII. Proc Natl Acad Sci USA 1986;83:2412.
34. De Grouchy J, et al. Regional mapping of clotting factors VII and X to 13q34: expression of factor VII through chromosome 8. Hum Genet 1984;66:230.
35. Nemerson Y. Tissue factor and hemostasis. Blood 1988; 71:1.
36. Rapaport SI. Regulation of the tissue factor pathway. Ann NY Acad Sci 1991;614:51.

37. Bajaj MS, Rana SV, Wysolmerski RB, Bajaj SP. Inhibitor of the factor VIIa–tissue factor complex is reduced in patients with disseminated intravascular coagulation but not in patients with severe hepatocellular disease. J Clin Invest 1987; 79:1874.

38. Wilcox JN, Smith KM, Schwartz SM, Gordon D. Localization of tissue factor in the normal vessel wall and in the atherosclerotic plaque. Proc Natl Acad Sci USA 1989;86:2839.

39. Drake TA, Morrissey JH, Edgington TS. Selective cellular expression of tissue factor in human tissues. Implications for disorders of hemostasis and thrombosis. Am J Pathol 1989; 134:1087.

40. Spicer EK, et al. Isolation of cDNA clones coding for human tissue factor: primary structure of the protein and cDNA. Proc Natl Acad Sci USA 1987;84:5148.

41. Scarpati EM, et al. Human tissue factor: cDNA sequence and chromosome localization of the gene. Biochemistry 1987;26:5234.

42. Morrissey JH, Fakhari H, Edington TS. Molecular cloning of the cDNA for tissue factor, the cellular receptor for the initiation of the coagulation protease cascade. Cell 1987;50:129.

43. Fisher K, et al. Cloning and expression of human tissue factor cDNA. Thromb Res 1987;48:89.

44. Marder VJ, Shulman NR. Clinical aspects of congenital factor VII deficiency. Am J Med 1964;37:182.

45. Ragni MV, Lewis JH, Spero JA, Hasiba U. Factor VII deficiency. Am J Hematol 1981;10:79.

46. Triplett DA, et al. Hereditary factor VII deficiency: heterogeneity defined by combined functional and immunochemical analysis. Blood 1985;66:1284.

47. Girolami A, et al. Factor VII Padua: a congenital coagulation disorder due to an abnormal factor VII with a peculiar activation pattern. J Lab Clin Med 1978;91:387.

48. O'Brien DP, et al. Purification and characterization of factor VII 304-Gln: a variant molecule with reduced activity isolated from a clinically unaffected male. Blood 1991;78:132.

CHAPTER 31

Factor VIII Defects

PETER S. SMITH

An account of an hemorrhagic disposition existing in certain families
—V. C. Otto, Medical Repository, 1803

Factor VIII, or antihemophilic globulin, is a trace glycoprotein circulating as a two-chain complex in the plasma bound to von Willebrand's factor in a ratio of one molecule per von Willebrand's monomer. It plays an indispensable role in coagulation by catalyzing the activation of factor X by activated factor IXa in the presence of calcium and phospholipid, thereby increasing the reaction rate ten thousandfold. Clinical conditions arising from the isolated deficiency of factor VIII are seen when its synthesis is impaired, as in hemophilia and von Willebrand's disease, and when it is neutralized by binding to an antibody. Although theoretically increased loss by catabolism or excretion could cause a deficiency, it is such a large molecule (approximately 300,000 daltons) that renal and gastrointestinal losses do not occur, and consumption is preceded by degradation of other factors. Factor VIII is synthesized in the hepatocyte, the spleen, and other tissues, and with von Willebrand's factor—a huge multimeric protein—it is stored in the Weibel-Palade bodies of the endothelial cell. Certain biogenic amines, such as vasopressin and catecholamines, can cause release of the factor VIII–von Willebrand's complex. An acute phase reactant, factor VIII, like fibrinogen, is increased in infection and inflammation. A meticulous review of the structure and molecular genetics of factor VIII is provided by the review article of White and Shoemaker (1). Three of the cases discussed below deal with common situations seen in factor VIII deficiency and von Willebrand's disease, while the last one, relatively rare, illustrates how difficult and therapeutically daunting autoimmune factor VIII deficiency can be in a nonhemophiliac.

Severe Hemophilia A

A 1-day-old infant was noted to ooze intermittently from a circumcision, and his thigh had become swollen and tense following a vitamin K injection. He was born at term to a 26-year-old gravida IV para III woman following an uneventful pregnancy. Delivery was vaginal over a small midline episiotomy, and he cried vigorously. The mother's health had always been excellent, and she denied any abnormal bleeding or bruising. Her family history was likewise unrevealing. Before the infant was transferred to the neonatal special unit, the following studies returned:

hemoglobin	*167 g/L*
hematocrit	*52%*
platelet count	*339 × 10⁹/L*
white blood cell count	*19.4 × 10⁹/L*
prothrombin time (PT)	*30 sec (nl 10–16 sec)*
activated partial thrombo-plastin time (aPTT)	*115 sec (nl 31–55 sec)*

On examination, the infant was pink, easily aroused, and had good muscle tone. Bright red blood discolored the circumcision dressing. The left thigh was swollen, its circumference measurably larger than the right. A repeat hematocrit several hours later was 37%, the aPTT was 105 sec, and the PT was 16 sec. Coagulation studies were as follows: factor XII, 60% (nl 13–93%); factor XI, 45% (nl 10–66%); factor IX, 39% (nl 15–91%); factor VIII, less than 1% (nl 40–180%); factor XIII screen, normal; fibrinogen, 2.55 g/L (nl 1.67–4.0).

Ten milliliter per kilogram fresh frozen plasma was infused because factor VIII concentrate was not readily available, and the oozing ceased. Thereafter, ultrapurified "monoclonal" factor VIII, 250 units daily, was used, with gradual improvement of the involved leg. Before discharge the infant received hepatitis B vaccine. His hemoglobin was 90 g/L, the reticulocyte count was 5.4%, and his left leg was of equal circumference to the right with a small area of induration. The bilirubin peaked on day 4 at 0.123 g/L.

Bleeding from the circumcision site as described here is the classical presentation of hemophilia, the earliest account of which goes back to the Babylonian Talmud in the 3rd century (2). With improvements in technique and circumcision devices and, above all, earlier (nonritual) circumcisions, this kind of presentation has become less common. Other kinds of neonatal presentations have been reported, such as intracranial hemorrhage or (as here) a thigh hematoma from an intramuscular injection (3). Sometimes a bleeding disorder is not suspected until the infant begins venturing out into its environment several months later, when trauma is more likely. This latency period, sometimes surprisingly long, has been wryly called "the hemophilia honeymoon." Once the toddler begins walking, running, and falling, bleeding events involving the joints and less commonly the muscles cause visits to the accident room.

Musculoskeletal bleeding characterizes hereditary clotting disorders, particularly, classical hemophilia (factor VIII deficiency) and Christmas disease (factor IX deficiency). While superficial bleeding may occur from the skin or the mouth, it more common andly generally follows deeper lacerations that involve larger and greater numbers of blood vessels. The distinction between disorders of **primary hemostasis** and those of **secondary hemostasis** is useful because these different presentations help lead to the likely cause of bleeding.

Disorders of *primary* hemostasis affect the skin, mucosa, and linings of the hollow organs, causing petechiae, bruises, oozing, and excessive menstrual losses. Such disorders are due to quantitative or qualitative platelet defects, an abnormal vasculature, or both. Bleeding occurs soon after trauma because formation of the platelet plug is delayed or inadequate. In secondary hemostasis disorders, bleeding is deep into the tissues, with a predilection for the joint spaces, muscles, and deep subcutaneous soft tissues. Because such hemorrhages are not easily seen, they are more difficult to detect early and are frequently misdiagnosed (e.g., as arthritis). Since secondary hemostasis encompasses the formation of the definitive fibrin-consolidated platelet plug through the activation of a series of plasma proteins, a disorder affecting this phase of hemostasis causes delayed bleeding from trauma. Hence a person with hemophilia will hemorrhage later from a dental extraction than will a person with thrombocytopenia or von Willebrand's disease. Figure 31.1, which depicts the events in primary hemostasis, and Figure 31.2, which represents the clotting cascade, help clarify these distinctions.

In the case narrated above, the combination of intermittent oozing, thigh swelling following an intramuscular injection, and a drop in the hematocrit suggests bleeding due to a clotting disorder causing anemia. The screening tests confirmed this. Although the prothrombin time was prolonged according to adult normal values and some of the factor levels appeared rather low, for an infant this age they were normal (4). The almost undetectable factor VIII level seen here is diagnostic of severe hemophilia A, or classical hemophilia, the most common type, occurring in approximately one in 7500 males. It accounts for nine out of ten cases of hemophilia, while Christmas disease and the rare and milder factor V, X, and XI deficiencies make up the remainder. Classical hemophilia and Christmas disease occur worldwide and are inherited in an X-linked recessive manner.

The mother's negative family history does not raise doubts about her son's hemophilia, since about one-third of all cases have uninformative family histories. Elaborate techniques have enabled researchers to pinpoint areas within the long arm of the X chromosome that are mutagenic "hot spots"—molecular aberrations culminating in the absence of the gene product (5).

In the two-thirds of cases in which the family is affected, the bleeding pattern in the relative is predictive of the probable course in the newly diagnosed child. Hence a crippled maternal uncle, hospitalized several times in the past, will no doubt also have an affected nephew with severe hemophilia. The severity of hemophilia is a clinical concept, but it is associated typically with characteristic ranges of factor VIII levels. In **severe hemophilia**, bleeding often occurs without the patient recalling any trauma; in fact, he will often wake up with a painful joint or relate it to stress. In such cases, the factor level is usually below 1%, and the bleeding frequency is as high as once or twice weekly. In **moderate hemophilia**, bleeding is more often associated with trauma; bleeding events depend upon the intensity of activity of the patient but occur much less often. The factor VIII level ranges between 1% and 5%. In **mild hemophilia**, bleeding is rare; it occurs following substantial trauma or after major surgery. In such patients, the factor VIII level ranges from 5% to 40% (normal range, 40–180%). Many such mild hemophiliacs are identified only because a presurgical aPTT is prolonged.

The choice of products to use in treating hemophilia has expanded considerably under the impetus of the AIDS epidemic, which devastated the hemophilia community (6). As a result of transfusions using concentrates, each lot of which derives from several thousand donors, over 70% of multiply-transfused persons have been HIV infected. Now with stringent donor selection criteria and several methods to rid concentrates of transmissible microorganisms, no new HIV infections have occurred in

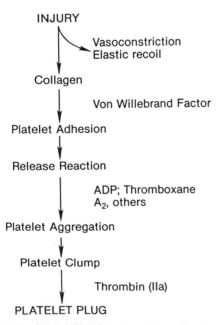

Figure 31.1. The factor VIII deficiencies. (From Corrigan JJ. Hemorrhagic and thrombotic diseases in childhood and adolescence. New York: Churchill Livingstone, 1985:6. With permission.)

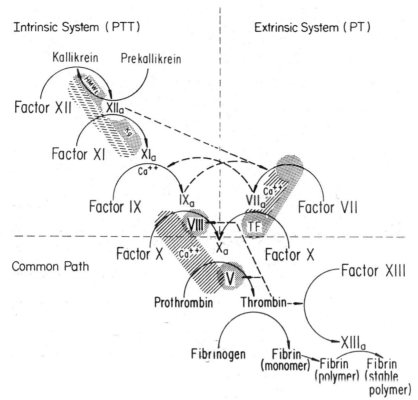

Figure 31.2. Mechanisms of clotting factor interactions. Clotting is initiated by either an *intrinsic* or *extrinsic* pathway, with subsequent factor interactions that converge upon a final *common path*. The clinical screening tests are indicated as *PTT* (partial thromboplastin time) and *PT* (prothrombin time). The factors circulate as *(a)* zymogens, which are activated by specific cleavages to highly specific serine proteases, *(b)* cofactors *(stippled* for protein and *hatched* for phospholipid), or *(c)* the precursor of the structural protein of the clot (fibrinogen). A separate enzymatic system, generation of factor XIIIa, follows for clot stabilization. Protein cofactors include high-molecular-weight kininogen *(HMWt Kg),* tissue factor *(TF),* and factors VIII and V; each of the latter two require modification by thrombin. Other interactions between the intrinsic and extrinsic systems *(arrows* and *dashed lines)* can be demonstrated under some conditions. (From Thompson AR, Harker LA. Manual of hemostasis and thrombosis. 3rd ed. Philadelphia: FA Davis, 1983:25.)

the U.S. in previously untransfused patients since 1985. In this infant the safest replacement therapy is with one of these highly purified products. Various methods isolate the factor VIII molecule, which is then lyophilized, after sterilization, to yield a specific dose. The factor in each vial is dissolved in water within a minute and is injected intravenously. The half-life of the factor VIII ranges from 8 to 12 hours. A recombinant factor VIII concentrate is commercially available.

When the exact clotting factor deficiency is not known initially and brisk bleeding demands immediate treatment, fresh frozen plasma is the product of first choice. By definition, one unit of any clotting factor is that amount present in 1 mL of pooled fresh frozen plasma (FFP). Since the FFP is from one donor, the exact amount of factor is not known exactly, but the risk of infection if untested is that of one unit of blood, i.e., approximately 0.04% for HIV and 0.8% for non-A, non-B hepatitis (7, 8). Cryoprecipitate, still the only available blood product in many parts of the world for factor VIII deficiency, is another option in this infant if a pure concentrate is not available. Each bag of cryoprecipitate is obtained by thawing a unit of FFP and resuspending the frozen precipitate, which is rich in factor VIII. Usually a bag contains 80–100 units of factor VIII in only 35–40 mL of plasma, thus yielding more factor on a volume per volume basis.

One unit per kilogram of infused factor VIII raises the plasma level approximately 2%. Hence, to achieve a hemostatic level (above 20%) in this infant, infusion of at least 40 mL of FFP is required, while the same volume of cryoprecipitate would achieve levels above 40%. Once this infant received concentrate—the smallest dose contains 250 units in 2 mL of water—the blood titer was 125% immediately, dropping to about 30% after 24 hours, high enough to need only one infusion daily.

Two months later this mother brought her baby to the emergency room because he had cried inconsolably all night. By that age he had attained the expected milestones and was generally an active, happy baby. The mother denied that he had any fever but noted that he did not use one arm at all. Any attempt to move it caused him to cry. On examination, none of his joints or muscles were swollen or tender, but trying to bend one elbow made him cry. Within an hour of infusing factor VIII concentrate, all symptoms subsided.

It is not clear exactly what initiates bleeding in severe hemophilia, nor do we know why some persons with severe hemophilia bleed less than others. Suffice it to emphasize that barring trauma, bleeding is unpredictable, and a high degree of suspicion is warranted when there is any discomfort or sparing of a limb. Limitation of motion always precedes tenderness and swelling. Radiographs are useless. Replacement therapy, as here, provides almost immediate relief of all symptoms. Treatment at this early stage requires small doses and avoids costly diagnostic procedures and hospitalizations and long-term complications such as contractures and hemophilic arthropathy.

Most often the large joints are involved, particularly those bearing weight, such as the ankles and knees. Bleeding originates from the vessels in the synovial villi, which have little protective basement membrane and supporting tissues. Synovial fluid, poor in thromboplastin and rich in heparinoids, inhibits hemostasis, which may contribute to the continued seeping of blood into the joint in hemophilia. Instead of normal hemostasis arresting this process, it is the pressure equilibration of joint fluid and countervailing capsule tension, a most painful and damaging alternative. The joint is poorly equipped to resorb large amounts of blood, and it does so slowly. This exposes the synovium and the cartilage to the damaging effects of blood, setting the stage for a succession of degenerative changes (9–11).

Bleeding into the muscles is less common than joint bleeding, involving mainly the calf, forearm, and iliopsoas. Unlike in hemarthrosis, pain is not perceived early, perhaps owing to the larger volume of blood required to stretch the pain receptors of the muscle sheath. Because of the blood volume loss, bleeding into large muscles causes anemia. Where nerves course next to distended muscles, they can sustain damage from pressure. Similarly, pressure necrosis of muscle fibers may occur, causing a compartment syndrome and permanent deformities if nothing is done. Muscles, which are richly supplied with blood vessels, are also more likely to rebleed; hence the rationale for replacement therapy for several days.

Toddlers with hemophilia often bleed from the mouth. It typically follows a tongue bite, a foreign body laceration, or a fall and is uncommon spontaneously. Oozing can last days, and large, imperfect "liver" clots protrude from the cut and spread it further. A small dose (10 units/kg) of AHF (VIII concentrate) is usually adequate to stop the bleeding and is all that is needed, provided an oral antifibrinolytic drug is also given for the first 3 or 4 days. Mouth blood clots are dissolved rapidly because of plasminogen normally present in significant amounts in the saliva. Blocking its conversion to plasmin with ϵ-aminocaproic acid (Amicar) syrup in a dose of 1 mL per 2.5 kg every 6 hours is usually effective. In older children or in adults, another such drug, tranexamic acid (Cyclokapron) can be used in tablet form in a dose of 20 mg/kg/day. (The tablets are easier to swallow than Amicar tablets, because they are smaller, and fewer are needed for treatment.)

Prolonged external bleeding, unlike, for example, intramuscular bleeding, causes iron deficiency anemia, best treated with oral iron supplementation. The iron deposited from internal bleeding is available for hemoglobin synthesis.

At age 6 years, the patient was seen at an annual multidisciplinary clinic for routine evaluation. At age 5, his parents began home care, injecting him with factor concentrates after thorough training by the hemophilia center staff. Now he is a bright, very active boy who seems to seek out precisely those games and stunts from which his parents have tried to discourage his participation. His infusions are at times difficult because he squirms. To avoid them he does not consistently inform his parents until pain is severe, or he begins to limp noticeably. A review of a year's infusion records reveals that he had 68 bleeding events requiring 78 infusions, mostly involving his knees and ankles. A disproportionate number involved his right ankle and were repeated the next day because of persistent pain and swelling. For the most part, pain began at school and his parents infused him at home, often hours later. In the clinic he appeared to walk normally, but his right ankle was swollen, nontender, but boggy to palpation. Its range of motion was slightly decreased. An x-ray revealed moderate demineralization of the adjacent bones but no narrowing of the joint spaces, subchondral cyst formation, or bony spurs. Pertinent laboratory studies showed only mildly elevated ALT, 65 U; AST, 72 U, (normal levels less than 40 U/mL).

At a routine comprehensive clinic visit, it is common to discover potentially disabling abnormalities in asymptomatic patients. *This school-age boy has the characteristic findings of chronic synovitis, as well as low-grade, probably non-A, non-B hepatitis.* Both require closer scrutiny and possibly aggressive therapy. Home care, now available and subsidized in many developed countries, has dramatically decreased crippling arthropathies, contractures, and palsies. Death from hemorrhage and pseudotumors are both preventable and rare catastrophes. Newer morbidities, less devastating in the short term, are taxing the ingenuity and resources of health care providers: HIV infection, chronic synovitis, and chronic hepatitis.

In this boy, a nontender swollen joint with a normal range of motion and radiographic appearance fulfills the criteria for chronic synovitis. Contributing to this complication are his high level of activity and deliberate delay in treatment.

Typically, chronic synovitis occurs in a large weight-bearing joint such as the knee or ankle, or the elbow of the dominant arm. Anatomic pathologic changes observed both in the human and in animal models are a rusty-colored, hypervascular, hypertrophied synovium that bleeds readily (10, 11). Over a period of months to years, the neglected joint will show iron deposition and necrosis of chondrocytes. Ulcerations covered by an adherent synovial pannus ensue, as in rheumatoid arthritis. In the end, demineralization, cystic degeneration, and fibrous or bony ankylosis immobilize the joint in a fixed, partially flexed position. Such joints hurt less or not at all.

Although very expensive and not necessary for diagnosis, magnetic resonance images in these situations show a hypertrophied synovium and loss of cartilage (12). The treatment of such chronic synovitis can be vexing, since its cause is multifactorial and calls for behavioral change and reversal of a process set in motion by blood in the joint space. Since the success rate is modest, there is no "treatment protocol." Most clinicians focus their management on preventing further bleeding by more frequent (even prophylactic) factor VIII infusions; decreasing motion by putting on a splint, orthosis, or cast; and inhibiting inflammation with corticosteroids. Prophylactic alternate-day infusions of approximately 30 units per kilogram may significantly decrease the swelling over a period of weeks, but venous access is frequently a problem, and relapses are common upon discontinuation. Similarly, prednisone at a therapeutic dose of 2 mg/kg over a week may only work temporarily. Joint immobilization is helpful but causes disuse atrophy of the supporting muscles. Combining intermittent immobilization and physical therapy may therefore be preferable.

Removing the diseased synovium yields encouraging results (13) by decreasing the amount of bleeding into the affected joint. Results are better if synovectomy is carried out before significant cartilage damage. Open synovectomy is more successful in removing more synovium, but invariably the postsurgery range of motion decreases. Also, the length of hospital stay and duration of rehabilitation are longer. Arthroscopic synovectomy addresses these drawbacks, but a second procedure is often required to remove residual synovium (14). Controlled studies are needed to indicate which therapeutic approach or, more likely, which combined modality is most effective in preventing hemophilic arthropathy. With proper care, total joint replacements should become as obsolete as the preventable end-stage conditions that call for them (15).

There is evidence of damage to the liver cells in this boy. Since he received a hepatitis B vaccine early on, the cause is most likely hepatitis C from his first treatment at birth.

Hepatitis C, constituting some 90% of cases of non-A, non-B hepatitis, can frequently cause chronic active hepatitis and liver cirrhosis in some 10% of cases (16). The seroprevalence of hepatitis C in persons with hemophilia who received many infusions is very high, even in those with normal transaminase levels (17, 18). This suspicion must be confirmed with repeated transaminase determinations and specific viral serologies. Efforts to inhibit or arrest the progression include using subcutaneous α-interferon injections (19). Its many side effects warrant careful monitoring.

Mild Hemophilia

Rodrigo, a 7-year-old Latino boy, was reported to the child welfare agency because of suspected child abuse. He had large bruises on his forehead and legs and painful swelling of one knee. In the hospital where he underwent evaluation, he was alert, but apprehensive. He did not communicate well in English. Like his younger brother, he had always bruised easily, accord-

ing to his family. The bruises were often very large, and he bled frequently from the nose. This was the first time his knee was swollen and painful. His left knee was distended in all directions, held in partial flexion, and warm and tender to touch. The rest of his examination was unremarkable.

An x-ray of the knee revealed soft tissue enlargement; a survey of the long bones and head revealed no fractures or periosteal elevation. The laboratory studies on admission were as follows:

hemoglobin	*100 g/L*
MCV	*85 fL*
WBC	*6.9 × 10⁹/L*
PMNs	*72%*
monocytes	*3%*
lymphocytes	*25%*
platelets	*270 × 10⁹/L*
aPTT	*40.4 sec*
PT	*16 sec*
factor VIII:C	*25%*
factor VIII:Ag	*85%*
von Willebrand's factor	*84%*
bleeding time	*7 min*
ferritin	*0.6 mg/L*

The physical findings and radiologic and laboratory studies did not support child abuse, infection, or immune-mediated cause for this boy's clinical presentation, although all are plausible. On the other hand, the history of large bruises, epistaxis, and a swollen, tender knee suggest a congenital bleeding disorder.

Bruising and nosebleeds (but not hemarthrosis) can occur with thrombocytopenia, a functional platelet defect, or von Willebrand's disease. The evaluation, therefore, must look into disorders of both primary and secondary hemostasis. The modified Ivy bleeding time using a commercial device (Simplate) to make a small incision of specific depth and length may commend itself for its simplicity and reproducibility (20). In disorders of primary hemostasis, the bleeding time may be prolonged. Here it was not. In contrast, the aPTT was prolonged, and the factor VIII level was low. These tests, together with normal levels of factor VIII antigen and von Willebrand's factor, support the diagnosis of hemophilia and rule out a more common mild bleeding disorder, von Willebrand's disease. Table 31.1 lists differentiating features of these two related disorders.

The laboratory allows distinction between these two disorders, which overlap clinically. The factor VIII antigen assay measures the amount of *immunogenic* factor VIII in the plasma when tested against antibodies from a sensitized animal. *Plasma from people with hemophilia A contains normal amounts of immunogenic factor VIII,* which implies a functionally abnormal protein. A property of factor VIII coagulant protein, called factor VIII:C, is its ability to shorten the activated partial thromboplastin time. Factor VIII:C has recently been purified and cloned. The disparity between a normal factor VIII:Ag level and factor VIII:C is pathognomonic

Table 31.1. Distinguishing Properties of von Willebrand's Disease and Mild Hemophilia

	Von Willebrand's Disease	Mild Hemophilia
Gender	Both sexes	Males
Inheritance	Autosomal dominant	X-linked recessive
Bruises	++	+
Ecchymoses	(+)	++
Epistaxis	+++	+
Hemarthrosis	–	++
Menorrhagia	++	–
Factor VIII:C	decr or nl	decr
Factor VIII:Ag	decr or nl	nl
Ristocetin cofactor (von Willebrand's) factor)	decr	nl

for hemophilia A. A normal titer of von Willebrand's factor, also called ristocetin cofactor, confirms the diagnosis. (In the presence of adequate amounts of von Willebrand's factor, the antibiotic ristocetin causes platelet aggregation, as described in chapter 30.)

The knee swelling in this boy is an acute hemarthrosis. There is little evidence to support aspiration, either for diagnosis in this setting or for therapy. Only a poor response to specific therapy would warrant it.

The treatment of mild factor VIII deficiency has changed recently with the commercial availability of desmopressin acetate, better known as DDAVP, which circumvents exposure of people with a mild bleeding disorder to the complications of blood products. A vasoactive amine related to vasopressin, DDAVP has few side effects. Given parenterally, DDAVP releases factor VIII into the blood from endogenous sites in the vascular endothelium where it is stored bound to von Willebrand's factor. A single dose of 0.3 μg per kilogram body weight will usually triple the level of factor VIII:C well beyond the hemostatic range. The drug may be given intravenously or intranasally, which is more concentrated than the spray used for diabetes insipidus. A peak level is attained within an hour, the half-life being the same as infused factor VIII. DDAVP regularly causes facial flushing, much less commonly headache and fluid retention. It is best to use it no more than once every 24 hours to avoid these side effects. Shorter intervals do not allow stores to be replenished. Thus, severe hemorrhage may demand supplemental factor VIII replacement. In such a case, an ultrapure concentrate or a single-donor product such as cryoprecipitate is preferred.

As in the previous case, this boy has evidence of iron deficiency, probably from recurrent nosebleeds. Hemophilia alone does not initiate epistaxis. Rather, it aggravates bleeding, the cause of which is usually a local factor, such as dryness, allergies, abnormal vessels, and irritation. Treating these causes should suf-

fice in most cases. Nasal packing and intravenous agents can be reserved for the rare cases of severe prolonged bleeding.

von Willebrand's Disease

Brenda, a 14-year-old girl, came to the emergency room with 18 days of profuse vaginal bleeding and with pallor and weakness. This was her second menstrual period, and because it was painful, she had taken several aspirins. She denied any recent sexual activity and said she had always been in perfect health. At age 12, however, she had bled so much after a tooth extraction that her dentist had to pack and suture the bleeding site. Like one of her younger brothers, she bruised easily. Her father had once required a blood transfusion after a tonsillectomy but had had an uneventful postoperation course following a herniorrhaphy.

Her blood pressure was 110/60 recumbent and 90/50 sitting up; her resting pulse was 100. She was dizzy and anxious when she was upright. Her abdomen was soft and nontender, and no masses were felt. On bimanual pelvic examination, the uterus was midline, anteverted, and normal in size; the adnexae were soft and nontender. There was much blood flowing from an intact cervical os to the vagina.

The laboratory findings were as follows:

hemoglobin	*60 g/L*
MCV	*85 fL*
WBC	*16.4 × 10⁹/L, with a normal differential*
aPTT	*39 sec (nl 33–27 sec)*
PT	*14 sec*
pregnancy test	*negative*

She was admitted to the hospital and received one unit of packed red blood cells and two 25-mg doses of conjugated equine estrogen, with some improvement. She later received a progestational agent. She was discharged on medroxyprogesterone for 10 days. At the next visit, a bleeding time was 12 minutes (nl less than 9 min), and the following clotting studies were obtained:

aPTT	*38.5 sec (nl 27–37 sec)*
PT	*14 sec (nl 11–14 sec)*
factor XII	*60% (nl 52–164%)*
factor XI	*72% (nl 67–127%)*
factor IX	*73% (nl 55–163%)*
factor VIII:C	*38% (40–149%)*
factor VIII:Ag	*35% (nl 40–149%)*
von Willebrand's factor (risocetin cofactor)	*45% (nl 50–150%)*

Brenda's presentation and past medical history offer clues such as bruising, excessive bleeding after oral surgery, and menorrhagia following a painful menses treated with aspirin. Her father's hemorrhage after a tonsillectomy and the brother's tendency to bruise also raise the suspicion of a familial disorder that is not sex-linked.

Postsurgical bleeding from the tonsillar fossa is not rare, even in hemostatically normal people. The pharyngeal tissues are vascular, and securing good surgical hemostasis is difficult. This is not so in a herniorrhaphy, which requires little tissue dissection for which wound edges can be tightly sutured together.

There are contributory factors in this case that may account in part for the severity of the blood loss. Anovulatory cycles in adolescents are common at the beginning of reproductive life because of the proliferation of the endometrium uninterrupted by the effects of progesterone, causing breakthrough bleeding from focal necrosis. The administration of a gestagen causes vasoconstriction and platelet plugging of the arterioles, followed by shedding of the endometrium (21).

Aspirin (acetylsalicylic acid) strongly impairs platelet function by blocking prostaglandin-mediated platelet adhesion and aggregation and worsens defective platelet plug formation in von Willebrand's disease, causing decompensated primary hemostasis. Some clinicians have even relied on an "aspirin tolerance test," which disproportionately prolongs the bleeding time, to screen for a mild hemostasis disorder (22).

The physical findings and laboratory studies were typical of an adolescent girl with von Willebrand's disease, probably the most common mild bleeding disorder of primary hemostasis. There was orthostatic hypotension from blood volume depletion, a normal abdominal and pelvic examination, severe anemia, and a moderately prolonged aPTT. A normal platelet count suggested that the problem was one of platelet function. The coagulation studies confirmed the condition.

A typical profile in von Willebrand's disease consists of a prolonged bleeding time, a moderately prolonged aPTT, and characteristic and variable decreases in factor VIII:C, factor VIII antigen, and von Willebrand's factor (ristocetin cofactor). There are three major subtypes, based upon the factor VIII–related activities; the most common is type I, which is inherited in an autosomal dominant manner, and the least common, type III, is a homozygous disorder. Further confusing the spectrum is an ever-increasing array of subtypes with few, if any, major clinical differences, but which differ significantly at the molecular level.

The distinction between von Willebrand's disease and mild hemophilia has perplexed students for generations, because in both conditions, factor VIII activity levels are decreased. It is useful to remember that von Willebrand's disease affects platelets primarily and hemophilia does not. Table 31.1 further highlights some distinctions. Readers are referred to review articles for greater detail (23, 24).

von Willebrand's disease is often mild enough to remain undetected until a critical event occurs, such as in Brenda's case. One who always bruises easily may consider it normal. Often, a severe nosebleed or hemorrhaging after a tonsillectomy prompts laboratory investigation. With improved automated and quality-controlled screening tests, mild and asymptomatic cases are routinely identified before surgery. The disorder may behave differently in members of the same family and even in the same patients over time. In contrast to factor VIII levels in hemophilia, the laboratory tests are poor predictors of severity.

Despite their increased level of activity, children with von Willebrand's disease rarely bleed severely, and reports of postcircumcision hemorrhage or of intracranial hemorrhage in the newborn are lacking. In a large survey in Italy (25), most symptomatic children had epistaxis and bruising, and a few bled excessively after a tooth was extracted or with menstruation. The most frequent symptoms in adults were epistaxis and menorrhagia.

Abnormal bleeding in von Willebrand's disease is due to the lack or abnormality of a very large adhesive plasma protein called von Willebrand's factor (vWF). It has binding sites for collagen, platelet surface receptors, and factor VIII:C, and it anchors platelets to vascular subendothelium, causing them to cluster (aggregation). In binding factor VIII:C, vWF both protects it from degradation and places it in a position to catalyze the clotting reaction, which yields the tight, fibrin-bound definitive platelet plug. Deficiency of vWF predictably impairs hemostasis wherever blood vessels are most exposed to disruption, usually on body surfaces. The sparing effect of vWF on VIII:C is rarely of clinical significance except in the rare type III variant, in which vWF is totally lacking. Factor VIII:C is then broken down rapidly, resulting in low plasma levels, often below 10%. Clinically, patients show features consistent with hemophilia (musculoskeletal bleeding) and von Willebrand's disease.

vWF is a multimer, the heaviest components of which are the best adhesives. In type I von Willebrand's disease, there is a balanced deficiency of all monomers; in type II von Willebrand's disease, the heavier monomers are lacking. There are subtypes of both type I and II variants because of altered conformation of the monomers, manifest by specific patterns on column chromatography and different factor VIII laboratory profiles (table 31.2). For instance, in type II$_B$, increased binding of the heavier monomers to platelets decreases their plasma level. When release of vWF from storage sites is increased by DDAVP, the platelets aggregate, and thrombocytopenia occurs. For this reason, DDAVP is contraindicated in type II$_B$ von Willebrand's disease.

Table 31.2. Factor VIII–related Activities in the Major von Willebrand's Disease Subgroups

	VIII:C	VIII:Ag	VIII:RC
Type I	↓	↓	↓
Type II	nl or ↓	nl or ↓	↓
Type III	↓↓	0	0

Blood levels of vWF and its "passenger" factor VIII:C are governed not only by biogenic amines but also by pregnancy, in which both factors tend toward normal levels. In vitro endothelium releases vWF when cultured with estrogens (26), which likely accounts for the uneventful deliveries in women with von Willebrand's disease.

The blood transfusion in this young woman was certainly appropriate because of her hypovolemia and orthostatic hypotension. Medicinal iron should have been prescribed on discharge. Because hormonal therapy was effective, treatment with DDAVP or cryoprecipitate was not necessary.

Indeed, the preferred treatment for menorrhagia in von Willebrand's disease is oral contraceptives, adjusting the amount of estrogen to achieve an acceptable menstrual blood loss. Should this be unsuccessful, DDAVP would be the next choice. As noted above, cryoprecipitate is rich in vWF and is generally administered in a dose of one bag per 10 kg body weight. Certain virus-attenuated concentrates (Humate-P and Koate HS) contain substantial amounts of vWF.

Aspirin and phenylbutazone are the most potent inhibitors of cyclooxygenase, an enzyme that converts arachidonic acid to the potent platelet aggregation mediator thromboxane. Both drugs must be avoided in bleeding disorders such as von Willebrand's disease. Although several other nonsteroidal antiinflammatory agents (NSAIDs) have a similar mechanism of action, studies in normal volunteers have not shown them to increase the bleeding time (27). If acetaminophen (paracetamol) fails to alleviate dysmenorrhea, a trial of such NSAIDS may be warranted.

Acquired Anticoagulant

Two weeks after the delivery of her third child, Mrs. Y, 32 years old, noticed large bruises on her limbs and along the pelvic brim. They grew rapidly to several centimeters in diameter, raising the skin surface, and were moderately tender. A day later, pain, swelling, and oozing from the midline episiotomy repair made sitting impossible.

On examination in the emergency room, she was alert, well nourished, and afebrile and had considerable localized pain. Her blood pressure was 130/80, her pulse was 110 per minute, her respiratory rate was 20 per minute. Ecchymoses were seen on her arms and legs, and the tissues around the episiotomy were suffused, bluish, and tender. There were no cervical tears. Upon release of the vaginal episiotomy sutures, large clots were evacuated from the episiotomy wound. Hemostasis with several mattress sutures to the deeper tissues was attempted. Brisk bleeding occurred throughout the procedure, and oozing continued from the repair site. Because of this, fresh whole blood was given, with no apparent effect on bleeding. A blood specimen obtained before the transfusion yielded the following results:

hemoglobin	*110 g/L*
hematocrit	*33%*
MCV	*83 fL*

white blood cells	*16.5 × 10⁹/L*
polymorphonuclear cells	*61%*
band forms	*3%*
monocytes	*5%*
lymphocytes	*31%*
platelets	*435 × 10⁹/L*
PT	*14 sec*
aPTT	*95 sec*
fibrinogen	*3 g/L*
fibrin degradation products	*>10 but <40 µg/mL (nl >10)*

Although postpartum hemorrhage from an episiotomy or a hematoma is not rare when surgical hemostasis is inadequate, it seldom occurs so late. The unexpected coincidence with ecchymoses raises the concern of a generalized hemorrhagic diathesis. Were this picture to occur in a febrile woman, one would strongly consider postpartum sepsis with disseminated intravascular coagulation. But such women are profoundly ill, often with accompanying mental changes and shock by the time generalized bleeding is apparent. The wound hemorrhage and large ecchymoses on pressure-prone spots in a previously well woman occurring so late after parturition suggests an acquired anticoagulant.

The normal prothrombin time with prolonged aPTT excludes a consumption coagulopathy and points to a deficiency in the intrinsic factor pathway.

Without exactly pinpointing a specific defect, Mrs. Y's physicians treated her with 2 units of FFP, but blood continued to ooze from the vagina. Her coagulation studies following the FFP were: aPTT, 81 sec; PT, 13 sec; factor VIII, 3%; factor IX, 85%; factor XI, 67%; vWF, 75%. A one-to-one mixture of her plasma and normal plasma yielded an aPTT of 70 sec.

Poor response to FFP, which at this dose would have sufficed to raise all plasma coagulation proteins to within the hemostatic range, suggests an inactivation process. This was confirmed by the mixture experiment, which should have normalized or greatly improved the aPTT (28). Such is the clinical and laboratory behavior of an **acquired inhibitor,** *in this case directed against factor VIII:C.*

Acquired anticoagulants are a more frequent finding in severe hemophiliacs whose immune system recognizes exogenous factor as foreign. In fact, a recent report of screening of persons attending hemophilia treatment centers documents inhibitors in 10–15% of those with factor VIII deficiency, fewer with factor IX deficiency (29). Persons without hemophilia may also develop such antibodies against a procoagulant, usually factor VIII:C. Unusual as it is in clinical practice, it must be recognized because of the spontaneous life-threatening hemorrhage that invariably follows, in contrast to inhibitors in persons with hemophilia, which do not cause more frequent hemorrhage. De novo inhibitors may arise within the context of another medical problem of suspect autoimmune etiology, such as rheumatoid arthritis or malignancy. In a review of 215 cases, 54% occurred in persons with an underlying medical condition known to cause autoimmune manifestations (30). Rheumatoid arthritis and the postpartum condition accounted for about 8% each, followed by malignancies. Men and women were equally affected, mainly adults, and hemorrhage was significant, involving the joints, the intestine, and the retroperitoneal and intracranial spaces.

Acquired autoimmune inhibitors are immunoglobulins of the IgG class. Those against factor VIII are directed against epitopes of the factor VIII coagulant protein. They show species specificity and are neutralized by serum against human IgG. They may last for months without treatment or they spontaneously disappear, particularly postpartum. Because inhibitors in this population are so dangerous, most cases require treatment.

In persons with hemophilia, inhibitors are most often detected shortly after institution of factor VIII infusions, and they tend to cluster in related persons. In "low responders," the inhibitor titer rises to a level that may remain stable despite continued infusions of factor; in "high responders," the anamnestic response is strong enough to completely inactivate any infused factor VIII. In measuring inhibitor titers, it is important to incubate the specimens at body temperature for 2 hours for maximum binding. The most commonly used measurement for antibodies is the Bethesda unit (BU), defined as the amount of antibody that neutralizes 50% of factor VIII:C in 1 mL of plasma after a 2-hour incubation at 37°C.

When bleeding from the episiotomy wound increased a few hours later, Mrs. Y received three vials of factor VIII concentrate with no appreciable improvement, either clinically or in laboratory responses. Meanwhile, an expedited shipment of porcine factor VIII arrived. The lyophilized product, a polyelectrolyte-purified product, was administered in the recommended dose of 50 units per kilogram. Bleeding subsided, and with repeat infusions every 6 hours, it ceased altogether. Factor VIII:C assays rose gradually. The consulting hematologist also ordered 1 g per kilogram of intravenous gamma globulin daily for 2 days to decrease the neutralization of factor VIII. Upon discharge 8 days later, Mrs. Y's factor VIII level was 45% (normal 40–160%); the inhibitor titer had decreased from a high of 65 BU when first measured to 4 BU.

The treatment of inhibitors is not standardized because no method invariably works. A rational approach based upon the pathophysiology would consist of achieving measurable levels of factor VIII to stop the bleeding, preventing factor neutralization, and decreasing antibody production. Reaching measurable levels is often impossible because of rapid binding of human factor VIII to the antibody. Because the anti–factor VIII antibody may show little affinity to porcine factor VIII, the latter is frequently effective, particularly when inhibitor titers are below 50 BU. There is, however, cross-reactivity when inhibitor levels are very high, and after several days, sensitization by porcine factor VIII. When inhibitor levels are less than 5 BU, one can administer an excess of human factor VIII,

enough to saturate the inhibitor and provide a hemostatic factor VIII level. Failing that, prothrombin complex concentrates, which contain factors II, VII, IX, and X and variable amounts of their activated congeners, often stop the bleeding. Prothrombin complex concentrates containing more activated factor are commercially available, but there are conflicting reports their efficacy over less expensive concentrates, generally known as factor IX concentrates (Konyne, Profilnine, etc.) The mechanism of action for securing hemostasis in inhibitor patients is thought to be direct activation of the common coagulation pathway, bypassing the step carried out by the IX_a–factor VIII–calcium–phospholipid complex. The best treatment may be recombinant activated factor VII, whose action is precisely the activation of factor X.

In treating the cause of the acquired anticoagulant, drugs directed against the cells responsible for the immune response to factor VIII:C would conceivably yield better long-term results. A scheme to do so by priming the immune cells with an infusion of factor VIII, causing them to enter a susceptible phase of the cell cycle, and then destroying them with cyclophosphamide has been successful in 11 of 12 subjects with acquired inhibitors (31). There are also several reports claiming cures with intravenous gamma globulins alone or in combination with cyclophosphamide (32). The effect of the immunoglobulins is believed to be the binding of factor VIII:C antibodies by anti-idiotype antibodies in pooled human IgG. In any case, it is difficult to establish with certainty that acquired inhibitors are cured with these measures, since they tend to disappear by themselves. If their disappearance very quickly follows therapy, one may more convincingly attribute success to an intervention.

The comments in principle apply largely also to classical hemophilia where improvements in current therapy and new strategies will alter the present outlook for hemophiliacs of all types.

REFERENCES

1. White GC, Shoemaker CB. Factor VIII gene and hemophilia A. Blood 1989;73:1–12.
2. Epstein I, ed. The Babylonian Talmud, Yebamath Sect. 64B. Slotki WI, trans. London: Soncino Press, 1936;1:431.
3. Smith PS. Congenital coagulation protein deficiencies in the perinatal period. Semin Perinatol 1990;14:384–392.
4. Andrew M, Pae B, Johnston M. Development of the hemostatic system in the neonate and young infant. Am J Pediatr Hematol Oncol 1990;12:95–104.
5. Antonarakis SE, Youssoufian H, Kazazian HH. Molecular genetics of hemophilia in man (factor VIII deficiency). Mol Biol Med 1987;4:81–94.
6. Pierce GF, et al. The use of purified clotting factor concentrates in hemophilia. JAMA 1990;261:3434–3438.
7. Peterson LR, Doll LS, et al. HIV type I infected blood donors: epidemiologic, laboratory, and donation characteristics. Transfusion 1991;31:698–703.
8. Richards C, et al. Prevalence of antibody to hepatitis C virus in a blood donor population. Transfusion 1991;31:109–113.

9. Gilbert MS. Musculoskeletal manifestations of hemophilia. Mount Sinai J Med 1977;44:339–358.

10. Madhok R, Bennet D, Sturrock RD, Forbes CD. Mechanisms of joint damage in an experimental model of hemophilic arthritis. Arthritis Rheum 1988;81:1148–1155.

11. Joist JH, Ameri A. Pathogenesis of hemophilic arthropathy. In: Gilbert MS, Greene WB, eds. Musculoskeletal problems in hemophilia. New York: National Hemophilia Foundation, 1991.

12. Yulish BS, et al. Hemophilic arthropathy: assessment with MR imaging. Radiology 1987;164:759–752.

13. Kay L, et al. The role of synovectomy in the management of recurrent hemarthroses in hemophilia. Br J Haematol 1981; 49:53–60.

14. Wiedel JD. Arthroscopy of the knee in hemophilia. In: Gilbert MS, Greene WB, eds. Musculoskeletal problems in hemophilia. New York: National Hemophilia Foundation, 1991.

15. Figgie MP, Goldberg VM. Total knee arthroplasty for the treatment of chronic hemophilic arthropathy. In: Gilbert MS, Greene WB, eds. Musculoskeletal problems in hemophilia. New York: National Hemophilia Foundation, 1991.

16. Randell RL, Holland PV. Transfusion-associated hepatitis. In: Smith DM, Dodd RY, eds. Tranfusion-transmitted diseases. Chicago: ASEP Press, 1991:115–131.

17. Rumi MG, et al. High prevalence of antibody to hepatitis C virus in multitransfused hemophiliacs with normal transaminase levels. Ann Intern Med 1990;112:379–380.

18. Makris SM, et al. Hepatitis C antibody and chronic liver disease in haemophilia. Lancet 1990;335:1117–1119.

19. Davis GL, et al. Treatment of chronic hepatitis C with recombinant interferon alpha: a multicenter randomized controlled trial. N Engl J Med 1989;321:1501.

20. Roper-Drewinko PR, et al. Standardization of platelet function tests. Am J Hematol 1981;11:183–203.

21. Cowan BD, Morrison JC. Management of abnormal genital bleeding in girls and women. N Engl J Med 1991;324: 1710–1715.

22. Stuart MJ, et al. The post-aspirin bleeding time: a screening test for evaluating hemostatic disorders. Br J Haematol 1979; 43:649–659.

23. Smith PS. Von Willebrand's disease: pathophysiology, diagnosis, and treatment. In: Hilgartner MW, Pochedly C, eds. Hemophilia in the child and adult. 3rd ed. New York: Raven Press, 1989.

24. Coller BS. Von Willebrand's disease. In: Ratnoff OD, Forbes CD, eds. Disorders of hemostasis. New York: Grune & Stratton, 1984:241–249.

25. Rodeghiero F, Castraman G, Dini E. Epidemiological investigation of the prevalence of von Willebrand's disease. Blood 1987;69:454–459.

26. Harrison RL, Mikee PA. Estrogen stimulates von Willebrand factor production by cultured endothelial cells. Blood 1984; 63:657–664.

27. Buchanan GR, et al. The effect of "anti-platelet" drugs on bleeding time and platelet aggregation in normal human subjects. Am J Clin Pathol 1977;68:355–359.

28. Kasper CK, Ewing NP. Measurement of inhibitors to factor VIII:C. In: Bloom AL, ed. The hemophilias. New York: Churchill Livingstone, 1982.

29. Gill J, et al. The natural history of factor VIII inhibitor in patients with hemophilia A. Prog Clin Biol Res 1984;150: 19–29.

30. Green D, Lechner K. A survey of 215 non-hemophilic patients with inhibitors to factor VIII. Thromb Haemost 1981;45:200–203.

31. Lian CY, Larcada AF, Chiu A. Combination immunosuppressive therapy following factor VIII infusion for acquired factor VIII inhibitor. Ann Intern Med 1989;110: 774–778.

32. Lionnet F, et al. Autoimmune factor VIII:C inhibitor durably responsive to immunoglobulins: a new case. Thromb Haemost 1990;64:488–489.

CHAPTER 32

Factor IX Defects

ELIZABETH M. KURCZYNSKI

If two sons of same mother died of uncontrollable bleeding following circumcision, subsequent offspring were not circumcised.
— Collection Putti, Hebrew Law, Bologna, 18th century

Christmas disease (hemophilia B) is an inherited clotting defect, named by Biggs and McFarlane after a family in Great Britain in early 1950. Their work (1) showed that hemophilia is actually two diseases, (a) so-called classical hemophilia and (b) Christmas disease. In the United States alone, there are in excess of 2800 proven cases with associated physical, psychologic, monetary, and iatrogenic complications.

Case 1

AS presented at 5 days of age with prolonged bleeding from a circumcision. He was a full-term infant from an uncomplicated pregnancy and vaginal delivery, but his mother had significant postpartum bleeding. His physical examination was normal except for a few bruises on his arms, scalp, and feet and oozing from his circumcision. A CBC was normal except for a hemoglobin of 8.0. A prothrombin time (PT) and partial thromboplastin time (PTT) were drawn, but "clotted." He was given 10 mL/kg fresh frozen plasma, and his bleeding site was sutured with no further oozing. The mother's factor VIII and factor IX levels were 208% and 54%, respectively.

The mother's first cousin (on her father's side) has classical hemophilia with less than 1% factor VIII. There is no other family history of bleeding disorders, and there are no other siblings.

He was seen 3 months later with scattered ecchymoses, and a large leg bruise from his first DPT immunization. Repeat blood studies: PTT, 95 sec (normal <37); bleeding time, 6 min (normal); factor IX <1%. His mother's factor IX level had fallen to 15%. At that time, AS received his first hepatitis B immunization. At 16 months of age, he fell on his chin and sustained a laceration of his palate, behind his upper central incisors. He received fresh frozen plasma and oral Amicar (ε-aminocaproic acid), but the bleeding persisted, and his hematocrit dropped to 25% and then to 15%. He was admitted to the hospital, placed NPO, and heavily sedated to prevent him from dislodging the clot with his tongue. He was treated with prothrombin complex concentrate for 4 days, and the bleeding stopped. He also received ferrous sulfate drops.

After that episode, he was fitted with a helmet, but at 23 months of age, without his helmet on, he fell off a porch. He vomited several times over the next 3 days and developed increasing lethargy. A head CT scan showed a 1.5-cm left frontal subdural hematoma, following which he was given 33 units/kg Konyne (a prothrombin-complex concentrate) plus 100 u heparin and taken to the operating room where the hematoma was removed. No abnormal bleeding occurred during surgery. He received 10 u/kg fresh frozen plasma 6 hours after surgery and another dose of Konyne 9 hours later. For the next 10 days, he was covered with Mononine, a monoclonal purified factor IX product that was supplied by Armour.

AS continues to require treatment 3 or 4 times a month for bleeding episodes, but he has no joint problems, and he is human immunodeficiency virus (HIV) negative with normal liver function tests. A review of the various processes associated with Christmas disease follows.

The Normal Coagulation Cascade

To evaluate a patient with excessive bleeding, an understanding of basic clotting mechanisms is necessary. The blood circulates in a fluid phase that is controlled through a series of coagulation proteins that are balanced by natural inhibitors. Once a blood vessel is injured, the vessel contracts, and platelets adhere to the site. The platelets then may undergo the aggregation and release reaction that is triggered by exposure to subendothelial collagen. A series of changes in platelets produces a platelet plug. The plasma coagulation system then is activated to form fibrin, the final result of the hemostatic mechanism.

The blood coagulation system (especially as it has recently been reconsidered) is reviewed in chapter 33. Factor IX is activated to IXa as a result of a series of reactions in the *intrinsic pathway* and also by the tissue factor (TF)/VII complex generated by the *extrinsic pathway*. The latter is probably physiologically more significant in activating Christmas factor, but factor XII (Hageman factor), factor XI, and other elements in the inflammatory/complement cascade and the endothelium itself (especially if damaged) may also play a part in pathologic situations. The role of factor IX is in the activation of X to Xa, pivotal to the formation of thrombin from prothrombin and, subsequently, fibrin from fibrinogen. Traditionally, the reactions pictured in Figure 32.1 reflect activity within the intrinsic and common pathways and are tested for by the activated partial thromboplastin time (aPTTs), while those in Figure 32.2, reflecting extrinsic and common pathways, affect the prothrombin time (PT). For the aPTTT, kaolin or a similar activating agent is added to partial thromboplastin, e.g., from a platelet source in the presence of calcium, and for the PT, calcium and a source of thromboplastin such as rabbit or human brain are added to the test plasma in a calcium-binding anticoagulant such as citrate. Clotting times are measured and compared with the standard of the day for the laboratory.

AS developed bleeding following a circumcision. It was necessary, therefore, to look for abnormalities in the various phases of blood coagulation by doing the following: a platelet count, aPTT, and PT. Unfortunately, the blood was not collected properly or an incorrect amount was put into the tube.

Errors in drawing and testing are common, and a markedly abnormal test should be repeated to insure that it is an accurate value. Clotting tests are usually abnormal in newborns, in contrast with older children and adults, because factors XII and XI are moderately low, and the vitamin K–dependent factors (II, VII, IX, and X) are markedly decreased. These four proteins plus proteins C and S (whose deficiencies can produce hereditary thrombotic disorders) are synthesized as precursors in the liver. They all require vitamin K to produce γ-carboxylation of the amino-terminal glutamic acid residue of the precursor to

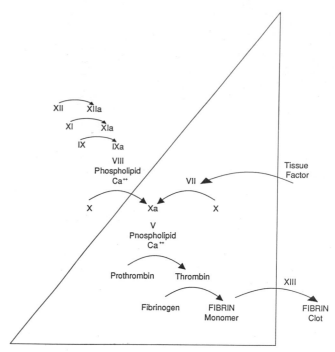

Figure 32.2. Prothrombin time (PT). Clotting factors measured by the PT are included within the *triangle*.

form the functional calcium-binding protein in the hepatic microsomes. Premature infants have even lower levels of these vitamin K–dependent factors than full-term newborns. Similar deficiencies in vitamin K factors can be seen in patients with chronic liver disease or malabsorption, or following long courses of antibiotics that impair bacterial production of vitamin K in the gastrointestinal tract, or following ingestion (accidental or therapeutic) of warfarin compounds such as Coumadin. This anticoagulant blocks the carboxylase reaction in vitamin K synthesis. Because of their low levels of vitamin K, all newborns in the United States receive an injection of vitamin K at delivery, to prevent **hemorrhagic disease of the newborn,** a disorder that was probably responsible for ancient laws requiring that circumcisions be delayed until the 8th day of life (1a).

The bleeding time, in addition to the PT and PTT, is frequently used as a screening test for coagulation disorders. Although convention has it that the bleeding time is normal in hemophilia, two studies have shown that about 25% of hemophiliacs have prolonged bleeding times for reasons that are unknown (2, 3).

In addition to hemophilia, several other disorders must be considered when a child develops bruising or bleeding. It is important to distinguish between congenital disorders, such as hemophilia or more rare coagulation factor deficiencies (dysfibrinogenemia, molecular defects in prothrombin, factor VII, factor XIII, congenital disorders of platelet production) and acquired abnormalities in a child who had never bruised before. The latter situation occurs with **immune thrombocytopenic purpura of childhood,** and disorders causing decreased production of platelets such as marrow replacement disorders (myelophthisis). Accidental ingestion of Coumadin-containing

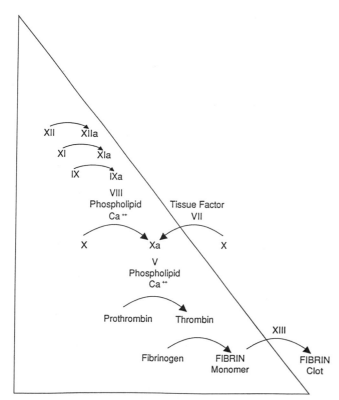

Figure 32.1. Activated partial thromboplastin time (PTT). Coagulation factors measured by the PTT are included within the *triangle*.

anticoagulants (present in some rat poisons) can cause sudden severe bleeding and should be considered when an otherwise healthy individual develops bleeding and has a prolonged PT and aPTT. **Disseminated intravascular coagulation** (DIC) is an acquired bleeding disorder in which factor IX levels are low, but it is usually seen in the context of a patient who is very ill with meningitis, sepsis, massive burns, amniotic fluid embolism, or other life-threatening problems. It is distinguished from hemophilia B by the low platelet count, fibrinogen, factor VIII, and factor V and often elevated FDPs.

At 3 months of age, repeat studies on AS showed a markedly prolonged PTT of 95 seconds, with a very low factor IX level, less than 1%. Normal values of the coagulation factors generally range from 50 to 250% and may increase with pregnancy, inflammation, and use of certain drugs. His mother is a carrier (see below), with a low level of factor IX. Her higher level at delivery was due to a pregnancy-induced rise in factor IX. Thus, the diagnosis of hemophilia B, or Christmas disease, is confirmed.

Factor IX Molecule

Factor IX is produced in the liver and has a molecular mass of 54 kDa and 415 amino acid residues, with a biologic half-life of 24 hours (4). The molecule contains exons I through VIII and introns A through G. The International Hemophilia Database Registry now contains 400 different factor IX mutations causing hemophilia B (5). These include 40 short deletions or additions and 206 unique mutations, confirming the molecular heterogeneity of Christmas disease.

The gene for factor IX is located near the tip of the X chromosome, confirming it as an X-linked disorder, the same as classical hemophilia. Thus males have the disease, and mothers are carriers of the abnormal gene, which arises as a spontaneous mutation in about one-third of cases.

Carrier Testing

For two decades, standard techniques of carrier testing in hemophiliacs have been based on the factor VIII or IX clotting assay. The hemophilic patient generally has less than 5% of circulating factor, compared with a normal level of 50–150%. A woman who is a carrier of the hemophilia gene would be expected to have a level between 5% and normal, since she has one normal and one abnormal gene directing factor VIII or IX synthesis. However, because of Lyonization of X chromosome inactivation, female carriers may have levels within the normal range or very low levels causing clinical bleeding. AS's mother has occasional menorrhagia, probably secondary to her low factor IX level. Because a significant number of carrier women have clinical bleeding (6), all potential carriers should have factor levels obtained. If the level is below 20%, they should receive hepatitis B vaccine because of possible ex-

posure to blood products at some time in their lives. Fortunately, factor VIII and IX levels increase during pregnancy, and carrier mothers rarely have severe bleeding during deliveries.

Antigenic factor VIII assays have been developed that allow comparisons between the functional and antigenic factor levels, and which define carrier states with greater than 95% accuracy (7). This test is readily available at most coagulation laboratories. However, such assays have not been developed for factor IX carrier testing. Many laboratories are now using restriction fragment length polymorphism techniques for carrier detection based on linkage analysis (8, 9). These techniques have limitations because they require several affected family members for testing, and they are not predictive in all families (10).

Prenatal testing for classical hemophilia in the first trimester of pregnancy by use of fetal blood sampling has been available for over a decade. This technique is less accurate in hemophilia B because factor IX levels in cord blood are much lower than factor VIII levels, and the factor IX antigen is present in amniotic fluid. The use of chorionic villus sampling to analyze fetal DNA for specific factor IX gene polymorphisms is a much more accurate method (11).

Hemophilia B

Clinical

Hemophilia B is classified as mild, moderate, or severe on the basis of the patient's factor level (table 32.1). The distinction is clinically important and is useful for educating families. Patients with mild hemophilia may be diagnosed at any age. A 15-year-old boy was recently diagnosed with 15% factor VIII when he bled from an arteriogram site 4 days after craniotomy to repair a ruptured aneurysm. Therefore, screening aPTT and PT studies are an important part of the preoperative workup prior to major surgical procedures. Patients with mild hemophilia may also present with bleeding if they receive drugs such as valproic acid or aspirin, both of which interfere with other parts of the coagulation pathway (aspirin interferes with platelet function, and valproic acid may actually cause thrombocytopenia).

There has been debate for years about whether hemophilia B is clinically different from hemophilia A. Data from the Hemophilia Center of Western New York show that for any given level of factor VIII and IX, hemophilia A patients bleed more frequently and have about 50% more episodes of joint bleeding than those with hemophilia B (12). Severe

Table 32.1. Severity of Hemophilia A and B

Severity	Factor Level	Symptoms
Mild	<1%	Frequent spontaneous bleeding
Moderate	1–5%	Bleeding with mild trauma
Severe	6–20%	Bleeding with severe trauma

hemophilia A patients bled an average of 45 times per year as compared with an average of 12 times per year in severe hemophilia B patients. This difference may be due to the longer half-life of factor IX.

Significant neonatal bleeding is not common but can be life threatening, particularly if labor is prolonged and difficult or if forceps delivery is necessary. Therefore, it is important for the obstetrician to know if a woman is a hemophilia carrier and if the fetus is a male, since cesarean section may be advisable. Types of neonatal bleeding are listed in Table 32.2, in order of decreasing frequency. In Ljung's survey of severe hemophilia in Sweden, 20% of patients had some type of bleeding in the neonatal period (13).

Patients with severe hemophilia usually do not have significant bleeding episodes until they begin to walk, i.e., once they pass beyond the problems of the neonatal period. This patient required hospitalization for persistent mouth bleeding, a common and frustrating problem in toddlers. Factor replacement often must be supplemented by soft diet or even parenteral nutrition, bed rest, and sometimes sedation to control the oral bleeding sites. Because saliva contains fibrinolysin, antifibrinolytic agents (ϵ-aminocaproic acid or tranexamic acid) are valuable adjuncts in the treatment of bleeding from oral lacerations, dental procedures, or tooth eruptions. They are usually given for 5–7 days, until the bleeding site heals. Patients with recurrent or prolonged mouth or nose bleeding require close monitoring of hematocrit levels and should be given oral iron therapy.

The most common type of bleeding in hemophilia is hemarthrosis, particularly of the weight-bearing joints, (knee, ankle, or elbow). Intraarticular blood causes cartilage damage. Recurrent bleeding produces hypertrophy and increased vascularity of the synovium, resulting in more frequent bleeding, leading to irreversible damage to the cartilage and underlying bone, plus bone overgrowth due to a prolonged increase in periarticular blood flow. The goal of comprehensive hemophilia treatment is to prevent permanent joint damage by treating joint bleeding early (within 2 hours of the first symptom), protecting the joint with good muscle strength via long-term exercise programs, and treating recurrent joint bleeding aggressively with limited courses of prophylactic factor replacement. Arthroscopic synovectomy of chronically inflamed synovium is useful to prevent permanent severe cartilage damage when conservative measures fail. A key factor in maintaining normal joint function is teaching families to recognize and treat joint bleeding immediately. School-age children can keep factor concentrates in

school and infuse themselves if they develop bleeding. By young adulthood, the frequency of joint bleeding decreases dramatically.

In the United States, the standard of care for hemophilia has been to treat bleeding when it occurs, but there are situations in which prophylactic treatment is indicated. A patient who has had recurrent frequent bleeding into a joint, resulting in chronic synovial thickening and joint effusion, frequently benefits from a 2–4 month period of prophylaxis to allow the inflamed synovium to heal and to break the cycle of recurrent bleeding. A dose of 30–40 u/kg given every 3 days or even once a week is used.

Arthroscopic synovectomy is being used more frequently for patients with chronic joint effusions and bleeding that recurs in spite of adequate prophylaxis. Such procedures are optimally done by a surgeon experienced in treating hemophiliacs and at a hemophilia center where coagulation factor levels can be frequently monitored to control bleeding.

Spontaneous hematuria is another common problem in hemophilia, second only to hemarthrosis as a cause of school or work absences in teens and young adults; 62% of patients experience this problem by age 21 (14). These episodes resolve spontaneously. Bed rest and a few days of oral prednisone are used to shorten the duration of bleeding, but these have never been proved to be of value in formal studies. An initial dose of factor concentrate should be given, but further doses are not useful.

Soft tissue bleeding is common in hemophilia B. It must be treated vigorously, since large amounts of blood can be lost into areas such as the thigh, and permanent nerve damage can occur if the bleeding is not controlled promptly. Other common sites are the iliopsoas or iliacus muscle in the abdomen, which cause abdominal pain, numbness in the lateral thigh from nerve compression, an inability to fully extend the hip, and in some instances femoral nerve damage. CT or MRI scans are very useful for diagnosing and monitoring bleeding in this area.

Hemophilia B Leyden

An unusual form of hemophilia B (hemophilia B Leyden) has been described in which boys have clinically severe bleeding with low levels of factor IX in infancy and childhood. When they reach puberty, the level of factor IX increases to low normal values and bleeding episodes stop, possibly related to increasing levels of testosterone (15). DNA analysis in three patients with this syndrome showed a mutation in the promoter region of the factor IX molecule at position +13 (16).

Treatment of Hemophilia B

Several different products are currently available to treat bleeding in hemophilia B (table 32.3). To determine which one to use in a given situation, the advantages and

Table 32.2. Types of Neonatal Bleeding in Hemophilia

Bleeding after injection or blood sampling
Intracranial hemorrhage
Cephalic or subgaleal hematomas
Orbital bleeding
Umbilical bleeding

Table 32.3. Products for Treatment of Hemophilia B

Available as of late 1991
Fresh frozen plasma
Prothrombin complex concentrates
Proplex, Konyne, Konyne 80
Contain factors II, VII, IX, and X
AlphaNine
Awaiting release in the U.S. or in testing
Monoclonal purified factor IX
Coagulation factor IX
Recombinant factor IX

disadvantages of each product must be weighed. These include availability, cost, risk of hepatitis and HIV seroconversion, risk of thrombotic complications, and the probability that the patient may require more than one dose of the product for a given episode. In addition, the patient's immune status and the products he or she has received in the past must be considered.

Fresh frozen plasma is readily available in any hospital and contains all clotting factors. Therefore, it may be indicated in a neonate when specific clotting assay results are not known and either hemophilia A or B may be involved. It has a small risk of transmitting hepatitis B or C. A dose of 10–15 u/kg will stop most bleeding, but it has the disadvantage of a large volume and high protein load if repeated treatment is necessary.

AS received plasma for his circumcision bleeding for the above reasons.

Prothrombin Complex Concentrates

Commencing in the late 1960s, prothrombin complex concentrates (PCCs) have been the most widely used products for the treatment of hemophilia B. They are made from pooled human plasma by a process involving Cohn fractionation, followed by DEAE Sephadex purification and fractional elution (17). These products have the advantage of being effective, cheap, and easily stored for home therapy. However, they carry a risk of viral transmission and thrombotic complications.

Factor IX is distributed into extravascular spaces, unlike factor VIII, which is a much larger molecule. Therefore, a dose of 1 unit/kg raises the blood level of factor IX by about 1%. Dosage of factor IX products for moderate bleeding such as early hemarthrosis or mouth bleeding should be 25–30 units/kg. This generally can be given once a day. For severe bleeding, such as head trauma, or for major surgery, 40–50 units/kg is the initial dose, followed by 30–40 units/kg every 12–18 hours. Continuous infusion of PCCs has been used for surgical coverage (18), although this may cause an increased risk of thrombotic complications.

Thrombosis related to PCC use was first reported several years after introduction of the product to the U.S. market (19). It is now well established that this severe, and sometimes fatal, problem usually occurs following multiple doses of PCCs, and in patients undergoing major (frequently orthopaedic) procedures. Seventy-two thrombotic

complications were recently documented in a 4-year period (20). The Factor IX Task Force of the International Society on Thrombosis and Hemostasis in 1974 recommended adding 5–10 I.U. of heparin to each milliliter of reconstituted PCC to try to prevent this problem (21), but thromboses have occurred even with the addition of heparin (22). Several possible mechanisms have been postulated: (a) PCCs contain small amounts of activated factors (IXa, Xa) that may trigger clotting, (b) individuals with low levels of antithrombin III may have slower removal of clotting intermediates from the circulation, or (c) the large amounts of prothrombin and factors VII and X with long half-lives may cause zymogen overload. Table 32.4 lists types of complications that have been described. Autopsies on several patients who died of myocardial infarctions have shown diffuse hemorrhage within the myocardium, with no evidence of emboli (23). Thromboses have occurred both with regular PCCs and with the activated products (Feiba and Autoplex) that are used for treating bleeding episodes in hemophilia A patients with inhibitors. Antithrombin levels should be checked prior to surgery, and patients with low or borderline levels should be given intermittent plasma infusions to replace antithrombin. Since the exact mechanism of this devastating complication is not known, prevention has been impossible. For this reason, many centers do not perform elective surgery on hemophilia B patients using PCCs.

Konyne-80 is a PCC that has been made more safe from viral contamination by dry heat treatment to 80°. Similar products have been tested in the United Kingdom and shown to be free of hepatitis viruses. However, Konyne-80 still carries the risk of thromboses.

Pure Factor IX Products

Several new products containing pure factor IX are now available.

Coagulation factor IX (AlphaNine, Alpha Therapeutic Corporation) was licensed in the United States on 12/31/90, the first pure factor IX product to be released. Because of its limited availability and high cost, it is being used mainly for patients who are undergoing surgery or who have had prior thrombotic complications. It is viral inactivated by heat treatment at 60°C for 20 hours and therefore may have a risk of transmission of hepatitis B or C. A pure factor IX product (Mononine) has been developed by Armour with monoclonal antibody purification techniques, and it has been used for both surgery and home care treatment with no evidence of thrombotic complications (24). The factor VIII products produced by sim-

Table 32.4. Thrombotic Complications from Prothrombin Complex Concentrates

Superficial phlebitis
Deep vein thromboses
Pulmonary emboli
Disseminated intravascular coagulation
Myocardial infarction
Cerebral thrombosis

ilar techniques have been on the market since 1987 and have not shown transmission of hepatitis or HIV. One final product, recombinant factor IX, is being developed by several companies.

Dosages of the pure factor IX products are currently being evaluated. Surgical patients may safely be given higher doses than those used for PCCs, while the long half-life may allow dosing intervals to be increased.

The number of products that will be available in the next few years for hemophilia B necessitates treatment decisions. The care provider will need to evaluate each new product for availability, risk of hepatitis transmission (all current products are HIV safe), thrombogenicity, cost, and suitability for home care use.

Comprehensive Care

The introduction of purified products for hemophilia in the early 1970s allowed home care programs to develop at hemophilia centers around the world. A patient or parent learns to evaluate bleeding episodes and then prepare and infuse concentrate at home, rather than traveling to an office or hospital for treatment. Careful records are kept each time treatment is given. These programs have been highly desirable because of their many benefits, including more rapid treatment of bleeding, less time lost from work or school, and increased independence, since the family can carry factor on trips and vacations. In addition, home care programs are safe and cost efficient (25). Most parents learn to give factor at home when the child is old enough to sit still for an infusion, usually at age 4 or 5, depending on venous access.

Home care programs are only a part of the comprehensive care that is given at hemophilia centers. This complicated, chronic disease requires a multidisciplinary team to help patients and their families achieve their maximum potential and deal with the many problems associated with hemophilia. The basic team consists of a hematologist and hemophilia center nurse coordinator, an orthopaedist skilled in evaluating hemophilic arthropathy, and a physical therapist. They evaluate patients on a routine basis with the goal of preventing irreversible joint damage. In addition, psychologists serve a necessary team role. A hereditary lifelong illness puts many psychologic stresses on families, including parental guilt at passing on a defective gene, overprotectivness with consequent acting-out behavior by the child or young adult patient, plus problems with peer relationships, dating, acceptance in school settings, and AIDS issues. Vocational guidance is critical for young boys who need to be trained for careers that do not require intense manual labor or prolonged standing and lifting that puts unnecessary stress on their joints. Social workers are also invaluable to the team, since school issues and insurance problems are a major concern. In the United States, families may reach lifetime insurance caps or be refused insurance for hemophilic individuals and their families.

Dentists are equally important in comprehensive hemophilia care, both to give direct patient care and evaluation and to educate community dentists and orthodontists about the proper management of dental procedures in hemophilia.

Many state hemophilia foundations offer summer camps for boys with hemophilia, to decrease the feeling of isolation that occurs with chronic disease and help boys learn to be active in sports that increase their strength and thus their joint protection. Such programs are an invaluable experience and a tremendous boost to the hemophilic boy's self esteem and independence.

Complications of Hemophilia Therapy

The products used to treat hemophilia for the past 30 years are made from human plasma and therefore have significant risk of transmission of viruses including hepatitis B and C and HIV. The two major therapy-related complications in hemophilia patients over the age of 10 are HIV infection and chronic hepatitis. Several cases of clinical illness due to parvovirus have been reported from factor VIII and IX concentrates (26). Table 32.5 lists the viruses that are known to be transmitted by blood products.

Hepatitis

The clotting factor concentrates given in the 1970s and 1980s contained large numbers of hepatitis viruses. Although most children under age 10 are hepatitis B negative, there is a large group of adolescents and adults who are positive. About 60% of adult hemophilia patients have antibody to both hepatitis B surface (HbSAg) and core antigen, indicating prior infection, with about 5% being chronic carriers of HbSAg. These latter individuals are susceptible to hepatitis delta virus infection. This virus depends on HbSAg to provide a surrounding envelope protecting the delta virus from hemolysis. Superinfection or coinfection (of hepatitis B and delta hepatitis) has a high incidence of fulminant hepatitis or slowly progressive chronic changes leading to cirrhosis.

A safe hepatitis B vaccine is readily available, and all newly diagnosed hemophilia patients should be vaccinated immediately, before receiving blood products. For the 5% of hemophiliacs who are chronic carriers of hepatitis B, it is important to vaccinate family members to prevent spread of the virus.

Hepatitis B contamination has been almost completely eliminated from all factor concentrates currently on the market, because of heat treating methods and because all plasma donors have been screened for the virus since 1975.

Hepatitis C is a more frequent cause of liver disease in hemophilia patients than is hepatitis B. A survey of 131 patients at the New England Hemophilia Center,

Table 32.5. Viruses Transmitted by Blood Products

Hepatitis A
Hepatitis B
Hepatitis C
Human immunodeficiency virus
Parvovirus
Cytomegalovirus

ages 3–71, showed 76% positivity for hepatitis C antibody (27). Of this group, 81% had chronic or intermittent elevations of alanine aminotransferase (ALT) and apparent chronic hepatitis C infection. This infection has caused, and will continue to cause, cirrhosis or hepatocellular carcinoma in some of these infected individuals, in whom mortality is a significant risk.

Most hemophilia patients with chronic ALT elevations have minor degrees of liver damage, but significant numbers have chronic active hepatitis or cirrhosis. Many groups have examined the predictive value of liver enzyme levels or other serum tests (28), but liver biopsy remains the only effective way to determine the extent of hepatocellular damage. Aledort et al. evaluated 155 liver biopsies collected by an ad hoc hemophilia study group and found a 15% incidence of cirrhosis and 7% chronic active hepatitis, a lower percentage than previously reported (29). Their series had a 12% incidence of serious bleeding following the biopsy.

A study of hepatitis C antibody in children found that those treated with unheated or dry-heat-treated concentrates had a 95% seropositivity rate, while those treated with single-donor blood products or vapor-heated factor concentrates had a rate of 0%. These data indicate that many of the available clotting concentrates are apparently hepatitis B and C free, but continued surveillance of these products is very important (30, 31).

HIV Infection

Contamination of the United States blood supply with HIV between 1978 and 1984 produced the devastating complications of HIV infection and AIDS in many hemophilia patients and their families. In a Pittsburgh study it was found that 74% of hemophilia A patients and 33% of hemophilia B individuals treated with concentrate were positive for HIV (32), compared with 14% of those treated with cryoprecipitate. The pediatric center at the Scottish Rite Hospital in Atlanta has a 57% seropositivity rate in 49 moderate and severe hemophilia A patients and 10% in hemophilia B.

All studies have shown a lower incidence of seropositivity in hemophilia B than in hemophilia A, and it has been suggested that the frequency of HIV transmission is lower in factor IX concentrates. Goldsmith et al. examined serum from 12 hemophilia B patients and found a 66% seropositivity rate (33). Their positive patients received significantly more concentrate than did negative patients. Thus, the difference in incidence between the two types of hemophilia is probably related to variation in the number of severe patients and the amount of concentrates given, rather than to increased safety of the PCCs themselves. This effect was also documented by the Worcester group (34).

In addition, HIV seroconversion in spouses and sexual partners is a growing problem. Hemophilia centers and the National Hemophilia Foundation have strongly emphasized risk reduction through education about HIV transmission and safe sex practices over the last 5 years.

However, there is no indication that such emphasis is changing behavior, and heterosexual transmission of the virus continues to be an enormous problem (35).

In general, HIV infection in hemophiliacs is similar to that in nonhemophilic groups, and treatment is the same. The reader is referred to the many texts on AIDS and HIV infection currently available for details.

Chronic growth failure has been described in HIV infection in hemophilic children (36). This is apparently caused by changes in growth hormone regulation (37). Brettler et al. use a decrease of 15 percentile points or more in height or weight as a predictive marker for symptom development and as an indication for starting antiretrovirus therapy.

Thrombocytopenia is another complication of HIV infection (38). It usually presents as an ITP-like picture because of antiplatelet antibodies but also can result from decreased bone marrow production, particularly with *Mycobacterium avium intracellulare* infection. Various treatments such as steroids, intravenous immunoglobulins, and even splenectomy are sometimes curative but carry the risk of additional immunosuppression in an already immunocompromised patient. Symptomatic bleeding in a thrombocytopenic hemophilic may be more severe than in otherwise normal individuals because of the additional underlying clotting deficit.

HIV-positive patients with joint prostheses are another group of hemophilia patients at increased risk. Improvements in joint replacement techniques and prostheses over the past 10 years have significantly decreased the rate of infectious complications. However, as CD4 cell counts drop, patients with prostheses may develop septic arthritis, and clinicians must be prepared to culture swollen joints promptly if there is any suspicion of infection. In general, HIV-positive patients tolerate surgery without increased problems. In the Scottish Rite institution 12 synovectomies have been carried out on seropositive hemophiliacs, many of whom were on AZT at the time. None of them had any infectious complications or progression of HIV infection.

HIV infection in the hemophilic population is a tragedy of enormous proportion, with widespread psychologic consequences for the patients, their spouses and families, and their relationships with employers, coworkers, schools, and insurance carriers. Patients like Ryan White and the Ray family in Florida have demonstrated unbounded personal courage by publicly fighting AIDS discrimination and ignorance of disease spread. Although current heat treatment of the blood supply has prevented HIV seroconversion in young patients such as AS, a large number of patients deal with HIV every day. It has been estimated that this infection may wipe out two generations of hemophilia patients.

Inhibitors to Factor IX

In classical hemophilia, 15–25% of patients develop inhibitors or antibodies to factor VIII at some time in their lives. The incidence of inhibitor formation in hemophilia B is significantly lower, 1–2% (39). Some patients with inhibitor have been shown to have subtotal or total deletions at the factor IX locus (40, 41). However, inhibitor patients have been described with no detectable gene deletions (42). It therefore appears that some inhibitors are produced when there is no immunologically recognizable factor IX protein so that the infused factor IX is interpreted by the body as "foreign." Others have different mechanisms not yet completely understood but perhaps related to modifier genes or linkage to other systems such as HL-A (43).

Inhibitors are classified as high or low titer, based on the level, which is usually reported in Bethesda units. Patients with only 1–3 units can generally be treated with regular factor concentrates and frequently will not develop higher titers following treatment. Individuals with high-titer inhibitors do not respond to factor IX concentrates, and treatment of bleeding episodes can be very difficult. Activated PCCs are frequently effective treatment. Newer agents (not yet licensed in the United States) are recombinant factor VII and recombinant tissue factor, both of which appear to be effective in factor IX–inhibitor patients.

Data are emerging from clinical trials with recombinant factor VIII that indicate that there may be an increased incidence of factor VIII inhibitors with the two products currently being tested. Alterations in the structure of the recombinant molecule may be the cause of the inhibitor formation. As purified and recombinant factor IX products become available, the incidence of inhibitors will be closely monitored.

Summary and Future Therapies

The case of a young child with Christmas disease was discussed to illustrate the presenting clinical manifestations. These symptoms must be differentiated from similar bleeding due to thrombocytopenia, from other congenital coagulation disorders causing an elevated PTT such as classical hemophilia or factor XI deficiency, and from factor VII deficiency, which would cause a prolonged PT rather than aPTT. Child abuse must always be considered as a cause of bruising. Other causes of low factor IX levels are chronic or acute liver disease or ingestion of a Coumadin compound, both of which interfere with factor IX synthesis in the liver. The genetics of hemophilia, including the molecular basis of current methods of carrier detection, have been described. In our case, the relative with classical hemophilia is irrelevant. He is a relative of the father and therefore could not have the same gene as our patient, since hemophilia is a sex-linked disorder.

Pure factor IX products that carry no viral contaminants and are free of thrombogenic potential are close to being available in the United States. This would make possible prolonged prophylaxis to prevent bleeding episodes, provided the cost of the new products is reasonable. Recombinant factor IX molecules could possibly be altered, for example, to increase the half-life by preventing degradation by specific proteins.

Liver transplantation is currently being performed on selected patients with end-stage liver disease. Several successful transplants have been performed on hemophilia patients and have resulted in cure of the hemophilia (44). If rejection problems can be solved, this treatment may be used more frequently in the future.

Gene replacement therapy may have promise for hemophilia B patients. The factor IX molecule is particularly well suited for such techniques because it is relatively small, it could be synthesized in any tissue, and factor IX would be clinically effective at a broad range of concentrations, from 2–3% to more than 200%, without toxicity. A Seattle group has introduced the factor IX gene into skin fibroblasts by use of a retrovirus vector (45) and showed that the factor IX produced is functionally identical to normal human factor IX. They then transplanted the fibroblasts into nude mice and detected normal factor IX in the circulation. Other laboratories are developing methods to introduce the gene into animals in utero, with continued gene expression after the animal is born.

REFERENCES

1. Biggs R, Douglas AS, McFarlane, et al. Christmas disease: a condition previously mistaken for haemophilia. Br Med J 1952;1:221.
1a. Corrigan JJ Jr. Acquired bleeding disorders. In: Hemorrhagic & thrombotic diseases in childhood & adolescence. New York: Churchill Livingston, 1985:88–89.
2. Buchanan GR, Holtkamp CA. Prolonged bleeding time in children and young adults with hemophilia. Pediatrics 1980;66:951–955.
3. Eyster ME, Gordon RA, Ballard JO. The bleeding time is longer than normal in hemophilia. Blood 1981;58:719–723.
4. Thompson AR. Structure, function, and molecular defects of factor IX. Blood 1986;67:565–572.
5. Minutes of the report of Factor XIII and IX Subcommittee meeting, June 29, 1991, Scientific & Standardization Committee, International Society on Thrombosis and Hemostasis, Amsterdam.
6. Mauser Bunschoten EP, van Houwelingen JC, Sjamsoedin-Visser EJM, van Dijken PJ, Kok AJ, Sixma JJ. Bleeding symptoms in carriers of hemophilia A and B. Thromb Hemost 1988;59:349–352.
7. Zimmerman TS, Ratnoff OD, Littel AS. Detection of carriers of classical hemophilia using an immunologic assay for antihemophilic factor (factor VIII). J Clin Invest 1971;50:255–258.
8. Hay CW, Robertson KA, Yong SL, Thompson AR, Growe GH, MacGillivray RTA. Use of a *Bam*HI polymorphism in the factor IX gene for the determination of hemophilia B carrier status. Blood 1986;67:1508–1511.
9. Poon M-C, Chui DHK, Patterson M, Starozik DM, Dimnik LS, Hoar DI. Hemophilia B (Christmas disease) variants and carrier detection analyzed by DNA probes. J Clin Invest 1987;79:1204–1209.

10. Graham JB, Green PP, McGraw RA, Davis LM. Application of molecular genetics to prenatal diagnosis and carrier detection in the hemophilias: some limitations. Blood 1985;66:759–764.

11. Mariani G, Chistolini A, Hassan HJ, Gallo E, Xigen G, et al. Carrier detection for hemophilia B: evaluation of multiple polymorphic sites. Am J Hematol 1989;1:1–7.

12. Sweeney JD, Fitzpatrick L, Holmberg RP. Clinical differences between hemophilia A and hemophilia B [Abstract]. National Hemophilia Foundation annual meeting, 15 Oct 1988, Anaheim, CA.

13. Ljung R, Petrini P, Nilsson IM. Diagnostic symptoms of severe and moderate hemophilia A and B. Acta Paediatr Scand 1990;79:196–200.

14. Stuart J, Davies SH, Cumming A, Girdwood RH, Darg A. Hemorrhagic episodes in hemophilia: a 5 year prospective study. Br Med J 1966;1624–1626.

15. Veltkamp J, Meiloff J, Remmelts HG, van der Vlerk D, Loeliger EA. Another genetic variant of hemophilia B: haemophilia B Leyden. Scand J Haematol 1970;7:82–90.

16. Crossley PM, Winship PR, Black A, Rizza CR, Brownlee GG. Unusual case of hemophilia B. Lancet 1989;8644:960.

17. Silvija Hoag M, Johnson FF, Robinson JA, Aggeler PM. Treatment of hemophilia B with a new clotting factor concentrate. N Engl J Med 1969;280:581–586.

18. Bona RO, Weinstein RA, Weisman SJ, Bartolomeo A, Rickles FR. The use of continuous infusion of factor concentrates in the treatment of hemophilia. Am J Hematol 1989;32:8–13.

19. Blatt PM, Lundblad R, Kingdom HS, McLean G, Roberts HR. Thrombogenic materials in prothrombin complex concentrates. Ann Intern Med 1974;81:766–770.

20. Lusher JM. Thrombogenicity associated with factor IX complex concentrates. Semin Hematol 1991;28(Suppl 6):3–5.

21. Menache D, Roberts HR. Summary report and recommendations of task force members and consultants. Thromb Haemost 1975;33:645–647.

22. Chavin SI, Siegel DM, Rocco TA Jr, Olson JP. Acute myocardial infarction during treatment with an activated prothrombin complex concentrate in a patient with factor VIII deficiency and a factor VIII inhibitor. Am J Med 1988;85:245–249.

23. Sullivan DW, Purdy LJ, Billingham M, Glader BE. Fatal myocardial infarction following therapy with prothrombin complex concentrates in a young man with hemophilia A. Pediatrics 1984;74:279–282.

24. Kim HC, Matts L, Eisele J, Czachur M, Saidi P. Monoclonal antibody purified factor IX—comparative thrombogenicity to prothrombin complex concentrates. Semin Hematol 1991;28(Suppl 6):15–19.

25. Smith PS, Keyes NC, Forman EN. Socioeconomic evaluation of a state-funded comprehensive hemophilia-care program. N Engl J Med 1982;306:575–579.

26. Lyon DJ, Chapman CS, Martin C, Brown KE, Clewley JP, et al. Symptomatic parvovirus B19 infection and heat-treated factor IX concentrate. Lancet 1989;May 13:1085.

27. Brettler DB, Alter HJ, Dienstag JL, Forsberg AD, Levine PH. Prevalence of hepatitis C virus antibody in a cohort of hemophilic patients. Blood 1990;76:254–256.

28. Hay CRM, Preston FE, Triger DR, Greaves M, Underwood JCE, Westlake L. Predictive markers of chronic liver disease in hemophilia. Blood 1987;69:1595–1599.

29. Aledort LM, Levine PH, Hilgartner M, Blatt P, Goldberg JD, et al. A study of liver biopsies and liver disease among hemophiliacs. Blood 1985;66:367–372.

30. Hollinger FB. Hepatitis B and delta hepatitis viruses in complications of hemophilia therapy: new strategies for risk reduction. Symposium sponsored by Armour Pharmaceutical Company, Scottsdale, AZ, September 1987.

31. Blanchette VS, Vorstman E, Shore A, Wang E, Petric M, Jett BW, Alter HJ. Hepatitis C infection in children with hemophilia A and B. Blood 1991;78:285–289.

32. Ragni MV, Tegtmeier GE, Levy JA, Kaminsky LS, Lewis JH, et al. AIDS retrovirus antibodies in hemophiliacs treated with factor VIII or factor IX concentrates, cryoprecipitate, or fresh frozen plasma: prevalence, seroconversion rate, and clinical correlations. Blood 1986;67:592–595.

33. Goldsmith JM, Variakojis D, Phair JP, Green D. The spectrum of immunodeficiency virus infection in patients with factor IX deficiency (Christmas disease). Am J Hematol 1987;25:203–210.

34. Brettler D, Brewster F, Levine PH, Forsberg A, Baker S, Sullivan JL. Immunologic aberrations, HIV seropositivity and seroconversion rates in patients with hemophilia B. Blood 1987;70:276–281.

35. Overby KJ, Lo B, Litt IF. Knowledge and concerns about acquired immunodeficiency syndrome and their relationship to behavior among adolescents with hemophilia. Pediatrics 1989;83:204–210.

36. Brettler B, Forsberg A, Bolivar E, Brewster F, Sullivan J. Growth failure as a prognostic indicator for progression to acquired immunodeficiency syndrome in children with hemophilia. J Pediatr 1990;117:584–588.

37. Kaufman FR, Gomperts ED. Growth failure in boys with hemophilia and HIV infections. Am J Pediatr Hematol Oncol 1989;11:292–294.

38. Karpatkin S. Immunologic thrombocytopenic purpura in HIV-seropositive homosexuals, narcotic addicts and hemophiliacs. Semin Hematol 1988;25:219–229.

39. Lusher JM. Diseases of coagulation: the fluid phase. In: Hematology of infancy and childhood. Philadelphia: WB Saunders, 1987:1312–1313.

40. Hassan HJ, Leonardi A, Guerriero R, Chelucci G, Cianetti L, et al. Hemophilia B with inhibitor: molecular analysis of the subtotal deletion of the factor IX gene. Blood 1985;66:728–730.

41. Matthews RJ, Anson DS, Peake IR, Bloom AL. Heterogeneity of the factor IX locus in nine hemophilia B inhibitor patients. J Clin Invest 1987;79:746–753.

42. Tanimoto M, Kojima T, Kamiya T, Takamatsu J, Ogata K, et al. DNA analysis of seven patients with hemophilia B who have anti-factor IX antibodies: relationship to clinical manifestations and evidence that the abnormal gene was inherited. J Lab Clin Med 1988;112:307–313.

43. Poon M-C. Patients with hemophilia B (Christmas disease) who have anti factor IX: genetic heterogeneity. J Lab Clin Med 1988;112:283–284.

44. Scharrer I, Encke A, Hottenrott C. Clinical cure of hemophilia A by liver transplantation. Lancet 1988;Oct 1:800.

45. Palmer TD, Thompson AR, Miller AD. Production of human factor IX in animals by genetically modified skin fibroblasts: potential therapy for hemophilia B. Blood 1989;73:438–445.

CHAPTER 33

Consumptive Coagulopathies

JOHN L. FRANCIS

I have heard William Harvey say, that after his book of the circulation of the blood came out, that he fell mightily in his practice, and that 'twas believed by the vulgar that he was crack-brained; and all the physicians were against his opinion.
—Aubrey, 1690

Disseminated intravascular coagulation (DIC) is an acquired disorder characterized by the formation of microthrombi, consumption of clotting factors, secondary activation of the fibrinolytic system and a variable, but often severe, bleeding diathesis. This potentially very serious condition may complicate a wide variety of conditions and therefore spans many medical and surgical specialities. DIC is also sometimes referred to as "consumption coagulopathy" but as this term does not accurately reflect the pathophysiology of the condition, it is best avoided. The term "defibrination syndrome" is more appropriate, especially in more florid cases, although DIC is in more common usage and better reflects the role of coagulation activation as the basic cause. Furthermore, as will become evident later, DIC may exist without marked reduction in plasma fibrinogen levels. It should also be emphasized that DIC is always a complication of an underlying disease process that initiates and maintains the inappropriate clotting activation. The basis of treatment therefore becomes the removal of the original triggering factor. Although the etiology of DIC is very varied, the basic pathophysiology of clotting activation is the abnormal presence in the blood of a procoagulant stimulus. In this chapter, the etiology, laboratory findings, and aspects of treatment are illustrated by reference to some typical cases.

Etiology of Acute Disseminated Intravascular Coagulation

Our present understanding of the evolution of DIC comes from experiments in which thromboplastic substances were injected into laboratory animals (1, 2). Extrapolation of such data to a wide range of clinical conditions has led to the assumption that clot-promoting (procoagulant) substances find their way into the circulating peripheral blood, resulting in widespread clotting activation and, ultimately, fibrin deposition.

Obstetric Accidents—Case 1

JB, a 26-year-old primigravida was admitted with a suspected intrauterine death at 24 weeks gestation. Five weeks previously, the pregnancy had apparently been proceeding normally, and fetal heart sounds could be heard. One week prior to admission, the fundal height was 20 cm, and no heart sounds were audible. On admission, vital signs were stable. Examination revealed a fundal height of 15 cm, a markedly reduced amount of amniotic fluid, and confirmed fetal death. Coagulation testing at this time showed (normal values in parentheses):

PT	*12.5 sec (11–13 sec)*
aPTT	*40 sec (35–50 sec)*
Thrombin time	*23 sec (20–25 sec)*
Platelet count	*201 × 10⁹/L (150–400 × 10⁹/L)*

The patient was transferred to the operating room 18 hours after admission for dilation and evacuation. A paracervical block was uneventful but on insertion of a 12-mm suction catheter into the intrauterine cavity she began coughing, became profoundly hypotensive, and developed severe peripheral cyanosis. She continued to deteriorate despite administration of epinephrine, losing consciousness and requiring intubation. Blood pressure was not measurable but eventually recovered following external chest compression, bicarbonate, and continuous pressor infusion. The patient regained consciousness and began breathing spontaneously. Products of conception were removed, and she was transferred to the intensive care unit. Coagulation studies at that time revealed:

Platelets	*105 × 10⁹/L*
PT	*180 sec*
aPTT	*245 sec*
Thrombin time	*70 sec*
Fibrinogen	*0.2 g/L (1.5–4.0 g/L).*
D-dimer	*4000 μg/mL (<200 μg/mL)*
Antithrombin	*35% (70–130%)*

She was given packed red cells and fresh frozen plasma but continued to ooze from venipuncture and intravenous line sites and had profuse vaginal bleeding. The platelet count fell to $30 \times 10^9/L$. Cryoprecipitate was given 4 hours postoperatively, and coagulation studies 2 hours later showed:

PT	*13 sec*
aPTT	*42 sec*
Fibrinogen	*1.5 g/L*
D-dimer	*1200 µg/mL*
Antithrombin	*65%*

She made an uneventful recovery and was discharged on the fifth postoperative day with a platelet count of $130 \times 10^9/L$ and fibrinogen of 2.9 g/L.

Discussion: Obstetric accidents are a common cause of DIC, and some examples of these are shown in Table 33.1. Amniotic fluid embolism is a relatively rare complication of pregnancy and, as illustrated by Case 1, is associated with acute respiratory failure, shock, circulatory collapse, and severe coagulopathy. In some cases, the condition is immediately fatal and is the principal cause of death during childbirth (3). The proposed trigger for DIC in amniotic fluid embolism is the entry into the maternal circulation of amniotic fluid. The latter contains a considerable amount of cellular material of varying origin that can be shown to contain procoagulant activity (4) and which has been identified as tissue factor or as a preformed tissue factor–factor VIIa complex (5, 6). Amniotic fluid may

also contain Cancer Procoagulant, a direct activator of factor X (7). The means by which these procoagulants activate coagulation are discussed in detail below. Amniotic fluid gains entry to the maternal circulation through tears in the placental/amniotic membrane, and its presence in the circulation can be demonstrated by detection of amniotic debris such as desquamated fetal epithelial cells. Onset of coagulopathy is sudden and dramatic, but given prompt and appropriate supportive therapy as in this case, recovery may also be rapid. However, the prognosis is generally poor, and mortality has historically been as high as 80% (8).

In **placental abruption**, thromboplastic material may again be released into the maternal circulation; placenta has a particularly high concentration of tissue factor (9). Premature separation of the placenta complicates about 0.5–1.0% of deliveries. In about one-quarter of these, the condition is accompanied by profound hypofibrinogenemia (<1 g/L) and a bleeding diathesis (3). In fatal cases, thrombi may be found occluding small vessels. Treatment consists of uterine evacuation and maternal circulatory support. The hypofibrinogenemia usually self-corrects within 12 hours of emptying the uterus. In the **retained dead fetus syndrome**, the incidence of DIC rises to almost 50% when the condition has persisted for more than 5 weeks and often begins as a chronic, compensated form that left untreated progresses to a more fulminant DIC with hemorrhagic and thrombotic manifestations. In this situation, the trigger for intravascular coagulation is presumed to be the release of necrotic, tissue factor–containing fetal tissue, although sepsis (see below) may also contribute.

Eclampsia may be accompanied by some of the hallmarks of DIC such as thrombocytopenia, but markedly reduced fibrinogen levels are unusual (3). Similar, but generally less marked, abnormalities may be present in **preeclampsia.** The origin of the hemostatic defect in these conditions is unclear. A profound coagulopathy occurs in **acute fatty liver of pregnancy** (3). This devastating condition is accompanied by acute liver failure and a severe bleeding disorder due to a combination of DIC and the failure of the diseased liver to synthesize clotting factors. Rarer causes of DIC in obstetric practice include septic abortion, leiomyoma of the uterus, and hydatidiform mole.

Table 33.1. Conditions That May Be Complicated by Acute Disseminated Intravascular Coagulation

Obstetric complications
   Aminotic fluid embolism
   Premature placental separation (abruptio placentae)
   Retained dead fetus syndrome
   Eclampsia
   Acute fatty liver of pregnancy
   Septic abortion (now rare)
Systemic infection
   Gram-negative organisms (endotoxinemia)
   Gram-positive organisms (mucopolysaccharides)
   Viremia (cytomegalovirus, hepatitis, Varicella)
Malignant disease
   Disseminated solid tumors
   Leukemia (especially acute promyelocytic leukemia)
Intravascular hemolysis
   Incompatible blood transfusion
   Massive blood transfusion
Miscellaneous
   Burns
   Crush injuries and major trauma
   Liver disease
   Vascular disorders
   Prosthetic devices (e.g., aortic balloon)
   Snake bite

Septicemia—Case 2

*AH, a 17-year-old female student, was admitted to the emergency room at 7:30 AM in a state of collapse. Her illness had apparently been brief; she started to vomit after lunch on the previous day. At 5:30 AM she was found at home unconscious and convulsing. However, she regained consciousness and was awake when admitted. She had a past medical history of **hereditary spherocytosis** for which she was splenectomized when aged 4 years. Three of her siblings underwent similar surgery.*

The patient's temperature was 101°F, respirations were 42/min, blood pressure was unrecordable, and she was in obvious shock. Her extremities were cold, and she had no radial pulse. Pinpoint purple petechiae were evident on the anterior chest wall, dorsum, and soles of the feet. Some blood was noted on rectal examination. Her neck remained supple. Blood was obtained by femoral arterial puncture 2 hours after admission:

Hematocrit	*0.45*
Platelets	*115 × 10⁹/L (150–400 × 10⁹/L)*
PT	*>180 sec (11–13 sec)*
aPTT	*>300 sec (35–55 sec)*
Thrombin time	*>180 sec (20–25 sec)*
Fibrinogen	*<0.1 g/L (1.5–4.0 g/L)*
Prothrombin	*12% (70–130%)*
Factor V	*2% (70–130%)*
Factor VIII	*25% (70–130%)*
Factor X	*25% (70–130%)*
Factor XII	*70% (70–130%)*
D-dimer	*5000 μg/mL (<200 μg/mL)*
Antithrombin	*25% (70–130%)*

Blood cultures and throat swabs taken at this time were subsequently found to contain Streptococcus pneumoniae. The patient was treated with transfusion of whole blood (2 units), 3 g fibrinogen and hydrocortisone but died approximately 5 hours after admission. Autopsy showed severe diffuse hemorrhage and focal necrosis of the adrenal glands together with generalized petechiae on the scalp and conjunctivae. She also had pulmonary edema, bilateral hydrothorax, and severe soft tissue edema of the thorax, abdomen, and mesenteries. Brain and adrenals also contained a few fresh thrombi.

Discussion: DIC is a common and often major complication of septicemia (table 33.1), especially that associated with gram-negative organisms and meningococcal infections. Septicemia, often combined with septic shock, is the most frequent disease state associated with DIC (10). As many as 60% of all cases of DIC are precipitated by infection. In this situation the trigger is considered to be the bacterial endotoxin, the lipopolysaccharide that forms the outer coat of the bacterial cell wall. Endotoxin has multiple deleterious effects on hemostasis and induces a whole body inflammatory response that in turn mediates organ damage, eventually leading to multiorgan failure (11). It may activate platelets and factor XII, cause endothelial injury with subsequent exposure of a thrombogenic surface, and activate granulocytes, causing release of potent proteinases such as elastase. Infectious agents may lead to vascular injury with damage, denudation, or perturbation of endothelial cells. Bacterial sepsis in particular is associated with endotoxin-induced endothelial injury. In addition, the widespread inflammatory response produces a variety of other mediators including tumor necrosis factor (TNF), interleukin-1,

platelet-activating factor (PAF), and activated complement products that contribute to endothelial cell injury (10). Release of elastase from activated granulocytes can also have multiple adverse effects on hemostasis. This potent proteinase degrades platelet membrane glycoproteins, interfering with adhesion and aggregation (12), and proteolyzes many of the coagulation factors including fibrinogen (13) and antithrombin (14). Elastase can also in-hibit platelet function by other means (15) and activate fibrinolysis, further upsetting the hemostatic balance (16). Finally, endotoxin is a very potent stimulator of tissue factor expression by blood monocytes (17) and endothelial cells (18), and this is thought to be an important cause of the clotting activation in such cases (see below).

As illustrated in this case, the DIC that accompanies the rapid onset, fulminant DIC that may occur in asplenia is especially catastrophic. The causative organism is usually *Streptococcus pneumoniae* but other bacteria, including *Neisseria meningitidis* and *Haemophilus influenzae*, may also be responsible. Routine vaccination of splenectomized patients against Pneumococcus does not always prevent this complication. The mortality rate is distressingly high, and death (as in this case) often occurs within hours of the onset of symptoms. Another striking example of DIC resulting from sepsis is that associated with meningococcal septicemia. Like our patient AH, these patients are characterized by marked shock, cutaneous bruising, and petechiae. At autopsy, visceral petechiae are especially prominent in the adrenal cortex, whose damage gives rise to the classic **Waterhouse-Friderichsen syndrome.**

Malignant Disease—Case 3

CS, a 66-year-old man, was admitted with abdominal pain and a 20-lb weight loss over the previous 9 months. He complained of urinary urgency, nocturia, and weak urinary flow. Physical examination was unremarkable except for an enlarged, nodular, and firm prostate. X-ray revealed lytic lesions involving multiple ribs, and subsequent open rib biopsy confirmed a poorly differentiated clear cell adenocarcinoma. This was followed by slow, but persistent, bleeding from the wound site. Blood tests revealed:

Total acid phosphatase	*55 IU/L (0–9 IU/L); prostatic fraction 43 IU/L (0–2 IU/L)*
Alkaline phosphatase	*180 IU/L (24–96 IU/mL)*
PT	*16.5 sec (11–13 sec)*
aPTT	*62 sec (35–50 sec)*
Thrombin time	*30 sec (20–25 sec)*
Fibrinogen	*5.1 g/L (1.5–4.0 g/L)*
Platelets	*199 × 10⁹/L (150–400 × 10⁹/L)*
D-dimer level	*500 μg/mL (<200 μg/mL)*
Antithrombin	*70% (70–130%)*
Prothrombin F1.2 level	*6.0 nM/L (0.4–1.1 nM/L)*

Cystourethroscopy revealed an obstructing prostate with extension of prostatic tissue into the trigone. The following day the patient experienced chills and fever and increased bleeding from biopsy and venipuncture sites and from the urinary tract. Escherichia coli was cultured from the urine. Repeat coagulation studies were performed and showed:

PT	27 sec
aPTT	85 sec
Thrombin time	50 sec
Platelets	97×10^9/L
Fibrinogen assay	2.1 g/L
D-dimer	2500 μg/mL
Antithrombin	65%

The bleeding did not subside spontaneously, and the patient was treated with antibiotics, 1500 IU heparin intravenously every 4 hours for 7 days, and begun on high-dose estrogen. The patient eventually recovered with total correction of the clotting defect.

This case illustrates a common pattern of presentation of DIC in the urologic patient. Clinical and laboratory findings were compatible with a preexisting, low-grade, chronic DIC associated with grade IV prostate cancer that had advanced to an acute bleeding diathesis following an episode of sepsis related to cystoscopy. The underlying disorders were treated with antibiotics and estrogen therapy. Heparin was also used until the coagulopathy was under control.

Malignant Disease—Case 4

A 10-week-old black male infant was admitted for investigation of an abdominal mass detected during routine physical examination. There was no history of illness; the child had had an uneventful vaginal delivery following a normal gestation. Examination on admission showed a healthy infant apart from some pallor of the mucous membranes and a firm, nontender mass in the upper abdominal quadrant. Skull and chest x-rays were normal. Laboratory studies showed:

Hematocrit	0.22
Reticulocytes	9.1%
WBC	10.0×10^9/L
Platelets	189×10^9/L ($150–400 \times 10^9$/L)
Blood film: marked variation in red cell size and shape with some schistocytosis	
Sickle cell test negative	
Coombs' test negative	
PT	30 sec (11–13 sec)
aPTT	65 sec (30–45 sec)
Liver function tests normal	

On day 2, oozing was noted from fingerprick and venipuncture sites. Further blood tests revealed:

Hematocrit	0.17
Reticulocytes	7.5%
Platelets	61×10^9/L

The child was given 1 mg vitamin K intramuscularly, and observation was continued. The following day (day 3), the abdomen became distended, and bleeding from puncture sites worsened. The hematocrit fell to 15%, and the blood film became more abnormal, with the appearance of normoblasts. Bone marrow aspiration confirmed marked normoblastic hyperplasia. Coagulation studies showed:

PT	120 sec
aPTT	250 sec
Thrombin time	110 sec (20–25 sec)
Platelets	20×10^9/L
Fibrinogen	<0.1 g/L (1.5–4.0 g/L)
Prothrombin	30% (70–130%)
Factor V	50% (70–130%)
Factor VIII	40% (70–130%)
Factor IX	59% (70–130%)
D-dimer	4500 μg/mL (<200 μg/mL)

The child was treated with 120 mL whole blood and 1 g fibrinogen, and the bleeding subsided. The fibrinogen level returned to normal (2.4 g/L). His clinical condition stabilized over the next few days, although further whole blood transfusions were required to maintain the hematocrit. Fibrinogen levels determined on days 5 and 6 had fallen to 0.6 and 0.3 g/L, respectively, and the D-dimer level remained markedly elevated (>4000 μg/mL). The patient deteriorated on day 9, although the laboratory parameters remained much as they were on day 3. He died on day 10.

Autopsy revealed enlarged adrenal glands, the medulla of which were completely replaced by tumor cells consistent with neuroblastoma. The liver was enlarged, and the cut surface was largely composed of tumor nodules. No clots were found in any organs or in the blood vessels examined.

Discussion: Malignant disease is often complicated by DIC. However, like the urologic patient illustrated by Case 3, many patients will have a subclinical coagulopathy that can only be detected by more sophisticated laboratory tests (see below). Acute DIC, such as that seen in Case 4, is rather less common and tends to be more thrombotic in nature than the condition associated with, for example, obstetric accidents (Case 1). The clinical picture is very variable and may consist of a combination of bleeding and thromboembolic phenomena, although clinically obvious thrombosis or bleeding is suffered by relatively few patients with malignant disease. A much greater number have a hemostatic defect detectable in the laboratory, although the exact incidence is directly proportional to the sensitivity of the laboratory techniques employed.

Laboratory evidence of intravascular activation of the coagulation and/or fibrinolytic mechanisms can be found in most cancer patients (19–25), although variations in the criteria for laboratory diagnosis have made the incidence of acute DIC in patients with malignant disease difficult to establish. Some 8–15% of patients may show thrombocytopenia, falling fibrinogen levels, and raised fibrin degradation products (FDP) (21, 26). However, these represent only the decompensated form of DIC, and a much larger proportion may exhibit signs of compensated DIC.

Thrombocytopenia is a useful indicator of DIC but, in patients with cancer, may also occur as a result of malignant infiltration of the bone marrow or as a side effect of radiotherapy or chemotherapy. Thrombocytopenia may be present in a quarter of patients with disseminated malignancy (21, 26, 27), although in one large study, the incidence was only 4% (28). Thrombocytosis is more common, between 10 and 57% of patients (21, 26–28), and platelet counts tend to increase before death (28). Most cancer patients are said to have decreased platelet survival, which improves during response to treatment (29); very short survival suggests a poor prognosis (29).

Qualitative platelet defects are reportedly common in cancer. Shortened bleeding times have been found in nearly half of patients with disseminated malignancy (27), although various other platelet function defects including reduced adhesion, impaired aggregation, and poor clot retraction have also been described (30, 31). Plasma β-thromboglobulin (β-TG) levels (see below) are elevated in most cancer patients and may be a useful indication of the tumor burden and response to treatment (32).

The PT is prolonged in approximately 14% of unselected cases (21, 28) but in rather more of those with established DIC (26). The incidence of a prolonged aPTT is very variable but is probably under 25% (21, 28). Again, it is much higher in those individuals with overt DIC (26). Shortened aPTTs are also not uncommon; the presence of DIC makes little difference to this finding (26). Prolongation of the thrombin clotting time is rather more common (21, 26) and is profoundly influenced by the presence of DIC (26).

Hypofibrinogenemia is surprisingly uncommon in cancer and is found in less than 5% of unselected patients (21, 26, 28, 31), although this figure is higher in patients with overt DIC (26). Hyperfibrinogenemia, in contrast, is found in 50–80% of patients (21, 28, 31), and fibrinogen levels increase during the terminal phase (28). As shown in Case 3, high fibrinogen levels may appear to mitigate against the presence of DIC, but rapidly falling levels certainly support the diagnosis. Acquired dysfibrinogenemia is rare in most malignant diseases (26). It occurs commonly in patients with hepatocellular carcinoma but is unusual with carcinoma from other sites that has metastasized to the liver (33).

Plasma fibrinopeptide A (FpA; see below) is a sensitive indicator of in vivo coagulation activation and is elevated in most patients with malignant disease (34–37). FpA increases as patients become terminally ill, and persistently raised levels suggest treatment failure and a poor outcome (37). Serial FpA measurements may therefore be a useful indicator of tumor progression or response to treatment. Other markers of clotting activation such as prothrombin F1.2 are also increased (38) and, as in Case 3, may be the only hard evidence of intravascular coagulation.

As intravascular activation of the blood coagulation pathway in cancer patients is virtually inseparable from activation of fibrinolysis, evidence of fibrinolytic activation is frequently observed. Shortened euglobulin clot lysis times, indicating increased fibrinolytic activity, may be seen (21), while plasminogen is decreased in about two-thirds of cases complicated by DIC and about one-quarter of individuals without DIC (26). FDPs are formed as a result of plasmin action on fibrinogen (fibrinogenolysis) or fibrin (fibrinolysis) (39). The presence of FDPs therefore represents direct evidence of the activation of the fibrinolytic pathway, and most, if not all, patients with malignancy and acute DIC have elevated FDP levels (23, 26). In the absence of overt DIC, however, the incidence of raised FDP levels is very variable (19, 21, 26, 28). Since the incidence is greater in patients with remote metastases than in those with localized disease, determination of FDPs may have some prognostic value (40). Even in acute DIC, some patients may not develop significantly raised FDP levels (23), and therefore normal or minimally raised FDP levels do not necessarily exclude DIC in the presence of other compelling evidence.

The etiology of DIC in malignancy is diverse (41, 42). Neovascularization of tissue may activate platelets and coagulation by virtue of an abnormal endothelial lining. There is also considerable evidence that tumor cells may produce procoagulant substances that can directly initiate the coagulation process (43). One extensively studied substance is known as Cancer Procoagulant (CP) (44). This protein is capable of activating factor X directly and is unusual for a clotting enzyme in that it is a cysteine, rather than a serine, proteinase. To what degree CP contributes to intravascular coagulation in cancer is not clear. It appears to be almost ubiquitous in malignant cells, but compared with tissue factor (discussed in more detail in the next section), CP is not a very potent clotting activator. Many tumor types express tissue factor (TF), sometimes in greater amounts than their normal tissue counterparts (45). The contribution of tumor-derived TF to intravascular clotting is difficult to establish, although the role of tumor procoagulants in the extravascular coagulation that occurs in the tumor vicinity seems more assured. Available evidence suggests that much of the intravascular coagulation activation associated with solid tumors is a result of expression of TF on the surface of circulating blood monocytes (see below).

Patients with most forms of leukemia, acute and chronic, may have evidence of DIC. Acute DIC, however, is usually observed in patients with acute promyelocytic leukemia (APL). The mechanism for this appears to be the release of TF from the granules of the malignant promyelocytes (46). Sudden release of this procoagulant from dying cells accounts for the observation that even if the APL patient does not have DIC on presentation, this will ensue on starting chemotherapy. Patients treated with all-trans-retinoic acid (ATRA) seem to fare rather better in this regard (47), and this may be due to a direct effect of this drug on TF synthesis in the abnormal cells (48).

Other Causes of DIC

Numerically, obstetric accidents, sepsis, and malignancy account for most cases of DIC. However, many other causes exist (table 33.1). One acute type may follow the bite of various **poisonous snakes** (49). Many snake venoms contain agents that cause vascular endothelial damage and bleeding. Others contain enzymes that activate clotting factors directly. Venom from the Malayan pit viper, *Ankistrodon rhodostoma*, is a thrombin-like enzyme that directly cleaves FpA from fibrinogen Aα-chains. The saw-scaled viper *(Echis carinatus)*, the Australian tiger snake *(Notechis scutatis)*, and the African Boomslang snake *(Dispholidus typus)* produce an enzyme that directly converts prothrombin to thrombin. The venom of the well-known Russell's viper activates factor X directly.

Transfusion of blood or blood products may also induce DIC. Red cell stroma is a fairly potent trigger for intravascular clotting, and incompatible blood transfusions, even in relatively small amounts, may bring about bleeding accompanied by laboratory evidence of DIC. Thrombosis has been reported after infusion of concentrates containing the vitamin K–dependent clotting factors (50). Near-drowning in fresh water results in intravascular hemolysis and a DIC similar to that of incompatible blood transfusion (51). Severe burns can also be associated with DIC, which may, at least in part, be due to hemolysis although trauma, shock, and sepsis must all play a role (52).

Severe head injury is a well-established cause of acute DIC. Brain tissue contains the body's highest concentration of TF, and this can presumably enter the circulation after cerebral trauma and activate coagulation. Severe trauma to any part of the body, especially that due to major crush injuries, may be followed by DIC for the same reason. DIC may also follow severe shock. This is multifactorial, but is probably largely associated with vascular damage due to tissue anoxia and other origins. Subsequent acidosis tends to enhance the thrombotic tendency in hypovolemic shock.

Differential Diagnosis of Disseminated Intravascular Coagulation

Formation of thrombi in small vessels may accompany a variety of disorders. These do not usually progress to DIC,

Table 33.2. Disorders Associated with Localized Intravascular Coagulation

Purpura fulminans
Thrombotic thrombocytopenic purpura
Hemolytic uremic syndrome
Renal disease
Malignant hypertension
Hemangiomas
Malignant hypertension

although there is some overlap in clinical and laboratory findings. The more common disorders characterized by localized clotting are presented in Table 33.2.

Purpura fulminans is a rare disorder that occurs almost entirely in children. It is characterized by the appearance of cutaneous gangrenous patches in apparently healthy individuals with a recent history of infections such as chickenpox or scarlet fever or following smallpox vaccination (53). Patients become febrile, hypotensive, and extremely ill. The gangrenous lesions are a result of thromboses in the affected area, and larger vessels may also become occluded, with dire results. The pathogenesis is not known. Although the precipitating event may be localized, patients may have a generalized bleeding problem with the laboratory picture of acute DIC.

Thrombotic thrombocytopenic purpura (TTP) is characterized by fever, severe thrombocytopenia, renal failure, and a microangiopathic hemolytic anemia. The latter is due to blockage of arterioles and capillaries by platelet-fibrin thrombi. Like purpura fulminans, the onset of TTP may follow an infectious illness but may also be associated with pregnancy or the puerperium (54). The laboratory findings are usually easy to distinguish from those of DIC, as markers of clotting and fibrinolytic activation are generally normal, while platelet-release proteins are markedly increased (table 33.3).

Hemolytic-uremic syndrome is an acute onset condition that superficially resembles TTP and also tends to follow some form of infectious episode (55). Patients suffer necrosis or infarction of the renal glomeruli, and there is deposition of fibrin-platelet thrombi in the small vessels of the kidney. There is thrombocytopenia, but hypofibrinogenemia and other evidence of DIC is rare.

Drug-induced thrombotic microangiopathy is a syndrome of microangiopathic hemolytic anemia that sometimes accompanies therapy with certain cytotoxic agents including cyclosporin A, cisplatin, bleomycin, and mitomycin C. The pathogenesis of this condition is not understood but may involve platelet aggregation and/or endothelial damage by circulating immune complexes. The prognosis is generally poor.

Henoch-Schönlein purpura is an acute vasculitis involving the skin, kidneys, gut, and joints, and its appearance is commonly preceded by a history of acute upper respiratory tract infection. The condition is readily distinguished from purpura due to intravascular coagulation, as hemostatic screening tests and appropriate molecular marker results are normal.

The Tissue Factor–Induced Pathway of Blood Coagulation

As discussed above, the primary trigger for DIC in many conditions appears to be the inappropriate and uncontrolled activation of coagulation by TF. At this point, therefore, some discussion of the mechanisms involved in TF-induced coagulation is merited.

Table 33.3. Differential Diagnosis of Disseminated Intravascular Coagulation (DIC), Thrombotic Thrombocytopenic Purpura (TTP), and Primary Fibrinogenolysis

	DIC	TTP	Primary Fibrinogenolysis
Thomboxane B2	Increased	Increased	Normal
β-Thromboglobulin	Increased	Increased	Normal
Prothrombin F1.2	Increased	Normal	Normal
Thrombin-antithrombin complex (TAT)	Increased	Normal	Normal
Fibrinopeptide A	Increased	Normal	Normal
Bβ15–42 peptide	Increased	Normal	Increased
D-dimer	Increased	Normal	Normal

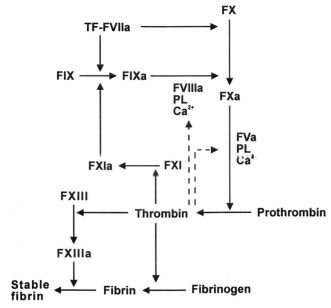

Figure 33.1. Modern concept of the blood coagulation mechanism.

Physiologic Mechanisms

TF is a membrane-bound protein that is found in a wide variety of tissues and cells throughout the body. The molecule consists of three portions: an intracellular domain (which probably has some signaling function), a transmembrane or anchoring domain, and a much larger extracellular domain that contains the clotting activity (56). The tissue distribution of TF has been likened to a "hemostatic envelope" ready to activate coagulation when vascular integrity is breached (57).

It is now generally accepted that TF is the major physiologic route for clotting activation. Recognition of this fact, coupled with the discovery of a natural inhibitor to TF-induced coagulation, has led to a major revision of the classic coagulation cascade (fig. 33.1) (58). In this scheme, TF exposed on a cell membrane forms a complex with factor VII, rapidly activating the latter. The TF-VIIa complex then activates some FIX to FIXa and some FX to FXa. Activated factor X, in the presence of FV, converts prothrombin to thrombin, which then forms fibrin from fibrinogen.

Activated factor X, formed initially by the action of the TF-FVIIa complex, binds to TF pathway inhibitor (TFPI). This complex then binds to and inhibits the TF-FVIIa complex, effectively preventing any further clotting activation via this route. However, thrombin formed in the initial burst of activation cleaves factor XI, which then feeds back to activate more factor IX. Further coagulation then proceeds through the action of factor IXa on factor X. This revised scheme of clotting thus places the major physiologic importance on TF; there is no place for factor XII in this hypothesis, since FXII-deficient patients have a thrombotic, rather than a bleeding, tendency.

As detailed above, DIC may be triggered by the release of TF into the circulation. This may arise from direct cell damage such as major trauma or obstetric accidents. However, there is increasing evidence that much of the intravascular coagulation associated with disease states is a result of inappropriate TF expression on the surface of circulating blood monocytes.

Pathologic Mechanisms—the Role of Monocyte and Endothelial Cell Tissue Factor

Under normal circumstances, TF is not exposed to the circulating blood. In this way, clotting is only activated when the vessel wall is damaged. However, in various pathologic situations, the blood monocytes may be stimulated to express TF on their cell membranes. TF expression may be induced by various cytokines such as the interleukins, by TNF, and by endotoxin (24, 59). As discussed above, the presence of endotoxin in the blood certainly forms part of the pathogenesis of DIC in septic patients (60), and several studies have demonstrated increased monocyte TF expression in such infected individuals. The effects of cytokines on monocyte TF expression and the relationship of this process to the inflammatory response is complex and is outside the scope of this chapter; the interested reader is referred to a recent review for more information (59). Cellular TF expression can be up-regulated by a wide variety of inflammatory mediators including interleukin-1, TNF, complement components, and prostacyclin (10). Monocyte TF has been shown to be elevated in a wide range of inflammatory conditions, and levels often correlate with other parameters of clotting activation, for example, FpA (61). Endothelial cells are also capable of synthesizing TF, but whether this actually occurs in vivo is more difficult to assess. Interestingly, mediators such as TNF that up-regulate TF expression in endothelial cells also act to down-regulate thrombomodulin (TM) expression (62, 63). This would have the additional effect of reducing clotting inhibition via the protein C pathway, since TM is an essential cofactor in the activation of this inhibitor.

Fibrinolysis and DIC

Activation of the fibrinolytic system almost inevitably follows that of the coagulation pathways in DIC. Indeed the degree of bleeding or thrombosis observed clinically depends on the relative balance between these two pathways (64). The central reaction in the fibrinolytic system is the conversion of circulating plasminogen to plasmin. The mechanism for this in DIC is not clear but may be due to release of tissue plasminogen activator from stimulated endothelial cells or via activation of factor XIIa. Generation of plasmin has a marked effect on the clinical and laboratory pictures in DIC, since this enzyme proteolyzes several of the clotting enzymes, including factors V and VIII and fibrinogen, and adversely affects platelet adhesion (65). Plasmin is also responsible for the generation of fibrin and fibrinogen degradation products, which have additional deleterious effects on the clotting process. Inappropriately rapid breakdown of clots in hemostatic plugs, for example in surgical wounds, venipuncture sites, etc., is a major cause of the oozing seen in acute DIC.

Laboratory Diagnosis of Acute DIC

The laboratory diagnosis of acute DIC is generally not difficult. In florid intravascular coagulation, the clinical picture is often sufficient to suggest the diagnosis, which is readily confirmed by routine hematologic and hemostatic evaluation (table 33.4).

The platelet count is typically markedly reduced, but actual values vary widely. Although very low counts (<10 ×

Table 33.4. Laboratory Tests for the Diagnosis of Acute DIC

Acute DIC
    Prothrombin time (PT)
    Activated partial thromboplastin time (aPTT)
    Thrombin time (TT)
    Platelet count
    Fibrinogen assay
    Antithrombin
Chronic DIC
    As above plus:
        Blood film
        Fibrinopeptide A[a]
        Prothrombin F1.2[a]
        Thrombin-antithrombin complex[a]
        Bβ15–42 (if available)
    Platelet factor 4 or β-thromboglobulin
    Plasminogen

[a]One of these markers usually suffices.

10^9/L) are not uncommon, values of 100–150 × 10^9 can occur and certainly do not exclude the diagnosis. The blood film can confirm a profound thrombocytopenia and may additionally show the presence of red cell fragmentation (schistocytosis) caused by physical damage to the red cells by strands of fibrin deposited in the microcirculation. Such patients may also have evidence of hemolysis (microangiopathic hemolytic anemia), and this situation was observed in Case 4. However, this is by no means an absolute finding, and about half the patients with acute DIC lack this feature.

The PT and aPTT are usually the first tests requested on patients suspected of having DIC. They are usually abnormal and may be infinitely prolonged. The major clotting defect in acute DIC is the *presence of very low, or even absent, fibrinogen levels.* Routine clotting tests such as PT and aPTT rely on the conversion of fibrinogen to fibrin as the endpoint of the test. Thus, very low levels will greatly prolong the clotting times, irrespective of abnormalities in other clotting factors measured by these assays. Conversely, in the presence of normal or near-normal levels of other clotting factors (≈60% of normal), fibrinogen levels would have to fall to under 0.9 g/L to prolong the PT and aPTT, and moderate hypofibrinogenemia would go undetected. Production of large amounts of fibrin(ogen) degradation products (FDPs; see below) additionally interfere with fibrin formation and thus contribute to the prolongation of the clotting times.

The PT is prolonged in about 75% of cases of acute DIC, while the aPTT is abnormal in approximately half such patients. To further complicate interpretation, *shortened* clotting times may occur in a significant proportion of patients. This is because some patients have circulating activated clotting factors, which, if the fibrinogen level is adequate, may actually speed clot formation. Furthermore, early degradation products of fibrinogen retain the ability to be clotted by thrombin and readily gel during the test. Because of the wide variation in the results of these tests and because they can be influenced by factors other than those they are designed to measure, the PT and aPTT are of only limited use in patients with suspected DIC.

The TT is rather more useful; it is only sensitive to the conversion of fibrinogen to fibrin and is not, therefore, affected by circulating clotting factors, activated or otherwise. With appropriate choice of thrombin concentration (the normal range should ideally lie within 20–25 sec). The TT is sensitive to both fibrinogen concentration (much more so than the PT and aPTT) and the inhibitory effects of FDP. However, the TT is also exquisitely sensitive to heparin, and if the patent is being treated with heparin or blood has inadvertently been taken through a heparinized line, it will be spuriously (and often infinitely) prolonged. The answer to this problem is the reptilase time (RT). Reptilase is a snake venom that, like thrombin, converts fibrinogen to fibrin, but it is totally insensitive to heparin. Thus, a prolonged TT but normal RT almost always indicates the presence of heparin. In the presence of hypofibrinogenemia and/or the inhibitory effects of FDP, the two tests are equally prolonged.

A useful and simple addition to the diagnostic powers of the TT is to observe periodically the clot formed in the test for the onset of lysis. In normal circumstances, the clot will remain intact for hours, but in acute DIC with active secondary fibrinolysis, the clot may dissolve within 10–30 minutes.

A specific fibrinogen assay is useful confirmation of the TT result and should be performed if possible. Clottable fibrinogen estimations are most useful and are generally rapid to perform. Typically, levels in acute DIC are less than 1 g/L (normal, 1.5–4.0 g/L) and may be unmeasurable. Serial fibrinogen levels are even more valuable, as a falling value is more informative than a single estimation, especially if the latter is not very low. This is illustrated by Case 3, in which a raised fibrinogen level on presentation rapidly fell as the DIC changed from a chronic, compensated form to a more acute variety. Fibrinogen, an acute-phase protein, may rise in disease states (e.g., cancer) and during pregnancy. A level of 2 g/L, for example, although apparently normal, may be distinctly abnormal in a pregnant or newly delivered woman who might have had a level of 5 g/L a few hours earlier. In these situations, therefore, a single normal fibrinogen level should not necessarily exclude the diagnosis of DIC.

Coagulation factor assays are not useful in the diagnosis of acute DIC. In the first place, as in Cases 2 and 4, levels of individual clotting factors are extremely variable and may often be in the normal range. Secondly, as noted above, the presence of circulating activated clotting factors may bypass the requirement for the factor under test in the assay, and thus a spuriously normal level may be reported by the laboratory. Finally, a battery of factor assays is time-consuming, and since DIC is a dynamic event, the clinical situation will have long since changed by the time the assay results are available.

FDPs are increased in most patients with acute DIC. Earlier assays measured a combination of fibrinogen- and fibrin-derived products, but many laboratories now use an assay for D-dimer. This fragment is derived specifically from cross-linked fibrin and is more specific for the presence (or absence) of DIC. Rapid slide-based latex agglutination tests for D-dimer are now widely available and are ideal for the emergency situation. D-dimer is elevated in a very high proportion of patients with acute DIC (>90%), but positive results are also found in, for example, deep vein thrombosis (DVT) and pulmonary embolism. Nevertheless, levels in DIC are typically much higher, often in excess of 2000 μg/mL (normal, <200 μg/mL), and the assay is probably one of the most useful means of differentiating DIC and non-DIC (66). High levels were observed in all four cases described above. Certainly, the D-dimer test provides more useful information than that given by older tests such as ethanol or protamine gelation tests for soluble fibrin monomers, and the FDP titer and should be used in preference.

The natural coagulation inhibitor antithrombin (AT) is consumed during clotting, and as expected, many patients with acute DIC will therefore have reduced levels. Pa-

tients with DIC secondary to cancer, however, tend not to fit this pattern for reasons that are not well understood. AT levels in Case 3, for example, were not as low as might have been expected. In general, AT levels do not add significantly to diagnostic efficiency but may help to determine the need for AT replacement therapy (see below).

Laboratory Diagnosis of Chronic DIC

Routine Tests

As stated above, the diagnosis of acute DIC is relatively simple and is based on the combination of clinical picture and a few simple clotting tests. In chronic DIC, however, the picture is very different. The underlying clinical condition may not be so obvious, and many of the more readily available hemostatic tests are normal or fall into a "gray area" just outside the normal range. Many such patients have what is termed a "compensated" DIC; that is to say that production of new clotting factors and platelets keeps pace with consumption in the clotting process. If measured, however, the turnover and survival of these components are abnormal.

Fibrinogen levels are usually normal but can be elevated due to the presence of underlying inflammatory disease. Levels of factors V and VIII behave in a similar fashion. The PT and aPTT are usually normal but may be shortened due to the presence of circulating activated clotting factors as described for acute DIC. The TT is variable, depending on the levels of circulating fibrinogen and FDPs. High fibrinogen levels can, paradoxically, result in prolonged TTs, and in patients with liver disease, acquired dysfibrinogenemia may also prolong this test.

The presence of schistocytosis in the peripheral blood film is more common in chronic DIC, mainly because these forms are more likely to be associated with a thrombotic diathesis. D-dimer is elevated, although levels are generally lower than those observed in the acute forms of DIC, and it may be difficult to distinguish between this and other causes of raised levels such as DVT and pulmonary embolism. However, elevations of D-dimer are generally more persistent.

Molecular Markers of Hemostatic Activation

The advent of monoclonal antibody technology and improvements in biochemical methods has led to the introduction of several methods for detecting low levels of clotting and fibrinolytic activation in vivo (67). These assays are based on one of two main principles (fig. 33.2).

First, when an activated clotting factor (e.g., thrombin) is neutralized by its natural inhibitor (e.g., AT), a complex is formed that persists in the circulation. Such complexes often create a "neoantigen" that is not expressed on either of the original components of the complex. Monoclonal antibodies raised against such antigens can therefore be used in a immunologic assay for the complex. Currently available examples of such assays are thrombin-antithrombin (TAT)

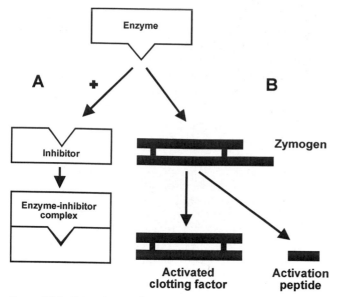

Figure 33.2. Principles involved in assays for molecular markers of clotting activation. *(A)* formation of an enzyme-inhibitor complex and *(B)* formation of an activation peptide during activation of a clotting protein.

and plasmin-antiplasmin (PAP). Second, activation of many of the clotting factors involves the release of a small peptide by enzymatic cleavage. Antibodies directed against such activation peptides can be used to measure their plasma concentrations, and this is a highly sensitive way to detect hemostatic activation (fig. 33.3). The most widely used activation peptide assays are for FpA (released from fibrinogen by the action of thrombin), prothrombin fragment 1.2 (prothrombin F1.2; released from prothrombin following activation by factor Xa), and Bβ15–42 (a fragment cleaved from the fibrinogen Bβ chain by plasmin). Other markers (e.g., for the activation peptides of factors IX, X, and XII) have also been described, and it is possible to distinguish accurately the degradation productions of fibrinogen and fibrin. Platelet activation can be assessed with assays for platelet release proteins such as platelet factor 4 (PF4) and β-TG. Recently, an assay has been described that measures the activated form of factor VII (FVIIa) (68). No results of this assay in DIC have yet been reported, but given that most cases of DIC are triggered by the TF–factor VII pathway, it seems likely to be a promising approach.

Patients with chronic DIC will certainly have increased levels of, for example, β-TG, prothrombin F1.2, and Bβ15–42, indicating degrees of activation of platelets, coagulation, and fibrinogenolysis, respectively. In the face of equivocal results from conventional hemostatic tests, these new assays are very useful and show great promise in understanding the balance between coagulation and fibrinolysis in a wide range of conditions (67). They are also potentially useful in monitoring therapy; prothrombin F1.2, for example, is reduced during heparin therapy, although research in this area is far from complete. The use of these markers has made it possible to detect accurately very small amounts of hemostatic activation and to distinguish

between DIC, TTP, and primary fibrinolysis (table 33.3). These markers are also markedly elevated in acute DIC but generally do not add to the diagnosis. Since they are also very expensive to detect, their use is best restricted to those situations in which conventional tests fail to provide the required information. Theoretically, molecular markers such as FpA and prothrombin F1.2 would give valuable information about the course of intravascular clotting. Unfortunately, the length of time these immunoassays take to perform also makes them useless in the emergency setting at present.

Soluble Tissue Factor in Plasma

As discussed elsewhere in this review, the major trigger for DIC in a wide range of clinical conditions is thought to be the exposure or release into the circulation of TF, although direct laboratory support for this hypothesis is lacking. Recently, immunologic methods have become available to measure circulating TF (69), and preliminary data (unpublished) indicate that this is elevated in many patients with acute DIC. However, the source of soluble (lacking transmembrane and intracellular domains) TF, whether such material remains active in initiating coagulation, and whether levels correlate with the degree of intravascular coagulation (measured by activation peptide levels) is not yet clear. Although potentially useful from the mechanistic standpoint, detection and measurement of plasma TF is currently unlikely to contribute to the diagnosis or management of DIC.

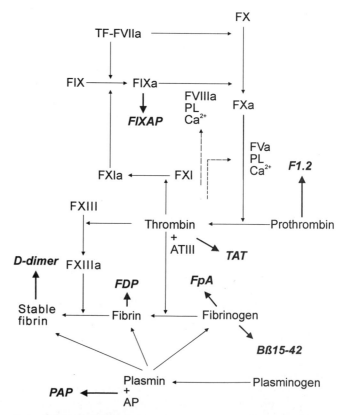

Figure 33.3. Generation of molecular markers of hemostatic activation during intravascular coagulation.

Treatment of DIC

The treatment of DIC has been a controversial issue in clinical hematology. The disease does not lend itself to clinical trials to support any particular treatment regimen, which has allowed debate, especially over the value of heparin, to rage unabated.

As discussed at length above, acute DIC is the result of a distinct triggering factor. Thus, the key to successful treatment is, when possible, to first treat or remove the triggering process. In retained dead fetus syndrome, for example, uterine evacuation is the top priority, although persuading a surgeon to operate in the face of infinitely prolonged clotting tests is seldom easy. Heparin treatment in obstetric complications is rarely necessary, although amniotic fluid embolism is an exception to this rule. Antibiotic treatment of septicemia, especially if this is combined with volume replacement therapy and antishock measures, may be successful in slowing the clotting process.

The second phase of treatment is to stop the process of intravascular coagulation. Many patients will benefit from the administration of subcutaneous low-dose heparin (70), especially if bleeding continues for more than 4 hours after attempts to remove the initial trigger. One authority (70) advocates giving subcutaneous calcium heparin, 80–100 U/kg every 4–6 hours, depending on the site and severity of bleeding. This approach seems more efficacious than larger intravenous doses of heparin and results in improvement in laboratory indices of DIC and cessation of bleeding and/or thrombosis in 3–4 hours. One of the major advantages of this approach is that low-dose heparin is unlikely to increase the chance of bleeding, and it is often difficult for a clinician to administer large doses of an anticoagulant to an already bleeding patient. Antiplatelet agents are generally ineffective in acute DIC but may be valuable in the chronic forms. AT concentrates have been shown to be effective in acute DIC, and further studies of this approach are warranted.

If the previous two steps fail to stop the clotting process and bleeding continues, it is probable that the patient has become depleted in one or more of the components of the hemostatic system. However, there is a potential danger in administering certain clotting components in patients with ongoing DIC; fibrinogen-containing replacement therapy should not be used in this situation (70). The use of fresh whole blood and fresh frozen plasma may be associated with potentiating bleeding and clotting in patients with continuing DIC. This is sometimes referred to as "fueling the fire." The only safe components in this situation are washed packed red cells, platelet concentrates, AT concentrates, and plasma volume expanders. This can be done as an exchange transfusion procedure.

If bleeding still persists, it may be due to continued activation of the fibrinolytic system, and antifibrinolytic drugs should be considered. It should be emphasized that such treatment should never be used in patients with ongoing intravascular coagulation, since this will enhance thrombosis by impairing the patient's ability to clear fibrin clots from the circulation. In these rare cases (about 3% of all instances of acute DIC), ϵ-aminocaproic acid (EACA) may be given. Other possibilities include tranexamic acid and aprotinin, although there is little published experience with these agents in acute DIC.

Summary

This chapter has sought to illustrate the etiology, pathophysiology, and some aspects of treatment of DIC by reference to four case reports. These cases demonstrate some of the more common situations in which DIC might present, but it should be emphasized that a very wide range of clinical conditions may be complicated by intravascular coagulation, and the present review is not exhaustive in this respect. Fortunately, diagnosis of this condition is now relatively straightforward, especially with recent advances in the detection and measurement of molecular markers of hemostatic activation. Appropriate treatment modalities, however, remain less well defined, mainly because of the lack of controlled clinical trials in this area.

REFERENCES

1. Mills CA. The action of tissue extracts in the coagulation of blood. J Biol Chem 1921;46:167.
2. Ratnoff OD, Conley CL. Studies on afibrinogenemia. II. The defibrinating effect on dog blood of intravenous injection of thromboplastic material. Bull Johns Hopkins Hosp 1950; 88:414.
3. Ratnoff OD. Disseminated intravascular coagulation during pregnancy. In: Greer IA, Turpie AGG, Forbes CD, eds. Haemostasis and thrombosis in obstetrics and gynaecology. London: Chapman & Hall Medical, 1992:117–142.
4. Phillips LL, Davidson EC. Procoagulant properties of amniotic fluid. Am J Obstet Gynecol 1972;113:911.
5. Pusey ML, Mende TJ. Studies on the procoagulant activity of human amniotic fluid. 2. The role of factor VII. Thromb Res 1985;39:571.
6. Lockwood CJ, et al. Amniotic fluid contains tissue factor, a potent initiator of coagulation. Am J Obstet Gynecol 1991; 165:1335.
7. Gordon SG, et al. Cysteine proteinase procoagulant from amnion-chorion. Blood 1985;66:1261.
8. Morgan M. Amniotic fluid embolism. Anaesthesia 1979; 34:20.
9. Edgington TS, et al. Isolation and characterisation of the human placental tissue factor molecule [Abstract]. Fed Proc 1986;245:1073.
10. Muller Berghaus G. Pathophysiologic and biochemical events in disseminated intravascular coagulation: dysregulation of procoagulant and anticoagulant pathways. Semin Thromb Hemost 1989;15:58.
11. Welbourn CRB, Young Y. Endotoxin, septic shock and acute lung injury—neutrophils, macrophages and inflammatory mediators. Br J Surg 1992;79:998.
12. Brower MS, Levin RI, Garry K. Human neutrophil elastase modulates platelet function by limited proteolysis of membrane glycoproteins. J Clin Invest 1985;75:657.
13. Bilezikian SB, Nossel HL. Unique pattern of fibrinogen cleavage by human leukocyte proteases. Blood 1977;50:21.
14. Carrell RW, Owen MC. Plakalbumin, alpha-2-antitrypsin, antithrombin and the mechanism of inflammatory thrombosis. Nature 1985;317:730.

15. Marcus AJ. Neutrophils inhibit platelet reactivity by multiple mechanisms: relevance to thromboregulation. J Lab Clin Med 1990;116:138.

16. Machovich R, Owen WG. The elastase-mediated pathway of fibrinolysis. Blood Coag Fibrinol 1990;1:79.

17. Rickles FR, Rick PD. Structural features of *Salmonella typhimurium* lipopolysaccharide required for activation of tissue factor in human mononuclear cells. J Clin Invest 1977; 59:1188.

18. Colucci M, et al. Cultured human endothelial cells generate tissue factor in response to endotoxin. J Clin Invest 1983; 71:1893.

19. Peck SD, Reiquam CW. Disseminated intravascular coagulation in cancer patients: supportive evidence. Cancer 1973; 31:1114.

20. Sun NCJ, et al. Blood coagulation studies in patients with cancer. Mayo Clin Proc 1974;49:636.

21. Sun NCJ, McAfee WM, Hum GJ, Weiner JM. Hemostatic abnormalities in malignancy, a prospective study of one hundred eight patients. Part 1. Coagulation studies. Am J Clin Pathol 1979;71:10.

22. Rasche H, Dietrich M. Hemostatic abnormalities associated with malignant disease. Eur J Cancer 1977;13:1053.

23. Bick RL. Alterations of haemostasis associated with malignancy. Etiology, pathophysiology, diagnosis and management. Semin Thromb Hemost 1978;5:1.

24. Rickles FR, Edwards RL. Activation of blood coagulation in cancer: Trousseau's syndrome revisited. Blood 1983;62:14.

25. Dvorak HF. Thrombosis and cancer. Human Pathol 1987; 18:275.

26. Kies MS, Posch JJ, Giolama JP, Rubin RN. Haemostatic function in cancer patients. Cancer 1980;46:831.

27. Miller SP, Sanchez-Avalos J, Stefanski T, Zuckerman L. Coagulation disorders in cancer. I. Clinical and laboratory studies. Cancer 1967;20:1452.

28. Edwards RL, et al. Anormalities of blood coagulation tests in patients with cancer. Am J Clin Pathol 1987;88:596.

29. Slichter SJ, Harker LA. Haemostasis in malignancy. Ann NY Acad Sci 1974;230:252.

30. Stiles CD. The molecular biology of platelet-derived growth factor. Cell 1983;33:653.

31. Davis RB, Theologides A, Kennedy BJ. Comparative studies of blood coagulation and platelet aggregation in patients with cancer and non-malignant diseases. Ann Intern Med 1969; 71:67.

32. Bidet JM, et al. Evaluation of β-thromboglobulin levels in cancer patients: effects of antitumor chemotherapy. Thromb Res 1980;19:429.

33. Francis JL. Acquired dysfibrinogenaemia. In: Francis JL, ed. Fibrinogen, fibrin stabilization and fibrinolysis. Chichester: Ellis Horwood, 1988:128–156.

34. Peuscher FW, et al. Significance of plasma fibrinopeptide A (FPA) in patients with malignancy. J Lab Clin Med 1980; 96:5.

35. Myers TJ, Rickles FR, Barb C, Cronlund M. Fibrinopeptide A in acute leukaemia: relationship of activation of blood coagulation to disease activity. Blood 1981;57:518.

36. Mombelli G, Roux A, Haeberli A, Staub PW. Comparison of ^{125}I-fibrinogen kinetics and fibrinopeptide A in patients with disseminated neoplasias. Blood 1982;60:381.

37. Rickles FR, Edwards RL, Barb C, Cronlund M. Abnormalities of blood coagulation in patients with cancer. Fibrinopeptide A generation and tumor growth. Cancer 1983; 51:301.

38. Seitz R, et al. Activation of coagulation and fibrinolysis in patients with lung cancer—relation to tumour stage and prognosis. Blood Coag Fibrinol 1993;4:249.

39. Collen D, Lijnen HR. Molecular and cellular basis of fibrinolysis. In: Hoffman R, et al., eds. Hematology: basic principles and practice. New York: Churchill Livingstone, 1991: 1232–1242.

40. Carlsson S. Fibrinogen degradation products in serum from patients with cancer. Acta Chir Scand 1973;139:499.

41. Bick RL. Coagulation abnormalities in malignancy—a review. Semin Thromb Hemost 1992;18:353.

42. Bick RL. Alterations of hemostasis in malignancy. In: Bick RL, et al., eds. Hematology. Clinical and laboratory practice. St Louis: Mosby-Year Book, 1993:1583–1602.

43. Gordon SG. Cancer cell procoagulants and their role in malignant disease. Semin Thromb Hemost 1992;18:424.

44. Gordon SG, Franks JJ, Lewis B. Cancer procoagulant: a factor X-activating procoagulant from malignant tissue. Thromb Res 1975;6:127.

45. Rao LVM. Tissue factor as a tumor procoagulant. Cancer Metast Rev 1992;11:249.

46. Gralnick HR, Abrell E. Studies of the procoagulant and fibrinolytic activity of promyelocytes in acute promyelocytic leukaemia. Br J Haematol 1973;24:89.

47. Dombret H, et al. Coagulation disorders associated with acute promyelocytic leukemia—corrective effect of all-*trans*-retinoic acid treatment. Leukemia 1993;7:2.

48. Rickles FR, et al. All-*trans* retinoic acid (ATRA) inhibits the expression of tissue factor in human progranulocytic leukemia [Abstract]. Thromb Haemost 1993; 69:107.

49. Minton S. Clinical hemostatic disorders caused by venoms. In: Ratnoff OD, Forbes CD, eds. Disorders of hemostasis. Philadelphia: WB Saunders, 1991:518–531.

50. Davey RJ, Shashaty GG, Rath CE. Acute coagulopathy following infusion of prothrombin complex concentrate. Am J Med 1976;60:719.

51. Culpepper RM. Bleeding diathesis in fresh water drowning. Ann Intern Med 1975;83:675.

52. McManus WF, Eurenius K, Pruitt BAJ. Disseminated intravascular coagulation in burned patients. J Trauma 1973; 13:416.

53. Forbes CD, Prentice CRM. Vascular and non-thrombocytopenic purpuras. In: Bloom AL, Thomas DP, eds. Haemostasis and thrombosis. Edinburgh: Churchill Livingstone, 1987:321–332.

54. Horger EO III. Thrombotic thrombocytpoenic purpura. In: Hematologic problems in pregnancy. Oradell, NJ: Medical Economics, 1987:353–359.

55. Brozovic M. Acquired disorders of coagulation. In: Bloom AL, Thomas DP, eds. Haemostasis and thrombosis. Edinburgh: Churchill Livingstone, 1987:519–534.

56. Brozna JP. Cellular regulation of tissue factor. Blood Coag Fibrinol 1990;1:415.

57. Drake TA, Morrissey JH, Edgington TS. Selective cellular expression of tissue factor in human tissues. Implications for disorders of hemostasis and thrombosis. Am J Pathol 1989; 134:1087.

58. Broze GJ. The role of tissue factor pathway inhibitor in a revised coagulation cascade. Semin Hematol 1992;29:159.

59. Edwards RL, Rickles FR. The role of leukocytes in the activation of blood coagulation. Semin Hematol 1992;29:202.

60. Rivers RPA, Cattermole HEJ, Wright I. The expression of surface tissue factor apoprotein by blood monocytes in the course of infections in early infancy. Pediatr Res 1992; 31:567.

61. Edwards RL, et al. Activation of blood coagulation in Crohn's disease. Increased plasma fibrinopeptide A levels and enhanced generation of monocyte tissue factor activity. Gastroenterology 1987;92:329.

62. Conway EM, Rosenberg RD. Tumor necrosis factor suppresses transcription of the thrombomodulin gene in endothelial cells. Mol Cell Biol 1988;8:5588.

63. Moore KL, Esmon CT, Esmon NL. Tumor necrosis factor leads to the internalization and degradation of thrombomodulin from the surface of bovine aortic endothelial cells in culture. Blood 1989;73:159.

64. Bennett B, Ogston D. Fibrinolytic bleeding syndromes. In: Ratnoff OD, Forbes CD, eds. Disorders of hemostasis. Philadelphia: WB Saunders, 1991:327–351.

65. Adelman B, et al. Plasmin effect on platelet glycoprotein IB–von Willebrand factor interaction. Blood 1985; 65:32.

66. Bick RL, Baker WF. Diagnostic efficacy of the D-dimer assay in disseminated intravascular coagulation (DIC). Thromb Res 1992;65:785.

67. Bauer KA. Laboratory markers of coagulation activation. Arch Pathol Lab Med 1993;117:71.

68. Morrissey JH, Macik BG, Neuenschwander PF, Comp PC. Quantitation of activated factor VII levels in plasma using a tissue factor mutant selectively deficient in promoting factor VII activation. Blood 1993;81:734.

69. Albrecht S, et al. An ELISA for tissue factor using monoclonal antibodies. Blood Coag Fibrinol 1992;3:263.

70. Bick RL. Disseminated intravascular coagulation and related syndromes. In: Bennett JM, et al., eds. Hematology. Clinical and laboratory practice. St Louis: Mosby-Year Book, 1993: 1463–1499.

CHAPTER 34

Thromboembolic States

JOHN L. FRANCIS

A pint of sweat will save a gallon of blood.
—Patton, War As I Knew It, 1945

Thromboembolic disease is a major clinical problem, and in many patients, a definable cause for the thrombotic episode cannot be determined. Traditionally, the investigation of thromboembolic states has been a "gray area" in hematology. While the laboratory investigation of bleeding disorders has advanced rapidly in the last 20 years, coagulationists have had relatively little to offer the clinician faced with a patient with thrombosis. Two things have happened to change this depressing picture. First, we now have a greater understanding of the coagulation system, which has permitted the recognition of patients whose thrombotic tendency is due to congenital deficiency of one of the natural coagulation inhibitors. Second, the identification of hypercoagulability has been greatly facilitated by the evolution of "molecular markers" of coagulation activation. Thus, the laboratory investigation of recurrent thrombosis now boasts a battery of tests to rival that offered to patients with a bleeding tendency.

This chapter discusses the thromboembolic states whose etiology can be traced to a distinct hemostatic abnormality. Laboratory diagnosis and treatment is illustrated by references to typical case studies, although as far as familial thrombophilia is concerned, these tend to be rather similar. To provide a foundation for this discussion, this chapter begins with a brief overview of the mechanisms and regulation of the hemostatic pathways.

The Blood Coagulation System

Classical blood coagulation theory has divided the clotting process into intrinsic and extrinsic pathways (fig. 34.1). Although it remains convenient to consider the process in these terms when interpreting the results of coagulation screening tests, it is now clear that these pathways are not independent.

The relatively recent discovery of tissue factor pathway inhibitor (TFPI), coupled with the need to explain the clinical effects of various coagulation factor deficiencies, has given rise to a revised concept of blood coagulation (fig. 34.2) (1). In this scheme, coagulation is initiated when factor VII or VIIa in flowing blood comes into contact with tissue factor (TF) constitutively expressed by subendothelial cells. Factor VII binds to TF where it is rapidly activated to FVIIa. The resultant TF-VIIa complex activates some factor X to Xa and some factor IX to IXa.

The generation of FXa results in the intervention of TFPI, which binds FXa and then forms a quaternary complex with FVIIa and TF, effectively blocking further FXa generation through this route. The coagulation process is maintained by feedback action of FIX through the action of FIXa. In this scheme of coagulation, factor XI is placed at the terminal end of the cascade where it acts as an alternative substrate for thrombin (2).

Factor XIa converts factor IX to FIXa, which then forms a complex with factors VIII and X, calcium ions, and phospholipid derived largely from platelet membranes. The resultant factor Xa then forms a similar complex with factor V and prothrombin. Factors V and VIII act as accelerators, the activity of which is greatly increased by trace amounts of thrombin. However, at higher thrombin concentrations, factors V and VIII are degraded, reducing the rate of reaction and slowing down the natural amplification of the process. The activated factor X complex, known as prothrombinase, converts the phospholipid-bound prothrombin to the active enzyme, thrombin, the primary function of which is the conversion of fibrinogen to fibrin. The removal of fibrinopeptides A and B from the fibrinogen molecule allows the spontaneous polymerization of the resultant fibrin monomers. The final stage of blood coagulation is the stabilization of the fibrin clot by thrombin-activated factor XIII, which catalyses the formation of $\epsilon(\gamma$-glutamyl)-lysine bonds between adjacent fibrin molecules (3).

TFPI-regulated feedback inhibition of the TF-FVIIa complex explains the clinical importance of both "intrinsic" and "extrinsic" coagulation factors. It appears that the TF-factor VII pathway is responsible for the rapid generation of thrombin sufficient to cause local platelet aggregation and activation of the critical cofactors V and VIII. Continuing hemostasis, however, certainly requires ongoing generation of factor Xa through the actions of factors VIII and IX, which explains the clinical importance of these clotting factors. The "contact" factors FXII, prekallikrein, and high-molecular-weight (HMW) kininogen have no role in this revised scheme of coagulation. It seems likely that their importance lies in orchestrating other inflammatory responses such as complement, kinin, and fibrinolytic activation.

Because of the natural amplification of the enzyme products of the coagulation cascade, there is always a

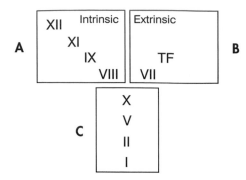

Figure 34.1. Classical cascade theory of blood coagulation.

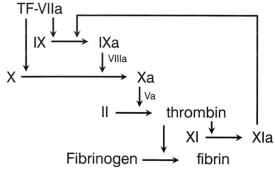

Figure 34.2. Modern concept of blood coagulation.

danger that the process may get out of hand and develop systemic proportions. Therefore, to contain the fibrin clot to the site of vessel damage, the hemostatic system provides a variety of inhibitory mechanisms (4). The major inhibitors of the blood coagulation pathway are antithrombin, activated protein C, and TFPI (these are discussed in more detail below). Clinical evidence suggests that these inhibitors are essential to prevent thromboembolic disease.

The Fibrinolytic System

The major function of the fibrinolytic system is the degradation and dissolution of formed fibrin within the circulation. It is assumed that fibrinolysis is normally required to degrade small quantities of fibrin that are continually being deposited within the circulation and is therefore the body's first line of defense against thrombosis. Although the evidence for this hypothesis remains equivocal, it is widely held that there is a balance between the coagulation and fibrinolytic pathways in vivo.

The fibrinolytic system has four main components: plasminogen activators, plasminogen, plasmin, and fibrinolytic inhibitors (fig. 34.3). Plasminogen activation can occur via an intrinsic pathway, possibly mediated by components of contact activation and protein C activation or via an extrinsic mechanism involving activators released from the blood vessel wall. Plasminogen activators are present in many different human and animal tissues and secretions. The major plasminogen activator in blood is known as tissue-type plasminogen activator (t-PA); the other major type is found predominantly in urine and is known as urokinase-type plasminogen activator (u-PA) (5).

t-PA is a serine proteinase whose main physiologic function is to cleave a specific arginine-valine bond in the plasminogen molecule, and it is distinguished from u-PA by the former's strong affinity for fibrin. In the absence of fibrin, t-PA activates plasminogen relatively slowly. At physiologic plasminogen concentrations, one molecule of t-PA takes approximately 30 minutes to activate one molecule of plasminogen. In the presence of fibrin, however, this process may take less than 5 seconds. Fibrin accelerates plasminogen activation by increasing the affinity of plasminogen for fibrin-bound t-PA and ensures that fibrinolysis is mainly localized to the fibrin clot (5, 6). Locally generated plasmin is then free to digest the fibrin with relatively little interference from circulating fibrinolytic inhibitors. This process ensures rapid and specific fibrinolysis with minimal degradation of circulating fibrinogen or other clotting factors. Urokinase (UK, u-PA) is a trypsin-like proteinase that occurs in both single chain (scu-PA, "prourokinase") and two-chain (tcu-PA) forms. Urokinase converts plasminogen directly to plasmin and does not require the presence of fibrin (6).

Fibrinolysis can be activated by several mechanisms that are closely linked to the activation of coagulation. t-PA released from the vessel wall binds to newly formed fibrin along with the fibrinolytic zymogen, plasminogen. Thus, the fibrin clot is produced already equipped with the mechanisms for its own dissolution. Plasminogen may also be activated by kallikrein and factor XIa, providing further links with the intrinsic clotting system. Plasminogen activation can be accelerated by leukocytes, a mechanism that may have particular relevance in vivo (7). Irrespective of the pathway involved, plasminogen activation results in the generation of plasmin. The main physiologic "target" of plasmin is fibrin, but if its action remains unchecked, plasmin will also cleave intact fibrinogen and other clotting proteins.

The breakdown of a fibrin clot results in the formation of fibrin degradation products (FDPs) (6). These are easily measured in plasma or urine and indicate activation of the coagulation and fibrinolytic pathways. The exact structure of FDPs varies according to whether the substrate for plasmin action is fibrinogen, non-cross-linked fibrin, or factor XIII–stabilized fibrin. In particular, plasmin degradation of cross-linked fibrin yields a unique fragment known as D-dimer comprising a pair of D-fragments from adjacent fibrin molecules. The development of specific monoclonal antibodies has made it possible to accurately distinguish between fibrin- and fibrinogen-derived degradation products, which may be useful in diagnosing thrombosis (8).

Uninhibited fibrinolytic activity is dangerous, and like the coagulation system, the fibrinolytic pathway is equipped with a variety of inhibitory mechanisms (9). The major physiologic inhibitor of plasmin is α_2-antiplasmin; additional plasmin activity is neutralized by α_2-macroglobulin. α_2-Antiplasmin is a serine proteinase inhibitor that forms a

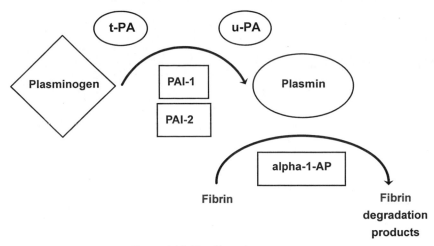

Figure 34.3. The fibrinolytic system.

1:1 complex with plasmin. α_2-Macroglobulin reacts more slowly with plasmin but, over a longer period, can inactivate a greater amount of enzyme. There is also a clearance mechanism, probably through the reticuloendothelial system, that can remove activated fibrinolytic (and coagulation) enzymes. The primary rapid-acting inhibitor of t-PA and u-PA in plasma is plasminogen activator inhibitor-1 (PAI-1). PAI-1 is released from platelet α-granules during platelet activation. As far as the hemostatic balance is concerned, anything that interferes with the normal fibrinolytic process is likely to cause or potentiate thrombosis.

Thrombosis

Virchow, with remarkable perception at the time, observed more than 100 years ago that there are three primary factors in the development of thrombosis: (a) changes in blood flow, (b) alterations in the composition of circulating blood, and (c) alterations in the nature of the vessel wall. In this chapter, however, only those disorders that result from an identifiable abnormality in a specific hemostatic protein leading to thrombosis are discussed.

Congenital Predisposition to Thrombosis

The importance of the natural inhibitors of blood coagulation in the pathogenesis of venous thrombosis has only become appreciated in the last 15 years. Estimates of the prevalence of familial thrombophilia have varied considerably, largely due to different methods of selecting patients. Simply identifying those patients with unusually low inhibitor levels is insufficient, as such individuals may be normal statistical outliers and may not in any case suffer from thrombosis. The presence of a positive family history does not detect all patients with a familial tendency to thrombosis (10), and there are differing views on what constitutes a positive family history (11). Familial thrombosis could theoretically result from a variety of abnormalities in the hemostatic system (table 34.1); a genuine rela-

Table 34.1. Possible Causes of Familial Thrombosis

Accelerated fibrin formation
 Increased procoagulant activity
 Diminished natural inhibitor activity
Defective fibrinolysis
 Reduction in profibrinolytic factors
 Increased levels of fibrinolytic inhibitors
Abnormal fibrin
 Congenital dysfibrinogenemia

tionship has, however, been demonstrated in relatively few of these (11). A laboratory abnormality in a patient with thrombosis does not necessarily indicate a causal relationship, and it is therefore essential to demonstrate the following (11):

1. That both the laboratory defect and the thrombotic tendency are inherited
2. That the laboratory defect coseggregates with the thrombotic tendency
3. That the association of the thrombotic state and the laboratory defect is statistically significant in a 2×2 table
4. That significance obtained in #3 persists when the proband has been eliminated from the analysis

Congenital Antithrombin Deficiency

Case Report

The propositus (IV-1, fig. 34.4) is an 18-year-old boy who had an unremarkable medical history until the age of 14, when he developed a right iliofemoral thrombosis during the course of a urinary tract infection. Two years later, he developed an acute pulmonary embolism, which responded poorly to heparin. Indeed, despite relatively high doses of heparin (40,000 units/day) he developed thrombophlebitis of the right calf. During this period, the whole blood clotting time, used to control heparin therapy, was in the range of 11–13 min, despite the hep-

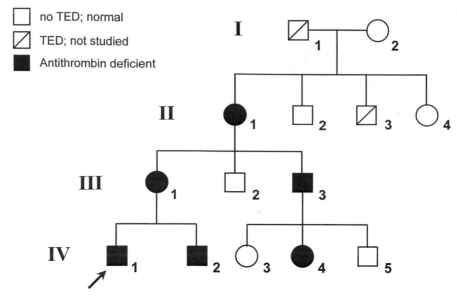

Figure 34.4. Four generations of a family with congenital antithrombin deficiency. The propositus is indicated by an *arrow* (IV-1).

arin infusion. Warfarin therapy was instituted, and the thromboembolic problems resolved. The patient was discharged and remains on continuous oral anticoagulant treatment.

Blood samples taken on admission revealed a normal full blood count and platelet count. The PT was 12 sec (11–13), aPTT was 43 sec (35–50), and thrombin time 19 sec (18–24). Plasma fibrinogen was 2.4 g/L (2–4). Levels of total and functional protein C and protein S were normal, and there was a normal aPTT response to activated protein C. Antithrombin (AT) activity, determined by a chromogenic (functional) assay was 42% (70–130). AT was also measured using an immunologic method (Laurell immunoelectrophoresis) and found to be 49% (70–130).

Family studies (34–fig. 34.4) revealed histories of thrombosis in the propositus' cousin (IV-4), mother (III-1), and maternal grandmother (II-1). These individuals also had reduced levels of AT activity. Several other family members also had a history of thromboembolic disease, and some were being treated with oral anticoagulants. A great-grandmother was known to have suffered from thrombosis and had died from pulmonary embolism some years previously. Affected family members had AT levels ranging from 40 to 54%; levels in unaffected relatives ranged from 82 to 106%.

The term "antithrombin" is rather a misnomer; AT is not only the main physiologic inhibitor of thrombin but also of all the other activated serine proteinase clotting enzymes (IXa, Xa, XIa, and XIIa). The importance of AT in the inhibition of blood coagulation is clearly demonstrated by the high incidence of venous thrombosis in patients with congenital AT deficiency (12). AT reacts irreversibly with thrombin and other serine proteinases to form a complex in which both components are inactivated. This reaction is greatly accelerated (about 2000-fold) by the presence of heparin, and this represents the molecular basis for the anticoagulant activity of heparin (13). Heparin promotes the formation of a ternary complex with antithrombin and thrombin in which the active site of the proteinase is brought into close contact with the reactive site of AT. The process of binding produces a conformational change in AT that further enhances heparin binding.

The reaction of heparin with AT is clearly of clinical significance in anticoagulant treatment. Thus, as in the case presented above, AT-deficient individuals do not respond well to heparin treatment, and heparin resistance may be a presenting feature of this condition. Heparin is not usually present in the vasculature, and the major physiologic role of AT must therefore be seen as regulating the generation of coagulation enzymes. Nevertheless, a similar mechanism may operate in vivo through heparan sulfate proteoglycans present on the surfaces of endothelial cells.

The first examples of congenital AT deficiency were reported in 1965 (14) in a Norwegian family with a history of recurrent venous thrombosis. Numerous other cases have since been identified. AT deficiency is inherited as an autosomal dominant and affects both sexes equally. The prevalence of this condition probably varies with the ethnic population studied but has been estimated to be of the order of 1/2000 to 1/5000 of the general population. The incidence of AT deficiency in young (<40 years) patients presenting with thrombosis is about 5%. Thrombosis is not universal among affected patients and about 40–50% are largely asymptomatic. Indeed, in one survey of Scottish blood donors, a sensitive heparin-binding assay revealed an incidence of AT deficiency of 1 in 350, most of whom were asymptomatic (15). In those with thrombosis, approximately 40% occurred spontaneously; the rest are related to specific events such as pregnancy, oral contraception, and surgery. Thrombosis in patients under 50 years of age is uncommon. The commonest sites for thrombosis are the deep leg veins, iliac and femoral veins, and the superficial veins of the legs. Arterial thrombosis is rare but can occur, especially in patients who are homozygous for AT variants with defective heparin-binding (see below).

There are two major forms of AT deficiency (12). Type I is the most common and, as illustrated by the case report above, is characterized by a parallel reduction of AT antigen and activity, typically to 40–60% of normal levels. Type II deficiency is a result of a specific molecular defect in the AT molecule; thus, circulating AT antigen levels are normal while the biologic activity is decreased. This classification can be expanded as shown in Table 34.2.

Molecular Basis of AT Deficiency

The polymerase chain reaction has given considerable impetus to the molecular definition of AT deficiency, and many different mutations have now been identified and characterized (16). Single-base substitutions within coding regions form the basis of all known type Ib and II variants. However, the nature and site of the amino acid substitution is critical in determining the resultant phenotype. Like the hemoglobinopathies, variant antithrombins are named after their place of discovery.

Type Ia deficiencies are due to mutations that result in a null allele. This is attributable to either a complete deletion of the entire gene or to other alterations such as nonsense mutations or base substitutions at splice sites. Type Ib variants often first appear to be type Ia but closer study shows that the AT antigen level is disproportionately higher than the activity level and that low levels of a variant molecule is present. The first of these variants to be described was AT Utah ($Pro_{407} \rightarrow Leu$) (17). Several other such variants have been identified and have a common defect in being unable to inactivate thrombin and having reduced heparin-binding affinity.

Table 34.2. Classification of Antithrombin Deficiency

Type I.   Reduced immunologic and functional AT
    Subtype Ia: Reduced levels of normal AT
    Subtype Ib: Reduced levels of AT and the presence of low levels of an AT variant
Type II. Normal immunologic but reduced functional AT
    Subtype IIa: Functional defect affecting both reactive and heparin-binding sites.
    Subtype IIb: Functional defect limited to the reactive site.
    Subtype IIc: Functional defect limited to the heparin-binding site.

Table 34.3. Some Examples of Type II Antithrombin Mutants Affecting Functional Activity

Functional Defect	Name	Thrombosis
Reduced heparin affinity	Rouen I	+
	Rouen III	+
Loss of heparin affinity	Toyama	+
	Geneva	+
Increased heparin affinity	Rouen II	−
	Truro	+
Defective thrombin inhibition	Glasgow III	−
	Hamilton	+
	Cambridge II	+

Type IIa and IIb variants are unable to inactivate proteinases. They generally have amino acid substitutions around the reactive site and can be further subdivided into two main groups. The first group comprises those cases with substitutions at the reactive site P1 position (e.g., ATs Northwick Park and Glasgow); the second involves the P12–P10 region (e.g., ATs Hamilton and Charleville). Some examples of type II mutants and the relationship of their functional defect to thrombosis are shown in Table 34.3.

Treatment of Antithrombin Deficiency

Since the biologic half-life of AT is relatively long (48 hours) plasma levels of this protein can be maintained by bolus injection (50 U/kg body weight) of commercially available AT concentrate. In congenitally deficient patients with baseline levels of about 50%, this procedure will elevate plasma levels to approximately 110–120%. Regular monitoring to maintain a level of at least 80% is advisable. Oral anticoagulants are very effective in preventing further thrombosis in congenital AT deficiency. Treatment should be continued for life. Individuals who are asymptomatic should not normally receive prophylactic anticoagulation unless they become predisposed to thrombosis by situations such as surgery and pregnancy.

Pregnancy poses a particular problem in management. Previously asymptomatic individuals should receive heparin therapy throughout pregnancy. Women with previous thrombotic episodes may benefit from AT replacement therapy; warfarin should not be given in the first 6 weeks of pregnancy. Thus, AT-deficient women receiving prophylactic warfarin should undergo regular pregnancy testing if conception is a possibility.

Congenital Protein C Deficiency

Protein C is one of the more recently discovered vitamin K–dependent hemostatic factors (18, 19). This protein plays a dual role in hemostasis by inhibiting blood coagulation on the one hand and stimulating fibrinolysis on the other. Protein C is activated by thrombin in the presence of calcium ions. However, this reaction takes place very slowly and is greatly accelerated by thrombomodulin on the surface of endothelial cells in a process analogous to the activation of the other vitamin K–dependent clotting factors. Thrombomodulin forms a complex with thrombin, which activates protein C. Once protein C is activated, it forms a 1:1 stoichiometric complex with another vitamin K–dependent protein, known as protein S, on endothelium, platelets, and possibly other cells (see below).

Activated protein C (APC) inhibits the coagulation cascade by proteolytically inactivating factors Va and VIIIa (18, 19). Initially, APC acts on factor Va bound to the platelet membrane, specifically cleaving peptide bonds in FVa and interfering with assembly of the prothrombinase complex. This process is modulated by FXa, which can bind to platelet-bound FVa and protect it from the action of APC. In addition to this effect, APC interferes with the regulation of the interaction between FIXa and FX on phospholipid membranes by destroying the biologic activity of FVIIIa.

Thus, APC prevents the generation of both FXa and thrombin, both key enzymes in the coagulation process. In addition, thrombin bound to thrombomodulin is no longer capable of activating factors V and VIII, cleaving fibrinogen, or aggregating platelets. Deficiency of protein C or its cofactor protein S (see below), therefore, allows coagulation to proceed relatively unchecked and thus predisposes to a thrombotic tendency.

Congenital deficiency of protein C was first described in 1981 (20), and numerous other cases have since been reported (21, 22). The defect is inherited as an autosomal dominant trait and, from a clinical standpoint, is virtually identical to congenital antithrombin deficiency. Approximately 75% of affected individuals have suffered one or more thrombotic episodes. Thrombosis occurs spontaneously in about 70% of patients; the remainder are triggered by risk factors such as pregnancy, oral contraceptives, and surgery. Clinical symptoms are rare in patients under 30 years of age, but the incidence of thromboembolic events climbs rapidly as subjects reach 50. Heterozygous protein C deficiency occurs in about 5% of patients with a previous history of thrombosis (23). The deficiency may be present in as many as 1/200–1/300 of the adult population, but relatively few of these individuals have a history of thromboembolic complications (24)—a finding borne out by family studies in protein C deficiency (25).

Protein C deficiency is also responsible for the occurrence of warfarin-induced skin necrosis, which typically, but rarely, occurs in the first few days of oral anticoagulant treatment. Interestingly, the dermal manifestations of this condition are very similar to those of infantile purpura fulminans, which is associated with very low levels of protein C (11).

Molecular Genetics of Protein C Deficiency

Using immunologic and functional assays for protein C, it is possible to classify patients as having type I or type II deficiencies. Type I is the most common and is characterized by a reduction in both antigenic and biologically active protein C. Patients with type II deficiency, in contrast, have normal total (immunologic) levels but reduced functional activity. In one study of 14 families with type I protein C deficiency, 3 had an entire deletion of the gene, while 2 had deletions or insertions of sequences. Most families probably have nonsense or missense point mutations (26).

Treatment of Protein C Deficiency

The acute management of thrombosis associated with protein C deficiency is the same as that in otherwise normal individuals. Large loading doses of oral anticoagulants, which may result in skin necrosis, should be avoided. Management of symptomatic subjects is via long-term oral anticoagulant therapy, and the indications and contraindications for this approach are the same as those for AT deficiency. Anabolic steroids such as stanozolol and danazol greatly increase protein C levels in patients with type I protein C deficiency (27). However, this does not prevent thrombosis, and there is evidence of increased clotting activation in protein C–deficient patients treated with stanazolol (28).

Congenital Protein S Deficiency

Congenital deficiency of protein S was described in 1984 in several families with a history of recurrent venous thrombosis (29, 30). The clinical presentation is similar to that in patients with protein C or antithrombin deficiencies. A slight majority of cases have spontaneous thrombotic episodes, while the remainder are apparently triggered by a recognizable risk factor in a similar manner to that seen in protein C deficiency.

Typically, affected individuals have approximately 50% of the normal level of protein S antigen and about 40% of normal levels of free protein S antigen and functional activity. A relatively high proportion of affected individuals have thromboembolic events including deep vein thrombosis (DVT), superficial thrombophlebitis, or pulmonary embolism.

Protein S is another member of the vitamin K–dependent clotting factors and has a molecular weight of 70,000. Functionally, protein S acts as a cofactor in the inactivation of factors Va and VIIIa by activated protein C. Normally, about 60% of the circulating protein S is bound to C4b-binding protein, and changes in the plasma level of the latter protein can alter the level of free, and thus anticoagulantly active, protein S. Since only this form can act as a cofactor for protein C, the C4-binding protein (C4b-BP) can regulate the function of this anticoagulant pathway.

Molecular Genetic Studies

Several workers have now cloned the human protein S cDNA, and the gene has been localized to chromosome 3 (31). There are two highly homologous genes for protein S. The active gene (PSalpha) contains 15 exons, while the pseudogene (PSbeta) contains a number of splice site, nonsense, and missense mutations that render gene expression impossible (11).

Protein S deficiency appears to be an important risk factor for venous thrombosis, and many reports have documented heterozygous (type I) protein S deficiency in association with recurrent thromboembolism (32). It is one of the more common known causes of familial thrombophilia, accounting for about 5% of subjects with a history of thrombosis. In type I deficiency, the total amount of protein S is reduced, which (as most is bound to C4b-BP) results in low levels of free protein S. Molecular genetic analysis has identified a partial protein S gene deletion in some kindreds. Another form of hereditary deficiency state (type II) has been reported in which total protein S antigen is normal, but levels of free protein S and protein S functional activity are reduced. The molecular basis of this defect remains unclear, but it may result from a molecular abnormality in either protein S or C4b-BP (33). Severe, homozygous protein S deficiency has also been reported. Parents of these individuals appeared to have the classic protein S deficiency state. Type III deficiency, which is less common, results from altered binding of C4b-BP and protein S. The equilibrium between free and bound protein S is shifted toward the bound form, resulting in low levels of free protein S (33).

Clinically, protein S deficiency is indistinguishable from that of protein C. Venous thromboembolism, thrombophlebitis, and deep vein thrombosis account for most of the thrombotic events. Thrombosis often occurs at a relatively young age; two-thirds of patients have experienced a thrombotic event by the age of 35. Warfarin-induced skin necrosis has been reported in several patients with protein S deficiency (34).

Treatment of Congenital Protein S Deficiency

Congenital protein S deficiency in patients with a history of thrombosis is effectively treated with prophylactic oral anticoagulants in a similar manner to deficiencies of antithrombin and protein C. Heparin therapy is useful in the management of acute thrombotic episodes. Steroids do not increase protein S levels (unlike those of protein C) and are therefore not useful in treatment.

Congenital Resistance to Activated Protein C

Case Report

A 49-year-old male was referred for investigations with a history of multiple venous thromboses, mainly affecting the deep veins of the legs, since he was 17 years old. These episodes were treated with oral anticoagulants for periods up to 6 months. Apart from the thrombotic events, his previous medical history was unremarkable. Family history revealed that several relatives also had histories of venous thromboses; both parents were deceased. Initial laboratory tests revealed:

Antithrombin	*102% (70–130)*
Protein C	*100% (70–130)*
Protein S	*94% (70–130)*
Plasminogen	*97% (70–130)*
Thrombin time	*23.5 sec (20–25)*
Lupus anticoagulant	*Not detected*

An aPTT-based method was used to assess the response of the patient's plasma to APC. Because of the anticoagulant action of APC, its addition to plasma normally prolongs the aPTT. Results are expressed as a ratio (with APC:without APC). In this case, the APC-resistance test gave a result of 1.5 (normal, 2.0–4.0). The poor anticoagulant response to APC is illustrated in Figure 34.5.

This patient had a strong personal and family history of venous thromboembolism but was negative for all the hitherto most common hereditary coagulation inhibitor defects. However, his plasma was not significantly anticoagulated by the addition of activated protein C. A similar defect was subsequently found in those family members with a similar history of DVT, thus establishing the familial nature of the defect.

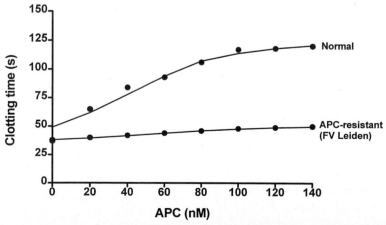

Figure 34.5. Poor anticoagulant response of the aPTT to the addition of activated protein C in a patient with congenital resistance to this inhibitor.

Congenital resistance to activated protein C is a relatively newly recognized cause of recurrent venous thrombosis (35) and now appears to be the single most common basis for congenital thrombophilia. Among patients presenting with thrombosis, APC resistance is present in approximately 20–40% (35–38); in subjects in whom deficiencies of AT, protein C, and protein S have already been excluded, the incidence may be as high as 50% (39). In women with thrombosis during pregnancy the incidence was 60% (40). There is also general agreement that this defect is present in about 4–5% of apparently normal individuals (41). In many cases, possession of the abnormal gene may be asymptomatic until some other triggering factor (e.g., surgery, pregnancy, oral contraceptives) is also present. The high prevalence also means that patients heterozygous for both APC resistance and other inhibitor defects (AT, protein C, etc.) can and do occur (42). Thus it is important to perform these investigations in patients shown to be APC-resistant.

The defect was originally thought to be due to the congenital deficiency of a previously unrecognized cofactor to protein C (35). However, it is now established that the molecular defect lies in an amino acid substitution at one of the APC cleavage sites on the factor V (FV) molecule. In APC-resistant individuals, the Arg residue at position 506 has been replaced by Gln (41, 43). Thus, APC does not recognize a major cleavage site on FV, and prothrombin activation continues relatively unchecked. This molecular defect has been termed FV Leiden (41) and accounts for approximately 90% of patients with APC resistance (44). Heterozygotes for FV Leiden have a 7-fold increase in their risk of thrombosis (36). Homozygotes appear to have a greatly increased (probably >20-fold) propensity to thrombosis. The high prevalence of the FV Leiden gene in the normal population suggests that it may have conferred some selective advantage during evolution (40).

Heparin Cofactor II Deficiency

Heparin cofactor II (HC II) is a plasma glycoprotein of molecular weight 65,500 that acts as an inhibitor of thrombin. Its activity is greatly stimulated by the presence of glycosaminoglycans such as dermatan sulfate and heparin (45). HC II appears to function as a "suicide" substrate by mimicking the cleavage site of thrombin and forming a stable stoichiometric complex with this serine proteinase.

The role of HC II in normal hemostasis remains to be determined. A role as a natural inhibitor of coagulation is suggested by the finding of thrombosis in two pedigrees with only 50% levels of HC II (46, 47). Others, however, have suggested that HC II deficiency is not a common cause of thrombosis (48). There is presently no evidence of an association between inherited HC II deficiency and a predisposition to thrombosis, and it would therefore not appear to be a risk factor for thrombophilia.

Tissue Factor Pathway Inhibitor Deficiency

The existence of an inhibitor of TF was suggested by the early observation that the procoagulant activity of tissue extracts could be inhibited by serum (49). It is now known that plasma contains an inhibitor that binds and inhibits factor Xa directly (50). Since 1991, this inhibitor has been known as TFPI, although in older literature it is also referred to as extrinsic pathway inhibitor (EPI) and lipoprotein-associated coagulation inhibitor (LACI).

In plasma, TFPI circulates bound to lipoproteins, mainly the low-density type. Platelets contain about 10% of the blood pool of TFPI, and this can be released by thrombin stimulation. Plasma TFPI levels increase 2- to 4-fold during heparin infusion. This additional TFPI appears to be bound to heparan sulfate and similar molecules on the surface of endothelial cells, the site of synthesis of this inhibitor. The liver does not appear to contribute significantly to the synthesis of TFPI.

TFPI works by binding to and inhibiting factor Xa activity. The TFPI-FXa complex then binds to the TF-FVIIa complex thereby blocking its proteolytic activity. Even in the absence of factor Xa, TFPI may bind and inhibit the TF-VIIa complex, but the reaction requires about 100 times more TFPI than in the presence of factor Xa. The role of TFPI in the modern concept of coagulation is discussed above; however, relatively little is known about the effect of TFPI deficiency on the hemostatic system. It seems surprising that despite extensive screening of individuals with thrombotic disease (51), no cases of TFPI deficiency have been identified. There may be several reasons for this: (*a*) congenital TFPI deficiency may be incompatible with life; (*b*) TFPI might not as important as is currently thought; and (*c*) current assays of TFPI might not permit the identification of the condition.

Whether TF is involved in the pathogenesis of venous thrombosis is not known. Even if TF is the initial trigger for this event, it may not play a role in its further propagation. TFPI may therefore not be important in preventing venous thromboembolism. In contrast, rupture of arteriosclerotic plaques exposes TF, and this is probably the trigger for subsequent arterial thrombosis (52). TFPI may therefore be an important control mechanism in this situation. Recombinant TFPI has been shown to prevent postthrombolysis reocclusion in a dog model of vascular-induced arterial thrombotic occlusion (53). TFPI appears to act more as a limiter of disseminated intravascular coagulation than of local thrombosis. TF exposed on the surfaces of activated blood monocytes is an important trigger of disseminated intravascular coagulation. Artificially induced TFPI deficiency greatly increases the susceptibility to TF-induced coagulopathy (54), whereas elevating plasma TFPI levels protects against the intravascular coagulation induced by infusion of tissue thromboplastin (55) or endotoxin (56).

Congenital Dysfibrinogenemia

Dysfibrinogenemia may be defined as a molecular defect of the fibrinogen molecule. Like the hemoglobinopathies, the dysfibrinogenemias are named after their place of discovery. Well over 100 cases of congenital dysfibrinogenemia have been described. Many of these are asymptomatic, but a proportion have been associated with a bleeding or a thrombotic tendency. Some authors have suggested that this condition accounts for approximately 1% of unexplained venous thrombosis in young adults (57). Thrombosis occurs in a minority of affected subjects, and it seems likely that this is related to the specific molecular defect involved. Thrombosis may be either venous or arterial, and some abnormal fibrinogens have been associated with both bleeding and thrombosis (58).

The reason(s) for thrombosis associated with congenital dysfibrinogenemia remains unclear. Fibrinogen Oslo I clots more rapidly with thrombin, but fibrinogen New York I is poorly clottable, despite its association with thromboembolic disease. However, the latter interacts poorly with t-PA or plasminogen, which could explain the thrombotic tendency. Other abnormal molecules, such as fibrinogens Dusard and Chapel Hill III, form clots that are poorly lysed. Despite the obvious interest in the congenital dysfibrinogenemias as structure-function models, it seems unlikely that they account for a significant proportion of cases of familial thrombophilia.

Factor XII Deficiency

Patients with congenital FXII deficiency have markedly prolonged aPTTs but exhibit a distinct lack of a hemorrhagic tendency. As illustrated by the original patient, John Hageman, these individuals may have a thrombotic tendency. This may be due to impaired fibrinolytic activation by the contact activation system, but detailed family and mechanistic studies are presently lacking.

Abnormalities of Plasminogen

Congenital plasminogen deficiency is a relatively rare disorder, inherited as an autosomal recessive trait. It occurs in both type I (absence of gene product) and type II (dysfunctional) forms. Clinically, the disorder is similar to deficiencies of AT and protein C. Thromboembolic complications seem to develop by about 20 years of age, and DVT and PE are the most common events.

Although levels of functional plasminogen below 40% appear to predispose toward thrombosis, the relationship of plasminogen defects to thrombosis remains ill-defined, since in all reported kindreds, thrombosis was confined to the propositus (11). In one study of unrelated families with type I plasminogen deficiency, only a few affected individuals had a history of thrombosis, and there was no differ-

ence in the incidence of thrombosis between normal controls and subjects with congenital plasminogen deficiency (59). This does not support a correlation between type I plasminogen deficiency and thrombosis. Similar criticisms can be leveled against type II deficiency (dysplasminogenemia). Thus, the congenital plasminogen defects do not satisfy the criteria required to establish a causal relationship between the laboratory abnormalities and familial thrombosis outlined earlier in this chapter.

Acquired Predisposition to Thrombosis

Acquired Deficiencies of Natural Anticoagulants

Antithrombin

AT is synthesized in the liver and is therefore decreased in a variety of hepatic disorders; most commonly, acute liver failure and cirrhosis. This is not usually associated with a thrombotic tendency, since levels of the procoagulant clotting factors are generally reduced in parallel. AT is often reduced in patients with disseminated intravascular coagulation (chap. 33) due to consumption coagulopathy and may be diagnostically useful in this condition. AT falls after surgical procedures, reaching a nadir around the third postoperative day, and is proportional to the degree of surgical trauma (60). Acquired AT deficiency may also arise in inflammatory bowel disease and protein-losing enteropathy (12). Such patients have other evidence of hypercoagulability and have a definite thrombotic tendency to which the AT deficiency contributes. AT is lost in the urine in patients with nephrotic syndrome, although the thrombotic tendency in this disorder is probably multifactorial. Other conditions in which acquired deficiencies of AT may occur include cardiopulmonary bypass and dialysis (dilutional effects), treatment with estrogens, heparin and L-asparaginase, diabetes, and malnutrition (12, 61).

Proteins S and C

The protein C inhibitor pathway may be altered by disease states in several ways. Protein C and S depend on vitamin K for their synthesis. They therefore tend to decrease together with factors II, VII, IX, and X in conditions of vitamin K absence or antagonism, thus maintaining the balance between procoagulant and anticoagulant effects. However, in major inflammatory events, agents such as interleukins, tumor necrosis factor, and endotoxin may suppress the express of thrombomodulin on the endothelial cell surface. Coupled with the production of TF stimulated by the same agents, this gives rise to a marked procoagulant state (62).

Lupus Anticoagulants

Lupus anticoagulants (LAs) are immunoglobulins that interfere with those coagulation reactions that depend on phospholipids, e.g., the activation of factor X and prothrombin. LAs may occur in up to 10% of patients with systemic lupus erythematosus (SLE). LAs are common in HIV-positive subjects and may be associated with scleroderma. They are also associated with recurrent fetal loss (63). Some patients with LAs develop a bleeding tendency, but a greater number have an increased tendency toward thrombosis. Thromboembolism occurs in about 10% of patients with SLE, but this incidence rises to 30–50% in those patients who also have LAs. Although LAs may be associated with renal microvascular thrombosis, they are more often associated with DVT and pulmonary embolism. LAs are most often detected in the laboratory by use of the aPTT. However, commercial aPTT reagents vary in their sensitivity, and a number of alternative tests for LA detection have been developed (table 34.4).

LAs appear to be related to antiphospholipid (aPL) antibodies (64) and can be difficult to distinguish from other inhibitors. aPL (or anticardiolipin) antibodies have been associated with both venous and arterial thrombosis, recurrent fetal loss, and thrombocytopenia and are distinct from LAs. Their mechanism of action is unknown but may include interference with (a) endothelial cell prostacyclin release, (b) protein C activity via thrombomodulin or protein S, (c) antithrombin, (d) platelet membrane phospholipid, (e) prekallikrein activation, and (f) endothelial release of t-PA (65). Many of these reactions depend on phospholipid. Understanding the mechanisms in autoimmune LA-related thrombosis may enable study of the great majority of unexplained thrombotic episodes not due to known risk factors such as deficiency of AT, proteins C and S, and resistance to activated protein C.

Malignant Disease

Abnormalities of hemostasis have been known to occur in association with malignant disease for over 100 years (66). An early study of blood changes in patients with cancer suggested that the bleeding time was accelerated in most cases (67). Since these classic observations, the literature on this subject has become considerable, and the interested reader is referred to several recent reviews for more detailed coverage of this area (68–72).

Thromboembolic events are common in patients with solid tumors (69, 72). Venous thrombosis, in one form or another, occurs in over 50% of affected patients (73) and may precede diagnosis of the malignant disease (74). Many patients may also suffer arterial thrombosis or embolic complications (73), commonly in cerebral vessels, spleen,

Table 34.4. Screening Tests for Lupus Anticoagulants

Surface-activated clotting times (aPTT, KCCT)
Contact product-activated aPTT
Dilute tissue thromboplastin inhibition test (DRVVT)
Dilute Russell's viper venom time (DRVVT)
Factor Xa–activated aPTT
Taipan venon time (TVT)

kidney, and peripheral arteries. The recognition that thrombosis may be an early symptom of malignant disease has prompted some authors to suggest that unexplained thrombophlebitis, especially in relatively unusual sites, should prompt regular searches for underlying cancer (75). It is certainly reasonable to strongly consider this possibility in patients with unexplained thrombosis in sites such as upper extremity or hepatic vein or in those with recurrent migratory thrombophlebitis, especially in younger individuals (under 40 years) (75). The clinical manifestations of clotting activation in patients with cancer are highly variable and range from diffuse multiple thrombosis on the one hand to acute hemorrhage on the other. Thrombotic complications are more common than bleeding, but many more patients have only laboratory evidence of coagulation activation.

In the clinical laboratory, hypercoagulability may be manifested by shortened prothrombin and activated partial thromboplastin times. However, this is relatively uncommon and does not correlate with any particular thrombotic event. Studies in the author's laboratory have revealed that a significant proportion of patients with breast (20%) and colon cancer (65%) had accelerated clotting of whole blood when assessed by a viscoelastic technique (76). More detailed laboratory workups will reveal evidence of clotting activation in an even higher proportion of patients. Fibrinogen and platelet survival is decreased, reflecting an increased catabolic rate (77), and this is accompanied by increased levels of molecular markers of clotting activation such as fibrinopeptide A, thrombin-antithrombin complexes, and prothrombin F1.2. (70, 78–81). These findings are compatible with the presence of low-grade and usually well-compensated disseminated intravascular coagulation (see also chap. 33). These abnormalities are frequently accompanied by decreases in the natural inhibitors of coagulation antithrombin, protein C, and protein S (71).

The mechanism of hypercoagulability in malignant disease is complex and variable. Many malignant tumors possess procoagulant activity that can accelerate coagulation in vitro (82–84), although the role of tumor-derived procoagulants in hypercoagulability in vivo is less easy to establish. Evidence from studies in the author's laboratory using animal models, however, suggests that this is a likely pathway of clotting activation (85). Peripheral blood monocytes in cancer patients may be "activated" and express TF on their surfaces, and this appears to correlate with the degree of clotting activation (86, 87). The role of monocyte TF expression in triggering intravascular coagulation is given more detailed consideration elsewhere in this volume. Most malignant tumor cells express *Cancer Procoagulant*, a cysteine proteinase that can activate factor X directly (88, 89). Whether this can contribute to hypercoagulability and thrombosis has not yet been proven.

Treatment of the coagulopathy associated with malignant disease depends on the clinical manifestation of the defect. Like other causes of DIC (chap. 33), successful treatment depends ultimately on removal of the underlying trigger. In the absence of clinical complications, treating the coagulopathy is not indicated. Heparin is useful for the treatment of thrombotic complications, while oral anticoagulants may be beneficial for patients with stable tumor burdens. Warfarin is not very efficacious in preventing recurrence of thrombosis in cancer patients, however (73). Thus, recurrent thrombosis, especially with increasing tumor load requires long-term heparin therapy. Antiplatelet agents may be helpful in individuals who do not respond well to heparin (90).

Laboratory Investigation of Thrombophilia

As alluded to above, the laboratory investigation of thrombophilia is rapidly becoming as comprehensive as that of a bleeding tendency. The initial work up is similar and consists of routine hematologic and coagulation screening. The diagnosis of congenital thrombophilia requires detailed medical and family histories and careful exclusion of secondary disease. It should be emphasized that laboratory investigation cannot reliably be undertaken during episodes of acute thromboembolism, when levels of natural coagulation inhibitors are often reduced, during pregnancy, or while the patient is receiving oral anticoagulants.

If underlying disease that may predispose to thrombosis can be excluded, it is worth proceeding to systematic assay of natural inhibitors and determining the patient's resistance to activated protein C. Commercial kits are available for this purpose and are readily automated. It should be emphasized that resistance to activated protein C may give falsely decreased levels of functional protein S (91, 92), and patients previously diagnosed with PS deficiency should therefore be reevaluated. This should be followed by a search for lupus anticoagulant and/or antiphospholipid antibodies. Only if these tests are negative is it worth attempting to exclude the more esoteric (and unlikely) causes of thrombophilia (table 34.5).

Summary

The laboratory investigation of thromboembolic states has recently received fresh impetus, and an increasing proportion of patients with familial thrombosis can now be identified as having a specific congenital defect of the hemostatic system. Numerically, the most important of these is the newly recognized resistance to activated protein C syndrome, and this may lead to the recognition of further players in this important inhibitory pathway. At our current level of understanding, approximately 60% of patients with familial thrombophilia can be explained. The remainder are still a diagnostic challenge, but it seems reasonable to suppose that other, presently unrecognized, defects exist and that study of such individuals will contribute to our understanding of the hemostatic mechanism.

Table 34.5. Laboratory Investigation of Thrombophilia[a]

Screening tests
   Full blood count and platelet count
   Routine coagulation screening (PT, aPTT)
   Thrombin and reptilase clotting times
   Fibrinogen assay
Specific (high-priority) assays
   Resistance to activated protein C (modified aPTT) assay)
      (confirmation of FV Leiden by PCR analysis)
   Protein C (functional and immunologic assays)
   Protein S (functional and immunologic assays)
   Antithrombin (functional and immunologic assays)
   Lupus anticoagulant and antiphospholipid antibodies
Specific (low-priority) assays
   Heparin cofactor II
   Tissue plasminogen-activator release from endothelium
   Plasminogen antigen and activity
   Tests for dysfibrinogenemia

[a]Antithrombin, protein C, and protein S assays should be performed by functional assays first; confirmation and classification (type I or type II) requires subsequent immunologic determinations. Assays of proteins C and S and the original aPTT-based method of APC resistance cannot be performed reliably in patients receiving oral anticoagulants. The diagnosis of APC resistance should always be confirmed and classified (heterozygote or homozygote) by the polymerase chain reaction (PCR) test 41.

REFERENCES

1. Broze GJ. Tissue factor pathway inhibitor and the revised hypothesis of blood coagulation. Trend Cardiovasc Med 1992; 2:72.
2. Broze GJ, Gailani D. The role of factor XI in coagulation. Thromb Haemost 1993;70:72.
3. Francis JL. Detection and measurement of factor XIII. In: Francis JL, ed. Fibrinogen, fibrin stabilization and fibrinolysis. Chichester: Ellis Horwood, 1988:203.
4. Roath S, Francis JL. Normal blood coagulation, fibrinolysis and natural inhibitors of coagulation. In: Uppington J, ed. International Anesthesiology Clinics. Coagulation disorders and the hemoglobinopathies. Boston: Little, Brown & Co, 1985:23.
5. Brommer EJP, Brakman P. Developments in fibrinolysis. In: Poller L, ed. Recent advances in blood coagulation. Edinburgh: Churchill Lingstone, 1991:17.
6. Collen D, Lijnen HR. Molecular and cellular basis of fibrinolysis. In: Hoffman R, et al. Hematology: basic principles and practice. New York: Churchill Livingstone, 1991:1232.
7. Machovich R, Owen WG. The elastase-mediated pathway of fibrinolysis. Blood Coag Fibrinol 1990;1:79.
8. Heijboer H, Tencate JW, Buller HR. Diagnosis of venous thrombosis. Semin Thromb Hemost 1991;17:259.
9. Henkin J, Marcotte P, Yang HC. The plasminogen-plasmin system. Prog Cardiovasc Dis 1991;34:135.
10. Heijboer H, Brandjes DPM, Buller HR, et al. Deficiencies of coagulation-inhibiting and fibrinolytic proteins in outpatients with deep vein thrombosis. N Engl J Med 1990; 323:1512.
11. Preston FE, Briet E. Familial thrombosis. In: Brenner MK, Hoffbrand AV, eds. Recent advances in haematology. Edinburgh: Churchill Livingstone, 1993:217.
12. Lane DA, Olds RR, Thein S-L. Antithrombin and its deficiency states. Blood Coag Fibrinol 1992;3:315.

13. Barrowcliffe TW, Thomas DP. Antithrombin III and heparin. In: Haemostasis and thrombosis. Edited by Bloom AL, Thomas DP, eds. Edinburgh: Churchill Livingstone, 1987:849.

14. Egeberg O. Inherited antithrombin deficiency causing thrombophilia. Thromb Diath Haemorrh 1965;13:516.

15. Tait RC, Walker ID, Perry DJ, Carrell RW, Islam SIA, et al. Prevalence of antithrombin III deficiency subtypes in 4000 healthy blood donors [Abstract]. Thromb Haemost 1991; 65:839.

16. Lane DA, et al. Antithrombin III: a database of mutations. Thromb Haemost 1991;66:657.

17. Bock SC, Marrian JA, Radziejewska E. Antithrombin III Utah: proline 407 to leucine mutation in a highly conserved region near the inhibitor reactive site. Biochemistry 1988; 27:6171.

18. Esmon CT. The protein-C anticoagulant pathway. Arterioscler Thromb 1992;12:135.

19. Walker FJ, Fay PJ. Regulation of blood coagulation by the protein-C system. FASEB J 1992;6:2561.

20. Griffin JH, et al. Deficiency of protein C in congenital thrombotic disease. J Clin Invest 1981;68:1370.

21. Bertina RM, Broekmans AW, Van der Linden IK, Mertens K. Protein C deficiency in a Dutch family with thrombotic disease. Thromb Haemost 1982;48:1.

22. Mannucci PM, Owen WG. Basic and clinical aspects of proteins C and S. In: Bloom AL, Thomas DP, eds. Haemostasis and thrombosis. Edinburgh: Churchill Livingstone, 1987:452.

23. Gladson CL, et al. The frequency of type I heterozygous protein S and protein C deficiency in 141 unrelated young patients with venous thrombosis. Thromb Haemost 1988; 59:18.

24. Miletich J, Sherman L, Broze G. Absence of thrombosis in subjects with heterozygous protein C deficiency. N Engl J Med 1987;317:991.

25. Bovill EG, et al. The clinical spectrum of heterozygous protein C deficiency in a large New England kindred. Blood 1989;73:712.

26. Bauer KA. Pathobiology of the hypercoagulable state: clinical features, laboratory evaluation, and management. In: Hoffman R, et al. Hematology. Basic principles and practice. New York: Churchill Livingstone, 1991:1415.

27. Gonzales R, Alberca I, Sala N, Vicente V. Protein C deficiency—response to danazolol and DDAVP. Thromb Haemost 1985;53:320.

28. Broekmans AW, et al. Treatment of hereditary protein C deficiency with stanozolol. Thromb Haemost 1987;57:20.

29. Comp PC, Esmon CT. Recurrent venous thromboembolism in patients with a partial deficiency of protein S. N Engl J Med 1984;311:1525.

30. Schwartz HP, et al. Protein S deficiency in familial thrombotic disease. Blood 1984;64:1297.

31. Ploos van Amstel JK, et al. Two genes homologous with protein S cDNA are located on chromosome 3. Thromb Haemost 1987;58:982.

32. Engesser L, et al. Hereditary protein S deficiency: clinical manifestations. Ann Intern Med 1987;106:677.

33. Comp PC, Doray D, Patton D, Esmon CT. An abnormal plasma distribution of protein S occurs in functional protein S deficiency. Blood 1986;67:504.

34. Moreb J, Kitchens CS. Acquired functional protein S deficiency, cerebral venous thrombosis and coumarin skin necro-

sis in association with antiphospholipid syndrome: report of two cases. Am J Med 1989;87:207.

35. Dahlback B, Carlsson M, Svensson PJ. Familial thrombophilia due to a previously unrecognized mechanism characterized by poor anticoagulant response to activated protein C: prediction of a cofactor to activated protein C. Proc Natl Acad Sci USA 1993;90:1004.

36. Koster T, et al. Venous thrombosis due to poor anticoagulant response to activated protein C: Leiden Thrombophilia Study [see comments]. Lancet 1993;342:1503.

37. Halbmayer WM, Haushofer A, Schon R, Fischer M. The prevalence of poor anticoagulant response to activated protein C (APC resistance) among patients suffering from stroke or venous thrombosis and among healthy subjects. Blood Coag Fibrinol 1994;5:51.

38. Svensson PJ, Dahlback B. Resistance to activated protein C as a basis for venous thrombosis [see comments]. N Engl J Med 1994;330:517.

39. Griffin JH, Evatt B, Wideman C, Fernandez JA. Anticoagulant protein C pathway defective in majority of thrombophilic patients. Blood 1993;82:1989.

40. Dahlback B. Physiological anticoagulation. Resistance to activated protein C and venous thromboembolism. J Clin Invest 1994;94:923.

41. Bertina RM, et al. Mutation in blood coagulation factor V associated with resistance to activated protein C [see comments]. Nature 1994;369:64.

42. Koeleman BPC, Reitsma PH, Allaart CF, Bertina RM. Activated protein C resistance as an additional risk factor for thrombosis in protein C-deficient families. Blood 1994; 84:1031.

43. Emmerich J, et al. A new cause of familial hypercoagulable state: activated protein C resistance. Presse Med 1994; 23:1285.

44. Dahlbüack B. Factor V gene mutation causing inherited resistance to activated protein C as a basis for venous thromboembolism. J Intern Med 1995;237:221.

45. Tollefson DM, Blank MK. Detection of a new heparin-dependent inhibitor of thrombin in human plasma. J Clin Invest 1981;68:589.

46. Sie P, Dupouy D, Pichon J, Boneu B. Constitutional heparin cofactor II deficiency associated with recurrent thrombosis. Lancet, 1985;ii:414.

47. Tran TH, Marbet GA, Duckert F. Association of hereditary heparin cofactor II deficiency with thrombosis. Lancet 1985; ii:413.

48. Betina RM, et al. Hereditary heparin cofactor II deficiency and the risk of development of venous thrombosis. Thromb Haemost 1987;57:196.

49. Schneider CL. The active principle of placental toxin: thromboplastin; its inactivation in blood: antithromboplastin. Am J Physiol 1947;149:123.

50. Broze GJ, et al. The lipoprotein-associated coagulation inhibitor that inhibits the factor VII-tissue factor complex also inhibits factor Xa: insight into its possible mechanism of action. Blood 1988;71:335.

51. Novotny WF, et al. Plasma antigen levels of the lipoprotein-associated coagulation inhibitor in patient samples. Blood 1991;78:387.

52. Wilcox JN, Smith KM, Schwartz SM, Gordon D. Localization of tissue factor in the normal vessel wall and in the atherosclerotic plaque. Proc Natl Acad Sci USA 1989; 86:2839.

53. Haskel EJ, et al. Prevention of arterial reocclusion after thrombolysis with recombinant lipoprotein associated coagulation inhibitor. Circulation 1991;84:821.

54. Sandset PM, Warncramer BJ, Maki SL, Rapaport SI. Immunodepletion of extrinsic pathway inhibitor sensitizes rabbits to endotoxin-induced intravascular coagulation and the generalized Shwartzman reaction. Blood 1991; 78:1496.

55. Day KC, Hoffman LC, Palmier MO, et al. Recombinant lipoprotein-associated coagulation inhibitor inhibits tissue thromboplastin induced intravascular coagulation in the rabbit. Blood 1990;76:1538.

56. Brenengard C, et al. The effect of two-domain tissue factor pathway inhibitor on endotoxin-induced disseminated intravascular coagulation in rabbits. Blood Coag Fibrinol 1993; 4:699.

57. Sakariassen KS, Barstad RM. Mechanisms of thromboembolism at arterial plaques. Blood Coag Fibrinol 1993; 4:615.

58. Mammen EF. Congenital coagulation protein disorders. In: Bick RL, et al., eds. Hematology. Clinical and laboratory practice. St Louis: Mosby—Year Book, 1993:1391.

59. Shigekiyo T, Uno Y, Tomonari A, et al. Type I congenital plasminogen deficiency is not a risk factor for thrombosis. Thromb Haemost 1992;67:189.

60. Hoffmann R. The thrombo-embolic risk in surgery. Hepatogastroenterology 1991;38:272.

61. von Kaulla E, Droegemueller W, von Kaulla KN. Conjugated estrogens and hypercoagulability. Am J Obstet Gynecol 1975;122:688.

62. Stern DM, Kaiser E, Nawroth PP. Regulation of the coagulation system by vascular endothelial cells. Haemostasis 1988;18:202.

63. Feinstein DI. Lupus anticoagulant, thrombosis and fetal loss. N Engl J Med 1985;313:1348.

64. McNeil P, Chesterman CN, Krilis SA. Immunology and clinical importance of antiphospholipid syndrome. Adv Immunol 1991;49:193.

65. Bick RL. Hypercoagulability and thrombosis. In: Bick RL, et al., eds. Hematology. Clinical and laboratory practice. St Louis: Mosby—Year Book, 1993:1555.

66. Trousseau A. Phlegmasia alba dolens. In: Clinique Médicale de l'Hôtel Dieu de Paris. London: The New Sydenham Society, 1865;3:94.

67. Morrison M. An analysis of the blood picture in 100 cases of malignancy. J Lab Clin Med 1932;17:1071.

68. Davis RB, Theologides A, Kennedy BJ. Comparative studies of blood coagulation and platelet aggregation in patients with cancer and non-malignant diseases. Ann Intern Med 1969; 71:67.

69. Dvorak HF. Thrombosis and cancer. Hum Pathol 1987; 18:275.

70. Rickles FR, Levine M, Edwards RL. Hemostatic alterations in cancer patients. Cancer Metastasis Rev 1992;11:237.

71. Bick RL. Alterations of hemostasis in malignancy. In: Bick RL, et al., eds. Hematology. Clinical and laboratory practice. St Louis: Mosby—Year Book, 1993:1583.

72. Naschitz JE, Yeshurun D, Lev LM. Thromboembolism in cancer—changing trends. Cancer 1993;71:1384.

73. Sack GH, Levin J, Bell WR. Trousseau's syndrome and other manifestations of chronic DIC in patients with neoplasms. Medicine 1977;56:1.

74. Gore JM, et al. Occult cancer in patients with acute pulmonary embolism. Ann Intern Med 1982;96:556.

75. Goldberg RJ, et al. Occult malignant neoplasm in patients with deep venous thrombosis. Arch Intern Med 1987; 147:251.

76. Francis JL, Francis DA, Gunathilagan GJ. Assessment of hypercoagulability in patients with cancer using the Sonoclot analyzer and thromboelastography. Thromb Res 1994; 74:335.

77. Slichter SJ, Harker LA. Haemostasis in malignancy. Ann NY Acad Sci 1974;230:252.

78. Peuscher FW, et al. Significance of plasma fibrinopeptide A (FPA) in patients with malignancy. J Lab Clin Med 1980; 96:5.

79. Edwards RL, et al. Activation of blood coagulation in Crohn's disease. Increased plasma fibrinopeptide A levels and enhanced generation of monocyte tissue factor activity. Gastroenterology 1987;92:329.

80. Gabazza EC, et al. Evaluating prethrombotic state in lung cancer using molecular markers. Chest 1993;103:196.

81. Seitz R, et al. Activation of coagulation and fibrinolysis in patients with lung cancer—relation to tumour stage and prognosis. Blood Coag Fibrinol 1993;4:249.

82. Francis JL, El-Baruni K, Roath OS, Taylor I. Factor X-activating activity in normal and malignant colorectal tissue. Thromb Res 1988;52:207.

83. El-Baruni K, Taylor I, Roath OS, Francis JL. Factor X-activating procoagulant in normal and malignant breast tissue. Hematol Oncol 1990;8:323.

84. Adamson AS, Luckert P, Pollard M, Snell ME, Amirkhosravi M, Francis JL. Procoagulant activity may be a marker of the malignant phenotype in experimental prostate cancer. Br J Cancer 1994;69:286.

85. Amirkhosravi M, Francis JL. Procoagulant effects of the MC28 fibrosarcoma cell line in vitro and in vivo. Br J Haematol 1993;85:736.

86. Edwards RL, Rickles FR, Cronlund M. Abnormalities of blood coagulation in patients with cancer. Mononuclear cell tissue factor generation. J Lab Clin Invest 1981;98:917.

87. Morgan D, Edwards RL, Rickles FR. Monocyte procoagulant activity as a peripheral blood marker of clotting activation in cancer patients. Haemostasis 1988;18:55.

88. Gordon SG, Franks JJ, Lewis B. Cancer procoagulant: a factor X-activating procoagulant from malignant tissue. Thromb Res 1975;6:127.

89. Gordon SG, Cross BA. A factor X-activating cysteine protease from malignant tissue. J Clin Invest 1981;67:1665.

90. Bick RL. Alterations of haemostasis associated with malignancy. Etiology, pathophysiology, diagnosis and management. Semin Thromb Hemost 1978;5:1.

91. Faioni EM, et al. Resistance to activated protein C in nine thrombophilic families: interference in a protein S functional assay. Thromb Haemost 1993;70:1067.

92. Cooper PC, et al. Further evidence that activated protein C resistance can be misdiagnosed as inherited functional protein S deficiency. Br J Haematol 1994;88:201.

CHAPTER 35

Fibrinolytic Disorders

KENNETH C. ROBBINS

In habitual or frequent bleeding at the nose, it will be necessary to give a brisk purgative, repeated occasionally, and make use of measures to equalize the circulation. Keep the feet warm and the head cool.
—John Gunn, M.D., *Home Book of Health*, 1880

During the pre-Columbian civilization common bleeding was controlled by placing masticated herbs over the bleeding sites.
—Anonymous

Clinical manifestations of fibrinolytic disorders are primarily thrombophilia and bleeding. Physiologic fibrinolysis is a balance between fibrin formation and dissolution. The coagulation and fibrinolytic systems influence the occurrence and clinical course of thrombotic disease. Disruption of the control of fibrinolysis can shift the balance of clot formation to dissolution and lead to bleeding or thrombosis.

Impairment of the fibrinolytic system, the *hypofibrinolytic state,* interferes with the hemostatic balance and leads to thrombosis by inhibiting clot resolution while clot formation continues. Thrombophilia may be due to both dysfunctional plasminogen and fibrinogen molecules. Congenital dysplasminogenemias are found in patients with both normal and lowered plasminogen antigen levels. Some congenital dysfibrinogenemias can lead to thrombotic disease. Defective activation of the fibrinolytic system may be due to defective synthesis and release of vascular plasminogen activator from the vessel wall (endothelial cell) or to increased plasma concentrations of the plasminogen activator inhibitor(s). Congenital protein C and protein S deficiencies may also produce a hypofibrinolytic state leading to thrombophilia.

The *hyperfibrinolytic state* leads to bleeding complications due to either defective inhibition or to excessive activation. Congenital bleeding disorders due to defective inhibition are decreased functional activity or deficiency of α_2-plasmin inhibitor and decreased functional activity or deficiency of the plasminogen activator inhibitor(s). Excessive activation of fibrinolysis may be due to excessive release of circulating plasminogen activator(s) from the vessel wall, a congenital defect. Thrombolytic therapy can also produce a hyperfibrinolytic state due to excess plasminogen activator and depletion of the plasminogen activator inhibitor(s).

Dysplasminogenemia with Thrombophilia

Case 1 (1)

The patient was a 31-year-old man (II-10) (Fig. 35.1) who had been in excellent health until age 15, when he developed severe thrombophlebitis in his left leg after sustaining a bruise on his left calf. Thrombophlebitis recurred several times over the next 2 years, and secondary varicose veins gradually developed in his left leg. At the age of 19, he developed thrombophlebitis in his right leg. Varicose veins developed in both legs. At the age of 21, he had a sudden onset of tinnitus, dizziness, headache, nausea, vomiting, and transient unconsciousness. Following admission to the hospital, intracranial hypertension of undetermined cause was diagnosed. He then developed dyspnea, chest pain, and cough with hemoptysis; workup revealed pulmonary embolism. At the age of 25, he suffered from sudden onset of chest pain, dyspnea, and hemoptysis. Pulmonary infarction was diagnosed by chest x-ray, pulmonary angiography, hemodynamic studies, and lung perfusion scan using ^{125}I-labeled macroaggregated albumin. At the age of 27, *he suffered cramping abdominal pain and was hospitalized. He underwent laparotomy; approximately the upper half of the small intestine was found to be swollen and discolored, and the superior mesenteric vein was occluded with thrombi that extended to the portal vein. The mesenteric artery appeared to be free of thrombi. There was no evidence of angiitis such as fibrinoid necrosis, leukocyte infiltration, or disruption of the elastica. At the age of 30, he suffered generalized urticaria associated with aggravation of the thrombophlebitis of both legs. In July of the same year, he was admitted to the hos-*

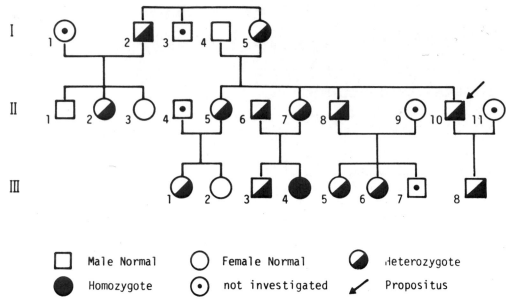

▢ Male Normal	◯ Female Normal	◐ Heterozygote
● Homozygote	⊙ not investigated	↙ Propositus

Figure 35.1. Pedigree of family Y with abnormal plasminogens. Each family member may be located in the pedigree by a roman numeral indicating generation and an arabic numeral indicating position within the generation. Subjects possessing approximately 5–6 U/mg plasminogen were considered to be heterozygotes. Subject III-4 was considered to be a homozygote because of her very low functional activity per milligram plasminogen (<1 U/mg).

pital with a diagnosis of acute abdomen and underwent laparotomy. A perforated duodenal ulcer was found, and a gastrojejunostomy was performed. Histologic examination showed a chronic duodenal ulcer that was perforated and the presence of intimal fibrosis of the small veins in the major omentum, suggestive of the presence of organized thrombi. Prophylactic treatment with an oral anticoagulant was instituted 5 months later.

Because of the striking thrombotic tendency of the patient, his family members were subjected to study. None of these family members (23 in 3 generations) reported any episode of thrombosis. Two sisters had two miscarriages each. There was no history of consanguinity.

Comment:

Coagulation/Fibrinolysis Parameters. *The propositus was evaluated for evidence of coagulation/fibrinolysis abnormalities. The results are presented in Table 35.1. The only abnormality found was a low functional activity of plasminogen (Plg), about half of normal, with normal antigen concentration.*

Evaluation of Patient's Plasminogen. *The plasma Plg specific enzyme activity (after activation with streptokinase (SK)) was calculated to be about 5.0 U/mg protein, which is about half of the normal control value of 10.7 U/mg protein. The plasma antigen (immunoreactive) concentration was 13.5 mg/dL, compared with normal values of 15.7 ± 1.3 mg/dL. Family members whose Plg specific activities were calculated to be above 8.3 U/mg protein (normal mean ±3 SE) were provisionally regarded as normal. The father and paternal uncles of the propositus were all normal, and the abnormality appeared to have been inherited from the maternal side. The Plg specific activity of the abnormal family members, except for one niece, was calculated to be 5.4 U/mg*

Table 35.1. Coagulation/Fibrinolysis Studies on the Propositus

	Propositus	Normal or Control
Prothrombin time (sec)	12	11–12
Activated partial thromboplastin time (sec)	25	24–32
Antithrombin III		
Activity (%)	95	90–110
Antigen concentration (mg/100 mL)	27	17–30
Fibrinogen (mg/100 mL)	190	150–400
Platelet count (per μL)	150,000	150,000–400,000
Platelet aggregation	Normal	
Plasminogen activity (U/mL)	0.69	1.3–2.1
Euglobulin lysis time (hr)	5	2–4
α_2-Plasmin inhibitor (mg/100 mL)	5.05	5–7
α_2-Maroglobulin (mg/100 mL)	210	150–300
α_1-Antitrypsin (mg/100 mL)	215	150–300

protein, approximately half of normal. One of the nieces of the propositus was found to have exceptionally low plasma functional activity (0.1 U/mg) with normal Plg antigen; her Plg specific activity was calculated to be 0.61 U/mg protein. Her parents both had half of normal Plg specific activities; her mother was a sister of the propositus. The results indicate that the niece is a homozygote, and her parents as well as other family members (10 descendants of the mother of the propositus) are heterozygotes. These studies suggest that the molecular abnormality of the propositus was inherited as an autosomal characteristic.

Purified Plg of the propositus and the other family member heterozygotes was found to have half the specific activity of that of the normal family members. The inactive Plg, half of the total Plg of the heterozygotes, can be converted to a nonfunctional two-chain plasmin (Pln) molecule by SK in the equimolar Plg · SK complex, similar to the conversion of the normal Plg to Pln. The total nonfunctional Plg of the homozygote is converted to the nonfunctional two-chain molecule. Gel isoelectrofocusing of the heterozygote purified Plg consisted of 10 normal bands and 10 additional abnormal bands (doublets), each of which had a slightly higher isoelectric point; the gel electrofocusing pattern of the homozygote consisted of abnormal bands only. The gene frequency of abnormal Plg (rare alleles) in the Japanese population is 0.02, compared with 0.01 in American and European populations.

Molecular Defect in Tochigi I Plasminogen. *Amino acid sequence analysis revealed that several individuals in the family had a substitution of Ala-601 by Thr in the active center region of the primary structure. This substitution is close to the active site His-603, Asp-645, and Ser-741 residues in the active center responsible for enzymatic activity. An abnormal gene coding for Plg was identified in this family; nucleotide sequencing showed that a guanosine in GCT coding for Ala-601 was replaced by an adenosine, resulting in ACT coding for Thr (in exon 15).*

Case 2 (2)

The propositus was a 48-year-old man (II-2) (Fig. 35.2) who was examined following an episode of chest pain, associated with nausea, vomiting, and diaphoresis; he had acute ECG changes. Emergency cardiac catherization revealed the left coronary artery to be normal but a 60% occlusion of the proximal right coronary artery. Intracoronary SK (40,000 IU) was given without any change in the occlusive lesion. He was given continuous heparin infusion and underwent angioplasty. During the procedure, a clot formed at the site of angioplasty, which was resistant to 240,000 IU SK, and the procedure was stopped. His condition progressed to a complete inferior wall MI. Coagulation/fibrinolysis tests carried out at this time (Table 35.2) showed low functional Plg activity with normal Plg antigen. His liver function tests were normal. Seven days later, he developed chest pain and had evidence for further myocardial necrosis by ECG and enzyme criteria. He was discharged 10 days later on an oral anticoagulant.

He was admitted 4 months later for mitral valve replacement, following which he developed progressive dyspnea and was found to have severe mitral regurgitation. Respiratory failure that required mechanical ventilation ensued. On admission, he required an intraaortic balloon pump for blood pressure support and oxygen for correction of hypoxemia. Because of his prior thrombosis during angioplasty, there was great concern regarding the heart valve surgery. He was placed on

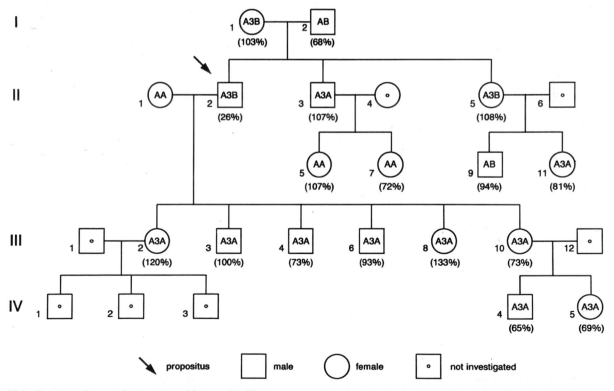

Figure 35.2. Family pedigree of propositus, Maywood I. The roman numeral indicates the generation and the arabic numeral the position within the generation. Plasminogen functional activity (%) is given for family each member (normal, 70–134%).

Plasminogen phenotypes are found in the symbols. The nomenclature is that proposed by the International Society of Blood Transfusion (10).

continuous-drip heparin. His low functional Plg activity was treated with plasma exchange (Fig. 35.3). Ten days later, he underwent mitral valve replacement with a Carpentier-Edwards porcine valve, and bypass graft to the right coronary artery. Continuous-drip heparin (500 U/hour) was begun 12 hours after surgery and increased to full dose 48 hours after surgery (Pt: 2–2.5 × control). He was started on an oral anticoagulant 24 hours after surgery and discharged on the 10th postoperative day.

Comment: *There was no family history of thrombosis or coronary artery disease; at age 25, the propositus developed a pulmonary embolism after knee surgery. The propositus's family members (Fig. 35.2) were tested for functional Plg activity; his father (I-2) and his grandchildren (IV-4, age 6) and (IV-5, age 5) had functional Plg activities of 68%, 65%, and 69%, respectively, and the propositus's daughter (III-10), the grandmother of the children, had a functional Plg activity of 73%. Assuming a normal functional range of about 70–134%, several family members had low normal levels. The*

propositus's father, one son, one daughter, and her children have structurally abnormal Plgs.

Plg phenotyping was carried out using isoelectric focusing and immunofixation methods with reference sera of known Plg phenotypes. The Plg phenotype of the propositus and his mother was A3B, abnormally migrating acidic forms; a brother and a sister gave phenotypes A3A and A3B, respectively. The propositus's father was phenotype AB (normal); however, his four sons and two daughters were type A3A (Fig. 35.2).

The propositus's plasma Plg antigen concentration was determined to be 9.5 mg/dL (normal range, 8.5–17.0 mg/dL), with a functional concentration of 26%. The Plg yield using affinity chromatography isolation with L-lysine-substituted Sepharose, was 8.6 mg/dL, about 88% of the plasma Plg antigen level; with normal plasmas, the yield was about 11.0–13.0 mg/dL. The specific activity was determined to be 24.4 IU/mg protein, compared with a specific activity of 28.5 IU/mg protein for normal plasma Plg. The protein was the native Glu-form, with isoelectric points between pH 6.40 and pH 5.45; it did not show a charge mutation. Titration of the equimolar Plg · SK complex gave 85% active sites, indicating a homogeneous population of molecules; therefore, the patient is a homozygote. Pln generation with SK, urokinase (u-PA), or tissue Plg activator (t-PA) plus fibrin, was less than 5% of that generated from normal Plg by the same activators. This variant Plg forms two equimolar complexes with SK, with different mobilities in PAGE, in equal amounts. Also, it showed substantially lowered kinetics of activation second-order rate constants with both SK and u-PA, primarily due to lower catalytic rate constants. This variant Plg, Maywood I, may be classified as a

Table 35.2. Coagulation and Fibrinolysis Studies on the Propositus, Maywood I

	Propositus	*Normal*
PT (sec)	12.4	11.5–13.5
APTT (sec)	29	23–31
Fibrinogen (mg/dL)	460	150–400
Antithrombin III activity (%)	89	85–125
Protein C antigen (%)	70	67–155
Protein S antigen (%)	108	60–150
α-Antiplasmin (%)	125	103–127
Plasminogen function (%)	26	70–134
Antigen (mg/dL)	9.5	8.5–17

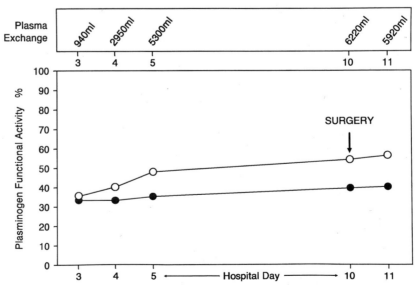

Figure 35.3. Plasminogen functional activity after plasmapheresis in the propositus with dysplasminogenemia, Maywood I. *Arrows* (↓) refer to plasmapheresis episodes. The volume of exchange is given above the arrow. *Closed circles* (●) represent prepheresis plasminogen levels. *Open circles* (○) represent levels after pheresis. Plasminogen functional activity is given on the y axis (normal, 70–134%). Hospital day is indicated on the x axis.

dysplasminogenemia with active center and kinetic defects, type 1c.

This case and the preceding case are examples of dysplasminogenemia and thrombosis. In case 2, the trauma of angioplasty was probably a precipitating event in the development of a clot refractory to lysis. Angioplasty or similar procedures should be avoided in patients with an established diagnosis of dysplasminogenemia because of the high risk of clot formation. The patient required mitral valve replacement and was probably at high risk for preoperative thrombosis. An increase in the functional Plg activity level was accomplished after plasma exchange. One cannot conclude from this case that the increase in functional Plg activity level was a major factor in keeping the patient free of thrombosis postoperatively. However, plasma exchange is a reasonable option for patients with dysplasminogenemia who demonstrate recurrent thrombosis and require vascular surgery, or when anticoagulants cannot be given continuously. This case suggests a role for normal Plg in preventing thrombosis; abnormal Plg can tip the balance toward thrombosis, but other events need finally occur to precipitate the acute thrombosis. Patients with dysplasminogenemia should have long-term treatment with an oral anticoagulant.

The Plasminogen-Plasmin System

The generation of Pln in plasma is regulated by (a) Plg, the zymogen precursor of Pln; (b) Plg activators, urokinase-type (scu-PA and tcu-PA) and tissue-type (sct-PA and tct-PA), synthesized and released from the liver and vascular endothelium into the circulation; (c) protein inhibitors that inactivate Pln, α_2-Pln inhibitor (α_2PI) and α_2-macroglobulin (α_2M), and the Plg activator inhibitor (PAI-1); and (d) the fibrin thrombus (Fig. 35.4) (3–6). Other factors that modulate the activation of the system are histidine-rich glycoprotein (HRG), which interferes with the binding of Plg to fibrin, and C1-inhibitor, which inactivates kallikrein, generated in a second activator pathway involving prekallikrein, factor XII, and high-molecular-weight (HMG) kininogen, which converts scu-PA to tcu-PA (5). α_2M is a scavenger protease inhibitor that intervenes only when α_2PI is markedly decreased, as during thrombolytic therapy and in patients with α_2PI deficiencies. The activators, u-PA and t-PA, are serine proteases formed from native proactivators by specific limited proteolysis, either in the circulation or at the surface of the cells secreting these activators. Activation of Plg can occur both in the fluid phase surrounding the thrombus and at the thrombus surface, involving both the fibrin clot, the platelet membrane, and circulating white cells (e.g., the monocyte). *The components of the system, such as Plg, Plg activators (scu-PA, tcu-PA and tct-PA), α_2PI, and PAI-1, when assembled at cell surface receptors (e.g., on endothelial cells and monocytes), are responsible for the regulation of the Plg-Pln system.*

Physiologic Fibrinolysis

The physiologic response to the formation of a hemostatic plug, or thrombus, requires a localized activation of Plg to Pln to remove the fibrin deposit without systemic activation of Plg, which causes the proteolytic degradation of many biologically active plasma proteins. The physiologic factors that influence thrombolysis are (a) Plg incorporation into the thrombus, and its binding to fibrin; (b) local release of both scu-PA and sct-PA by endothelial cells and their binding to fibrin; (c) the enhanced u-PA and t-PA activity in the presence of fibrin and proteolytically degraded fibrin; and (d) the protection of fibrin-bound Pln from inhibition by α_2 PI (6). Other important factors that influence clot lysis are (a) fibrin cross-linking by factor XIIIa, (b) the binding of α_2PI to fibrin through factor XIIIa, and (c) the inhibition of free Pln by α_2PI, impairing its binding to fibrin.

The binding of native Plg (Glu-form) to the fibrin thrombus is an important consideration in clot dissolution. Glu-Plg does not bind to fibrin to any extent. Therefore, the circulating Plg in contact with the thrombus needs to be activated to Pln, which binds to the fibrin. The fibrin thrombus–containing cellular elements, such as platelets and monocytes, may be able to assemble the Plg and Plg activators at their surfaces through their respective receptors and thus regulate thrombolysis (7). A well-defined partially degraded form of Plg (Lys-form) binds with high affinity to fibrin and cell-surfaces and is also a more efficient substrate for Plg activators than is the native Plg. Lys-Plg is not formed from Glu-Plg in the circulation but may be formed at cell surfaces from the native form and may provide an important physiologic mechanism for localizing proteolytic activity on the surface of the fibrin thrombus.

Plg activators are released from endothelial cells contiguous to the thrombus, perhaps in response to high local concentrations of thrombin or other stimuli associated with venous stasis. The released activators have a high affinity for fibrin or degraded fibrin-bound Plg, and with t-PA, increased activity in the presence of fibrin. The fast-acting inhibitors of Pln and the Plg activators, α_2PI and PAI-1, respectively, are much more efficient in the plasma milieu than are the bound forms, thus preventing both physiologic and pathologic concentrations of the enzymes from circulating in their active forms. Also, fibrin-bound Pln, in situ, is protected from α_2 PI, and fibrin-bound t-PA increases the binding of Plg. Dissolution of a pathologic thrombus is slow and incomplete because of the small surface of endothelium and limited amount of activators released onto the thrombus. Acceleration of pathologic thrombus dissolution, as achieved by Plg activator administration, is a desired clinical effect. Control mechanisms regulate plasma fibrinolytic activity as well, tending to restrict its action to sites of fibrin deposition and to prevent systemic activation. Normal plasma has a low concentra-

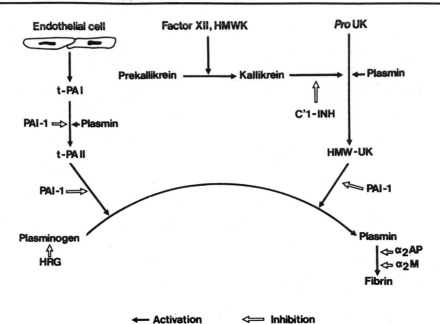

◄── Activation   **⇐══ Inhibition**

Figure 35.4. The fibrinolytic system of human plasma. t-PA I, single-chain tissue-type plasminogen activator, also called sct-PA; t-PA II, two-chain t-PA (tct-PA); PAI-I, plasminogen activator inhibitor-I (endothelial type); HMWK, high-molecular-weight kininogen; Pro UK, prourokinase, also called single-chain urinary-type PA (scu-PA); HMW-UK, high-molecular-weight urokinase, also called two-chain u-PA (tcu-PA); C′1-INH, C1-inhibitor; α_2AP, Alpha$_2$-antiplasmin; α_2-M, Alpha$_2$-macroglobulin.

tion of Plg activators, most of which is either inactive zymogen or bound to inhibitor. Plasma Plg activity increases transiently with exercise, epinephrin, DDAVP, nicotine, and venous occlusion, suggesting release from storage sites. A more sustained elevation of Plg activator could result from persistent stimuli such as a prolonged surgical procedure or a neoplasm. Plasma fibrinolytic activity reflects the PAI-1 level.

Pathologic Fibrinolysis

Coagulation and fibrinolysis are carefully coordinated physiologically, providing prompt control of bleeding with eventual resolution and healing. Fibrin formation and dissolution are thought to occur simultaneously during hemostasis, with the balance of these forces influencing the occurrence and clinical course of thrombotic disease. *Bleeding* complications may result from either *excessive activation,* or *defective inhibition,* of the fibrinolytic system. Excessive activation may be due to excessive release of Plg activators, impaired clearance of activator, localized excess activator, or deficiency of PAI-1; defective inhibition may be due to a molecular defect of the α_2PI protein or the PAI-1 protein. *Thrombotic* complications may also be due to *defective activation* of Plg resulting from an inadequate release of activators, a molecular defect of the Plg molecule, or *excessive inhibition* of the fibrinolytic system by elevated blood levels of PAI-1 (8–10).

The **hyperfibrinolytic state** (bleeding) may be due to excessive amounts of Plg activators (a) released into the blood by a generalized response of the entire vascular system (a lifelong bleeding disorder) or (b) released by neo-

plasms or (c) administration of exogenous activators (thrombolytic therapy). The hyperfibrinolytic state may also be due to defective inhibition of the system, as seen in patients with (a) congenital deficiency of α_2PI or (b) a congenital deficiency of PAI-1 (a lifelong bleeding disorder). Acquired increased endogenous PA activity is found in liver disease (cirrhosis), primary amyloidosis, acute promyelocytic leukemia with concomitant disseminated intravascular coagulation (DIC), solid tumors, and some snakebites (venoms). This increased fibrinolytic activity with bleeding usually responds well to ϵ-aminocaproic acid (EACA).

The **hypofibrinolytic state** (thrombosis) resulting in defective fibrinolysis has been difficult to evaluate (8–12). Specific congenital defects in this system have been associated with abnormalities of both Plg (10–12) and fibrinogen (13, 14). Familial Plg deficiency accounts for 2–3% of unexplained thrombotic disease in young adults. Hypoplasminogenemia, with a parallel reduction in both functional and antigen (immunoreactive) Plg levels (with a 1:1 molar ratio) below 65%, usually 50%, has been described in fewer than 20 families, usually discovered after a single family member had presented with thrombovascular disease (10–12). In most cases, family members with Plg levels similar to the propositus are asymptomatic. The inheritance pattern is autosomal dominant; about 30% of the heterozygotes are symptomatic. The absence of circulating Plg (i.e., aplasminogenemia), has not been described; it is apparently not compatible with life. **Dysplasminogenemia** with a reduced functional Plg level and a normal antigen level (from 0.88:1 to 0.2:1, molar ratios), with defective activation to Pln, and abnormalities in the Plg molecule, has been described (12). Abnormal, variant, Plgs have been described in 12 families, with only a single family member manifesting recurrent thromboembolic disease. Again, family members with similar reduced functional Plg levels and normal antigen levels are asymptomatic. The inheritance pattern is autosomal dominant; most of the heterozygotes and several of the homozygotes are asymptomatic. Abnormal Plgs has been described in two families with hypoplasminogenemia, with variants also found in asymptomatic family members. The propositus and mother in only one family were symptomatic. Fullterm newborns have also been found with reduced functional Plg levels and normal antigen levels (50% of normal adult Plg levels). Acquired, reduced Plg levels have been found in liver disease and sepsis and in Argentine hemorrhagic fever. Familial thrombotic disease has also been associated with defective release of Plg activators and increased release of PAI-1 inhibitor.

Plasminogen

Structure

Human Plg is a single-chain zymogen synthesized in the liver and present in plasma in a concentration of about 2 μM (3, 4). It is about 92 kDa and contains 2% carbohydrate. The native molecule, Glu-1-Plg, contains 791 amino acids, 24 disulfide bonds, and 5 regions of sequence homology, triple-loop structures called kringles, in the NH$_2$-terminal region of the molecule. There is a well-defined plasmin-degraded form of Plg, designated Lys-78-Plg, and an elastase-degraded form of Plg, designated Val-443-Plg (mini-Plg). The native plasma Glu-1-Plg can be separated into two forms by affinity chromatography; form 1 contains two oligosaccharide chains, whereas form 2 contains only one of the two oligosaccharide chains. Native Plg has 10–13 isoelectric forms, with isoelectric points between 6.2 and 6.6.

All Plg activators (e.g., u-PA, t-Pa, and SK) convert Plg to the proteolytic enzyme, Pln, by cleavage of a single Arg-561-Val peptide bond. The two polypeptide chains, A and B, are connected by two disulfide bonds. The COOH-terminal light (B) chain, Arg-561-Pln contains the serine protease active site. The NH$_2$-terminal heavy (A) chain contains the lysine/fibrin binding sites located on the five kringle structures, which regulate the binding of fibrin, α_2PI, HRG, and thrombospondin. Specific binding of Plg, via lysine binding sites, to Plg receptors on endothelial cells, monocytes, and monocytoid cells, results in enhanced rates of activation by u-PA and t-PA.

The organization and structure of the gene coding for Plg has been determined (Fig. 35.5) (15). The gene spans

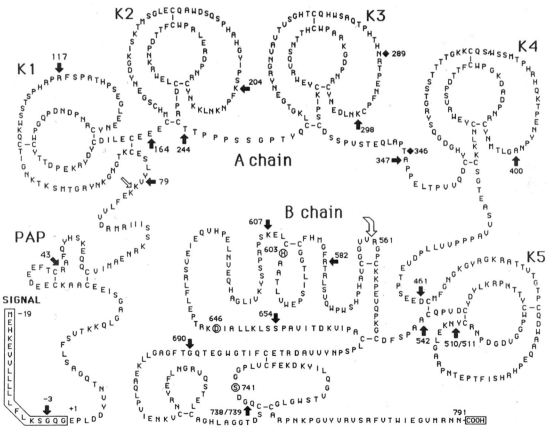

Figure 35.5. Amino acid sequence for human plasminogen and the location of the 18 introns in the gene coding for plasminogen. The positions of the introns (A–R) are indicated by *solid arrows* at or between specific amino acids. The amino acid residues are numbered starting with the amino-terminal glutamic acid residue as number 1 and ending with residue 791. The signal peptide (PAP) is generated primarily by the cleavage between Lys-77 and Lys-78 *(open straight arrow)* by plasmin. The conversion of the plasminogen to plasmin occurs by the cleavage between Arg-561 and Val-562 *(open curved arrow)*. K1–K5 refer to kringles 1–5 in the A chain; the active site His, Asp, and Ser residues in the B chain are *circled*. Carbohydrate attachment sites (Asn-289, Thr-346) are shown by *diamonds*.

about 52.5 kilobases of DNA and consists of 19 exons, separated by 18 introns. The five kringle structures are coded by two exons. The Plg gene, closely related to apolipoprotein(a), was mapped to the long arm of chromosome 6 at bands q26–q27. Polymorphism of Plg has been described (3). The plasma forms can be detected by isoelectric focusing–immunofixation and isoelectric focusing–zymography methods in polyacrylamide gels. Plg is coded by an autosomal gene with two common alleles, Plg A and Plg B, and a large number of rare alleles; a nomenclature has been proposed for the designation of the rare Plg variant alleles (16). The allele frequencies differ substantially in various racial groups but are fairly constant within one race. Rare Plg alleles occur with a frequency of about 0.01–0.02; it is in this group of rare alleles that variant Plgs may be found.

Variant Plasminogens

The major components of the plasma fibrinolytic system can be measured by both enzymatic and immunologic methods. Plg can be measured functionally with excess SK, by titrating the equimolar Plg · SK active site with a chromogenic substrate, and immunochemically using either rocket immunoelectrophoresis, immunodiffusion, or a nephelometric method. The concentration of Plg in plasma is about 20 mg/dL (functional/antigen). Measurement of the plasma Pln generation rates with two or three different activators is a useful method for the identification of variant Plgs. The determination of u-PA and t-PA and their inhibitor, PAI-1, is of little value in the identification of variant Plgs. Identification of rare Plg phenotypes by use of polyacrylamide gels may be a useful screening method for finding variant Plgs.

Purified Plasminogen

Characterization of the dysfunctional Plg and determination of the molecular defect must be carried out with the highly purified protein. Affinity chromatography with L-lysine-substituted Sepharose is used for the isolation of Plg from plasma. This purified Plg is characterized by (a) the determination of specific proteolytic activity; (b) Pln generation rates; (c) rate of generation of the active site in the Plg · SK equimolar complex; (d) kinetic parameters of Plg activation; (e) formation, conversion, and degradation of the equimolar Plg · SK complexes as studied by PAGE and SDS-PAGE; (f) polymorphisms detected by isoelectric focusing techniques; and (g) electrophoretic mobility. The molecular defect can be determined by both amino acid sequence analysis and nucleotide sequence analysis of genomic DNA and RNA.

Classification of Dysfunctional Plasminogens

A classification of abnormal Plgs has been proposed (Table 35.3) (12). The type 1 dysplasminogenemias can

Table 35.3 Classification of Abnormal Plasminogens: Dysplasminogenemias

		Plasma	
		Functional Level[a] (% of Normal)	Antigen Level[b]
Dysplasminogenemia: type 1			
a. Active center defect	Heterozygotes[c]		
Tochigi I		46	N
Tochigi II		45	N
Nagoya		45	N
Paris I		28	N
Tokyo		20	N
b. Active center defect and charge mutation	Heterozygotes		
Frankfurt I		48	N
San Antonio		44	N
c. Active center and kinetic defects	Homozygotes[d]		
Chicago I		41	N
Chicago II		88	N
Chicago III		80	N
Maywood I		26	N
Dysplasminogenemia-hypoplasminogenemia: type 2			
a. Active center defect			
Frankfurt II		62	66[e]

[a]Functional: % of normal value, not % of normal range values.
[b]Range 70–130%, varies in different laboratories. Abbreviation: N, normal.
[c]Heterozygotes: normal and abnormal plasminogen molecules, mainly 50% each; Tochigi I has homozygote niece, 6% normal and 94% abnormal molecules, the abnormal molecules do not form active enzyme.
[d]Homozygotes: homogeneous population of abnormal plasminogen molecules with more than 85% forming active molecules.
[e]Percentage of mean of normal range and below lowest value in normal range.

be subdivided into three classes: *(a)* active center defects: e.g., Tochigi I and II, Nagoya, Paris I, and Tokyo, both heterozygotes and homozygotes; *(b)* active center defect and charge mutation: e.g., Frankfurt I and San Antonio, heterozygotes; and *(c)* active center and kinetic defects: e.g., Chicago I, II, and III, and Maywood I, homozygotes. The type 2 dysplasminogenemias-hypoplasminogenemias: *(a)* active center defect: e.g., Frankfurt II. The Ala-601 to Thr substitution and a Val-355 to Phe substitution have been found only in Japanese families, in which heterozygotes and homozygotes have been identified (Fig. 35.6) (17). Two types of mutations, I and II, were identified in these abnormal genes, in exons X and XV, respectively.

Many patients with thrombophilia have been found to have abnormal, variant, Plgs. Laboratory diagnosis of normal Plg antigen levels and lower-than-normal Plg functional levels in plasma indicates that an abnormal Plg is present. Patients with congenital Plg deficiencies (less than 70% of normal) with functional:antigen ratios of 1:1 may also have dysfunctional Plgs. In most patients with variant Plgs, some of the major thrombosis risk factors (e.g., AT III deficiency, and protein C and S deficiencies) were not found. Patients have been found with combined dysplasminogenemia–protein C deficiency and combined dysplasminogenemia–AT III deficiency.

In patients with abnormal Plgs, the factors involved in the precipitation of the thrombotic event are not known. Most family members, who also have variant Plgs, do not have a history of recurring thromboembolic disease. The Tochigi I homozygote, with neglible functional Plg activity, has no history of thrombotic disease. Perhaps, the problem is with the assembly of Plg, Plg activators, and their inhibitors on the fibrin thrombus/endothial cell surface, where defective assembly is the predisposing factor to thrombophilia (Fig. 35.7). Poor binding of Plg to its cellu-

lar receptors, preventing the generation of Pln, may be responsible for the thrombotic event.

Dysfibrinogenemia with Thrombophilia
Case 3 (18)

The propositus was a 49-year-old man (II-6) (Fig. 35.8) who had experienced spontaneous deep vein thrombosis (DVT) at the age of 45. His mother had recurrent venous thrombosis starting at an early age, and four of his siblings had experienced venous thrombotic events. All four had died at a relatively young age. His eldest sister (II-1) had developed a malignant disease and subsequently suffered from DVT as well as myocardial infarction (MI); she died at the age of 46. One brother (II-3) had experienced spontaneous DVT as well as a cerebrovascular accident, from which he died at the age of 27. A second brother (II-5) developed DVT and died at the age of 33. His younger brother (II-9) died at the age of 41, following DVT complicated by pulmonary embolism (PE) and a cerebrovascular accident. Arterial occlusions without venous thrombosis also occurred in this family; two brothers (II-2, II-4) had experienced MI at a young age and their father (I-1) had a history of peripheral arterial occlusion as well as cerebral thrombosis. They were treated with heparin and an oral anticoagulant. Two sisters, one brother, and the propositus's children, nieces, and nephews were asymptomatic. A concomitant disorder in this family is familial hypercholesterolemia type IIb, which could be demonstrated in all of the investigated individuals of the second generation (range of cholesterol levels: 6–12 mmol/L). This abnormality is probably related to the arterial thrombotic events in II-2 and II-4.

Coagulation/Fibrinolysis Parameters: The patient was evaluated for evidence of coagulation/fibrinolysis abnormalities (Table 35.4). The only abnormality revealed was a prolongation of the thrombin and reptilase

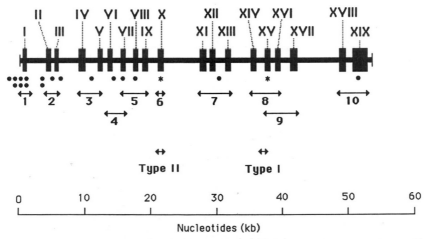

Figure 35.6. Regions of the genomic DNA coding for plasminogen that were amplified by the polymerase chain reaction. To detect the molecular defect in abnormal plasminogen, all 19 exons of the plasminogen gene were amplified, employing 10 pairs of oligonucleotide primers. For analysis of type I or type II mutations, exons X and XV were amplified separately. *Asterisks* represent sites of type I and II mutations, and *solid circles* indicate additional sites of nucleotide substitutions.

clotting times. Fibrinogen was low when measured functionally by the Clauss method, in contrast to the fibrinogen antigen levels. Hereditary dysfibrinogenemia was suggested by a prolonged thrombin clotting time, which was also found in 5 of the 10 investigated family members.

Evaluation of Patient's Fibrinogen: Fibrinogen was purified from the propositus, his sister, and a normal control. Thrombin clotting times and reptilase clotting times, measured on the purified fibrinogen preparations, were found to be prolonged, when compared with the normal. This suggested that the two siblings could have abnormal fibrinogens. SDS-PAGE analysis showed an identical pattern for all three fibrinogens in the two siblings and the normal, indicating that no gross deletions were present. Clottability was determined by measuring

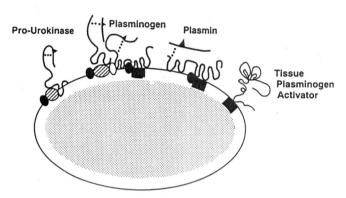

Figure 35.7. Assembly of the fibrinolytic system on cell surfaces. Cells can express specific receptors for the plasminogen activators, tissue-type plasminogen activator and urokinase-type plasminogen activator, and for plasminogen. As a consequence of colocalization of activators and zymogen, plasminogen is converted to plasmin, and plasmin is retained on the cell surface. Cell-bound plasmin may convert single-chain u-PA to its two-chain form, which, in turn, propagates plasmin formation. By virtue of its broad substrate recognition, cell-bound plasmin may be used to execute a variety of cellular functions.

residual fibrin(ogen) in the supernatant of thrombin-induced fibrin clots after 1 hour. These fibrinogens were clottable; the propositus's level was 92%, the sister was 93.%, and the normal was 97%. Thrombin-induced release of fibrinopeptides A and B was normal. The rate of polymerization of fibrin monomers showed that fibrin aggregation appeared to be abnormal in the propositus and his sister; the abnormality was more pronounced in thrombin monomers (Des AABB-fibrin) than in reptilase monomers (Des AA-fibrin), in the presence or absence of calcium ions.

To investigate whether these variant fibrinogens might influence the process of fibrinolysis, clot lysis experiments were performed with whole blood from the propositus, his sister, and normal healthy volunteers. With t-PA, blood clots of the propositus and his sister lysed more slowly than those of the controls, and the lysis curves of the propositus and his sister appeared to be different from the normals. In the propositus and his family members, soluble Des AA-fibrin showed a decreased stimulation of Plg activation with t-PA. This

Table 35.4. Coagulation and Fibrinolysis Parameters in the Propositus's Plasma

	Propositus	*Normal Range*
Thrombin clotting time (sec)	20.2	14.3–18.5
Reptilase clotting time (sec)	22.7	<20
Fibrinogen (Clauss) (mg/mL)	1.2	1.8–4.9
Fibrinogen antigen (mg/mL)	3.5	1.6–5.0
Antithrombin III activity (%)	92	75–120
Protein C antigen (%)	112	75–135
Protein S antigen (%)	86	67–125
Plasminogen activity (%)	76	70–140
t-PA antigen (%)	78	65–169
μ-PA antigen (%)	113	44–184
α_2-Antiplasmin activity (%)	101	80–136
PA-inhibitor activity (IU/mL)	11.3	1.7–34.0

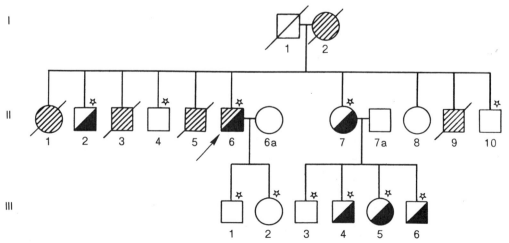

Figure 35.8. Pedigree of the family (↗ = propositus). Family members with a history of venous thrombosis are indicated (▨,◪). Prolonged thrombin clotting time (◣,◐) was found in 6 of the 11 investigated individuals of two generations (II-2, II-6, II-7, III-4, III-5, III-6). Other symbols: male (□); female (○); decreased (▨,⊘); investigated (✶).

could not be attributed to defective binding of Plg to the fibrin. However, the binding of t-PA to the fibrin of the propositus and his sister was significantly reduced when compared with the control. This impairment of fibrinolysis might explain the thrombosis in the patient.

Fibrinogen to Fibrin Conversion

The normal hemostatic mechanism prevents blood loss from intact vessels and stops excessive bleeding from severed vessels. This process involves the vessel wall, blood platelets, the blood coagulation and fibrinolytic systems, and the kininogen and complement pathways. The major function of the blood coagulation system is the generation of insoluble fibrin at a site of injury to limit the amount of blood loss. When this aim has been achieved and tissue repair is under way, it is the function of the fibrinolytic system to remove the fibrin deposits and restore the patency of the blood vessel. Fibrin deposition and degradation occurs continually in the circulation of normal individuals. Thus, the hemostatic process may be viewed as a fine balance between the blood coagulation and fibrinolytic systems.

Soluble plasma fibrinogen is converted by thrombin to soluble fibrin, a relatively unstable molecule. For the clot to survive until tissue repair has been effected, it is necessary for this fibrin to be cross-linked and stabilized by factor XIIIa, the fibrin-stabilizing factor (19, 20).

Lack of circulating fibrinogen, afibrinogenemia, presents as a bleeding disorder; its genetic basis remains unknown. Hypofibrinogenemia is the term used for patients with low levels of fibrinogen; sometimes, congenitally low fibrinogen levels may be associated with the presence of abnormal molecules. Congenital dysfibrinogenemia may be defined as a qualitative abnormality of plasma fibrinogen, a functional defect, most often manifested by a prolonged thrombin clotting time (Table 35.5) (21–24). A genetic defect has caused the production of fibrinogen molecules with structural alterations affecting fibrinogen to fibrin conversion. Many dysfibrinogenemias are clinically asymptomatic, one-third have a bleeding tendency, and about one-sixth have a tendency to develop throm-

bosis. It seems paradoxical that thrombotic tendencies have been reported in patients with defective clotting caused by dysfibrinogenemia. In recent years, increasing effort has been made to correlate molecular and functional variations in fibrinogen with clinical symptoms. In patients with thrombosis and dysfibrinogenemia, such a link is not easy to make.

Fibrinogen

The fibrinogen concentration of normal plasma is approximately the same, varying from 1.5 to 4.0 g/L, regardless of the type of assay (i.e., functional or immunologic assay). The fibrinogen molecule, 340 kDa, is a covalently linked dimer consisting of three pairs of nonidentical disulfide-linked polypeptide chains: Aα (67 kDa), Bβ (56 kDa), and y (47 kDa) (Fig. 35.9) (25–27). Each molecule has four carbohydrate chains, one on each Bβ-chain and one on each y-chain, while the Aα-chains are devoid of carbohydrate; it makes up 2.6% of the fibrinogen mass. Fibrinogen is synthesized by the parenchymal cells of the liver, and the constituent polypeptide chains are assembled within the rough endoplasmic reticulum; the fibrinogen is secreted into the circulation. Each fibrinogen subunit is encoded by single copies of genes located on the long arm of human chromosome 4 in the q23–q32 region (28). Within this region is a 50-kilobase (kb) span that contains the three genes for Aα-, Bβ-, and (gy)-chains; they are arranged in the order (gy)-Aα-Bβ. The α and β genes give rise to single gene products; (gy)-gene expression results in two different polypeptide chains, (gy)- and (gy)'-chains. About 10% of the normal circulating fibrinogen contains the (gy)' variant, which consists of a 16–amino acid extension at the carboxyl terminus. The variant fibrinogen contains one (gy)-chain and one (gy)'-chain. The genes for the Aα, Bβ, and (gy) chains are 5.4, 8.2, and 8.4 kb in length. The Aα gene consists of 5 exons, the Bβ gene has 8 exons and 7 introns, and the y gene has 10 exons and 9 introns. They are derived from a single ancestral gene.

The conversion of soluble fibrinogen by thrombin into an insoluble polymer, fibrin, can be considered a three step process. Fibrinopeptide A is cleaved from

Table 35.5. Abnormal Laboratory Results in Patients with Congenital Fibrinogenopathies

	Homozygous	*Heterozygous*	*Afibrinogenemia*	*Hypofibrinogenemia*
Activated partial thromboplastin time	P[a]	N or P	P	N
Prothrombin time	P	N or P	P	N
Thrombin time[b]	P	P	P	N or P
Reptilase time[c]	P	P	P	N or P
Fibrinogen (functional)	D	D	Absent	D
Fibrinogen (antigen)	N or D	N or I	Absent	D
Bleeding time	N	N	P†	N

[a]N, normal: P, prolonged; D, decreased; I, increased.
[b]Thrombin time is shortened with fibrinogen Oslo I. Reptilase time is normal with fibrinogen Milano II. Most heterozygotes display either prolonged thrombin time or reptilase time but rarely both.
[c]Approximately 30% of patients have prolonged bleeding times.

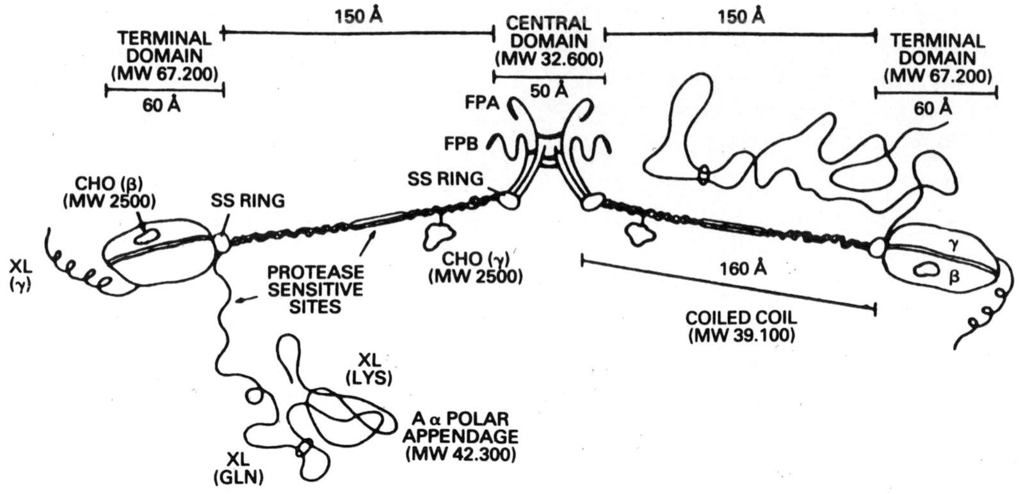

Figure 35.9. Schematic model of fibrinogen molecule according to Doolittle (1984). The central domain contains the amino termini of all 6 polypeptide chains. Fibrinopeptides A (FPA) and B (FPB) are located at the amino-terminal ends of Aα- and Bβ-chains, respectively. The 2 terminal nodules are connected to the central domain by coiled coils, 112 residues in length (160 Å). The half-dimers of the molecule are connected by a single disulfide bridge between Aα-chains and a double disulfide bond between γ-chains. Disulfide rings are shown on both ends of the coiled coil connector, holding all 3 chains in register. There are 4 oligosaccharides (CHO), 2 located on the γ-chains close to the central domain and 2 on the Bβ-chains within each distal domain. Cross-linking sites (XL) are situated at the carboxyl termini of the γ-chains. On each Aα-chain, there are 2 cross-linking acceptor sites (XL, GLN) and 5 potential donor sites (XL, LYS). Two characteristic protease-sensitive segments are shown: cleavage of the carboxyl-terminal Aα-chain protuberance results in formation of fragment X, while plasmin attack on the susceptible peptide bonds in the coiled coils splits fragment X into Y and D, and fragment Y into D and E.

the NH_2-terminus of the A chains, resulting in formation of the fibrin monomer. Des-AA-fibrin forms end-to-end polymers, and then the fibrinopeptide B is released. This is followed by side-to-side association forming protofibrils (oligomers); the protofibrils associate to form fibrin fibers, which join into bundles of larger widths twisted helically (fibrin gel). Calcium binding sites are integral parts of the fibrinogen molecule, and calcium ions are important for fibrin monomer polymerization.

Polymerization and gelation of fibrin is stabilized by introduction of covalent bonds between neighboring fibrin monomers by a calcium-dependent, sulfhydryl-type transglutaminase, factor XIIIa. Factor XIII, a proenzyme, is activated by the thrombin to factor XIIIa, which covalently links specific lysine and glutamine residues denoted as donors and acceptors, respectively. Cross-links are formed between carboxy-terminal segments of adjacent y-chains, antiparallel reciprocal cross-linking. Up to six cross-links per mole of fibrin monomer may be introduced under optimum conditions. The resulting stabilized fibrin is insoluble in strong acids and denaturing solvents (e.g., urea, guanidine · HCl). Cross-linked fibrin is mechanically stronger and more resistant to lysis by Pln than is non-cross-linked or nonstabilized fibrin.

Binding sites on fibrin have been localized for thrombin, calcium ions, Plg, Plg activator, α_2PI, and fibronectin (Fig. 35.10). There appear to be several thrombin-binding sites on the Aα-chain; thrombin can be released when fibrin is lysed by Pln. Bound thrombin appears to be partially protected from inactivation by the antithrombins. Calcium ions are required for normal fibrin polymerization; human fibrinogen has three high-affinity binding sites for calcium ions and many low-affinity binding sites. Calcium ions and other divalent cations may affect the confirmation of the fibrinogen molecule, leading to an enhanced rate of fibrin polymerization as well as protection against proteolytic degradation. Native Plg binding sites are hidden in fibrin(ogen); however they are uncovered following Pln degradation of fibrin. Partially degraded Lys-Plg has a high affinity for fibrin. Plg binding sites are found on both the Aα and Bβ chains. Cross-linked fibrin has a lower affinity for Plg than does non-cross-linked fibrin. Histidine-rich glycoprotein and α_2PI both interact with the high-affinity o-aminocarboxylic acid binding sites of Plg, its lysine binding sites, and fibrin binding sites. Plg binding to fibrin is inhibited by α_2PI. The Plg activators, u-PA and t-PA, mediate the binding of native Plg to fibrin. Apolipoprotein(a) (Apo(a)), a member of the Plg-Apo(a) gene family, inhibits the binding of native Plg to fibrin. There is also a cooperative association of native Plg with fibrinogen. Fibrin serves as a surface on which Plg and t-PA are associated. t-PA has a high affinity for fibrin; the binding site is located on the Aα-chain, particularly after degradation of fibrin by Pln. α_2PI binds to fibrin, and can be covalently cross-linked to fibrin by factor XIIIa. Fibronectin is also incorporated (cross-linked) into the fibrin network during clotting; fibronectin provides the glutamine acceptors, and the fibrin Aα-chains provide the lysine donors.

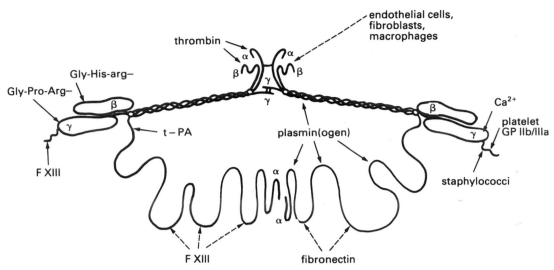

Figure 35.10. Schematic diagram of the domain structure and of interactions of human fibrinogen with other molecules and cells. *Full arrows* denote binding sites, the location of which has been confined to specific domains of the fibrinogen molecule. *Dashed arrows* point to the tentative binding sites. The positions of bind-ing sites for the following ligands have not been included in the diagram: α_2-plasmin inhibitor, collagen, von Willebrand factor, histidine-rich glycoprotein, thrombospondin, protamine, ristocetin, and acidic polyaccharides (several are unknown).

Dysfibrinogenemias

Congenital. Most individuals with congenital dysfibrinogenemia are asymptomatic. Most are also heterozygotes, with approximately half normal and half abnormal fibrinogen molecules. This may be the principal reason for the absence of symptoms in many. If the concentration of normal fibrinogen is greater than 100 mg/dL, there appears to be a decreased tendency for bleeding problems. The few who appear to be homozygous for a fibrinogen abnormality (e.g., fibrinogens Detroit, Metz, Giessen II) have a hemorrhagic diathesis, but their heterozygous kindred do not. The seeming paradox of poorly clottable fibrinogen and associated thrombosis, both venous and arterial, has been reported. The first report of an abnormal fibrinogen was of Oslo I. This fibrinogen was characterized by an abnormally short thrombin time, abnormally fast polymerization, and enhanced support of platelet aggregation with ADP. The other fibrinogen variants with thrombotic complications have normal to prolonged thrombin and reptilase times, defective thrombin binding, and disordered, delayed, fibrin polymerization. They include fibrinogens New York I, Malmo, and Milan II. Fibrinogens New York I, Dusard, Chapel Hill III, and Nijmengen have defects in their interaction with the fibrinolytic system. Their clinical presentation is DVT and PE. Impaired Plg activation has been reported for fibrinogens New York I and Dusard. Fibrinogen Dusard shows a reduced binding of Plg, about half, to fibrin, and fibrin-mediated enhancement of Plg activation by t-PA is strongly reduced. Fibrinogen New York I gives abnormal fibrin structure and abnormal binding of t-PA, resulting in abnormal Plg activation. This dysfibrinogenemia has a large deletion in the Bβ chains and consequently abnor-mal release of fibrinopeptide B. Fibrinogen Nijmengen shows impaired binding of t-PA to fibrin, with defective fibrin polymerization, and prolonged blood clot lysis. With fibrinogen Chapel Hill III, the fibrin gel is highly rigid, and it cannot be digested by Pln. None of these abnormal fibrinogens shows (*a*) defects in fibrinopeptide A release or (*b*) fibrin cross-linking defects. There is great difficulty in establishing relationships between the clinical symptom—a thrombotic tendency—and molecular defects in the dysfibrinogenemias. A molecular defect has been found in only one patient with an abnormal fibrinogen in whom a thrombotic disease has been found; a deletion defect was established in fibrinogen New York I, where a 64-residue (9–72) deletion was found in the β-chain, corresponding exactly to exon 2 of this chain.

The congenital dysfibrinogenemias are classified according to the stage of fibrin formation primarily affected by the defect: (*a*) impairment of fibrinopeptide release, (*b*) impairment of fibrin monomer polymerization, and (*c*) impairment of fibrin stabilization, and also to abnormal Plg activation.

Acquired. The acquired dysfibrinogenemias are classified according to the clinical condition of the patient in which they occur (22–23). Abnormal fibrinogens are found in patients with hepatocellular disease (e.g., cirrhosis, hepatitis, liver failure, and hepatomas) with properties similar to those of the congenital variants (Table 35.6), including elevated bound sialic acid. In newborn infants, qualitative differences between neonatal and adult fibrinogens are found. The existence of a distinct fetal fibrinogen has been postulated but not proven. The dysfibrinogenemia found in normal newborn infants and in liver disease appear to be functionally similar.

Table 35.6. Fibrinogenopathies

I.   Quantitative abnormalities
   A.   Congenital
      1.   Afibrinogenemia (autosomal recessive)
      2.   Hypofibrinogenemia (autosomal dominant)

   B.   Acquired
      1.   Hypofibrinogenemia
         a.   Disseminated intravascular coagulation
         b.   Liver failure
         c.   Snake bit
         d.   L-Asparaginase
         e.   Thrombolitic therapy
      2.   Hyperfibrinogenemia
         a.   Inflammation
         b.   Neoplasia

II. Qualitative defects
   A.   Congenital
      1.   Dysfibrinogenemia (autosomal dominant)
         a.   Associated with bleeding
         b.   Associated with thrombosis
         c.   Asymptomatic
      2.   Hypodysfibrinogenemia
         (autosomal dominant)
   B.   Acquired
      1.   Liver disease (hepatitis, cirrhosis)
      2.   Hepatoma, renal cell carcinoma
      3.   Diabetes mellitus
      4.   Antifibrinogen antibodies
      5.   Paraproteinemia (multiple myeloma)

Thrombophilia Due to Defective Release of Vascular Plasminogen Activator: Increased Concentration of Plasminogen Activator Inhibitor

Case 4 (29)

The propositus was a 14-year-old boy (IV-26) (Fig. 35.11) who was admitted to the hospital because of a swollen left leg. Phlebography revealed thrombosis occluding the deep venous system, including the left iliac vein. Chest x-ray, pulmonary scintigram, and angiography, showed signs of bilateral embolism. Treatment was started with SK, followed by heparin and an oral anticoagulant.

Analysis of Case 4: Coagulation/Fibrinolysis Parameters: *Laboratory studies revealed that the release of fibrinolytic activity from the vessel wall was deficient. The fibrinolytic activity of resuspended euglobulin precipitates on unheated fibrin plates was determined after 20 min of venous occlusion; the fibrinolytic response to venous occlusion was abnormally weak, as was the stimulation with DDAVP. The number and function of platelets, the coagulation factors, Plg, AT III, PAI-1, and α_2M, were normal.*

Evaluation of Propositus and Family Members' Fibrinolytic System: *Many of the propositus's relatives had a history of thromboembolic disease. The pedigree includes a marriage between cousins. The propositus's elder brother (IV-22), at age 28, had an attack of DVT of unknown cause. Since then, he has regularly taken an oral anticoagulant and has had no recurrence. He too had a defective fibrinolytic release mechanism. Among their 21 cousins and second cousins in generation IV, 8 had episodes of DVT, 6 on two or more occasions. A cousin (IV-3) had his first episode at 11 years of age and has since had DVT of an arm. Of the 12 cousins and second cousins investigated, 6 with a history of DVT, 9 had*

an isolated defective fibrinolytic release mechanism after venous occlusion. The patient's father (III-7) had recurrent DVT in his twenties and thirties, probably complicated by PE. Examination revealed a defective release of fibrinolytic activity but otherwise nothing remarkable. Moreover, four of his six siblings had had DVT. Thus, of the 17 family members investigated, 13 had had DVT; among these 13 individuals, the fibrinolytic activity response to venous occlusions and/or DDAVP was weak in 12.

Case 5 (Group of Cases) (30)

One hundred patients with recurrent DVT or PE without any other known disease were investigated 3 months after their latest thrombotic episode. In every case, diagnosis had been verified by phlebography, pulmonary scintigraphy, or angiography. At the time of the investigation, 73% of the patients were taking an oral anticoagulant; the study included 60 men and 40 women, aged 14–70 years (mean, 43 years). Fifty-seven volunteers, aged 20–60 years (mean, 33 years) of whom 27 were women, served as controls. All were apparently healthy, and none had any history of superficial thrombophlebitis, DVT, or any other disease in which thrombosis is a complicating factor. None of the women in the control group was taking a contraceptive drug, and both groups were studied in parallel.

Analysis: Coagulation/Fibrinolysis Parameters: *All patients had normal platelet counts, activated PTT, one-stage PT, factor V, factor VIII clotting activities, factor VIII–related antigen, AT III, α_2PI, and protein C.*

Fibrinolytic Systems: *t-PA values, after release by venous occlusion, showed wide variation in the controls with three different assay methods: functional fibrin plate, amidolytic assay, and antigen assay (Table 35.7). The patients could be divided into three groups. Group 1 consisted of 67 patients, all of whom had normal t-PA values after venous occlusion. The concentration of*

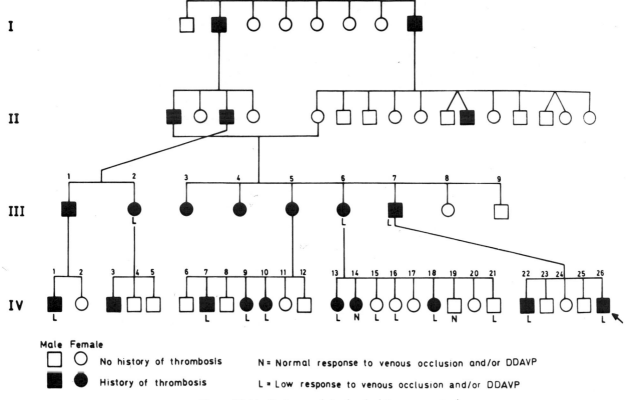

Figure 35.11. Pedigree of the family (✗ = propositus).

Table 35.7 Mean (SD) [range] Values of Fibrinolytic Components after Venous Occlusion and Tissue Plasminogen Activator (t-PA) before Venous Occlusion in 100 Patients with Recurrent Deep Venous Thrombosis or Pulmonary Embolism and 57 Controls, (Patients Divided into Groups on Basis of Results)

		Patients		
	Controls (n = 57)	Group 1 (n = 67)	Group 2 (n = 22)	Group 3 (n = 11)
Fibrin plates	18 (5)	18 (4)	4 (4)	6 (4)
(mm)	[8.4–21.9]	[9.7–22.6]	[0–12.1]	[0–11.7]
t-PA S-2551	18 (2)	23 (18)	1 (1)	1 (1)
(U/mL)	[4–47]	[5.7–59]	[0–4.2]	[0.1–4.1]
t-PA antigen	15 (10)	20 (11)	22 (11)	2 (1)
	[4.9–37]	[2.8–61]	[10–75]	[1.9–7.6]
t-PA inhibitor	8 (2)	8 (3)	45 (20)	7 (4)
(U/mL)	[4.7–11]	[1–16]	[17–109]	[2.5–14]

PAI-1, always determined in the samples taken before venous occlusion, was also within the normal range. A defective fibrinolytic system was found in 33 patients, and two different groups could be distinguished. Group 2 comprised 22 patients, all with normal concentrations of released t-PA after venous occlusion, as measured by the antigen assay, but with a poor response when measured by the functional assays. These patients had significantly increased PAI-1 inhibitor values, which in three patients was 7–10 times higher than that of normal plasma. Group 3 consisted of

11 patients, all with low concentrations of released t-PA after venous occlusion, as measured by both functional and antigen assays. The values for t-PA antigen differed significantly from those of patients in group 2. Ten patients had normal PAI-1 values. The age of the patients in group 1 varied between 14 and 67 years (mean, 41 years), in group 2 between 30 and 73 years (mean, 53 years), and in group 3 between 15 and 72 years (mean, 35 years).

Plasminogen Activators

Plasma Plg activators activate circulating Plg to Pln (see case 1, Fig. 35.1) (6, 31). The physiologic Plg activators are u-PA and t-PA, both direct activators. SK, a bacterial protein that is an indirect activator, combines with Plg to form an equimolar complex, which is a direct activator. These Plg activators are serine proteases that can cleave a single specific Arg-561–Val peptide bond in Plg, a single-chain molecule, to form Pln, a two-chain molecule. Pln, a serine protease with trypsinlike specificity can degrade biologically active plasma proteins, particularly the coagulation and complement proteins.

Urokinase. Pro-u-PA, the zymogen precursor of u-PA, is found in endothelial, kidney, and tumor cells and most mammalian tissues and is released from these cells as an inactive proenzyme (6, 31, 32). It is converted to the active enzyme by limited proteolysis. The zymogen is a single-chain protein (scu-PA), without an active center and without Plg activator activity. It is converted to the fully enzymatically active two-chain u-PA (tcu-PA), a serine protease, by Pln. Pro-u-PA (scu-PA) and u-PA (HMW-u-PA) have identical Mrs of about 54,000; a low-molecular-weight partially degraded form of u-PA (LMW-u-PA), approximately 32 kDa, has been found in urine and tissue culture systems and is derived from the HMW form. On a molar basis, the two u-PA forms have similar specific activities. The complete primary amino acid and cDNA sequences of pro-u-PA have been determined, and the cDNA gene has been expressed in *Escherichia coli* and mammalian cells. The human urokinase gene structure has been elucidated and assigned to chromosome 10. Several types of cells, both normal and transformed, possess specific receptor sites for pro-u-PA and u-PA.

Tissue Plasminogen Activator. t-PA has been found in many mammalian tissues, including endothelial and tumor cells (6, 31, 33). It is released into the circulation following exercise and venous occlusion as a single-chain active enzyme (sct-PA) and is easily converted by Pln to a two-chain enzyme (tct-PA). Both sct-PA and tct-PA are serine proteases with kDas of about 68,000 and similar specific activities. Both t-PAs bind to fibrin, and their Plg activator activities are markedly potentiated in the presence of fibrin. The complete primary amino acid and cDNA sequences of t-PA have been determined, and the cDNA gene expressed in *E. coli* and mammalian cells. The human t-PA gene structure has been elucidated and assigned to chromosome 8. Specific receptors have been identified in both normal and transformed cells.

Streptokinase. SK, about 50 kDa, forms an equimolar, irreversible, activator complex with Plg and Pln (Plg · SK/Pln · SK) with a serine protease active center (6, 31, 34, 35). It is species restricted, forming equimolar activator complexes only with human, cat, and dog Plgs. The human Plg · SK/Pln · SK complexes are called preformed complexes. The complete primary amino acid and cDNA sequences have been determined, and the SK gene has been elucidated.

An important property of Plg activators is their catalytic efficiency (by kinetic analysis: second-order rate constants) in the activation of native Plg (3). SK and its complexes with Plg and the Pln-derived carboxyl-terminal B-chain have the highest catalytic efficiencies. Fibrin greatly influences the catalytic efficiency of t-PA, perhaps 10-fold, but minimally influences the catalytic efficiencies of either u-PA or SK. Plg activators are assayed for fibrinolytic potency, or activity, in a clot lysis assay in which the response depends only on the concentration of the activator species, referenced against WHO International Reference Preparations (u-PA, t-PA, and SK) in international units (IU) (36). The activator assay response is dependent on the Plg substrate concentration, the Plg form (Glu or Lys), and the fibrinogen milieu (plasma or purified fibrinogen). Similar parallel curves are obtained with u-PA (both HMW and LMW preparations) and with the SK and Plg · SK forms, permitting a comparison between u-PA and SK; however, the t-PA curves are not parallel to either the u-PA or the

SK curves, and, therefore, they are not comparable. The t-PA IU is based on a longer lysis time and cannot be compared with either the u-PA or SK IUs. Also, u-PA and SK cannot be compared with each other because the mechanisms of Plg activation are different and the definitions of the IU in the WHO International Reference Preparations are not the same. The IU is an in vitro assessment of potency. The specific activities (IU/mg protein) of highly purified/pure preparations of HMW-u-PA, LMW-u-PA, SK, and t-PA are approximately 100,000, 200,000, 100,000, and 600,000, respectively. When Plg activators are used as thrombolytic agents in patients, the dose (IU) is not related to clinical efficacy, and their IUs cannot be compared; also, each activator has a different mechanism of Plg activation in the fibrin thrombus (32, 37, 38). Therefore, in clinical trials, it is not possible to compare the Plg activators with one another.

Plasminogen Activator Inhibitors

The activity of the physiologic Plg activators (u-PA and t-PA) is controlled in plasma by specific inhibitors (6, 31, 39, 40). These inhibitors play an important role in regulating u-PA- and t-PA-dependent fibrinolysis in situ; they prevent premature fibrinolysis at the adhesion site of clots on the endothelial cell before wound healing, and they prevent and modulate the destruction of vascular walls. Impairment of fibrinolysis may be due to deficient synthesis and/or release of PAI-1 from the vascular wall.

PAI-1. The specific rapid-reacting inhibitor of u-PA and t-PA, about 52 kDa, is found in plasma, platelets, endothelial cells, fibroblasts, smooth muscle cells, hepatocytes, and tumor cells (31, 39, 40). In normal human plasma, it is the primary inhibitor of u-PA and t-PA, forming irreversible 1:1 stoichiometric complexes. It appears to be synthesized in an active form that forms a stable complex with the activator, but it is a relatively unstable molecule and rapidly decays into a latent, inactive, form that can be reactivated by treatment with denaturing agents. Platelets release the latent form. The PAI-1 activity of plasma is associated with a binding protein, vitronectin, in a complex that stabilizes PAI-1 in the plasma. PAI-1 is a member of the serpin family of protease inhibitor proteins. The complete primary amino acid and cDNA sequences of PAI-1 have been determined, and the cDNA expressed in *E. coli* and mammalian cells. The PAI-1 gene structure has been elucidated and assigned to chromosome 7.

PAI-2. The placental-type inhibitor of u-PA and t-PA found in pregnancy plasma is also found in other cells and tissues and in tumor cells (39, 41). There are two forms of this inhibitor: an HMW form (approximately 70 kDa) and an LMW form (approximately 47 kDa). These two forms form 1:1 complexes with both u-PA and t-PA; the u-PA complexes are irreversible, whereas the t-PA complexes are weaker and reversible, particularly the sct-PA-PAI-2 complex. PAI-2 inhibits u-PA about 10 times better than it inhibits tct-PA and is a poor inhibitor of sct-PA. In contrast to PAI-1, PAI-2 is a stable inhibitor. The reaction rate of PAI-2 is at least one order of magnitude slower than that of PAI-1. The complete primary amino acid and cDNA sequences of PAI-2 have been determined. It is also a member of the serpin family of protease inhibitor proteins.

PAI-3. The plasma heparin-dependent activated protein C inhibitor is similar to the heparin-dependent u-PA inhibitor, PAI-3, which is also found in human urine. It is a much less effective inhibitor than either PAI-1 or PAI-2. However, the plasma concentration of PAI-3 is at least two orders of magnitude higher than that of PAI-1, and it is also an inhibitor of both u-PA and t-PA.

Pathophysiologic Relevance of t-PA and PAI-1 in Hemostasis

Impairment of fibrinolysis due to deficient synthesis and/or release of t-PA from the vessel wall or to increased levels of PAI-1 is associated with a tendency to thrombotic disease. Defective release of t-PA from the vessel wall during venous occlusion and/or a decreased t-PA content in the walls of superficial veins was found in about 70% of a large series of patients with idiopathic venous thrombosis. This association of recurrent venous thrombosis with a defect in the fibrinolytic system is more frequent than with any other known disturbance of hemostasis. Phenformin combined with ethylestrenol stimulates the release of fibrinolytic activity from the vessel wall and diminishes the frequency of thrombotic episodes. A defective capacity to release fibrinolytic activity from the vessel wall after venous occlusion and/or infusion of DDAVP was found in a large family with a high incidence of thrombosis (case 4). The fibrinolytic activity of the vessel wall was normal in all cases. In a large series of 100 consecutive patients with recurrent DVT (case 5), two different mechanisms responsible for a poor fibrinolytic response could be distinguished. Twenty-two patients in whom the response was poor after venous occlusion released normal amounts of t-PA, both functional and antigen, into the plasma but had appreciably increased concentrations of plasma PAI-1. The 11 other patients in whom the response was poor after venous occlusion had low t-PA functional and antigen activities but normal concentrations of PAI-1. In another study, 120 patients with spontaneous or recurrent DVT were investigated for fibrinolytic response to venous occlusion (before and after 10 min) (42). They were classified into three groups: (a) good responders (76 patients), with less than 2-fold increase in euglobulin fibrinolytic activity; (b) poor responders (12 patients), with deficient t-PA release and high risk for recurrent DVT; and (c) poor responders (32 patients), with normal t-PA release but increased levels of PAI-1. In these studies, AT III, heparin cofactor II, protein C, and protein S levels were normal.

Protein C and Protein S Pathway Deficiencies with Thrombophilia

Case 6 (Protein C Deficiency) (43)

A 29-year-old woman (III-1) (Fig. 35.12) presented with suspicion of pulmonary embolism. At the age of 20, she experienced an unexplained DVT of the left leg, complicated by PE, and was treated with an oral anticoagulant for 6 months. Later, she developed a postthrombotic syndrome of her left leg and was again treated with an oral anticoagulant. She did not use oral contraceptives during the study. A brother of the propositus (III-2), at age 16, developed DVT and secondary varicose veins during immobilization following trauma of the left calf. Two years later, the left long saphenous vein was removed; postoperatively, he had a superficial thrombophlebitis. The same year he experienced superficial thrombophlebitis of the right long saphenous vein and DVT of the right leg. He was treated for 3 months with an oral anticoagulant. One year later, he had a recurrence of the DVT of the right leg; long-term treatment with an oral anticoagulant was instituted. A second brother of the propositus (III-3), at age 18, suffered an unexplained superficial thrombophlebitis of the right long saphenous vein and was anticoagulated. The father (II-2), at age 48, developed unexplained DVT complicated by PE; he was treated with an oral anticoagulant. At ages 54 and 56, he suffered from myocardial infarctions and died suddenly at age 57. The mother (II-1) died at age 33, 20 days postpartum, due to consequences of a hemorrhagic infarction of the small bowel. Her previous medical history was not significant.

Analysis: The propositus (III-1) and her two brothers (III-2 and III-3) with a history of thrombotic disease showed a deficiency of PC antigen: levels of 0.51, 0.14, and 0.15 U/mL, respectively (normal range, 0.75–1.35 U/mL), and a third half-brother (different mother) was found to have normal PC antigen, 0.92 U/mL (Tables 35.8 and 35.9). No other coagulation abnormalities were found; a detailed analysis of fibrinolytic system components was not made. Because the father and mother of the propositus had died by the time of the study, the in-

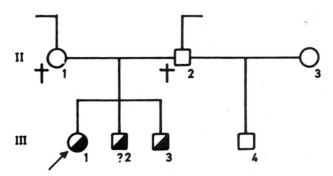

Figure 35.12. Pedigree of the family (↗ = propositus). The symbols indicate males (□); females (○), patients with protein C deficiency (◪,◑), heterozygotes (◪,◑), suspected heterozygotes (□,○).

Table 35.8. Plasma Coagulation Factor Concentrations of Propositus (III, 1)

Protein C antigen	0.51 U/mL
Factor VII:C	1.00 U/mL
Factor II:C	1.12 U/mL
Factor IX:C	0.90 U/mL
Factor X:C	0.94 U/mL
Factor VIII:C	1.95 U/mL
Fibrinogen	3.1 g/L
Antithrombin III	1.13 U/mL
Plasminogen	0.83 U/mL
α_2-antiplasmin	0.83 U/mL

Table 35.9. Plasma Coagulation Factor Concentrations of the Brothers of Propositus

	III,2[a]	III,3[a]	III,4
Protein C antigen (U/mL)	0.14	0.15	0.92
Factor II antigen (U/mL)	0.50	0.56	0.88
Factor X antigen (U/mL)	0.36	0.28	0.88
Antithrombin III (U/mL)	0.87	0.95	1.17
Protein C antigen/ factor X antigen	0.28	0.27	1.04
Protein C antigen/ factor II antigen	0.39	0.53	1.04
Thrombotest (sec)	92	157	40

[a]both patients were under stable oral anticoagulant treatment.

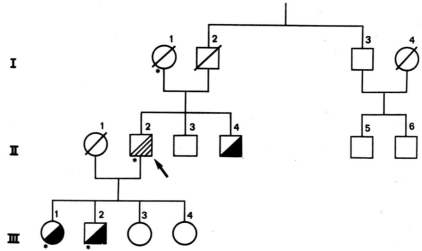

Figure 35.13. Pedigree of the family (✓ = propositus). The symbols indicate males (□); females (○), patients with protein S deficiency (◼, ◖), propositus treated with vitamin K antagonist (◩), patients with episodes of thrombosis (∗).

heritance pattern in this family was not established. However, it is highly unlikely that the occurrence of three such patients in one such family is accidental. The propositus is probably a heterozygote, and her affected brothers are homozygotes; their parents were probably heterozygotes. Congenital deficiency of protein C is inherited as an autosomal dominant disease.

Case 7 (Protein S Deficiency) (44)

A 37-year-old man (II-2) (Fig. 35.13) presented with spontaneous DVT in both legs; he was treated with an oral anticoagulant during the subsequent 3 months. Two years later, he developed a new spontaneous thrombotic event, including a left-sided DVT and a superficial thrombophlebitis of the left antebrachial vein. The patient was again treated an with an oral anticoagulant and for 6 years did not suffer new episodes of thromboembolism. The mother of the propositus (I-1) had an episode of clinically suspected DVT. Most of the patient's brothers, an uncle, cousins, and two of his four children have a history of thrombophlebitis. One of the proposi-

tus's daughters (III-1) suffered spontaneous DVT at the age of 15. Long-term treatment with an oral anticoagulant was instituted. At the age of 21, this daughter became pregnant, and she was immediately changed from Coumadin to subcutaneous heparin (5000 IU every 12 hours). A spontaneous abortion occurred after 3 months of pregnancy. The propositus's son (III-2), at the age of 13, had an appendectomy; the postoperative period was complicated by a DVT and PE. Long-term oral anticoagulant therapy was instituted. This son, at ages 14 and 19, suffered new episodes of DVT associated with noncompliance with anticoagulant therapy.

Analysis: Four of the family members—propositus (II-2), and brother (II-4), and children (III-1, and III-2)—with a history of thrombotic disease showed a deficiency of PS antigen of 28%, 51%, 51%, and 56%, respectively, with normal PC antigen. Two of the three PS-deficient patients suffering from episodes of thrombosis had low t-PA activity (Table 35.10); the one PS-deficient patient without signs of thrombotic disease had very high t-PA activity. One PS-deficient family member (III-2) also had high PAI-1 activity. Functional and anti-

gen Plg, α₂PI, and HRG were normal in the four family members with PS deficiency. These data are compatible with an autosomal dominant pattern of inheritance. The origin of the defect, the PS deficiency, is probably the mother and perhaps the father, both heterozygotes; the PS-deficient patients are both homozygotes (II-2) and heterozygotes (II-4, III-1, III-2), with the possibility of dysfunctional protein C molecules in the propositus, his brother, and his son. The present data did not definitively indicate a relationship between the PS deficiency and a defective fibrinolytic system, but the possibility exists.

Table 35.10 Variables of the Fibrinolytic System in 4 Patients with Inherited Protein S Deficiency

	Patients				
	II-2[a]	*II-4*	*III-1*	*III-2*	*Reference Intervals*
t-PA Act (IU/mL)[b]	0.05	12.3	<0.01	0.12	0.00–0740
PAI Act (IU/mL)[b]	8.6	7.6	6.1	30.6	1.7–12.7
Plg Ag (%)	106	104	98	121	74–136
Plg Act (%)	100	105	94	114	86–124
HRG Ag (%)	118	122	119	145	61–145
α₂-AP Act (%)	96	98	106	114	85–110
C1-INA Ag (%)	98	141	94	104	68–140

[a]Blood sample obtained during oral anticoagulant treatment.
[b]The reference intervals of the t-PA Act and PAI Act have been calculated on the basis of the median values and the 95% interpercentiles of the observations in the reference population and the other reference intervals were expressed as mean (2 SD).

Protein C/S Deficiency: Hypofibrinolysis

Patients who have a congenital deficiency of protein C or protein S frequently exhibit severe recurrent thromboembolic disease, indicating that the main function of the protein C pathway is to regulate intravascular blood coagulation (45–52). Protein C is activated by a complex formed between thrombin and thrombomodulin on the vascular wall, assembles with protein S on the surface of platelets and endothelial cells, and then inhibits the prothrombinase and tenase complex (Fig. 35.14). The profibrinolytic and anticoagulant activity of activated protein C (APC) depends upon the same cofactors. Stimulation of fibrinolysis was observed after infusion of APC into cats and dogs (51). In these species, the level of fibrinogen/fibrin degradation products was increased, and in the dog, an increase in PA was observed. In in vitro studies, human and bovine APC induced the lysis of blood clots, plasma clots, and euglobulin clots (52). One possible mechanism for the profibrinolytic effect of APC is that it neutralizes PAI-1 (50). Consumption of PAI-1 by APC probably elevates the PA level in plasma.

Protein C

Protein C is a vitamin K–dependent plasma zymogen that is activated to APC, a serine protease. It is synthesized in the liver as a single-chain glycoprotein with 407 amino acid residues, about 62 kDa. The primary structure has been established by both amino acid sequence analysis and cDNA cloning. The PC gene, 11.2 kilobases in length, is

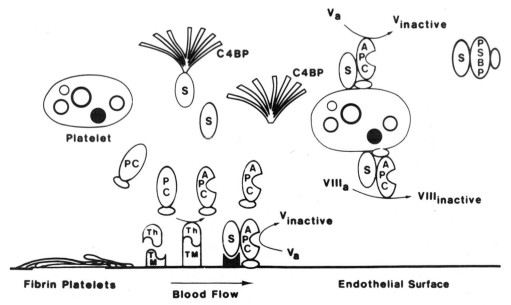

Figure 35.14. Vascular injury leads to thrombin (Th) formation. Thrombin is carried by blood flow downstream where it binds thrombomodulin (TM). Protein C (PC) is converted to activated protein C (APC) by this complex. Activated protein C complexes with protein S (PS) to form the functional complex responsible for factor Va and VIIIa inactivation. Protein S is in a reversible complex with C4bBP, and in normal individuals, approximately 40% is free. Only the free form is functional, shown here in complex with activated protein C on either endothelial or platelet surfaces.

divided into 9 exons and 8 introns and has been localized on chromosome 2 q14–q21.

PC is a two-chain enzyme connected by a single disulfide bond. The first 11 glutamate (Gla) residues are γ-carboxylated. The heavy chain (approximately 41 kDa) contains the serine protease domain. PC is converted to APC by thrombin in the presence of thrombomodulin. APC inactivates factors Va and VIIIa by limited proteolysis. PS is a cofactor required for the stimulation of the APC-catalyzed inactivation of factor Va by enhancing the binding of APC to phospholipids. APC is inhibited by both PC inhibitor (53) and α_1AT. The PC inhibitor, which is heparin-dependent, appears to be similar to the urinary Plg activator inhibitor (PAI-3).

Protein S

Protein S is another vitamin K–dependent plasma single-chain glycoprotein, about 84 kDa, with 635 amino acid residues. It is not a serine protease. It contains 11 glutamate (Gla) residues, which are γ-carboxylated, in the NH_2-terminal domain. It is synthesized in the liver, vascular endothelial cells, and megakaryocytes and is stored in the platelets. The PS gene contains 15 exons; it has been localized on chromosome 3.

In plasma, PS is present in two forms in about equal amounts: a free form and a complex with the C4b-binding protein. The free PS can function as a cofactor for APC but the complex cannot, and the C4b-binding protein inhibits the cofactor activity of PS in vitro. The C4b-binding protein is a regulatory protein in the classical complement system acting as a cofactor in the dissociation of C3 convertase (C4bC2a complex) into C4b and C2a. C4b is a glycoprotein of about 500 kDa. It is thought that the complexed PS competitively inhibits APC binding to free PS.

Protein C and Protein S Deficiencies

Patients who have congenital deficiencies of PC or PS frequently exhibit severe recurrent venous thromboembolic disease, indicating that the main function of the PC pathway is to regulate intravascular blood coagulation (see chapter 34). Many of these patients in families with PC and PS deficiencies have a history of thrombotic disease, with superficial thrombophlebitis, DVT, and PE; they develop these conditions without an apparent cause at a relatively young age. Such patients with thrombotic disease have been effectively treated with an oral anticoagulant. Normal levels of t-PA and PAI-1 were found in all of the patients with PC deficiencies.

The mechanism for the profibrinolytic effect of APC has not been definitively established. However, profibrinolysis appears to depend upon APC with Gla domains, Ca^{2+}, platelets, and other blood cells. A congenital abnormal protein C with a dysfunctional Gla domain was found in a 60-year-old man with recurrent thrombotic disease (54); however, family members with the same abnormality were asymptomatic. The PC anticoagulant activity and the antigen level measured by an ELISA, utilizing a calcium-dependent monoclonal antibody that recognizes the Gla-domain, was half of normal, indicating a structural defect in the Gla-region and heterozygosity.

Most reported cases have half-normal PC levels, and the deficiency is transmitted from parents to children of both sexes, suggesting heterozygosity for an autosomal gene with variable penetrance. At least seven unrelated families in which newborns had very low, or unmeasurable, levels of PC, while their parents had half-normal levels, have been described, suggesting homozygosity for these cases. Infants with severe homozygous protein C deficiency and neonatal purpura fulminans have been treated with highly purified protein C concentrates (55). Two types of PC deficiency have been described: (a) type I, characterized by a concomitant decrease in PC functional activity and antigen, and (b) type II, characterized by disproportionately low functional activity compared with antigen (e.g., a dysfunctional molecule) (56).

A congenital, probably homozygous, deficiency of protein C (<5% antigen) combined with a heterozygous Plg abnormality (50% functional, 86% antigen) has been described in a 21-year-old man (57). The propositus survived his neonatal period without any clinical manifestation of thromboembolic disease. However, he has been suffering from recurrent and persistent venous thrombotic disease since the age of 14. His clinical condition greatly improved following oral anticoagulant therapy. Both parents were PC heterozygotes (50% antigen), and the father and aunt had a heterozyous abnormality of Plg (38% functional, 86% antigen) (dysplasminogenemia). A hypoplasminogenemia-dysplasminogenemia was described in a 33-year-old man (45% functional, 56% antigen), and his 72-year-old mother (58% functional, 58% antigen) with a history of massive DVT following minor surgery; the 77-year-old father was normal, and a 34-year-old sister was found to have the Plg abnormality (48% functional, 52% antigen) (58). This family also showed a PC deficiency in the propositus (38% functional, 38% antigen), the mother (44% functional, 57% antigen), and sister (53% functional, 40% antigen), with normal PC levels in the father. Both the Plg abnormality and the PC deficiency suggested heterozygosity in the mother. Although PC molecular abnormalities have been postulated, they have not yet been described.

The profibrinolytic effect of APC appears to be involved in the neutralization of PAI-1, which could lead to the stimulation of profibrinolysis by elevating the relative PA level in plasma; but, the Scandinavian family with the PS deficiency and recurrent venous thromboembolism (case 7) showed t-PA activities in the lower normal range for 3 family members (II-2, III-1, III-2). One family member (11–4), a 38-year-old with no history of thrombotic disease, had a high plasma level of t-PA. Three of four family members had normal plasma PAI-1 levels, but one family member (III-2), a 15-year-old young man, had a high plasma level of PAI-1. Another mechanism for the stimulation of profibrinolysis may be reduction of thrombin generation due to APC-PS-induced inactivation of factors Va and VIIIa, which may lead to a decrease in the thrombin-stimulated secretion of PAI-1 from the endothelial cell.

Acquired Deficiencies of Protein C and Protein S

Since PC and PS are vitamin K–dependent proteins, oral anticoagulants decrease the synthesis of both proteins and lead to the formation of an acarboxylated protein with decreased calcium-binding capacity. Long-term anticoagulant therapy of patients reduces the PC antigen to about half-normal levels. PC levels (functional and antigen) are low in patients with chronic hepatitis or liver cirrhosis, and vitamin K deficiency. In clinical conditions associated with DIC and in renal failure, PC levels are low. After plasma exchange, PC decreases to half of the normal level but returns to normal within 24 hours. Acquired PS deficiency is observed during oral anticoagulant therapy and in the nephrotic syndrome, DIC, and other conditions associated with an increase in the C4b-binding protein.

Bleeding Disorder Due to an α_2-Plasmin Inhibitor Deficiency

Case 8 (59)

A 15-year-old young man (III-6) (Fig. 35.15) was referred for evaluation of easy bruisability from early childhood. He had umbilical bleeding at birth, and after minor trauma, subcutaneous hematomas easily developed. There was no prolonged hemorrhage from small cuts but sometimes bleeding started again after 24 hours. At age 4, following tonsillectomy, he began to bleed; bleeding persisted for 2 days and ceased after a blood transfusion. At age 8, there was bleeding for some hours following a tooth extraction. At age 14, he suffered again from prolonged bleeding after a dental extraction. Epistaxis, spontaneous gingival bleeding, and muscle or joint bleeding did not occur. His 5-year-old sister (III-8) bruised easily but had not had any operative procedures or injuries. Both siblings had normal growth and development. There were no signs suggesting liver disease, and routine liver function tests were normal. Besides mild bleeding after a tooth extraction, the father of the

siblings had no bleeding tendency. The other family members did not have any signs of a hemorrhagic diathesis.

Analysis: Identification of the Defect: Assessment of propositus's coagulation and platelet functions in general tests showed no defects in either system (Table 35.11). In the fibrinolysis assays (Table 35.12), all factors were found to be normal except for the functional activity of α_2PI, which was 4% for the propositus and 2% for his sister. On the other hand, the concentrations of α_2PI antigen were found to be 83% and 92%, respectively, in the plasmas of the propositus and his sister (normal range, 64–145%). The siblings also had reduced dilute

Table 35.11. Results of Hemostasis Tests

	Propositus	Normal Range
Prothrombin time (sec)	12.0	10.3–12.3
Activated partial thromboplastin time (sec)	40	32–42
Thrombin time (sec)	22.7	19.5–25.5
Reptilase time (sec)	22.3	19.3–22.3
Fibrin monomer test	Negative	Negative
Urea test	Normal	
Antithrombin III activity (%)	130	80–120
Protein C antigen (%)	76	67–140
Bleeding time (min)	5.15	3–8
Platelet count (μL^{-1})	271,000	150000–320,000
Platelet aggregation studies	Normal	
Whole blood clot lysis (hr)	>36	>36
Dilute blood clot lysis, 10% (min)	87	>162
Plasma on fibrin plates, 30 μL (mm)	6.7	0
Euglobulin activity on fibrin plate (mm)	15.0	9–15
FDP (Wellco test) (μg/mL)	<10	<10

Table 35.12. Results of Fibrinolysis Assays

	Propositus	Propositus's Sister	Normal Range
Plasminogen (%)	80	88	75–125
Histidine-rich glycoprotein (%)	84	85	60–140
t-PA activity (mU/mL)	118	5	0–250
t-PA antigen (ng/mL)	11.8	16.1	10–30
Fast-acting t-PA inhibition (%)	64	133	20–350
Plasma urokinase activity (BAU/mL)	51	53	35–60
Factor XII–dependent activator activity (BAU/mL)	49	47	35–60
C1-inactivator activity (%)	78	125	80–120
α_2-Macroglobulin activity (%)	225	250	80–120
α_2-AP activity (%)	4	2	85–140

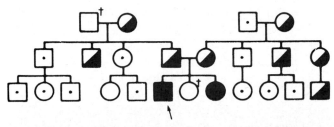

Figure 35.15. Pedigree of the family ($\nearrow$ = propositus). Male normal (□); female normal (○); heterozygotes (◨, ◐) homozygotes (■,●); not tested (□,○); deceased (†).

blood clot (10%) lysis times. The propositus's plasma exhibited spontaneous lysis on fibrin plates. The fibrin-bound α_2PI of the propositus did not inhibit Pln. It was concluded that the propositus and his sister have a functional α_2PI deficiency.

Family Studies: Analysis revealed normal α_2PI antigen levels in all family members. Eight members of the family showed approximately half-normal functional α_2PI activity levels in their plasma, including the propositus's father and mother. These family members are classified as heterozygotes, and the inheritance pattern is apparently autosomal recessive. None of the inhibition patterns showed a significant difference between heterozygotes from the paternal or maternal family. Both families have lived for generations in the eastern part of the Netherlands; the family history was obtained by interview and examination of official registration dating back to 1780, but no (official) consanguinity was found in six generations. The dysfunctional molecule was designated α_2PI Enschede (the city of birth of the propositus).

α_2-Plasmin Inhibitor Deficiency: Hyperfibrinolysis

Two plasma proteins are involved in the inhibition and clearance of the proteolytic enzyme Pln, α_2PI and α_2M. α_2-PI is the major inhibitor of Pln (10, 60); α_2M binds the enzyme but does not inhibit it. Pln formed from Plg by physiologic and pathologic activators is responsible for the degradation of fibrin both in wound healing and in the fibrin thrombus. α_2PI in normal plasma is heterogeneous and consists of functionally active and inactive proteins. Complete activation of the Plg present in normal plasma converts only 70% of the α_2PI antigen into a complex with Pln; 30% of the inhibitor-related antigen appears to be functionally inactive. Human plasma also contains two forms of the inhibitor, which differ in their binding to Plg. The form that does not bind well remains an active Pln inhibitor but reacts much more slowly with Pln. This form lacks a 26-residue peptide from the COOH-terminal end of α_2PI, which inhibits the interaction of α_2PI with Pln, suggesting that it contains the Pln (Plg)-binding site. The weak-binding form is converted from the strong-binding form in the circulation.

α_2-PI has three functional sites: (a) the Pln (Plg) binding site, (b) the reactive site, and (c) the cross-linking site. It has a strong affinity for Pln (Plg) and preferentially binds to sites on the Pln (Plg) molecule called lysine-binding sites (LBS) or fibrin-binding sites (kringles 1, 2, 3, 4, and 5). α_2PI competitively inhibits the binding of Plg to fibrin. The naturally occurring fibrinolytic process is caused by fibrin-associated Plg activation and depends on the amount of both Plg and Plg activators bound to fibrin. Therefore, inhibition of Plg binding to fibrin by α_2PI results in retardation of the initiation of the

fibrinolytic process. The Pln (Plg) binding site in α_2PI is located in the COOH-terminal end, at Lys-436 and Lys-452. This binding site plays an important role in the inhibition of Pln. α_2PI rapidly forms a reversible complex with Pln through noncovalent binding between the LBS in Pln and the Pln (Plg) binding site of α_2PI. This step in the reaction can be competitively inhibited by Plg fragments containing the LBS or by EACA, which binds to the LBS. The partially degraded form of α_2PI, without the Pln (Plg) binding site, reacts less readily with Pln, indicating a significant contribution of the Pln (Plg) binding site to the efficient inhibition of Pln. In the second step, a covalent bond is formed between the active-site serine of Pln and the reactive site of α_2PI, resulting in the loss of Pln proteolytic activity. The reactive site of α_2 PI is located at Arg-364.

Another important function of α_2PI is its cross-linking to fibrin. When blood clots, part of the α_2PI in plasma is rapidly cross-linked to the fibrin α-chain by activated factor XIII. While clot retraction is progressively taking place, the fibrin-bound α_2PI becomes condensed in the clot and contributes to the resistance of the clot against lysis. Fibrin-fibrin cross-linking is of only minor importance in endowing the clot with resistance to lysis. The α_2PI cross-linking site is located at the second amino acid from the N$_2$-terminus, glutamine. The residue in the fibrin(ogen) molecule where the glutamine residue of α_2PI cross-links is Lys-303 of the Aα-chain. No other serine protease inhibitor has a factor XIIIa–catalyzed cross-linking site under physiologic conditions. When homologous amino acid sequences of α_2PI and the other members of the serine protease inhibitor family (serpins) (e.g., AT III, α_1AT, PAI-1) are aligned, α_2PI extends 50–52 amino acids beyond the COOH-terminal ends of the other members of the serpin family. This extra COOH-terminal end, which is specific for α_2PI, contains the Pln (Plg) binding-site.

Although the cross-linking reaction proceeds rapidly, maximum cross-linking is limited to only 20–25% of the α_2PI present in plasma before clotting. Most of the α_2PI cross-linked to the α-chain of fibrin is in the form of the α-chain monomer–α_2PI complex, which is gradually transformed to the α-chain polymer–α_2PI complex as polymerization proceeds. Another plasma protein, fibronectin, is also cross-linked to the fibrin α-chain by activated factor XIII when blood coagulation takes place. However, these two proteins, α_2PI and fibronectin, are independently cross-linked to fibrin, without affecting the cross-linking of the other. Although the amount of α_2PI cross-linked to fibrin is low, it is significant in the inhibition of clot lysis. However, the inhibitory effect of free α_2PI on clot lysis is limited. The absence of cross-linking of α_2PI to fibrin, in addition to an increased affinity of non-crossed-linked fibrin for Pln (Plg), may contribute to the instability of hemostatic plugs in factor XIII deficiencies by increasing the susceptibility of fibrin clots to naturally occurring fibrinolytic process. The congenital deficiency of α_2PI results in a lifelong severe hemorrhagic tendency due to the premature degradation of hemostatic plugs by the physiologically occurring fibrinolytic process.

α_2-Plasmin Inhibitor

α_2PI. α_2PI, also called α_2-antiplasmin, is a single-chain glycoprotein with a carbohydrate content of 13–14% and two disulfide bridges, of about 58 kDa (10, 60). Its concentration in plasma is about 1 μM, corresponding to 7 mg/dL. DNA and protein sequencing revealed that it contains 452 amino acids and four Asn-linked glycosylation sites.

Molecular Basis for α_2PI Deficiency: The α_2PI gene contains 10 exons and 9 introns distributed over approximately 16 kilobases of DNA. A restriction fragment length polymorphism found in the gene can be attributed to the presence of two alleles, A and B. The minor allele, B, is due to the deletion of about 720 base pairs in intron VIII. The two alleles A and B were distributed with frequencies of 73.5% and 26.5%, respectively, in 77 unrelated Caucasian individuals, or with frequencies of 51.0% and 49.0% respectively, in 50 unrelated Japanese individuals. The α_2PI gene is located on chromosome 18 p11.1–q11.2. α_2PI-Enschede's molecular defect consists of the insertion of an extra Ala residue (GCG) somewhere between amino acid residues 350 and 357, 7–10 positions Nα_2-terminal from Arg-364 in the reactive site. This three base pair insertion within the gene was identified in two true heterozygotes and in their two homozygous children. The α_2PI genes from two Japanese families with congenital deficiencies showed a nucleotide insertion in exon X in α_2PI-Nara and a trinucleotide deletion of Glu-137 in exon VIII in α_2PI-Okinawa. In α_2PI-Nara, an elongated mutant, 178 COOH-terminal amino acid residues were substituted for the 12 COOH-terminal amino acid residues of native α_2PI.

Congenital α_2PI Deficiency. Six families with congenital deficiencies and clinically severe bleeding tendencies have been reported. Severe bleeding in these families occurred only in the homozygotes; the molecular defect has been established in three of these families. The heterozygotes, with 40–60% α_2PI levels, showed no discernible, or mild, bleeding. Four additional families with congenital α_2PI deficiency and mild bleeding have been reported.

Acquired α_2PI Deficiency. The plasma level of α_2PI is significantly decreased in liver cirrhosis, other liver diseases, DIC, and some forms of renal disease and in patients undergoing thrombolytic therapy.

Bleeding Disorder Due to Excess Plasminogen Activator

Case 9 (61)

The propositus is a 43-year-old man with a history of recurrent bleeding after trauma since birth. As a child, he had prominent bruising on participation in contact sports and frequent episodes of knee swelling after playing soccer. The propositus had been told that he has "mild hemophilia." As an adolescent, he had minor orthopaedic surgery to correct a deformity of the right great toe; this was followed by severe and prolong bleeding, and the patient recalled that his leg was "black from the knee down" due to subcutaneous blood. Many dental extractions were followed by bleeding, which often ceased immediately following the extractions; but bleeding recurred after a day or two, when it would continue for many days, apparently unmodified by transfusion of fresh frozen plasma.

There was no family history of abnormal bleeding; the propositus's father and paternal grandfather had died at ages 38 and 55, respectively, of MI, without showing any bleeding tendencies. He had been known, since 1974, to have hyperlipidemia, for which he had initially received clofibrate. His mother, paternal grandmother, and two brothers were free of symptoms of bleeding and ischemic heart disease. No specific treatment was given. At age 46, he was admitted to the hospital with nausea, vomiting, and severe headache. A CAT scan revealed a hematoma in the right parieto-occipital region. Treatment with EACA was started at once. His clinical condition stabilized for several days. On the sixth day, signs of raised intracranial pressure with features of early brainstem compression arose; craniotomy with evacuation of the clot was undertaken, but the propositus died within 24 hours of surgery.

Routine hemostatic studies (Table 35.13) showed normal platelet function. Plasma coagulation pathways were normal. Clot solubility in either monochloracetic acid or urea was not increased, suggesting that levels of factor XIIIa were adequate for cross-linking; factor XIII subunits a and b antigen levels were about 30%, more than the 5% or less sufficient for normal hemostasis.

Screening of the fibrinolytic pathway revealed grossly abnormal indices of overall fibrinolytic activity (rapid whole blood and euglobulin lysis and extensive lysis of a Plg-containing fibrin plate by plasma), evidence of breakdown of fibrin and/or fibrinogen, but no depletion of plasma Plg. This excessive fibrinolytic activity, invariably present on repeated study over 3 years, was not due to a deficiency of known inhibitors. Plasmin inhibitor levels, α_2PI (functional and antigen) and α_2M (antigen) and the Plg activator inhibitor, PAI-1 (antigen), level were normal. The HRG level was normal. No free Pln was found, but Pln-α_2PI complexes were found that were rapidly cleared. C1-inactivator, which inhibits the generation of Plg activator by the factor XII/ prekallikrein activation pathway, was normal. The patient's plasma activator was not identified, except for preliminary qualitative biochemical studies. In neutralization experiments with an antibody to PA, isolated from human uterine tissue (probably to t-PA), the patient's plasma PA after venous occlusion and the PA

Table 35.13. Routine Hemostatic Studies

	Patient[a]	Mean Normal Value or Range[a]
(1) Platelet function		
Bleeding time	4.0 min	4.5 ± 1.3 min
Platelet count	70–130 × 10⁹L	>100 × 10⁹/L
Platelet aggregation		
ADP	Normal	
Collagen	Normal	
Ristocetin	Normal	
(2) Coagulation		
Thrombin time	10.8 sec	9–11 sec
Prothrombin time	15.5 sec	11–14 sec
Partial thromboplastin time	39.0 sec	38–45 sec
Fibrinogen level	210 mg/dL	300 ± 70 mg/dL
Factor VIII activity	104%	100%
Factor-VIII-related antigen	86%	100%
Factor XII (immunoassay)	100%	100%
Factor XIIIa (immunoassay)	33%	100%
Factor XIIIb (immunoassay)	30%	100%
Ethanol gelation test	Normal	
(3) Fibrinolysis		
Whole blood clot lysis time	<6 hr	>48 hr
Plasma euglobulin lysis time	<50 min	80–240 min
Plasma lysis of fibron plate containing plasminogen	15 mm	0 mm
Plasma lysis of plasminogen-free fibrin plate	0 mm	0 mm
Euglobulin lysis of fibrinplate containing plasminogen	19.7 mm	6.2–16.5 m
Euglobulin plus CI-inactivator lysis of fibrin plate containing plasminogen	13.0 mm	0–8.8 mm
Plasminogen (caseinolysis)	4.5 CU/mL	4.1 CU/mL
Plasminogen (immunoasssay)	130%	100%
Serum fibrin/fibrinogen-related antigens (FDP)	>40 µg/mL	<5 µg/mL
Protein C	100%	100%

[a]Values expressed as percentages refer to those observed in a plasma pool that was prepared from 25 normal healthy male subjects between 20 and 40 years old and that was stored at −70°C.

present in normal plasma were quenched, indicating its similarity to t-PA.

The observation on the propositus with a lifelong bleeding disorder due primarily to an excess of a PA, probably t-PA, with possibly normal levels of PAI-1, represents a genuine excess of extrinsic, or vascular, activator. Whether this reflects increased synthesis or decreased clearance of activator from the circulation is unknown. With the single exception of his final episode of intracerebral hemorrhage, this man did not exhibit spontaneous bleeding but bled severely only after trauma. Nonetheless, he showed evidence of continuously enhanced fibrinolytic activity, with consistently very high levels of PA, grossly elevated levels of fibrin/fibrinogen-related antigens, and Pln-α₂PI complexes, indicating continuous Pln generation, in the blood. There was no deficiency of Plg, or α₂PI, and only a slight reduction in fibrinogen. The patient's lipid disorder may have played a role in altering his fibrinolytic disorder. However, hyperlipidemia has been associated with depressed, rather than enhanced, fibrinolysis.

Excess Plasminogen Activator: Hyperfibrinolysis

Lifelong bleeding disorders due to enhanced fibrinolysis are rare. They can be due to (*a*) excess activator (62, 63), (*b*) deficiency of α₂PI, (*c*) decreased functional activity of PAI-1, (*d*) deficiency of PAI-1, or (*e*) deficiency of factor XIII.

Activity of Type I Plasminogen Activator Inhibitor: Dysfunctional PAI-I

Case 10 (64)

The propositus is a 76-year-old man with persistent bleeding after transurethral resection of the prostate. He had a long history of bleeding after surgery. At age 56, severe postoperative bleeding occurred after total hip replacement. At age 65, revision of his hip prosthesis was associated with postoperative bleeding requiring 10 units of packed red blood cells. Five episodes of upper gastrointestinal bleeding occurred during the following 3 years, requiring multiple blood transfusions. No specific site of bleeding was identified despite upper gastrointestinal x-ray series and endoscopy. At age 71, the propositus fell on his side and developed a massive hematoma. Two years later, he developed obstructive urinary symptoms and underwent a transurethral resection of the prostate for benign hyperplasia. The postoperative course was complicated by bleeding, requiring four units of packed red blood cells. Bleeding resolved, but he was readmitted 3 days after discharge with persistent gross hematuria. Cystoscopy was negative, and the clot was evacuated. He continued to bleed and was treated with eight units of packed red blood cells and eight units of fresh frozen plasma without cessation of bleeding.

Analysis: Routine coagulation studies were normal, including the PT and PTT. There was no evidence of ongoing DIC, with normal fibrinogen (0.256 g/L; normal range, 0.160–0.350 g/L), normal thrombin and reptilase times, and normal D dimer, with only modestly elevated fibrin degradation products (20–40; normal, <10). The bleeding time and vW factor antigen, ristocetin cofactor, and factor VIII coagulant activities were normal, suggesting that a diagnosis of von Willebrand's disease was unlikely. Although routine coagulation tests were normal, there was evidence of ongoing fibrinolysis with a shortened euglobulin clot lysis time (50 min; normal, no lysis at 2 hr), which partially corrected in vitro after the addition of EACA. Additionally, serum Plg (40%; normal range, 72–128%) and α_2PI (55%; normal range, 70–145%) were persistently decreased. He was presumed to have a hyperfibrinolytic state of undetermined etiology and was treated empirically with EACA, with prompt resolution of his bleeding. When seen in the clinic over the next 2 weeks to 10 months, he continued to have laboratory evidence of hyperfibrinolysis, with decreased levels of α_2PI and Plg, despite no clinical evidence of bleeding. His plasma u-PA level was normal; his AT III level was normal. His α_2PI (55%) and Plg (68%) levels continued to be abnormally low 2 years after his diagnosis of disordered fibrinolysis, while his AT III levels continued to be in the normal range.

Both of his parents were deceased, and he had no siblings. His mother had no siblings. She had had an unexplained severe hemorrhage after a hysterectomy. The propositus has two children; both sons are alive and well and have no history of a bleeding dyscrasia. However, neither son has undergone any surgical procedure or experienced severe trauma. Both sons have normal serum levels of α_2PI and Plg.

The propositus's serum was assayed on three separate occasions by an IRMA assay for t-PA antigen; his t-PA antigen level (4.7 ± 0.9 ng/mL) was within the normal range (3.5–7.2 ng/mL). His PAI-1 antigen level (31.8 ± 5.4 ng/mL), by an IRMA assay, was also within the nor-

mal range (19.6–42.2 ng/mL); however, his PAI-1 activity was found to be 0.36 ± 0.12 units/mL, lower than normal (0.87–1.81 units/mL), by an IRMA t-PA binding assay. Normal plasma contains quite low levels of PAI-1, whereas normal serum and platelets have high levels of this inhibitor. The propositus had a reduced PAI-1 functional activity and, in addition, slower formation of normal complexes with t-PA. This decreased PAI-1 functional activity was found in both serum and plasma and in platelet lysates (0.01 units/mL vs. 0.09–0.11 units/mL in control lysates). However, the PAI-1 antigen levels were normal in plasma and platelet lysates. His circulating t-PA-PAI-1 complexes were modestly reduced (1.9 ng/mL vs. 2.5–5.3 ng/mL in control plasma).

Disordered fibrinolysis has infrequently been associated with a bleeding diathesis. Homozygous α_2PI deficiency causes a severe hemorrhagic diathesis and is associated with almost no plasma α_2PI functional activity and little detectable α_2PI antigen. The propositus's α_2PI antigen and activity levels ranged from 52% to 65%. Patients with heterozygous α_2PI deficiency infrequently have a history of excessive bleeding and, in contrast to this patient, have normal serum Plg levels. The propositus has normal circulating levels of t-PA antigen, normal levels of u-PA antigen, and no increase in circulating levels of t-PA–PAI-1 complexes. Additionally, excess release of PAs would not be expected to deplete functional PAI-1 compartmentalized in platelets, nor would a primary excess release of t-PA be likely to explain low platelet PAI-1 activity, coupled with normal PAI-1 antigen.

Low PAI-1 activity in combination with normal levels of t-PA and PAI-1 antigen suggests a qualitative defect in PAI-1. The explanation for the decreased functional activity of the propositus's PAI-1 is unclear. PAI-1 interacts with both PAs and a variety of other proteases.

It was thus possible that excessive protease activity in the propositus's blood might have inactivated PAI-1 before assay, by either proteolytic cleavage or by formation of inactive protease–PAI-1 complexes. This possibility was eliminated after it was shown that the propositus and control PAI-1s migrated similarly in SDS-PAGE. Since circulating inhibitors to PAI-1 were not found in the propositus, the data suggests an abnormality in his PAI-1 molecule or a defect in the PAI-1 gene. His bleeding diathesis, controlled with EACA, is most likely due to hyperfibrinolysis and deficient PAI-1 activity. The decreased PAI-1 activity results in an increase of free t-PA, which in turn causes Pln generation and predisposes to excessive bleeding. The evidence for persistent accelerated fibrinolysis in the propositus (moderate consumption of both Plg and α_2PI as well as a shortened euglobulin lysis time) suggests that ongoing production of functionally active PAI-1 is necessary to complex with small amounts of continuously released free PA.

Defective Plasminogen Activator Inhibitor, PAI-1: Hyperfibrinolysis

The specific plasma inhibitor of both u-PA and t-PA, which rapidly inactivates physiologic concentrations of these activators, is PAI-1, called the endothelial cell inhibitor (see cases 4 and 5) (6, 39). Enhanced fibrinolysis has been associated with excessive release of endothelial Plg activator (t-PA).

Bleeding Disorder Due to a Plasminogen Activator Inhibitor, PAI-1, Deficiency

Case 11 (65)

The propositus, a 29-year-old man, first presented for a major hemarthrosis after meniscectomy. He had a lifelong history of epistaxis and delayed bleeding after surgery and trauma (e.g., an appendectomy and a head injury). He also experienced hematuria 2 days after a renal contusion. After two dental extractions, bleeding stopped rapidly but resumed 24 hours later, and on one occasion, dental extraction was complicated by a sublingual hematoma. None of these hemorrhagic episodes required a blood transfusion, and on all occasions, bleeding stopped spontaneously. After the diagnosis of the fibrinolytic state was made, the patient was treated with EACA before other dental extractions, and in contrast to previous minor traumas, no delayed bleeding was noted.

Analysis: *The coagulation parameters were all within the normal range (Table 35.14), except for fibrinogen, which was at the lower limit. On all five occasions over a 7-year period, basic fibrinolytic activity was elevated as measured by the ECLT (80–105 min; normal, >140 min). However, no evidence of systemic fibrin-(ogen) lysis was noted. The levels of Plg, α_2PI, and fibrin degradation products were normal, and no Pln-α_2PI complexes were detected. At rest, plasma t-PA antigen was normal (5 ng/mL; normal range, 3–13 ng/mL), but t-PA activity was elevated (3.2 units/mL; normal range, 0.2–2 units/mL) (Table 35.15). A t-PA specific activity, at rest, of 640,000 IU/mg was calculated, a value similar to that given for the International t-PA standard (83/517; National Institute for Biological Standards and Con-*

Table 35.14. Coagulation Parameters in the Patient with Bleeding and Deficient PAI-1

	Patient	Normal
Bleeding time (Ivy method, min)	5	<8
Platelet count (G/L)	2.3	1.5–4
Prothrombin time (sec)	12	11–13
APTT (sec)	34	30–37
Fibrinogen (g/L)	1.7	1.8–4
Thrombin time (sec)	17	16–20
Factor XIII (IU/mL)	1.0	0.7–1.5

Table 35.15. Fibrinolytic Parameters in the Patient with Bleeding and Deficient PAI-1

		Patient	Normal
ECLT (min)	Before stasis	80–105	>140
	After stasis	10–15	10–90
t-PA antigen (ng/mL)	Before stasis	5	3–13
	After stasis	43	10–38
t-PA activity (IU/mL)	Before stasis	3.2	0.2–2
	After stasis	20.7	1.4–14
PAI-1Ag (ng/mL)			
ELISA	Before stasis	<2[a]	4–43
RIA	Before stasis	<6[b]	12.5–39
PAI activity (U/mL)	Before stasis	<1[c]	4.8–17.2
α_2-Antiplasmin (%)		100	80–120
Plasminogen			
antigen (g/L)		0.1	0.1–0.2
activity (%)		80	80–120
Fibrin degradation			
products (µg/mL)		<0.5	<0.5

[a]Lower limit of detection for PAI-1 Ag by ELISA method is 2 ng/mL.
[b]Lower limit of detection by RIA is 6 ng/mL.
[c]The detection limit for PAI activity is 1 U/mL. The patient PAI-1 antigen and activity were measured at 10 AM and 4 PM.

trols, South Mims, Herts, England). These results suggest that all of the circulating t-PA was in a free active form, in contrast to normal healthy people, in whom most of the t-PA at rest is complexed to PAI-1. In agreement with this finding, plasma PAI-1 antigen and activity levels were below the limits of detection (antigen: RIA, <6 ng/mL, and ELISA, <2 ng/mL; activity <1 unit/mL). In contrast to plasma, serum PAI-1 antigen was within the normal range (70–330 ng/mL); the difference between serum and plasma PAI-1 activity was 7.8 units/mL, a value close to the median obtained for three healthy individuals of the same age (9.2 units/mL), indicating that the PAI-1 pool in platelets and the release of PAI-1 from platelets was normal. The propositus has a good response to venous stasis (10 min): t-PA antigen increased from 5 to 43 ng/mL, and t-PA activity from 3.2 to 20.7 units/mL, somewhat higher than the upper limit of the normal range (1.4–14 units/mL). The high specific activity of t-PA and the low PAI-1 antigen levels make it likely that in the propositus's plasma, all PAI-1, if any, is complexed to t-PA.

The propositus has a lifelong history of delayed bleeding after minor trauma; high plasma fibrinolytic activity was measured on five occasions over 7 years; plasma PAI-1 antigen and activity were undetectable; and all of the plasma t-PA is active. This deficiency of plasma PAI-1 associated with a high potential release of t-PA led to uncontrolled t-PA activity on fibrin clots and a bleeding diathesis.

Plasminogen Activator Inhibitor, PAI-1, Deficiency: Hyperfibrinolysis

Hyperfibrinolysis can be caused either by (*a*) a deficiency of α_2PI, (*b*) excess Plg activators, or (*c*) a dysfunctional

PAI-1 (defective inhibitor). The specific, rapid, PAI-1 inhibitor of t-PA and u-PA has assumed an important role in patients with both thrombotic diseases and bleeding disorders. (See cases 4, 5, and 10) (6, 39).

Conclusions

An impaired fibrinolytic system characterized by either **thrombophilia, or a bleeding state,** is described in a variety of clinical disorders. These pathologic hypofibrinolytic and hyperfibrinolytic states are due to both congenital and acquired disorders and are associated with dysfunctional molecules, deficiencies, and defective or excessive activation and inhibition of the components of the fibrinolytic system. These disorders involve primarily the conversion of Plg by specific activator(s) to Pln and the inhibition of both Pln and the activators(s) by specific plasma inhibitors. They also involve defective biosynthesis and release of activator(s) from the vessel wall and the liver.

The diagnosis of fibrinolytic disorders requires the use of a sophisticated battery of laboratory tests for both plasma coagulation and fibrinolysis and platelet function tests. Isolation and characterization of the dysfunctional molecules are essential for an understanding of these disorders.

The current methods used for treating the *thrombotic* diseases—thrombolytic agents, followed by oral anticoagulants—are, in most cases, effective. The *bleeding* states can be prevented and controlled with EACA and related drugs.

REFERENCES

1. Aoki N, et al. Abnormal plasminogen. A hereditary molecular abnormality found in a patient with recurrent thrombosis. J Clin Invest 1978;61:1186–1195.
2. Robbins KC, Boreisha I, Godwin JE. Abnormal plasminogen Maywood I. Thromb Haemost 1991;66:575–580.
3. Robbins KC. The plasminogen-plasmin enzyme system. In: Colman RW, Hirsh J, Marder VJ, Salzman EW, eds. Hemostasis and thrombosis: basic principles and clinical practice. Philadelphia: JB Lippincott, 1987:340–357.
4. Henkin J, Marcotte P, Young H. The plasminogen plasmin system. Prog Cardiovasc Dis 1991;34:135–164.
5. Kluft C, Dooijewaard G, Emeis JJ. Role of the contact system in fibrinolysis. Semin Thromb Hemost 1987;13:50–68.
6. Bachmann F. Fibrinolysis. In: Verstraete M, Vermylen J, Lijnen R, Arnout J, eds. Thrombosis and haemostasis. Leuven: Leuven University Press, 1987:227–265.
7. Plow EF, Felez J, Miles LA. Cellular regulation of fibrinolysis. Thromb Haemost 1991;66:32–36.
8. Francis CW, Marder VJ. Physiologic regulation and pathologic disorders of fibrinolysis. In: Colman RW, Hirsh J, Marder VJ, Salzman EW, eds. Hemostasis and thrombosis: basic principles and clinical practice. 2nd ed. Philadelphia: JB Lippincott, 1987:358–379.
9. Francis RB. Clinical disorders of fibrinolysis: a critical review. Blut 1989;59:1–14.
10. Lijnen HR, Collen D. Congenital and acquired deficiencies of components of the fibrinolytic system and their relation to bleeding or thrombosis. Fibrinolysis 1989;3:67–77.
11. Dolan G, Preston FE. Familial plasminogen deficiency and thromboembolism. Fibrinolysis 1988;2(Suppl 2):26–34.
12. Robbins KC. Dysplasminogenemias. Prog Cardiovasc Dis 1992;34:1–15.
13. Southan C. Molecular and genetic abnormalities of fibrinogen. In: Francis JL, ed. Fibrinogen, fibrin stabilisation, and fibrinolysis. Clinical, biochemical and laboratory aspects. Chichester, England: Ellis Horwood, 1988:65–99.
14. Dang CV, Bell WR. The normal and morbid biology of fibrinogen. Am J Med 1989;87:567–576.
15. Petersen TE, Martzen MR, Ichinose A, Davie EW. Characterization of the gene for human plasminogen, a key proenzyme in the fibrinolytic system. J Biol Chem 1990;265:6104–6111.
16. Skoda V, et al. Proposal for the nomenclature of human plasminogen (Plg) polymorphisms. Vox Sang 1986;51:244–248.
17. Ichinose A, Espling ES, Takamatsu J, Saito H. Two types of abnormal genes for plasminogen in families with a predisposition for thrombosis. Proc Natl Acad Sci USA 1991;88:115–119.
18. Engesser L, et al. Fibrinogen Nijmengen: congenital dysfibrinogenemia associated with impaired t-PA mediated plasminogen activation and decreased binding of t-PA. Thromb Haemost 1988;60:113–120.
19. Hantgan RR, Francis CW, Scheraga HA, Marder VJ. Fibrinogen structure and physiology. In: Colman RW, Hirsh J, Marder VJ, Salzman EW, eds. Hemostasis and thrombosis: basic principles and clinical practice. 2nd ed. Philadelphia: JB Lippincott, 1987:269–288.
20. Miloszewski KJA, Losowsky MS. Fibrin stabilization and factor XIII deficiency. In: Francis JL, ed. Fibrinogen, fibrin stabilisation, and fibrinolysis. Clinical, biochemical and laboratory aspects. Chichester, England: Ellis Horwood, 1988:175–202.
21. McDonagh J, Carrell N. Disorders of fibrinogen structure and function. In: Colman RW, Hirsh J, Marder VJ, Salzman EW, eds. Hemostasis and thrombosis: basic principles and clinical practice. 2nd ed. Philadelphia: JB Lippincott, 1987:301–317.
22. Southan C. Molecular and genetic abnormalities of fibrinogen. In: Francis JL, ed. Fibrinogen, fibrin stabilization, and fibrinolysis. Clinical, biochemical and laboratory aspects. Chichester: England, Ellis Horwood, 1988:65–99.
23. Dang CV, Bell WR. The normal and morbid biology of fibrinogen. Am J Med 1989;87:567–576.
24. Francis JL. Acquired dysfibrinogenemia. In: Francis JL, ed. Fibrinogen, fibrin stabilisation, and fibrinolysis. Clinical, biochemical and laboratory aspects. Chichester: England, Ellis Horwood, 1988:128–156.
25. Doolittle RF. Fibrinogen and fibrin. In: Bloom AL, Thomas DP, eds. Haemostasis and thrombosis. 2nd ed. Edinburgh: Churchill Livingstone, 1987:192–215.
26. Furlan M. Structure of fibrinogen and fibrin. In: Francis JL, ed. Fibrinogen, fibrin stabilisation, and fibrinolysis. Clinical, biochemical and laboratory aspects. Chichester: England, Ellis Horwood, 1988:17–64.
27. Doolittle RF. The structure and evolution of vertebrate fibrinogen: a comparison of the lamprey and mammalian proteins. In: Liu CY, Chien S, eds. Fibrinogen, thrombosis, coagulation, and fibrinolysis. New York: Plenum, 1990:25–37.

28. Chung DW, Harris JE, Davie EW. Nucleotide sequences of the three genes coding for human fibrinogen. In: Liu CY, Chien S, eds. Fibrinogen, thrombosis, coagulation, and fibrinolysis. New York: Plenum, 1990:39–48.

29. Johansson L, Hedner U, Nilsson IM. A family with thromboembolic disease associated with deficient fibrinolytic activity in vessel wall. Acta Med Scand 1978;203:477–480.

30. Nilsson IM, Ljungner H, Tengborn L. Two different mechanisms in patients with venous thrombosis and defective fibrinolysis: low concentration of plasminogen activator or increased concentration of plasminogen activator inhibitor. Br Med J 1985;290:1453–1456.

31. Bachmann F. Plasminogen activators. In: Colman RW, Hirsh J, Marder VJ, Salzman EW, eds. Hemostasis and thrombosis: basic principles and clinical practice. 2nd ed. Philadelphia: JB Lippincott, 1987:318–339.

32. Gurewich V. Activation of fibrin-bound plasminogen by pro-urokinase and its complimentariness with that by tissue plasminogen activator. Enzyme 1988;40:97–108.

33. Lijnen HR, Collen D. Strategies for the improvement of thrombolytic agents. Thromb Haemost 1991;66:88–110.

34. Robbins KC, Markus G. The interaction of human plasminogen with streptokinase. In: Gaffney PJ, Balkuv-Ulutin S, eds. Fibrinolysis: current fundamental and clinical concepts. London: Academic Press, 1978:61–75.

35. Jackson KW, Esmon N, Tang J. Streptokinase and staphylokinase. Methods Enzymol 1981;80:387–394.

36. Robbins KC, Barlow GH, Nguyen G, Samama MM. Comparison of plasminogen activators. Semin Thromb Hemost 1987;13:131–138.

37. Lijnen HR, Collen D. Mechanisms of plasminogen activation by mammalian plasminogen activators. Enzyme 1988; 40:90–96.

38. Robbins KC. Fibrinolytic therapy: biochemical mechanisms. Semin Thromb Hemost 1991;17:1–6.

39. Kruithof EKD. Plasminogen activator inhibitors—a review. Enzyme 1988;40:113–121.

40. Sakata Y, Tanaka T. Regulation of fibrinolysis system by plasminogen activator inhibitor. In: Tanaka K, ed. Recent advances in thrombosis and fibrinolysis. Tokyo: Academic Press, 1991:109–121.

41. Astedt B, Lecander I, Ny T. The placental type plasminogen activator inhibitor, PAI-2. Fibrinolysis 1987;1:203–208.

42. Johan-Vague I, et al. Deficient t-PA release and elevated PA inhibitor levels in patients with spontaneous or recurrent deep venous thrombosis. Thromb Haemost 1987;57: 67–72.

43. Bertina RM, Broekmans AW, van der Linden IK, Mertens K. Protein C deficiency in a Dutch family with thrombotic disease. Thromb Haemost 1982;48:1–5.

44. Jespersen J, Gram J, Bertina RM. The risk of thrombosis in hereditary protein S deficiency in a Scandinavian family. Fibrinolysis 1989;3:37–40.

45. Esmon CT. Protein C. Prog Hemost Thromb 1984;7:25–54.

46. Bertina RM. Protein C and related proteins. Edinburgh: Churchill Livingstone, 1988.

47. Green D. Protein C and protein S. In: Kwaan HC, Samama MM, eds. Clinical thrombosis. Boca Raton, FL: CRC Press, 1989:243–253.

48. Owen WG. Protein C. In: Colman RW, Hirsh J, Marder VJ, Salzman EW, eds. Hemostasis and thrombosis: basic principles and clinical practice. 2nd ed. Philadelphia: JB Lippincott, 1987:235–241.

49. Mannucci PM, Owen WG. Basic and clinical aspects of proteins C and S. In: Bloom AL, Thomas DP, eds. Haemostasis and thrombosis. 2nd ed. Edinburgh: Churchill Livingstone, 1987:452–464.

50. Suzuki K. Anticoagulant protein C pathway. In: Tanaka K, ed. Recent advances in thrombosis and fibrinolysis. Tokyo: Academic Press, 1991:29–46.

51. Comp PC, Esmon CT. Generation of fibrinolytic activity by infusion of activated protein C into dogs. J Clin Invest 1981; 68:1221–1228.

52. De Fouw NJ, Haverkate F, Bertina RM. Protein C and fibrinolysis: a link between coagulation and fibrinolysis. In: Liu CY, Chien S, eds. Fibrinogen, thrombosis, coagulation, and fibrinolysis. New York: Plenum, 1990:235–243.

53. Geiger M. Protein C inhibitor/plasminogen activator inhibitor 3. Fibrinolysis 1988;2:183–188.

54. Iijina K, et al. A new hereditary abnormal protein C (protein C Yonago) with a dysfunctional Gla-domain. Thromb Res 1991;63:249–257.

55. Dreyfus M, et al. Treatment of homozygous protein C deficiency and neonatal purpura fulminans with a purified protein concentrate. New Engl J Med 1991;325:1565–1568.

56. Marlar RA, Adcock DM, Madden RM. Hereditary dysfunctional protein C molecules (type II): assay characterization and proposed classification. Thromb Hemost 1990;63: 375–379.

57. Manabe S, Matsuda M. Homozygous protein C deficiency combined with heterozygous dysplasminogenemia found in a 21-year-old thrombophilic male. Thromb Res 1985;39: 333–341.

58. Kozlowski KA, Berlet A, Mondorf W, Scharrer I, Robbins KC. M-family dysplasminogenemia: assembly of these variant plasminogens and urokinase on U937 cell receptors. Fibrinolysis 1992;6:57.

59. Kluft C, et al. α_2-Antiplasmin Enschede: dysfunctional α_2-antiplasmin molecule associated with an autosomal recessive hemorrhagic disorder. J Clin Invest 1987;80: 1391–1400.

60. Aoki N. Alpha 2-plasmin inhibitor. In: Tanaka K, ed. Recent advances in thrombosis and fibrinolysis. Tokyo: Academic Press, 1991:91–107.

61. Booth NA, Bennett B, Wijngaards G, Grieve JHK. A new life-long hemorrhagic disorder due to excess plasminogen activator. Blood 1983;61:267–275.

62. Aznar J, et al. Inherited fibrinolytic disorder due to an enhanced plasminogen activator level. Thromb Haemost 1984; 52:196–200.

63. Pizzo SV, et al. Releasable vascular plasminogen activator and thrombotic strokes. Am J Med 1985;79:407–411.

64. Schleef RR, Higgins DL, Pillemer E, Levitt LJ. Bleeding diathesis due to decreased functional activity of type 1 plasminogen activator inhibitor. J Clin Invest 1989;83: 1747–1752.

65. Dieval J, et al. A lifelong bleeding disorder associated with a deficiency of plasminogen inhibitor type 1. Blood 1991;77: 528–532.

EXERCISES AND TOOLS FOR HYPOCOAGULABLE AND HYPERCOAGULABLE STATES

Hemostasis is so finely tuned and so exquisitely balanced that one perceives neither spontaneous bleeding nor spontaneous clotting.

1. Blood clotting *in vivo* is promoted through (*a*) the rheology of flow; (*b*) the chemistry of vascular competence; (*c*) presence, adherence and activation of platelets; (*d*) adequacy of coagulant levels, and (*e*) interactions with leukocytes.

2. Under normal circumstances hemostasis is only tentatively complete at birth, at which time even mild hemostatic disorders may be severely debilitating (e.g., thrombocytopenia, hemophilia) or may be incompatible with life (e.g., homozygous protein C deficiency.

3. Construct a paradigm that accounts for the clinical expression of the molecular arrangements that result in arterial thrombosis in an individual without intrinsic defects of hemostasis. Follow this line of reasoning to explain why certain individuals are more prone to venous thrombosis.

4. Through its secretory activities and unique anatomical landmarks, endothelium plays a dominant role in hemostasis. Platelets especially can be either attracted to or repelled by its products. Damaged endothelium may lead to cellular diapedesis, which in microseconds is repaired by arachidonate-initiated vasoconstricting and platelet attractant chemistry. Construct the components of a primary vascular defect using as an example the Ehlers-Danlos syndrome. Consider differences in venous and arterial systems in this disorder.

5. Construct a paradigm that shows how platelets complete the endothelial role via the adherence, aggregation, spreading, and synthesis of both pro- and anticoagulants.

6. Review the clotting cascade with its complex feedback systems and its manifold epithelial, platelet, and protein interaction; recognize the seminal role of tissue factor as a trigger of both normal and pathological clot formation and regard this system in terms of interacting biological events as the ultimate process of inflammation. Feed all the components of inflammation into this construct.

7. Account for the variation in intensity in the hemophilias. Consider the importance of factor levels in terms of X chromosome activation along with level and functional impairment. Explain the presence of the occasional female with classical hemophilia.

8. Develop a paradigm that explains the abnormalities encountered in DIC. In developing a schema to account for the biological processes that follow trauma (e.g., infections, surgery, neoplasia, etc.) take into account the events that must be initiated in order to minimize the chances of morbidity or mortality. Note the role of anticoagulants and volume control in these initiatives.

9. Consider the broad range of iatrogenic events. Develop a construct that shows the mechanisms of drug-induced bleeding or hypercoagulation and where in the pathways these events take place. Include aspirin, penicillin, thiazide diuretics, quinine, corticosteroids, coumadin, heparin, and l-asparaginase in this construct.

10. Diagram the mechanisms of action of the various anticoagulants.

SECTION V APPENDIX

Appendix 1. Types and Frequency of Platelet Alloantigens

HPA-1A	Common	>95%
HPA-1B	Rare	<30%
HPA-2A	Common	>95%
	Rare	<20%
HPA-3A	Intermediate	70–90%
HPA-3B	Intermediate	65–70%
HPA-4A	Common	>95%
HPA-4B	Very rare	<1%
HPA-5A	Common	>95%
HPA-5B	Rare	<25%

Appendix 3. Clinical and Laboratory Features of Thrombocytosis and Thrombasthenia

	Thrombocytosis	Thrombasthenia
Megakaryocytes	4+	+
Platelet numbers	(>1000 × 10^9/L)	(<1000 × 10^9/L)
Platelet survival	N	N
Embolism	3+	+
Splenomegaly	2+	−
Bleeding time	N	A

N, Normal; A, Abnormal.

Appendix 2. Disorders with Either Thrombocytosis or Thrombocytopenia

	Thrombocytosis	Thrombocytopenia
Chronic inflammatory disease	✓	
Cushing's syndrome	✓	
Early iron deficiency	✓	
Glycogen storage disease	✓	
Intensive exercise	✓	
Myeloproliferative disease	✓	
Postsplenectomy	✓	
Renal cysts	✓	
Acute and chronic leukemias		✓
Bernard-Soulier syndrome		✓
Deficient platelet factor-3 activity		✓
Disseminated intravascular coagulation		✓
Chemoradiotherapy		✓
Immune suppression		✓
Liver failure		✓
Megakaryocytic hypoplasia		✓
Renal failure		✓
Polycythemia vera		✓
Postinfection states		✓
Storage pool/release disorder		✓
Thrombotic thrombocytopenic purpura		✓

Appendix 4. Platelet-Function Disorders

	Storage Pool Diseases	Bernard-Soulier Syndrome
Platelet morphology/count	Normal/Normal	Giant platelets/Normal
Bleeding time	+/− Prolonged	Prolonged
Clot retraction	Abnormal	Normal
Platelet adhesion	Normal	Abnormal
Platelet aggregation [5 mm ADP]	Normal	Normal
Platelet aggregation [<1.5 mm ADP]	Deficient second phase	Normal first phase +/− second phase
Platelet aggregation [Dilute collagen] [5 mm epinephrine]	Abnormal/Abnormal	Normal/Normal
Platelet aggregation [Ristocetin]	Normal	Deficient
Storage nucleotide pool	Diminished	Normal

Appendix 5. Quantitative Platelet Disorders

	Primary	Secondary
Bernard-Soulier syndrome	✓	
Chronic myelocytic leukemia		✓
Deficient platelet factor-3 activity	✓	
Disseminated intravascular coagulation		✓
Drugs		✓
Inflammatory liver disease		✓
Polycythemia vera		✓
Storage pool/related release mechanism diseases	✓	
Thrombasthenia	✓	
Uremia		✓

Appendix 6. Bleeding Disorders Secondary to Vascular Defects

Autoerythrocyte sensitization
Connective tissue defects
    Cachetic purpura
    Cushing's disease
    Ehlers-Danlos syndrome
Drug-induced vasculitis
Immune vasculitis
Infection-induced vasculitis
Paraproteinemias
Snake venom intoxication
Telangiectatic purpura

Appendix 7. Synthesis Sites and Pathway/Activity of Protein Coagulation Factors

Common Name and Number	Synthesis Site	Activity/Pathway
Fibrinogen (I)	Liver	C
Prothrombin (II)	Liver	K, C
Thromboplastin (III)	Tissues	—
Proaccelerin (V)	Liver	C
Proconvertin (VII)	Liver	K, E
Antihemophilic factor (VIII)	Red Cells, Megakaryocytes, Endothelium	I
Christmas factor (IX)	Liver	K, I
Stuart Prower factor (X)	Liver	K, C
Plasma thromboplastin antecedent (XI)	Liver	K, I
Hageman factor (XII)	Unknown	I
Fibrin stabilizing factor (XIII)	Liver, Megakaryocytes	C
Fletcher factor (Prekallikrein)	Liver	I
High molecular weight kininogen [Fitzgerald, Williams, Flaujec factors)	Liver	I

K, Vitamin K dependent; C, Common pathway; I, Intrinsic pathway; E, Extrinsic pathway.
Protein S and C are also liver synthesized and Vitamin K dependent.

Appendix 8. Lowest Clotting Factor Levels Capable of Sustaining Stable Coagulation

Factors	Percentage
I	>50%
II, V, VII, X	>35%
XI	>20%
XII, XIII, Prekallikrein	>1%
High molecular weight kallikrein	>1%
Platelet count	$>80 \times 10^9$/L

Appendix 9. Inherited Patterns of Coagulation Disorders

Factor	Inheritance
VIII	XL
IX	XL
I	AR
II	AR
V	AR
VII	AR
X	AR
XI	AR
XII	AR
XIII	AR
Protein C	AR
Prekallikrein	AR
Von Willebrand	
Types IIC, III	AR
Types I, II A,B	AD
Platelet type	AD

XL, X-Linked recessive; *AR,* Autosomal recessive; *AD,* autosomal dominant.

Appendix 10. Clotting Disorders, Related Tests and Standard Results

Disorder	Tests	Normal Values
Group I		
Afibrinogenemia	Fibrinogen	150–400 mg/dl
Hypofibrinogenemia	Plasma prothrombin time	10–15 seconds
Thrombin inhibitors	Plasma thrombin time	13–17 seconds
Dysfibrinogenemia		
Group II		
Dis. intra. coag. (DIC)	Fibrin degradation products	2–10 mg/dl
Dysfibrinogenemia		
Fibrinogenolysis		
Liver disease		
Thrombolysis		
Group III		
Hemophilia A	Factor VIII assay	50–150 IU/dl
Von Willebrand's	Activated PTT	30–35 seconds
Factor VIII antibodies		
Group III		
Inhibitors/deficiencies	Activated PTT	
Factors I, II, V, VI, VII, IX, X	PT	11–13 seconds
	Factor assays	50–150 IU/dl
Group IV		
Thrombocytopenia	Platelet count	$150–450 \times 10^9$/L
	Ivy bleeding time	1–9 minutes
Thrombocytosis	Platelet count	
Von Willebrand's platelet dysfunction +/− vascular diseases	Ivy bleeding time	
	Aggregation, adhesion	See above

Appendix 11. Laboratory Data and Treatment Modalities for Clotting Disorders

Factor Deficiency	BT	PT	PTT	TT	Therapy
VIII	N	N	↑	N	Plasma, rF
IX	N	↑	↑	N	Plasma, Rf
V	N	N	↑	N	Plasma
VII	N	↑	↑	N	Plasma, serum
X	N	N	↑	N	Plasma, serum
XI	N	N	↑	N	Plasma, serum
XII	N	N	T	N	Plasma, serum
XIII	N	N	N	N	Plasma, serum
Von Willebrand	↑	N	↑	N	Plasma, serum
I	↑	↑	↑	↑	Serum
II	N	↑	↑	N	Plasma, serum

N, Normal; ↑, Prolonged; *rF*, Recombinant factor; *PT*, Prothrombin time; *PTT*, Partial thromboplastin time; *BT*, Bleeding time; *TT*, Thrombin time.

CHAPTER 36

Chemotherapy

RICHARD F. BAKEMEIER

Extracts of the periwinkle plant, *Vinca rosea*, fed to rats produced severe granulocytopenia. These observations initially designed to study diabetes led to the development of vinblastine and vincristine.
—R. L. Noble, Biochem Pharmacol, 1958

Chemotherapy is the youngest of the three standard forms of cancer therapy: surgery, radiotherapy, and chemotherapy; but from its modest beginnings in the 1940s, when nitrogen mustard was converted from a devastating wartime vesicant to a promising antineoplastic agent, to the early 1990s, when the microtubule inhibitor paclitaxel was added to the armamentarium for ovarian and breast cancer, massive strides have been made in the understanding and utilization of a wide range of chemically and biologically based anticancer agents. The following material serves as a basis of understanding the interrelationships of cell growth and drug-cell interactions.

Case 1

The patient is a 53-year-old white female nurse who had noticed an enlarged, nontender, left midcervical lymph node for several weeks. Otherwise she had felt generally well, noticing no change in her chronic hot flashes associated with the menopause. She consulted her primary care physician who referred her to a medical oncologist/hematologist. The patient denied any weight loss, change in appetite, known fever, cough, or shortness of breath. There was mild early satiety. Physical examination revealed bilateral enlarged 1–2 cm cervical and axillary lymph nodes and a palpable spleen. Peripheral blood counts included an hematocrit of 36% with a normochromic, normocytic smear; a white cell count of 5.5 × 10⁹/L with a normal differential; and a platelet count of 130 × 10⁹/L. A cervical lymph node biopsy was interpreted as a follicular mixed cleaved cell lymphoma. Immunohistochemistry showed monoclonal surface immunoglobulin with lambda light chains, and CD10, CD19, and CD20 expression. Southern blot analysis indicated unique JH rearrangement, and flow cytometry revealed a normal DNA index and a low S phase. Further staging workup included a CT scan, which showed slightly enlarged periaortic lymph nodes, an enlarged spleen, and a normal-appearing liver. A bone marrow biopsy revealed increased lymphoid cells similar to those in the lymph node.

Multidisciplinary discussion between the medical oncologist/hematologist, primary care physician, patholo-gist, diagnostic radiologist, radiation oncologist, and surgeon led to a consensus that the patient had stage IV follicular mixed, non-Hodgkin's (B-cell) lymphoma, that no additional staging was necessary at this time, and that if therapy were to be initiated, the recommendation would be for chemotherapy.

Comments

Chemotherapy of non-Hodgkin's lymphomas embraces virtually the entire scope of principles of chemotherapy of malignant diseases. This ranges from when to treat or not to treat; which of many active chemotherapeutic agents to use, including biologic response modifiers; what combinations of drugs to employ, based on mechanisms of action, mechanisms of resistance, and toxicities; dose intensity, timing, and route of administration; potentiation of antitumor effects with noncytotoxic drugs; use of combined modality therapy, such as chemotherapy and radiation therapy; control of drug-associated toxicities; and evolution of chemotherapeutic regimens through controlled clinical trials.

Indications for Treatment

One of the most important aspects of clinical chemotherapy of malignant disease is developing skill in determining whether to treat a given patient, in addition to determining how to treat the patient. Thorough knowledge of the natural history of individual malignancies is an important foundation for such skill. Some disseminated neoplastic diseases, including low-grade non-Hodgkin's lymphomas, may be essentially asymptomatic for prolonged periods and may progress very slowly. If such indolent malignancies are considered incurable by currently available methods, a period of observation may be preferable to exposing the patient to the inconvenience, expense, and toxicity of therapy immediately upon diagnosis. As symptoms and signs of progressive disease are observed through careful follow-up, appropriate therapy can be initiated with palliation as its goal. At the other end of the spectrum is the patient with a far advanced disseminated malignancy when diagnosed and with a low performance status (e.g., Karnofsky Performance Status <40% or ECOG Performance Status 4) (1, 2). Especially if the disease is one with generally poor response rates to chemotherapy, such as pancreatic carcinoma or malignant melanoma, the side effects of meaningful doses of most cytotoxic drug regimens may not be warranted. Palliation in such instances may be more effective through attention to nutrition, pain relief, and psychologic support. However, strong motivation of the patient to enter into more specific therapy and the availability of either (a) a therapeutic regimen with a relatively high response rate associated with relatively limited toxicity or (b) a well-conceived Phase I, II, or III clinical trial (see below) for which the patient is eligible may justify chemotherapy in such circumstances, with careful attention to informed consent procedures.

This complex subject of indications for treatment may be summarized by listing topics that should be thoughtfully addressed with the patient and the patient's family before initiating therapy:

1. Natural history of the disease
2. Patient's symptoms and performance status
3. Patient's general health, age, and life expectancy from other factors
4. Patient's motivation for therapy
5. Goals of therapy: cure, palliation, prolonged survival
6. Response rates with available regimens
7. Toxicities (severity of side effects)
8. Measurability of effects of therapy: accurate monitoring of tumor response or progression
9. Psychosocial aspects: nature of patient's support systems, transportation (time and distance), costs of therapy, effects on other family members
10. Availability of appropriate clinical trial(s)

The clinician should consider each of these topics, assigning to each a net indication or contraindication for the initiation or continuation of antineoplastic therapy in a sort of conceptual "balance sheet," arriving at a summation that can assist in advising the patient.

Principles of Antineoplastic Chemotherapy

Important concepts contributing to the effective application of antineoplastic chemotherapy can be classified as

1. Tumor biologic aspects of chemotherapy
2. Pharmacologic aspects of chemotherapy
3. Clinical aspects of chemotherapy

Tumor Biologic Aspects of Chemotherapy

Most currently used antineoplastic chemotherapeutic agents have been developed through an empiric approach based initially on their ability to inhibit experimental animal tumors in a screening process rather than being cho-

sen because of a priori knowledge of their mechanisms of action on specific biologic functions of tumor cells. Nevertheless, eventually the effects of most promising new agents are clarified in relation to cellular and molecular biologic events, and the clinical chemotherapist must have a working knowledge of current concepts of tumor cell biology to use these agents optimally. This includes cell kinetics, membrane structure and function, macromolecular synthesis, molecular genetics, drug activation and inactivation, and mechanisms of drug resistance, both genetic and those due to cell kinetic phenomena.

An important conclusion from decades of research in tumor biology is that the genotypic and phenotypic alterations in tumor cells, as contrasted to their normal counterparts, result in primarily *quantitative* differences rather than major therapeutically exploitable *qualitative* differences. Although the biologic behavior of cancer cells, in terms of abnormal proliferation, invasion, and metastasis, may be strikingly aberrant, the coexisting responses to the effects of chemotherapeutic agents are unfortunately similar to those of nonneoplastic cells (3, 4). The activation of proto-oncogenes in a variety of human neoplasms through mutation, translocation, or gene amplification has been demonstrated. As the products of the resulting oncogenes become clarified in cancer cells, more specific targets for chemotherapeutic agents should become available, with the anticipated result of more tumor cell killing with less normal cell toxicity. These targets may include growth factors or their receptors, enzymes such as tyrosine-specific protein kinases, and nuclear proteins involved in chromatin activation. Even without such specific targets, the design of effective chemotherapeutic regimens can be enhanced by a general understanding of the biologic processes involved, providing an appreciation of the known mechanisms of action of currently available therapeutic agents.

The **kinetic basis of cancer chemotherapy** involves the concept of tumor cell burden. Figure 36.1 presents a simplified growth curve, with the tumor cells in logarithmic (exponential) growth with a constant doubling time preceding the development of a tumor of a billion (10^9) cells. Such a tumor is potentially detectable as a 1-cm mass, generally a lethal body burden in mouse models (5). If this constant doubling continued to a total of 40 doublings, a body burden of approximately a trillion (10^{12}) cells would result, which might be lethal in man, depending on their location. This idealized situation is rarely seen, particularly in solid tumors in man, in which only a portion, perhaps less than 15%, of the total tumor cell population is proliferating (6). These proliferating tumor stem cells are actively progressing through the mitotic cycle (Fig. 36.2) and constitute what is termed the growth fraction (7). Human leukemias and high-grade lymphomas may have higher growth fractions than the more common human solid tumors such as breast cancer. Associated doubling times may vary from about 4 weeks for high-grade lymphomas to 14 or more weeks for breast cancer (8). The nonproliferating cell fraction consists of cells that have differentiated or have become deprived of nutrients and may

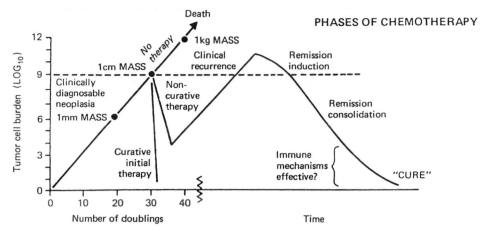

Figure 36.1 The relation of tumor cell burden to various outcomes resulting from cancer chemotherapy.

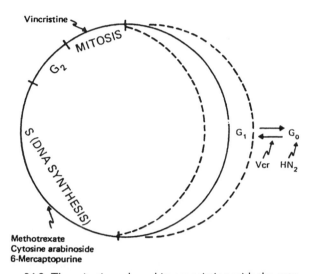

Figure 36.2 The mitotic cycle and its association with the cytotoxic effects of various antitumor agents that act in specific phases of the cycle. The gaps before and after DNA synthesis are termed G_1 and G_2, respectively. G_0 refers to cells that are not dividing but retain the capacity, between mitosis and DNA synthesis.

be dead or dying, particularly toward the center of tumor nodules. These kinetically mixed populations of cells result in human tumors demonstrating a sigmoid-shaped Gompertzian growth curve with an early lag phase and progressively slower growth after attaining a clinically apparent size (9). The clinical application of flow cytometry has made available specific information about the kinetic state of human tumors, with increasingly useful predictive value of the S-phase fraction and DNA content per cell (ploidy).

This discussion is relevant to the basic principles of cancer chemotherapy in several respects. Most anticancer drugs are more effective against proliferating cells than against nonproliferating cells. This is often related to their mechanisms of action affecting one or more phases of the mitotic cycle (e.g., the S phase or DNA synthesis phase as indicated in Fig. 36.2). The decreased sensitivity of nonproliferating cells may also be related to decreased drug

delivery to the less well vascularized central portions of tumor cell masses. Other changes occurring during successive tumor doublings that may affect chemosensitivity include progressive accumulation of mutant cells that are genetically resistant to chemotherapy through several mechanisms that will be considered later (10–13). This line of reasoning leads to the conclusion that early treatment, at a time of low tumor cell burden and maximal growth fraction, is more likely to result in favorable outcomes of chemotherapy.

Figure 36.1 depicts various outcomes of tumor treatment, including curative initial therapy with killing of all potentially proliferating cells. The work of Skipper and Schabel (5) demonstrated that proliferating cells are killed by chemotherapeutic agents according to first-order kinetics; i.e., a given dose of drug kills a constant fraction of tumor cells. This "log-kill" model indicates that a 5-log kill (reduction of 10^9 cells to 10^4 cells or killing of 99.999%) can result in an apparent clinical remission followed by a recurrence, with the interval determined by the doubling time of the residual tumor cell burden. This rate of doubling depends on the summation of tumor cell divisions and cell death. It remains a challenge to the chemotherapist to determine the choice of drugs, their doses, and the timing of their administration to maximize tumor cell kill and to minimize the emergence of populations of resistant cells.

Adjuvant chemotherapy, administered to eliminate distant micrometastases after local treatment of breast carcinoma with surgery or radiation therapy, is a good example of the application of these tumor kinetic principles in the planning of clinical chemotherapy. The generally observed inverse relationship between tumor size and tumor cell growth fraction in experimental animal systems suggests that micrometastases in human breast cancer may have a higher growth fraction than in the primary tumor or in clinically apparent metastases. Since many of the drugs employed in clinical chemotherapy are more active against dividing than against nondividing cells (i.e., they are somewhat cell cycle–specific), it has been speculated that administering these agents in the period following primary local tumor therapy, in the absence of demonstrable metastases, is likely to delay or prevent recurrences and improve survival. This concept has been strongly supported by a variety of animal tumor model experiments. Adjuvant chemotherapy appears to provide benefit in breast carcinoma, particularly in premenopausal women; in carcinomas of the colon, rectum, and anus; in osteosarcoma; and in certain pediatric malignancies including Wilm's tumor, neuroblastoma, rhabdomyosarcoma, and Ewing's sarcoma (14). Adjuvant chemotherapy administere d prior to surgery or radiation therapy is referred to as **primary** (or "neoadjuvant") chemotherapy. It has the potential advantage of not only dealing with any micrometastases but also reducing the extent of the primary tumor, thereby possibly reducing the morbidity of surgery or radiation therapy. This approach has been employed widely in certain pediatric tumors and in adult lung and head and neck cancers. Analogous reasoning from kinetic principles has been used in developing postremission therapy for acute leukemia, both in children and in adults. This may involve **consolidation** chemotherapy with the same agents used in induction or additional agents; **intensification** chemotherapy, often defined as additional therapy to patients in continuous complete remission for 6 or more months; and **maintenance** chemotherapy, which is usually low-toxicity therapy administered over a long period of time to delay the proliferation of residual tumor cells. These approaches employ concepts of cell kinetics, dose intensity, and development of drug resistance (discussed below).

Pharmacologic Aspects of Chemotherapy

The **pharmacologic basis of cancer chemotherapy** involves an appreciation of principles of pharmacokinetics (drug absorption, distribution, metabolism, and excretion) and of pharmacodynamics (dose-response relationships) (15–17).

Absorption characteristics determine whether a given antineoplastic agent is given orally, intramuscularly, intravenously, or intrathecally. Some agents, such as cyclophosphamide, can be given either orally or intravenously. The choice may depend primarily on the therapeutic benefits of large intermittent intravenous pulse doses that result in high drug gradients across cell membranes and more intense exposure of tumor cells to the drug. It may depend on other factors such as less toxicity in normal tissues with intravenous pulse doses, including gastrointestinal tract and bone marrow, than with prolonged oral intake. It may even depend on increased patient compliance resulting from a known intravenous dose under observation contrasted with daily oral administration over an unobserved 7- to 14-day course. Other agents, however, such as doxorubicin, are too irritating to be administered orally, intramuscularly, or intrathecally and thus must be given intravenously.

Distribution of chemotherapeutic agents may be restricted, even after intravenous administration. For example, the central nervous system and the pleural or peritoneal space may be "sanctuary sites" into which drugs cannot penetrate in high concentrations unless directly instilled by intrathecal, intrapleural, or intraperitoneal administration, respectively. Systemically administered nitrosoureas may also penetrate the central nervous system better than other drugs because of increased lipid solubility. Intraarterial infusions, such as into the hepatic artery, or perfusions with controlled efflux, such as in an extremity, are other approaches to enhancing the local distribution of a drug into an affected site.

Metabolism of certain agents is necessary for their activation. This includes the phosphorylation of 5-fluorouracil (5-FU) and the action of mixed-function oxidases in the liver on cyclophosphamide. Metabolism also inactivates certain drugs. An example is the catabolism of the purine analogue 6-mercaptopurine (6-MP) by the enzyme xanthine oxidase. Since this enzyme is inhibited by allopurinol, a drug used to prevent hyperuricemia in malignant diseases such as lymphomas and leukemias, 6-MP doses must be decreased when used together with allopurinol.

Excretion characteristics of cancer chemotherapeutic agents must be kept in mind, particularly when excretory organ systems are impaired either by the neoplasm or by previous treatment. For example, methotrexate is largely excreted by the kidney, and if there is renal impairment, doses should be reduced. Methotrexate itself may compound the problem, since it may precipitate in renal tubules and increase renal impairment, especially in acid urine. The liver helps to excrete vincristine and doxorubicin, both commonly used in the treatment of lymphomas. In the presence of liver dysfunction or biliary obstruction, doses of these two drugs may need to be reduced.

Mechanisms of Action

Anticancer drugs may be conveniently categorized by their mechanisms of action (18). The following is a brief classification. Virtually every class of drugs has one or more member that is in common use in the treatment of lymphomas. Table 36.1 lists some of the more widely used of these agents (19).

1. Alkylating agents (cross-link DNA strands)
2. Topoisomerase II inhibitors
3. DNA intercalators
4. Mitotic spindle poisons
5. Antimetabolites (enzyme inhibitors)
6. Hormones and antihormones
7. Biologic response modifiers
8. Miscellaneous agents

The approximately 30 currently available antineoplastic drugs can generally be classified in one of these groups. The choice of an antitumor agent is generally not based on a logical a priori process but on empiric clinical trials. Single agents do not, in general, produce cures or even significant long-term remissions. Therefore, more than one agent is

Table 36.1 Chemotherapeutic Agents Used in Cancer Treatment

Alkylating agents	
Nitrogen mustards	Mechlorethamin, cyclophosphamide, melphalan, chlorambucil, ifosfamide
Nitrosoureas	BCNU (carmustine), CCNU (lomustine), streptozotocin, chlorozotocin
Miscellaneous	Thiotepa, busulfan, dacarbazine, mitomycin C
Topoisomerase inhibitors	
Antibiotics	Doxorubicin, daunorubicin, mitoxantrone, epirubicin
Podophyllotoxins	Etoposide, teniposide
DNA intercalators	Doxorubicin, dactinomycin, mithramycin, bleomycin
Mitotic spindle poisons	
Vinca alkaloids	Vinblastine, vincristine, vindesine, paclitaxel
Antimetabolites (enzyme inhibitors)	
Thymidylate synthase	5-fluorouracil, 5-fluoro-2′-deoxyuridine (FUDR)
Dihydrofolate reductase	Methotrexate
DNA polymerase	Cytarabine hydrochloride
Ribonucleotide reductase	Hydroxyurea
Phosphoribosylpyrophosphate aminotransferase	6-Mercpatopurine, 6-thioguanine
Hormones and antihormones	
Hormones	Estrogens, androgens, progestational agents, corticosteriods
Antihormones	Aminoglutethimide, tamoxifen, leuprolide, flutamide
Biologic response modifiers	BCG, interferons, interleukins, levamisole
Miscellaneous agents	Cisplatin, carboplatin, L-asparaginase, procarbazine

Modified from Yarbro JW. The scientific basis of cancer chemotherapy. In: Perry MC, ed. The chemotherapy sourcebook. Balitmore: Williams & Wilkins, 1992:2–14.

used concurrently. The design of **combinations of agents** into new chemotherapeutic regimens requires an appreciation of their mechanisms of action. In general, it is preferable to choose a drug from each of several of these groups in an effort to damage several different biochemical sites in the tumor cells, to reduce the survival and proliferation of genetically resistant tumor cells, and to minimize toxicity to normal tissues. Ideally, the major toxicity of each of the components of a drug combination will be different so they will not be additive. However, so many agents share myelosuppression as a side effect that it is difficult not to have more than one drug with this toxicity. Principles observed in designing combinations of agents are

1. Include only agents that have shown activity against the malignancy involved when used alone
2. Include agents that differ in their mechanisms of action
3. Include agents that differ in their major toxicities

4. Use optimal doses and timing for each agent, based on both tumor cell and normal cell kinetics

The application of these principles can be illustrated by the four-drug combination widely used in the treatment of non-Hodgkin's lymphomas and referred to as "CHOP" from the first letters of its constituents: *c*yclophosphamide, *h*ydroxydaunorubicin (doxorubicin), *O*ncovin (the commercial name for vincristine), and *p*rednisone. Cyclophosphamide is an alkylating agent whose major toxicity is myelosuppression. Doxorubicin is an antibiotic that intercalates in DNA and stabilizes DNA–topoisomerase II complexes, preventing repair of DNA breaks. Its major toxicities are myelosuppression and cardiac toxicity. Vincristine is a mitotic spindle poison with peripheral nerve toxicity but little myelosuppression. Prednisone is a synthetic corticosteroid hormone that is lympholytic and immunosuppressive and whose side effects include alterations of glucose metabolism and bone matrix. This four-drug combination can be augmented by adding other agents with still other mechanisms of antitumor action. Nonmyelosuppressive drugs such as the antibiotic bleomycin or the antimetabolite methotrexate combined with leucovorin (folinic acid) rescue can be used during the periods of leukopenia resulting from doses of cyclophosphamide and doxorubicin. These principles have been widely used in developing effective and tolerable combinations for the treatment of a wide variety of malignant diseases.

Development of New Agents and Combinations

Because many neoplastic diseases are not satisfactorily treated with current methods, development of new agents and combinations is an important aspect of cancer chemotherapy. In the United States, this endeavor involves the cooperative interaction of the National Cancer Institute, the pharmaceutical industry, academic researchers, and the Food and Drug Administration. Screening of potential chemotherapeutic agents begins with a panel of human tumor cell lines in vitro (20). Promising agents are then administered to animals carrying human tumor cell lines corresponding to the positive in vitro lines. Implanted animal tumor models are also used in tests examining host tolerance of the agent. Animal toxicology and pharmacokinetic studies follow, first in mice, then in rats and in dogs, assessing the maximum tolerable doses for various schedules. Clinical trials are begun at a fraction of the doses causing significant toxicity in test animals. **Phase I** clinical trials seek to determine the maximum tolerable dose of an agent in patients with a malignancy for which there is no effective standard therapy, who have good performance status, good bone marrow, renal, and liver function, and who have given written informed consent. A predetermined dose escalation scheme is followed, with each dose level being administered to a small number of patients until significant toxicity is observed. Pharmacokinetic studies are usually performed, including determination of peak plasma drug concentrations or areas under the concentration × time curves. Tumor response is assessed, although this is not the primary purpose of Phase I studies. **Phase II** clinical trials are designed to determine the tumor types against which the agent has activity and the extent of that activity. Subjects generally are required to have very good performance status, to have had no previous chemotherapy except perhaps adjuvant chemotherapy, and to have measurable disease. Complete and partial remissions are documented, as well as stable disease and tumor progression. Toxicity is also assessed, and dosing strategy is further considered. **Phase III** clinical trials compare promising new agents from Phase II trials with a standard treatment, usually in a randomized, stratified design. The predetermined sample size is usually large because of anticipated small differences in the activities of the two regimens. Therefore, these trials are generally conducted through multiple institutions organized into cooperative groups supported by grants from the National Cancer Institute or other funding sources.

Clinical Aspects of Chemotherapy

Some of the important clinical aspects of cancer chemotherapy have been introduced in the earlier section "Indications for Treatment," including the importance of physiologic and psychosocial factors in determining whether to, and when to, treat a given patient. Performance status of the patient is important in making these decisions, influencing both the likelihood of response and the selection of appropriate therapeutic regimens. Assessment and control of pain, associated nonneoplastic disorders influencing general health, nutritional status, and emotional status all require attention by the medical oncologist/hematologist to optimize the chances for a satisfactory response to chemotherapy. Another facet of the clinical challenge presented by cancer chemotherapy is drug toxicity and the importance of the clinician anticipating and counteracting its various manifestations. A subsequent section considers this topic that unfortunately often overshadows the beneficial results of cancer chemotherapy, reflecting the depths of the physiologic and emotional problems associated with side effects.

The patient and her medical oncologist/hematologist discussed management options, which included observation, or combination chemotherapy. Her background as a nurse provided her with an excellent grasp of the general nature of her disease and the likely consequences of therapy. Although her symptoms were minimal and it was explained to her that this histologic diagnosis (nodular mixed cleaved-cell lymphoma) was not felt to be curable with even intensive therapy, it was mutually decided to proceed with combination chemotherapy. The indications were felt to be the splenomegaly, which was contributing to early satiety, the bone marrow involvement, and her strong desire to be treated. No other causes of her anemia and borderline thrombocytopenia were demonstrable. She was eligible for a clinical trial being conducted by a major cooperative oncology group involving randomization between CHOP chemotherapy with alpha interferon versus CHOP chemotherapy alone. After thorough discussion and written informed consent, she was randomized to CHOP chemotherapy without interferon.

She received as an outpatient 10 cycles of intravenous cyclophosphamide, doxorubicin, and vincristine at approximately 3-week intervals and 5 days of oral prednisone with each cycle, over the next 9 months. There were occasional delays of 1 week and moderate attenuation of drug doses (cyclophosphamide and doxorubicin only) because of low platelet counts. Her lowest recorded platelet count was $80 \times 10^9/L$, and the lowest recorded leukocyte count was $3.2 \times 10^9/L$ with a normal differential. Nausea was mild to moderate, usually occurring about 6 hours after drug infusion. Hair loss was considerable, but regrowth was noted within 5 months. She had mild paresthesias in the fingertips, attributed to the vincristine. Her chronic hot flushes did not change. When receiving her treatments she occasionally missed a day of work in the doctor's office that she supervised. Abdominal CT scan after 7 months showed normal-sized periaortic nodes and spleen. Peripheral lymphadenopathy had disappeared after two cycles of treatment. Repeat bilateral bone marrow biopsies showed no increase in lymphoid cells. She entered the observation phase of the trial.

Commentary. A clinical complete remission was considered achieved. More extensive pathologic staging was not required by the trial protocol nor by standards of good clinical management. Complete cure of this lymphoma was not considered to be the goal of therapy, considering the natural history of the disease, the stage of the disease, and the age of the patient. The intent of the trial was to assess the effect on remission duration and survival of the added alpha interferon, and the patient had been assigned to the control group. It was assumed that a significant body burden of lymphoma cells probably still persisted after the induction of a clinical complete remission, although without a sensitive tumor marker, analogous to β-human chorionic gonadotrophin or α-fetoprotein in non-seminomatous germ cell tumors of the testes, subclinical tumor cell burdens would be difficult to document. The growth fraction of her tumor was not determined, although there were not large numbers of mitoses in the histologic sections. Studies by flow cytometry have reported 4–9% S-phase fractions in low- and intermediate-grade lymphomas and 24% in high-grade lymphomas (8). The design of the CHOP regimen administered to the patient has been described in the section above on combination chemotherapy, and it contains drugs active against most lymphomas, given in standard doses. Cyclophosphamide, doxorubicin, and vincristine demonstrate selectivity for proliferating cells. These observations suggest further that residual, possibly nonproliferating, lymphoma cell deposits were likely.

Myelotoxicity. The drugs in the CHOP regimen were administered intermittently to provide drug-free intervals in which normal bone marrow, gastrointestinal, and hair follicle cells might repair drug-induced damage. Hematopoietic stem cells are mostly nonproliferating at any given time. With damage to more mature cells, the stem cells are recruited into the mitotic pool, with maximum activity at about the time of the peripheral blood granulocyte nadir, or about 10 days following administration of most myelosuppressive agents. Cell cycle–specific agents should be avoided at this time to minimize damage to the proliferating stem cells and should be delayed if possible to 17–21 days after the previous cycle, when the stem cells have returned to the resting state (Fig. 36.3) (21). Nitrosoureas and phenylalanine mustard show a biphasic suppression of peripheral blood granulocytes and platelets, the first at about 10 days and the second at about 30 days. Intervals between treatments with these drugs should be extended to about 6–8 weeks to protect the hematopoietic stem cells. Intermittent large doses of cell cycle–specific agents can be administered over many months without excessive myelosuppression by observing these principles. The inclination to attenuate or delay doses significantly because of moderate cytopenias should be resisted during induction regimens because of the apparent importance of dose intensity in reducing the tumor cell burden in a variety of malignant diseases. Firm guidelines are difficult to define, however. Clinical judgment, experience, and a clear understanding of the goals of treatment are important (6, 22).

Nausea and Vomiting. Although the patient had no major problems with nausea and vomiting from the CHOP regimen, with the assistance of antinausea medications, these symptoms can be severe and can limit therapy in some patients. However, nausea control has evolved impressively in the past decade. Various chemotherapeutic agents, especially cisplatin, nitrogen mustard, and dacarbazine (imidazole carboxamide), can cause significant nausea, primarily through stimulation of chemoreceptors in the brainstem as well as direct effects on the gastrointestinal tract. 5-hydroxytryptamine 3 (5-HT3) receptors in the brain, in addition to dopamine receptors, are involved. The availability of ondansetron, a 5-HT3 receptor inhibitor, as well as phenothiazines and metoclopramide, both dopamine receptor inhibitors, have contributed to the improved control of chemotherapy-induced nausea (16, 23, 24).

Alopecia. Since about 90% of hair follicles are normally in the growth phase of the hair cycle, they are highly at risk for chemotherapy-induced damage with consequent hair loss. This is virtually unavoidable, but the patient should be reassured that hair will regrow, especially after termination of the chemotherapy. Some patients actually prefer the hair that returns after the alopecia to that which preceded it. This patient was pleased with the reappearance and quality of her hair in less than a year after chemotherapy was completed. Scalp hypothermia has met with limited success in reducing alopecia, and it introduces the risk of providing a sanctuary for metastatic tumor cells by reducing blood flow during drug administration (25).

Second Malignancies. The potential mutagenic activity of a number of commonly used cancer chemotherapeutic agents appears to be associated with the occurrence of second malignancies such as acute myelogenous leukemia, and lung, stomach, and bone cancers in patients with long remissions or cures following chemotherapy, particularly when accompanied by radiation therapy. Alkylating agents seem to be most commonly implicated. This has been well documented in long-term survivors of Hodgkin's disease and non-Hodgkin's lymphoma. The mean interval from di-

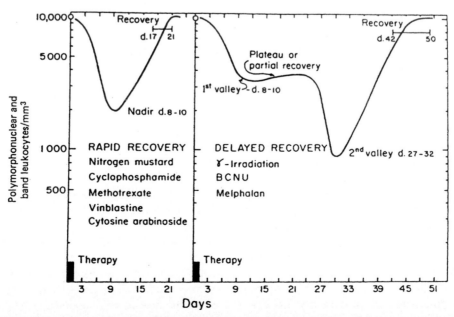

Figure 36.3 Recovery patterns of peripheral blood granulocyte counts following pulse doses of common antitumor drugs. (From Bergsagel DE. An assessment of massive-dose chemotherapy of malignant disease. Can Med Assoc J 1971;104:31–36. With permission.)

agnosis of Hodgkin's disease to that of acute leukemia has been about 6 years. The risk is about 10% at 10 years, with patient age over 40 increasing the risk significantly (26, 27) (see chapter 27).

Cardiac Toxicity. This side effect is discussed below.

Other Organ Toxicities. The reader is referred to reviews of these topics (28).

The 53-year-old nurse with non-Hodgkin's lymphoma described previously first complained of abdominal bloating and dysphagia one month after completing the 9-month CHOP chemotherapy program. She was found to have tachycardia with a gallop rhythm and nonspecific T wave changes on electrocardiogram, tender hepatomegaly, and cardiac enlargement on chest x-ray, leading to the diagnosis of congestive heart failure. Radionuclide angiocardiography revealed an ejection fraction of 23%, and there was diffuse hypokinesis of both ventricles. Review of her records indicated she had received 701 mg of intravenous doxorubicin in 10 fractions over the 9-month period, or 440 mg/m². Evaluation of lymph nodes by physical examination and CT scan revealed no enlargement.

The anthracycline antibiotics most commonly used in cancer chemotherapy, doxorubicin and daunorubicin, have been recognized as associated with cardiotoxicity since the 1970s. Doses of drug associated with this potentially life-threatening side effect usually exceed 500 mg/m² of doxorubicin, although congestive heart failure has been recognized in patients receiving less than 100 mg/m² of body surface area. As much as 5000 mg/m² has been administered without signs of cardiac problems (29). Acute changes within 24 hours after a dose of doxorubicin include hypereosinophilia of cardiac myocytes, accumulation of hyaline material, and cytoplasmic granulation. Chronic changes include a predictable stepwise loss of myofibrils and vacuolization. Diagnosis can be suspected by radionuclide angiocardiography and confirmed by endomyocardial biopsy, although the histologic findings are also seen in other cardiomyopathies. The mechanism of doxorubicin cardiotoxicity is not understood, although it may involve the known occurrence of free radical formation. It appears less likely to involve the DNA intercalation of doxorubicin, which has been implicated in tumor cell killing, particularly since myocytes are nondividing. The more recently recognized binding to topoisomerase II raises the possibility of interference with the function of critical enzymes in the myocytes. Prediction of cardiotoxicity and consequent early discontinuance of the drug can be assisted by performing a baseline radionuclide angiocardiogram prior to reaching a dose of 100 mg/m², repeating it at 400 mg/m², and stopping treatment at 450 mg/m² or at most 550 mg/m². It appears that smaller weekly doses may be associated with a lower incidence of cardiotoxicity.

The patient was treated with digoxin, diuretics, and an inhibitor of angiotensin I–converting enzyme. Her tachycardia with mild exercise has persisted for over 5 years, but she has maintained generally normal activity for her age, without strenuous exercise. Her latest left ventricular ejection fraction was 42%.

Seven months after her latest CHOP chemotherapy and 6 months after the onset of congestive heart failure, the patient noticed progressively poorer appetite, early satiety, and possibly an increase in night sweats (confounded by her chronic hot flashes). Abdominal CT scan showed probable increased spleen size during the preceding 5 months and slight increase in periaortic node size. She was felt to be in an early relapse. Extensive discussions with the patient, her cardiologist, and her husband led to the decision to reinstitute combination chemotherapy, avoiding the use of any doxorubicin. The combination consisted of intravenous cyclophosphamide, vincristine, etoposide, and cytosine arabinoside, with 5-day courses of oral prednisone with each cycle every 3 weeks. She tolerated the regimen fairly well, with moderate, short-lived nausea and satisfactory blood counts. After 3 months a repeat CT scan still showed persistent splenomegaly, although the periaortic lymph nodes were within normal limits. Intravenous methotrexate with leucovorin rescue at 24 hours was added at the midpoint between the next two cycles of combination chemotherapy. Chemotherapy was terminated after that point, and she has been observed for 3 years with the only additional antitumor chemotherapy being a 6-month course of single-drug chlorambucil, an alkylating agent. There has been periodic waxing and waning of a left cervical lymph node, and serial CT scans have shown stable periaortic nodes and spleen. She has continued to have some hot flushes but has had no known fever, weight loss, or change in appetite. She continues to work full time in the doctor's office.

Because of persistent splenomegaly, a liver biopsy was performed, which showed micronodular cirrhosis, considered to be posthepatitic, and she is felt to have an element of congestive splenomegaly from portal hypertension, with minimal, if any, current apparent progression of her lymphoma.

Drug Resistance. The apparent relapse of the patient's lymphoma in spleen and probably in lymph nodes 7 months after completion of the CHOP chemotherapy was interpreted to suggest resistance of some cells of her lymphoma to the four-drug combination of which she had received 10 cycles. Since the lymphoma had mixed large and small cell histology, it was considered possible that a transition to a more aggressive, large cell population might have occurred, associated with elimination by the chemotherapeutic agents of the more chemosensitive cells in the original population. The CHOP combination had been developed to provide a variety of mechanisms of drug action, theoretically increasing biochemical damage in tumor cells, killing a broader range of tumor cells, and thereby decreasing the likelihood of surviving cells having the opportunity to undergo genetic changes that might lead to drug resistance. This concept has been expressed by Goldie and Coldman, whose hypothesis suggests that drug-resistant cells arise spontaneously at measurable mutation rates, and that the earlier and more intensively a tumor is treated, the less likely is the development of multiple clones of drug-resistant tumor cells (10).

A number of mechanisms demonstrated in tumor cells convey resistance to commonly used anticancer agents. These include decreased drug uptake by the tumor cells; decrease in drug-activating enzymes; increase in drug-degrading enzymes; increased DNA repair; alternative biochemical pathways bypassing the drug inhibition; increased levels of the inhibited target enzyme, often associated with gene amplification; altered affinity of the target enzyme for the drug; inactivation of the drug by sulfhydryl compounds; increased levels of topoisomerase II, resulting in decreased drug-induced DNA damage; inhibition of apoptosis; and increased drug removal from tumor cells. This last mechanism has been associated with increased levels of a 170-kDa membrane glycoprotein (P-glycoprotein) that confers resistance to a variety of structurally diverse drugs, including doxorubicin, etoposide, vincristine, actinomycin D, and other related drugs. The P-glycoprotein is encoded by *mdr* genes, which can transfer this multidrug (pleiotropic) resistance to drug-sensitive cells by transfection. Resistant cells have been observed to pump out increased amounts of the drugs involved, a process that can be inhibited by calcium channel blockers (verapamil), calmodulin inhibitors (quinidine, chloroquine), and cyclosporin A (12).

The induction of apoptosis (programed cell death) by cancer chemotherapeutic agents is now well recognized, although the causative mechanisms are not well understood (30, 31). Certain instances of tumor cell drug resistance may occur in association with the inhibition of apoptosis resulting from the increased expression of the *bcl-2* proto-oncogene. Activation of the *bcl-2* proto-oncogene has been observed in association with chromosomal translocations in certain human B-cell lymphomas. The resultant deregulation of *bcl-2* expression may contribute to suppression of apoptotic deletion of tumor cells, which otherwise would occur following exposure to chemotherapeutic agents (30). Furthermore, there is growing evidence that expression of the *p53* tumor suppressor gene is required for efficient activation of apoptosis following exposure of tumor cells to chemotherapeutic agents. Cellular resistance may, therefore, be linked to absence of *p53* gene expression in tumor cells (32).

Increased understanding of these mechanisms of drug resistance may lead to the development of other potentiators of chemotherapy that counteract the processes contributing to the resistance (19). Such approaches, if relatively specific for tumor cells, would avoid the increased normal tissue toxicity associated with current methods of countering drug resistance. Those methods include the use of greater dose intensity, with or without subsequent bone marrow transplantation or other "rescue" procedure such as leucovorin (folinic acid) following high doses of methotrexate, and larger numbers of drugs in alternating, non-cross-resistant combinations. The ready availability of reliable predictive in vitro assays of tumor cells for drug resistance before exposing patients to ineffective drugs has been a point of interest for years. Unfortunately, not all tumors can be cultured successfully, and clinically significant predictions frequently do not occur, even when in vitro growth is achieved.

The patient has been in a stable, although perhaps only partial, remission for over 3 years since her latest chemotherapy. The regimens with which she had been treated over a 19-month period included an alkylating agent, an antibiotic, two antimetabolites, an epipodophyllotoxin, a vinca alkaloid (metabolic spindle poison), and a synthetic hormone. Treatment was fairly intensive from the beginning, although severe levels of hematologic, gastrointestinal, or neurologic toxicity were not reached. The persistence, or development, of a resistant population of lymphoma cells was not conclusively documented, but the appearance of low-grade lymphadenopathy periodically, not uncommon in the natural history of low-grade non-Hodgkin's lymphomas, suggests that such chemoresistant cells continue to persist. Their eradication by even more intensive therapy, different agents, and possibly the application of autologous bone marrow transplantation was not chosen, either by the patient or by her physicians. Biologic response modifiers, such as alpha interferon, which she has not yet received, may offer an acceptable approach to a future relapse if symptoms warrant. To return to the subject discussed at the beginning of this chapter, indications for treatment continue to be a primary concern in this patient's case. A balance is being sought between the potential contributions of scientific, clinical, and investigational chemotherapy to her survival and the equilibrium she seems to have established with her disease.

REFERENCES

1. Karnofsky DM, Abelmann WH, Craver LF, Burchenal JH. The use of the nitrogen mustards in the palliative treatment of carcinoma. With particular reference to bronchogenic carcinoma. Cancer 1948;1:634–669.
2. Bakemeier RF, Qazi R. Basic concepts of cancer chemotherapy and principles of medical oncology. In: Rubin P, ed. Clinical oncology. A multidisciplinary approach for physicians and students. 7th ed. Philadelphia: WB Saunders, 1993:105–116.
3. Mendelsohn J, Howley PM, Isreal MA, Liotta LA, eds. The molecular basis of cancer. Philadelphia: WB Saunders, 1995.
4. Hill RP, Tannock IF. Introduction: cancer as a cellular disease. In: Tannock IA, Hill RP, eds. The basic science of oncology. 2nd ed. New York: McGraw-Hill, 1992:1–4.
5. Skipper HE. Laboratory models: the historical perspective. Cancer Treat Rep 1986;x70:3–7.
6. Tannock IF. Biological properties of anticancer drugs. In: Tannock IA, Hill RP, eds. The basic science of oncology. 2nd ed. New York: McGraw-Hill, 1992:302–316.
7. Mendelsohn ML. The growth fraction: a new concept applied to tumors. Science 1960;132:1496.
8. Tannock IF. Cell proliferation. In: Tannock IA, Hill RP, eds. The basic science of oncology. 2nd ed. New York: McGraw-Hill, 1992:154.
9. Norton L. The Norton-Simon hypothesis. In: Perry MC, ed. The chemotherapy sourcebook. Baltimore: Williams & Wilkins, 1992:36.

10. Goldie JH, Coldman AJ. The genetic origin of drug resistance in neoplasms: implications for systemic therapy. Cancer Res 1984;44:3643.

11. Goldie JH. Drug resistance. In: Perry MC, ed. The chemotherapy sourcebook. Baltimore: Williams & Wilkins, 1992: 54–66.

12. Tannock IF. Experimental chemotherapy. In: Tannock IA, Hill RP, eds. The basic science of oncology. 2nd ed. New York: McGraw-Hill, 1992:338–359.

13. Ling V, Gerlach JH, Chan HSL, Thorner PS, Gariepy J, Bradley G, Georges E. P-glycoprotein and resistance to anticancer drugs. In: Bergsagel DE, Tak WM, eds. Molecular mechanisms and their clinical application in malignancies. San Diego: Academic Press, 1991:17–34.

14. Gilewski T, Bitran JD. Adjuvant chemotherapy. In: Perry MC, ed. The chemotherapy sourcebook. Baltimore: Williams & Wilkins, 1992:67–89.

15. Ratain MJ, Schilsky RL. Principles of pharmacology and pharmacokinetics. In: Perry MC, ed. The chemotherapy sourcebook. Baltimore: Williams & Wilkins, 1992: 22–35.

16. Erlichman C. Pharmacology of anticancer drugs. In: Tannock IA, Hill RP, eds. The basic science of oncology. 2nd ed. New York: McGraw-Hill, 1992:317–337.

17. Chabner BA, Myers CE. Clinical pharmacology of cancer chemotherapy. In: DeVita VT, Hellman S, Rosenberg SA, eds. Cancer. Principles and practice of oncology. 3rd ed. 1989:349–391.

18. Pratt WB, Ruddon RW, Ensminger WD, Maybaum J. The anticancer drugs. 2nd ed. New York: Oxford University Press, 1994.

19. Yarbro JW. The scientific basis of cancer chemotherapy. In: Perry MC, ed. The chemotherapy sourcebook. Baltimore: Williams & Wilkins, 1992:2–14.

20. Conley BA, VanEcho DA. Antineoplastic drug development. In: Perry MC, ed. The chemotherapy sourcebook. Baltimore: Williams & Wilkins, 1992:15–21.

21. Bergsagel DE. An assessment of massive-dose chemotherapy of malignant disease. Can Med Assoc J 1971;104:31–36.

22. Hoagland HC. Hematologic complications of cancer chemotherapy. In: Perry MC, ed. The chemotherapy sourcebook. Baltimore: Williams & Wilkins, 1992:498–507.

23. Hesketh PJ, Gandara G. Serotonin antagonists: a new class of antiemetic agents. JNCI 1991;l:83:613–620.

24. Mitchell EP, Schein PS. Gastrointestinal toxicity of chemotherapeutic agents. In: Perry MC, ed. The chemotherapy sourcebook. Baltimore: Williams & Wilkins, 1992: 620–634.

25. DeSpain JD. Dermatologic toxicity. In: Perry MC, ed. The chemotherapy sourcebook. Baltimore: Williams & Wilkins, 1992:531–547.

26. Blayney DW, Longo DL, Young RC, Greene MH, Hubbard SM, et al. Decreasing risk of leukemia with prolonged follow-up after chemotherapy and radiotherapy for Hodgkin's disease. JAMA 1987;316:710–714.

27. Kyle RA, Gertz MA. Second malignancies after chemotherapy. In: Perry MC, ed. The chemotherapy sourcebook. Baltimore: Williams & Wilkins, 1992:689–702.

28. Perry MC, ed. The chemotherapy sourcebook. Baltimore: Williams & Wilkins, 1992.

29. Allen A. The cardiotoxicity of chemotherapeutic drugs. In: Perry MC, ed. The chemotherapy sourcebook. Baltimore: Williams & Wilkins, 1992:582–597.

30. Kerr JFR, Winterford CM, Harmon BV. Apoptosis. Its significance in cancer and cancer therapy. Cancer 1994; 73:2013.

31. Meyn RE, Stephens LC, Hunter NR, Milas L. Apoptosis in murine tumors treated with chemotherapy agents. Anticancer Drugs 1995;6:443.

32. Lowe SW, Ruley HE, Jacks T, Housman DE. p53-Dependent apoptosis modulates the cytotoxicity of anticancer agents. Cell 1993;74:957.

CHAPTER 37

Radiation Therapy and Hematologic Malignancies

ROBERT B. MARCUS, JR.

. . . bury the radium to obtain the greatest efficiency in its use, as otherwise more than half the Gamma rays are lost. This can be done by the use of exploring needles containing the radium or its emanation in fine capillary tubes.
—Walter Clegg Stevenson, 1914

In 1931 radium dial workers were shown to have an excessive number of cancer cases.
—Martland, 1931

With the exception of Hodgkin's disease and some of the adult non-Hodgkin's lymphomas (NHLs), most hematopoietic malignancies are primarily treated with chemotherapy. However, there are a number of indications for localized radiation therapy. This chapter covers some of these, with particular emphasis on the leukemias. There are separate chapters regarding the treatment of Hodgkin's disease and adult NHLs in which radiotherapy is discussed. The pediatric NHLs are closely related to leukemia, and most applications in treatment for leukemia are appropriate for this group of diseases as well.

Case 1

A 6-year-old Caucasian male presented with acute lymphoblastic leukemia (ALL). His initial white blood cell count was 10 × 109/L, and he phenotyped as a pre-B-cell ALL. There was no clinically significant adenopathy or organomegaly and no leukemia cells present in the CSF. As part of the initial workup, he was sent to a radiation oncologist for consideration of cranial irradiation (CrI) as part of his CNS prophylactic therapy.

Commentary. In 1965, because of the significant incidence of CNS failure in leukemia patients, it was proposed that lymphoblasts invaded the meninges in essentially all patients before any treatment was given and that standard chemotherapy as given in that era was not sufficient to penetrate the meninges in adequate concentrations (1). Because of this theory, as well as data from mice with L1210 leukemia successfully treated with cyclophosphamide and CrI (2), a number of trials that included some form of preventative CNS therapy were begun at St. Jude Children's Research Hospital. CrI doses of 6 Gy, then 12 Gy, were tried without success, but in 1972 it was reported that 24 Gy plus intrathecal

methotrexate (IT-MTX) given simultaneously early in remission helped prevent CNS relapse and increased survival (3). A number of other early studies using craniospinal irradiation (CSI) or CrI plus IT-MTX also showed a drop in CNS relapse rates from over 50% to under 10% and an improvement in survival from near zero to about 50% (4). Since those studies in the early 1970s, all patients with ALL have received some form of preventative therapy to the CNS.

In the 1970s, most patients received CrI and IT-MTX. Over the next two decades, treatment philosophies changed. Even though most chemotherapy agents do not achieve adequate dose levels in the cerebrospinal fluid, it is clear that a number of drug alternatives, such as triple intrathecal therapy (Ara-C, methotrexate, prednisone), do exist to potentially prevent the development of overt CNS disease. So, which patients therefore need irradiation?

A number of factors are associated with a high risk of CNS leukemia relapse, including an initial WBC over 50 × 109/L, age less than 2 or greater than 9 years, and a T-cell immunophenotype. If none of these factors are present, as in the case presentation, CNS prophylactic therapy can be achieved without CrI. The Pediatric Oncology Group has used triple intrathecal chemotherapy throughout the entire course of treatment and shown it to be as effective as 24 Gy of CrI plus IT-MTX (5). In a similar trial, the Children's Cancer Study Group (CCSG) showed that IT-MTX with intensive systemic chemotherapy is as effective as 18 Gy CrI in standard-risk patients less than 10 years of age (6).

The data for patients at high risk for CNS relapse are more controversial. The risk of CNS relapse is lower in patients who receive CrI and IT-MTX, but there is no definite advantage in survival (7, 8). A number of institutions and cooperative groups still give CrI for T-cell disease or initial high WBC. Others believe that intensive systemic chemotherapy in addition to triple intrathecal chemotherapy can give equivalent results. There are no unequivocal data to prove that either approach is superior. Currently in the Pediatric Oncology Group (POG), only patients with T-cell disease receive CrI. All other pediatric patients are managed with chemotherapy alone.

Adult patients may be managed differently. Many institutions still employ CrI with IT-MTX in the treatment of adults. As noted before, the elimination of CrI in children, particularly those with high-risk features, requires the substitution of intensive systemic chemotherapy and usually triple intrathecal therapy as well. Adults, particularly older adults, may not tolerate the necessary drug doses, and it may be less toxic to include CrI as the CNS preventive therapy instead.

Other lymphoproliferative disorders rarely require the use of radiation therapy as part of the CNS preventative therapy. Although used in some cooperative group protocols in the 1970s for acute myelogenous leukemia (AML), this practice is not necessary because of the low risk of CNS relapse in this disease. Likewise, NHLs (adult and pediatric) are not routinely given CrI.

If localized radiotherapy is to be used as part of the CNS preventative therapy in an ALL patient with no detectable CNS disease at diagnosis, it is now accepted that CrI with IT-MTX is adequate to prevent CNS relapse in over 90% of patients. About 95% of the arachnoid tissue is contained in the cranial vault, and methotrexate injected into the lumbar sac reaches acceptable levels in the spinal fluid. It is, of course, necessary to give at least a portion of the intrathecal drugs during the course of CrI so that the entire CSF pathway is covered at one time. **Spinal irradiation** is not necessary in this setting and is contraindicated because the large amount of bone marrow irradiated (when treating both the cranium and the spine) can subsequently prevent the delivery of appropriate doses of chemotherapy.

The target volume of the cranial field should include the entire intracranial subarachnoid space. The inferior margin of the field is at the bottom of C2. At least a 1-cm margin should be given around the base of the skull, paying particular attention to the temporal fossa and cribriform plate. The most common mistake seen in cooperative group protocols is failure to adequately cover these two areas, and inadequately treated patients are more likely to relapse in the CNS (9). Although intraocular relapses are exceedingly rare, it is conventional to treat the posterior half of the globe, and a portion of the superior globe is often treated when the cribriform plate is covered. To do this and not irradiate (with the divergence of the beam) the anterior half of the opposite eye, the gantry can be angled 5° posteriorly or the central axis of the beam can be placed at the equator of the eye, with a shaped block designed to shield the face. A small amount of flash around the skull is necessary but is more critical for 60Co than for accelerator beams.

Low-energy megavoltage photons are the beam of choice, since the primary goal of treatment is the meninges, and they often lie as superficial as 1 cm below the surface of the scalp in young children. The beam energy of choice is therefore 6 MV; for teenagers and adults, an 8 MV beam can be used, though few institutions have this. The wide penumbra of the 60Co beam makes it difficult to treat the cribriform plate adequately without also irradiating a large portion of the anterior half of the eye. For years, the standard dose to the cranial meninges has been 24 Gy (usually given in fractions of 1.5–2.0 Gy), based on the original studies by Aur et al. (3), but recent data from the CCSG indicate that a dose of 18 Gy (in 10 fractions) is equally efficacious (10). Both regimens are used today, but the lower dose should result in less late morbidity and is therefore recommended.

Even lower doses have been reported to be successful in less-than-high-risk patients. The German BFM group reported no difference in CNS relapse or survival between 18 Gy and 12 Gy when intensive systemic therapy was used, including intermediate-dose methotrexate (7). No studies have duplicated this in high-risk patients.

For children under 3 years of age at diagnosis, a dose of 12–15 Gy at 1.5 per day is used.

It was decided that CrI was not required in the 6-year-old boy presented above as he did not fall into a high-risk category. He received 3 years of chemotherapy on a POG protocol. At the end of treatment he was in complete remission, with a negative bone marrow and spinal tap. He did well for 3 months off treatment; then his mother noticed that his left face was not moving normally, and he was found to have a left seventh cranial nerve palsy. An MRI of the brain and bone marrow biopsy were normal, but the spinal tap revealed numerous lymphoblasts in the CSF. The parents were referred to a radiation oncologist to discuss the need for irradiation as part of the treatment for his relapse.

Commentary. Whereas CrI is no longer used in most preventative CNS regimens, it is considered a necessary part of the treatment for CNS relapse. In the case presented, the first consideration with regard to treatment is the cranial nerve palsy. The most common cranial nerve to be affected is the VIIth nerve, with cranial nerves II, III, and VI also involved relatively commonly (11–14). Multiple cranial nerve involvement occurs in about a third of patients (11, 14). Whether it occurs at the time of the initial diagnosis of leukemia or lymphoma or at the time of relapse, a cranial nerve palsy needs to be managed acutely, as quickly after diagnosis as possible, since resolution of cranial nerve dysfunction has been reported to occur more frequently if radiotherapy is started within 24 hours of the onset of symptoms (11). This is best done with small fields localized to the track of the cranial nerve involved, to a dose of 6–10 Gy at 1.5–1.8 Gy per day. This dose can be essentially disregarded when more definitive CNS irradiation is to be given later in treatment. In one report, 70% of patients experienced resolution of the cranial nerve dysfunction (11). Cranial nerve involvement is more common in childhood NHL than in ALL, and extremely rare in AML. The treatment is similar, no matter which process is the cause.

Definitive irradiation for a CNS relapse is given after the patient obtains a complete bone marrow and CSF remission using intrathecal as well as systemic chemotherapy. Data (15, 16) indicate that CSI is superior to CrI and IT-MTX. In one study, 7 of 16 patients remained in secondary continuous remission for more than 6 years after therapy with CSI versus 1 of 11 patients after IT-MTX and CrI (15). The Southwest Oncology Group (SWOG) trial 7712, reported a 3% second CNS relapse rate after CSI, versus 31% after CrI and IT-MTX, and a secondary continuous complete response (CCR) of 44% for CSI, versus 7% for CrI and IT-MTX (Fig. 37.1) (16). It is always necessary to clear the CSF with IT chemotherapy before the use of CSI.

Standard doses of CSI are 24 Gy at 1.8–2.0 Gy per day to the cranial field and 15 Gy at 1.5 Gy per day to the spinal field. Lower doses are used to the spinal field because of the previous IT-MTX employed in all protocols. Currently, trials with lower doses (18 Gy to the cranium, 12 Gy to the spine) are under way, but no definite data exist indicating that these doses are as efficacious as the more standard ones.

For patients with overt CNS disease, the data are less clear. Some trials employ CSI, while others use only intrathecal drugs and CrI. Based on the results of the above trials treating CNS relapse patients, one would think that CSI would be a superior treatment in this setting as well, but there are no available data directly comparing the two methods.

After completing his CSI, the child continued on maintenance chemotherapy. In follow-up, however, he had a small white infiltrate in the anterior chamber of his right eye, though he denied any visual symptoms. Suspecting an anterior chamber relapse, an extensive physical examination, MRI of the brain and spine, and a bone marrow biopsy and spinal tap were carried out. All were negative. No treatment was given, but within 2 weeks the infiltrate had filled the anterior chamber, and vision was dramatically decreased to finger movements only.

Because the optic nerve and retina of the eye are embryologically outgrowths of the brain, an occasional patient with overt CNS disease will also develop infiltration of the retina, anterior chamber, or even the orbits.

Radiation therapy is the treatment of choice for an anterior chamber relapse. Since the advent of successful CNS preventative treatment (both radiotherapeutic and chemotherapeutic), eye relapses have become much less common, since they are usually a sign of CNS relapse. Most occur in patients with previous CNS relapse (17). In any case, the CNS should be considered at risk, and the patient treated as if a CNS relapse has occurred. If CrI has already been given, treatment of the eye with doses of 20–24 Gy at 1.5–2.0 Gy per day is rapidly effective, with systemic chemotherapy and appropriate chemotherapeutic CNS treatment. If CrI has never been given, then a short course of 3–10 Gy to the eye can be given to relieve any symptoms. Following induction chemotherapy, CSI should be given, including the previous area of anterior chamber involvement. All this assumes the patient is still considered to be "curable." If palliation is the goal, then a

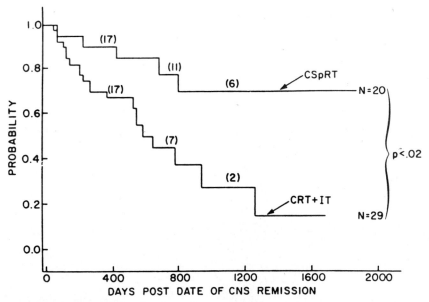

Figure 37.1. Duration of complete clinical response by treatment (cranial irradiation plus intrathecal therapy (CRT + IT) versus craniospinal irradiation (CSpRT)) for patients with CNS relapse only treated on SWOG protocol 7712. (From Land VJ, Thomas PR, Boyett JM, Glicksman AS, Culbert S, et al. Comparison of maintenance treatment regimens for first central nervous system relapse in children with acute lymphoblastic leukemia. A Pediatric Oncology Group study. Cancer 1985;56:81–87. With permission.)

course of 10–15 Gy to the eye is sufficient to achieve this in most patients.

In the event of retinal or orbital infiltration (fig. 37.2), localized radiotherapy may also be of benefit. Since these events are a manifestation of overt CNS involvement, CrI or CSI should be part of the overall plan of treatment if the patient is still being treated for cure. If so, a short course of emergent radiotherapy to the orbits (up to 10 Gy at 1.5–2.0 Gy per day) will relieve the symptoms. At a later time, after induction chemotherapy and a CR, the CrI can be given in conjunction with more radiation to the orbits. For that reason, the dose of the emergent radiotherapy should be as low as possible. The other alternative is to initiate the CrI with the emergent orbital irradiation at the beginning of treatment. The disadvantage of this is that CrI is more effective if given when there is no detectable leukemia, to minimize the risk of reseeding the CNS after the completion of radiation therapy. If palliation is the only goal, then there is no contraindication to giving the entire course of radiotherapy immediately after diagnosis. The total dose in this case depends upon the estimated length of survival of the patient. A total dose of 10–15 Gy will provide

short-term palliation. Higher doses are needed for long-term control.

Leukostasis

Emergent whole brain irradiation at the beginning of treatment is recommended by some authors in those cases with very high white counts ($>100 \times 10^9$/L) because of the risk that thrombi leading to infarction and intracranial hemorrhage may develop. While this may be appropriate, there are actually no data to indicate that this approach is superior to chemotherapy and supportive measures to decrease the risk of thrombi until chemotherapy decreases the WBC. The disadvantage is that the CrI is given at a time (before complete remission) when it is less effective as CNS preventative therapy. Standard doses of CrI are used.

Testicular Relapse

Instead of relapsing in the CNS, assume that our patient, now 9 years old, relapses in the right testicle 1 year off therapy. Is there a role for radiotherapy?

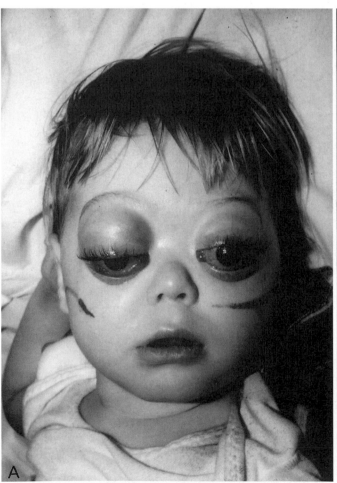

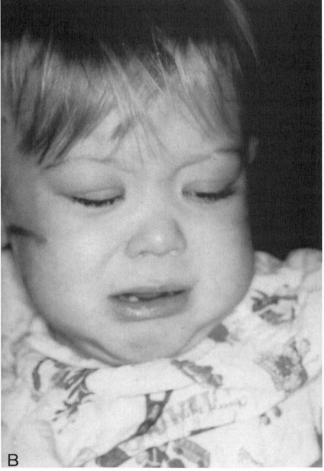

Figure 37.2. An 18-month-old white female who presented with a 3-month history of proptosis secondary to ALL (A). Though her spinal tap was unremarkable, she also had a left VIIth nerve palsy, and it was decided that she had CNS disease with infiltration into her retina and orbit bilaterally. Her proptosis did not respond initially to induction chemotherapy, and she was started on emergent cranial RT with coverage of both orbits as well. B, A rapid response to radiotherapy was noted, with resolution of her cranial nerve palsy and proptosis by the end of 20 Gy in 10 fractions.

When testicular relapse occurs off treatment, conventional therapy includes a course of bilateral testicular irradiation, in concert with reinduction systemic chemotherapy. In general, doses of 24 Gy at 1.5–2.0 Gy/day with a single anterior field are employed. Electrons or low-energy photons are used, but to obtain a homogeneous distribution, a bolus is usually required. This course of radiation can be given as soon as the patient is back in remission, since, unlike with CSI, there is no bone marrow suppression (18, 19).

Testicular involvement during the initial course of chemotherapy probably represents a different clinical situation. In general, it is a very poor prognostic sign and is more likely an indicator that the disease is resistant to the systemic therapy than a sign of a relapse in a sanctuary site. Because of this, it is not clear that radiation therapy helps at all in this setting (20). If radiotherapy is used, similar doses to those previously mentioned are given.

Splenic Involvement

Symptomatic splenic involvement occurs primarily in CML and CLL but can occur in other diseases such as myelofibrosis or myeloid metaplasia. Although splenic irradiation for CML was first reported in 1903 (21), currently it is usually reserved for patients with that and other myeloproliferative or lymphoproliferative disorders who continue to be symptomatic despite chemotherapy.

The primary indications for splenic irradiation are symptoms arising from splenomegaly: splenic pain, early satiety, and thrombocytopenia from platelet trapping (sequestration). For malignant diseases such as CML and CLL, pain and discomfort from the enlarged spleen are the most common reasons.

The mechanism of action of splenic irradiation in CLL is thought to be destruction of neoplastic B cells, which are more sensitive to irradiation when blocked in their maturation, and selective destruction of one well-defined T subset, identified as T-γ OKT8+, OKT17+ suppressor cells (22).

Several different fractionation schemes have been successful. The safest regimen to start with is 0.25–0.5 Gy per day, 2–3 days a week. Some authors report that total doses of 2–4.5 Gy at these slow fractionations are effective (22–26). Other authors recommend increasing the dose to 1 Gy per day if the initial fractions are well tolerated, to a total dose of 10–15 Gy (27). However, most reports do not show an improved response rate to higher doses (22, 23, 25).

A reduction in palpable splenomegaly by at least 50% occurs in about one-third to two-thirds of patients; it is rare to not achieve some shrinkage in CLL, CML, or B-prolymphocytic leukemia, the diseases in which it is used most (23, 26, 28). Of those patients who have splenic pain, at least two-thirds note significant improvement (23, 26). Byhardt et al. (26) reported improvement in platelet

counts in 18 of 23 courses of splenic irradiation, and stabilization or improvement of hemoglobin levels in 21 of 23 courses, but other authors have not reported such good results for thrombocytopenia in myeloproliferative-associated splenomegaly (22, 23, 25). The average time for response of the platelet count was 48 days, and 42 days for hemoglobin (26). In patients with a good hematologic response, the median duration of response was 9 months (22). It is not clear from evaluating the reports available in the literature that there is any significant difference between the response rates of CLL and CML.

The toxicity of splenic irradiation is primarily hematologic, though nausea, vomiting, and malaise also occur. The nausea and vomiting can usually be controlled with modern antiemetics. Significant thrombocytopenia requiring a break in treatment occurs in 10–20% of patients (22).

Low-dose hydroxyurea is being tried to improve the response rate of splenic irradiation for CML, but there are no firm data to show that it is superior to radiation therapy alone (23).

In the event of a good response but subsequent progression, a second course of splenic irradiation can be given (22).

Other Extramedullary Sites

Symptomatic involvement of other organs is possible with any of the leukemias or NHLs, particularly those that occur in childhood. Mediastinal involvement, with airway obstruction or superior venocaval syndrome (SVC) syndrome, and renal involvement are probably the most serious. The dose and volume to be treated depend upon the treatment goal: curative or palliative. Since patients with these diseases generally receive chemotherapy as their primary curative treatment, radiation is usually given to these sites only as a palliative measure. Certainly there are no data showing that consolidative therapy to bulky disease with radiotherapy adds to the cure rate for patients with leukemia or pediatric NHLs (29). This statement does not apply to adult NHLs or Hodgkin disease.

In a palliative setting, a dose of 10–15 Gy at 1.5–3.0 Gy per fraction will achieve significant shrinkage of the lesions in most cases. The shorter courses should be given to patients with the shortest life expectancy, unless a large mucosal surface will be in the field. In this case, the fractionation should be protracted to minimize acute side effects.

If the patient has a long life expectancy or is still being treated with a curative goal, total doses up to 20–30 Gy should be given to try to achieve more lasting control.

Chloromas

Chloromas represent skin infiltration by leukemic cells. They occur primarily in AML but can occur in other leukemias. Although they can present early in the course of the disease, usually they present after the patient fails primary systemic therapy. In this setting, palliative irradi-

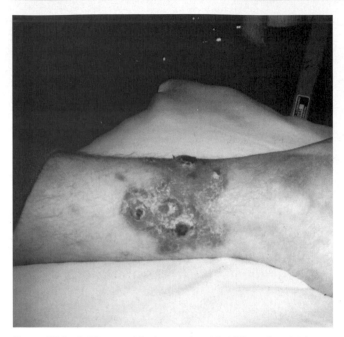

Figure 37.3. A 72-year-old white male with AML and multiple chloromas. Shown here is a lesion on his forearm. Complete resolution was achieved with 20 Gy in 10 fractions.

ation may be required to achieve relief of symptoms. The course of irradiation depends upon the goal of therapy and the life expectancy of the patient. Palliation can be achieved with very short courses of irradiation: 10–15 Gy in 2–3 fractions. If the lesion is over a mucosal surface or another anatomic area where a rapidly fractionated course might produce considerable acute effects, a more prolonged fractionation can be used, such as 15–20 Gy at 1.5–2.0 Gy per fraction. If the patient is still a candidate for curative therapy, a more prolonged course of radiation is also preferable, with a total dose of 20–30 Gy (fig. 37.3).

Summary

Localized regional radiotherapy plays an important, if often adjunctive, role in the management of myeloproliferative and lymphoproliferative disorders. The techniques for delivery and the sources of ionizing radiation continue to improve, and there is every reason to suppose that the considered use of this therapy will continue to be of value in cure and palliation of such disorders. Table 37.1 is an example of dosimeters for localized therapy.

Table 37.1 Recommended Doses for Hodgkin's Disease and Multiple Myeloma

Disease	Age	Clinical Setting	Total Dose (Gy)	Dose (Gy)/Fraction
Hodgkin's disease	>15	Involved site (RT alone)	25–35°	1.5–1.8
	>15	Uninvolved site (RT alone)	20–30°	1.5–1.8
	<15	Involved site	24–35°	1.5
	<15	Uninvolved site	15–30°	1.5
Plasmacytoma	—	Localized	40–50	1.8
Multiple myeloma	—	Disseminated	20–25	2.0–2.5

°Lower doses to be used after full dose chemotherapy, higher doses for RT alone.

REFERENCES

1. George P, Pinkel D. CNS radiation in children with acute lymphocytic leukemia in remission. Proc AACR 1965;6:22.
2. Johnson RE. An experimental therapeutic approach to L1210 leukemia in mice: combined chemotherapy and central nervous system irradiation. JNCI 1964;32:1333–1340.
3. Aur RJ, Simone JV, Hustu HO, Verzos MS. A comparative study of central nervous system irradiation and intensive chemotherapy early in remission of childhood acute lymphocytic leukemia. Cancer 1972;29:381–391.
4. Dritschilo A, Cassady JR, Camitta B, Jaffe N, Furman L, Traggis D. The role of irradiation in central nervous system treatment and prophylaxis for acute lymphoblastic leukemia. Cancer 1976;37:2729–2735.
5. Sullivan MP, Chen T, Dyment PG, Hvizdala E, Steuber CP. Equivalence of intrathecal chemotherapy and radiotherapy as central nervous system prophylaxis in children with acute lymphatic leukemia. A Pediatric Oncology Group study. Blood 1982;60:948–958.
6. Turbergen DG, Gilchrist GS, O'Brian RT, Coccia PF, Sather HN, Waskerwotz MJ, Hammond GD. Prevention of CNS disease in intermediate acute lymphoblastic leukemia: comparison of cranial radiation and intrathecal methotrexate and the importance of systemic therapy. A Children's Cancer Group report. J Clin Oncol 1993;11:520–526.
7. Riehm H, Gadner H, Henze G, et al. Results and significance of six randomized trials in four consecutive ALL-BFM studies. In: Buchner T, Schellong, Hiddeman, Ritter, eds. Haematology and blood transfusion 33: Acute leukemias II. Berlin: Springer-Verlag, 1990:439–450.
8. Niemeyer CM, Hitchcock-Bryan S, Sallan SE. Comparative analysis of treatment programs for childhood acute lymphoblastic leukemia. Semin Oncol 1985;12:122–130.
9. Kun LE, Camitta BM, Mulhern RK, Lauer SJ, Kline RW, et al. Treatment of meningeal relapse in childhood acute lymphoblastic leukemia. I. Results of craniospinal irradiation. J Clin Oncol 1984;2:359–364.
10. Nesbit ME Jr, Sather HN, Robison LL, Ortega J, Littman PS, D'Angio GJ, Hammond GD. Presymptomatic central nervous system therapy in previously untreated childhood acute lymphoblastic leukaemia: comparison of 1800 rad and 2400 rad. A report for Children's Cancer Study Group. Lancet 1981;1:461–466.
11. Paryani SB, Donaldson SS, Amylon MD, Link MP. Cranial nerve involvement in children with leukemia and lymphoma. J Clin Oncol 1983;1:542–545.

12. Nieri RL, Burgert EO, Groover RV. Central nervous system complications of leukemia: a review. Mayo Clin Proc 1968; 43:70–79.

13. Pochedly C. Neurologic manifestations in acute leukemia. II. Involvement of cranial nerves and hypothalamus. NY State J Med 1975;75:715–721.

14. Ingram LC, Fairclough DL, Furman WL, Sandlund JT, Kun LE, Rivera GK, Pui CH. Cranial nerve palsy in childhood acute lymphoblastic leukemia and non-Hodgkin's lymphoma. Cancer 1991;67:2262–2268.

15. Willoughby MLN. Treatment of overt meningeal leukaemia in children: results of second MRC meningeal leukaemia trial. Br Med J 1976;1:864–867.

16. Land VJ, Thomas PR, Boyett JM, Glicksman AS, Culbert S, et al. Comparison of maintenance treatment regimens for first central nervous system relapse in children with acute lymphoblastic leukemia. A Pediatric Oncology Group study. Cancer 1985;56:81–87.

17. Harnett AN, Plowman PN. The eye in acute leukemia. 2. The management of solitary anterior chamber relapse. Radiother Oncol 1987;10:203–207.

18. Hustu HO, Aur RJ, Verzosa MS, Simone JV, Pinkel D. Prevention of central nervous system leukemia by irradiation. Cancer 1973;32:585–597.

19. Sullivan MP, Perez CA, Herson J, Silva-Sousa M, Land VJ, et al. Radiotherapy (2500 rad) for testicular leukemia: local control and subsequent clinical events. A Southwest Oncology Group Study. Cancer 1980;46:508–515.

20. Kim TH, Hargreaves HK, Brynes RK, Hawkins HK, Lui VK, Woodard J, Ragab AH. Pretreatment testicular biopsy in childhood acute lymphocytic leukaemia. Lancet 1981;2: 657–658.

21. Senn NS. Case of splenomedullary leukemia successfully treated by the use of roentgen ray. Med Record 1903; 64:282.

22. Chisesi T, Capnist G, Dal Fior S. Splenic irradiation in chronic lymphocytic leukemia. Eur J Haematol 1991;46: 202–204.

23. Wagner H Jr, McKeough PG, Desforges J, Madoc-Jones H. Splenic irradiation in the treatment of patients with chronic myelogenous leukemia or myelofibrosis with myeloid metaplasia. Results of daily and intermittent fractionation with or without concomitant hydroxyurea. Cancer 1986;58: 1204–1207.

24. Parmentier C, Charbord P, Tibi M, Tubiana M. Splenic irradiation in myelofibrosis: clinical findings and ferrokinetics. Int J Radiat Oncol Biol Phys 1977;2:1075–1081.

25. Guiney MJ, Liew KH, Quong GG, Cooper IA. A study of splenic irradiation in chronic lymphocytic leukemia. Int J Radiat Oncol Biol Phys 1989;16:225–229.

26. Byhardt RW, Brace KC, Wiernik PH. The role of splenic irradiation in chronic lymphocytic leukemia. Cancer 1975;35: 1621–1625.

27. Wilson JF, Johnson RE. Splenic irradiation following chemotherapy in chronic myelogenous leukemia. Radiology 1971; 101:657–661.

28. Oscier DG, Catovsky D, Errington RD, Goolden AW, Roberts PD, Galton DA. Splenic irradiation in B-prolymphocytic leukaemia. Br J Haematol 1981;48:577–584.

29. Link MP, Donaldson SS, Berard CW, Shuster JJ, Murphy SB. Results of treatment of childhood localized non-Hodgkin's lymphoma with combination chemotherapy with or without radiotherapy. N Engl J Med 1990;322: 1169–1174.

CHAPTER 38

Radiation Therapy and Marrow Transplantation

ROSS A. ABRAMS, MICHAEL G. HERMAN

> Radol, prepared by Dr. Rupert Wells, as a critic said, contained "exactly as much radium as dishwater" did and had the same therapeutic powers when treating cancer.
> —Samuel Hopkins Adams, The Great American Fraud, Chicago, 1906

Although radiation treatments are generally given in radiation suites geographically removed from bone marrow transplant (BMT) units, the impact of radiation on the outcome of the transplant patient's experience may be substantial. Unfortunately, the clinical use of ionizing irradiation may not be well understood by clinicians who are not radiation oncologists. Radiation physics and radiation biology are not well integrated into most medical school basic science curricula. Thus, both the basis for, and the process of, radiation treatment remain beyond the experience of many physicians during their training.

For the radiation oncologist, the use of ionizing irradiation as part of the preparative regimen prior to the infusion of hematopoietically reconstituting stem cells can be seen as a highly specialized example of a very general clinical problem; namely, what is the "best" radiation therapy prescription that can be written in an effort to optimize the patient's clinical management. "Best" is placed in quotations to acknowledge its subjectivity. In this case, best is an integrated concept reflecting chance of treatment success as defined by disease eradication, hematopoietic reconstitution, extent and risk of complications, both immediate (i.e, within days to weeks) and late (i.e., after months or years), following the transplant experience, the expected acute and long-term quality of life for the proposed transplant candidate, and the risks of inducing subsequent secondary neoplasia (Table 38.1). Of course, the outcomes experienced by the patient during and following the transplant process depend on factors (Table 38.2) other than the preparative regimen and the radiation component of the preparative regimen. Even so, the preparative regimen clearly contributes to these outcomes and represents a component of the transplant process readily subject to physician control and modification.

Case Presentation

A 22-year-old man with no prior history of radiation treatment is referred for consideration of total body irradiation (TBI) as part of marrow ablative treatment prior to infusion of allogeneic bone marrow cells from his 26-year-old HLA-identical MLC-negative brother. Five months prior to referral he had been diagnosed with acute myelocytic leukemia (AML) (FAB class M2). Bone marrow–documented complete remission occurred following two cycles of induction therapy. Induction was followed by consolidation. In the 2 weeks prior to being seen, CBC, urinalysis, chemistries, lumbar puncture, chest x-ray, pulmonary function testing, radionuclide assessment of left ventricular function, and bone marrow aspiration and biopsy were performed. These studies documented continued complete remission, and no other problems or concerns were identified. Physical examination is similarly unrevealing. Following the evaluation the patient and his family asked the following questions:

1. *How long will the irradiation take? Will there be noticeable or unpleasant sensations or side effects during the irradiation? What position will he be in during irradiation?*
2. *Why is irradiation being incorporated into his management now? What are the immediate and late consequences of receiving TBI? Could these consequences be avoided by using a preparative regimen not incorporating irradiation? To what extent does the irradiation damage critical organs such as the lungs or liver?*
3. *What will be the source of the irradiation?*

The bone marrow transplant trainee fellow also has questions:

4. *He has heard that not only is the total dose of irradiation important but also the number of irradiation treatments, the number of treatments per day, the interval between treatments, the point at which the dose is specified, and the dose rate. He would like some clarification.*
5. *He has also heard that "blocking" of lungs and/or liver is done in some centers and would like comments about what blocking is, how it is done, and whether it is advisable.*

Table 38.1. Desirable and Undesirable Outcomes of Bone Marrow Transplantation Potentially Influenced by TBI Regimen

Desirable	Undesirable
Permanent disease control	Persistence or relapse
Full functional engraftment of reconstituting lymphohematopoietic stem cells	Failure to engraft
Benign posttransplant course	
No severe acute or subacute sequelae	Interstitial pneumonitis
	Hepatic veno-occlusive disease
	Renal failure
No severe late sequelae	Chronic lung disease
	Cataracts
	Endocrinopathy (thyroid, pituitary)
	Induction of secondary malignancy

The arrival of the transplant fellow jostles the memory of the patient's fiancee. Reaching into her purse, she retrieves a typed list of questions from her father, a radiation physicist at a major medical center. He would like to know:

6. *What steps have been taken to verify the dosimetry of the TBI setup, how you ensure maximal dose homogeneity, and whether the calculated dose is verified by monitoring during treatment. Everyone else present would like to know what "dosimetry" and "dose homogeneity" refer to and why there should be any need to actually measure the dose administered during treatment.*

With the exception of some referral centers that utilize radiation equipment and rooms specifically dedicated for performing TBI (1, 2), most facilities use radiation equipment and rooms designed for more conventional radiation treatments (3, 4). (Given the costs of designing and constructing adequately protected and shielded radiation facilities and the costs of modern linear accelerators, this approach is consistent with fiscal reality, especially since most transplant centers will not be able to use all of the potentially available time slots for a dedicated TBI unit).

Conventional non-TBI radiation treatments are delivered with fields usually no larger than 30 cm by 30 cm or perhaps 40 cm by 40 cm at dose rates (i.e., number of units of irradiation per minute) of 200–300 cGy per minute. (A centigray (cGy) is one hundredth of a gray. The gray (one joule/kg) is the standard unit of energy absorbed from radiation into matter (e.g., tissue). In older terminology, dose was expressed in rads (radiation ab-

sorbed dose). One cGy equals one rad. For ease of localization and daily reproducibility, therapy machines and treatment rooms are constructed so that the axes of rotation of the machine gantry, the collimating head of the treatment machine, and the treatment couch intersect at a common point in space, called the isocenter. Most modern therapy machines are designed so that the distance from the source of the irradiation beam to the isocenter will be 100 cm, and treatment field size is normally defined at this distance.

Although the pioneering work in TBI for purposes of bone marrow transplantation was done with cobalt-60, utilizing the naturally occurring high energy x-rays (gamma rays) emitted by this substance (1), more recently linear accelerators have been used for TBI. The physical and biologic effects of the radiation treatment depend on the physical characteristics of the treating beam but are otherwise independent of whether the beam is emitted by natural radioactive decay or from accelerating electrons in a linear accelerator. In the linear accelerator, the x-ray beam is generated as a secondary phenomenon by directing the beam of electrons into a dense heavy metal target, resulting in the production of the x-ray beam as the electrons are stopped there.

To accommodate the physical size of most adult transplant patients for TBI, it is necessary to take advantage of the fact that x-ray beams emerging from a source diverge with distance just like flashlight beams. In some cases, this divergence can be attained by lowering the treatment couch to the floor, but more commonly, adequate divergence requires distances achievable only by directing the radiation beam horizontally across the room (parallel to the floor and ceiling) toward a distant wall of the treatment room with the patient placed as close as possible to this wall. In most treatment rooms, this provides a distance of 3–4 meters and a field size of nearly 1.5 meters. This degree of divergence, coupled with flexion of knees and hips to a definite but comfortable extent, allows the entire body to be encompassed within the treatment beam and results in a significant reduction in dose rate (5–50 cGy/min). For most adult patients, it may also be necessary to rotate the collimator to line up the diagonal of the treatment field with the long axis of the patient's body (Fig. 38.1). Different centers have adopted various approaches to patient po-

Table 38.2. Factors Independent of Conditioning Regimen That May Impact on Outcome of Bone Marrow Transplant

Nature and extent of prior treatment
Age
Presence of comorbid conditions
Demonstrated development of disease resistance to nonablative levels of therapy
Source of reconstituting stem cells
Development of severe acute or chronic graft versus host disease (GVHD)
Drugs used for GVHD prophylaxis

TBI Radiation Field Geometry

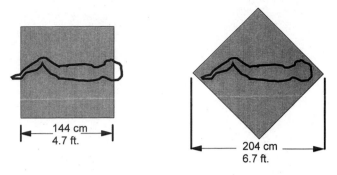

a) Unrotated   b) Rotated 45°

Figure 38.1. Outline of field size; effect of collimator rotation. A 40-cm square field is allowed to diverge a distance of 3.6 meters from the treatment machine to the far wall of the treatment room. Its effective size is now a square 144 cm (4.7 feet) on each side. By rotating the collimator 45°, the diagonal of the square, 204 cm (6.7 feet), is made available. With comfortable hip and knee flexion, most patients will fit along this diagonal for TBI.

Dose Homogeneity

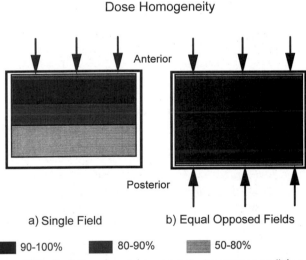

a) Single Field   b) Equal Opposed Fields

■ 90-100%   ■ 80-90%   ▨ 50-80%

Figure 38.2. Radiation dose inhomogeneity in a treatment "phantom" from a), single 4-MV x-ray field (AP only) showing large dose gradients and b), equally weighted opposing (AP, PA) 4-MV x-ray fields showing reduced dose gradient with the 90–100% dose region covering almost the entire phantom.

sitioning, with some using special stands on which patients sit or stand and others using portable gurneys or beds with patients lying either supine or on their sides (37). In all cases, patient comfort and stabilization are essential. Radiation treatments for TBI may require from 10–15 minutes to as long as an hour or more, depending on the total number of radiation treatments (fractions), dose rate, and dose per fraction (see below).

For the most part, there is no sensation associated with TBI, although patients are generally aware of machine sounds and movements. For longer treatments and/or higher dose rates, there is an increasing risk of nausea during treatment, requiring premedication with antiemetics (3).

At the midpoint in the treatment, patient position is usually reversed when single source treatment is being administered (i.e., treatment from a single linear accelerator or cobalt machine). This movement is necessary to even out the dose distribution in the patient (i.e., assure dose homogeneity, see below). This improvement is shown in Figure 38.2, where *a* shows a large variation in dose in different areas of the patient from a single radiation beam, and *b* shows the homogeneity obtained with equal weighted opposing beams. Position reversal means treating first from the right side and then from the left if patients are being treated supine with the beam entering from the side; if patients are being treated lying on their sides, position reversal means treating with the patient facing toward the machine (AP treatment) and then facing away from the machine (PA treatment). With specially designed treatment rooms utilizing two simultaneous radiation sources, patient position may not require this adjustment.

Additional Considerations Regarding the Physics and Dosimetry of TBI

Although TBI doses are generally specified as if they were completely uniform throughout the entire body (e.g., 1200 cGy TBI), the actual dose absorbed at any specific site in the body may vary substantially from the stated dose. In fact, the stated dose, as far as the radiation oncologist or radiation physicist is concerned, is specified only at a single point in the patient; for example, the point of midseparation between the entry and exit points of the radiation beams at a precise level in the patient such as the umbilicus. This may seem confusing at first but is readily clarified.

Consider the pharmacology of administering a drug. The amount of drug in the bloodstream at any point in time depends on the route of administration (oral, intramuscular, or intravenous) as will the kinetics of drug appearance in the blood stream and ultimate peak levels. Tissue concentrations will vary based on organ site, related to factors such as molecular weight, protein binding, lipophilicity, and state of ionization. Thus, the concentration of drug and duration of drug exposure "seen" in cerebrospinal fluid, aqueous humor, blood, or tissues such as lung, liver, bone, or kidney may vary substantially for any stated dose, such as 100 mg intravenously (or, if you will, 100 mg total body dose).

Similarly, with respect to external beam irradiation, there are factors that cause variation (heterogeneity) of absorbed dose. Instead of being pharmacologic, these factors are physical. Such factors include the extent to which the beam is uniform across its entire width or length, the extent to which dose is absorbed at the surface (high-energy x-ray beams transfer their energy to tissue maximally only

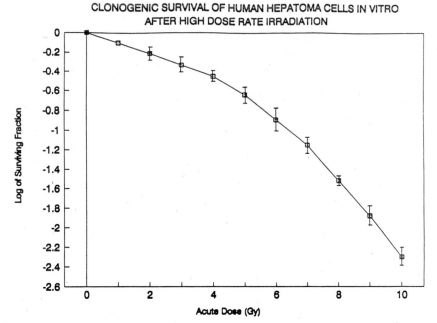

Figure 38.3. Typical mammalian dose response curve to irradiation in vitro (Courtesy of Dr. Jerry Williams, Professor of Radiobiology, Johns Hopkins Oncology Center, Baltimore, Maryland)

Table 38.3. Patient Dose Inhomogeneity and Dose Modified by Compensators for AP-PA TBI with 300 cGy Prescribed to Patient Midplane (see Fig. 38.4)

Site	Unmodified Dose (cGy)	Modified Dose (cGy)
Head	343	292
Neck	364	272
Shoulder	318	318
Mediastinum	289	289
Umbilicus	291	291
Hip	320	320
Thigh	318	318
Knee	395	330
Ankle	331	282

after interacting with some initial thickness of tissue. Depending on the energy of the x-ray beam, this thickness may range from a few millimeters to several centimeters), and the extent to which the x-ray beam is attenuated as it continues through the patient's body. To a certain extent, these factors can be modeled for purposes of dose calculation by precise consideration of treatment geometry and distances, utilizing pretreatment physical measurements of the uniformity of the emitted beam (beam profiles) and beam attenuation within tissue-equivalent material (water chambers or treatment "phantoms"), and measured patient separation at many different levels. In general, the simplest, most effective regimen is selected. However, calculations incorporating the physical characteristics of the patient and the treatment beam will show substantial dose inhomogeneity (8, 9).

For example, using a 4-mV linear accelerator operating at a distance of 360 cm from the midplane of the patient's umbilicus, one can find calculated dose variations in the range of 20–30%, with the greatest variability in the thinnest regions of the body, namely, head, neck, knees, and ankles (Fig. 38.3, Table 38.3).

This variation can be modified and reduced. "Tissue equivalent" rice bags can be placed around the neck to increase its effective thickness, compensating material made from sheets of lexan plastic can be interposed between the patient and the x-ray beam to reduce the dose in critical regions such as from the head to the shoulders or from the knees to toes (Fig. 38.4).

For critical structures such as the lungs or liver, anatomically selective blocking can be utilized (Fig. 38.5) to reduce risk of life-threatening damage, minimize the need for precise calculation of dose variation due to tissue inhomogeneity, and permit more extensive irradiation of other body sites. Depending on the specifics of the overall treatment plan, full-thickness blocks (which permit only about 3% transmission of the x-ray beam) or partial-thickness blocks (designed to attenuate the beam by precise partial amounts) may be used.

Because of the complexity of these factors and the potentially narrow dose window between desired therapeutic effect and unacceptable toxicity, measured dose verification during treatment is essential. In the setting of fractionated TBI, this can readily be accomplished using strategically placed thermoluminescent dosimeters (TLDs) or on-line diodes during the first treatment session.

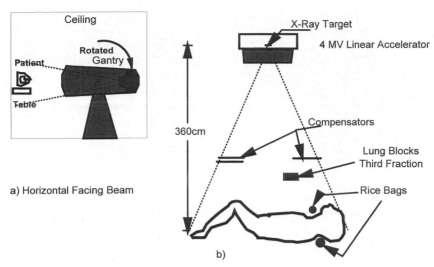

Figure 38.4. Patient setup from TBI as used at Johns Hopkins Oncology Center. Beam modified by rice bags and compensators made of lexan plates. Lung blocks are used on the third day of treatment.

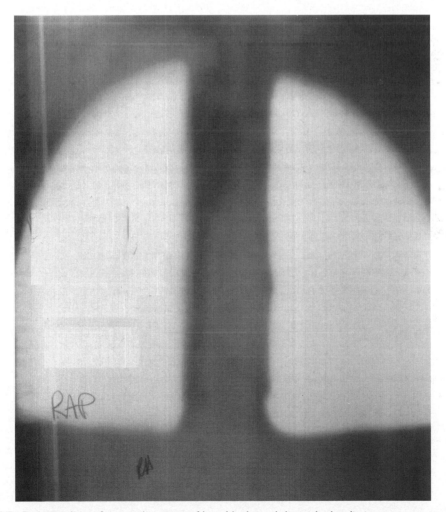

Figure 38.5. Radiograph confirming placement of lung blocks and diminished radiation exposure to lung regions due to lung blocking. Patient identification has been blocked out.

Radiobiologic and Therapeutic Considerations in the Use of TBI

Initially, TBI was selected for inclusion in the "Seattle preparative regimen" for patients with refractory acute leukemia because it was an effective cytocidal modality not normally utilized in the management of leukemia. It was effective in eradicating leukemic cells in chemotherapy sanctuary sites such as the CNS and testicle, and there was good basis in an animal (dog) model for anticipating that tolerable acute doses in the range of 1000 cGy would sufficiently eliminate recipient hematopoietic stem cells and lymphoid cells mediating marrow rejection to allow engraftment of transfused allogenic marrow cells (1, 10, 11). A lower dose of 500 cGy (single fraction) was found in animal models to be hematopoietically ablative but not sufficiently immunosuppressive (11). Initial efforts in man using TBI alone at the higher dose of 1000 cGy were associated with early relapse of leukemia, and cyclophosphamide was added to the conditioning regimen with improved results (11).

Because of the complexity of the bone marrow transplant experience it is difficult to identify effects specific to TBI alone. Beyond the desired effects of immunosuppression and spontaneously irreversible bone marrow ablation, TBI has been associated with variable degrees of nausea, diarrhea, mucositis, fever, and parotid gland swelling and tenderness within the first 7–11 days of its initiation. Based on irradiation outcomes outside the TBI/BMT context, TBI would be expected to contribute (in the subacute context) to the incidence of alopecia, interstitial pneumonitis, and hepatic veno-occlusive disease. The dosing regimen of the TBI can have profound impact on these toxicities, as can other factors such as extent and severity of graft versus host disease and the extent and nature of chemotherapy and radiotherapy prior to the bone marrow transplant experience. For example, when giving 750 cGy midplane dose at 26 cGy/min, Kim et al. (3) observed severe nausea or vomiting during irradiation sessions in 47% of patients, but when giving 1320 cGy in eight sessions (two per day over 4 continuous days; daily sessions separated by 4–6 hr) at 10 cGy/min, these authors observed severe nausea or vomiting in only 11% of patients ($P \le .001$).

Bearman et al. (12) made a major contribution to quantifying the importance of regimen-related toxicity and the factors contributing to it for patients receiving BMT for leukemia. Using a comprehensive scoring system for each organ system, they observed that survival probability was diminished with increasing regimen-related toxicity, that increasing the dose of TBI from 12 Gy in 6 fractions (1 fraction per day) to 15.75 Gy in 7 fractions (1 fraction per day) substantially increased the incidence of severe toxicity in liver (2.7% to 12.4%), kidney (1.4% to 6.6%), and mucosa (39.2% to 70.2%), with the overall incidence of life-threatening or fatal toxicity rising

from 8.1% to 19.8% ($P \le .028$). Other factors that correlated with severe toxicity were relapsed disease status, nature of graft versus host disease prophylaxis, and source of reconstituting marrow (none for autologous, 14.6% for matched allogeneic, 25.4% for mismatched allogeneic).

A similar analysis by the same group of 95 patients with lymphoma undergoing bone marrow transplant did not find increased toxicity with the higher dose of fractionated TBI (15.75 Gy vs. 12.0 Gy) or with the source of reconstituting marrow (13); however, severe toxicity could be correlated with lower initial performance status, prior mediastinal irradiation of 20 Gy or more, or the inclusion of cytosine arabinoside in the preparative regimen instead of or in addition to cyclophosphamide.

Interstitial pneumonitis and hepatic veno-occlusive disease deserve special comment. Both are formidable BMT complications that are frequently associated with fatal outcomes (14–18). Risk of interstitial pneumonitis has been shown to correlate with a number of irradiation-related variables including radiation dose, fractionation, and dose rate (14–18) in addition to non-radiation-related factors such as patient age, nature of graft versus host disease prophylaxis, duration between initial diagnosis of leukemia and bone marrow transplant, and pretransplant performance status. The overall risk of interstitial pneumonitis varies, depending on the number of risk factors present. Since roughly two-thirds of interstitial pneumonitis cases prove fatal, the importance of considering total dose, fractionation scheme, and dose rate is readily apparent.

The possible association of irradiation in producing hepatic veno-occlusive disease is less clear than the association with interstitial pneumonitis (17, 18). However, in nontransplant settings, radiation alone can produce hepatic veno-occlusive disease. Interestingly, workers at Johns Hopkins have found a strong association between the occurrence of hepatic veno-occlusive disease and interstitial pneumonitis (19).

With respect to the question of chemotherapy-based preparatory regimens that exclude TBI, a number of centers have examined various regimens in both autologous and allogenic settings (20–26). These regimens have been variably successful in eradicating acute leukemia or lymphoma. As is the case in radiation-based regimens, disease status prior to treatment and patient condition are major prognostic factors. Regimen-related toxicity is substantial with non-TBI regimens, and there is thus far no suggestion that these regimens are less toxic than TBI-based regimens, although in some cases, the organ pattern of toxicity may vary. Interstitial pneumonitis and hepatic veno-occlusive disease are seen with non-TBI-based regimens; more commonly in allogenic rather than autologous settings (just as with TBI-based regimens). At the Johns Hopkins Hospital (26), patients with relapsed Hodgkin's disease were found to have comparable rates of disease control and type and severity of regimen-related toxicity, independent of whether their conditioning regimen was busulfan-cyclophosphamide or cyclophosphamide-TBI. (Busulfan-cyclophosphamide regimen: busulfan 1 mg/kg orally q6h × 16 doses followed by cyclophosphamide 50 mg/kg i.v. daily for 4 days. Cyclophosphamide-TBI regimen: cyclophosphamide 50 mg/kg daily i.v. for 4 days followed by TBI 300 cGy daily for 4 days with lungs blocked on day 3 of the TBI. Dose rate of TBI 4–5 cGy/min.) Conditioning regimen assignment was based on extent of prior irradiation, with patients previously irradiated to 3000 cGy or more to the mediastinum receiving the busulfan-cyclophosphamide regimen.

The general rationale for fractionating treatment with radiation (giving more than one fraction per day) and modifying dose rate is based on an extensive body of preclinical and clinical radiobiologic study (27–29). In brief, as reviewed by Peters (30), and by Travis et al. (31) and discussed above, the dose-limiting organs for bone marrow transplant appear to be lung, gut, kidney, and liver for TBI-based regimens. The original use of single large fractions of TBI for patients with relapsed, refractory leukemia was based on the desire to compress the treatment regimen to the least amount of time possible, rather than specific radiobiologic considerations. The general shape of the curve resulting from a plot of in vitro cell survival versus increasing dose of irradiation reveals a relatively flat portion followed by a relative steep portion (Fig. 38.3). In general, curves of nonhematopoietic normal cells are believed to have broader shoulders than those of either malignant or nonmalignant hematopoietic cells. In addition nonhemopoietic normal cells are believed to have shallower slopes in the postshoulder region of their survival curves than hematopoietic cells. The shoulder region of the curve reflects a cell's ability to absorb radiation without lethality. If time is allowed for repair mechanisms to operate (e.g., 4–6 hr), this sublethal damage may be largely repaired and, with reirradiation, the shoulder region of the curve is repeated. In general, cells or cell lines showing large curve shoulders also show the most substantial sparing, with decreasing dose rates between 50 and 1 cGy/min (30). In treating hematologic neoplasms, these considerations suggest that (a) fractionated irradiation will produce less normal tissue toxicity without sacrificing antineoplastic effect, (b) that a substantial number of days can be saved by giving two (or more) fractions per day separated by *minimal* intervals of 4–6 hours, and (c) that reductions in dose rate will further enhance normal tissue tolerance, one hopes without sacrificing antineoplastic effect (Table 38.4).

These concepts as applied to the bone marrow transplant context should not be accepted without reservation. For example, Song et al. (32) pointed out in a critical review of available in vitro and animal data that the inability of hematopoietic cells to repair sublethal damage was probably relative rather than absolute, and more recently, Fitzgerald et al. have shown that expression of oncogenes *c-fms*, *v-abl*, or *c-raf* in a transfected hematopoietic murine cell line conveyed both increased radiation resistance and increased repair capability (33). Similarly, while the salutary effects of decreased dose rate and increasing fractionation on sparing late tissue effects in nonhematopoietic tissues have been confirmed in both murine and canine models (31, 34, 35), so also has the concern that hematopoietic and lymphatic cells would be partially spared by these dose rate and fraction modifications (36, 37). Clinically, workers in Genova have observed a suggested increase in relapse of AML and CML after TBI and allogeneic bone marrow transplant, if the TBI dose rate was less than 4 cGy/min (38).

Late Complications of Bone Marrow Transplant: Correlations with TBI

In non-TBI clinical contexts, radiation therapy is well known to produce complications that may require months or years to appear. When searched for, a number of late effects, potentially related to TBI, have been observed, including restrictive or obstructive lung disease, hypothyroidism, renal failure, retarded growth, infertility and induction of menopause, cataracts, and secondary neoplasms (39, 40). The occurrence of restrictive lung disease may be related more to the occurrence of interstitial pneumonitis than to TBI (39). Hypothyroidism has generally been subclinical, that is, asymptomatic elevations of TSH (39). Renal failure was predicted to be a risk based on animal results following TBI (41) and subsequently observed in the subacute posttransplant period (3–6 months) in pediatric patients whose conditioning regimen also included *cis*-platinum, a known nephrotoxic agent (40).

Strong correlations between TBI administration and effect have been observed with ovarian failure and cataract formation. Sanders et al. (42) reported that following cyclophosphamide alone, all of 27 patients under age 26 recovered ovarian function, compared with only 9 of 76 women who received cyclophosphamide and

Table 38.4. Effect of Dose Rate on Dose Required to Produce 50% Lethality (LD 50) for Hematopoietic Death (No Bone Marrow Rescue) and Nonhematopoietic Death (Syngeneic Bone Marrow Rescue) in BALB/C Mice following TBI

Dose Rate (cGy/min)	1.0	2.5	5	12	25
Approximate LD50: hematopoietic (Gy)	7.5	7.3	6.6	5.8	5.5
Approximate LD50: Nonhematopoietic (Gy)	19.6	16.6	11.8	10.9	9.1

Data from Travis EL, et al. Effect of dose rate on total body irradiation: lethality and pathologic findings. Radiother Oncol 1985;4:341.
Note that decreasing the dose rate from 25 cGy/min to 1 cGy/min results in more than doubling the dose required for nonhematopoietic lethality, while changing the dose for hematopoietic lethality relatively little.

TBI. Menopausal symptoms developed in 74% of women older than 25 at the time of TBI, and virtually all transplanted women showed menopausal levels of FSH and LH after cyclophosphamide and TBI, compared with only 35% after cyclophosphamide alone. With respect to cataracts, Deeg et al. (43), have found that BMT with single-dose TBI produces an 80% incidence of cataracts by 5 years, of which at least 60% are sufficiently severe to require surgical correction. In contrast, fractionated TBI produced an incidence of cataracts of only 18%, not different from the frequency seen in aplastic anemia patients transplanted without TBI, and of these 18% only about one-fifth (of the postfractionated TBI patients) have required surgical correction.

Finally, with respect to secondary cancers, Witherspoon et al. (44) observed 35 patients with this occurrence out of 2246 at risk (crude incidence, 1.6%). Of these 35, 32 had received TBI. The risk of developing a new malignancy was roughly 6- to 7-fold higher in the transplant population than in the general population. Risk was highest in the first posttransplant year (1.2 cases per 100 exposure years) and declined there after. The malignancies observed included non-Hodgkin's lymphoma, leukemia, and solid tumors. Risk factors in addition to TBI included acute graft versus host disease and the use of antithymocyte globulin or anti-CD3 monoclonal antibody.

Conclusions and Future Developments

TBI administered by external beam techniques has an established role in the clinical practice of bone marrow transplantation. Optimal utilization and results require precise attention to the same principles of physics and radiobiology that dominate radiation oncologic practice in other contexts. With respect to TBI, this requires careful attention to dosimetry, treatment planning, fractionation schedules, and dose rate.

A promising development in the systemic use of radiation has been the growth and development of radioimmunotherapy (45). This field promises to allow precise targeting of small clinical or subclinical foci of hematogenously disseminated malignancy by antibodies conjugated with therapeutic amounts of radionuclides. This approach may increase therapeutic efficacy while adding minimal toxicity. For example, based on previous work at our institution (46), we are now beginning to engage in this transplant approach for patients with refractory Hodgkin's disease by adding yttrium-90-conjugated polyclonal antiferritin to our standard non-TBI transplant regimen of busulfan and cyclophosphamide. Our hope is that this precisely targeted irradiation will permit continued use of full doses of busulfan and cyclophosphamide and result in enhanced therapeutic effect.

REFERENCES

1. Thomas ED, Storb R, Buckner CD. Total body irradiation in preparation for marrow engraftment. Transplant Proc 1976; 8:591.
2. Lutz WR, Dougan PW, Bjarngard BE. Design and characteristics of a facility for total body and large-field irradiation. Int J Radiat Oncol Biol Phys 1988;15:1035.
3. Kim TH, Khan FM, Galvin JM. A report of the work party: comparison of total body irradiation techniques for bone marrow transplantation. Int J Radiat Oncol Biol Phys 1980; 6:779.
4. Shank B. Techniques of magna-field irradiation. Int J Radiat Oncol Biol Phys 1983;9:1925.
5. Engler MJ. A practical approach to uniform total body photon irradiation. Int J Radiat Oncol Biol Phys 1986; 12:2033.
6. Lawton CA, et al. Technical modifications in hyperfractionated total body irradiation for T-lymphocyte depleted bone marrow transplant. Int J Radiat Oncol Biol Phys 1989; 17:319.
7. Breneman JC, et al. A technique for delivery of total body irradiation for bone marrow transplantation in adults and adolescents Int J Radiat Oncol Biol Phys 1990;18:1233.
8. Lam W-C, et al. The dosimetry of ^{60}Co total body irradiation. Int J Radiat Oncol Biol Phys 1979;5:905.
9. Lam W-C, Order SE, Thomas ED. Uniformity and standardization of single and opposing cobalt 60 sources for total body irradiation. Int J Radiat Oncol Biol Phys 1980;6:245.
10. Thomas ED. Total body irradiation regimens for marrow grafting. Int J Radiat Oncol Biol Phys 1990;19:1285.
11. Thomas ED, et al. Bone marrow transplantation (first of two parts). N Engl J Med 1975;292:832.
12. Bearman SI, et al. Regimen-related toxicity in patients undergoing bone marrow transplantation. J Clin Oncol 1988; 6:1562.
13. Bearman SI, et al. Regimen-related toxicity and early posttransplant survival in patients undergoing marrow transplantation for lymphoma. J Clin Oncol 1989;7:1288.
14. Bortin M, Kay HEM, Gale RP, Rimm AA. Factors associated with interstitial pneumonitis after bone marrow transplantation for acute leukemia. Lancet 1982;1:437.
15. Bortin MD, Gale RP, Kay HEM, Rimm AA. Bone marrow transplantation for acute myelogenous leukemia—factors associated with early mortality. JAMA 1983;249:1166.
16. Weiner RS, et al. Interstitial pneumonitis after bone marrow transplantation—assessment of risk factors. Ann Intern Med 1986;104:168.
17. Rollins BJ. Hepatic veno-occlusive disease. JAMA 1986; 81:297.
18. Jones RJ, et al. Veno-occlusive disease of the liver following bone marrow transplantation. Transplantation 1987; 44:778.
19. Wingard JR, et al. Association of hepatic veno-occlusive disease with interstitial pneumonitis in bone marrow transplant recipients. Bone Marrow Transplant 1989;4:685.
20. Ayash LJ, et al. Hepatic veno-occlusive disease in autologous bone marrow transplantation of solid tumors and lymphomas. J Clin Oncol 1990;8:1699.
21. Nevill TJ, et al. Regimen related toxicity of busulfan-cyclophosphamide conditioning regimen in 70 patients undergoing allogeneic bone marrow transplantation. J Clin Oncol 1991;9:1224.

22. Phillips GL, et al. Busulfan, cyclophosphamide, and melphalan conditioning for autologous bone marrow transplantation in hematologic malignancy. J Clin Oncol 1991;9:1880.

23. Lotz JP, et al. Phase I-II study of two consecutive courses of high dose epipodophyllotoxin, ifosfamide, and carboplatin with autologous bone marrow transplantation for treatment of adult patients with solid tumors. J Clin Oncol 1991;9:1860.

24. Jagannath S, et al. High dose cyclophosphamide, carmustine, and etoposide and autologous bone marrow transplantation for relapsed Hodgkin's disease. Ann Intern Med 1986; 104:163.

25. Copelan EA, Kapoor N, Berliner M, Tutschka PJ. Bone marrow transplantation without total body irradiation in patients aged 40 and older. Transplantation 1989;48:65.

26. Jones RJ, et al. High dose cytotoxic therapy and bone marrow transplantation for relapsed Hodgkin's disease. J Clin Oncol 1990;8:527.

27. Hall EJ. Time, dose and fractionation in radiotherapy. In: Hall EJ, ed. Radiobiology for the radiologist. 3rd ed. Philadelphia: JB Lippincott, 1988.

28. Hall EJ. Radiation damage and the dose-rate effect. In: Hall EJ, ed. Radiobiology for the radiologist. 3rd ed. Philadelphia: JB Lippincott, 1988.

29. Withers HR. Biologic basis of radiation therapy. In: Perez CA, Brady LW, eds. Principles and practice of radiation oncology. 2nd ed. Philadelphia: JB Lippincott, 1992.

30. Peters L. Discussion: the radiobiological basis of TBI. Int J Radiat Oncol Biol Phys 1980;6:785.

31. Travis EL, et al. Effect of dose rate on total body irradiation: lethality and pathologic findings. Radiother Oncol 1985; 4:341.

32. Song CW, et al. Radiobiologic basis of total body irradiation with different dose rate and fractionation: repair capacity of hemopoietic cells. Int J Radiat Oncol Biol Phys 1981; 7:1695.

33. Fitzgerald TJ, et al. The *v-abl, c-fms,* or *v-myc* oncogene induces gamma radiation resistance of hematopoietic progenitor cell line 32d CL 3 at clinical low dose rate. Int J Radiat Oncol Biol Phys 1991;21:1203.

34. Deeg HJ, et al. Single dose or fractionated total body irradiation and autologous marrow transplantation in dogs. Effects of exposure rate, fraction size, and fractionation interval on acute and delayed toxicity. Int J Radiat Oncol Biol Phys 1988; 15:647.

35. Tarbell NJ, et al. Fractionation and dose rate effects in mice: a model for bone marrow transplantation in man. Int J Radiat Oncol Biol Phys 1987;13:1065.

36. Salomon O, et al. Induction of donor-type chimerism in murine recipients of bone marrow allografts by different radiation regimens currently used in treatment of leukemia patients. Blood 1990;76:1872.

37. Storb R, et al. Comparison of fractionated to single-dose total body irradiation in conditioning canine littermates for DLA-identical marrow grafts. Blood 1989;74:1139.

38. Scarpati D, et al. Total body irradiation in acute myeloid leukemia and chronic myelogenous leukemia: influence of dose and dose rate on leukemia relapse. Int J Radiat Oncol Biol Phys 1989;17:547.

39. Deeg HJ, Storb R, Thomas ED. Bone marrow transplantation: a review of delayed complications. Br J Haematol 1984; 57:185.

40. Tarbell NJ, et al. Late onset of renal dysfunction in survivors of bone marrow transplantation. Int J Radiat Oncol Biol Phys 1988;15:99.

41. Moulder JE, Fish BL. Late toxicity of total body irradiation with bone marrow transplantation in a rate model. Int J Radiat Oncol Biol Phys 1989;16:1501.

42. Sanders JE, et al. Ovarian function following marrow transplantation for aplastic anemia or leukemia. J Clin Oncol 1988; 6:813.

43. Deeg HJ, et al. Cataracts after total body irradiation and marrow transplantation: a sparing effect of dose fractionation. Int J Radiat Oncol Biol Phys 1984;10:957.

44. Witherspoon RP, et al. Secondary cancers after bone marrow transplantation for leukemia or aplastic anemia. N Engl J Med 1989;321:784.

45. Order SE. Presidential address: systemic radiotherapy—the new frontier. Int J Radiat Oncol Biol Phys 1990;18:981.

46. Vriesendorp HM, et al. Phase I-II studies of yttrium labeled antiferritin treatment for end stage Hodgkin's disease, including Radiation Therapy Oncology Group 87-01. J Clin Oncol 1991;9:918.

EXERCISES AND TOOLS FOR CHEMOTHERAPY AND RADIATION THERAPY

Apoptosis is a way of life

1. In developing a therapeutic paradigm on the use of therapeutic radiation, note that:
   a. Ionization permanently destabilizes target molecules by releasing energetic electrons, which, in turn, produce short-lived free radicals that effect single and double strand breaks in DNA;
   b. Nucleoproteins are much more radiosensitive than cytosol proteins;
   c. The effects are dose dependent.
   Build into this paradigm the nature of DNA reparative mechanisms, differences between normal and malignant cells, dividing and nondividing cells, cells with or without oncogenes, and the development of resistance.
2. Develop a construct on the effects of radiation therapy on cytokines, enzymes, and specific cell protein activation. Conversely, examine the effects of cytokines, drugs, radiation sensitizers, and growth factors on ionizing radiation. Note the clinical correlations following these activities.
3. Review radiation doses and fractions in terms of efficacy and morbidity to target organs and systems. Pay particular attention to the skin.
4. Develop a construct that addresses short, medium, and long-term complications of radiation therapy and consider the complications of nausea, vomiting, mucositis, pneumonitis, veno-occlusive disease, cataracts, sterility, and secondary malignancies.
5. Note the differences in radiation delivered from cobalt sources, other radiation emitting isotopes, and linear accelerators. Relate these forms to specific tumor types. Use as an example the use of linear accelerators and radiolabeled P in the treatment of splenomegaly in various malignancies.
6. Consider the hazards of the various natural sources of radiation and their quantifiable features.
7. In constructing a working model for chemotherapeutic drugs, refer to the cell cycle in terms of therapeutic efficacy, the role of Go, and "checkpoints" in the cycle.
8. Given the likelihood that the potential for successful therapy with drugs is almost inexhaustible, develop a schema that shows how such therapy interferes with either protein synthesis or cell division (a process that includes separation and arrangement of chromosomes, spindle formation, and the creation of the new cell entities). Determine also how alterations in structure and cytoskeleton, growth characteristics, and anchorage (adhesion) can effect changes in the immediate environment, e.g., neoangiogenesis.
9. Develop a schema that distinguishes between upstream and downstream acting drugs (the site of action in the cell cycle). Use as clues the conclusion that DNA synthesis is upstream and the organization and separation of DNA is downstream.
10. Determine how drugs actually reach their intracellular sites of action: inwardly diffused, actively internalized; the control of drug resistance; the advantage of microsomal forms of drugs; efficacy of bolus versus slow release and therapeutic intervals.
11. Describe the pharmacokinetic value of multimodal, continuous therapy.
12. Develop a schema that encompasses drug dose and toxicity, the role of biological response modifiers, drugs as toxins, targeted therapy, and the mechanisms of secondary malignancies.
13. Develop an apoptosis therapeutic model using radiation therapy and drug therapy.

Bone Marrow Infusion and Transplantation

CHAPTER 39

HLA Testing

LEE ANN BAXTER-LOWE, JAMES T. CASPER

The first inkling of an HLA system appeared in 1936 with Peter Gorer's discoveries of antibodies to mouse H_2 antigens.
—British Medical Bulletin, 1936

Ten years ago, donors for bone marrow transplant recipients were essentially limited to HLA-matched siblings. Recently, the advent of the National Marrow Donor Program and other large international registries have allowed successful transplants when the donor is not a matched sibling. However, class I and class II HLA typing is now more critical because there is a high likelihood of HLA disparity between two unrelated individuals. The DNA technology now used has allowed more precise determination of HLA specificities and, for most transplant centers, has alleviated the need to perform mixed lymphocyte culture assays. However, as the technology continues to improve, more disparities between unrelated donors and recipients will be elucidated. The challenge for the future will be to determine which disparities can be overcome.

Case 1

J.C. is a 4-year-old white male diagnosed with acute lymphocytic leukemia (ALL) in May of 1991. He was considered to have standard risk features by Pediatric Oncology Group (POG) criteria, which include age of 3–6 years, WBC below 10,000, and DNA index above 1.16. He was initially treated with prednisone, vincristine, and L-asparaginase. On day 28, he attained a complete hematologic remission. However, the initial chromosomal studies revealed the presence of a Philadelphia chromosome (Ph+) in the lymphoblasts. Treatment of Ph+ ALL with present chemotherapy has been very disappointing (1). Therefore, the current recommendation at our institution and others has been to proceed with a bone marrow transplant when the patient is in a first complete remission (2).

Selection of a histocompatible donor has been a key factor in the success of bone marrow transplants. Early experience suggested that a sibling with identical human leukocyte antigens (HLA) was the only acceptable donor. Since an HLA-identical sibling is available for only about 30% of patients (3), considerable effort has been devoted to exploring the use of unrelated bone marrow donors who are closely HLA matched. These donors have recently been successfully utilized for patients such as J.C. who lack an HLA-identical sibling (4–7).

In this case, conventional serologic HLA typing was performed for J.C. and immediate family members to identify suitable donors within the family. HLA-A, -B, and -C typing (class I HLA) was successful for J.C., but HLA-DR and -DQ (class II HLA) typing failed, most likely because of his leukemia. Since the class I HLA typing revealed that J.C.'s sibling had different HLA-A and -B types, the only sibling was not a suitable donor. DNA-based HLA typing was used to determine J.C.'s HLA-DR and -DQ types. J.C.'s HLA types were then used to initiate a search for an unrelated marrow donor.

Comment: *What follows is an overview of the strategies currently available for selection of bone marrow donors and the means by which these strategies enable one to identify a donor.*

Selection of Donors for Bone Marrow Transplantation

Identifying an unrelated donor who is HLA matched can be difficult because there is extreme diversity of HLA in the population (8). Each individual expresses several polymorphic HLA proteins that are likely to be important in bone marrow transplantation. HLA molecules are peptide receptors that bind a variety of peptides and present them on the cell surface. T lymphocytes recognize these HLA-peptide complexes, and this recognition underlies immunologic discrimination between donor and host in bone marrow transplantation (9). HLA proteins are divided into two major categories, class I HLA (HLA-A, -B, -C) and class II HLA (HLA-DR, -DQ, and -DP). Class I HLA proteins consist of an HLA heavy chain that is noncovalently bound to β_2-microglobulin (10). Class II HLA proteins contain two HLA chains, designated α and β (11); the genes encoding the α and β chains are designated A and B (8). For example, an HLA-DR molecule consists of an α and a β chain that are encoded by loci designated HLA-DRA and HLA-DRB, respectively. The α and β chains of class II HLA proteins are polymorphic, with the most extensive polymorphism in the β chains. As a result, recent molecular HLA typing methods detect polymorphism in the B loci.

Several additional proteins may play a role in histocompatibility. For example, there are additional HLA-like genes (Fig. 39.1), but the exact role of the protein products has not yet been determined (12). Several other poly-

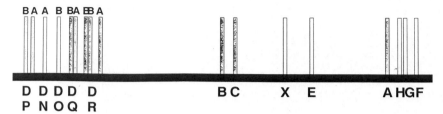

Figure 39.1. Map of HLA and HLA-like genes identified in the human major histocompatibility complex. Genes encoding proteins that are identified by routine HLA typing are shown as *solid* rectangles. Recently discovered HLA-like genes are *open rectangles*. Genes located between HLA-DQ and -DP (not shown) are involved in proteolytic generation and transport of peptides.

morphic proteins (e.g., proteins involved in proteolytic cleavage, peptide transporters, and HLA-DM) play a role in the assembly and loading of HLA molecules and may also affect histocompatibility (13). In addition, there are polymorphic proteins that can be recognized as peptides presented by HLA proteins, which are referred to as minor histocompatibility antigens (14). There is too little known about HLA-like proteins, proteins that affect HLA-expression, and minor histocompatibility antigens to delineate their importance in allogeneic transplantation. There is considerable evidence suggesting that HLA disparity is related to immunologic complications (4–7). Since genes encoding proteins associated with proteasomes, peptide transporters, and HLA-like molecules are located near the HLA genes in the major histocompatibility complex (MHC) (15), it is possible that matching for HLA-A, -B, -C, -DR, and -DQ alleles may result in matching of alleles of polymorphic genes located in the MHC.

HLA Typing

Conventional HLA typing uses alloantibodies whose binding is detected in complement-mediated cytotoxicity assays (15). This method detects HLA types or "specificities" that are designated by the World Health Organization (WHO) (8). Sometimes subtypes or "splits" of serologic specificities have been added when reagents become available to further subdivide a particular specificity (8, 15). For example, the HLA-DR2 specificity was resolved into two specificities, designated HLA-DR15 and HLA-DR16. Thus, an individual who is typed as HLA-DR2 is potentially HLA-DR matched with another individual who is typed as HLA-DR15.

Although serologic typing has been extremely useful, particularly in the transplant setting, other methods have shown that most of the serologic specificities encompass several different HLA molecules (8, 15). Thus the number of alleles for a particular locus is always greater than the number of serologically defined types. For example, there are 23 HLA-A serologic specificities and there were 59 HLA-A alleles known in June 1995, and for the common HLA specificity HLA-A2, there are at least 17 different alleles (8). The number of established HLA alleles continues to increase each month. Molecular HLA typing methods have been developed to resolve most, if not all, HLA alleles (15, 16). Further, there are several commercial products for molecular typing of HLA, -B, -DR, -DQ, and -DP,

and these typically provide greater resolution than conventional serologic typing.

Several cellular assays have been used to supplement HLA typing. One cellular test that was popular for many years is the mixed lymphocyte culture (MLC) (15, 17). This assay involves lymphocyte recognition of differences in the HLA molecules expressed on the cells of another individual (stimulator cells). Cells from one individual are treated with mitomycin C or x-irradiation to prevent cell division while allowing the HLA molecules on the cell surface to be recognized by lymphocytes from a second individual. If the lymphocytes recognize the HLA molecules of the stimulator cells as foreign, the cells proliferate, and this is usually the endpoint of the assays. Although the MLC was widely used for many years, its clinical use has recently diminished because many assays are not interpretable for technical reasons and the relationship to graft-versus-host disease (GVHD) remains controversial (17). These observations are probably not the result of a fundamental flaw in the method but rather an inability to control factors that can influence the MLC in clinical settings. For example, patients with chronic myelogenous leukemia (CML) have a very high "resting" background that makes it difficult to assess the response of donor cells, and cells from individuals with aplastic anemia often fail to stimulate in an MLC (17).

Another cellular method that has been used for HLA typing is a variation of the MLC that is often referred to as HLA-Dw typing (15). This technique takes advantage of a panel of homozygous testing cells or clones to serve as stimulator cells in an MLC. If the responder cell expresses the same determinant as the homozygous stimulator cell, it should not proliferate. These results are used to assign specificities (1 through 26) that begin with "Dw." The HLA-Dw specificities represent clusters of antigenic determinants predominantly attributable to HLA-DR, -DQ, and -DP. One example of the use of this typing is subdivision of the HLA-DR4 serologic specificity into five cellular specificities: Dw4, Dw10, Dw13, Dw14, and Dw15 (Table 39.1).

More recently, the frequency of donor-directed cytotoxic T lymphocyte precursors has been reported to be predictive of GVHD (18). This test is relatively new, and its clinical utility remains to be established by more extensive study.

In the past, most transplant programs used serologic HLA typing of HLA-A, -B, and -DR along with the MLC assay to evaluate potential bone marrow donors. Beyond this basic testing, the use of additional assays varied considerably and sometimes included serologic typing of HLA-C and -DQ as well as some cellular tests. However, a recent

Table 39.1. Typing Methods Provide Variable Levels of Resolution

Level of Resolution	Molecular Typing	Cellular Typing	Serological Typing
Low	DRB1-04	4	4
Intermediate	DRB1-0401	Dw4	N/A
	DRB1-0402	Dw10	
	DRB1-0403	Dw13	
	DRB1-0404	Dw14	
	DRB1-0405	Dw15	
High	DRB1-0401	N/A	N/A
	DRB1-0402		
	DRB1-0403		
	DRB1-0404		
	DRB1-0405		
	DRB1-0406		
	DRB1-0407		
	DRB1-0408		
	DRB1-0409		
	DRB1-0410		
	DRB1-0411		
	DRB1-0412		
	DRB1-0413		
	DRB1-0414		
	DRB1-0415		
	DRB1-0416		
	DRB1-0417		
	DRB1-0418		
	DRB1-0419		
	DRB1-0420		
	DRB1-0421		
	DRB1-0422		

proliferation of molecular approaches to HLA typing has resulted in dramatic changes in histocompatibility testing.

Several studies have shown that nucleic acid–based methods of HLA typing substantially improve accuracy, resolution, sensitivity, and success rate (19–21). These improvements are in part attributable to technical failure of about 10–30% for serologic typings. Specimens that are more than 1 day old or derived from patients are most often associated with technical problems, because factors such as low levels of HLA expression, insufficient numbers of normal viable lymphocytes, and medication can adversely affect the assays. Fortunately, most molecular biologic typing methods are not affected by these factors, and it is currently possible to obtain reliable class II HLA types using nucleic acid–based typing methods. Nucleic acid–based methods are not subject to another problem common to serologic methods—cross-reactivity of reagents. Because nucleic acid–based methods provide significant improvements in HLA typing, they are increasingly used in research and clinical settings (19).

One of the first molecular biologic methods used for HLA typing detected the presence of restriction fragment length polymorphism (RFLP) in the HLA genes (19). This method provided a means to type specimens that were difficult or impossible to type using serologic methods. In addition, several reports showed that RFLP typing was more accurate than serologic typing, including one large study that suggested that the assignment of 25% of HLA-DR serologic specificities was incorrect (20). Although RFLP typing provides certain improvements in HLA typing, most laboratories have replaced conventional RFLP typing with methods that use selective amplification of HLA genes.

HLA genes can be selectively amplified by use of the polymerase chain reaction (PCR), which provides sufficient quantities of material for a variety of molecular methods of HLA typing (15, 16, 21). The first amplification-based HLA typing method was oligotyping, which used PCR to selectively amplify targeted HLA genes followed by hybridization with a panel of oligonucleotide probes to detect key polymorphic sequences in the amplified products (15, 16, 21, 22). Other names for this method include SSOP, SSOPH, PCR-SSO, and oligonucleotide genotyping. Oligotyping methods have been reported for HLA-A, -B, -C, -DR, -DQ, and -DP. Commercial products for class II HLA oligotyping are currently available, and it is expected that class I HLA typing reagents will be commercially available in the near future.

Many other amplification-based methods have been reported; the most popular of these is PCR-sequence-specific primers (PCR-SSP), which uses the specificity of the PCR to determine HLA types (15, 16, 23). This method uses a different combination of primers to amplify each HLA type. The presence of a product for a particular primer mixture detects the presence of the HLA type. If no product is present, it is assumed that the type is not present. Approximately 125–150 primer mixtures are currently required for a low-resolution HLA-DR typing. The advantage of this method is that typing can be completed in less than 1 day. Disadvantages of PCR-SSP include practical issues related to achieving stringent thermal cycling of large numbers of tubes and limitations in use of internal controls. It is possible that the molecular methods described above will ultimately be supplanted by nucleotide sequencing.

The resolving power of individual molecular methods varies (Table 39.1). For example, the resolving power of oligotyping is determined by the specificity and number of amplification steps as well as the number and sequence of oligonucleotide probes included in the assay. Some oligotyping methods identify only 16 oligotypes that approximate the 16 HLA-DR serologic specificities. This is sometimes called "low-resolution" or "generic" oligotyping. The most comprehensive methods can assign types corresponding to all known alleles (e.g., the 137 HLA-DRB alleles currently recognized by the WHO) (8). Other oligotyping methods provide an intermediate level of resolution. The term "high resolution" is often used to describe any method that resolves more types than those identified by conventional serologic typing. There can be dramatic differences in the number of types identified by "high-resolution" methods. Table 39.1

illustrates different levels of resolution that have been used for HLA-DR4. Some typing methods that have been referred to as high resolution divide the HLA-DR4 type into five subtypes that can be correlated with the cellular specificities Dw4, Dw10, Dw13, Dw14, and Dw15. The most comprehensive methods for high-resolution oligotyping detect polymorphic sequences that differentiate all known alleles, provided that the sequences are publicly available. In the case of HLA-DR4, 22 alleles are currently recognized by the WHO, and sequences are available for all of these alleles. Many of the recently discovered alleles are generated by new combinations of known polymorphic sequences. In this case, existing typing reagents may detect a new allele without prior knowledge of the sequence. As additional HLA-DR4 alleles are discovered, typing methods must be modified to continue to detect and resolve all known alleles.

At the current time there is no official nomenclature for molecular typing methods. Since each laboratory establishes a local nomenclature system, it is sometimes incorrect to directly compare types assigned by two different laboratories. Most laboratories use nomenclature that is based upon the official WHO designation for alleles. The official nomenclature for alleles has a designation for the locus followed by a number containing four or more digits. The first two digits indicate similarity of the sequence to others with the serologic specificity with that number, and the next two numbers indicate the chronologic order of official recognition by the WHO Nomenclature Committee. For example, the first of the HLA-DR4 alleles was assigned the name HLA-DRB1*0401. The locus is HLA-DRB1, the serologic type is DR4, and it was the first HLA-DR4-associated allele. The "*" located between HLA-DRB1 and 0401 denotes that this is the name of an allele (unique nucleotide sequence). As stated above, 22 HLA-DR4 associated alleles have been recognized by the nomenclature committee, and the names range from HLA-DRB1*0401 to HLA-DRB1*0422. If another allele is recognized, it will receive the official name of HLA-DRB1*0423. A fifth number is used to distinguish alleles that encode an identical protein (silent mutations), and two additional numbers are used to name intron and flanking sequence polymorphism.

Low-resolution types assigned using DNA-based methods usually correspond to the first two numbers of the allele designation. For example, an HLA-DR4 type is assigned to this group of alleles (Table 39.1). If typing resolves all known HLA-DR4 alleles, the types are sometimes differentiated from allele designation by substituting a "-" for the "*" in the name. Thus, the HLA-DRB1-0401 type would be assigned to the HLA-DRB1*0401 allele (Table 39.1). Some nucleic acid–based methods provide an intermediate level of resolution. For example, a common intermediate-level oligotyping method assigns the same type to alleles HLA-DRB1*0403, 0406, 0407, 0411, 0417, and 0420. In this case, the oligotype HLA-DRB1–0403 is sometimes used to represent the group. Thus, some methods assign an oligo-

type of HLA-DRB1-0403 that corresponds to one allele, HLA-DRB1*0403, while others assign an oligotype of HLA-DRB1-0403 that corresponds to any one of a group of alleles, HLA-DRB1*0403, 0406, 0407, 0411, 0417, and 0420. One must be aware of these differences when using nucleic acid–based typing to evaluate potential donors.

Nomenclature of HLA alleles was initially based on the serologic specificities. This facilitates the correlation of types assigned by each method, but the correlation is not absolute. The serologic specificities of many recently discovered alleles are uncertain or blank. These alleles are classified with those that have the most similar sequences in certain key positions of the molecule. In routine practice, other inconsistencies exist because cross-reactivity of serologic reagents may contribute to assignment of a type that differs from that assigned using molecular methods. For example, certain antigens are often assigned HLA-DR11 by routine serologic typing, but the genetic sequence detected by nucleic acid–based methods is classified in the HLA*DR13 group. Therefore, it is important to use the same typing method for comparison of HLA types of donor-recipient pairs.

Highest-resolution HLA oligotyping currently provides the most detailed information, but the testing usually requires additional time and expense. Low-resolution oligotyping is usually adequate for typing family members or for an initial screening of many potential unrelated donors. High-resolution molecular typing is particularly useful for selecting the best-matched unrelated donor after several well-matched donors have been identified. One report suggests that high-resolution oligotyping is useful for donor selection because HLA-DR disparity detected using this method is associated with increased risk of GVHD (24).

Although HLA-C and HLA-DP molecular typing methods are currently available, the importance of matching these HLA products is not yet well established. One study describing HLA-DP typing of 129 patients and their donors suggests that HLA-DP disparity does not have a significant impact on the probability of developing grades II–IV acute GVHD (25). However, undetected HLA disparity at other loci may obscure the affect of HLA-DP. Additional studies using precise molecular methods of HLA typing are required to understand the relationship between HLA disparity and transplant outcome.

Future Directions

The initial experience with molecular methods for HLA typing has provided dramatic improvements in practical aspects of HLA typing such as improved accuracy, ability to type poor-quality samples, and more sensitive detection of HLA disparity. Perhaps the most important advance provided by molecular typing methods is the opportunity to compare different HLA alleles at the level of primary sequence. For example, a patient with an HLA-DRB1*1301 allele may lack matched donors, but there may be several potential donors with HLA-DR13 oligotypes. Comparison of the key polymorphic sequences for this group of alleles shows that one oligotype, HLA-DR-1302, is identical in primary sequence with the exception of a single amino acid difference, glycine or valine (15). Other HLA-DR13 oligotypes have more significant differences, with several disparate residues located at functionally important positions (11, 26). For example, HLA-DRB1-1101 (a member of a different serologic group) has three amino acid differences, while HLA-DRB1-1303 has six amino acid differences in functionally important positions (11, 26).

Sequencing of HLA genes has revealed other surprising relationships. For example, HLA-B12 is split into two serologic specificities, B44 and B45. Analysis of the sequences revealed that these alleles are quite different (27). Apparently, the serologic specificity is attributable to a single amino acid residue that is shared by B12 molecules. Analogous relationships have been demonstrated for other specificities. Since structurally and functionally diverse molecules have the same serologic specificity, a new nomenclature that better reflects the functionality of HLA molecules may be developed in the future. Research efforts are currently under way to identify HLA disparities that are strongly immunogenic compared with those that are nonimmunogenic. This may result in development of approaches that match highly immunogenic epitopes rather than the HLA types that are used today.

HLA typing methods have undergone a technologic explosion in recent years, but the evolution of HLA typing methods is not yet complete. Many laboratories are currently investigating the use of automated nucleotide sequencing for HLA typing (16). Anticipated improvements in automated sequencing technology may make sequencing of HLA genes the most cost-effective and rapid method of "HLA typing," while providing absolute information about the structure of each HLA molecule. These changes will provide a dramatic improvement in the ability to detect HLA disparity between two individuals and to use detailed information regarding the structure and function of HLA molecules to select the optimal donor for a patient who lacks an HLA-identical sibling.

Searching for an Unrelated Donor

Using the simplest classification of HLA types (serologic specificities shown in Table 39.2), the random distribution of types for HLA-A, -B, and DR would yield millions of combinations of HLA types. Fortunately, HLA types are not randomly distributed in the population. Certain types are linked together in a large number of individuals, and these linkages are characteristic of different racial and ethnic groups. This was clearly demonstrated in recent studies from the 11th International Histocompatibility Workshop (28), which estimated frequencies and linkage disequilibria for three-locus haplotypes (HLA-A, -B, and -DR) for several racial and ethnic groups (Table 39.3).

Table 39.2. Recognized HLA Specificities

A	B	C	D	DR	DQ	DP
A1	B5	Cw1	Dw1	DR1	DQ1	DPw1
A2	B7	Cw2	Dw2	DR103	DQ2	DPw2
A203	B703	Cw3	Dw3	DR2	DQ3	DPw3
A210	B8	Cw4	Dw4	DR3	DQ4	DPw4
A3	B12	Cw5	Dw5	DR4	DQ5(1)	DPw5
A9	B13	Cw6	Dw6	DR5	DQ6(1)	DPw6
A10	B14	Dw7	Dw7	DR6	DQ7(3)	
A11	B15	Dw8	Dw8	DR7	DQ8(3)	
A19	B16	Dw9(w3)	Dw9	DR8	DQ9(3)	
A23(9)	B17	Cw10(w3)	Dw10	DR9		
A24(9)	B18		Dw11(w7)	DR10		
A2403	B21		Dw12	DR11(5)		
A25(10)	B22		Dw13	DR12(5)		
A26(10)	B27		Dw14	DR13(6)		
A28	B35		Dw15	DR14(6)		
A29(19)	B37		Dw16	DR1403		
A30(19)	B38(16)		Dw17(w7)	DR1404		
A31(19)	B39(16)		Dw18(w6)	DR15(2)		
A32(19)	B3901		Dw19(w6)	DR16(2)		
A33(19)	B3902		Dw20	DR17(3)		
A34(10)	B40		Dw21	DR18(3)		
A36	B4005		Dw22			
A43	B41		Dw23	DR51		
A66(10)	B42					
A68(28)	B44(12)		Dw24	DR52		
A69(28)	B45(12)		Dw25			
A74(19)	B46		Dw26	DR53		
	B47					
	B48					
	B49(21)					
	B50(21)					
	B51(5)					
	B5102					
	B5103					
	B52(5)					
	B53					
	B54(22)					
	B55(22)					
	B56(22)					
	B57(17)					
	B58(17)					
	B59					
	B60(40)					
	B61(40)					
	B62(15)					
	B63(15)					
	B64(14)					
	B65(14)					
	B67					
	B70					
	B71(70)					
	B72(70)					
	B73					
	B75(15)					
	B76(15)					
	B77(15)					
	B7801					
	Bw4					
	Bw6					

If a patient has two haplotypes that are common, there is a high likelihood of locating a well-matched unrelated donor. For example, before large donor registries were available, it was calculated that a patient with common

Table 39.3. Haplotype Frequencies (HF) and Linkage Disequilibria (LD) for HLA-A, -B, and -DR Haplotypes[a]

Sample Population	HLA-A	HLA-B	HLA-DR	HF(%)	LD(%)	N
Brazilian	2	35	11	1.8	1.3	286
	2	44	7	1.7	1.4	
	1	8	3	1.5	1.5	
French	1	8	3	3.7	3.6	244
	29	44	7	2.3	2.2	
	3	7	15	2.1	2.0	
German	1	8	3	6.1	5.9	203
	3	7	4	2.2	2.0	
	2	44	11	1.7	1.3	
Greek	2	18	11	4.0	3.6	176
	2	51	11	2.8	1.8	
	1	8	3	2.2	2.2	
Italian	1	8	3	3.7	3.6	483
	2	51	11	2.3	1.7	
	3	35	11	2.2	1.6	
Japanese	24	52	15	8.2	7.5	893
	33	44	13	5.2	5.1	
	24	7	1	3.6	3.5	
Korean	33	44	13	4.5	4.3	235
	33	44	7	3.8	3.7	
	30	13	7	3.4	3.4	
North	30	42	8	1.6	1.5	312
American	36	53	11	1.3	1.2	
Negroid	3	53	8	1.1	1.0	
Spanish	29	44	7	3.5	3.2	192
	1	8	3	2.3	2.3	
	30	18	3	2.0	2.0	
Thais	2	46	9	4.7	4.3	238
	33	44	7	3.1	3.1	
	11	75	15	2.3	1.7	
U.S.A.	1	8	3	6.6	6.4	226
	2	7	15	1.8	1.6	
	2	44	4	1.5	1.1	

[a]Three most common haplotypes for sample populations ≥150 determined during the 11th International Histocompatibility Workshop (13).

types such as HLA-A1,3; B7,8; DR2,3 would have an 80% chance of finding a matched donor among 1000 unrelated individuals (3). A relatively rare HLA type, A1,24; B35,50;DR5,7 was predicted to have only a 40% chance of having a match among 100,000 potential donors. It is now conceivable to locate well-matched donors for such patients because the number of potential donors listed in registries throughout the world exceeds 2,000,000 individuals. *Bone Marrow Donors Worldwide*, 22nd edition (29), lists HLA-A and -B types of more than 2,000,000 volunteers, and HLA-DR types are available for more than 30% of these. A search of a registry to approximately 1,000,000 individual using the types HLA-A1,24;B35,50;DR5,7 (Fig. 39.2) revealed that many individuals are either HLA matched or have broad specificities, A9 or B21, corresponding to A24 or B50, respectively, or are subtypes of DR5, DR11. There are donors who are potentially matched for A, B, and DR antigens (Fig. 39.2). It is possible to estimate the likeli-

hood that donors without HLA-DR typing will be matched for HLA-DR5,7 by determining the proportion of HLA-A,B-matched individuals who are HLA-DR matched or mismatched. In this example, there are 17 HLA-A and -B matched donors with HLA-DR typing. Two of the 17 are potentially HLA-DR matched. Thus one would predict that about 12% of those donors without HLA-DR typing are likely to be HLA-DR matched at the level of serologic typing. If a matched donor is not available, it is sometimes beneficial to confirm the typing of closely matched donors who may have been incorrectly typed for one specificity. In this example, one might consider confirming the typing of individuals who are HLA-A23 or -B49.

Although the combined registries contain HLA types of more than 2,000,000 individuals, certain patients have rare combinations of HLA types, and an unrelated matched donor cannot be found. For these patients, the likelihood of locating a perfectly matched donor is very low (less than 1 in 2,000,000). For this reason, it is sometimes beneficial to perform HLA typing of the patient's extended family. This approach is best suited to patients who have one common haplotype and one rare haplotype. In this circumstance, the HLA types of family members related to the parent with the rare haplotype are determined with the hope that one of the relatives may have inherited the common haplotype along with the rare haplotype. If this alternative is not successful, one can consider transplantation using a partially matched family member or a mismatched unrelated donor. The risk of transplant-related morbidity and mortality increases along with HLA disparity between a recipient and donor (4–7, 30–34). If the best available donor is substantially mismatched, alternative treatments should be carefully considered before performing a high-risk transplant. Alternatively, recent transplant approaches developed for HLA-mismatched family members might be considered (35).

Studies involving the effect of donor-recipient HLA disparity on transplant outcome have focused on the HLA-A, -B, and -DR products because typing of these products has been routinely available. HLA disparity between donor and recipient has been associated with graft failure, GVHD, and poor reconstitution of immunity (4–7, 30–34). Clearly, HLA disparity has an adverse effect on transplant outcome, but transplants can be successful even with HLA disparity between marrow recipients and donors (4–7, 30–35). Considerable investigation is required to better understand this relationship. Until this information becomes available, a variety of tests can be used to select the donor who is most closely matched with the patient. Until recently, most unrelated donors were selected on the basis of serologic typing and MLC, often supplemented with additional tests including IEF, Dw typing, and other cellular assays. At our institution, the selection of donors is based upon serologic typing of HLA-A and B in conjunction with high-resolution oligotyping of HLA-DR and -DQ.

A	A	B	B	D	D	AUS	B	CH	CND	CS	DK	E	F	GB	GR1	GR2	H	IL	IRL	NL	NR	SLO	USA1	USA2	n	
1	9	21	35			·	·	·	1	·	·	·	6	1	·	·	·	1	·	·	·	·	1	·	8	♦
1	9	49	35			·	·	·	·	1	·	·	·	2	·	·	·	·	·	·	·	·	1	·		
1	9	50	35			·	·	1	·	·	·	·	·	·	·	·	·	·	·	·	·	·	1	·	1	♦
1	23	21	35			·	·	1	·	1	·	·	·	·	1	·	·	·	1	·	·	·	1	9	3	
1	23	49	35			·	1	·	·	·	2	·	·	·	1	·	·	1	·	1	·	·	5	·		
1	23	50	35			·	1	·	·	·	·	·	·	·	·	·	·	·	1	·	·	·	1	·		
1	24	21	35			·	2	·	·	1	·	4	·	1	1	·	·	5	·	·	·	·	9	5	1	♦
1	24	49	35			·	2	·	·	1	·	·	·	1	1	·	·	5	·	·	1	·	9	5		
1	24	50	35			·	1	·	·	1	·	·	·	·	·	·	·	·	·	·	1	·	9	1	13	♦
1	9	21	35	1	5	·	·	·	·	·	·	·	3	·	·	·	·	·	·	·	·	·	·	·		
1	9	21	35	1	8	·	·	·	·	·	·	·	1	·	·	·	·	·	·	·	·	·	·	·		
1	9	21	35	2	5	·	·	·	·	·	·	·	1	·	·	·	·	·	·	·	·	·	1	·		
1	24	50	35	2	7	·	·	·	·	·	·	·	·	·	·	·	·	·	·	·	·	·	1	·		
1	9	21	35	4	5	·	·	·	·	·	·	·	1	·	·	·	·	·	·	·	·	·	·	·		
1	9	49	35	4	11	·	·	·	·	·	·	·	·	1	·	·	·	·	·	·	·	·	·	·		
1	9	21	35	4	6	·	·	·	·	·	·	·	1	·	·	·	·	·	·	·	·	·	·	·		
1	9	21	35	4	7	·	·	·	·	·	·	·	1	·	·	·	·	·	·	·	·	·	·	·		
1	24	49	35	4	7	·	·	·	1	·	·	·	·	·	·	·	·	·	·	·	·	·	·	·		
1	9	21	35	5		·	·	·	·	·	·	·	2	·	·	·	·	·	·	·	·	·	1	·		
1	24	49	35	5		·	·	·	·	·	·	·	·	·	·	·	·	·	·	·	·	·	·	·		
1	24	49	35	11		·	·	·	·	·	·	·	·	·	1	·	·	·	·	·	·	·	1	·		
1	23	49	35	11	13	·	·	·	·	·	·	·	·	·	2	·	·	·	·	·	·	·	1	·		
1	24	49	35	5	6	·	·	·	·	·	·	·	·	·	·	·	·	·	·	·	·	·	·	·		
1	9	21	35	5	7	·	·	·	·	·	·	·	1	·	·	·	·	·	·	·	·	·	1	1		*
1	24	50	35	11	7	·	·	·	·	·	·	·	·	·	·	·	·	·	·	·	·	·	1	1		*
1	9	21	35	5	8	·	·	·	·	·	·	·	1	·	·	·	·	·	·	·	·	·	·	·		
1	9	21	35	6		·	·	·	·	·	·	·	1	·	·	·	·	·	·	·	·	·	·	·		
1	9	21	35	7		·	·	·	·	·	·	·	2	·	·	·	·	·	·	·	·	·	·	·		

Figure 39.2. Section of *Bone Marrow Donors Worldwide,* 9th edition, containing donors who are closely HLA matched to an patient with HLA-A1,24;B35,50,DR5,7. Abbreviations for donor registries are listed at the *top,* reported types are listed at the *left,* and the number of donors is shown in the grid. Some donors (*solid diamond*) have types that correspond to broad specificities detected in the patient sample (i.e., HLA-A24, HLA-B50, and HLA-DR11 are subtypes of HLA-A9, HLA-B21 and HLA-DR5, respectively). There are two donors who are potentially matched for HLA-A, -B, and -DR (*).

Serological Specificities   ## Oligotypes

	A	B	C	DR	DQ	DRB1	DRB3	DRB4	DRB5	DQB1
a	2	8	w7	17(52)	2	0301	0101			0201
b	25	18	-	4(53)	8	0401		0101		0302
c	3	7	w7	4(53)	8	0404		0101		0302
d	32	-	-	15	1	1501			0101	0602

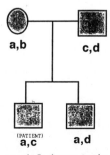

Figure 39.3. Family pedigree. The haplotypes (*a, b, c,* and *d*) shown in the *top* were determined by serologic typing and oligotyping of the parents and children. The pedigree of the patient's family is shown in the *bottom.*

Selection of an Unrelated Donor for J.C.

As mentioned in the initial clinical description, serologic HLA typing was performed to evaluate J.C.'s parents and sibling as potential donors (Fig. 39.3). There was no problem in identifying the HLA-A and B antigens, but the class II HLA specificities of the patient's specimen could not be determined, presumably the result of factors related to the patient's underlying leukemia.

This is not unusual and occurs in about 20–30% of all leukemia patient referrals.

Oligotyping was used to compare class II HLAs of family members. Unfortunately, the patient has only one

Table 39.4. Serological Typing and Oligotyping of Potential Unrelated Donors

	Serological Typing					Oligotyping			
	HLA-A	HLA-B	HLA-C	HLA-DR	HLA-DQ	HLA-DRB1	HLA-DRB3	HLA-DRB4	HLA-DQB1
Patient	2,3	7,8	-,-	-,-	-,-	0301,0404	0101	0101	0302
Donor 1	2,3	7,8	7,-	4,17	2,8	0303,0401	0101	0101	0302
Donor 2	1,2	7,8	7,-	4,17	2,8	0301,0404	0101	0101	0302
Donor 3	3,28	7,8	7,-	4.17	2,7	0301,0404	0101	0101	0301
Donor 4	1,2	7,8	-,-	4,17	2,8	0301,0401	0101	0101	0302
Donor 5	2,7	7,8	7,-	4,17	2,7	0301,0407	0101	0101	0301
Donor 6	1,2	7,8	7,-	4.17	2,7	0301,0401	0101	0101	0301
Donor 7	1,2	7,8	7,-	4,17	2,7	0301,0401	0101	0101	0301
Donor 8	1,2	7,8	7,-	4,17	2,8	0301,0401	0101	0101	0302

sibling who shares a single haplotype with the patient (Fig. 39.3). Although serologic typing suggested that the patient's mother is matched for the shared haplotype plus HLA-DR and -DQ, oligotyping revealed that the unshared haplotype was actually HLA-DR disparate as well (Fig. 39.3).

Since none of the immediate family members were HLA matched, a search for an unrelated donor was initiated. Eleven potential donors were identified, and samples were requested for further histocompatibility testing. Samples from eight of the potential donors were received between 2 and 10 weeks later. Serologic typing revealed one donor matched for all specificities and seven donors with a single HLA-A disparity (Table 39.4). MLCs were performed for five of the donors. Two patient samples were tested in the MLC, and both failed to stimulate or to respond to any of the samples, including HLA-disparate controls.

This circumstance is common for patients with leukemia or aplastic anemia.

High-resolution oligotyping detected HLA-DR disparity between the patient and seven of the unrelated donors (Table 39.4). The serologically matched donor proved to be HLA-DR disparate (Table 39.4, donor 1). One donor was HLA-DR and -DQ matched, but disparate for one HLA-A specificity (Table 39.4, donor 2). Since HLA-DR disparity has been associated with severe GVHD (24), donor 2 was selected for transplantation. This donor was requested through the National Marrow Donor Program, and the transplant was performed 5 months after the initial request for donor samples. The patient received pretransplant conditioning with cyclophosphamide, cytosine arabinoside, and total body irradiation as previously described (4). GVHD prophylaxis included in vitro T-cell depletion with a single monoclonal antibody (CD3) and cyclosporine, 3 mg/kg/day posttransplant. He attained a PMN above 500/mm³ on day 21 and maintained an untransfused platelet count above 25,000/mm³ on day 27. He developed mild GVHD of the skin (total grade I) on day 22, which responded very well to methylprednisolone. Currently, he is disease free more than 4 years posttransplant.

Summary

More than 150 unrelated-donor transplants have been carried out in pediatric patients in this and related centers. The results, which mimic those performed with matched siblings (33, 34), would not have been possible without advances in molecular-based HLA typing and the creation of the National Marrow Donor Program. As the technology for typing has advanced and the size of the donor file increased, the length of time to identify a donor has decreased to 2–3 months. The challenge for the immediate future is to further refine the selection of unrelated and/or mismatched donors, while the ultimate challenge is to overcome histocompatibility barriers.

REFERENCES

1. Fletcher JA, et al. Translocation (9;22) is associated with extremely poor prognosis in intensively treated children with acute lymphoblastic leukemia. Blood 1991;77:435.
2. Casper JT, et al. Bone marrow transplantation for Philadelphia chromosome positive (Ph+) acute lymphocytic leukemia (ALL) using alternative donors. Blood 1992;80(Suppl 1):249a.
3. Beatty PG, et al. Probability of finding HLA-matched unrelated marrow donors. Transplantation 1988;45:714.
4. Ash RC, et al. Successful allogeneic marrow transplantation from closely HLA-matched unrelated donors using T-cell depletion. N Engl J Med 1991;322:485.
5. Camitta B, et al. Bone marrow transplantation for children with severe aplastic anemia: use of donors other than HLA-identical siblings. Blood 1989;74:1852.
6. Beatty PG, et al. Marrow transplantation from HLA-matched unrelated donors for treatment of hematologic malignancies. Transplantation 1991;51:443.
7. Kernan N, et al. Analysis of 462 transplantations from 462 unrelated donors facilitated by the National Marrow Donor Program. N Engl J Med 1993;328:593.
8. Bodmer JG, et al. Nomenclature for factors of the HLA system, 1991. Hum Immunol 1995;43:149.
9. Sherman L, Chattopadhyay S. The molecular basis of allorecognition. Annu Rev Immunol 1995;11:385.
10. Bjorkman PJ, et al. Structure of the human class I histocompatibility antigen. HLA-A2. Nature 1987;329:506.
11. Brown JH, et al. Three-dimensional structure of the human class II histocompatibility antigen HLA-DR1. Nature 1993;364:33.

12. Campbell RD, Trowsdale J. Map of the human MHC. Immunol Today 1993;14:349–352.
13. Monaco J. Pathways for the processing and presentation of antigens to T cells. J Leukocyte Biol 1995;57:543.
14. Goulmy E, et al. The role of minor histocompatibility antigens in GVHD and rejection: a mini-review. Bone Marrow Transplant 1991;7:49.
15. Dyer P, Middleton D. Histocompatibility testing: a practical approach. Oxford: Oxford University Press, 1993.
16. Baxter-Lowe LA. Molecular techniques for typing unrelated marrow donors: potential impact of molecular typing disparity on donor selection. Bone Marrow Transplant 1994; 14(Suppl 4):S42–50.
17. Mickelson EM, et al. Role of the mixed lymphocyte culture reaction in predicting acute graft-versus-host disease after marrow transplants from haploidentical and unrelated donors. Transplant Proc 1993;25:1239.
18. Spencer A, et al. Cytotoxic T lymphocyte precursor frequency analyses in bone marrow transplantation with volunteer unrelated donors. Value in donor selection. Transplantation 1995;59:1302.
19. Noreen HJ, et al. HLA class II typing by restriction fragment length polymorphism (RFLP) in unrelated bone marrow transplant patients. Transplant Proc 1989;21:2968.
20. Opelz G, et al. Survival of DNA HLA-DR typed and matched cadaver kidney transplants. Lancet 1991;338:461.
21. Ng J, et al. The accuracy, specificity and reliability of large-scale oligonucleotide typing for HLA-DR and HLA-DQ. Tissue Antigens 1993;42:473.
22. Baxter-Lowe LA, Hunter JB, Casper JT, Gorski J. HLA gene amplification and hybridization analysis of polymorphism: HLA matching for bone marrow transplantation of a patient with HLA-deficient SCID. J Clin Invest 1989;613.
23. Olerup O, Zetterquist H. HLA-DR typing by PCR amplification with sequence-specific primers (PCR-SSP) in 2 hours: an alternative to serological DR typing in clinical practice including donor-recipient matching in cadaveric transplantation. Tissue Antigens 1992;39:225.
24. Petersdorf E, et al. The significance of HLA-DRB1 matching on clinical outcome after HLA-S, -B, DR identical unrelated donor marrow transplantation. Blood 1995; 86:1606.
25. Petersdorf EW, et al. The role of HLA-DPB1 disparity in the development of acute graft-versus-host disease following unrelated donor marrow transplantation. Blood 1993;81:1923.
26. Marsh SGE, Bodmer JG. HLA class II nucleotide sequences. Tissue Antigens 1995;46:258.
27. Hildebrand W, et al. Serologic cross-reactivities poorly reflect allelic relationships in the HLA-B12 and HLA-B21 groups. Doninant epitopes of the alpha 2 helix. J Immunol 1992; 149:3563.
28. Tsuji K, Aizawa M, Sasazuki T, eds. HLA 1991. Oxford: Oxford University Press, 1992.
29. van Rood JJ, ed. Bone marrow donors worldwide. Compiled by the editorial board. 22nd ed. 1991.
30. Atkinson K, et al. Analysis of late infections after human bone marrow transplantation: role of genotypic nonidentity between marrow donor and recipient and of nonspecific suppressor cells in patients with chronic graft-versus-host disease. Blood 1982;60:714.
31. Anasetti C, et al. Effect of HLA compatibility on engraftment of bone marrow transplants in patients with leukemia or lymphoma. N Engl J Med 1989;320:197.
32. Anasetti C, et al. Effect of HLA incompatibility on graft-versus-host disease, relapse, and survival after marrow transplantation for patients with leukemia or lymphoma. Hum Immunol 1990;29:79.
33. Weisdorf D, et al. Treatment of moderate/severe acute graft-versus-host disease after allogeneic bone marrow transplantation: an analysis of clinical risk features and outcome. Blood 1990;75:1024.
34. Casper J, Truitt R, Baxter-Lowe L, Ash R. Bone marrow transplantation for severe aplastic anemia in children. Am J Pediatr Hematol/Oncol 1990;12:434.
35. Henslee-Downey PJ, Parrish R, MacDonald JS, Romand EH et al. Combined in vitro and in vivo T lymphocyte depletion for the control of graft-versus-host disease following haplidentical marrow transplant. Transplantation, 1996;61:738.
36. Casper J, et al. Unrelated donors for bone marrow transplantation in children. Keystone symposia. J Cell Biochem 1993;16(Suppl):208 (#503).

CHAPTER 40

Autologous Reinfusion

KAREL A. DICKE

My students are dismayed when I say to them, "Half of what you are taught as medical students will in ten years have been shown to be wrong, and the trouble is, none of your teachers knows which half."

In this chapter, the role of autologous bone marrow transplantation (auto-BMT) is discussed in acute myelogenous leukemia (AML) and in acute lymphocytic leukemia (ALL). Since AML and ALL are two distinctly different diseases, this chapter is subdivided into the following sections: "Case Reports," "Introduction to Bone Marrow Transplantation," "Results of Auto-BMT in AML," and "Results of Auto-BMT in ALL."

Case Reports

Case 1

A 52-year-old white male visited his family physician because of fatigue and several nosebleeds. A blood count revealed a white cell count of 50×10^9/L, a red cell count of 2.3×10^{12}/L, hemoglobin of 79 g/L, and a platelet count of 12×10^9/L. The differential count was 90% immature cells, 7% lymphocytes, and 2% eosinophils. Acute leukemia was suspected, and the patient was referred to a hematolo-gist who did a marrow aspiration and biopsy, which confirmed the high percentage of blast cells (90%with lack of differentiation into mature myeloid elements), lack of red cell precursors, and lack of megakaryocytes. Auer rods were noted in some of the blast cells. The biopsy revealed a cellularity of 80%. His-tological staining was peroxidase positive, periodic acid–Schiff (PAS) negative, and esterase negative. The immunophenotypes of the blast cells by flow cytometry revealed 80% CD33+, 70% DR+, 85% CD45+, less than 5% CD4+, less than 5% CD8+, less than 5% CD3+, and less than 5% CD19+. The chromosome analysis revealed a diploid karyotype. A diagnosis of acute myeloblastic leukemia M2 was made. The patient was treated for induction of remission with a combination of cytarabine arabinoside (Ara-C), 100 mg/m²/day by continuous infusion for 7 days, and idarubicin, 12 mg/m² intravenously over 2 hours on days 1, 2, and 3. Prophylactic antibiotics were started immediately and consisted of vancomycin (1 g i.v. q12h), ciprofloxacin (750 mg p.o. q12h), Diflucan (100 mg p.o. q24h), and amphotericin (20 mg i.v. q.o.d.). No in-fectious complications occurred. The patient received allopurinol (100 mg t.i.d.) to avoid uric acid toxicity. Uric acid levels rose from 4.5 to 20 mg/100 mL during induction treatment. The patient was transfused with platelets and packed red cells to maintain his platelets over 20×10^9/L and hemoglobin over 80 g/L.

Within the first 10 days, the blast cells disappeared from the peripheral blood. A bone marrow aspiration on day 14 after starting treatment revealed an empty marrow; the biopsy revealed less than 5% cellularity. A bone marrow aspiration 3 days later showed red blood cell precursors and a single myelocyte. A subsequent marrow on day 20 revealed 40% RBC precursors, 10% myeloblasts, 15% myelocytes, and 15% mature myeloid cells. The WBC count in the peripheral blood was less than 0.2×10^9/L on day 14 and rose to 3×10^9/L on day 21, with 50% neutrophils, 10% monocytes, 25% lymphocytes, 5% eosinophils, 3% basophils, and 7% (normal?) blasts. The platelet count increased to 200×10^9/L, and the hemoglobin stabilized at 101 g/L. Electrolytes and chemistry profile, including BUN/creatinine, remained unremarkable throughout the induction treatment. There was a transient increase in uric acid during the first week, as noted.

Within 3 weeks of starting chemotherapy, the patient achieved complete remission after one course of induction therapy. Ten days later, remission intensification treatment, consisting of Ara-C (100 mg/m² continuous infusion over 7 days) and mitoxantrone (12 mg/m² i.v. on days 1, 2, and 3), was started. The neutropenic phase lasted 5 days, and prophylactic antibiotics, similar to those used during induction, were administered intravenously. Full hematopoietic recovery was achieved after 24 days. A second intensification course was started a week later with the use of 18 g of Ara-C (3 g over 2 hr q12h for six doses) in combination with mitoxantrone (12 mg on days 1, 2, and 3). Granulocyte colony-stimulating factor (G-CSF) was started on day 8 after initiation of chemotherapy, to reduce the neutropenic phase. Full WBC recovery was obtained on day 19, and platelet recovery (over 150×10^9/L) on day 24.

The patient consulted our clinic regarding auto-BMT. In addition, two other treatment modalities, continuation of "conventional-dose" chemotherapy and allogeneic bone marrow transplantation (allo-BMT) preceded by cyclophosphamide (60 mg/kg × 2), VP-16 (1800 mg/m²), and total body irradiation (TBI) (1200 rads in 6 fractionated doses) were discussed. After explaining that there is a trend toward better disease-free survival (DFS) after auto-BMT than with conventional chemotherapy and that the treatment-related mortality of allo-BMT is 20–30% versus less than 5% with auto-BMT, the patient opted for auto-BMT, even though he had an HLA-identical brother. The bone marrow was harvested shortly after remission intensification ("in vivo" purge)—a time when residual disease would be minimal. After marrow harvest, the patient was treated with one additional course of high-dose Ara-C and mitoxantrone, followed 4 weeks later with CBV and auto-BMT. The CBV program consisted of cytoxan (6 g/m²), BCNU (300 mg/m²), and VP-16 (600 mg/m²). Marrow was infused 2 days after the last dose of cytoxan.

Hematopoietic recovery was relatively slow; on day 30, the neutrophils were 0.5 × 10⁹/L, and on day 40, the platelets increased to 50 × 10⁹/L. Prophylactic antibiotics were administered, and the patient experienced no infectious complications during the posttransplant period. The patient is 2.5 years posttransplant and 3 years after onset of first complete remission (CR1). His chances for a 5-year DFS are greater than 80%.

Case 2

A 30-year-old black female visited her physician because of a persistent cough and fatigue. The cough continued even after 10 days of antibiotic treatment, and a chest x-ray revealed an enlarged mediastinum. A CT scan of the chest revealed several enlarged lymph nodes in the mediastinum. Peripheral blood examination showed a WBC count of 80 × 10⁹/L, predominantly immature lymphoid cells; a platelet count of 90 × 10⁹/L, and a hemoglobin of 95 g/L. A bone marrow aspiration showed 80% blast cells that were PAS stain positive, peroxidase negative, and esterase negative. Immunophenotyping revealed that the bone marrow cells were CD3+, CD4+, CD8+, CD45+ in 90% of the cells, CD33+ in 25% of the cells, and CD34−.

The diagnosis of T-cell ALL was made, and induction chemotherapy was initiated. The patient was treated with VAD: vincristine (2 mg/m² i.v. [total dose not to exceed 2 mg] as a continuous infusion over 4 days), Adriamycin (50 mg/m² i.v. continuous infusion over 3 days), and dexamethasone (40 mg/m² intravenously for 4 days and on days 8–12 and 16–20). Allopurinol (100 mg t.i.d.) was administered to minimize excessive increase in serum uric acid. Blast cells disappeared from the peripheral blood within 10 days. On day 18, the bone marrow showed return of myeloid, erythroid, and megakaryocytic elements, but there were persistent abnormal cells. It was decided to treat the patient with an

additional course of VAD to which was added 1 g/m² of Cytoxan (C-VAD).

Hematologic complete remission was achieved 25 days after the second course. The total duration of remission induction lasted 45 days. Lymph node enlargement disappeared in the mediastinum. It was decided to start remission consolidation treatment consisting of 5 courses of methotrexate (120 mg/m²) followed 24 hours later by L-asparaginase (15,000 U/m²) with a 10-day interval between the five courses. This was followed by one course of Ara-C (18 g total divided over six doses of 3 g/m²) and mitoxantrone (12 mg/m²). The last course was given because some of the ALL blast cells appeared to be CD33+ and thus had B-lineage features (lymphoid as well as myeloid). During the consolidation treatment, 100 mg of Ara-C was administered intrathecally once a week for 4 weeks. Also during consolidation, the patient received 3000 rads of x-radiation to the mediastinum.

After finishing consolidation therapy, the patient was referred to our center for consideration for autologous marrow transplantation; she had no HLA-identical siblings. She was presented with the options of either intensifying remission with cyclophosphamide, TBI, and autologous marrow rescue followed by maintenance chemotherapy or continuing the same maintenance program without BMT. She opted for the latter but requested that her bone marrow be harvested and stored. She was treated with C-VAD followed by the methotrexate/L-asparaginase program as mentioned earlier and afterward by another course of Ara-C and mitoxantrone. After that, she received a maintenance program of methotrexate (20 mg/m² weekly) and 6-mercaptopurine (150 mg p.o. daily for 9 months).

Relapse in the bone marrow occurred 6 months after she finished chemotherapy; the total duration of her CR1 was 21 months. She achieved second remission after four weekly courses of methotrexate (120 mg/m²) and L-asparaginase (15,000 U/m²) and was again referred to our unit for evaluation of auto-BMT. This time she received cyclophosphamide (120 mg/kg) and TBI (1200 rads, 200 rads b.i.d. for 3 days) followed by infusion of her own stored marrow. She received G-CSF from day 1 after BMT to day 16. On day 21, her neutrophil count was over 1.5 × 10⁹/L, and platelets were 33 × 10⁹/L. Full platelet recovery, over 100 × 10⁹/L, was achieved by day 35. She is still in complete remission 24 months after transplant. The second remission has exceeded the first remission, which is a change in the usual treatment course of the disease.

Autologus Bone Marrow Transplantation

The cellular components of blood comprise several specified cell types. These include erythrocytes, involved in oxygen transport, platelets that initiate clotting, and white blood cells (lymphocytes, granulocytes, basophils, eosinophils, and monocytes) that are involved in immune and inflammatory responses. The mature blood cells develop from pluripotent stem cells capable of reconstituting the entire blood cell system. These cells are found in embryonic yolk sac, fetal liver, and adult marrow. These cells are also recognized in the peripheral blood in quantities of about 10–20% less than in the marrow. The functionally specialized mature cells are generally short-lived and are constantly replaced. For example, approximately 1–2 million erythrocytes and 0.5 million white cells are replaced per second in the steady state, and these rates are increased after bleeding and during an inflammatory or immune response. This process is called hematopoiesis, and it is maintained by the hematopoietic stem cells (HSCs). The frequency of the HSC population in the bone marrow is 0.05–0.1%.

Most of the current knowledge on hematopoiesis and the practice of BMT originates from the observations of Jacobson et al. (1, 2) and Lorenz et al. (3) showing that spleen and bone marrow cell suspensions, respectively, protect lethally irradiated animals against death. Both groups originally ascribed their findings to a humoral factor capable of stimulating the regeneration of blood-forming tissue. It took more than 5 years to reject this hypothesis. Three groups, using four different procedures, independently demonstrated the protective effect due to replacement of the host's hematopoietic system by donor-type cells (4–6). Although these findings were basic to the notion of HSCs, identification of the effective cell type was not immediately successful (7). In retrospect, Till and McCulloch (8) showed, another 5 years later, that only a small proportion of the injected bone marrow cells effectively contribute to the repopulation of the spleen of an irradiated host. They observed a small number of macroscopically visible colonies, composed of proliferating hematopoietic cells, in the spleen of lethally irradiated mice that had been injected with isogeneic bone marrow. The link between these spleen colonies and the protective effect of bone marrow suspensions was established in 1963, when Trentin and Fahlberg (9) demonstrated the development of a complete hematopoietic system out of the progeny of a single spleen colony. The clonal nature of the spleen colonies and the occurrence of colony-derived lymphoid cells was further demonstrated in studies employing chromosomal markers (10, 11). Irrevocable evidence for the inclusion of lymphoid cells in the progeny of a single spleen colony was obtained by Nowell et al. (12) in 1970. Thus, the cells that give rise to spleen colonies fulfill the requirements of pluripotentiality and extensive self-renewal and can therefore, by definition, be considered pluripotent HSCs. However, the notion that all spleen colonies are derived from pluripotent stem cells has recently been challenged (13, 14).

The production of blood cells in the normal mammalian organism is tightly controlled; the peripheral numbers fluctuate only slightly despite the large daily replacement. First evidence for a humoral control mechanism of hematopoiesis dates back to 1906. A few years after

Bayliss and Starling (15) had given their definition of a hormone, Carnot and Deflandre (16, 17) observed that injection of the serum of bled rabbits rapidly increased the number of blood corpuscles in a normal rabbit. After 50 years, this observation was confirmed by several independent studies (18–22); again, Jacobson's group (23) was among the first to provide conclusive evidence. The plasma factor that increased erythropoiesis had been termed "hemopoietine" by Carnot and Deflandre. However, when it appeared to be involved exclusively in red cell production, the name erythropoietin (24) was rapidly adopted. Erythropoietin was first isolated and identified as a glycoprotein in 1961 (25); it was not purified until 1977 (26).

In the last 25 years, there has been a rapid advance in the techniques required to grow hematopoietic cells as clones in semisolid or viscous cultures and in the knowledge of specific regulatory molecules similar to erythropoietin that are required for their proliferation and maturation. After the initial description of hematopoietic colonies composed of neutrophilic granulocytes and macrophages in agar (27, 28), other systems have been developed for progenitor cells of erythrocytes (29, 30), eosinophils (31), and megakaryocytes (32, 33) and for colonies composed of lymphocytes (34, 35). The bone marrow cells that give rise to colonies in culture are mostly restricted in their proliferation and differentiation capacity, whereas their physical properties are, with a few exceptions, distinct from those of pluripotential stem cells detected by the spleen colony assay. These differences have been strongly emphasized in the past 10 years. It is, however, not justified to conclude that pluripotential stem cells cannot form colonies in vitro or that some early pathway-restricted progenitor cells do not have the capacity to form a macroscopically visible spleen colony.

The process of hematopoiesis is, in part, regulated by a family of glycoproteins called colony-stimulating factors (CSFs). Erythropoietin belongs to that family. In the last several years, it has been shown that these "hematopoietic growth factors" are involved in regulating the survival, proliferation, and differentiation of hematopoietic progenitor cells in vivo as well as in vitro. The classical CSFs are G-CSF and M-CSF (CSF-1), which are relatively specific for end-stage progenitors of the granulocytic and monocytic lineages, respectively, and GM-CSF and interleukin-3 (IL-3), which are capable of acting on earlier progenitors to produce cells of not only granulocytic and monocytic lineages, but also eosinophils, megakarayocytes, mast cells, and erythroid cells under the right conditions (36, 37). More recently, the picture of growth-factor control of hematopoiesis has become increasingly complex, with demonstrations that several other polypeptide factors are capable of acting on hematopoietic precursors (38–41).

In man, bone marrow cells are collected by multiple aspiration from the posterior iliac crest of the pelvis. After removal of bone particles from the harvested cells, the cells are infused intravenously. After infusion, marrow cells circulate and within 24 hours home into the bone marrow cavity, provided that it is empty. Space in the marrow cavity is obtained by myeloblative chemotherapy with or without TBI. As in the rodent (mouse and rat) and also in the primate (man and monkey), the population in the marrow transplant that is responsible for hematopoietic recovery is the pluriopotent HSCs. Usually the first neutrophils and red cell precursors are visible within 2 weeks after marrow infusion. Full recovery to normal numbers of neutrophils, lymphocytes, and monocytes is within 2–3 weeks; platelets recover 1 week later. The use of hematopoietic growth factors after transplantation has markedly reduced the time to full hematopoietic recovery (42, 43). Recently, peripheral blood has been used to a source of HSC. Körbling et al. (44) and Kessinger et al. (45) used peripheral blood mononuclear cell suspensions for protection against myeloablative chemotherapy. The number of HSCs in steady state peripheral blood is a factor of 10–20 lower than that in the bone marrow, so more mononuclear cells are needed for transplantation. This picture has changed with pretreatment with hematopoietic growth factors that mobilize stem cells into the peripheral blood, increasing the circulating number of stem cells to values equivalent to that in the bone marrow. Insufficient information was available about the stability of engraftment, but recently obtained results were very promising in this respect (46).

BMT can be considered a special form of tissue transplantation. Four different types of grafts can be distinguished according to the immunogenetic relation between the host and the donor: (a) autologous bone marrow grafts: the marrow to be grafted is taken from the same individual; (b) isogeneic transplantation: host and donor are genetically identical; in this case, the marrow is derived either from an identical twin (in humans) or from an animal of the same inbred strain (e.g., in mice); (c) allogeneic bone marrow grafts: host and donor are genetically different but still belong to the same species; and (d) xenogeneic transplantation: donor and recipient belong to different species.

Acute Myelogenous Leukemia

Leukemic cell kill follows first order kinetics, as has been described by Skipper (47). The higher the dose of chemotherapy, the higher the fraction of cells killed, independent of the total number of tumor cells. These findings in experimental leukemia models form the basis of high-dose therapy in leukemia. Thomas et al. started treating leukemia patients on a large scale with a combination of cyclophosphamide and TBI, in conjunction with bone marrow cells from histocompatible sibling donors (48). Results of this approach are described in chapter 41. Limited availability of identical sibling donors (only in 25–30% of patients) and the morbidity of graft-versus-host disease (GVHD) prompted several groups to explore the use of

autologous marrow for reconstitution of hematopoiesis after high-dose cytoreduction (49, 50). A major consideration against the use of the patient's own bone marrow is the probability of contamination by residual leukemic cells, even though the marrow is harvested during the remission phase. Within 6 months after achieving remission, the number of leukemic cells in the marrow is estimated to be between 10^6 and 10^8 cells. If one assumes a homogenous distribution of leukemic cells in the marrow cavity, and if the total number of bone marrow cells harvested for transplantation is estimated to be 1–2% of the entire bone marrow reserve, the number of leukemic cells in the marrow graft may range from 10^4 to 10^6. Consequently, one of the major research areas in the field of autologous marrow transplantation has been the *eradication of residual leukemic cells*. The principle of an "in vivo purge" by harvesting marrow cells after remission intensification therapy was introduced to address the minimal numbers of leukemic cells present in the marrow (51). Methods have also been developed for in vitro purging of leukemic cells from the marrow cell suspension after harvesting. Currently several different in vitro methods are used: (a) incubation of marrow cells with cytotoxic agents, such as 4-hydroperoxycyclophosphamide (4-HC) and mafosfamide (52,53), (b) physical removal, (c) complement lysis after incubation with monoclonal antibodies against surface antigens on the leukemic cells, and (d) monoclonal antibodies attached to magnetic microspheres and directed against leukemic cell antigens (54).

Despite concerns about residual disease in the harvested marrow, there was a need to explore the potential role of auto-BMT. Patients who failed second-line chemotherapy were treated with a pretransplant regimen consisting of combination piperazinedione and TBI. Piperazinedione is a fermentation product of *Streptomyces*, has alkylating activity, and is cell cycle–nonspecific (50). With this regimen, 32 relapsed patients were treated with marrow that was harvested in first remission. The treatment-related mortality was 8%. Of these patients, 80% achieved complete remission, although none lasted beyond 18 months (50). These results were still encouraging, since hematopoietic recovery could be obtained with a low treatment-related mortality rate and without immediate recurrence of leukemia. These and related studies formed the basis of further exploration of the role of auto-BMT in AML.

Results of Auto-BMT in First Remission AML

Results from 9 groups established in the treatment of acute leukemia are listed in Table 40.1. A total of 470 patients were transplanted. In 4 series of patients, marrow was purged with either 4-HC or mafosfamide. As noted, none of the treatment or purging methods were consistent among the teams. The outcome was not influenced by the presence or absence of TBI. (Yeager's results may change, since the median follow-up is short, 18 months. This is in contrast with the more than 7-year follow-up

Table 40.1. Overall Results of Individual Teams of Auto-BMT in AML CR1

Group	Number of Patients	Follow-up Median (range)	Interval[a] onset CR/BMT	Pre-BMT Regimen	DFS (%)	Relapse (%)
Haas (55)	35	39 (4–85)	6	Cy + TBI	58	32
Keating (92)	21	28 (NA)	10	Mel + TBI	58	39
Rizzoli (93)	125	50 (4–90)	6	CyTBI	58	40
Dicke (51)	18	96 (84–108)	6	CBV	56	44
Gorin (55, 94)	45	105 (60–120)	5	CY + TBI	56	31
Yeager (95)	48	18 (1–132)	2.5	BuCy	51	49
Carella (55, 96, 97)	55	29 (2–92)	6	Cy + TBI	49	43
Goldstone (55)	82	31 (12–96)	6	BACTD	48	48
Schaefer (98)	41	44 (2–72)	5	BuCy	45	50
Total	470				56 (45–58)	44 (31–50)

[a]Median in months.

in Gorin's and our studies.) Overall, the median DFS of the 470 patients was 56 ± 11%, with a median relapse rate of 44 ± 12%.

From January 1980 to 31 December 1991, 1040 autotransplants in CR1 were reported to the European Bone Marrow Transplant Registry (EBMTR) by 130 transplant teams in 22 countries. The data were analyzed by Gorin and presented at the 18th EBMTR meeting in Stockholm in 1992 (55). The projected 8-year DFS rate was 49 ± 4%. Gorin studied the respective roles of patient, disease, and treatment characteristics on outcome after auto-BMT. Table 40.2 contains a list of these characteristics. It appeared that sex and age of the patients, as well as FAB classification and pretransplant regimen had no influence on outcome after auto-BMT. On the other hand, time to achieve remission had a significant impact on DFS after auto-BMT. In 414 patients, remission was achieved within 40 days after initiation of treatment. The DFS rate in this patient group was 51 ± 3%, which was significantly higher than the 35 ± 3% in 522 patients in whom remission induction lasted longer than 40 days (P < .0001).

The interval between onset of CR and autotransplantation also had a significant bearing on DFS rate after BMT (Table 40.2). One hundred eighty patients were transplanted within 3 months after achieving complete remission, 453 patients within 3–6 months, and 313 after 6 months. The DFS rates were 23 ± 6%, 44 ± 4%, and 48 ± 4%; the relapse rates were 64 ± 5%, 45 ± 3%, and 46 ± 4%, respectively. The differences were statistically significant between the patients transplanted within 3 months and patients transplanted after 3 months (P < .0001, Table 40.3).

Gorin also explored the role of in vitro purging by using the EBMTR data. He compared the DFS of patients receiving mafosfamide-purged marrow with that of patients given unmanipulated marrow (55). In two subsets of patients who received TBI in their transplant conditioning regimen, the outcome using in vitro purged marrow was significantly better. As shown in Table 40.4, these subsets included patients who had been harvested early and transplanted within 6 months of achieving CR1

Table 40.2. Influence of Patient and Disease Characteristics on Outcome after Auto-BMT in AML CR1 (European Bone Marrow Transplant Registry)

No Influence	Influence
Age, sex	Interval onset CR and auto-BMT
Pretransplant regimens	Time to achieve CR
FAB classification	

Table 40.3. Results of Early versus Late BMT in AML CR1 Obtained by the EBMT

Time Interval Onset CR-BMT	5-Year DFS	Number of Patients
<3 months	23 ±6%	181
3–6 months	44 ±4%	453
>6 months	48 ±4%	303

Table 40.4. Definition of Patient Subpopulations in AML CR1 Who Benefit from Purged Marrow (EBMT results)

| Patient Population | Relapse Rate | | P |
	Purged	Unpurged	
Remission induction longer than 40 days	37 ±6	58 ±5	.01
BMT within 6 months	35 ±6	54 ±4	.02

as well as patients who took longer than 40 days to achieve CR1. TBI is effective in eradicating endogenous residual leukemic cells in first remission, which might logically explain the difference in outcome in terms of residual leukemic cells in the harvested marrow. In these patient subsets, unpurged marrow is still contaminated with leukemic cells, so that the risk of relapse is directly related to the number of malignant cells infused. Conversely, reduction of leukemic cells by in vitro purging reduces the relapse rate. According to the EBMTR results, the outcome of patients who achieved CR1 in less than 40 days and patients transplanted later than 6 months is not influenced by mafosfamide purging (55).

Results of Auto-BMT in Second-Remission AML

Second remission is a later stage than first remission; the remissions are shorter, and the cells are more resistant to chemotherapy. Any treatment that prolongs second remission beyond duration of CR1 has changed the usual history of the disease. These "CR duration inversions" can be used as indicators for effectivness of treatment. Using this analytical approach, patients can be used as their own controls.

Table 40.5 lists the results of auto-BMT of three individual groups. In these studies, unpurged marrow was used. The best results have been obtained by Meloni et al., who reported 49% DFS with a 40% relapse rate at 5 years. In this study, the remissions after auto-BMT were of the inversion type. In 3 of the 5 patients in the study by Bjorkstrand et al., no inversion had been reached, which reduces the adjusted DFS rate to 30% and is in sharp contrast to the author's study of only 14% due to a high early relapse rate. Although patient selection was a possible reason, the high relapse rate was likely due to the relatively mild cytoreductive program regimen of Cytoxan, BCNU, and VP-16. While this program is sufficiently cytoreductive in AML CR1 (see Table 40.1), in a setting in which leukemic cells are more resistant, it is clearly less effective.

Table 40.6 lists the individual studies in which in vitro purged marrow was used for transplantation. In the adult AML patients, the DFS rate is 30–34%, with a relapse rate of 58–66%, which is no better than the results with unpurged marrow listed in Table 40.5. The low relapse rate of 33% in the studies of Ball et al. (54) might be due to mortality from causes other than leukemia. The pediatric AML study from Lenarsky's group awaits more patients for more definitive conclusions. In this latter study, the remissions were inverted, in contrast to studies by Yeager et al. (53), which included several patients with a relatively short follow-up.

Analysis of the EBMTR data resulted in a DFS rate of $33 \pm 3\%$ in 305 patients registered (55). In that group, the relapse rate was $60 \pm 4\%$. The interval from diagnosis to ABMT in CR2 patients was found to have a significant influence on outcome. Patients transplanted in CR2 18 months or longer after diagnosis had a significantly higher DFS rate and lower relapse rate than those with a shorter time interval: DFS, $39 \pm 4\%$ versus $26 \pm 4\%$ ($P < .01$); relapse rate, $51 \pm 5\%$ versus $68 \pm 5\%$ ($P = .0001$). Also, in CR2 transplant patients, the interval from remission to ABMT was significant for outcome. Patients autografted after 6 months or longer from onset from second remission had a $48 \pm 6\%$ DFS rate. This was significantly higher than the $31 \pm 4\%$ in the patients transplanted within 3–6 months and $24 \pm 2\%$ in the patients transplanted within 3 months after onset of CR ($P = .03$). The EBMTR analysis, like the individual studies, did not show a significant influence of purging on DFS. After marrow puring, relapse rates where high ($63 \pm 6\%$ vs. $52 \pm 5\%$ in the unpurged group) when marrow was collected in CR2. However, when marrow was collected in CR1, puring tended to have a favorable influence on relapse rate ($35 \pm 16\%$ in the purged group vs. $69 \pm 8\%$ in the unpurged group). Results were not satistically significant (55).

Comparison of Auto-BMT with Chemotherapy

Auto-BMT takes place after remission induction at a time when there is minimal residual disease. When the auto-BMT results are compared with the results of chemotherapy, two factors need to be taken into account: patient selection and time censoring. Outcome in AML is influenced by prognostic factors, of which cytogenetics and time to achieve complete remission are most signifi-

Table 40.5. Unpurged Auto-BMT Results of Individual Teams in AML CR2

Group	Number of Patients	Age (years)	CR1 Duration[a]	Time CR/BMT[a]	DFS (%)	Follow-up[a]	Relapse (%)	Conditioning
Bjorkstrand (99)	10	15–60	—	6 (2–14)	50	26 (5–49)	40	BuCy
Meloni (100)	50	26 (1–51)	15 (1–44)	2 (1–13)	49.6	96	42	BAVC
Dicke (101)	14	31 (21–55)	10 (2–29)	3 (1–6)	14	84 (72–96)	70	CBV
Total	74				49.6 (14–50)		42 (40–70)	

[a]Months

Table 40.6. Purged Auto-BMT results of individual teams in AML CR2

Group	Number of Patients	Age (years)	CR1 Duration[a]	Time CR/BMT[a]	DFS (%)	Follow-up[a]	Relapse (%)	Conditioning
Lenarsky (102)	13	5 (1–21)	12 (2–60)	1 (1–12)	53	34 (22–39)	46	BuCy
Haas (55)	37	38 (16–51)	—	3 (1–24)	34	41 (1–80)	66	Cy + TBI
Ball (103)	26	38 (11–53)	—	2 (0–15)	33	42 (11–71)	33	Cy + TBI
Yeager (95)	82	30 (1–56)	—	3 (1–8)	30	46 (1–106)	58	BuCy
Total	158				33 (30–53)		52 (33–66)	

[a]Months.

cant. Patients need to be matched for these parameters. With regard to time censoring, the relapse rate decreases with duration of complete remission, so that the chance of DFS increases. In other words, the chance of 5-year DFS of a patient increases from 32% immediately after onset of CR to 43% when the patient is 7 months in CR, to 53% when 12 months in CR, to 63% when the remission is 24 months (54). Therefore, when the time interval between onset of CR and auto-BMT is 7 months, outcome after ABMT should be compared with results of chemotherapy-treated patients already 7 months in CR. Patients transplanted in CR1 compared with matched chemotherapy-treated patients did not show statistically significant outcome differences, although there was a trend in favor of auto-BMT (55). Three randomized studies (56–58) reported similar results, a trend of improved DFS in the auto-BMT group. Only in the EORTC trial was auto-BMT statistically superior to chemotherapy alone (Table 40.7). Marrow was harvested shortly after the first intensification course, so that it was subjected to in vivo purging. A problem in the randomized studies was the relatively small percentage of patients, less than 20%, randomized in each treatment arm because of high dropout, protocol violation, toxicity, and relapse prior to randomization. Outcomes after auto-BMT are consistent in the three trials, 48%, 48%, and 49%; outcomes in the chemotherapy-treated patient group varied: 49%, 42%, and 30%. The largest randomized trial, organized by the MRC in Great Britain, is still in progress (59). In the EORTC trial, also the results after allogeneic BMT were significantly superior. The overall survival of the patients in the 3 arms did not differ significantly, as more patients who relapsed following chemotherapy entered into a second remission and were then salvaged by auto-BMT. In addition, the analysis has shown other differences between the treatment arms, with a higher treatment-related mortality and more time spent in the hospital with allo-BMT and delayed hematologic recovery after auto-BMT. The results of this prospective study, the most important so far in terms of number of patients included, may help in decision making about therapeutic main options in AML.

Concluding Remarks

In first remission, auto-BMT results in approximately 50% long-term DFS. Compared with outcomes of chemotherapy-treated patients, outcomes are statistically superior in 1 of the 3 randomized studies; in the other 2 studies, there is a clear trend in favor of auto-BMT. The outcome after auto-BMT is influenced by factors such as length of remission induction and time interval between onset of CR and auto-BMT. The role of in vitro purging is not yet elucidated, but there seems to be an outcome advantage of certain patient subpopulations.

In second remission, auto-BMT induces long-term DFS. The DFS rate has not been compared with that of patients treated with chemotherapy alone. However, the results are promising and certainly warrant randomized prospective trials. Currently, the role of in vitro purging in CR2 is unclear.

Acute Lymphocytic Leukemia

Adult ALL is a hemotologic malignancy characterized by an uncontrolled proliferation and accumulation of immature lymphocytes and their progenitors. ALL is the most common leukemia in children; however, a substantial proportion of cases occur in adolescents and adults. Approximately 25% of the acute leukemia cases in adults are ALL. This review is limited to adult ALL.

ALL is a heterogeneous disease. Morphologic and immunologic features are useful in classifying patients with ALL. A French-American-British (FAB) morphologic classification of ALL has been established. This system recognizes three types of lymphoblasts, termed L1, L2, and L3 (60). The FAB classification is based on a spectrum of cell properties such as the size ratio of nucleus to cytoplasm, the number and size of nucleoli, and the degree of cytoplasmic basophilia. Adults with ALL have a predominance of L2 morphology. L2 cells are typically large with an irregular nuclear outline. The nucleus may be cleft, and it contains one or more large nucleoli. The cytoplasm is deeply basophilic and may be abundant. The L3 morphology, resembling that in Burkitt's lymphoma, is occasionally present in adult ALL. In addition, cytochemical reactions such as periodic acid–Schiff reaction (PAS) and acid phosphatase are useful for confirmation.

A second approach in the classification of adult ALL is based on the immune features of leukemic cells (61, 62). Subtypes of ALL include the common, T, B, and null phenotypes. The nomenclature is based on detection on the cell surface of one of the following: the common ALL antigen, a 100-kDa glycoprotein; receptors for sheep red blood

Table 40.7. Results of three Randomized Trials in AML CR1

Patients	BGMT 87 (Reiffers[56])	GOELAM (Harousseau[57])	EORTC (Zittoun[58])
Age	39 (18–52)	36 (15–50)	35 (10–60)
No. at onset	204	305	988
No. at consolidation	162	150	581
No. at randomization	135	106	239
Auto-BMT			
No. of patients	39	45	119
DFS (4 year)	**48%**	**48%**	**49%**
Relapse rate (4 year)	47%	51%	
Chemo			
No. of patients	38	50	120
DFS (4 year)	**42%**	**49%**	**30%**
Relapse rate (4 year)	58%	50%	
Significance	N.S.	N.S.	P = .026

cells (RBCs) or T-cell antigens; and immunoglobulin T (Ig) molecules. Null cells lack these surface features. Recent data indicate that most cases of common ALL are committed to the B-lymphocyte lineage, based on detection of surface Ig and immunoglobulin gene rearrangements (63–65). In adults, 50% of cases are of the common phenotype, T-ALL accounts for 20%, and B-ALL for 2–7%. In earlier studies more than 20% of cases were null-ALL, but with the use of monoclonal antibodies, most of the null-ALL cases appear to be B-lineage ALL. Monoclonal antibodies can also subdivide, (a) B-ALL into pre-pre-B, pre-B, and B and (b) T-ALL divided into pre-pre-T, pre-T, and T-ALL.

Treatment of ALL is generally divided into two phases, induction and postremission therapy. The latter is subdivided into consolidation, intensification, and maintenance. Usually there is also a phase of CNS prophylaxis. The objective of induction chemotherapy is to achieve remission, that is, eradication of leukemia detectable by conventional techniques. Consolidation and intensification refer to either high-dose chemotherapy, the use of multiple new agents, or less often, readministration of the induction regimen. These measures are aimed at eliminating clinically undetectable leukemia and thereby preventing relapse as well as emergence of drug-resistant cells. Maintenance involves less-intensive chemotherapy.

The first autologous transplants in ALL were reported by McGovern et al. in 1959 (66). Marrow was harvested shortly after remission, stored at −80°C, and transplanted within 3 months after achievement of remission. The pretransplant regimen was 500 rads of TBI. Hematopoietic recovery was obtained, but the remissions did not last longer than 3 months. These results were very interesting, since marrow cells remained viable and could induce hematopoietic recovery even though they had been, apparently, suboptimally stored. Since the level of TBI was not myeloablative, it is likely that endogenous stem cells survived the TBI and contributed to hematopoietic recovery. The early re-

lapses after BMT are not surprising. In the first place, remissions were induced with single-agent chemotherapy, and marrow cells were harvested immediately after achieving remission, a time when the leukemic cell population in the marrow was large. Secondly, the leukemic cell reduction power of 500 rads of TBI is estimated to be 1–2 logs (66).

Not until the late seventies and early eighties was auto-BMT reintroduced in the treatment of ALL (50, 67). At that time, remission induction had greatly improved, and more was known about high-dose cytoreductive therapy. Successful application of autologous transplantation requires the collection and cryopreservation of enough hematopoietic progenitor cells to allow prompt hematologic and immunologic reconstitution after the stem cells are thawed and reinfused. Additionally, measures to address potential contamination of the harvested marrow inoculum with viable leukemic progenitor cells must be undertaken. These measures consist of ex vivo bone marrow purging after harvest and before cryopreservation, using either leukemia-associated antigen–directed immunologic purging techniques or ex vivo chemotherapy of the harvested autologous marrow. Additionally, successful leukemia control after autologous transplantation requires effective antileukemic pretransplant conditioning therapy and, in some recent approaches, posttransplant adjunct treatment to prevent leukemia relapse. Clinical studies to date have variably addressed all these elements in the search for optimal autologous marrow transplantation for ALL (68, 69). In the following section, the results of auto-BMT in CR1 and CR2 are presented as well as future directions in posttransplantation treatment modalities.

Clinical Results of Auto-BMT in CR1 in Adults

The results of 11 major groups have been listed in Table 40.8. A total of 400 patients were transplanted. The median

Table 40.8. Results of Autologous BMT in ALL in CR1[a]

Author, year (ref)	N (total)	Conditioning	Purging	DFS (%)	Time post-BMT (years)	Relapse (%)
Blaise, 1990 (85)	(22)	TBI + Cy or melphalan	—	40	3	52
Buckner, 1989 (83)	14 (37)	TBI + Cy	MoAb + C'	54	2	36
Carey, 1991 (91)	(15)	Melphalan + TBI	—	48	3	N.R.
Gilmore, 1991 (71)	(27)	Cy + TBI + Ara-C	MoAb + C'	32	>5	67
Meloni, 1990 (67)	9 (30)	Busulfan + Cy	Asta-Z or mafosfamide	33[b]	—	55[b]
Santos, 1989 (68)	12 (31)	TBI + Cy	4HC	25%		71
Simonsson, 1989 (76)	21 (54)	TBI + Cy ± multidrug	MoAb + C'	65	>2	30[b]
Spinolo, 1990 (70)	(26)	Cy, BCNU, VP-16	—	54	4	40[b]
Stoppa, 1990 (104)	6 (12)	TBI ± melphalan ± Cy	Immunomagnetic beads (CD10, 19)	50[b]	1	50[b]
Weisdorf, 1992 (105)	14 (155)	fTBI + Cy or Ara-C	MoAb + C' or i immunotoxin + 4HC	24	>5	69
Zintl, 1990 (84)	6 (15)	TBI + Cy	—	43	2.5	54
Gorin, 1990 (69)	233 (438)	Variable	Variable	41	>3	~53

[a]Abbreviations: MoAB, monoclonal antibody; Cy, cyclophosphamide; N.R., not reported; C, complement; EBMTG, European Bone Marrow Transplant Group.
[b]Not Kaplan-Meier projection.

DFS rate is 42 ± 2%. The follow-up of patients differs between the groups, so that the length of DFS per group is different. This makes comparison of data between the groups difficult. In many studies, detailed descriptions of disease, age, cytogenetics, duration of remission induction, and WBC at diagnosis have not been reported, which makes interpretation of results difficult. In two studies, Spinolo et al. (70) and Gilmore et al. (71), prognostic factors of the patient population were available. It appears that the same factors that determine outcome after chemotherapy influence the BMT results. Gorin analyzed the EBMTR data and found that the major prognostic factors were length of remission induction and time interval between onset of CR and BMT (table 40.9). Cytogenetic data were not available in the EBMT registry. It can be noted from Table 40.8 that the main stumbling block is recurrence of disease: the median relapse rate is 53% (30–71%). Gorin studied the effect of purging and only found a difference in T-ALL between patients receiving monoclonal antibody–treated marrow and those transplanted with unfractionated marrow. Patients receiving the purged marrow had a significantly higher DFS rate (40 ± 7% vs. 26 ± 6%).

Clinical Results of Auto-BMT in CR2 in Adults

The results of auto-BMT in CR2 are outlined in Table 40.10. A total of 182 patients were transplanted by 9 groups. The median DFS rate is 28 ± 15%, which is less than the DFS in first remission. The relapse rate is 65% (36–88), the main factor for failure after BMT. Analysis of the EBMTR results revealed that time interval between initial diagnosis and BMT as well as the time between onset of CR and BMT were determining factors influencing outcome.

Clinical Results of Randomized Studies between Auto-BMT and Chemotherapy

The French group Therapy of Adult ALL designed a study to evaluate the use of auto-BMT as intensification of remission in ALL (72). After consolidation therapy, patients with ALL under 50 years of age were randomized between a chemotherapy regimen and intensive consolidation, with auto-BMT. With a median follow-up of 30 months, the projected 3-year DFS is 49 ± 5% for the auto-BMT-treated patients and 42 ± 5% for the chemotherapy-treated patients. The relapse rate in the auto-BMT arm is 57%, versus 61% in the chemotherapy arm. These results are not statistically significant. In this study, patients with a related HLA-identical matched donor received an allogenic transplant, and the projected 3-year DFS is 55 ± 5%. In this arm, the relapse rate was 33%, significantly less than the relapse rate in the chemotherapy- and auto-BMT-treated patient groups.

Purging of Marrow in ALL

Leukemic blasts may differ in certain characteristics from the clonogenic leukemia progenitor cells capable of sustaining clinically active malignancy. During morphologically confirmed remission, marrow blasts are not recognizable microscopically, but it is generally accepted that viable clonogenic leukemia progenitor cells might proliferate and result in relapse if reinfused along with the cryopreserved autologous marrow (73). Most clinical experience to date has, therefore, utilized ex vivo marrow purging to deplete or eliminate leukemic progenitors from the marrow inoculum.

Marrow purging techniques in ALL have used primarily immunologic methods directed toward leukemia-associated antigens expressed on the cell surface. Monoclonal antibodies against B-lineage antigens (CD9, CD10, CD19, CD20, CD22, CD24) or T-lineage antigens (CD5, CD7) have been used to opsonize cells and trigger the lytic capacity of exogenous complement. Alternatively, such antibodies have been combined with chemical toxins (e.g., ricin, pokeweed antiviral protein) as biochemical or recombinant immunoconjugates. These immunotoxins use the specificity of the monoclonal antibody and are able to selectively poison cells expressing the leukemia-associated antigen while sparing hematopoietic progenitors (73–75).

Ex vivo incubations of marrow with low-dose chemotherapy designed to exploit the therapeutic window leukemic cell sensitivity and hematopoietic progenitor sensitivity have been used as well. Most frequently, 4-HC has been used either alone or in combination with immunologic purging techniques, but in some studies, combination ex vivo chemotherapy purging has been tested as well. Some reports have correlated the number of clonogenic leukemia progenitors present after purging with the clinical results of autologous transplantation (68, 74, 76, 77). Such correlations have been interpreted as support for the efficacy of ex vivo marrow purging (78).

There are important conceptual limitations to these techniques (79). Firstly, these methods rarely eliminate more than 3–4 logs of leukemia cells. Secondly, leukemia cells are heterogeneous in cell surface-antigen expression (and drug sensitivity). Although antibodies or drugs may eliminate most leukemia cells, they may not affect putative leukemia progenitor cells (80, 81). The efficacy of leukemia

Table 40.9. Identification of Factors Influencing the Outcome of Auto-BMT in CR1 by the EBMTR Database Analysis

Prognostic Factors	DFS (5 years) (%)	
FAB classification		
L3	78	
L1, L2	40	$P = .02$
Interval diagnosis-CR		
<40 days	50	
>40 days	35	$P = .008$
Interval onset CR–BMT		
<6 months	58	
>6 months	42	$P = .02$

Table 40.10. Results of Autologous BMT in ALL CR2[a]

Author, Year (ref)	N	Conditioning	Purging	DFS (%)	Time Post-BMT	Relapse (%)
Buckner, 1989[83]	23	TBI + Cy	MoAb + C'	17	2 years	75
Dicke, 1990[101]	14	CBV	—	14	8 years	70
Meloni, 1990[67]	16	Busulfan + Cy	Asta-Z or mafosfamide	40	—	40
Santos, 1989[68]	19	TBI + Cy	4HC	10		88
Schroeder, 1991[106]	7	Melphalan + TBI	Campath-1	50[b,c]	25 months	N.R.
Simonsson, 1989[76]	29	TBI + Cy ± multidrug	MoAb + C'	31	>2 years	60
Soiffer 1990[107]	48	Cy + fTBI ± Ara-C	MoAb + C'	34	4 years	36
Gorin, 1990[69] (EBMTG survey)	205	Variable	Variable	27	>3 years	~70

[a]Abbreviations: MoAb, monoclonal antibody; N.R., not reported; Cy, cyclophosphamide; C', complement; EBMTG, European Bone Marrow Transplant Group.
[b]Survival, not disease free.
[c]Not Kaplan-Meier projection.

cell depletion is difficult to evaluate in vitro, since assays of leukemia progenitor cells are imperfect and of unproven biologic import. The clinical value of ex vivo treatment of the graft to prevent leukemia relapse following an autotransplant is unproven so far and will be difficult to evaluate until more effective pretransplant antileukemia conditioning is developed.

Pretransplant Conditioning

Autologous transplantation produces less transplant-related morbidity and mortality than does allografting. In most studies, similar pretransplant conditioning has been used for autologous and allogeneic transplants (82–87). However, the additional safety of autologous transplantation might justify using more intensive, and possibly more effective, conditioning regimens, but this approach has not been fully explored. Pretransplant conditioning has most often included TBI in single or multiple fractions delivered at varying dose rates, energies, and total doses. Fractionated TBI is often used and reportedly induces less acute toxicity. Techniques to protect vulnerable tissues (lung shielding) and intensify antileukemic radiation (chest wall boosting) as well as high-energy techniques designed to increment the marrow dose have also been evaluated. Imaginative delivery techniques including radioimmunoconjugates or radiochemicals that accumulate in the marrow cavity are being developed experimentally to more effectively deplete the body leukemia burden. Though high-dose cyclophosphamide (100–200 mg/kg) has been the standard chemotherapy agent used with TBI before transplantation, some recent reports have shown favorable results using cytarabine, etoposide, melphalan, or combination-drug chemoradiotherapy (78).

Adjunct Antileukemia Therapy After Autologous BMT

The first reports of curative therapy for childhood ALL emphasized that extended-duration maintenance therapy

is critical for long-term disease control. However, the compromised marrow reserve of autograft recipients has impaired attempts to test maintenance therapy after transplantation. In one small controlled trial at the University of Minnesota, post-BMT maintenance (after allogeneic and autologous transplantation) was both difficult to deliver and ineffective at preventing or delaying leukemia relapse (88). In the M.D. Anderson series, in adult ALL after transplantation with CBV in first remission with unmanipulated marrow cells, maintenance chemotherapy could be administered, and even the extra cycle of first intensification could be repeated after BMT (69).

In the Powles' study (89), 38 patients with poor-risk ALL in first remission (age 3–41 years; median, 21 years) received maintenance chemotherapy following auto-BMT. Patients were conditioned for auto-BMT with high-dose melphalan and single-fraction TBI (TBI). Maintenance chemotherapy was commenced in a total of 26 patients and was tolerated to a median daily dose of 6-mercaptopurine of 40.5 mg/m² and a median weekly methotrexate dose of 8.3 mg/m². Twenty patients remain alive still in first remission with a projected DFS of 50% and a median follow-up in survivors of 200 weeks (range, 48–387 weeks). Eleven patients have relapsed, at a median of 4.5 months from auto-BMT. This group of auto-BMT patients was compared with remission patients with ALL receiving conventional chemotherapy in the United Kingdom Medical Research Council trials UKALL X and XA. After stratifying for major risk factors and allowing for the delay from remission to transplant, a significant reduction in the risk of relapse after auto-BMT could be demonstrated ($P = .04$). DFS was not significantly increased because of transplant-related toxicity. This study strongly suggests that maintenance chemotherapy to prevent relapse after auto-BMT for ALL is well tolerated and warrants assessment in a formal controlled study (89).

Modern approaches to adjunct therapy have focused on nonspecific immunotherapy or immunotoxins directed at leukemia-associated antigens. Activation of cytotoxic T lymphocytes (CTLs) or natural killer (NK) cells with recombinant interleukin 2 (IL-2) has received considerable interest in recent years. IL-2 has been given in high doses, often in conjunction with exogenously cultured lymphokine-activated killer (LAK) cells, and has demonstrated antineoplastic activity in various human tumors including some lymphoid neoplasms. However, the excess toxicity associated with high-dose IL-2/LAK cell therapy has stimulated interest in more modest and, one hopes, less toxic applications of IL-2 after autologous transplantation. No reports have yet demonstrated clinically useful antineoplastic activity of IL-2 given after autologous transplantation; however, immune activation (either CTL, NK, or LAK) has been observed. A recent Minnesota trial of IL-2 given immediately post-autologous-transplantation for ALL resulted in enhancement of CTL activity against ALL targets (90). In another report, low-dose, long-duration IL-2 therapy induced potent NK/LAK activation activity in autologous BMT recipients (91). Further studies will be required to test the clinical utility of immune effectors induced by IL-2 therapy.

Monoclonal antibodies or immunotoxins (74, 76) have also been considered for in vivo use in the post-BMT setting. Because of their immune specificity in targeting leukemia-associated antigens and because they are nonmyelosuppressive, this therapy is well suited to the treatment of posttransplant minimal residual disease.

These and other adjunct therapies offer great promise in enhancing the effectiveness of autologous transplantation in preventing leukemic relapse. They may substitute for the missing graft-versus-leukemia effect that accounts for some of the antileukemic potential of allogeneic transplantation. Because the toxicity of conventional chemotherapy conditioning is near maximal, these novel alternative therapies might be added to allogeneic transplantation as well. Future experimental and clinical studies have great potential to expand the applicability and effectiveness of autologous transplantation for ALL.

Induced GVHD

In allo-BMT, graft-versus-leukemia (GVL) is known to reduce relapse rates following transplantation (108). Patients with leukemia who develop GVHD following allo-BMT have lower relapse rates (109). Patients who relapse following allo-BMT for CML may enter remission after GVHD is induced by reducing immunosuppression or infusing donor leukocytes (110). These observations provide a rationale for inducing GVHD following auto-BMT (111). Cyclosporine can induce GVHD in rodent models as well as in some patients undergoing auto-BMT (112, 113). Mild-to-moderate cutaneous GVHD has been induced after auto-BMT for AML, but the clinical significance of this must await results of large prospective studies (114).

Concluding Remarks

The results with auto-BMT are not superior to those with chemotherapy, although a trend of higher DFS rates is apparent, and long-term DFS with auto-BMT in disease after first relapse has been reported by various groups. Although very promising, it needs to be seen if the DFS rate is *significantly* better than alternate treatment with chemotherapy alone.

Not only is there progress in transplants for ALL, but chemotherapy is also improving. Consequently, the greatest immediate challenge is to determine how to best use these modalities to cure ALL.

ACKNOWLEDGEMENTS

The author gratefully acknowledges the assistance of Kathy White and Deborah Hood in the preparation and editing of this chapter.

REFERENCES

1. Jacobson LO, Marks EK, Robson MJ, Gaston EO, Zirkle RE. The role of the spleen in radiation injury. Proc Soc Exp Biol Med 1949;70:740.
2. Jacobson LO, Simmons EL, Marks EK, Eldredge JH. Recovery from radiation injury. Science 1951;133:410.
3. Lorenz E, Uphoff DE, Reid TR, Shelton E. Modification of irradiation injury in mice and guinea pigs by bone marrow injections. JNCI 1951:12:197.
4. Ford CE, Hamerton JL, Barnes DWH, Loutit JF. Cytological identification of radiation chimaeras. Nature 1956; 177:452.
5. Vos O, Davids JAG, Weyzen WWH, van Bekkum DW. Evidence for the cellular hypothesis in radiation protection by bone marrow cells. Acta Physiol Pharmacol Ned 1956; 4:482.
6. Nowell PC, Cole LJ, Habermeyer JG, Roan PL. Growth and continued function of rat marrow cells in X-radiation mice. Cancer Res 1956;16:258.
7. van Bekkum DW, de Vries MJ. Radiation chimaeras. London: Logos/Academic, 1967.
8. Till JE, McCulloch EA. A direct measurement of the radiation sensitivity of normal mouse bone marrow cells. Radiat Res 1961;14:213.
9. Trentin JJ, Fahlberg WJ. An experimental model for studies of immunologic competence in irradiated mice repopulated with "clones" of spleen cells. In: Conceptual advances in immunology and oncology, 16th Annual Symposium (1962), Texas. New York: Harper & Tow, 1966:66.
10. Becker AJ, McCulloch EA, Till JE. Cytological demonstration of the clonal nature of spleen colonies derived from transplanted mouse marrow cells. Nature 1963;197:452.
11. Micklem HS, Loutit JF. Tissue grafting and radiation. New York: Academic Press, 1966.
12. Nowell PC, Hirsch BE, Fox DH, Wilson DB. Evidence for the existence of multipotential lympho-hematopoietic stem cells in the adult rat. J Cell Physiol 1970;75:151.
13. Abramson S, Miller RG, Phillips RA. The identification in adult bone marrow of pluripotent and restricted stem cells of the myeloid and lymphoid systems. J Exp Med 1977; 145:1567.
14. Magli MC, Iscove NN, Odartchenko N. Transient nature of early hemopoietic spleen colonies. Nature 1982;295:527.
15. Bayliss WM, Starling EE. The mechanism of pancreatic secretion. J Physiol London 1902;28:325.
16. Carnot P, Deflandre C. Sur l'activité hémopoiétique du serum au cours de la régénération du sang. C R Acad Sci 1906;143:384.
17. Carnot P, Deflandre C. Sur l'activité hémopoiétique des différents organes au cours de la régénération du sang. C R Acad Sci 1906;143:432.

18. Reissmann KR. Studies on the mechanisms of erythropoietic stimulation in parabiotic rats during hypoxia. Blood 1950; 5:372.

19. Borsook HA, Graybriel A, Keighley G, Windosr E. Polycythemic response in normal adult rats to a non-protein plasma extract from anemic rabbits. Blood 1954;9:734.

20. Erslev AJ. Humoral regulation of red cell production. Blood 1953;8:349.

21. Gordon AS, Piliero SJ, Medici PT, Siegel CD, Tannenbaum M. Attempts to identify site of production of circulating "erythropoietin." Proc Soc Exp Biol Med 1956;92:598.

22. Hodgson G, Tohá J. The erythropoietic effect of urine and plasma of repeatedly bled rabbits. Blood 1954;9:299.

23. Plzak LF, Fried W, Jacobson LO, Bethard WF. Demonstration of stimulation of erythropoiesis by plasma from anemic rats using Fe^{59}. J Lab Clin Med 1955;46:671.

24. Bonsdorff E, Jalavisto E. A humoral mechanism in chronic erythrocytosis. Acta Physiol Scand 1948;16:150.

25. White WF, Gurney CW, Goldwasser E, Jacobson LO. Studies on erythropoietin. Recent Prog Hormone Res 1960; 16:219.

26. Miyake T, Kung CKH, Goldwasser E. Purification of human erythropoietin. J Biol Chem 1977;252:5558.

27. Pluznik DH, Sachs L. The cloning of normal "mast" cells in tissue culture. J Cell Comp Physiol 1965;66:319.

28. Bradley TR, Metcalf D. The growth of mouse bone marrow cells in vitro. Aust J Exp Biol Med Sci 1966;44:287.

29. Stephenson JR, Axelrad A, McLeod DL, Schreeve MM. Induction of colonies of hemoglobin-synthesizing cells by erythropoietin in vitro. Proc Natl Acad Sci USA 1971; 68:1542.

30. Axelrad AA, et al. Properties of cells that produce erythrocytic colonies in vitro. In: WA Robinson, ed. Proceedings of the Second International Workshop on Hemopoiesis in Culture. DHEW Publ no. NIH 74205. Washington, DC: 1974:226.

31. Metcalf D, Parker J, Chester HM, Kincade PW. Formation of eosinophilic granulocytic colonies by mouse bone marrow cells in vitro. J Cell Physiol 1974;84:275.

32. Nakeff A, Dicke KA, Van Noord MJ. Megakaryocytes in agar culture of mouse bone marrow. Ser Haematol 1975; 8:1.

33. Metcalf D, MacDonald HR, Odartchenko N, Sordat B. Growth of mouse megakaryocyte colonies in vitro. Proc Natl Acad Sci USA 1975;72:1744.

34. Metcalf D, Warner NL, Nossal SJV, Miller JFAP, Shortman K, Rabellino E. Growth of B lymphocyte colonies in vitro from mouse lymphoid organs. Nature 1975;255:630.

35. Rosenzajn LA, Shoham D, Kalechman I. Clonal proliferation of PHA-stimulated human lymphocytes in soft agar culture. Immunology 1973;29:1041.

36. Metcalf D. The molecular biology and functions of granulocyte-macrophage colony stimulating factors. Blood 1986; 67:257.

37. Clark S, Kamen R. The human hematopoietic colony-stimulating factors. Science 1987;236:1229.

38. Mochizuki DY, Eisenman JR, Conlon PJ, Larsen AD, Tushinski RJ. Interleukin-1 regulates hematopoietic activity, a role previously ascribed to hemopoietin 1. Proc Natl Acad Sci USA 1987;84:5267.

39. Peschel C, Paul WE, Ohara J, Green I. Effects of B cell stimulatory factor-1/interleukin 4 on hematopoietic progenitor cells. Blood 1987;70:254.

40. Ikebuchi K, Wong GG, Clark SC, Ihle JN, Hirai Y, Ogawa M. Interleukin 6 enhancement of interleukin 3-dependent proliferation of multipotential hemopoietic progenitors. Proc Natl Acad Sci USA 1987;84:9035.

41. Sanderson CJ, Warren DJ, Strath M. Identification of a lymphokine that stimulates eosinophil differentiation in vitro. Its relationship to interleukin 3 and functional properties of eosinophils produced in culture. J Exp Med 1985; 162:60–74.

42. Brandt SJ, Peters WP, Atwater SK, et al. Effect of recombinant human granulocyte-macrophage colony-stimulating factor on hematopoietic reconstitution after high-dose chemotherapy and autologous bone marrow transplantation. N Engl J Med 1988;318:869.

43. Nemanaitis J, Singer JW, Buckner CD, et al. Preliminary analysis of a randomized, placebo-controlled trial of rhGM-CSF in autologous bone marrow transplantation (ABMT) [Abstract]. Proc Am Soc Clin Oncol 1990;9:10.

44. Körbling M, Dorken B, Ho AD, Pezzuto A, Hunstein W, Fliedner TM. Autologous transplantation of blood-derived hemopoietic stem cells after myeloblative therapy in a patient with Burkitt's lymphoma. Blood 1986;67:529.

45. Kessinger A, Armitage JO, Smith DM, Landmark JD, Bierman PJ, Weisenburger DD. High dose therapy and autologous peripheral blood stem cell transplantation for patients with lymphoma. Blood 1989;74:1260.

46. Körbling M, Fliedner TM, Holle R, Magrin S, Baumann M, Holderman E, Eberhardt K. Autologous blood stem cell (ABSCT) versus purged bone marrow transplantation (pABMT) in standard risk AML: influence of source and cell composition of the autograft on hematopoietic reconstitution and disease-free survival. Bone Marrow Transplant 1991;7:343.

47. Skipper HE, Schabel FM Jr, Wilcox WS. Experimental evaluation of potential anti-cancer agents. XII. On the criteria and kinetics associated with "curability" of experimental leukemia. Cancer Chemother Rep 1964; 35:1.

48. Thomas ED, Storb R, Clift RA, et al. Bone marrow transplantation. New Engl J Med 1975;292:832.

49. Gorin NC, Najman A, Duhamel G. Autologous bone marrow transplantation in acute myelocytic leukemia. Lancet 1977;14:1050.

50. Dicke KA, Zander AR, Spitzer G, Verma D, Peters L, Vellekoop L, McCredie KB. Autologous bone marrow transplantation in adult acute leukemia in relapse. Lancet 1979;1(8115):514–517.

51. Spinolo JA, Dicke KA, Horwitz LJ, Jagannath S, Zander AR, Auber ML, Spitzer G. Double intensification with amsacrine/high dose ara-C and high dose chemotherapy with autologous bone marrow transplantation produces durable remissions in acute myelogenous leukemia. Bone Marrow Transplant 1990;5;111–118.

52. Gorin NC, Douay L, LaPorte JP, et al. Autologous bone marrow transplantation using marrow incubated with Asta Z 7557 in adult acute leukemia. Blood 1986;67:1367.

53. Yeager AM, Kaizer H, Santos GW, et al. Autologous bone marrow transplantation in patients with acute non lymphoblastic leukemia using ex vivo marrow treatment with 4-hydroxperoxycyclophosphamide. N Engl J Med 1986; 315:141.

54. Ball ED. In vitro purging of bone marrow for autologous marrow transplantation in acute myelogenous leukemia

using myeloid specific monoclonal antibodies. Bone Marrow Transplant 1988;3:387.

55. Gorin NC, Dicke K, Löwenberg B. high dose therapy for acute myelocytic leukemia treatment strategy: what is the choice? Ann Oncol 1993;4:59.

56. Reiffers J, Stoppa AM, Attal M, Michallet M, Marit G, et al. Randomized trial comparing autologous stem cell transplantation and chemotherapy in adult patients with acute myeloid leukemia in first remission: the BGMT Group experience. In: Dicke KA, Keating A, eds. Proceedings of the Sixth International Symposium on Autologous Bone Marrow Transplantation, Houston, Texas, December 2–3. 1992:11–15.

57. Harousseau JL, Cahn JY, Pignon B, Mignard D, Witz F, et al. Comparison of intensive consolidation chemotherapy (ICC) and unpurged autologous bone marrow transplantation (ABMT) as post remission therapy in adult acute myeloid leukemia (AML). In: Dicke KA, Keating A, eds. Proceedings of the Sixth International Symposium on Autologous Bone Marrow Transplantation, Houston, Texas, December 2–3. 1992:16–19.

58. Zittoun R, Mandelli F, Willemze R, de Witte T, Labar B, et al. Prospective phase III study of autologous bone marrow transplantation (ABMT) vs short intensive chemotherapy (IC) vs allogeneic bone marrow transplantation (allo-BMT) during first complete remission (CR) of acute myelogenous leukemia (AML). Results of the EORTC-GIMEMA AML 8A Trial. Blood 1993;82(Suppl 1):85a.

59. Burnett AK, Goldstone AH, Stevens RF, Hann I, Rees J, Gray R, Wheatley K. UK MRC10: evaluation of auto-BMT in acute myeloid leukaemia. In: Dicke KA, Keating A, eds. Proceedings of the Sixth International Symposium on Autologous Bone Marrow Transplantation, Houston, Texas, December 2–3. 1992.

60. Bennett JM, Catovsky D, Daniel MT, et al. Proposals for the classification of the acute leukemias. Br J Haematol 1976;33:451–458.

61. Foon KA, Todd RF. Immunologic classification of leukemia and lymphoma. Blood 1986;68:1–31.

62. Foon KA, Gale RP, Todd RF. Recent advances in the immunologic classification of leukemia and lymphoma. Semin Hematol 1986;23:257–283.

63. Korsmeyer SJ, Arnold A, Bakhsi A, et al. Immunoglobulin gene rearrangement and cell surface antigen expression in acute lymphocytic leukemias of T cell and B cell precursor origins. J Clin Invest 1983;71:301–313.

64. Korsmeyer SJ, Hieter PA, Ravetch JV, et al. Developmental hierarchy of immunoglobulin gene rearrangements in human leukemia pre-B-cells. Proc Natl Acad Sci USA 1981;78:7096–7100.

65. Vogler LB, Crist WM, Bockman DE, et al. Pre-B-cell leukemia. A new phenotype of childhood lymphoblastic leukemia. N Engl J Med 1987;298:872–872.

66. McGovern JJ, Russell PS, Atkins L, Webster EW. Treatment of terminal leukemic relapse by total body irradiation and intravenous infusion of stored autologous bone marrow obtained during remission. N Engl J Med 1959;260:675–683.

67. Meloni G, De Fabritiis P, Carella AM, et al. Autologous bone marrow transplantation in patients with AML in first complete remission. Results of two different conditioning regimens after the same induction and consolidation therapy. Bone Marrow Transplant 1990;5:29–32.

68. Santos GW, Yeager AM, Jones RJ. Autologous bone marrow transplantation. Annu Rev Med 1989;40:99–112.

69. Gorin NC, Aegerter P, Auvert B. Autologous bone marrow transplantation for acute leukemia in remission: an analysis of 1322 cases. In: Buchner T, Schellong G, Hiddemann W, Ritter J, eds. Hematology and blood transfusion, vol 33. Acute leukemias II. Berlin: Springer-Verlag, 1990:660–666.

70. Spinolo JA, Dicke KA, Horwitz LJ, et al. High dose chemotherapy and ABMT for adult acute lymphoblastic leukemia in remission. In: Dicke KA, Armitage JO, Dicke-Evinger MJ, eds. Autologous bone marrow transplantation. Proceedings of the Fifth International Symposium, vol 5, Omaha: University of Nebraska, 1990:151–160.

71. Gilmore MJML, Hamon MD, Prentice HG, et al. Failure of purged autologous bone marrow transplantation in high risk acute lymphoblastic leukaemia in first complete remission. Bone Marrow Transplant 1991;8:19–26.

72. Fiere D, LePage E, Sebban C. Adult acute lymphoblastic leukemia: a multicentric randomized trial testing bone marrow transplantation as postremission therapy. The French Group on Therapy for Adult Lymphoblastic Leukemia. J Clin Oncol 1993;11(10):1990–2001.

73. Uckun FM, Gajl-Peczalska K, Meyers DE, et al. Marrow purging in autologous bone marrow transplantation for T-lineage acute lymphoblastic leukemia: efficacy of ex vivo treatment with immunotoxins and 4-hydroperoxycyclophosphamide against fresh leukemic marrow progenitor cells. Blood 1987;69:361–366.

74. Uckun FM, Kersey JH, Vallera DA, et al. Autologous bone marrow transplantation in high risk remission T-lineage acute lymphoblastic leukemia using immunotoxins plus 4-hydroperoxycyclophosphamide for marrow purging. Blood 1990;76:1723–1733.

75. Roy DC, Ish C, Blattler W, et al. Anti-B4 blocked ricin: a new immunotoxin for purging of acute lymphoblastic leukemia cells prior to autologous bone marrow transplantation. In: Proceedings of the Annual meeting of the American Association for Cancer Research, vol 31. 1990:A1737.

76. Simonsson B, Burnett AK, Prentice HG, et al. Autologous bone marrow transplantation with monoclonal antibody purged marrow for high risk acute lymphoblastic leukemia. Leukemia 1989;3:631–636.

77. Uckun FM, Kersey JH, Haake R, et al. Autologous bone marrow transplantation (BMT) in high risk remission B-lineage acute lymphoblastic leukemia using a cocktail of three monoclonal antibodies (BA-1/CD24, BA-2/CD9, BA-3/CD10) plus complement and 4-hydroperoxycyclophosphamide for ex vivo bone marrow purging. Blood 1992;79:1094–1104.

78. Zhang MJ, Hoelzer D, Weisdorf DJ, et al. Long-term follow-up of adults with acute lymphoblastic leukemia in first remission treated with chemotherapy or bone marrow transplantation. The Acute Lymphoblastic Leukemia Working Committee. Ann Intern Med 1995;123(6):428–431.

79. Gale RP. Bone marrow purging: current status, future directions. Bone Marrow Transplant 1987;2(Suppl 2):107–115.

80. Hagenbeek A, Martens AC. On the heterogeneity of minimal residual disease in acute leukemia. Bone Marrow Transplant 1989;4(Suppl 1):9–12.

81. Greaves MF. Differentiated-linked leukemogenesis in lymphocytes. Science 1986;234:796–802.

82. Kersey JH, Weisdorf D, Nesbit ME, et al. Comparison of autologous and allogeneic bone marrow transplanation for

treatment of high risk refractory acute lymphoblastic leukemia. N Engl J Med 1987;317:461–467.

83. Buckner CD, Sanders JE, Hill R, et al. Allogeneic versus autologous marrow transplantation for patients with acute lymphoblastic leukemia in first or second marrow remission. In: Dicke KA, Spitzer G, Jagannath S, Evinger-Hodges MJ, eds. Autologous bone marrow transplantation. Proceedings of the Fourth International Symposium. The University of Texas, M. D. Anderson Cancer Center, 1989:145–149.

84. Zintl F, Hermann J, Fuchs D, et al. Comparison of allogeneic and autologous bone marrow transplantation for treatment of acute lymphocytic leukemia in childhood. In: Buchner T, Schellong G, Hiddemann W, Ritter J, eds. Haematology and blood transfusion, vol 33. Acute leukemias II. Berlin: Springer-Verlag, 1990:692–698.

85. Blaise D, Gaspard MH, Stoppa AM, et al. Allogeneic or autologous bone marrow transplantation for acute lymphoblastic leukemia in first complete remission. Bone Marrow Transplant 1990;5:7–12.

86. Uderzo C, Colleselli P, Dini G, et al. An Italian study comparing allogeneic and autologous BMT in childhood acute lymphoblastic leukemia using HD-vincristine, F-TBI and cyclophosphamide. Bone Marrow Transplant 1991; 7(Suppl 3):19–21.

87. Cahn JY, Bordigoni P, Souillet G, et al. The TAM regimen prior to allogeneic and autologous bone marrow transplantation for high risk acute lymphoblastic leukemias: a cooperative study of 62 patients. Bone Marrow Transplant 1991; 7:1–4.

88. Weisdorf D. Nesbit ME, Ramsay NKC, et al. Allogeneic bone marrow transplantation for acute lymphoblastic leukemia in remission: prolonged survival associated with acute-graft-vs-host disease. J Clin Oncol 1987;5:1348–1355.

89. Tiley C, Powles R, Treleaven J, et al. Feasibility and efficacy of maintenance chemotherapy following autologous bone marrow transplantation for first remission acute lymphoblastic leukaemia. Bone Marrow Transplant 1993;12(5): 449–455.

90. Weisdorf DJ, Anderson P, Blazar B, et al. Interleukin-2 immediately after autologous marrow transplantation toxicity, T cell activation and engraftment. Blood 1991;78 (Suppl 1):226a.

91. Carey PJ, Proctor SJ, Taylor P, et al. Autologous bone marrow transplantation for high-grade lymphoid malignancy using melphalan/irradiation conditioning without marrow purging or cryopreservation. The Northern Regional Bone Marrow Transplant Group. Blood 1991;77:1593–1598.

92. Keating A, Crump M. High dose etoposide melphalan, total body irradiation and ABMT for acute myeloid leukemia in first remission. Leukemia 1992;6(Suppl 4):90–91.

93. Rizzoli V, Mangoni L. Pharmacological-mediated purging with mafosfamide in acute and chronic myeloid leukemias. In: Gross S, Gee AP, Worthington-White DA, eds. Bone marrow purging and processing. New York: Alan Liss, 1989;333.

94. Gorin NC, Labopin M, Meloni G, et al. Autologous bone marrow transplantation for acute myelocytic leukemia in Europe. Further evidence of the role of marrow purging by mafosfamide. Leukemia 1991;5(10):896–904.

95. Yeager AM, Rowley SD, Jones RJ, Kaizer H, Davis JM, Colvin OM, Santos GW. Autologous transplantation with chemopurged bone marrow in patients with acute myelocytic leukemia in second and third remission. In: Dicke KA,

Armitage JO, Dicke-Evinger MJ, eds. Autologous bone marrow transplantation. Proceedings of the Fifth International Symposium, vol 5, Omaha: University of Nebraska, 1990:151–160.

96. Carella AM, Gaozza E, Santini G, et al. Autologous unpurged bone marrow transplantation for acute non-lymphoblastic leukemia in first complete remission. Bone Marrow Transplant 1988;3:537–541.

97. Carella AM, Berman E, Maraone MP, Ganzina T. Idarubicin in the treatment of acute leukaemias: an overview of preclinical and clinical studies. Haematologica 1990;75: 1–11.

98. Beelen DW, Quabeck K, Graeven U, Sayer HG, Mahmoud HK, Schaefer UW. Acute toxicity and first clinical results of intensive postinduction therapy using a modified busulfan and cyclophosphamide regimen with autologous bone marrow rescue in first remission of acute myeloid leukemia. Blood 1989;74(5):1507–1516.

99. Bjorkstrand B, Ljungman P, Malm C, Vikrot O, Robert KH, Gahrton G. Autologous bone marrow transplantation with unpurged marrow in acute nonlymphoblastic leukemia. In: Dicke KA, Armitage JO, Dicke-Evinger MJ, eds. Autologous bone marrow transplantation. Proceedings of the Fifth International Symposium, vol 5. Omaha: University of Nebraska, 1990:151–160.

100. Meloni G, De Fabritiis P, Petti MC, Mandelli F. BAVC regimen and autologous bone marrow transplantation in patients with acute myelogeneous leukemia in second remission. Blood 1990;75(12):2282–2285.

101. Spinolo JA, Dicke KA, Horwitz LJ, Jagannath S, McCredie K, et al. High dose chemotherapy and unpurged autologous bone marrow transplantation for acute leukemia in second or subsequent remission. Cancer 1990;66:619–626.

102. Lenarsky C, Weinberg K, Petersen J, Nolta J, Brooks J, et al. Autologous bone marrow transplantation with 4-hydroperoxycyclophosphamide purged marrow for children with acute non-lynphoblastic leukemia in second remission. Bone Marrow Transplant 1990;6:425–429.

103. Selvaggi KJ, Wilson J, Mills LE, Cornwell III GG, Hurd D, et al. Improved outcome for high-risk AML using autologous bone marrow transplantation and monoclonal antibody purged bone marrow. In: Dicke KA, Keating A, eds. Proceedings of the Sixth International Autologous Bone Marrow Transplantation, Houston, Texas, December 2–3. 1992.

104. Stoppa AM, Hirn J, Blaise D, et al. Autologous bone marrow transplantation for B cell malignancies after in vitro purging with floating immunobeads. Bone Marrow Transplant 1990;6:307–307.

105. Weisdorf DJ, Kersey JH, Ramsay NKC. Unpublished data, 1992.

106. Schroeder H, Pinkerton CR, Powles RL, et al. High dose melphalan and total body irradiation with autologous marrow rescue in childhood acute lymphoblastic leukaemia after relapse. Bone Marrow Transplant 1991;7:11–15.

107. Soiffer RJ, Billett AL, Roy DC, et al. Autologous bone marrow transplantation for acute lymphoblastic leukemia in second or subsequent complete remission: ten years experience at Dana Farber Cancer Institute. In: Dicke KA, Armitage JO, Dicke-Evinger MJ, eds. Autologous bone marrow transplantation. Proceedings of the Fifth International Symposium, vol 5. Omaha, University of Nebraska, 1990: 151–160.

108. Aurer I, Gale RP. Are new conditioning regimens for transplants in acute myelogenous leukemia better? Bone Marrow Transplant 1991;7:255–261.

109. Weiden PL, Sullivan KM, Flournoy N, Storb R, Thomas ED. Anti-leukemic effect of chronic graft versus host disease. Contribution to improved survival after allogeneic bone marrow transplantation. N Engl J Med 1979;304: 1529–1533.

110. Weiden PL, Sullivan KM, Flournoy N, Storb R, Thomas ED. Antileukemia effects of graft-verus-host disease in human recipients of allogeneic-marrow grafts. N Engl J Med 1979;300;1068–1073.

111. Drobyski WR, Keever CA, Roth MS, et al. Salvage immunotherapy using donor leukocyte infusions as treatment for relapsed chronic myelogenous leukemia after allogeneic bone marrow transplantation: efficacy and toxicity of a defined T-cell dose. Blood 1993;82(8):2310–2318.

112. Jones RJ, Vogelsang GB, Hess AD, et al. Induction of graft versus host disease after autologous bone marrow transplantation. Lancet 1989;1:754–757.

113. Talbot DC, Powles RL, Sloane JP, et al. Cyclosporin-induced graft versus host disease following autologous bone marrow transplantation for acute myeloid leukemia. Bone Marrow Transplant 1990;6:17–20.

114. Yeager AM, Vogelsang GB, Jones RJ, Farmer ER, Hess AD, Santos GW. Cyclosporin-induced graft-versus-host disease after autologous bone marrow transplantation for acute myeloid leukemia. Leuk Lymphoma 1993;11:215–220.

CHAPTER 41

Allogeneic Transplantation

SAMUEL GROSS, FRED APPLEBAUM*

> For extreme diseases, extreme strictness of treatment is most efficacious.
> —Hippocrates, 480 BC

Bone marrow transplantation (BMT) is not a hematologic disease entity, but its therapeutic application has such profound influence on our understanding of the biology of so many hematologic disorders that it stands alone in any modern text. Its efficacy is truly outstanding and is underscored by more than 5000 procedures/year involving allogeneic (including syngeneic) bone marrow transplants in the 1990–1995 interval. Even more impressive is the fact that the number of transplants performed during this period probably reflects approximately 50% of all eligible candidates (fig. 41.1).

This modality, pioneered by the relentless efforts of E. Donnall Thomas and colleagues (1), has had a profound effect on a broad range of hematologic disorders. As improvements in efficacy permit further expansion of BMT into new investigative areas, so, too, will we expand our knowledge of the biology of hematopoiesis.

Allogeneic Bone Marrow Transplantation

A 16-year-old Caucasian male had a 2-week history of low-grade fevers, malaise, dry cough, and increasing neck size. At the physician's office, he appeared to be moderately ill and had the following vital signs: T, 39°C; P, 100/min; R, 28/min. He had enlarged, nontender, anterior cervical, submandibular, and submental lymph nodes; nonexudative, enlarged pharyngeal tonsils; and a slightly protuberant abdomen with nontender, enlarged liver and spleen. The remainder of his examination, including the cardiopulmonary evaluation, was normal. There were no obvious neurologic abnormalities and no evidence of papilledema.

His past medical history was unrevealing. His immunizations were up to date, and he had no unusual illnesses or exposures to real or possible leukemogens (e.g., benzene, cigarettes, high-tension wires). He lived with his mother, his stepfather, and his stepfather's biologic children. He had no related siblings, and his biologic father's whereabouts were unknown.

Laboratory values were as follows: Hgb, 127 g/L; Hct, 37%; red blood cell count, 4.45×10^{12}/L; platelet count, 147×10^9/L; white blood cell count, 97×10^9/L. His peripheral blood film contained 48% "primitive forms,"

most of which appeared to be L2 lymphoblasts. (Actual ratio 80% L2 :20% L1 (2–4).)

His urinalysis was normal, and the only untoward chemistries were an LDH of 3200 IU/dL and a serum uric acid level of 15.3 mg/dL. His chest films revealed impressive anterior confluency in the hilar area, typical of lymph node enlargement. All viral studies, including the human immunodeficiency virus (HIV), cytomegalovirus (CMV), and hepatitis screen, were negative.

The presumptive generic diagnosis of acute lymphocytic leukemia (ALL) was confirmed by a bone marrow aspirate that was 80% replaced by peroxidase- and esterase-negative and periodic acid–Schiff and terminal deoxytransferase-positive FAB L2 cells. On flow cytometry, the cells immunotyped positive for CD-2, CD-5, and CD-7. Cell cycle analysis revealed a tetraploid population, 14% of which were in S phase. Chromosomal typing revealed pseudodiploidy and a clonal abnormality of t(11;14). His DNA index was 1.2.

The cerebrospinal fluid contained numerous cells with cytologic and immunologic characteristics identical to the primitive elements in the marrow.

Blood, sputum, urine, and cerebrospinal fluid cultures were negative for bacterial growth.

The working diagnosis was acute T-cell lymphoblastic leukemia, ostensibly originating in the thymus, with spread to lymphatic tissue, bone marrow, and leptomeninges. The markedly increased uric acid and LDH levels underscored the rapidity of cell turnover and breakdown.

Because of his age and the excessive tumor burden, he was considered to be at high risk for early relapse; and preparations were made to follow induction therapy with a BMT. The induction therapy consisted of daily oral prednisone, every-other-day subcutaneous L-asparaginase for 9 doses, and four consecutive weekly intravenous doses of vincristine and daunomycin. Marrow reevaluation was planned for days 14 and 28 of the induction initiative. Combination intrathecal methotrexate, cytosine arabinoside, and hydrocortisone was scheduled for four weekly doses followed by monthly doses thereafter, depending on the time sequence of marrow transplantation. Craniospinal irradiation, which is appropriate for all newly diagnosed patients with CNS disease at presentation, was designed to be included in the total body irradiation (TBI) portion of the BMT preparative regimen.

*Section on Multiple Myeloma

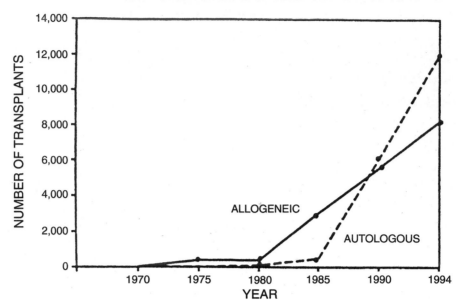

Figure 41.1. Annual numbers of allogenic and autologous transplants worldwide.

Table 41.1. HLA of Propositus and Step Relationship Compared with Theoretical Full-Sibling Relationships

		Stepparent and Sibling Relationships			
Mother	Stepfather	Patient	Step Sibling[a]	Step Sibling[a]	
A_2/A_{11}	A_1/ACW_{19}	A_2/A_9	$A_1/—$	AW_{19}/A_{28}	
B_{15}/BW_{46}	B_5/B_{14}	B_{15}/B_{35}	B_5/B_{12}	B_{14}/B_7	
DR_5/DR_9	DRW_6/DR_9	DR_5/DR_9	DRW_6/DRW_{10}	DR_9/DR_2	
		Theoretical Full Biologic Relationships			
Mother	Father	Patient	Sibling A	Sibling B	Sibling C
A_2/A_{11}	A_1/Aw_{19}	A_2/A_1	A_{11}/AW_{19}	A_2/A_1	A_2/AW_{19}
B_{15}/BW_{46}	B_5/B_{14}	B_{15}/B_5	BW_{46}/B_{14}	B_{15}/B_5	B_{15}/B_{14}
DR_5/DR_9	DRW_6/DR_9	DR_5/DRW_6	$DR_9/—$	DR_5/DRW_{16}	DR_5/DR_9

[a]The stepfather's first wife, the mother of the propositus' step siblings, was an A_9/A_{28}, B_{12}/B_7, DRW_{10}/DR_2 genotype.

The serious likelihood of chemotherapy-induced urate nephropathy occurring in a highly susceptible host prompted the initiation of aggressive pretherapy use of oral allopurinol and intravenous alkalinization to block further uric acid production and increase solubility, respectively. Despite these efforts, along with chemotherapy dose reductions, renal failure ensued, and hemodialysis was required to continue with the planned therapeutic regimens.

Over the ensuing 2 weeks, his course was marked by hypertensive swings, seizures, high fevers, and severe depression, as well as therapy-induced pancytopenia and painful mouth ulcers. All were treated symptomatically and without interruptions in chemotherapy. Six weeks later he was in complete hematologic, CNS, and clinical remission. Moreover, he had neither disease nor treatment-related organ dysfunction. In the remote likelihood that he would be haploidentical with his mother, the entire family was HLA typed. The results of the (non)match compared with a theoretic sibling match prompted a search for a matched unrelated donor (table 41.1).

HLA Typing and Histocompatibility

Although tissue typing is detailed in the HLA-typing chapter (39), a brief recapitulation is in order. The antigenic material of the major histocompatibility complex (MHC) resides in three regions, or classes (I, II, and III), on the short arm of chromosome 6. The polymorphic multiply-allelic forms of the class I genes, designated HLA-A, -B, and -C, are, like the class III genes, identified by serologic assays, or when batched, by isoelectric focusing. Class I group, HLA-E, -F, and -G, are as yet functionally unknown. The class II genes, which encode for HLA-DR, -DQ, and -DP, as well as a number of lesser-known histocompatibility genes, are identified by restriction length polymorphism fragment (RLPF) or polymerase chain reaction (PCR) assays. The class III region, positioned between the class I and II sites, contains the genes for tumor necrosis factor (TNF-α) certain of the complement factors, and a number of non-histocompatibility-related genes (5–10). Figure 41.2 is a map of the histocompatibility complex area.

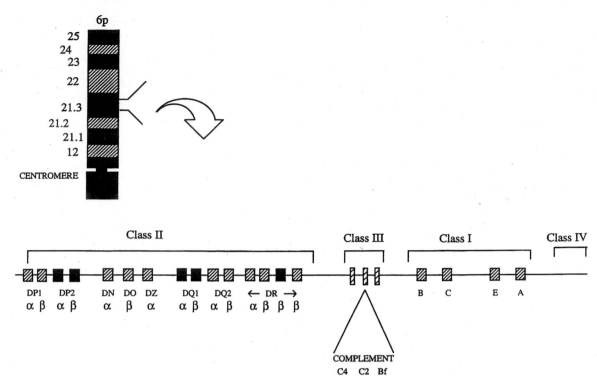

Figure 41.2. Human histocompatibility complex. Gene map of the human major histocompatibility complex on the short arm of chromosome 6. Genes that encode for class I or class II molecules are shown in black; cross-hatched areas are either pseudogenes (such as DP2α and β) or their function is uncertain, the area between DP and DQ is a high mutation and cross-over region.

Inheritance of the HLA haplotype, the genetic unit on the chromosome, is codominant. The HLA genotype is, in effect, a paired haplotype, and each offspring is a composite of one maternal and one paternal haplotype.

Alloreactivity, the generic term for the mixed leukocyte reaction/culture (MLR/MLC), is the capacity of class II material (HLA-D region) to induce T-cell activation (11–14). In this context, peripheral blood mononuclear cells from the antigen-presenting donor (stimulator) cells are irradiated to prevent proliferation (activation); cell proliferation in the responder cells is measured by labeled thymidine uptake. The direction deliberately chosen in the mixed leukocyte reaction determines the direction of action: recipient cell proliferation supports graft rejection; donor cell proliferation supports graft-versus-host disease (GVHD). However, greater predictive reliability is provided by RLPF and/or PCR sequence-specific oligonucleotide probes (SSOP), which eliminate the need for the MLC test and, in the process, streamline the unrelated donor screening time (15, 16).

The minor histocompatibility antigens (mHs) play a major reactivity role and must be reckoned with in every allo-BMT, particularly in unrelated, matched BMTs because of their role in contributing to the severity of GVHD. Fully compatible sibling matches share upward of 50% of the mH antigens, compared with no more than 10% in the unrelated matches (17).

While awaiting the results of the donor search, consolidation therapy was instituted. The rationale for con- *solidation therapy prior to BMT and as a constitutive process in non-BMT regimens is discussed further.*

Pre-BMT Induction and Consolidation Therapy

Other than the need to initiate tumor reduction therapy and the time involved in identifying a donor, the rationale for induction therapy is based on the assumption that a lesser tumor burden will enhance the effectiveness of the BMT preparative regimen and thereby increase the efficacy of the BMT. This rule applies whether the process involves first or later pre-BMT remission plans, and in principle it is sound. At the time of diagnosis, a fairly constant number of tumor cells, 25–30%, not to be confused with a much smaller number of multidrug-resistant cells (MDRs), is in G_0. It is postulated that in newly diagnosed and possibly in second remission patients as well, approximately 4–6 weeks of highly aggressive, albeit nonmarrow ablative, therapy will reduce the tumor mass by more than 90% (18–20). An additional 90% kill follows upon the transplantation treatment, which includes the effects of both (a) the preparative regimen on circulating cells and cells reentering from G_0 and (b) immune-modulated killing by donor lymphocytes, the latter presumably capable of also eliminating MDR cells. There are no easily interpreted concurrent studies that compare allo-BMT immediately following the diagnosis of ALL, or other hematopoietic malignancies, with BMT following induction of remission. The only suggestive evidence in support of the latter comes from data that show greater BMT cure rates following successful induction therapy in second remissions than in those transplanted after multiple relapses or with "resistant" disease (21). However, resistant disease is not the same as untreated early relapse, a condition that is probably no different than an apparent remission. In all likelihood, therefore, BMT is not the sole factor in effecting cure but rather the combination of both transplantation of leukemia-free cells and an antileukemic process as in a graft-versus-leukemia (GVL) effect (22).

Consolidation (or intensification) therapy, therefore, in the non-pre-BMT mode, is a mop-up process designed to rid tumor-burdened patients of residual tumor cells that may escape induction therapy. There are sufficient studies in support of such an approach in high-risk patients who do not go to BMT.

In this case, however, the intensification therapy offered little that the BMT per se could offer. It was essentially "filler" therapy designed to serve as a bulwark while waiting for the successful conclusion of the unrelated-donor search.

At the completion of 4 weeks of consolidation therapy, maintenance-dose-escalating treatment with weekly methotrexate, daily 6-mercaptopurine, in addition to intrathecal medication, was initiated. Six weeks into maintenance therapy a 45-year-old, HLA-identical, nonparous, female donor was identified, and preparations were made to start the BMT countdown.

Transplantation and Environmental Factors

Certain intangibles, including differences between health care providers, contribute to outcome differences; for example, large- versus small-volume programs, the variable use of laminar flow rooms, gut sterilization, response to fevers, use of cytokines, and GVHD prophylaxis/control. For example, studies of clinical outcome in children with acute myelogenous leukemia (AML) revealed the best event-free survival when treatment was carried out in protocol-driven studies by physicians with expertise in treating such diseases. This also applies to adolescents treated in pediatric cooperative group programs. Standardization of survival reports is also a much-needed process. Event-free survival and leukemia-free survival are terms that should be used consistently and appropriately so as not to lend obscurity or uncertainty to the data. The environment can affect treatment. Aspergillus is a constant companion of the hospital duct system in the southern (subtropical) areas and in all sites of construction-produced dust. Air flow facilities must always be calculated in determining risk, not so much in terms of the decision to transplant or not, but how to handle the patient in the transplantation site. In summary, the conditions under which data are obtained must be identified and kept constant to develop a well-characterized risk factor profile in

every therapeutic phase and in every therapeutic arena, with programs carried out by experienced personnel working in stable high-volume sites.

The Decision to Transplant: Predictive Factors

The decision to transplant following relapse is a powerful factor in virtually every hematologic malignancy, but the role of BMT as *initial* therapy is a far more selective process.

In this instance, the decision to transplant in first remission was based on the following information:

1. A teenager with karyotypic pseudodiploidy, t(11;14) and high-volume FAB L2 T-cell ALL has
    a. A less than 30% chance for a 3-year disease-free survival (DFS) with chemotherapy or combination chemoradiotherapy.
    b. A greater than 60% chance for long-term DFS leading to cure following allo-BMT in first remission.
2. In the decades commencing in 1975
    a. Knowledge of GVHD and toxicity control, as well as GVL exploitation, had a positive impact on allo-BMT outcome.
    b. The unrelated (especially Caucasian) donor pool had expanded to such an extent that finding a donor in less than 4 months (often within 2 months) is readily achievable.
    c. Autologous reinfusion of either purged or unpurged marrow (auto-BMT) offered a significantly lesser chance than allo-BMT for long-term DFS in second or later remission.

The choice also preceded recent promising studies on (a) the use of "positively" selected marrow precursors and (b) mechanisms of GVL induction in auto-BMT (23, 24).

The outcome data on allo-BMT in first and later remissions in both malignant and nonmalignant hematopoietic disorders are reviewed below.

The Rationale for BMT: Outcome Analyses

ALL

The overall mean DFS for ALL patients in early relapse or second remission treated with allo-BMT is 45% (range, 15–60%). ALL patients in third or greater remission or with resistant relapse can expect a less than 20% DFS (range, 10–30%). The results are much better for patients who receive allo-BMT in first remission (i.e., >60% DFS). Age is a factor, however. For patients above 17 years of age at diagnosis, the 5-year DFS is 45%; and for those under 17 years of age, DFS approaches 70%. In essence, all adults and approximately one-third (slightly more if 21 years is the pediatric age cutoff) of the pediatric patients are first remission allo-BMT candidates. The reason for the age-related difference in outcome, all other factors being consistent, is unclear. Other factors that play a favorable role include presence of GVHD (GVL), minimal residual toxicity from prior therapy, infection-free BMT transplant interval, and possibly hyperfractionation of the irradiation regimen (25–41). Figures 41.3 and 41.4 show the result of allo- and auto-BMT for ALL.

AML

BMT is the treatment of choice for all pediatric AML patients in first remission and is no less preferred for newly diagnosed adult AML (less than 60 years of age) as well. Aggressive chemotherapy programs in adult AML approach, but are not on par with, the efficacy of BMT. Overall, DFS is 55%: more than 60% in children, less than 45% in adults versus approximately 30% for solely chemotherapy-treated individuals (42–58). Figures 41.5 and 41.6 show the result of allo- and auto-BMT for AML.

Myelodysplasia and Myeloproliferative Diseases

The myelodysplasias, in accordance with the FAB classification, include refractory anemia, refractive anemia with

ringed sideroblasts, refractory anemia with excess blasts, refractory anemia with excess blasts in transformation (as well as the hypoplastic form of these disorders). Most of the myelodysplasias terminate as AML within months to several years, and because of the dyspoietic nature of these disorders, conventional chemotherapy is rarely if ever effective. The use of granulocyte and granulocyte-monocyte cytokines to induce hematopoietic maturation has met with variable success at best in all but refractory anemia and refractory anemia with ringed sideroblasts (59–61). Erythropoietin has been even less successful in decreasing transfusion requirements in most of these disorders (62). As noted in Chapter 24, danazol, interleukin-3 (IL-3), and cis-retinoic have also been used with minimal-to-average success (63–65).

Overall, the treatment of choice, with specific exceptions, is allo-BMT, with which the subgroup-dependent DFS rate is approximately 50% (40–65%). However, patients with refractory anemia with excess blasts do not respond as well to allo-BMT as do those in the other subgroups (66, 67). Among the most effective preparative regimens are fractionated TBI (fTBI) with either cyclophosphamide and etoposide, fTBI with cytosine arabinoside (Ara-C), or busulfan in combination with cyclophosphamide (BuCy) (68–72).

Myeloproliferative disorders include (adult and juvenile forms of) chronic myelogenous anemia, essential thrombo-

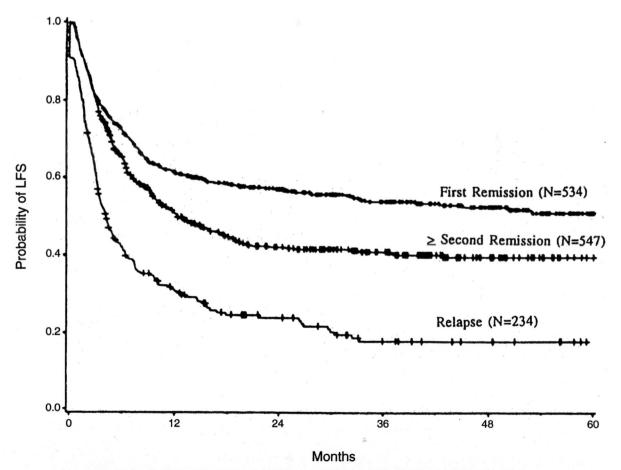

Months

Figure 41.3 Probability of LFS after HLA-identical sibling bone marrow transplants for ALL.

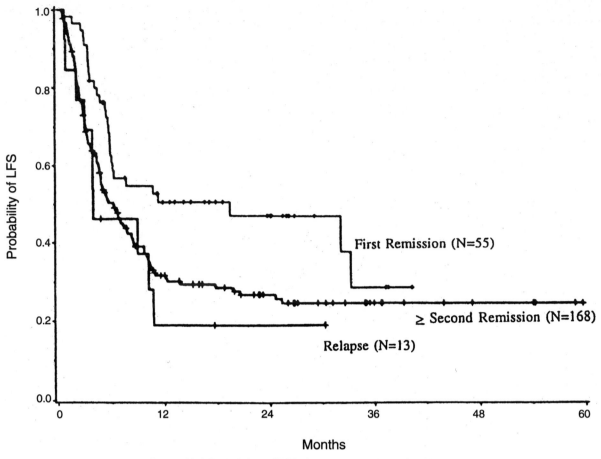

Figure 41.4 Probability of LFS after autotransplants for ALL.

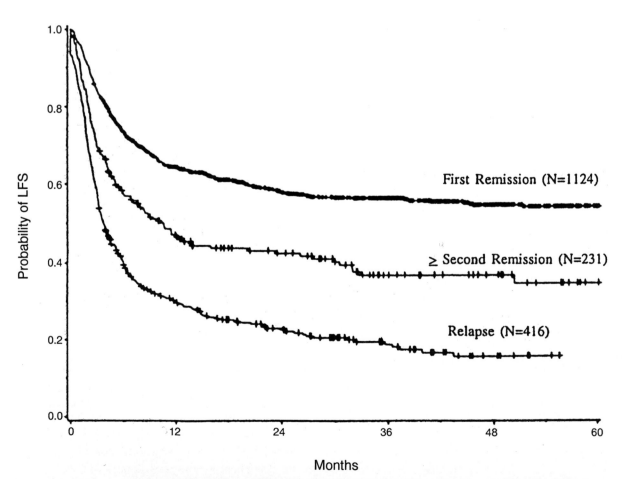

Figure 41.5 Probability of LFS after HLA-identical sibling bone marrow transplant for AML.

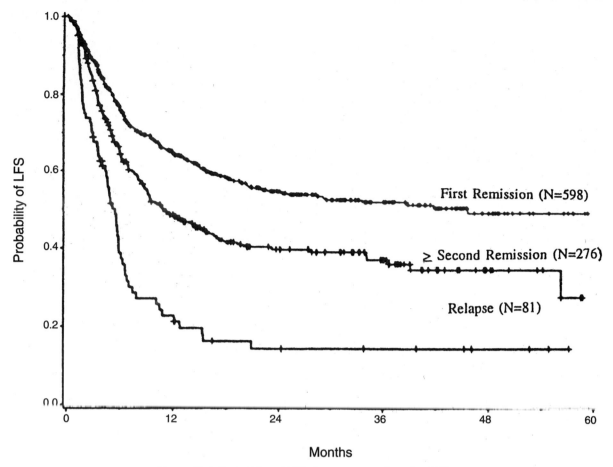

Figure 41.6 Probability of LFS after autotransplants for AML.

cytosis, agnogenic myeloid metaplasia/myelofibrosis, and polycythemia vera, most or all of which ultimately convert to an acute myelogenous type of leukemia. Because of the later average age of onset for all but the chronic myelogenous leukemia (CML) groups and the fact that supportive therapy is moderately effective in this older group of patients, allo-BMT is more commonly used in CML (73–77).

The juvenile and adult forms of CML are detailed in the chapter on chronic myelogenous leukemia. In brief, allo-BMT is the treatment of choice for CML, with best results in first chronic phase (fig. 41.7) (78–80). Patients transplanted less than 1 year after diagnosis have an 80% chance for 5-year DFS, compared with 62% for those transplanted more than 3 years after diagnosis. As in all leukemic disorders, the younger the patient, the better the overall post-allo-BMT outcome. Preparative regimens that include fTBI and control the severity of GVHD tend to be most effective. Table 41.2 summarizes the features of allo-BMT in first chronic phase CML.

In terms of GVHD control, ex vivo purging of donor marrow with anti CD-8 monoclonal antibody–coated microspheres effectively reduces the incidence of GVHD without apparent loss of the GVL effect, a process that is further enhanced by the use of cyclosporine A during the immediate posttransplant interval. On the other hand, pan-T-cell removal, either by elutriation or immunologic techniques, is more likely to induce greater frequency of graft failure.

Matched unrelated donor (MUD) transplants have also been successfully carried out in CML, but GVHD-related complications continue to be a major issue (81–95).

Multiple Myeloma

Allo-BMT

Less than 5% of conventionally treated patients live 10 years (96), and among these, almost all have suffered multiple relapses. Among the first seven patients treated in Seattle with cyclophosphamide (CY) and TBI, two remained alive without evidence of disease 8 and 15 years after transplant. Both long-term survivors had failed conventional therapy with prednisone and alkylating agents prior to transplant, thereby providing the first compelling evidence that high-dose therapy made possible with marrow transplantation may, indeed, cure multiple myeloma (97).

Table 41.3 summarizes several recently published studies of marrow transplantation for myeloma. Among 90 patients transplanted in the European Group for Bone Marrow Transplantation (EBMT) and followed for up to 7 years, the complete response (CR) rate was 43%, the overall survival at 5 years was 40%, and the DFS was 31% (98). Patients who were chemosensitive prior to transplant and those who had received only one previous regimen fared better than those who had failed multiple

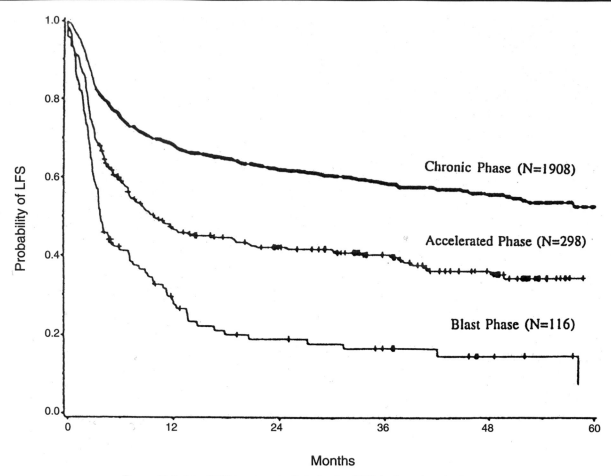

Figure 41.7 Allo-BMT treatment of choice for CML in first chronic phase.

Table 41.2. Allogeneic BMT in First Chronic Phase CML

1. >70% chance for long-term DFS if BMT carried out ≤1 year postdiagnosis with HLA-matched sibling donor
2. Same risk factors apply for matched unrelated donors, but with overall lower DFS
3. Syngeneic BMT and pan T depletion in allo-BMT result in 3-fold increase in risk for relapse
4. T cell subset (CD-8) depletion decreases risk of GVHD; it also increases risk of engraftment failure but does not increase risk of relapse.
5. f TBI/cyclophosphamide, f TBI-etoposide, and busulfan/cyclophosphamide are commonly used preparative regimens with essentially similar results

regimens. Similar results have been published by others. For example, in a Seattle study of allo-BMT for 50 patients with recurrent myeloma using a BuCy preparative regimen, the overall survival at 50 months was 30% and the DFS, 34%. The average age of these 50 patients was 43 years. The group included 3 recipients of unrelated marrow (1 alive at 4.6 years) and 5 recipients of 1-antigen-mismatched marrow (3 alive at 6.0, 4.4, and 1.6 years) (99). As in other situations, survival was better for patients transplanted in untreated first relapse or with chemotherapy-responsive disease, who have a probability of survival of 52% at 5 years. Of particular importance is the observation that both the EBMT report and the Seattle data suggest a plateau in DFS for patients beyond 3 years from transplant. Similar results have been reported from Italy and Vancouver (100, 101).

Unpurged Auto-BMT

Based on encouraging results achieved with high-dose alkylating agents alone or combined with syngeneic or allogeneic marrow, trials of high-dose therapy followed by unpurged auto-BMT were initiated in the early 1980s. Gore (101) and Jagannath (102), in separate studies, showed that high-dose melphalan, either alone or combined with TBI, followed by autologous marrow, could achieve CR rates of 10–30% in patients with recurrent myeloma. A summary from the French Registry reported on 120 patients treated with several regimens, mostly melphalan and TBI, with autologous marrow support, and showed a 35% CR rate with 50% partial responses and 3-year survival and DFS of 65% and 21%, respectively (103). As with allogeneic transplantation, responses were

Table 41.3. Selected Studies of Marrow Transplantation for Multiple Myeloma

Source	No.	Disease Status		Regimen		Outcome	
Allo-BMT							
EBMT 98	90	Responsive	57	Chemo + TBI	81	CR	= 43%
		Resistant	33	Chemo	9	DFS at 3 years	= 31%
Seattle 99	50	Responsive	16	BuCy	50	CR	= 42%
		Resistant	44			DFS at 4 years	= 34%
Italian 100	27	Responsive	13	Chemo + TBI	19	CR	= 58%
		Resistant	14	Chemo	8	DFS at 2 years	= 38%
Vancouver 101	17	Responsive	13	Chemo + TBI	4	CR	= 48%
		Resistant	4	BuCy	13	DFS at 3 years	= 44%
ABMT							
Barlogie 102	169	"Good risk"	114	Chemo + TBI	57	CR	= 18%
		"Poor risk"	55	Melphalan	112	Median survival	
						Good risk, 52 months	
						Poor risk, 18 months	
MD Anderson 104	49	Responsive	11	Chemo + TBI	31	Responses	= 61%
		Resistant	38	Chemo	18	Median remission	
						duration	= 12 months
Attal 105	35	Newly diagnosed		Chemo + TBI	35	CR	= 43%
						Survival at 42 months	= 81%
Attal 106	88	Newly diagnosed		Combined chemo	50	DFS at 30 months	= 10%
				Chemo + ABMT	38	DFS at 30 months	= 67%
APBT							
Fernand 109	43	Responsive	19	Chemo + TBI	43	CR	= 19%
		Resistant	24			Overall survival at 4 years	= 73%

more frequent in patients transplanted earlier in the disease course. The Royal Marsden Hospital Group, for example, used high-dose melphalan with autologous marrow support as consolidation therapy for 53 patients with myeloma and reported a very low treatment-related mortality (2%), a 5-year survival of 63%, and a DFS of 36% at 36 months (101). Similar results were published by Attal et al. The French Intergroup randomized 200 newly diagnosed patients to treatment with either conventional chemotherapy or chemotherapy followed by auto-BMT and reported significantly higher response rates (P < .01) and response duration (P < .01) in the transplant group and a trend toward longer overall survival (P = .08). None of these trials, however, showed a plateau on the disease-free survival curve (104–106). In contrast, others have failed to identify a survival benefit in a comparison of outcomes of auto-BMT in patients with refractory myeloma late in the course of the disease with those of nonrandomized controls (107).

Purged Auto-BMT

Studies using monoclonal antibodies, immunotoxins, or 4-hydroperoxycylophosphamide as purging agents, despite their ability to remove several logs of phenotypically obvious myeloma cells without loss of engraftment, have not demonstrated a lower incidence of tumor recurrence (108).

Peripheral Blood Stem Cells

Fernand et al. (109), in a study of 43 patients given TBI together with one or more alkylators followed by peripheral blood stem cell transplants, cite projected 4-year survival and DFS rates of 73% and 55%, respectively. Marit, Gianni, and Barlogie have reported similar results, albeit in smaller numbers of patients and with more-limited follow-up.

Marrow transplantation should be a consideration for every patient under age 55 for whom a matched related (and, probably, unrelated) donor can be found with a reasonable approach that (a) considers transplantation up front for patients with prognostic factors that predict a poorer response to conventional therapy (i.e., light-chain disease, high Durie stage, high β2-microglobulin, high DNA labeling index, or plasmablast morphology) and (b) delays transplantation until first relapse for patients with favorable prognostic factors.

There is also evidence that autologous transplantation can be carried out with relative safety and results in a substantial antitumor response, making continued study of this approach appropriate, both as consolidation therapy in patients without donors with high-risk disease and in those with responsive but recurrent disease. However, there is mounting evidence that autologous transplantation for patients with resistant disease more than 1 year from diagnosis is of little benefit, at least given the current state of the art. Future directions include the development of preparative regimens with greater antitumor effects, including the use of targeted therapy employing, for example, antibody-radionuclide conjugates or aminophosphonic acid–radionuclide conjugates. In animal models and in phase I studies in man, it has been demonstrated that severalfold more radiotherapy can be delivered to tumor with this approach than with routine external-beam TBI. Other approaches include the development of posttransplant immunotherapy using alpha interferon (IFN-α), IL-2, or immunotherapy directed against a specific myeloma idiotype (96–109).

Lymphomas and Chronic Lymphocytic Leukemia

Although many more autografts than allografts have been carried out in lymphomas, allo-BMT appears to be more beneficial than auto-BMT for the same reasons that allo-BMT is preferred to auto-BMT in the leukemias, that is, the problems of residual disease and lack of GVL effect, respectively. This approach applies both to aggressive non-Hodgkins and relapsed Hodgkins lymphomas. Data on the efficacy of allo-BMT for chronic lymphocytic leukemia (CLL) are incomplete at present, but in theory at least, they may well prove to be the treatment of choice in all but poor risks and the elderly (110–116). Support for this assumption is forthcoming from recent data on the use of allo-BMT for CLL comparing all patients with patients in stages 0–III and those who are stage IV (fig. 41.8).

AIDS

The role of BMT in patients affected with HIV is not auspicious. However, there is ample reason to pursue its use as a therapeutic modality. The underlying rationale is the theoretic possibility of allografting a clone of immunocompetent cells in a manner similar to that effected in patients with severe combined immunodeficiency diseases (SCID) (117, 118). Unfortunately, residual virus continues to be a major obstacle.

Nonmalignant Disorders of Hematopoietic Tissue

As indicated in other chapters, allo-BMT is the treatment of choice for thalassemia major, high-risk sickle cell disease, refractory red cell and platelet hypoplasias/aplasias, paroxysmal nocturnal hemoglobinuria, congenital or ac-

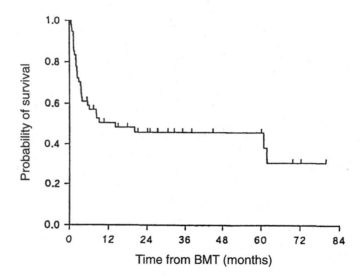

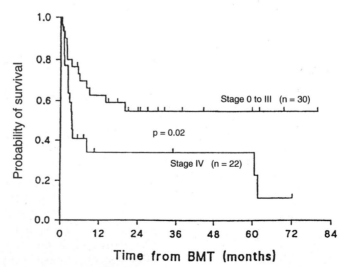

Figure 41.8 Probability of leukemia-free survival after HLA-identical sibling BMT for chronic lymphocytic leukemia.

quired aplastic anemias, certain of the storage disorders unresponsive to enzyme replacement therapy, and a host of lymphocytic- and granulocytic-related immune deficiency disorders including SCID, DiGeorge syndrome, Wiskott-Aldrich syndrome, leukocyte adhesion deficiency syndrome, Omenn's syndrome, etoposide-resistant familial erythrophagocytic lymphohistiocytosis, congenital agranulocytosis and Chediak-Higashi syndrome (119–155). Tables 41.4–41.7 list the features of allo-BMT for these disorders.

BMT-related toxicity continues to be the major limiting factor in all patients, irrespective of the diagnosis, with lesser toxicity outcome in patients 17 years of age and younger.

Table 41.4. Allo-BMT for Granulocyte Disorders[a]

Familial etoposide-resistant erythrophagocytic lymphohisto-
cytosis
Severe chronic granulomatous disease
Chediak-Higashi syndrome, granule-deficiency diseases
Congenital agranulocytosis resistant to cytokine therapy

[a]All require aggressive conditioning regimens.

Table 41.5. AlloBMT for Hematologic Disorders[a]

Thalassemia major
Refractory red cell aplasia
Amegakaryocytic disease
Severe aplastic anemias
Severe sickle cell disease[b]
Paroxysmal Nocturnal Hemoglobinuria[c]

[a]All require aggressive conditioning regimens.
[b]One major stroke and/or repeated infections requiring hospitalization; multiple transfusion to correct aplasias or hyperhemolytic disorders.
[c]Leukemic transformation.

Table 41.6. Allogeneic BMT for Storage Disorders

Type	Remarks[a]
Leukodystrophies	
Metachromatic leukodystrophy (MLD)	Conditioning required for all types; results variable
Global cell leukodystrophy	Results better than MLD[b]
Adrenoleukodystrophy	Results variable[b]
Mucopolysaccharidoses (MPS) MPS types I, II, III, IV, and VI	Conditioning required for all types
	Best results in types I and III[b]
Lipodoses	
Gaucher disease (clinically severe type only)	Conditioning required for all types; results favorable[b]
Niemann-Pick	Results variable
GM-1 gangliosidosis	Results poor
Osteoclast malfunction disorder	Conditioning required; results variable

[a]Conditioning regimens must be aggressive.
[b]BMT to be carried out in "responsive" cases once the diagnosis is established.

Table 41.7. Allogeneic BMT for Lymphocyte Deficiency Disorders

Type	Conditioning
Severe combined immune deficiency (SCID) T negative T positive	Conditioning not required for HLA-matched patients
Adenosine deaminase deficiency	BuCy
Full-expression leukocyte adhesion deficiency	BuCy
Major histocompatibility class II deficiency	BuCy, prednisone, Antithymocyte globulin (ATG)
SCID with maternal engraftment	BuCy, prednisone, ATG
Alloresponsive T-positive SCID	BuCy, prednisone, ATG
Less severe combined immune deficiency (CID)	Require aggressive conditioning
B lymphocyte proliferation disease	Etoposide/fTBI
Purine nucleotide phosphorylase deficiency	BuCy
Omenn's disease	Monoclonal Aby
DiGeorge syndrome	ATG/prednisone
Wiskott-Aldrich syndrome	

The Transplant Type: Donor Selection

This patient had no family matched donor, and the decision to seek an unrelated matched donor rather than undertake the use of processed autologous marrow was based on the following information.

Allo-BMT Sources and Auto-BMT

As noted, the ideal donor is an HLA fully matched sibling. The possibility of auto-BMT effectively serving as the appropriate therapeutic arm for first remission ALL is as yet unlikely, because of the proven greater efficacy of allo-BMT. Among the reasons for the excessive relapse rate in the auto-BMT group is lack of GVL effect, although measures (i.e., use of cyclosporine A (CSA) and/or (IL-2)) designed to initiate autocytotoxicity in auto-BMT, may one day eliminate the need for allo-BMT. Syngeneic BMT is similar to auto-BMT in terms of efficacy and lack of GVL effect.

Unrelated Donor Marrow

The first successful use of unrelated-donor BMT was in a child with severe combined immune deficiency (153). In short order this was followed by effective use of unrelated HLA-matched marrow in acute leukemia. Over the ensuing years, additional reports surfaced on the successful use of matched unrelated BMTs in a variety of malignant and nonmalignant hematopoietic disorders including severe congenital or acquired aplastic anemia, a variety of immunologic disorders and certain of the hemoglobinopathies, namely, thalassemia and sickle cell disease (154–160).

Nonconcurrent comparison of matched-unrelated and matched-related donor data derived from the IBMTR on more than 4000 allo-BMTs between 1985 and 1990 (400+ unrelated transplants) showed a 2-year DFS of 44% in the unrelated group versus 50% in the related group. Of particular value was the finding that significant differences in the incidence of severe GVHD (32% in the related group and 57% in the unrelated group) carried over to toxicity-related mortality: 26% related, 45% unrelated. Numerous additional studies have essentially confirmed these observations and, further, showed improved results with improved techniques (161).

Use of unrelated donors phenotypically matched for either 6 of 6 or 5 of 6 HLA-A, -B, -C, and -DR antigens in a variety of high-risk disorders (including advanced-stage leukemia and refractory relapse), second chronic phase CML, blast crisis CML, refractory cytopenia of myelodysplastic diseases, and severe aplastic anemia, continue to provide encouraging data. Patients with 6 of 6 matches have a 25% probability of DFS versus a 15% probability in the 5 of 6 match group. The inordinately high incidence of graft failure (17%) is likely due to underlying problems; that is, it is most commonly seen in patients with aplastic anemia, followed in succession by 4th remission acute leukemias, refractory leukemias, and accelerated chronic-phase CML. As in other similar studies, there were pronounced increases in both severity and frequency of GVHD, with 50% of the deaths as direct consequences of acute GVHD.

Mismatched bone marrow transplants have even less favorable outcomes. In a pooled data study of 102 consecutive CML (first chronic phase) patients (58 mismatched, related; 44 matched, unrelated), there was a 65% DFS for matched and 27% for mismatched donors. The incidence of severe (grades II–IV) GVHD in both unrelated matched and related mismatched groups was, as anticipated, high: 82% and 95%, respectively (83, 162, 163).

Donor Registries and Processing

When an unrelated, matched donor is sought through a donor registry, the results of the class I group testing (HLA-A, -B, and -C) are first transmitted for a computer-generated match that, if successful, is followed by a full match (164).

For a matched sibling donor, marrow may be drawn from the donor, processed (or modulated in accordance with protocol-generated studies), and then either used directly or DMSO treated and stored in liquid nitrogen for later use. Processing may include red cell removal, serum replacement, T-cell depletion, or even stem cell

selection. The physical properties of the frozen tissue renders it less process amenable after thawing. When needed, the marrow sample is thawed at the bedside in a 37°C sterile water bath and reinfused immediately via an indwelling venous catheter at a rate of 125 mL/hr.

When the marrow source is an unrelated donor, all the planned preevents must be carried out at the donor institution following detailed communication between all parties, including the registry, because donor anonymity cannot be violated. Unrelated-donor marrow is usually obtained and processed 36 hours or less prior to infusion and then taken to the BMT site in a 4°C container or, if drawn more than 48 hours prior to BMT, frozen in liquid nitrogen.

Preparation of the Donor and Recipient

Information required from both donor and recipient includes detailed history and laboratory data about pregnancy, prior surgery, anesthesia problems, seizures, bleeding, and genetic, metabolic, immune, infectious (including syphilis, hepatitis, HIV, Epstein-Barr virus (EBV), CMV, TORCH, HTL V I and II) disorders, or transfusion reactions, as well as complete blood counts and detailed red cell immunotyping, urinalysis, renal and metabolic profiles, and dental, cardiac (radionuclide scan or echocardiogram for recipient only), and pulmonary and ophthalmologic studies, along with a thorough physical examination.

Preparation of the Recipient

Information about the recipient includes all of the above as well as the current problem-based data to reduce, when appropriate, the use of agents that would severely compromise the health of the recipient.

For patients who fail allo-BMT, the success rate for second allo-BMT is marginal at best, and such efforts should be undertaken only at centers that devote research time to such endeavors (165–169).

Allogeneic BMT: Donor/Recipient Review

In sibling BMT, there is little difference in toxicity between a one-antigen mismatch and full match. This distinction does not carry over to either parental or unrelated donors. Overall, the comparison favors HLA-matched, younger age, same sex, or male-to-female donors. The above, in effect, refers to control of GVHD without loss of a GVL effect. Once methods are developed that obviate the untoward events of unfavorable matches, disparate effects will become a textbook footnote.

Syngeneic donors (complete identity at both MHC and mH sites) rarely induce GVHD or GVL. This is borne out by the less than favorable outcome in such efforts; patients who receive syngeneic BMT experience the same high relapse rate that occurs in patients treated with autoBMT for treatment of hematopoietic malignancies (170). Although one may choose to use the (chromium-release) cytotoxic T cell assay to predict GVHD, MLR/MLC testing is not consistently reliable, and it is more prudent, therefore, to use class I, II, and III DLR typing as a predictor of GVHD (171).

On the basis of controlled GVHD without loss of alloimmune-mediated antileukemic effects, the preferential list of ideal BMT donors is (a) fully matched sibling, (b) one-antigen-mismatched sibling, (c) fully matched parent donor, (d) matched unrelated donor, and (e) haploidentical parent.

Bone Marrow Harvest

The favorable anatomic sites for marrow harvest are the iliac crests. Depending on patient preference, the procedure can be carried out under general or local (spinal) anesthesia. The preferred volume is arrived at by multiple 5-mL aspirates of heparinized samples added to a doubly filtered, anticoagulated, marrow collection bag designed to collect $1–3 \times 108$ cells/kg of recipient body weight or approximately 15 mL/kg of recipient weight. To carry out modulation technologies etc., more cells are required. Aspirates as high as 25 mL/kg are appropriate. Most donors are functionally capable of returning home with minimal analgesic support on the day of marrow donation. On the (steadily increasing) occasions of donor peripheral blood use, collections follow cytokine stimulation, a process that readily overcomes the one-log deficit in peripheral blood stem cells and then decreases the frequency of peripheral blood harvesting.

Conditioning Regimens

The most frequently used conditioning regimens are CY and fTBI, cytosine arabinoside and fTBI, or combinations of the two. Less commonly used regimens are a busulfan-CY combination (used for AML and myeloma in some institutions and in certain of the infant leukemia protocols, the latter in an effort to reduce irradiation-induced CNS toxicity) and low-dose CY (for Fanconi's anemia, to reduce drug-related toxicity). Table 41.8 contains a list of the various combinations.

The first drug to be used in combination with irradiation was CY, and in a real sense that combination has become the yardstick against which others have been measured. Among the many agents that have joined CY in the pharmaceutical armamentarium are cytosine arabinoside, busulfan, etoposide, melphalan, prednisolone, platinum, and vincristine, all of which have been used in drug-drug combinations, in association with irradiation, or without. Factors that contribute to the selection solely of pharmaceutical combinations include difficulties in accessing radiation equipment and concern about possible untoward effects of TBI on the incompletely developed neurologic systems of infants (72, 172–179).

Table 41.8. AlloBMT Preparative Regimens

1.	Chemotherapy[a] only	
	A. Busulfan	750 mg/m²
	Cyclophosphamide	6,000–10,000 mg/m²
	B. BNCU ⇌ (carmustine)	300–600 mg/m²
	Cyclophosphamide	6,000–7,200 mg/m²
	Etoposide (VP-16)	600–2,400 mg/m²
2.	Total body irradiation[a,b] plus single-agent chemotherapy	
	A. Cyclophosphamide	6,000 mg/m²
	B. Etoposide	3,000 mg/m²
	C. Cytosine arabinoside	36 g/m²
	D. Melphalan	110 mg/m²
3.	Total body irradiation with two chemotherapy agents	
	A. Cyclophosphamide	3,000–6,000 mg/m²
	Cytosine arabinoside	6–36 g/m²
	B. Cyclophosphamide	2,500 mg/m²
	Busulfan	350 mg/m²
	C. Cyclophosphamide	4,500 mg/m²
	Etoposide	2,500 mg/m²

[a]Dose/m².
[b]12 Gy (6 Gy with top cytosine arabinoside dose fractionated b.i.d. or t.i.d.).

Irradiation

The fact that animals subjected to lethal doses of irradiation could be salvaged with BMT was a major factor in the use of this modality as a preparative regimen for BMT in humans. Details of TBI usage (e.g., dose, time, fractionation) are presented in the chapters on radiation therapy. The following is a brief summation. Single-dose irradiation delivered at an average rate of 26 cGy/min cannot exceed 850 cGy because of risk of severe tissue toxicity. By fractionating the total dose, the limits of toxicity can be extended to 1600 cGy without loss of efficacy. Fractionated doses generally consist of 200 cGy delivered at differing rates 2–3 times a day. Hyperfractionation usually consists of approximately 160 cGy administered 3–4 times daily. Seminal studies on (a) mechanisms protecting against deliberate, irradiation-induced marrow injury and (b) analyses of irradiation "accidents" were used to develop TBI regimens capable of suppressing both normal and abnormal hematopoiesis.

Failure to effect long-term, DFS solely with TBI in all but one patient was characteristic of the earliest BMT studies in Seattle (1). In that setting, however, all of those patients, including those with "resistant" disease, had experienced multiple relapses, which of itself lent powerful support to the efficacy of TBI. The process of combining TBI with chemotherapy has matured into a number of effective combinations, but it was only with the passage of time and carefully controlled studies that this has occurred. Examples of this approach include a University of Genoa study in the early 1980s, that compared the effects on survival of daily 330 cGy irradiation doses, the total of which were either slightly greater or slightly less than 990 cGy. Age, sex, diagnosis, FAB classification, and T-cell depletion were equally distributed in both groups. Of the 105 leukemic patients (61 AML, 44 CML), a significantly more favorable outcome with lesser toxicity was found in the above 990 cGy group. Actuarial survivals for the two groups were 74% and 38%, respectively. One year later, a Seattle study found no differences in actuarial 3-year DFS (58% vs. 59%) in a randomized trial of 1200 cGy versus 1575 cGy (200 cGy daily for 6 days vs. 225 cGy daily for 7 days) in 72 consecutive newly diagnosed AML patients. The 1200-cGy group had a higher probability of relapse, a lower probability of transplantation-related mortality, and greater likelihood of severe GVHD than the 1575-cGy group. Both of these studies confirmed the efficacy and established the limits of TBI. In effect, 800–1600 cGy TBI in delivery doses of 5.0–100.0 cGy/min, in combination with single- or multiple-drug regimens, has consistently brought about more than 90% engraftment in matched sibling donor transplants. As suggested, the desired effects are best achieved when fTBI is combined with chemotherapeutic agent(s). The busulfan (for marrow ablation)-CY (for immunosuppression) regimen was designed to be a less toxic (in terms of GVHD, pneumonitis, and VOD) but no less effective alternative to CY and fTBI. The antileukemic benefit of the busulfan-CY regimen was further enhanced by reducing the toxic effects brought about by the high CY concentration, a process that did not unfavorably affect the 70% 2-year DFS (180–187).

The preparative regimen of cytosine arabinoside (3 g/m2 i.v. every 12 hours × 12 doses followed by 200 cGy TBI every 12 hours × 6 doses) used in this patient was part of an ongoing study designed to identify the most efficacious means of (a) total leukemic cell kill, (b) rendering the host sufficiently immune suppressed to impede graft rejection without toxic risk or loss of GVL, and (c) providing an optimal physical environment for marrow engraftment. In addition to the cytosine arabinoside–fTBI preparative regimen, he also received booster irradiation to the testes to sterilize potentially high-risk occult sites of disease, capable of repopulating the marrow.

Prior to the countdown, he received an additional course of intrathecal antileukemic prophylaxis with methotrexate and hydrocortisone. Cytosine arabinoside was omitted from the IT regimen because of its high-dose usage in the preparative regimen.

The underlying issues in developing preparative regimens for BMT concern patient toleration and therapeutic efficacy, both of which are derived from phase II–III toxicity and dose-escalation studies. In the final analysis, dose toleration depends on a variety of factors including patient age, the extent of prior therapy, knowledge of drug kinetics, and clearance. Interacting factors include the dose and duration of irradiation: single bolus, frequency of fractionation and, possibly, the temporal relationship between irradiation and chemotherapy schedules. Therapy-related toxicity plays a significant outcome role irrespective of the transplantation process per se. The fine line between toxicity and therapeutic efficacy is

such that one rarely achieves minimal toxicity and maximal efficacy as a routine. In developing preparative regimens, it is advisable to prepare a toxicity scale that is both realistic and workable. A highly workable program is the toxicity scale developed at the Fred Hutchison Cancer Research Center, with grade I mild and (non-therapy-related) reversible; grade II, moderate with measurable organ damage, often requiring intervention and interference with other therapy; grade III, life threatening, not readily tolerated, often requiring intensive support (e.g., dialysis or assisted ventilation); and grade IV, fatal. This elegant schema enables the physician to evaluate individual toxicity as well as cumulative toxicity, with the latter a more precise predictor of outcome (188).

Toxicity Grading Scale

The following systems are included in the Fred Hutchison grading scale program: oropharynx, gastrointestinal tract, liver, heart, kidney, bladder, lungs, and CNS. Examples of grade I–III toxicity in each of these systems follow.

Oropharynx. Minimal irritation requiring minimal pain control to severe ulceration and mucositis requiring extensive narcotic use.

Gastrointestinal tract: liquid stools of 2000 mL/day to 5000 or more mL/day as well as hemorrhage controlled supportively and with surgical intervention, as required; seemingly minimal changes in bilirubin and liver enzymes ranging to severe malfunctions leading both to ascites and encephalopathic changes.

Liver: veno-occlusive disease (VOD) (189) is an example of a singularly serious liver-induced toxicity. This disorder occurs more commonly in adults than in children, and in patients treated with CY, but other agents have also been implicated, and it may actually occur before marrow infusion. Its pathogenesis is based on an initial tissue insult, most likely chemotherapy induced, which leads to activation of the clotting cascade and is followed in turn by intimal proliferation and subsequent obstruction to venous blood flow. Cytokine release following tissue injury accelerates the entire coagulation process, which is further complicated by the release of TNF-α. This, in turn, up-regulates factors V and VIII and platelet-activating factors and down-regulates certain of the less critical anticoagulant factors. Attempts at controlling VOD with heparin (by blocking clot propagation) and/or pentoxiphylline (by down-regulating TNF-α production) have not been effective (190). The use of leukotrienes such as prostaglandin E₁, designed to overcome thrombosis by inducing vasodilation, is encumbered by numerous side effects that render its efficacy less than desirable. Possible merit may be found in the use of cholagogues, agents designed to minimize cell membrane damage by increasing bile flow.

Kidney: changes ranging from increased creatinine levels to anuria, and bladder changes ranging from microscopic hematuria to massive hemorrhagic cystitis requiring surgical intervention.

Cardiac: nonspecific ECG changes to blatant heart failure.

Pulmonary: mild respiratory difficulty with minimal asymptomatic interstitial involvement to changes requiring ventilatory support.

Central nervous system: symptoms ranging from intermittent and arousable somnolence to coma, irrespective of the origin.

Although most of these symptoms occur during the transplantation interval, some may occur weeks or months later. An example of a condition whose origins are insidious and only apparent early or when scrupulously sought is bronchiolitis obliterans, which, untreated, leads to bronchiolar fibrosis and death (191).

Any of the agents used in the preparative regimens may provoke the aforementioned symptoms, and it is also likely that underlying host conditions accelerate the extent of damage. Examples of conditions that are often worsened by the conditioning regimens include Fanconi's anemia and ectodermal dysplasia.

On the 60th day of his illness, the countdown to an HLA-identical, red cell–incompatible, unrelated marrow transplantation from a nonparous 45-year-old female began. Differences in patient's red cell type, O, C– D– E– (Rh negative), and donor, B, C– D– E– (Rh negative), necessitated removal of donor red cells from the graft and suspension of the buffy coat in AB,CDE-compatible plasma before being frozen.

Isolation Techniques

The patient began the countdown in a laminar flow unit [to which medical support personnel had access with rigorous hand washing and clean gowns.]

Mask and gloves are used for all open tissue procedures, but along with slippers, they do not prevent infection during routine bedside evaluation. However, total surface (and gut) sterilization along with total surface sterilization is best reserved for programs involved in studying GVHD control in the mismatched BMT patient.

Total Nutrition

Total parenteral hyperalimentation was begun on day +2. This patient had a 16-hour hyperalimentation program and an 8-hour window designed to serve blood transfusion and other support activities.

The single most effective way to provide the 50–70% increase in energy demands of a patient undergoing BMT is via parenteral nutrition administered through a central venous catheter (192). The regimens can be readily individualized to address the broader aspects of nutritional support.

Infection Prophylaxis

The patient's herpes zoster titer was less than 1:8.

Acyclovir

Some programs do not initiate acyclovir prophylaxis in patients whose titers are below 1:4 (193). Others routinely administer acyclovir on the presumption that its activity extends beyond herpes, despite the fact that there are no data in support of acyclovir in any but zoster-type infections. For patients with active herpetic lesions, including "mouth sores," the countdown to BMT does not begin until therapy has eradicated all evidence of the active process.

In addition to acyclovir, he also received the following:
Nystatin Mouth Washes: Anticandidal/fungal oropharyngeal care is a well-established, effective control measure.

Peridex Dental Care: Aggressive oral cleanliness and dental prophylaxis is fundamental to the control of oropharyngeal-initiated bacterial and often viral illness.

Trimethoprim-Sulfa Prophylaxis: The control of Pneumocystis infection in the immunocompromised host is readily achievable with oral or parenteral trimethoprim sulfate or by parenteral or aerosolized pentamidine. Either one of these agents is a mandated part of the prophylaxis program.

Hyperimmune Gamma Globulin: Adjunct passive immune therapy may be valuable in control of infections in general. There are no data to support its use in prevention of cytomegaloviral disease, for which CMV-negative blood products (administered to CMV-negative recipients) is the single best control measure). For CMV + patients prophylactic gancyclovir has effected a significant decrease in the critical 100-day post-BMT period.

Blood Products

See under Blood Product Support.

On day −6, he developed photophobia. Examination revealed nonpurulent conjunctivitis without any scleral disease, which slowly cleared following the use of systemic analgesics and local steroidal solutions.

On day −4, he experienced erythema, swelling, and tenderness of his fingers and toes, and he developed ataxia to the extent that he lost control of his eating utensils. Two days after completing the preparative therapy, the ataxia abated, and it had completely disappeared by the time TBI was completed. The skin changes progressed to bullae and desquamation, followed by slowly progressive epidermal repair.

Among the various toxicities induced by high-dose cytosine arabinoside are conjunctivitis, with photophobia, dermatitis, cerebritis, and VOD. The eye findings are the most common; but none are regularly predictable, and all but VOD are readily reversible (194).

Antinausea Control

The various combinations used in an effort to control nausea are protean. The general maxim is that which works best is the preparation that should be used, providing obtundation and somnolence do not supervene.

The patient received a cocktail of intravenous Thorazine, Benadryl, and Solu-Medrol, which was discontinued at his request when neither nausea nor vomiting were persistent problems.

On day − 2, 500 mL of processed donor marrow arrived frozen in liquid nitrogen. On day 0, 12 hours after the last TBI dose and following a 1-hour thaw in a sterile 37°C water bath at the bedside, the donor marrow was infused at 150 mL/hr.

Had there been an episode of RBC transfusion incompatibility, he would have experienced hemoglobinemia leading to hemoglobinuria with subsequent and permanent clearing following aggressive hydration. This usually happens, but to a far lesser degree, in allotransplants following the thawing process wherein excretion of hemoglobin (as methemoglobin) follows on the heels of intravascular lysis of freeze-thawed (fragile) erythrocytes.

Engraftment

GVHD, when present, is a hallmark of alloengraftment. In most allo-BMTs, the first indication of engraftment is a rise in white cell numbers sometime between 10 and 18 days post-BMT. Lack of evidence of white cell production after 21 days may well presage engraftment failure, and only rarely is a stable or rising platelet count a first predictor of engraftment. Once cellular elements appear, one may confirm the donor source if the allograft is sex or red cell mismatched (195, 196). If neither is present, chimerism (recipient containing donor tissue except for marrow) can be determined by RLPF probes for karyotyping, by DNA sequence, and by white cell isoenzymes (197–202).

The commonest cause of graft failure is alloimmune rejection, the result of either persistence of radioresistant recipient T cells or antidonor antibodies (203). Pre-BMT steroid administration may help the former; irradiation, plasmapheresis, or the use of antithymocyte globulin (120, 204) may correct the latter. HLA-mismatched BMTs are a greater risk factor for graft failure as well as GVHD. The marrow dose, per se, only affects engraftment when fewer than 10^8 cells/kg are infused into the recipient. On the other hand, a patient at

risk for graft failure from other causes is not at less risk by having the number of donor marrow cells increased. Although there are no data that support the early use of cytokines post-BMT to prevent graft rejection, granulocyte-monocyte cloning stimulating factor (GM-CSF) has been shown to help prevent graft failure (205). T-cell depletion, designed to overcome or minimize GVHD, may also increase the risk of graft failure (206). Methods designed to control GVHD with pharmacologic agents, namely CSA and methotrexate (MTX), appear to have salubrious effects on engraftment as well (207).

A 1985 study by the University of Minnesota bone marrow transplantation group identified a curious phenomenon: the deleterious effects of histoincompatibility on engraftment in nonmalignant hematopoietic disorders (aplastic anemia) compared with malignant hematopoietic disorders (leukemia). The seemingly lesser frequency of GVHD in the aplastic anemias was the result of engraftment failure.

A contributing factor in the genesis of graft failure in both fully and partially matched allo-BMT is inadequate "ablative" therapy, very likely mediated by persistence of recipient T cells (208). Patients who experience graft failure following administration of marrow of variable genetic disparity (HLA haplo-mismatched siblings, phenotypically matched parental donors, and HLA matched–unrelated donors depleted of CD-8 lymphocytes), often show increased numbers of recipient HLA-DR + and CD-3,CD-8 lymphocytes (209). Multiply-transfused patients also are at greater risk for graft failure (210). Although failure to engraft is often a host-induced process, best controlled with marrow ablative regimens designed to suppress host lymphocyte competency, overzealous efforts to remove donor T cells in an attempt to control GVHD will also impair engraftment (207).

In effect, graft failure and/or GVHD occur more frequently in mismatched transplants. Once therapy-related toxicity is eliminated (i.e., once probes are developed that can identify minor histocompatibility antigens while maintaining antileukemic cytotoxicity), the number of patients engrafting and maintaining nontoxic durable survivals will markedly increase.

Infection Control

In the early BMT days, the three leading causes of failure were disease recurrence, infection, and complications secondary to GVHD. Of all of the infections, CMV was probably the most deadly but not the most common. Its 90%+ mortality rate was the highest of all identifiable infectious agents. Combination hyperimmune gamma globulin and gancyclovir appear to have reduced the mortality by well over 50% (211). The single most effective way to prevent CMV in the CMV-negative recipients is by the use of CMV-negative blood. Hyperimmune gamma globulin has become an integral part of allo-BMT therapy, but the rationale for its use continues to be unclear. It was initiated early on as a means of decreasing the frequency of all infections, including CMV, but evidence for the same is lacking.

This patient received hyperimmune gamma globulin (IVIG) weekly.

On day +7, his temperature rose to 39°C, and after throat, blood, and urine cultures were obtained, broad-coverage antibacterial agents were initiated. Three days later, amphotericin was added to the antibiotic regimen, because the temperature elevation persisted in the absence of culture-positive material. Cultures remained negative. He experienced little amphotericin-induced toxicity (fever, shaking, chills, excessive potassium wasting), in part because he received Tylenol, hydrocortisone, Benadryl, potassium supplementation as needed, and Demerol at infusion time.

Rapid use of antibiotics capable of covering resistant staphylococcal and microaerophilic infections is an established necessity when temperature elevation supervenes. Many institutions initiate antifungal therapy at the same time as antibacterial therapy; others wait 3–7 days. There are no data to support one approach over the other. Once initiated, antibiotics are not discontinued until the absolute granulocyte count reaches 350–500 × 10⁹/L if an organism is not isolated. Empirical antiinfective therapy consists of broad-spectrum, including microaerophilic, coverage. One example of an effective antibacterial spectrum would include ceftazidime and vancomycin.

On day 17+, a faint macular rash appeared on his forearms and abdomen. Two days later, it became more extensive and erythematous and was followed in short order by diarrheal stools. A skin biopsy was consistent with GVHD. Liver studies were negative for hepatitis screen and positive for elevated direct and indirect bilirubin, LDH, and liver enzymes. High-dose prednisone (i.v., 5 mg/kg) was initiated. His stools, rash, and liver function studies worsened over the next 3 days. His diarrheal output was such that it required almost 4 liters of parenteral fluid per day to maintain total energy and fluid balance. On day 19+ his total white cell count was 6×10^9/L. By day 27+, his rash began to fade, and his stool volume diminished to 2500 mL/24 hr; by day +32, it fell to 500 mL/24 hr. By day 30, his white cell count had risen to 14×10^9/L, with an absolute granulocyte count of 5×10^9/L on 2 consecutive days. All antibiotics were discontinued over the subsequent 3 days, following which, steroid dose reduction of 25% every 5 days was initiated.

Graft-versus-Host Disease Prophylaxis

The GVHD prophylaxis regimen administered to this patient included MTX and cyclosporine A (CSA) in the following schedule: 15 mg/m² intravenous MTX on day +1, followed by 10 mg/m2 on days 3, 6, 11, and 18, and 5 mg/kg intravenous CSA daily; the latter designed to maintain a therapeutic level in the range of 300–400 ng/100 mL. CSA was to be administered orally for 4 additional months following discharge.

Neither CSA nor MTX administered as single agents is as effective in controlling GVHD as both administered together, both of which eclipse prednisone or antithymocyte globulin (ATG) for prophylactic acute GVHD therapy (216–219). Treatment of severe GVHD occurring in patients who received prophylaxis includes slowly tapered high-dose prednisone with or without CSA (216, 217). ATG, anti-CD-3, IL-2, TNF-α, anti CD-5, UV irradiation, and, for chronic GVHD, total nodal irradiation and possibly macrolide (FR506) have gained moderate success when used following failure of "traditional" pharmaceutical therapy (218–225).

Measures designed to T-cell deplete the grafts, either as subset or total T reductions, alone or in combination with pharmaceutical agents (i.e., MTX and/or CSA), have been successfully employed in a number of institutions carrying out studies for GVHD control in patients at high risk of GVHD development (226–233). In the earliest studies of BMT, GVHD occurred at an unacceptable rate. Once refinements in T-cell removal were instituted, GVHD became more readily controlled without loss of the GVL effect.

No single aspect of BMT has been more intensively studied than GVHD. In 1955, Barnes and Loutit coined the term "secondary disease" to describe the epidermal desquamation along with hepatodegenerative changes and severe debilitation in mice transplanted with histoincompatible spleen cells (234). The process became known as "graft-versus-host disease" after Dutch studies on host cell–mediated recognition of recipient tissue. Ongoing studies identified a direct correlation between the number of infused mature lymphocytes and the severity of GVHD (235), and in the late 1960s, the pathophysiology of GVHD was well established: (a) immunologically competent cells present in the graft; (b) transplantation isoantigens present in the host but not in the graft; and (c) a finite or secure time interval during which the host is incapable of attacking the graft (236). Table 41.9 summarizes GVHD development.

It is a notable coincidence that at the time that information on the nature of GVHD was unfolding, so too was the identification of the histocompatibility antigens in mice and humans (237–240). Once these data were fully accepted, it was possible to establish guidelines for the development of both prophylactic and therapeutic modalities. Before doing so, organ dysfunction staging criteria were developed (241). The major organ involvement of GVHD includes skin, the gastrointestinal tract (and its hepatic derivative), and the lungs. Assessment of all but the pulmonary system is relatively easy, and although it is not routinely included in the categorization criteria, this in no way suggests that its involvement is less damaging. Table 41.10 contains GVHD staging and grading criteria.

Early on, the rash involves the palms and soles, often with itching and burning. It usually extends to the ears and thence to the thorax before spreading diffusely. As it expands geographically, it tends to change from a relatively mild maculopapular appearance to a generalized erythroderma, which, in its most advanced stage, forms bullae and then epidermal separation. In its early clinical stages, it is virtually indistinguishable from drug eruptions or viral exanthems. At this crucial interval, a punch biopsy must be examined by a skilled dermatopathologist to determine whether the exanthem exhibits characteristic lesions of focal vacuolar degeneration and perivenule lymphocytic infiltration. Early on, the distinction may not be readily

made, but in advanced stages, the pathologic appearance is easily recognizable. Fortunately, with the advent of aggressive prophylaxis, grade IV GVHD is now an uncommon event except for mismatched transplantation. Skin infiltration by lymphocytes may involve minimal damage to the subepidermal layers or be so massive as to cause bullous changes and ultimately loss of epidermal and dermal layers (242). Later-occurring or chronic skin GVHD may develop into an intractable sclerodermatous process (see "Chronic GVHD") (243).

So many factors contribute to the clinical expression of hepatic malfunction during the transplant interval that an unequivocal diagnosis of liver GVHD mandates an examination of biopsy material. VOD, infections, drugs, and parenteral hyperalimentation may cause elevations in bilirubin and liver enzymes otherwise indistinguishable from those of GVHD (244). The typical pathologic findings of hepatic GVHD involve portal and bile duct lymphocyte infiltration culminating in ductal obliteration (245, 246). Healing is considered complete when lymphocytic infiltration of the ductal basement membrane is no longer apparent.

Crampy abdominal pain, diarrhea, and bloody discharge, sometimes accompanied by tissue fragments, are the hallmarks of the progression of gastrointestinal GVHD. Diarrhea, per se, may be the consequence of the marrow transplantation preparative therapy, in which case it occurs in the first 10–14 days, or it may follow a variety of gut infections, including retroviral, adenoviral, enteroviral, or cytomegaloviral as well as protozoal (Giardia) or bacterial (Clostridium difficile, Escherichia coli, and Campylobacter) infections (247). The secretory type of diarrhea characteristic of gut GVHD is the result of inflammatory changes leading first to edema, then to localized and diffuse ulcers, and finally to denudation and intraluminal hemorrhage. The severity of the disease is much less apparent in the stomach than it is in the remaining bowel or rectum. Impaired infection control renders the gut easily accessible to the final destructive

---

Table 41.9. Known and Interacting Features in the Development of GVHD

1. Recognition of recipient class I & II antigens by donor CD-4 and CD-8 cells
   A. Major and minor antigen mismatches
   B. Autoimmune disorders involving class II antigens
2. IL-2 is both complementary and regulatory[a]
   A. T-cell expansion requires IL-2
   B. Increased dosage IL-2 pre-BMT protects against GVHD in MHC-mismatched mice
3. Effector (toxicity initiating) cells and proteins include CD-4, CD-8, NK cells; tumor necrosis factor (TNF), γ interferon (INF-γ).
4. Affector (tissue damaged) cells
   A. Basilar epidermis
   B. Biliary tract
   C. Bone marrow
   D. Intestinal mucosa
   E. Lymphoid tissue
   F. Lung tissue

[a]Both IL-2 and CSA induce chronic GVHD-like skin eruption in humans.

Table 41.10. Acute Graft-Versus-Host Disease: Clinical Stage (+→++++) and Grade (I→IV)[a]

Grade	Skin	Liver (bilirubin)	GI Tract (diarrhea)
I	(+) Maculopapular rash <25% body surface to (++) 25–50% body surface	0	0
II	(+) to (+++) Generalized erythroderma	Bilirubin (+) 2–3 mg/dL	Diarrhea (+) 500–1000 mL/day
III	(++) to (+++)	(++) 3–6 mg/dL to (+++) 6–15 mg/dL	(++) 1000–1500 mL/day to (+++) 1500 mL/day ± micro blood
IV	(+++) to (++++) Desquamation, blistering	(++) to (++++) >15 mg/dL	(++) to (++++) >1500 mL/day Pain/ileus; ± gross blood

[a]I, mild; II, moderate; III, severe; IV, life threatening (see toxicity scale).

processes brought about by microbial invasion. Lymphocyte infiltration of the gut mucosa may be massive enough to lead to total mucosal denudation. Minimalization of the severity of GVHD in histoincompatibly transplanted mice maintained in a sterile environment is the basis for the use of strict gut sterility–laminar flow isolation programs for patients at high risk for the development of severe GVHD. However, not all programs engaged in the study of mismatched BMT use such total isolation/sterilization procedures.

Acute GVHD involving the lungs is the result of bronchial lymphocytic infiltration with resultant loss of ciliary integrity and an increased likelihood for the development of opportunistic infections (248).

Over the ensuing 10 days, there was a steady improvement in liver function in association with an increase in granulocytes, fewer platelet transfusions, skin clearing, and a significant decrease in stool production. Steroid tapering continued, and by day 60, he was ready for discharge, at which time all cultures remained negative, stools were formed, small amounts of solid foods were being consumed, and he was maintained on oral anti-Pneumocystis therapy, oral CSA, and continuously (albeit slowly) tapered prednisone.

Hematopoietic Control

Platelet Support

More than 50% of multiply-transfused patients become refractory to pooled random-donor platelets. The most effective way to minimize exposure to incompatible material is to use single-donor platelet transfusions of antigencompatible platelets and, whenever possible, reduce the frequency of transfusions. In this regard, HLA-matched apheresis platelets are no better than random single-donor apheresis-obtained platelets.

Because of the difference in locale of class I and class II HLA antigens on transfused cells and the likely possibility that transfused leukocytes may result in cytotoxic antibodies directed against platelets, it has been proposed that leukocyte-poor blood be used to overcome platelet alloimmunization. To date there are no studies that confirm the efficacy of this approach. UV radiation of blood products may be more efficacious than filtration in that it tends to paralyze the antigenic material without harming the functional components (249–251). In the persistently platelet-refractory patient, there may be a role for the use of IVIG, but there are no data to support plasma exchange or the administration of ϵ-aminocaproic acid (EACA) as an antifibrinolytic in chronic thrombopenic states.

Transfusion-induced CMV is best prevented by using CMV-negative donors for CMV-negative recipients. However, there are no data to support the use of CMV-negative blood for CMV-positive recipients. In effect, the single best approach to minimizing CMV reactivation is to provide leukocyte-poor blood products.

Blood Component Support

An hematocrit between 20 and 25% and a platelet count above 20×10^9/L will likely suffice to maintain the integrity of the vascular system during the BMT recovery phase.

There are no data to support the use of granulocyte transfusions as a means of preventing infection during the same period, although any patient with a granulocyte count below 20×10^9/L is at risk for untoward infection. Attempting to control granulocytopenic-induced infections would require infusing granulocytes every 6 hours.

Platelet and red cell volumes were maintained at physiologically stable levels with a 20/25 formula: platelet transfusion at a level of 20×10^9/L and red cell transfusions at hematocrit levels of 25%.

Because of the red cell incompatibility, all initial packed, irradiated, and white cell–filtered transfusions were type O, Rh− (C− D− E−). He engrafted as a B, Rh− chimera, following which all subsequent transfusions were B, Rh−.

Irradiation and leukocyte depletion of all transfused blood products were carried out to avoid transfusion-induced GVHD and (phagocyte-transmitted) CMV disease, respectively. Of note is the fact that leukocyte-poor material does not prevent the transmission of hepatitis.

Platelet support at a count of 20×10^9/L was based on the greater likelihood of spontaneous bleeding at that level. The volume transfused followed on the knowledge that a platelet concentration of approximately 5×10^{10}/kg body weight is an easily calculated dose based on desired postinfusion levels. To test for refractoriness, irrespective of the cause, platelet counts were obtained 1 hour postinfusion and every 12 hours thereafter. Patients who fail to obtain a 1-hour response are clearly refractory. Crossmatching was carried out with a radiolabeled antiglobulin test. Single-donor platelets compatible in toto with the red cell type were always preferred when available.

Because platelet transfusion practices are common, patients are routinely premedicated with antihistamines and hydrocortisone.

The patient did not develop platelet refractoriness.

Cytokine Support

The administration of G-CSF or GM-CSF can shorten granulocyte recovery time just as erythropoietin (Epo) appears to shorten red cell recovery time. (Both factors may also increase allogeneic donor yield and reciprocal recovery time as well.) Carefully controlled trials are needed to establish the precise time and sequencing of these agents if improved survivals or shortened hospitalization time is to be borne out.

He received neither G-CSF, GM-CSF, nor Epo.

Although GM-CSF theoretically has a greater range of action, it is somewhat more toxic than G-CSF because of the greater frequency of GM-CSF-induced capillary leak syndrome. Details of these cytokines are presented in the chapter on cytokines.

Reconstitution Time

Red cells: approximately 4–5 weeks post-granulocyte-recovery, 1–2 weeks earlier with erythropoietin support.

Platelets: usually the last to recover; may stay below 50×10^9/L for many months.

Granulocyte/monocyte group: approximately 14–20 days post-marrow-infusion and somewhat earlier with G-CSF or GM-CSF; qualitative function on rare occasions lags behind by approximately 2–4 weeks.

Lymphocytes: approximately 8–10 weeks following infusion, with NK cells the earliest, B cells intermediate; and T cells the slowest of the group; complete functional recovery may take as long as 8–12 months.

Table 41.11 summarizes the hematopoietic recovery periods and the temporal relationships with potential infective agents.

Discharge Planning

At day +62, he was discharged to a clean abode. Discharge instructions included the use of oral trimethoprim sulfa, a decreasing dose schedule of intravenous prednisone, and magnesium and multivitamin supplements. CSA was discontinued when the steroids were ini-

Table 41.11. Post-Allo-BMT Hematopoietic Recovery and Time Sequences of Infections

Recovery

	Onset (Days)	Complete (Months)
Erythrocytes	20–30	1–3
Monocytes	30–45	1–3
Granulocytes	30–45	1–3
Platelets	40–50	3–6
B Lymphocytes	45–60	8–12
T Lymphocytes	45–60	8–12
CD-4	45–60	5–9
CD-8	45–60	5–9
NK cells	30–45	5–9

	Peak (Days)	Duration (Months)
Fungal infections	+15	4
Herpes	+60	4
CMV	+60	4
Hepatitis A, B, C	+45	4
Viral infections[a]	+30	4
Parasitic infections	+20	12
Bacterial infections	+1	12

[a]Other than CMV, hepatitis.

tially administered but readministered orally during the late stages of tapering, to minimize the risk of seizures. Plans were made to return to the BMT outpatient clinic on a regularly scheduled basis for blood, urine, and laboratory studies as well as platelet and red cell support as needed. Acyclovir was discontinued at discharge. IVIG administration was decreased to a 2-week schedule to be discontinued on day 100.

Schooling was carried out via telephone, and the patient was instructed to avoid contact with direct sunlight and, whenever outside, to wear sunscreen; ingestion of raw fruits, vegetables, meats, poultry, and fish was forbidden, and attendance at any crowded site was discouraged for the first 6 months post-BMT.

On day 1 82, he developed a dry raspy cough, and his temperature rose to 39°C. A complete blood count did not show evidence of leukemic cells, and except for platelet numbers in the low normal range, the remainder of his counts were normal. He had a 1;40 CMV IgM titer and a 1;100 hepatitis C IgM titer. A chest film showed minimal, albeit diffuse, interstitial pneumonic changes, and a PCR-assisted assay of his granulocytes was positive for CMV. HIV titers remained negative. At that point, the records of every blood donor were examined. Two donors were found to be equivocally positive for CMV and hepatitis, respectively, and on recall, both tested positive. Apparently both donors were in the process of converting at the time of donation, but the titers were too low to be readily detected. Ironically, it occurred in the last inpatient week.

Careful evaluation, including liver biopsy, failed to reveal evidence of chronic GVHD, which has a frequency of 80% in MUD BMT. Half of these patients go on to develop chronic GVHD. This patient did not have chronic GVHD. His biopsy was consistent with low-grade hepatitis.

Chronic GVHD (252)

Chronic GVHD (cGVHD) may be localized or diffuse and follow acute GVHD or occur for the first time weeks or even months after engraftment.

Localized cGVHD includes limited skin involvement with hepatic dysfunction and normal blood studies. Diffuse cGVHD includes extensive skin disease and sicca syndrome, with hepatic dysfunction and occasionally mild thrombocytopenia. Severe consequences of the above may lead to scleroderma, hepatic fibrosis, and/or bronchiolitis obliterans. Other involvement includes eyes, oropharynx, and neuromuscular and vaginal systems. Table 41.12 lists the features of GVHD.

The single most effective therapy for cGVHD includes high-dose corticosteroids and CSA. For steroid failure (253, 254), ATG and/or total nodal irradiation is a helpful alternative (224, 225).

He was readmitted to the hospital, where a transbronchial lung biopsy revealed typical necrotic-induced CMV changes. The organism was identified by PCR. He received intravenous gancyclovir daily and intravenous

Table 41.12. Chronic Graft-versus-Host Disease

Site	Clinical Expression	Investigation
Skin	Alopecia, depigmentation, erythema (anychodystrophy, scleroderma)	Biopsy
Mouth	Lichen planus, xerostomia	Biopsy
Eyes	Sicca, keratitis	Shirmer's test
Liver	Icterus	Elevated SGOT, alkaline phosphatase
Lungs	Obstructive/restrictive disease	Pulmonary function/blood gas studies
Vagina	Sicca, atrophy	Biopsy
Nutrition	Protein calorie malnutrition	Tissue losses, edema

With permission

IVIG weekly. Seven days later, he defervesced, and his temperature remained normal. He was discharged on the 11th hospital day to the outpatient clinic for follow-up ambulatory gancyclovir/IVIG therapy. His anti-CMV therapy was reduced to half-dose 3 months later and discontinued after 6 months. At that time, his CMV and hepatitis C titers had both converted to IgG. Early elevations in liver enzymes fell to normal over 4 months. Initial plans to consider the use of gamma interferon (INF-γ) to treat hepatitis C were abandoned because of both a lack of symptoms and an awareness of the potential severity of INF-γ toxicity. One year later, he remained in solid remission and off all therapy. There was no clinical evidence of any active CMV or hepatitis C, although serologic evidence for both disorders persisted.

Treatment of CMV with a combination of gancyclovir and IVIG has improved the previously devastating effects of this disorder in the immunosuppressed host, and, as stated, studies clearly support the use of gancyclovir alone for prophylaxis against CMV+ recipients.

For hepatitis C, the efficacious role of INF-γ awaits substantiation (255). However, in every case of suspected viral hepatitis C (VHC), one must be certain that the liver function abnormalities attributable to hepatitis C are not, in fact, due to chronic cGVHD, the effects of which may be severely worsened by the use of INF-γ. More to the point, hepatitis C is not necessarily a fatal downhill disorder; it may well dissipate.

In this case, the latter occurred. Two years post-BMT, he complained of bilateral hip pain radiating to the knees. CT scanning identified severe bilateral aseptic necrosis of the femoral heads, both of which were corrected with sequential bone graft surgery.

Aseptic necrosis occurs post-BMT following prolonged high-dose steroid therapy, which underscores the need for every post-BMT patient to undergo extensive organ system examinations in search of therapy-induced abnormalities including growth failure (in the preadolescent), pulmonary failure, hypothyroidism, chronic renal disease, heart disease, gonadal hypofunction, and psychologic disturbances (256).

Other Stem Cell Sources for Allo-BMT

Sources of stem cells, other than bone marrow itself, include peripheral (PB) and umbilical cord (CB) blood. PB has one log fewer, and CB one log more, stem cells per unit volume than does marrow. Unaltered cord blood has a low volume and limited capacity to mount an unassisted GVL response. The first successful CB transplants were carried out in patients with Fanconi's anemia in whom GVL was an undesirable event (257). However, CB GVL can, in fact, be turned on by biologic response modifiers (i.e., CSA, IL-2).

As information accrues on the nature of pluripotential cytokines, it is likely that CB and/or PB stem cells will be used more frequently in allo-BMT. Such endeavors will likely encompass the use of cytokines to enhance stem cell volume and the subsequent development of modulated banks of stem cells. In patients who receive stem cell infusion following marrow ablative preparation therapy, residual disease continues to be a major concern. Current methods for detection of residual disease are listed in Table 41.13. The other question, as always, is the role GVL plays in ridding the patient of residual tumor cells. Until the issue of residual disease is resolved, irrespective of the efficacy in controlling infection or the source of stem cells, BMT will continue to be a less than ideal therapeutic approach for the treatment of malignant hematologic disorders.

Conclusions

Early concerns regarding cost, efficacy, and ethical considerations in use of such alternate stem sources as PB or CB appear to be resolved. For a PB stem cell harvest, donor pretreatment with cytokines reduces the frequency of cytophereses, and it will likely do the same for CB in long-

Table 41.13. Minimal Residual Disease Detection

Technique	Activity Site	Sensitivity
Light microscopy	Cytology	10^{-1}
Fluorescent in situ hybridization	Chromosomes	10^{-2}
Cytogenetics	Chromosomes	10^{-2}
Fluorescent cell sorting	Antigen markers	10^{-3}
Gene rearrangement	DNA composition	10^{-3}
Polymerase chain reaction	DNA/RNA structures	10^{-5}
Clonogenic cultures asays	In vitro assays	10^{-5}

term culture. Moreover, newly emerging pluripotent cytokines will likely enhance primitive cell replication in culture, to which a variety of modulating activities, designed to enhance yield, reduce antigenicity, reconfigure its genomic constitution, support efficient engraftment, and direct cytotoxic activities, will be an additional factor. In effect, what is now a transplantable heterogeneous mononuclear cell mass will likely one day consist of pristine cultures of programmably modulated pluripotent stem cells consisting of no more than 3–4 mL of material; and at that stage, allo-BMT, as we know it now, will have become an historic event.

REFERENCES

1. Thomas ED, Lochte HL, Lu WC, et al. Intravenous feeding of bone marrow in patients receiving radiation and chemotherapy. N Engl J Med 1957;264:257.
2. Bennett JM, Catovsky D, Daniel MT, et al. Proposals for the classification of the acute leukemias. Br J Haematol 1976;33:451.
3. Bennett JM, Catovsky D, Daniel MT, et al. Proposed revised criteria for the classification of acute myeloid leukemia. Ann Intern Med 1985;103:626.
4. Bennett JM, Catovsky D, Daniel MT, et al. Criteria for the diagnosis of acute leukemia of megakaryocytic lineage (M7). Ann Intern Med 1985;103:460.
5. Yunis EJ, Awdeh Z, Raum D, et al. The MHC in human bone marrow transplantation. Clin Haematol 1983;12:641.
6. Bach FH, Sachs DH. Current concepts: immunology. Transplantation immunology. N Engl J Med 1987;317:489.
7. Bach FH, van Rood JJ. The major histocompatibility complex: genetics and biology. N Engl J Med 1976;295:806.
8. Stheim BG, Moller E, Ferrone S, eds. HLA class II antigens: a comprehensive review of structure and function. New York: Springer, Verlag, 1986.
9. Dorak MT, Chalmers EA, Sproul AM, et al. MHC class III polymorphisms in selection of donors for BMT. Bone Marrow Transplant 1993;11:37.
10. Bjorkman PJ, Saper MA, Samraoui M, et al. The foreign antigen binding site and T cell recognition regions of class I histocompatibility antigens. Nature 1987;329:512.
11. Wallny HJ, Rammensee HG. Identification of classical minor histocompatibility antigen cell-derived peptide. Nature 1990;343:275.
12. Germain RN. Immunology: the ins and outs of antigen presentation and processing. Nature 1986;322:687.
13. Bevan MJ. Antigen recognition: class discrimination in the world of immunology. Nature 1987;325:192.
14. Adorini L, Appella E, Doris E, et al. Competition for antigen presentation in living cells involves exchange of peptides bound by class II MHC molecules. Nature 1989;342:800.
15. Bodmer JG, Marsh SEG, Albert ED, et al. Nomenclature of factors of the HLA system, 1990. Hum Immunol 1991;31:196.
16. Hansen JA, Choo SY, Geraghy DE, et al. The HLA system in clinical marrow transplantation. Hematol Oncol Clin North Am 1990;4:507.
17. Martin PJ. Increased disparity for minor histocompatibility antigens from unrelated donors compared with related donors. Bone Marrow Transplant 1991;8:217.
18. Skipper HE, Schabel FM Jr, Wilcox WS. Experimental evaluation of potential anticancer agents. XIV. Further study of certain basic concepts underlying chemotherapy of leukemia. Cancer Chemother Rep 1965;45:5.
19. Skipper HE, Schabel FM Jr, Wilcox WS. Experimental evaluation of potential anticancer agents. XII. On the criteria and kinetics associated with "curability" of experimental leukemia. Cancer Chemother Rep 1964;35:1.
20. Goldie JH, Coldman AJ, Guduskas GA. Rationale for the use of alternating non-cross-resistant chemotherapy. Cancer Treat Rep 1982;66:439.
21. Brochstein JA, Kernan NA, Groshen S, et al. Allogeneic bone marrow transplantation after hyperfractionated total-body irradiation and cyclophosphamide in children with acute leukemia. N Engl J Med 1987;317:1618.
22. Bortin M, Rimm A, Saltzstein E. Graft versus leukemia: quantification of adoptive immunotherapy in murine leukemia. Science 1973;179:811.
23. Civin CI, Strauss LC, Brovall C, et al. Antigenic analysis of hematopoiesis. III. A hematopoietic progenitor cell surface antigen defined by a monoclonal antibody raised against KG-la cells. J Immunol 1984;133:157.
24. Porter D, Roth M, McGarigle C, et al. Adoptive immunotherapy induces molecular remission in relapsed CML following allogeneic bone marrow transplantation (BMT). Proc Am Soc Clin Oncol 1993;12:303.
25. Kersey J, Weisdorf D, Nesbit ME, et al. Comparison of autologous and allogeneic bone marrow transplantation for treatment of high risk refractory acute lymphoblastic leukaemia. N Engl J Med 1987;317:461.
26. Doney K, Buckner CD, Kopecky KJ, et al. Marrow transplantation for patients with acute lymphoblastic leukaemia in first marrow remission. Bone Marrow Transplant 1987;2:355.
27. Blume KG, Forman S J, Snyder DS, et al. Allogeneic bone marrow transplantation for acute lymphoblastic leukaemia during first complete remission. Transplantation 1987;43;389.
28. Blume KG, Forman SG, O'Donnell MR, et al. Total body irradiation and high-dose etoposide a new preparatory regimen for bone marrow transplantation in patients with advanced haematological malignancies. Blood 1987;69:1015.
29. Herzig RH, Bortin MM, Barrett AJ, et al. Bone marrow transplantation in high risk acute lymphoblastic leukaemia in first and second remission. Lancet 1987;1:786.
30. Brochstein JA, Kernan NA, Groshen S, et al. Allogeneic marrow transplantation after hyperfractionated total body irradiation and cyclophosphamide in children with acute leukaemia. N Engl J Med 1987;317:1618.
31. McCarthy DM, Barrett AJ, MacDonald D. Bone marrow transplantation for adults and children with poor risk acute lymphoblastic leukaemia in first complete remission. Bone Marrow Transplant 1988;3:315.
32. Vernant JP, Marit G, Maraninchi D, et al. Allogeneic bone marrow transplantation in adults with acute lymphoblastic leukemia in first complete remission. J Clin Oncol 1988;6:227.
33. Barrett AJ, Horowitz MM, Gale RP, et al. Factors affecting relapse and survival after bone marrow transplantation for acute lymphoblastic leukaemia: importance of regimens used for prophylaxis against graft-versus-host disease. Blood 1989;74:826.

34. Barrett AJ. Progress in allogeneic and autologous bone marrow transplantation for acute lymphoblastic leukaemia (ALL). Bone Marrow Transplant 1991;7(Suppl 2):59.

35. Barrett AJ, Locatella F, Treleaven JG, et al. Second marrow transplants for leukaemic relapse after bone marrow transplantation; high early mortality but favorable effect of chronic GvHD on continued remission. A report by the EMBT leukaemia working party. Br J Haematol 1991; 79:567.

36. Barrett AJ, Horowitz MM, Ash RC, et al. Bone marrow transplantation for Philadelphia chromosome-positive acute lymphoblastic leukaemia. Blood 1992;79(11):3067.

37. Torres A, Alonso MC, Gomez-Villagran JL, et al. No influence of numbers of donor CFU-GM on granulocyte recovery in bone marrow transplantation of acute leukemia. Blut 1985;50:89.

38. Torres A, Martinez F, Gomez P, et al. Allogeneic bone marrow transplantation versus chemotherapy in the treatment of childhood acute lymphoblastic leukemia in second complete remission. Bone Marrow Transplant 1989;4:609.

39. Chao NJ, Forman SJ, Schmidt GM, et al. Allogeneic bone marrow transplantation for high-risk acute lymphoblastic leukemia during first complete remission. Blood 1991; 78:1923.

40. Doney K, Fisher LD, Appelbaum FR, et al. Treatment of adult acute lymphoblastic leukemia with allogeneic bone marrow transplantation. Multivariate analysis of factors affecting acute graft-versus-host disease, relapse, and relapse-free survival. Bone Marrow Transplant 1991;7:453.

41. Blaise D, Gaspard AM, Stoppa AM, et al. Allogeneic or autologous bone marrow transplantation for acute lymphoblastic leukemia in first complete remission. Bone Marrow Transplant 1990;5:7.

42. Appelbaum FR, Clift RA, Buckner CD, et al. Allogeneic marrow transplantation for acute nonlymphoblastic leukemia after first relapse. Blood 1983;61:949.

43. Clift RA, Buckner CD, Thomas ED, et al. The treatment of acute non-lymphoblastic leukemia by allogeneic marrow transplantation. Bone Marrow Transplant 1987;2:243.

44. Zander AR, Dicke KA, Keating M, et al. Allogeneic bone marrow transplantation for acute leukemia refractory to induction chemotherapy. Cancer 1985;56:1374.

45. Mannoni P, Vernant JP, Rodet M, et al. Marrow transplantation for acute nonlymphoblastic leukemia in first remission. Blut 1980;41:220.

46. McGlave PB, Haake RJ, Bostrom BD, et al. Allogeneic bone marrow transplantation for acute nonlymphocytic leukemia in first remission. Blood 1988;72:1512.

47. Weisdorf DJ, McGlave PB, Ramsay NK, et al. Allogeneic bone marrow transplantation for acute leukaemia: comparative outcomes for adults and children. Br J Haematol 1988; 69:351.

48. Aschan J, Ringden O, Tollemar J, et al. Improved survival in marrow recipients above 30 years of age with better prevention of graft-versus-host disease. Transplant Proc 1990; 22:195.

49. Preisler HD, Anderson K, Rai K, et al. The frequency of long-term remission in patients with acute myelogenous leukemia treated with conventional maintenance chemotherapy: a study of 760 patients with a minimal follow-up time of 6 years. Br J Haematol 1989;71:189.

50. Wolff SN, Herzig RH, Fay JW, et al. High-dose cytarabine and daunorubicin as consolidation therapy for acute myeloid leukemia in first remission: long-term follow-up and results. J Clin Oncol 1989;7:1260.

51. Marmont A, Bacigalupo A, Van Lint MT, et al. Bone marrow transplantation versus chemotherapy alone for acute nonlymphoblastic leukemia. Exp Hematol 1985; 13(Suppl 17):40.

52. Appelbaum FR, Fisher LD, Thomas ED, et al. Chemotherapy versus marrow transplantation for adults with acute nonlymphocytic leukemia: a five-year follow-up. Blood 1988;72:179.

53. Reiffers J, Stoppa AM, Rigal-Huguet F, et al. Allogeneic versus autologous bone marrow transplantation versus chemotherapy for treatment of myeloid leukemia in first complete remission. Bone Marrow Transplant 1991; 7(Suppl 2):36.

54. Champlin RE, Ho WG, Gale RP, et al. Treatment of acute myelogenous leukemia: a prospective controlled trial of bone marrow transplantation versus consolidation chemotherapy. Ann Intern Med 1985;102:285.

55. Schiller GJ, Nimer SD, Territo MC, et al. Bone marrow transplantation versus high-dose cytarabine-based consolidation chemotherapy for acute myelogenous leukemia in first remission. J Clin Oncol 1992;10:41.

56. Zander AR, Keating M, Dicke K, et al. A comparison of marrow transplantation with chemotherapy for adults with acute leukemia of poor prognosis in first complete remission. J Clin Oncol 1988;6:1548.

57. Conde E, Iriondo A, Rayon C, et al. Allogeneic bone marrow transplantation versus intensification chemotherapy for acute myelogenous leukaemia in first remission: a prospective controlled trial. Br J Haematol 1988;68:219.

58. Dahl GV, Kalwinsky DK, Mirro J, et al. Allogeneic bone marrow transplantation in a program of intensive sequential chemotherapy for children and young adults with acute nonlymphocytic leukemia in first remission. J Clin Oncol 1990; 8:295.

59. Doll DC, List AF. Myelodysplastic syndromes. Semin Oncol 1992;19:1.

60. Vadham Raj-S, Keating M, LeMaistre A, et al. Effects of recombinant human granulocyte macrophage colony stimulating factor in patients with myeloplastic syndromes. N Engl J Med 1987;317:1545.

61. Negrin RS, Haeuber DH, Nagler A, et al. Treatment of myelodysplastic syndromes with recombinant human granulocyte colony-stimulating factor. Blood 1990;76:976.

62. Stein R, Abels R, Krantz S. Pharmacologic doses of recombinant human erythropoietin in the treatment of myelodysplastic syndromes. Blood 1991;78:1658.

63. Koeller HP, Heitjan D, Mertelsmann R, et al. Randomized study of 13-cis retinoic acid v placebo in the myelodysplastic disorders. Blood 1988;71:703.

64. Cines DB, Cassileth PA, Kiss JE. Danazol therapy in myelodysplasia. Ann Intern Med 1985;103:58.

65. Ganser A, Seipelt G, Lindemann A, et al. Effects of recombinant human interleukin-3 in patients with myelodysplastic syndromes. Blood 1990;76:455–462.

66. Marmount AM, Horowitz MM for the International Bone Marrow Transplantation Registry (IBMTR). Outcome of allogeneic bone marrow transplantation for myelodysplastic syndromes. Bone Marrow Transplant 1990; 5(Suppl 2):71.

67. Gale RP, Champlin RE. How does bone marrow transplantation cure leukaemia? Lancet 1984;2:28.

68. Cheson BD. Chemotherapy and bone marrow transplantation for myelodysplastic syndromes. Semin Oncol 1992; 19:85.

69. Kolb HJ, Holler E, Gender-Gotze C, et al. Myeloblative conditioning for marrow transplantation in myelodysplastic syndromes and paroxysmal nocturnal haemoglobinuria. Bone Marrow Transplant 1989;4:29.

70. Longmore G, Buinan EC, Weinstein HJ, et al. Bone marrow transplantation for myelodysplasia and secondary acute nonlymphoblastic leukemia. J Clin Oncol 1990;8:1707.

71. Bunin NJ, Casper JT, Chitambar C, et al. Partially matched bone marrow transplantation in patients with myelodysplastic syndromes. J Clin Oncol 1988;6:1851.

72. Santos GW, Tutschka PJ, Brookmeyer R, et al. Marrow transplantation for acute nonlymphocytic leukaemia after treatment with busulfan and cyclophosphamide. N Engl J Med 1983;309:1347.

73. Berk PD, Goldbert JD, Donovan PB, et al. Therapeutic recommendations in polycythemia vera based on Polycythemia Study Group protocols. Semin Hematol 1986; 23:132.

74. Talpaz M, Kurzrock R, Kantarjian H, et al. Recombinant interferon-alpha therapy of Philadelphia chromosome-negative marrow proliferative disorders with thrombocytosis. Am J Med 1989;86:554.

75. Manoharan A. Myelofibrosis: prognostic factors and treatment. Br J Haematol 1988;69:295.

76. Rajantic J, Sale GE, Deeg HJ, et al. Adverse effect of severe marrow fibrosis on hematologic recovery after chemoradiotherapy and allogeneic bone marrow transplantation. Blood 1986;67:1693.

77. Dokal I, Jones L, Deenmamode M, et al. Allogeneic bone marrow transplantation for primary myelofibrosis. Br J Haematol 1989;71:158.

78. Sanders JE, Buckner CE, Thomas ED, et al. Allogeneic marrow transplantation for children with juvenile chronic myelogenous leukemia. Blood 1988;71:1144.

79. Thomas ED, Clift RA. Indications for marrow transplantation in chronic myelogenous leukemia. Blood 1989;73:861.

80. Clift RA, Buckner CD, Applebaum FR, et al. Allogeneic marrow transplantation in patients with chronic myeloid leukemia in the chronic phase; a randomized trial of two irradiation regimens. Blood 1991;77:1660.

81. Clift RA, Martin PJ, Fisher L, et al. Allogeneic marrow transplantation for CML in accelerated phase—risk factors for survival and relapse. Blood 1987;70(Suppl 1):291. (Abstr no 1019).

82. Sanders JE, Buckner CD, Stewart P, et al. Successful treatment of juvenile chronic granulocytic leukemia with marrow transplantation. Pediatrics 1979;63:44.

83. Goldman JM, Gale RP, Horowitz MM, et al. Bone marrow transplantation for chronic myelogenous leukemia in chronic phase: increased risk for relapse associated with T cell depletion. Ann Intern Med 1988;108:806.

84. McGlave PB, Beatty P, Ash R, et al. Therapy for chronic myelogenous leukemia with unrelated donor bone marrow transplantation: results in 102 cases. Blood 1990;75:1728.

85. Apperley JF, Mauro F, Boldman JM, et al. Bone marrow transplantation for chronic myeloid leukaemia in chronic phase; importance of a graft-versus-leukaemia effect. Br J Haematol 1988;69:239.

86. De Witte T, Hoogenhout J, De Pauw B, et al. Depletion of donor lymphocytes by counterflow centrifugation successfully prevents graft-versus-host disease in matched allogeneic marrow transplantation. Blood 1986;67:1302.

87. Heit W, Bunges D, Wiesneth A, et al. Ex vivo T cell depletion with the monoclonal antibody Compath-1 plus human complement effectively prevents acute graft-versus-host disease in allogeneic bone marrow transplantation. Br J Haematol 1986;53:479.

88. Beatty PG, Clift RA, Micleson EM, et al. Marrow transplantation from related donors other than HLA-identical siblings. N Engl J Med 1985;313:765.

89. Ash RD, Casper JT, Chitambar CR, et al. Successful allogeneic transplantation of T cell depleted bone marrow from closely HLA-matched unrelated donors. N Engl J Med 1990;322:485.

90. Snyder DS, McGlave PB. Treatment of chronic myelogenous leukemia with bone marrow transplantation. Hematol Oncol Clin North Am 1889;4:535.

91. Fefer A, Cheever MA, Greenberg PD, et al. Treatment of chronic granulocytic leukemia with chemoradiotherapy and transplantation of marrow from identical twins. N Engl J Med 1982;306:63.

92. Martin PJ, Clift RA, Fisher LD, et al. HLA-identical marrow transplantation during accelerated-phase chronic myelogenous leukemia: analysis of survival and remission duration. Blood 1988;72:1978.

93. Copelan EA, Grever MR, Kapoor N, et al. Marrow transplantation following busulfan and cyclophosphamide for chronic myelogenous leukaemia in accelerated or blastic phase. Br J Haematol 1989;71:487.

94. Roth MS, Antin JH, Ash R, et al. Prognostic significance of Philadelphia chromosome-positive cells detected by the polymerase chain reaction after allogeneic bone marrow transplant for chronic myelogenous leukemia. Blood 1992; 79:276.

95. Champlin R, Ho W, Gajewski J, et al. Selective depletion of CD8 + T-lymphocytes for prevention of graft-versus-host disease after allogeneic bone marrow transplantation. Blood 1990;76:418.

96. Kyle RA. Long-term survival in multiple myeloma. N Engl J Med 1983;308:314.

97. Buckner CD, Fefer A, Bensinger WI, et al. Marrow transplantation for malignant plasma cell disorders: summary of the Seattle Experience. Eur J Haematol 1989;43:186.

98. Cahrton G, Tura S, Ljungman P, et al. Allogeneic bone marrow transplantation in multiple myeloma. Bone Marrow Transplant 1991;325:1267.

99. Bensinger WI, Buckner CD, Clift RA, et al. A phase I study of busulfan and cyclophosphamide in preparation for allogeneic marrow transplant for patients with multiple myeloma. J Clin Oncol 1992;10(9):1492.

100. Cavo M, Tura S, Rostig A, et al. Bone marrow transplantation for multiple myeloma (MM): the Italian experience. Bone Marrow Transplant 1991;7(Suppl 2):31.

101. Gore ME, Selby PJ, Viner C, et al. Intensive treatment of multiple myeloma and a criteria for complete remission. Lancet 1989;2:879.

102. Jagannath S, Barlogie B. Autologous bone marrow transplantation for multiple myeloma. Hematol Oncol Clin North Am 1992;6:437.

103. Harosseau JL, Attal M, Reiffers J, et al. Autologous hemopoietic stem cell transplantation in multiple myeloma. A report of the French registry [Abstract]. Blood 1992; 80(Suppl 1):361.

104. Montes A, Cunningham D, Paz-Ares L, et al. High dose melphalan and autologous bone marrow transplant in multiple myeloma: long-term follow-up [Abstract]. Abstracts 19th annual meeting of the EMBT Group, Garmisch-Partenkirchen, Germany. 1993:68.

105. Attal M, Huguet F, Schlaifer D, et al. Intensive combined therapy for previously untreated aggressive myeloma. Blood 1992;79:1130.

106. Attal M, Harousseau IL, Stoppa AM, et al. High dose therapy in multiple myeloma: a prospective randomized study of the Intergroupe Francais de Myeloma (IFM) [Abstract]. Blood 1993;82(Suppl 1):198.

107. Alexanian R, Dimopoulos M, Smith T, et al. Limited value of myeloablative therapy for late multiple myeloma. Blood 1994;83(2):512.

108. Anderson KC, Barut BA, Ritz J, et al. Monoclonal antibody-purged autologous bone marrow transplantation therapy for multiple myeloma. Blood 1991;77:712.

109. Fernand JP, Chevret S, Levy Y, et al. The role of autologous blood stem cells in support of high-dose therapy for multiple myeloma. Hematol Oncol Clin North Am 1992;6:451.

110. Appelbaum FR, Sullivan KM, Buckner CD, et al. Treatment of malignant lymphoma in 100 patients with chemotherapy, total body irradiation, and marrow transplantation. J Clin Oncol 1987;5:1340.

111. Jones RJ, Piantadosi S, Mann RB, et al. High-dose cytotoxic therapy and bone marrow transplantation for relapsed Hodgkin's disease. J Clin Oncol 1990;8:527–537.

112. Jones RJ, Ambinder RF, Piantadosi S, et al. Evidence of a graft-versus-lymphoma effect associated with allogeneic bone marrow transplantation. Blood 1991;77:649.

113. Copelan EA, Kapoor N, Biggins B, et al. Allogeneic marrow transplantation in non-Hodgkin's lymphoma. Bone Marrow Transplant 1990;5:47.

114. Lundberg JH, Hansen RM, Chitambar CR, et al. Allogeneic bone marrow transplantation for relapsed and refractory lymphoma using genotypically HLA-identical and alternative donors. J Clin Oncol 1991;9:1848.

115. Phillips GL, Reece DE, Barnett MJ, et al. Allogeneic marrow transplantation for refractory Hodgkin's disease. J Clin Oncol 1989;7:1039.

116. Nademanee AP, Forman SH, Schmidt GM, et al. Allogeneic bone marrow transplantation for high risk non-Hodgkin's lymphoma during first complete remission. Blut 1987;55:11.

117. Vilmer E, Rhodes-Feuilette A, Rabian C, et al. Clinical and immunological restoration in patients with AIDS after marrow transplantation using lymphocyte transfusions from the marrow donor. Transplantation 1987;44:25.

118. Lane HC, Zunich KM, Wilson W, et al. Syngeneic bone marrow transplantation and adoptive transfer of peripheral blood lymphocytes combined with zidovudine in human immunodeficiency virus (HIV) infection. Ann Intern Med 1990;113:512.

119. van Bekkum DW, Bach FH, Bergan JJ, et al. Marrow transplants from histocompatible, allogeneic donors for aplastic anemia. A report from the ACS/NIH bone marrow transplant registry. JAMA 1976;236:1131.

120. Champlin RE, Ho WG, Nimer SD, et al. Bone marrow transplantation for severe aplastic anemia. Transplantation 1990;49:720.

121. Gluckman E, Devergie A, Dutreix J. Bone marrow transplantation for Fanconi's anemia. In: Schroeder-Kurth TM,

Aeurbach AD, Obe G, eds. Fanconi anemia, clinical cytogenetic and experimental aspects. Berlin: Springer-Verlag, 1989:60.

122. Camitta B, Ash R, Menitove J, et al. Bone marrow transplantation for children with severe aplastic anemia: use of donors other than HLA-identical siblings. Blood 1989;74:1852.

123. Aeurbach AD, Liu Q, Ghosh R, et al. Prenatal identification of potential donors for umbilical cord blood transplantation for Fanconi's anemia. Transfusion 1990;30:682.

124. Gluckman E, Broxmeyer HE, Auerbach AD, et al. Hematopoietic reconstitution in a patient with Fanconi's anemia by means of umbilical cord blood from an HLA identical sibling. N Engl J Med 1989;321:1174.

125. Flowers MED, Doney KC, Storb R, et al. Marrow transplantation for Fanconi anemia with or without leukemia transformation: an update of the Seattle experience. Bone Marrow Transplant 1992;9:167.

126. Auborg P, Blanche S, Jambague I, et al. Reversal of early neurologic and neuroradiological manifestations of X-linked adrenoleukodystrophy by bone marrow transplantation. N Engl J Med 1990;322:1860.

127. Harris RE, Harron D, Vogler C, et al. Bone marrow transplantation in type IIa glycogen storage disease. Birth Defects 1986;22:119.

128. Hobbs JR, Hugh-Jones K, Shaw PL, et al. Wolman's disease corrected by displacement bone marrow transplantation with immunoprophylaxis. Bone Marrow Transplant 1986;1(Suppl):347.

129. Moser HW, Tutschka PJ, Brown FR III, et al. Bone marrow transplantation in adrenoleukodystrophy. Neurology 1984;34:1410.

130. Yeager A, Moser HW, Tutschka J, et al. Allogeneic bone marrow transplantation in adrenoleukodystrophy: clinical, pathological and biochemical studies. In: Krivit W, Paul N, eds. Bone marrow transplantation for treatment of lysosomal storage disorders. New York: Alan R Liss, 1986.

131. Krivit W, Shapiro E, Kennedy E, et al. Treatment of late infantile metachromatic leukodystrophy by bone marrow transplantation. N Engl J Med 1990;332:28.

132. Shapiro E, Lockman L, Kennedy W, et al. Bone marrow transplantation as treatment for globoid cell leukodystrophy. In: Desnick RJ, ed. Treatment of genetic disease. New York: Churchill Livingstone, 1991:221.

133. Saunders EF, Kirby MA, Solh HS, et al. Enzyme replacement in Hurler's syndrome using bone marrow transplantation. Keystone Symposium, UCLA BMT, Jan 1992.

134. Lucarelli G, Polchi P, Izzi T, et al. Allogeneic marrow transplantation for thalassemia. Exp Hematol 1984;12:676.

135. Lucarelli G, Polchi P, Galimberti M, et al. Marrow transplantation for thalassemia following busulfan and cyclophosphamide. Lancet 1985;1:1355.

136. Frappaz D, Gluckman E, Souillet G, et al. Allogeneic bone marrow graft in thalassemia major. The French experience. Arch Fr Pediatr 1990;47:97.

137. Fischer A, Friedrich W, Fasth A, et al. Reduction in graft failure by a monoclonal antibody (Anti LFA-1, CD11a) after HLA-nonidentical bone marrow transplantation in children with immunodeficiencies, osteopetrosis and Fanconi's anemia. Blood 1990;77:249.

138. Fischer A, Cerf-Bensussan A, Blanche S, et al. Allogeneic bone marrow transplantation for erythrophagocytic lymphohistiocytosis. J Pediatr 1986;108:267.

139. Fischer A, Landais P, Friedrich W, et al. European experience of bone marrow transplantation for severe combined immunodeficiency. Lancet 1990;11:850.

140. Goldsobel A, Haas A, Stiehm E. Bone marrow transplantation in DiGeorge syndrome. J Pediatr 1987;111:40.

141. Kapoor N, Kirkpatrick D, Blaese RM, et al. Reconstitution of normal megakaryocytopoiesis and immunologic function in Wiscott-Aldrich syndrome by marrow transplantation following myeloblation and immunosuppression with busulfan and cyclophosphamide. Blood 1981;57:692.

142. Kazmierowski JA, Elin RJ, Reynolds HY, et al. Chediak-Higashi syndrome: reversal of increased susceptibility to infection by bone marrow transplantation. Blood 1976; 47:555.

143. Levinsky RJ, Tiedeman K. Successful bone marrow transplantation for reticular dysgenesis. Lancet 1983;1:671.

144. Fischer A, Friedrick W, Levinsky R, et al. Bone-marrow transplantation for immunodeficiencies and osteopetrosis: European survey, 1968–1985. Lancet 1986;2:1080.

145. Foroozonfar N, Hobbs JR, Hugh-Jones D, et al. Bone marrow transplant from an unrelated donor for chronic granulomatous disease. Lancet 1977;1:210.

146. Rappeport JM, Parkman R, Newburger C, Camitta BM, Chusid MJ. Correction of infantile agranulocytosis (Kostmann's syndrome) by allogeneic bone marrow transplantation. Am J Med 1980;68:605.

147. LeDeist F, Blanche S, Keable H, et al. Successful HLA nonidentical bone marrow transplantation in three patients with the leukocyte adhesion deficiency. Blood 1989;74:512.

148. Fischer A, Descamps-Latscha B, Gerota I, et al. Bone marrow transplantation for inborn error of phagocytic cells associated with defective adherence, chemotaxis and oxidative response during opsonized particle phagocytosis. Lancet 1983;2:473.

149. Kodish E, Lantos J, Stocking C, et al. Bone marrow transplantation for sickle cell disease: a study of parents' decisions. N Engl J Med 1991;325:1349.

150. Mentzer W C, Kalinyak AK, Sulivan KM, et al. Bone marrow transplantation in sickle cell anemia: the United States experience. Am J Pediatr Hematol Oncol 1994;16:22.

151. Ferster A, De Valck D, Azzi N, et al. Bone marrow transplantation for severe sickle cell anaemia. Br J Haematol 1992;80:102.

152. Vermylen C, Cornu G. Bone marrow transplantation in sickle cell anemia: the European experience. Am J Pediatr Hematol Oncol 1994;16:18.

153. O'Reilly RJ, Dupont B, Pahwa S, et al. Reconstitution in severe combined immunodeficiency by transplantation of marrow from an unrelated donor. N Engl J Med 1977; 297:1311.

154. Ash RC, Horowitz MM, Gale RP, et al. Bone marrow identical siblings: effect of T-cell depletion. Bone Marrow Transplant 1991;7:443.

155. Beatty PG, Clift RA, Michekson EM, et al. Marrow transplantation from related donors other than HLA-identical siblings. N Engl J Med 1985;313:765.

156. Speck B, Zwaan FE, van Rood JJ, Ernisse JG. Allogeneic bone marrow transplantation in a patient with aplastic anemia using a phenotypically HLA-A identical unrelated donor. Transplantation 1973;16:24.

157. LaDeist F, Blanch S, Keable H, et al. Successful HLA nonidentical bone marrow transplantation in three patients with leukocyte adhesion deficiency. Blood 1989;74:512.

158. McCullough J, Bach FH, Coccia P, et al. Bone marrow transplantation from unrelated volunteer donors: summary of conference on scientific, ethical, legal, financial, and other practical issues. Transfusion 1982;22:78.

159. McGlave P, Scott E, Ramsay N, et al. Unrelated donor bone marrow transplantational therapy for chronic myelogenous leukemia. Blood 1987;70:877.

160. Beatty PG, Ash R, Hows JM, et al. The use of unrelated bone marrow donors in the treatment of patients with chronic myelogenous leukemia: experience of four marrow transplant centers. Bone Marrow Transplant 1989;4:287.

161. Ash RC, Horowitz NN, Gale RP, et al. Bone marrow transplantation from related donors other than HLA-identical sibling: effect of T-cell depletion. Bone Marrow Transplant 1991;7:415.

162. Beatty PG, DiBartolomeo P, Storb R, et al. Treatment of aplastic anemia with marrow grafts from related donors other than HLA genotypically-matched siblings. Clin Transplant 1987;1:117.

163. Anasetta C, Beatty PG, Storb R, et al. Effect of HLA incompatibility on graft-versus-host disease, relapse, and survival after marrow transplantation for patients with leukemia or lymphoma. Hum Immunol 1990;29:79.

164. McCullough J, Scott EP, Halagan N. Effectiveness of a regional bone marrow donor program. JAMA 1988;259:3286.

165. Frassoni F, Barrett AJ, Granena A, et al. Relapse after allogeneic bone marrow transplantation for acute leukaemia: a survey by the E.B.M.T. of 117 cases. Br J Haematol 1988; 70:317.

166. Atkinson K, Biggs J, Concannon A, et al. Second marrow transplants for recurrence of haematological malignancy. Bone Marrow Transplant 1986;1:159.

167. Sanders JE, Buckner CD, Clift RA, et al. Second marrow transplants in patients with leukemia who relapse after allogeneic marrow transplantation. Bone Marrow Transplant 1988;3:11.

168. Wagner JE, Santos GW, Burns WH, et al. Second bone marrow transplantation after leukemia relapse in 11 patients. Bone Marrow Transplant 1989;4:115.

169. Spinolo JA, Yau JC, Dicke KA, et al. Second bone marrow transplants for relapsed leukemia. Cancer 1992;69:405.

170. Fefer A, Sullivan K, Weiden P, et al. Graft versus leukemia effect in man; the relapse rate of acute leukemia is lower after allogeneic than after syngeneic marrow transplantation. In: Truitt R, Gale RP, Bortin MM, eds. Cellular immunotherapy of cancer. New York: Alan R Liss, 1987;401.

171. Kaminski E, Sharrock C, Hows J, et al. Frequency analysis of cytotoxic T lymphocyte precursors–possible relevance to HLA-matched unrelated donor bone marrow transplantation. Bone Marrow Transplant 1988;3:149.

172. Blume KG, Forman SJ, O'Donnell MR, et al. Total body irradiation and high-dose etoposide: a new preparatory regimen for bone marrow transplantation in patients with advanced hematological malignancies. Blood 1987; 69:1015.

173. Brochstein JA, Kernan, NA, Groshen S, et al. Allogeneic bone marrow transplantation after hyperfractionated total body irradiation and cyclophosphamide in children with acute leukemia. N Engl J Med 1987;317:1624.

174. Helenglass G, Powles RL, McElwain TJ, et al. Melphalan and total body irradiation (TBI) versus cyclophosphamide and TBI as conditioning for allogeneic matched sibling

bone marrow transplants for acute myeloblastic leukaemia in first remission. Bone Marrow Transplant 1988;3:21.

175. Herzig RH, Coccia PF, Lazarus HM, et al. Bone marrow transplantation for acute leukemia and lymphoma with high-dose cytosine arabinoside and total body irradiation. Semin Oncol 1985;12(Suppl 3):184.

176. Kanfer E, Buckner CD, Fefer A, et al. Allogeneic and syngeneic marrow transplantation following high-dose dimethylbusulfan, cyclophosphamide and total body irradiation. Bone Marrow Transplant 1987;1:339.

177. McCarthy D, Kanfer E, Samson D, et al. BMT after conditioning with lomustine, cytosine, arabinoside, etoposide and cyclophosphamide. Bone Marrow Transplant 1990;5(Suppl 2):124.

178. Petersen F, Buckner CD, Appelbaum FR, et al. Busulfan, cyclophosphamide and fractionated total body irradiation as a preparatory regimen for marrow transplantation in patients with advanced hematological malignancies: a phase I study. Bone Marrow Transplant 1989;4:617.

179. Slavin S, Or R, Weshler Z, et al. The use of total lymphoid irradiation for abrogation of host resistance to T-cell depleted marrow allografts. Bone Marrow Transplant 1986;1(Suppl 1):98.

180. Thomas ED, Ferrebee JW. Transplantation of marrow and whole organs; experiences and comments. Can Med Assoc J 1962;86:435.

181. Johnson F, Thomas ED, Buckner CD, et al. The current status of bone marrow transplantation in cancer treatment. Can Treat Rev 1974;1:81.

182. Thomas ED, Bucker CD, Clift RA, et al. Marrow transplantation for thalassemia. Lancet 1982;301:597.

183. Thomas ED, Clift RA, Hersman J, et al. Marrow transplantation for acute nonlymphoblastic leukemia in first remission using fractionated or single-dose irradiation. Int J Radiat Oncol Biol Phys 1982;8:817.

184. Frassoni F, Scarpati D, Bacigalupo A, et al. The effect of total body irradiation dose and chronic graft-versus-host disease on leukaemic relapse after allogeneic bone marrow transplantation. Fr J Haematol 1989;73:211.

185. Brochstein JA, Kernan NA, Groshen S, et al. Allogeneic bone marrow transplantation after hyperfractionated total-body irradiation and cyclophosphamide in children with acute leukemia. N Engl J Med 1987;317:1618.

186. Vitale V, Scarpati D, Frassoni F, Corvo R. Total body irradiation: single dose, fractions, dose rate. Bone Marrow Transplant 1989;4(Suppl 1):223.

187. Thomas ED, Clift RA, Hersman J, et al. Marrow transplantation for acute nonlymphoblastic leukemia in first remission using fractionated or single-dose irradiation. Int J Radiat Oncol Biol Phys 1982;8:817.

188. Bearman SI, Applebaum FR, Bucker CD, et al. Regimen-related toxicity in patients undergoing bone marrow transplantation. J Clin Oncol 1988;6:1562.

189. Jones RJ, Lee KSK, Beschorner WE, et al. Veno-occlusive disease of the liver following bone marrow transplantation. Transplantation 1987;44:778.

190. Bianco JA, Appelbaum FR, Nemunaitis J, et al. Phase I-II trial of pentoxifylline for the prevention of transplant related toxicities following bone marrow transplantation. Blood 1991;78:1205.

191. Sullivan KM, Mori M, Sanders J, et al. Late complications of allogeneic and autologous marrow transplantation. Bone Marrow Transplant 1992;10:127.

192. Reed MD, Lazarus HM, Herzig RH, et al. Cyclic parenteral nutrition during bone marrow transplantation in children. Cancer 1983;51:1563.

193. Meyers JD, Flournoy N, Thomas ED. Infection with herpes simplex virus and cell-mediated immunity after marrow transplantation. J Infect Dis 1980;142:338.

194. Vogler WR, Winton EF, Heffner LT, et al. Ophthalmological and other toxicities related to cytosine arabinoside and total body irradiation as preparatory regimen for bone marrow transplantation. Bone Marrow Transplant 1990;6:405.

195. Lawler SD, Baker MC, Harris H, et al. Cytogenetic studies on recipients of allogeneic bone marrow using the sex chromosomes as markers of cellular origin. Fr J Haematol 1984;56:431.

196. Van Dijk BA, Drenthe-Schonk AM, Bloo A, et al. Erythrocyte repopulation after allogeneic bone marrow transplantation, analysis using erythrocyte antigens. Transplantation 1987;44:650.

197. Blazer BR, Orr HT, Arthur DC, et al. Restriction fragment length polymorphisms as markers of engraftment in allogeneic marrow transplantation. Blood 1985;66:1436.

198. Meera Khan P, Winjen JT, Hagenbeek A, et al. Isozymes as host-donor blood cell "tracers" in bone marrow transplantation. In: Isozymes: current topics in biological and medical research, vol 16. New York: Alan R Liss, 1987:125.

199. Grahovac B, Labar B, Stavljenic A. Subtyping of erythrocyte phosphoglucomutase-1 as a genetic marker for bone marrow engraftment and hematopoietic chimerism after allogeneic bone marrow transplantation in a patient with acute lymphoblastic leukemia. Clin Chem 1988;34:2586.

200. Sadamori N, Ozer H, Higby DJ, et al. Chromosomal evidence of donor B-lymphocyte engraftment after bone-marrow transplantation in a patient with multiple myeloma. N Engl J Med 1983;308:1423.

201. Durnam DM, Anders KR, Fisher L, et al. Analysis of the origin of marrow cells in bone marrow transplant recipients using a Y-chromosome-specific in situ hybridization assay. Blood 1989;74:2220.

202. Ugozzoli L, Yam P, Petz LD, et al. Amplification by the polymerase chain reaction of hypervariable regions of the human genome for evaluation of chimerism after bone marrow transplantation. Blood 1991;77:1607.

203. Kernan NA, Flomenberg N, Dupont B, et al. Graft rejection in recipients of T-cell-depleted HLA-nonidentical marrow transplants for leukemia. Transplantation 1987;43:842–847.

204. Smith BR, Guinan EC, Parkman R, et al. Efficacy of a cyclophosphamide-procarbazine-antithymocyte serum regimen for prevention of graft rejection following bone marrow transplantation for transfused patients with aplastic anemia. Transplantation 1985;39:671.

205. Nemunaitis J, Singer JW, Buckner CD, et al. Use of recombinant human granulocyte-macrophage colony-stimulating factor in graft failure after bone marrow transplantation. Blood 1990;76:245.

206. Kernan NA, Collins NH, Juliano L, et al. Clonable T lymphocytes in T-cell-depleted bone marrow transplants correlate with development of graft-v-host disease. Blood 1986;68:770.

207. Bacigalupo A, Van Lint MT, Congiu M, Marmont AM. Bone marrow transplantation (BMT) for severe aplastic anaemia (SAA) in Europe: a report of the ABMT-SAA Working Party. Bone Marrow Transplant 1988;3:44.

208. Beatty, PG, DiBartolomeo P, Storb R, et al. Treatment of aplastic anemia with marrow grafts from related donors other than HLA genotypically matched siblings. Clin Transplant 1987;1:117.

209. Kernan NA, Flomenberg N, Dupont B, et al. Graft rejection in recipients of T cell depleted HLA non-host derived antidonor allocytotoxic T-lymphocytes. Transplantation 1987; 43:482.

210. Loughran TP, Storb R. Treatment of aplastic anemia. Hematol Oncol Clin North Am 1990;413:559.

211. Reed EC, Bowden R, Dandiker PS, et al. Treatment of cytomegalovirus (CMV) pneumonia in bone marrow transplant patients with gancyclovir and CMV immunoglobulin. Blood 1987;70(Suppl 1):313.

212. Lazarus HM, Coccia PF, Herzig RH, et al. Incidence of acute graft-versus-host disease with and without methotrexate prophylaxis in allogeneic bone marrow transplant patients. Blood 1984;64:215.

213. Ramsay NK, Kersey JH, Robison LL, et al. Acute graft-host disease in recipients of bone marrow from identical twin donors. Lancet 1979;2:717.

214. Storb R, Deeg HJ, Pepe M, et al. Methotrexate and cyclosporine versus cyclosporine alone for prophylaxis of graft-versus-host disease in patients given HLA-identical marrow grafts for leukaemia: long term follow up of a controlled trial. Blood 1989;73:1729.

215. Santos GW, Tutschka PJ, Brookmeyer R, et al. Cyclosporine plus methylprednisolone as prophylaxis for GvHD: a randomized double blind study in patients undergoing bone marrow transplantation. Clinical Transplant 1987;1:21.

216. Kendra J, Barrett AJ, Lucas C, et al. Response of graft versus host disease to high doses of methylprednisolone. Clin Lab Haematol 1981;46:125.

217. Deeg HJ, Henslee-Downey PJ. Management of acute graft-versus-host disease. Bone Marrow Transplant 1990;6:1.

218. Deeg HJ, Loughran TP Jr, Storb R, et al. Treatment of human acute graft-versus-host disease with anti-thymocyte globulin and cyclosporine withor without methylprednisolone. Transplantation 1985;40:162.

219. Gratama JW, Jansen J, Lipovich RA, et al. Treatment of acute graft-versus-host disease with monoclonal antibody OKT3. Clinical results and effect on circulating T lymphocytes. Transplantation 1984;38:469.

220. Gleixner B, Kolb HJ, Holler E, et al. Treatment of GVHD with OKT3: clinical outcome and side-effects associated with release of TNFα. Bone Marrow Transplant 1991; 8:93.

221. Byers VS, Henslee PJ, Kernan NA, et al. Use of an anti-pan T-lymphocyte ricin A chain immunotoxin in steroid-resistant acute graft-versus-host diseae. Blood 1990; 75:1426.

222. Hervé P, Wijdenes J, Bergerat JP, et al. Treatment of corticosteroid resistant acute graft-versus-host disease by in vivo administrtion of anti-interleukin-2 receptor monoclonal antibody (B-B10). Blood 1990;75:1017.

223. Hervé P, Flesch M. Tiberghien J, et al. Phase I-II trial of a monoclonal anti-tumor necrosis factor α antibody for the treatment of refractory severe acute graft-versus-host disease. Blood 1992;79:3362.

224. Socie G, Devergie A, Cosset JM, et al. Low-dose (one gray) total-lymphoid irradiation for extensive, drug-resistant chronic graft-versus-host disease. Transplantation 1990; 49:657.

225. Tzakis AG, Abu-Elmagd K, Fung JJ, et al. FK 506 rescue in chronic graft-versus-host disease after bone marrow transplantation. Transplant Proc 1991;23:3225.

226. Reisner Y, Kirkpatrick D, Dupont B, et al. Transplantation for acute leukemia with HLA-A and B nonidentical parental marrow cells fractionated with soybean agglutinin and sheep red blood cells. Lancet 1981;2:327.

227. Antin JH, Bierer BE, Smith BR, et al. Selective depletion of bone marrow T lymphocytes with anti-CD5 monoclonal antibodies: effective prophylaxis for graft-versus-host disease in patients with hematologic malignancies. Blood 1991; 78:2139.

228. Prentice HG, Janossy G, Sketts D, et al. Use of anti-T-cell monoclonal antibody OKT3 to prevent acute graft-versus-host disease in allogeneic bone marrow transplantation for acute leukemia. Lancet 1982;1:700.

229. Filipovich AH, Youle RJ, Neville DM, et al. Ex-vivo treatment of donor bone marrow with anti-T-cell immunotoxins for prevention of graft-versus-host disease. Lancet 1984; 1:469.

230. Martin PJ, Hansen JA, Torok-Storb B, et al. Effects of treating marrow with a CD3-specific immunotoxin for prevention of acute graft-versus-host disease. Bone Marrow Transplant 1988;3:437.

231. Vartdal F, Albrechtsen D, Ringden O, et al. Immunomagnetic treatment of bone marrow allografts. Bone Marrow Transplant 1987;2:94.

232. Noga SJ, Donnenberg AD, Schwartz CL, et al. Development of a simplified counterflow centrifugation elutriation procedure for depletion of lymphocytes from human bone marrow. Transplantation 1986;41:220.

233. Champlin R, Ho W, Gajewski J, et al. Selective depletion of CD8 × T lymphocytes for prevention of graft-versus-host disease after allogeneic bone marrow transplantation. Blood 1992;79:3380.

234. Barnes DWH, Loutit JF. Spleen protection: the cellular hypothesis. In: Bacq ZM, ed. Radiobiology symposium. London: Butterworth, 1955.

235. Kersey JH, Meuwissen HJ, Good RA. Graft-versus-host reactions following transplantation of allogeneic hematopoietic cells. Hum Pathol 1971;2:389.

236. Billingham RE. The biology of graft-versus-host reactions. In: The Harvey Lectures. New York: Academic Press, 1966;62:21.

237. Santos GW. Syngeneic or autologous graft-versus-host disease. Int J Cell Cloning 1989;7:92.

238. Hess AD, Horwitz L, Beschorner WE, Santos GW. Development of graft-vs-host disease-like syndrome in cyclosporine-treated rats after syngeneic bone marrow transplantation. I. Development of cytotoxic T lymphocytes with apparent polyclonal anti-Ia specificity, including autoreactivity. J Exp Med 1985;161:718.

239. Gluckman E, Devergie A, Sohier J, et al. Graft-versus-host disease in recipients of syngeneic bone marrow. Lancet 1980;1:253–254.

240. Hood AF, Vogelsang GB, Black LP, et al. Acute graft-vs-host disease. Development following autologous and syngeneic bone marrow transplantation. Arch Dermatol 1987; 123:745.

241. Glucksberg H, Storb R, Fefer A, et al. Clinical manifestations of graft-versus-host disease in human recipients of marrow from HLA-matched sibling donors. Transplantation 1974;18:295.

242. Lerner KG, Kao GF, Storb R, et al. Histopathology of graft-versus-host reaction (GVHR) in human recipients of marrow from HLA matched sibling donors. Transplant Proc 1974;6:389.

243. Shulman HM. Pathology of chronic graft-vs-host disease. In: Burakoff SJ, Deeg HJ, Ferrara J, Atkinson K, eds. Graft-vs-host disease: immunology, pathophysiology and treatment. New York: Marcel Dekker, 1990:587.

244. McDonald GB, Shulman HM, Wolford JL, et al. Liver disease after human marrow transplantation. Semin Liver Dis 1987;7:210.

245. Shulman HM, Sharma P, Amos D, et al. A coded histologic study of hepatic graft-versus-host disease after human bone marrow transplantation. Hepatology 1988;8:463.

246. Snover DC, Weisdorf SA, Ramsay NK, et al. Hepatic graft-versus-host disease: a study of the predictive value of liver biopsy in diagnosis. Hepatology 1984;4:123.

247. Beschorner WE. Destruction of the intestinal mucosa after bone marrow transplantation and graft-versus-host disease. Surv Synth Pathol Res 1984;3:264.

248. Beschorner WE, Saral R, Hutchins GM, et al. Lymphocytic bronchitis associated with graft-versus-host disease in recipients of bone marrow transplants. N Engl J Med 1978;299:1030.

249. Saarinen UM, Kekomaki R, Simes MA, et al. Effective prophylaxis against platelet refractoriness in multitransfused patients by use of leucocyte-free blood components. Blood 1990;75:512.

250. Kekomaki R, Elfenbein G, Gardner R, et al. Improved response of patients refractory to random-donor platelet transfusions by intravenous gamma globulin. Am J Med 1984;76:199.

251. Fisher M, Chapman JR, Ring A, et al. Alloimmunization to HLA antigens following transfusion with leucocyte poor and purified platelet suspension. Vox Sang 1985;49:331.

252. Atkinson K, Horowitz MM, Gale RP, et al Consensus among bone marrow transplanters for diagnosis, grading and treatment of chronic graft-versus-host disease. Bone Marrow Transplant 1989;4:247.

253. Sullivan KM, Shulman HM, Storb R, et al. Chronic graft-versus-host disease in 52 patients: adverse natural course and successful treatment with combination immunosuppression. Blood 1981;57:267.

254. Sullivan KM, Witherspoon RP, Storb R, et al. Prednisone and azathioprine compared with prednisone and placebo for treatment of chronic graft-v-host disease: prognostic influence of prolonged thrombocytopenia after allogeneic marrow transplantation. Blood 1988;72:546.

255. Goodrich JM, Mori M, Gleaves CA, et al. Early treatment with gancyclovir to prevent cytomegalovirus disease after allogeneic bone marrow transplantation. N Engl J Med 1991;325:1601.

256. Sullivan KM, Mori M, Sanders J, et al. Late complications of allogeneic and autologous marrow transplantation. Bone Marrow Transplant 1992;10(Suppl 1):127.

257. Gluckman E, Broxmeyer HE, Auerbach AD, et al. Hematopoietic reconstitution in a patient with Fanconi anemia by means of umbilical cord blood from an HLA identical sibling. N Engl J Med 1989;321:1174.

SECTION 8

Immunohematology and Blood Banking

CHAPTER 42

Immunohematology and Blood Banking

NAOMI L. C. LUBAN

Blood is life.
—Empedocles, 5th century BC

All human cells carry surface configurations peculiar to the species, organ or tissue, and individual: many are shared with other animals, races, and family members; some are unique to small groups (private antigens) or more commonly found (public antigens). Red blood cells (RBCs) are historically the best studied cells, and the practical importance of their surface character, the blood group, has been defined in some detail. The cases presented reflect the complexities of the blood group systems and instances in which disorders related to these can be biologically defined.

Case 1

A 15-month-old African American male presented to the emergency room with a history of passing dark urine, lethargy, and listlessness. Two weeks earlier, he had an upper respiratory tract infection and otitis media treated with oral penicillin with good clinical response. Two days prior to admission, the child's grandmother noted tea-colored urine staining in the boy's diaper but ascribed it to poor fluid intake; she also noticed a muddy appearance to his sclera.

On examination the child had poor skin turgor, blood pressure of 90/palpable, a pulse rate of 180, and respiratory rate of 26/min. His sclera were yellow, and mucous membranes pale. There was no nuchal rigidity, and his T° was 37.6°C. The liver was palpable at the costal margin, and his spleen was 5 cm below the left rib cage.

Pertinent laboratory investigation showed: Hb, 60 g/L, hematocrit, 18%; MCV, 120 fL; platelets, 512; nucleated cell count, 28; and WBC, 10.5×10^9/L, with a normal WBC differential. The reticulocyte count was 28%. The blood film demonstrated many nucleated RBCs, spherocytes, poikilocytes, anisocytosis, and polychromasia. A sickle cell test was negative, and screening assay for G-6-PD deemed adequate, though not corrected for the reticulocytosis. Total bilirubin was 16 mg/dL, direct 0.9 mg/dL. Serologic studies for hepatitis A, B, C, and human immunodeficiency virus (HIV), Epstein-Barr virus (EBV), cytomegalovirus (CMV), and syphilis were initiated. Chest x-ray showed cardiomegaly.

It was suspected that the child might have an acute hemolytic episode; in the absence of an obvious provocative underlying biology, a blood sample was referred not only for crossmatching for possible transfusion but also for assessment of a possible hemolytic anemia. Mixed-field reactions prevented accurate grouping. The direct antiglobulin test (DAT) showed 3+ agglutination in both serum and in EDTA. The DAT with an anticomplementary reagent was negative. The indirect DAT was negative in immediate spin in saline, 2+ when incubated at 37°C and with antihuman globulin (AHG). A cell panel assessment was performed with 24 cells, all of which gave essentially the same result. All attempts at crossmatching resulted in incompatibility. Treatment with high-dose corticosteroids was begun, but as the child began to show signs of cardiac decompensation, crossmatch-incompatible group O-negative blood was released; the first aliquot of 5 mL/kg of such washed warmed blood was transfused without incident, but a second transfusion was followed by passage of burgundy-colored urine. Cardiac asystole developed, which did not respond to resuscitation, and death ensued.

Basic Immunohematology

Blood Group Antigens

Blood group systems consist of antigens produced either directly or indirectly by alleles at a single genetic locus or at loci linked in such a fashion that crossing-over between loci rarely occurs. Antigen expression on the red blood cell membrane may be influenced by genes inherited independently at other blood group loci. For example, the antigens A and B are affected by the action of the I gene and by alleles that determine the H blood group locus. The ABO, H, P, I and Lewis blood group antigens are produced by addition of specific sugars to the ends of oligosaccharide chains through the action of specific transferases. The oligosaccharide chain may be attached to either a glycoprotein or a glycosphinoglipid carrier molecule. Glycosphingolipids form part of the red blood cell membrane and the membranes of endothelial cells and are present in soluble form in plasma. Glycoproteins are present in red blood cell membranes, as well as in many other body cells; the soluble glycoproteins are present in plasma and serous and mucous fluids through active secretion.

Over 300 red blood cell antigens exist. Antigens carried by most individuals are called public, or high-incidence, antigens; those of low incidence are called private antigens. The frequencies of antigens vary among racial groups. The two most important blood group systems are the *ABO* and *Rh* antigen systems. Three separate genetic loci control the localization of the A and B antigens: the ABO, Hh, and Sese loci. The A and B genes encode for glycosyltransferases that produce A and B antigens upon the H antigen substrate. The H antigens are constructed on precursor oligosaccharide chain endings called type 1 and type 2. The Se gene is directly responsible for the expression of H and indirectly responsible for the expression of A and B in the glycoproteins in epithelial secretions such as saliva.

The Rh system is genetically complex and has at least three nomenclatures. At least 40 Rh antigens have been identified. Genes determining Rh antigens are transmitted as haplotypes; one Rh haplotype is inherited from each parent. If the genes inherited from each parent are identical, then the gene will be expressed as a "double dose." When the genes from each parent are not identical, the product of both genes will be expressed on the infant's RBCs. While this sounds straightforward, when RBCs are tested with specific Rh antisera, the reaction patterns may not parallel the concept of antigen dose.

The five most important antigens in the Rh system are D, C, E, c, and e. A single gene or gene complex determines the production or nonproduction of D, together with the production of either C or c and E or e. Rh antigens are likely part of the transmembrane protein band 3 (1). (For a more complete review of dosage and D^u and Rh variants, see (2).)

Anti-A and anti-B production begins after the first few months of life and continues throughout the adulthood. Results of ABO grouping obtained with newborn sera may well represent acquired transplacental passage of maternal IgG anti-A or anti-B. Anti-A produced by group B persons and the anti-B produced by group A persons are predominantly IgM. Group O individuals have IgG anti-A and anti-B; this antibody is designated as anti-A, B. ABO hemolytic disease is, therefore, seen predominantly in group O mothers with transplacental passage of IgG anti-A or anti-B; it is rare in infants born of group A or group B mothers.

In contrast to the naturally occurring anti-A and anti-B, most Rh antibodies result from immunization by pregnancy or transfusion. D antigen is the most potent immunogen; c, E, C, e are potent immunogens in decreasing order. Rh antibodies may occur together—anti-E and c, for example, may be found together because of the inheritance pattern of the Rh phenotype.

Pretransfusion Testing

Pretransfusion testing includes testing for ABO, Rh, and unexpected antibodies. Direct, or forward, grouping involves determination of the presence of A and B antigens on RBCs by use of commercially manufactured anti-A and anti-B reagents. Reverse grouping confirms the presence in the serum of the corresponding anti-A or anti-B with commercially prepared reagent cells of A, A_1, and B phenotypes. Tube tests, microplate, and automated devices may be used to detect the endpoint of agglutination. Discrepancies between forward and reverse typing must be resolved before dispensing blood. Although five Rh reagent antisera are available (anti-D, C, E, c and e), routine pretransfusion testing includes only tests for D. Anti-D reagents can be used in slide, tube, or microplate tests or in automated systems. Several different kinds of reagents exist, both pooled plasma, chemically modified IgG, and monoclonally prepared, making it mandatory to carefully follow manufacturers directions with appropriated controls.

Clinically significant antibodies are detected by use of the serum or plasma of a recipient and single-donor suspensions of group O reagent RBCs. Cells are selected that contain blood group antigens likely to detect the most clinically significant unexpected antibodies that might result in a hemolytic transfusion reaction, hemolytic disease of the newborn, or shortened in vivo survival of transfused RBCs. Two or three cell suspensions are used.

Bovine saline albumin or low-ionic-strength saline (LISS) enhances agglutination of antibody red cell antigen reactions and is frequently used to improve the sensitivity of the hemagglutination. Because antibodies reactive at 37°C or in the antiglobulin phase are likely to cause hemolysis, the antiglobulin phase of testing is required. As a control, IgG-coated RBCs are used to make sure there is no inactivation of anti-IgG in the antiglobulin reagent.

Antibody detection tests are done either in advance of or together with a crossmatch between patient sera and donor RBCs. The reagent RBCs must have strong expression of antigens and have at least D, C, E, c, e, M, N, S, s, P1, Le^a, Le^b, K, k, Fy^a, Jk^a, and Jk^b. In some blood banks, careful antibody detection tests that result in no demonstrable antibody obviate the need to perform an antiglobulin crossmatch (see below). If the patient has a prior history of a clinically significant antibody, most blood banks will proceed with a full crossmatch. A major crossmatch consists of mixing the recipient's plasma or serum with a saline suspension of donor RBCs with donor serum or plasma with an antiglobulin test. A minor crossmatch includes recipient RBCs with donor serum or plasma with an antiglobulin test. This phase of pretransfusion testing is no longer required, at least in part because antibody detection tests would have been done in the donor blood; blood from a donor with a clinically significant antibody would not be used for transfusion.

The antiglobulin test may be performed with either anti-IgG with the major component being antibody to human γ chains or polyspecific antiglobulin reagent containing anti-IgG and anti-C3d. Some blood group antibodies bind complement to the red cell membrane and may cause in vivo lysis. These include anti-A, -B, -Tjª, -Jk^b, and Leª. In certain circumstances, the IgG coating is weak while the complement binding is strong (e.g., anti-Jk^a and anti-Jk^b). In these circumstances, use of polyspecific antigloublin reagent is necessary.

The two types of antiglobulin tests used are the DAT and the indirect antiglobulin test (IAT). The DAT is positive when RBCs are coated with red blood cell antibodies and/or complement. It is used to diagnose autoimmune and transfusion-induced alloimmunization. The IAT is positive when antibodies directed against RBCs are in the plasma and react with RBCs. The IAT techniques are used in antibody identification and detection, blood grouping, and compatibility tests. Several factors affect the sensitivity of the IAT. These include the incubation temperature, ionic strength of the medium in which the RBCs are suspended, incubation time, and the proportion of serum to cells in the incubation mixture. For example, when one uses LISS reagent, the antigen-antibody molecules associate more tightly and reach equilibrium in 15 minutes, while in saline medium, 30 minutes is required. There are many technical factors that may produce false-positive or false-negative DAT and IAT reactions (reviewed in (3)).

In most cases, the antibody screen is negative and the crossmatches are compatible. A compatible crossmatch should be interpreted as meaning that at a single point in time, the serum did not contain RBC antibodies that reacted with the screening cells or donor cells by routine techniques. If the antibody screen is positive and crossmatches are incompatible, the presence of an allo- or autoantibody should be suspected. This is done by identifying the specificity of the antibody by use of panels of cells and determining whether there is an allo- or autoantibody. If the autologous control cells are positive, the recipient either has an autoantibody or may have been transfused within the preceding several months. Alloantibody reacting with circulating donor cells is sometimes misinterpreted as autoantibody. In these cases, several different techniques may be used to distinguish allo- and autoantibodies. The serum may be reacted against panel cells that have been treated with enzymes to increase their reactivity to Rh antibodies, anti-Leª, and anti-Jk^b. Alternatively, an eluate of the antibody coating the RBCs may be used with the panel cells. A distinct pattern of reactivity should permit alloantibody identification, especially when different temperatures and test conditions are used. Absorption studies may be needed to establish the presence of autoantibodies masking a coexisting alloantibody. The end result of all of the testing is to identify the offending antibody(ies), which will permit selection of blood that is antigen-negative for the offending antibody(ies). Once multiple antibodies are identified, it often becomes necessary to use a rare donor file to identify donors of appropriate antigen phenotype. In such cases, transfusion may need to be delayed until antigen-negative blood is obtained.

Hemolytic Disease of the Newborn

Case 2

A 10-day-old infant was admitted to the NICU from the Emergency Room because of hyperbilirubinemia. The infant was a 38-week-gestation, white female, appropriate for gestational age, born to a gravida 4, para 3, ab 1, 38-year-old white female whose previous infants also had hyperbilirubinemia at birth; one infant required exchange transfusion. The mother had poor prenatal care at different institutions but had at least one positive DAT, with a documented anti-D titer of 1:32. Because of insurance issues, the infant had been discharged at day 2 postdelivery. Although the mother noted deepening yellow coloration and poor feeding, she did not bring the infant to the emergency room until day 10. She did not know the cause of the jaundice in her previous infants.

Pertinent positives on physical examination included poor skin turgor in an arousable but sleepy infant with yellow sclera, mucous membranes, and skin. The liver was palpable 3 cm below the right costal margin, and the spleen tip was palpable.

Pertinent laboratory evaluation included Hgb, 112 g/L; hematocrit, 33%; MCV, 109 fL; WBC, 15.6 × 10^9/L, corrected to 11.4 × 10^9/L. Differential: 23% segs, 2% bands, 65% lymphocytes, 5% monocytes, 5% eosinophils. Platelet count was 175 × 10^9/L. Reticulocyte count was 43%, with 35 NRBC/100 WBC, with a total bilirubin of 28.5 mg/dL and direct, 1.7 mg/dL. Smear demonstrated 2+ spherocytes, 2+ anisocytosis, 3+ poikilocytosis, and polychromatophilia.

The infant was admitted and begun on intravenous hydration and blue-range banked bilirubin lights. Blood serologies for toxoplasmosis, rubella, CMV, herpes, (TORCH), syphilis, HIV, and hepatitis A, B, and C were obtained. Blood and urine cultures were obtained.

The liver and spleen were increased in size, and a chest x-ray revealed patchy diffuse lower lobe infiltrates. The hemoglobin fell to 90 g/L while the heart rate increased to 185 beats/min. A specimen was sent to the blood bank to obtain emergency uncrossmatched RBCs; the DAT and IAT were both positive. The blood bank refused to provide uncrossmatched blood and proceeded with its evaluation, which included an RBC ficin panel that demonstrated anti-D and anti-Kell. Antigen typing revealed the infant's RBCs to be Rh positive (CDe/cde) and Kell antigen positive. crossmatch-compatible, O Rh-negative (Cde/Cde) Kell antigen–negative blood was provided and transfused without incident.

The bilirubin continued to fall with treatment with bilirubin lights and hydration. The infant was discharged on day 5 with a hemoglobin of 118 g/L and a bilirubin of 6.5 mg/dL. Serologic studies, blood, urine, and CSF cultures were negative. Specimens from both parents failed to reveal anemia or spherocytes; the mother was group O, Rh negative, Kell antigen negative, while the father was group O, Rh positive (CDe/CDe), Kell antigen positive.

Analysis

Hemolytic disease of the newborn (HDN) is caused by hemolysis of infant RBCs coated with IgG alloantibody of maternal origin directed against an antigen of paternal origin present on the fetal cells. IgG-coated cells undergo accelerated destruction, resulting in variable clinical severity ranging from death to a simple laboratory abnormality in an otherwise healthy newborn. Intravascular hemolysis and anemia result in extramedullary hematopoiesis in the liver and spleen, hyperbilirubinemia, and anemia. Inadequate compensation for the anemia may result in high-output cardiac failure and hypoproteinemia, a condition called **hydrops fetalis,** which may be fatal in utero or result in a stillborn infant. Infants surviving to delivery may have varying degrees of heart failure, anemia with evidence of erythroblastic peripheral blood smears, extramedullary hematopoiesis, and hyperbilirubinemia. Lipid-soluble unconjugated bilirubin crosses the blood-brain barrier and particularly affects the nuclei of the basal ganglia and cerebellum; this is seen in pathologic specimens as bilirbuin staining. Clinically, one may see death, ataxia, deafness, or mental retardation. This clinical-pathologic condition is called kernicterus. The more free bilirubin unbound to albumin, the higher the likelihood for bilirubin toxicity. Factors affecting bilirubin-albumin binding include anoxia, metabolic acidosis, presence of free fatty acids, and competition for albumin by certain drugs. If adequate serum albumin is available for bilirubin binding, less bilirubin will be circulating, and the risk of kernicterus is reduced. Milder cases of hyperbilirubinemia may be confused with other congenital hemolytic anemias, congenital heart disease, or primary hepatic disorders like galactosemia or neonatal hepatitis, and sepsis.

HDN is classified into three categories based on serologic specificity. These include, in order of severity:

1. Rh hemolytic disease due to anti-D or anti-D with anti-C or anti-E
2. Rh hemolytic disease due to other Rh system antigens such as anti-c, anti-E, or anti-e or due to other blood system antibodies such as anti-K, anti-JK^a, or anti-Fy^a
3. ABO HDN occurring in a group O woman delivering an infant of blood group A or B

Maternal immunization occurs from the entry of small numbers of fetal cells into the maternal circulation.

While this can occur throughout pregnancy, the usual immunizing event occurs at delivery, due to placental separation. It occurs more frequently with toxemia, cesarean section, or with manual removal of the placenta. It may also occur after amniocentesis, therapeutic or spontaneous abortion, ectopic pregnancy, and/or transfusion. Immunization via transfusion can occur with the small amount of RBC contamination in platelet concentrates; therefore, female Rh-negative recipients of Rh-positive platelets are candidates for Rh prophylaxis. The incidence of D sensitization in multiparous D-positive mothers is 18%. Immunization to anti-D during pregnancy can occur with as little as 0.1 mL of fetal D-positive cells; there is a greater likelihood of development of Rh sensitization with RBC transfusion and greater fetal-to-maternal bleeding. The risk of immunization in an ABO-compatible pregnancy is 3% with 0.1 mL of bleeding, increasing to 50–65% with bleeding of 5 mL or more (4).

Rh immunization is less frequent when there is ABO incomptability between mother and fetus. Presumably, circulating anti-A,B in the O mother attaches to fetal A and B antigens and causes them to lyse, so that fewer cells circulate to produce an immunizing event. In one series, 0.05 mL or more of fetal RBCs were found when the fetus was ABO incompatible versus 23.1 mL when the maternal-fetal unit was ABO compatible (4).

ABO hemolytic disease occurs in only 3% of pregnancies despite a possible association that would result in ABO disparity in 15% of pregnancies. The low frequency is due at least in part to the RBC membrane of the newborn; because of the wide distances between A antigen sites, fewer anti-A molecules can bind firmly to the membrane to result in hemolysis. In addition, antibody is further diluted by binding to cells that contain A and B substance but are not RBCs. Therefore, ABO hemolytic disease causes less intravascular and extravascular lysis and has a more benign presentation and outcome.

Severity of Fetal Hemolytic Disease

Several measures are used to predict the severity of fetal hemolytic disease. These include maternal history of previous severity of disease, maternal alloantibody titer, amniotic fluid spectrophotometry, fetal ultrasound, and percutaneous fetal blood sampling. The pregnancy history is helpful only if there is a past history of hydrops fetalis; there is a high likelihood of hydrops in each subsequent pregnancy. While severity of disease is thought to increase with subsequent pregnancies, this may not hold if the husband is heterozygous for the offending antigen. In this case, any fetus may be antigen negative and be nonaffected.

Amniotic fluid spectrophotometry is a method to measure the deviation from linearity at 450 nm of the absorption of bilirubin. By using the curves first described by

Liley that compare bilirubin concentration to gestation, disease; zone II, moderate disease; and zone III, severe disease or hydrops fetalis (fig. 42.1). The readings more accurately reflect severity of disease in the third trimester than in the second trimester (5). Amniocentesis can produce placental trauma resulting in fetomaternal transplancental hemorrhage. This may further expose the mother to more fetal RBC antigens, thereby increasing her alloantibody titer and the severity of HDN. **Rh prophylaxis is indicated when an Rh-negative mother with a known or suspected Rh-positive infant undergoes amniocentesis.** By combining amniocentesis with ultrasound techniques, placental localization has improved dramatically. In addition, the status of the fetus can be assessed serially on the basis of hepatic size, presence of ascites, cardiac contractility, and fetal movement, using a safe and noninvasive technique.

Percutaneous umbilical blood sampling (PUBS) is a technique that became feasible in the mid-1980s. An umbilical cord vessel is punctured under ultrasound visualization. PUBS permits direct assessment of fetal anemia (hemoglobin, hematocrit), red cell sensitization (ABO group, Rh typing, typing for offending antigen to which mother is sensitized, antiglobulin testing), and clinical status (bilirubin, total protein, and platelet and nucleated RBC counts); fetal blood gases and other measurements can also be made in fetuses as early as 18 weeks. A maternal blood bank specimen should be tested in parallel to assess purity of the fetal sample; I and i RBC antibody typing and MCV analysis by electronic cell counting are particularly helpful.

In one study, PUBS produced a greater increase in anti-D titer than when amniocentesis or fetoscopic blood was collected. This group advised use of PUBS only when anti-D titers reached a critical high titer or in the case of a severely affected previous pregnancy (6).

Every pregnant woman should be tested for ABO, D and have an antibody screen for unexpected antibodies (7). Any Rh-negative, Rh-immunized woman or Rh-positive woman with an unexpected antibody should have the antibody identified with commercial panel cells, and the titer of the antibody determined. Samples should be tested at 18 weeks of gestation and every 2–4 weeks, depending on the antibody titer. In the case of an anti-D titer at or above 16 in a woman with a history of a previously affected fetus, amniocentesis should be offered to evaluate the severity of hyperbilirubinemia through amniotic fluid analysis of bile pigment(s) by a change in optical density at 450 nm and the degree of fetal maturity through lecithin/sphingomyelin (L/S) and phosphotidylglycerol (PG) measurements. The amniocentesis may need to be repeated frequently. The accuracy of predicting severity of Rh or ABO of illness increases with repeated measurements (8). If it is determined that the infant has severe disease, intrauterine transfusion may be recommended.

If the mother is known to be Rh D negative, the infant's cord blood should be tested at least for hemoglobin, hematocrit, ABO group, Rh group, and direct and indirect antiglobulin. If the DAT is positive, an eluate from the infant cells should be made, and the antibody identified with commercial panel cells. If there is a discrepancy between the maternal and infant samples, with the mother's serum being negative, one should consider an antibody to a low-incidence antigen not present in the panel cells. If the mother's serum is ABO incompatible with the infant's cells, the IgG antibody is likely causing ABO HDN. The eluate from the infant's cells tested against A and B cells will help confirm the diagnosis. Occasionally, the DAT is negative

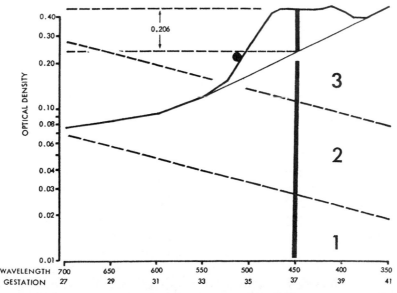

Figure 42.1 Spectrophotometry of amniotic fluid bilirubin. (From Zipursky A. Isoimmune hemolytic anemias. In: Nathan DG, Oski FA, eds. Hematology of infancy and childhood. Philadelphia: WB Sanders, 1994. With permission.)

but anti-A and anti-B can be eluted from the infant's cells. The eluate should be tested against A, B, and O cells with a sensitive antiglobulin technique. Other potential serologic conditions that cause confusion include low-frequency antigens and false-positive DATs (not discussed further).

Management of the Infant with Hemolytic Disease

Since the early 1940s, transfusion has been the primary therapy for the infant with HDN. However, the timing and nature of the transfusion has changed dramatically. Exchange transfusion of the affected infant will replace the infant's antibody-coated, antigen-positive sensitized RBCs with cells that do not have the offending antigen. In addition, exchange transfusion will remove the bilirubin and maintain the infant's hemoglobin level and total serum protein concentration, thereby preventing or attenuating progression of the neurologic and cardiac decompensation. Several laboratory methods have developed over the years to define precisely the risk of kernicterus. These include measurement of bilirubin-albumin binding and free bilirubin. Phototherapy with blue-region (420–460 nm) light changes the configurational isomer of bilirubin from the 4Z, 5Z isomer to a less toxic, unstable water-soluble form and into lumibilirubin, which is also water soluble and rapidly excreted in urine and bile. While phototherapy does not decrease either the hemolysis or anemia resulting from HDN, it does alleviate the complications of hyperbilirubinemia.

The decision to perform an exchange transfusion is based on a number of parameters including both the laboratory values and an assessment of the infant's clinical status. Rate of rise of bilirubin and hemoglobin concentration are the primary criteria, but they are attenuated when the infant has acidosis, hypoxia, or sepsis or is premature. Methods for performing an exchange are reviewed in (9).

Management of the Fetus with HDN

Serial amniotic fluid ΔOD 450 readings in the top of zone II or zone III or a single zone III measurement suggests imminent fetal demise. If the fetus is less than 32 weeks gestation, intrauterine fetal transfusion should be performed. If more than 33 weeks, delivery may be induced, particularly if the fetal lung maturity is adequate, based on the L/S ratio.

Intrauterine fetal transfusion can be performed by introducing a catheter under ultrasound guidance into the fetal peritoneal cavity. Transfused blood is absorbed via the lymphatic duct into the venous circulation. Direct intravascular transfusion is now more commonly used. In this technique, under ultrasound guidance, a 20–22-gauge needle is introduced into an umbilical blood vessel (artery or vein) at its insertion into the placenta. The advantages of this technique are that it allows direct fetal blood sampling to assess fetal anemia and degree of sensitization and it provides direct vascular access for transfusion. It does not depend upon diaphragmatic movement to assure in-

traperitoneal absorption of blood; in addition, the 8–10 days needed for absorption of transfused blood is shortened by using this direct route. Intraperitoneal transfusion may be necessary when cord vessels are too small for successful venipuncture or after 30-weeks gestation, when increased fetal size obscures the cord vessel insertion. Advantages and disadvantages of the different methods are reviewed in (10).

Red cell units selected for fetal transfusion should be group O, D negative, antigen negative for the offending antigen and crossmatch compatible with the maternal serum. By convention, the RBCs chosen are usually as fresh as possible to ensure in vivo survival. In addition, the RBCs should be CMV negative to avoid complications from posttransfusion CMV and irradiated to prevent graft-versus-host disease (GVHD), as the fetus is immunologically naive and, in part, immunocompromised. To reduce any possible complications from the metabolic sequences of an acidic anticoagulant and red cell leakage of K^+, the RBCs are washed, and the transfused blood has a hematocrit of 75%.

Rh Immunoprophylaxis

In the 1960s, trials using high-titer anti-D contained in immune serum globulin were very successful in the prevention of Rh immunization. During the last two decades, the dose and timing of administration has been the focus of much investigation. Administration of Rh immune globulin (Rh IG) will prevent Rh immunization if it is administered in adequate dosage before Rh immunization has begun. Rh IG is made by the Cohn cold ethanol method and contains small amounts of IgA and IgM. It is prepared from the plasma of hyperimmunized D-negative volunteers. It is pasteurized and therefore assumed to be relatively free of viral transmission. Monoclonally prepared or recombinant anti-D is not yet available. The usual dose is 50 µg Rh IG administered within 72 hours following abortion, and 300 µg is administered within 72 hours following delivery of an Rh-positive infant. More recently, a dose of 300 µg of Rh IG has been administered at 28-weeks gestation, followed by a dose at delivery; this is based on data suggesting that 9% of women receive an antigenic stimulus early in pregnancy and develop anti-D by 29 weeks. The half-life of Rh IG is 23 days; 20–30 µg of the 300-µg dose administered at 28 weeks is likely to be circulating at delivery.

Women who are Rh negative and undergo amniocentesis in the first trimester should receive 300 µg at first amniocentesis. A second dose should be administered 12 weeks later or at 28-weeks gestation, and a third dose at delivery if the infant is Rh positive. For amniocentesis performed in the second or third trimester, Rh-negative women should receive 300 µg Rh IG. If a subsequent amniocentesis is done more than 21 days later, an additional dose should be given (3). Larger doses at delivery are required in the setting of massive fetal-maternal hemorrhage. Careful monitoring of the mother with quantitative tests of hemorrhage is required. Rosette tests, quantitative

Kleihauer-Betke tests, and other modifications of these two tests yield quantiative data that help one decide when to administer more than 300 µg of Rh IG.

There are several theories about the mechanism(s) of action of Rh IG, which have been detailed by Bowman (11). One theory is called the "immunostat" hypothesis. When Rh IG is injected intramuscularly, it enters the circulation via the lymphatics. Depending on the dose of anti-D and the volume of Rh-positive cells, only a fraction of the fetal red cells will be bound. As antibody-coated red cells are filtered in the fetal spleen and lymph nodes, they set up a series of immunologic phenomena that depend upon the presence or absence of Fc receptor function. Fc receptors bound to antigen-antibody complexes stimulate suppressor T-cell response, prevent antigen-induced B-cell proliferation, and convert B cells to antibody-producing plasma cells (11).

Certain women are not candidates for Rh IG. They include Rh-negative women who deliver Rh-negative infants, Rh-positive women delivering Rh-positive or Rh-negative infants, and Rh-negative women who are known to be immunized to anti-D. Anti-D may be present in the maternal postpartum specimen, and there may be confusion as to its origin. Active immunization to anti-D would be suggested by the anti-D being reactive in saline or inactivated with 2-mercaptoethanol or dithiothreitol. Passive immunization is suggested by weak reactivity in the antiglobulin phase and a titer of 4 or less (3).

Neonatal Alloimmune Thrombocytopenia

RBC systems are not the only ones involved in immuno-hemotologic pathology.

Case 3

A 2000-g 39-week-gestation male infant was delivered following epidural anesthesia by uncomplicated vaginal delivery to a gravida 1, para 1, healthy 31-year-old lawyer who had excellent prenatal care and denied significant positive alcohol, tobacco, and medication history. The infant had Apgar scores of 9 and 10 and was taken to the term nursery. Six hours postdelivery, the infant was brought to the mother for breast-feeding. When the child was unwrapped, petechiae and a large hematoma at the right side of the head were noted. The chart was reviewed, and mother and obstetrician were questioned and could not document a positive history of preeclampsia, collagen vascular disease, or drug ingestion. The infant was taken to the intensive care nursery, where a sepsis workup and blood for TORCH serologies was obtained. A complete blood count on the infant revealed a hemoglobin of 122 g/L (decreased from the cord hemoglobin of 156 g/L), hematocrit of 36%, platelet count of 15×10^9g/L, and a unremarkable blood film for a newborn except for the low platelets. PT and PTT were appropriate for age, FDP

was negative, and fibrinogen was 250 mg/dL. A tibial bone marrow aspirate on the infant revealed normal megakaryocyte number, no evidence of atypical cells, and no increase in histiocytes. Platelet sizing revealed a mean platelet volume of 10 fL. The mother's platelet count was 210×10^9/L.

The infant did well until day 5 of life; all cultures were negative, and TORCH titers were negative. A nurse inadvertently dropped him against the side of the bassinet; this was followed by lethargy and poor sucking. The diagnosis of intracranial hemorrhage was made by CT scan. Platelet count was 10^9/L at the time. A random-donor platelet transfusion was given, which resulted in a posttransfusion count of 58×10^9/L, falling to 4×10^9/L by 4 hours. Specimens were collected and sent to a reference laboratory for platelet-specific antibodies from the mother, father, and infant. Maternal platelets were collected, washed, resuspended in thawed AB plasma, and transfused to the infant, resulting in a count of 20×10^9/L, which was sustained over 2 days. Every 2 days, washed maternal platelets were transfused, until day 15 of life. By 8 weeks, the platelet count was 50×10^9/L, increasing to 145×10^9/L by 12 weeks of life. At 4 years of age, a neurodevelopmental evaluation confirmed a right hemiparesis with delay in language skills and fine and gross motor coordination.

Etiology and Clinical Presentation

Neonatal alloimmune thrombocytopenia (NAIT) has similar pathophysiology to that of HDN. It occurs in 1 in 2000 live births and accounts for 20% of all neonatal thrombocytopenias (12). It is caused by destruction of fetal platelets by maternal alloantibodies directed against platelet-specific antigens inherited by the fetus from the father. The maternal IgG platelet antibodies pass transplacentally, bind to fetal platelets, and cause accelerated destruction. There are several different platelet-specific antibodies known to cause NAIT (table 42.1); anti-HLA alloantibodies also develop during pregnancy but have not been associated with NAIT. In contrast to HDN, NAIT occurs during the first

Table 42.1. Platelet-Specific Alloantigens

Traditional	Antigens	Glycoprotein		Phenotype Frequency (%) (Whites)
Zw, Pl^A	HPA-1a	Zw^a, Pl^A1	IIIc	97.9
	HPA-1b	Zw^bPl^A2		26.5
Ko, Sib	HPA 2d	Ko^b	Ib	99.3
BaK, Lek	HPA 2b	Ko^a, Sib		14,6
BaK, Lek	HPA 3a	Bak^a, Lek^a	IIb	87.7
	HPA 3b	Bak^b		64.1
Pen, Yuk	HPA 4a	Pen^a, Yuk^b	IIIa	99.9
	HPA 4b	Pen^b, Yuk^a		0.2
Br, Zav, Hc	HPA 5a	Br^b, Zav ^b	Ia	99.2
	HPA 5b	Br^a, Zav^a,Hc^a		20.6

Adapted from Goldman M, Filion M, Proulx C, Chartrand P, Decary F. Neonatal alloimmune thrombocytopenia. Transfus Med Rev 1994;8:123.

pregnancy in 50% of cases; as in HDN, previous abortion as well as pregnancy or transfusion may sensitize the mother. For subsequent pregnancies, the recurrence rate is above 80%, and the infants have a more severe clinical course. In contrast to HDN, transfusion is a rare cause of NAIT (12).

The severity of the thrombocytopenia that develops depends on the concentration and subclass of the maternal IgG alloantibody and the antigen density on the fetal platelet. Additional determinants include the ability of the fetal reticuloendothelial system to sequester the platelet-antibody complex and the capacity of the fetal bone marrow to compensate for the thrombocytopenia. Postdelivery, the laboratory diagnosis depends upon documentation of fetomaternal incompatibility for specific platelet surface antigen(s) and the presence of maternal alloantibodies reacting with both neonatal platelets and father's platelets.

Infants born with NAIT may present with only mucocutaneous bleeding or may present in extremis. In one large study, 25% of the children either died (6.5%) or had neurologic sequelae (19%) (13). Intracranial hemorrhage (ICH) may occur in 10% of cases, usually between 30 and 35 weeks of gestation, and is the basis for aggressive antenatal management of selected pregnancies (see below).

> The one consistent finding in NAIT is thrombocytopenia and bleeding within the first 24 hours of life. While the differential diagnosis of thrombocytopenia in the newborn is long, certain clinical features make NAIT unique. These include severe isolated thrombocytopenia in an infant who is otherwise well with no known cause of thrombocytopenia. Absence, of hemangiomas (Kasabach-Merritt syndrome), limb abnormalities (TAR syndrome), hepatosplenomegaly (TORCH), and toxic appearance (sepsis) are important to rule out when making the diagnosis of NAIT (see Chapter 21).

Alloimmunization to Pl^{A1} is HLA class II restricted, with strong association to HLA-DR3. More recently, de Waal et al. found that all immunized women had the supertypic determinant DRw 52, implying that this HLA class II chain is responsible for presenting the Pl^{A1} peptide to antigen-specific T cells (14).

Platelets express ABO-, HLA-, and platelet-specific antigens on their surfaces. HLA antibodies are commonly found in pregnant women and are commonly associated with other immune-mediated thrombocytopenias but are a rare cause of NAIT. This is likely due to neutralization by the HLA antigens present on placental tissue; therefore, little antibody passes to the fetus. Maternal platelet-specific antibodies, on the other hand, are not absorbed by placental antigens and pass to the fetus.

Several assays are available to confirm the laboratory diagnosis of NAIT, which use immunofluorescence, enzyme-linked immunosorbent assays (ELISA), antigen-capture ELISA, and radioimmunoassays. Some assays are now commercially available in kit form, making the tests more widely available, with rapid turnaround times. Most assays allow titration of the antibody. Platelet antigen typing uses test platelets incubated with typing antisera, wash steps, and incubation with labeled antihuman IgG. Platelet antibody typing uses platelets of known antigen types (PL^{A1} positive and negative, Bak^a positive/PL^{A1} negative, Bak^a negative/PL^{A1} positive, etc.) with maternal and neonatal sera. Some test systems use monoclonal antibody immobilization of platelet antigens. Reaction patterns usually confirm the diagnoses unless (a) platelet-specific and HLA alloantibodies coexist; (b) allo- and autoantibodies coexist; or (c) the assays fail to detect maternal antibody (15). In the first two cases, the mother's reactivity to the platelet panel will suggest the coexistence of more than one kind of antibody. In the third case, elution of the antibody and enrichment techniques or immunoblotting may prove successful (16).

It is important to predict whether second or subsequent siblings will be affected, so that subsequent pregnancies can be more carefully managed. Cesarean section may be indicated, or antenatal management might include treatment of the mother or fetus with intravenous immunoglobulin (IVIG) or fetus with platelet transfusion. Zygosity testing of the father for the implicated platelet antigen system often helps in this regard. Heterozygosity for PL^{A1} and PL^{A2}, for example, produces a 50% chance that the father will not pass the PL^{A1} gene to a subsequent offspring, while homozygosity for PL^{A1} almost certainly predicts an affected fetus. Serial maternal platelet-specific antibody titers predict neonatal thrombocytopenia, but the severity of thrombocytopenia may not be predicted by rise in titer (17) (table 42.2). (Other aspects of NAIT are referred to in chap. 28.)

Management of NAIT in Infants

> Because NAIT is caused by passive transfer of maternal IgG alloantibodies, one can expect that the disorder will regress over time as these and other maternal alloantibodies disappear. The half-life of IgG is 2–3 weeks, thereby defining this disorder as self-limiting. Despite the expected disappearance of the offending antibody, the thrombocytopenia that results from this disorder puts these infants at risk for intracranial hemorrhage and its sequela.

Unexpected NAIT

If there is no history of a previously affected infant, the diagnosis of NAIT has to be made as it was in the case history. Once the diagnosis is confirmed by serologic testing, infants at risk for ICH should receive maternal platelets or those obtained from a platelet donor known to be antigen-negative for the offending antibody. Maternal family members of appropriate antigen phenotype may serve as donors. If maternal platelets are used, they should be washed free of maternal antibody with manual or automated washing techniques and resuspended in saline or AB plasma prior to transfusion. A modified apheresis platelet collection using bags that allow 5-day storage provides more than one transfusion from the same donor. If

Table 42.2. Typical Reaction Patterns in Testing for NAIT

		Antigenic Type of Test Platelets (Platelet Panel)				
Pl^A1	+	+	−		−	
	Bak^a	+	−	+	−	Interpretation
Patient's serum (antibody status unknown)	3+	3+	−	0		Pl^A1 alloantibody
		3+	0	3+	0	Bak^1 alloantibody
		2+	2+	2+	2+	Probable HLA alloantibody (presence of platelet-specific alloantibodies cannot be excluded)
		3+	3+	1+	1+	Probable platelet-specific (Pl^A1) plus HLA antibody or platelet autoantibody

From Blanchette V. Neonatal alloimmune thrombocytopenia. In: Stockman JA, Pochedly C, eds. Developmental and neonatal hematology. New York: Raven Press, 1988. With permission.

[a]In this assay, positive reactions are graded 1+ to 4+, and negative reactions as 0.

the mother is used, washing and resuspension is still required. In addition, platelets obtained from the mother or first- or second-degree relatives should be irradiated to abrogate posttransfusion GVHD (18).

There are several other therapeutic approaches to the treatment of NAIT. These include the use of steroids to inhibit reticuloendothelial sequestration of antigen-antibody complexes, exchange transfusion to remove maternal alloantibodies, and high-dose IVIG to nonspecifically inhibit RE function. Certain investigators recommend using IVIG only (a) if antigen-negative platelets are delayed or unavailable (19) or (b) adjunctively if response to the platelet transfusions is delayed or inadequate. Doses range from 0.4 g/kg per day for 5 days to 1 g/kg per day for 2 days (20, 21).

Expected NAIT

The subsequent pregnancy of a woman with a previously affected infant with a homozygous platelet-antigen-positive father warrants careful antenatal management. While management of such pregnancies is not standardized, it might include serial fetal blood sampling for both diagnosis and quantitation of fetal platelet count, maternal treatment with IVIG and/or steroids, fetal platelet transfusions, and cesarean section to avoid the trauma of vaginal delivery.

Fetal blood sampling may be performed to obtain serial platelet counts by PUBS. The purity of the sample is critical, as small amounts of amniotic fluid will cause platelet clumping and spurious results. Expression of Pl^A1 antigen can occur as early as 19-weeks gestation, so that fetal sampling can be done as early as 20-weeks gestation to determine fetal platelet antigen phenotype and fetal platelet count. Some argue that fetal platelet transfusion can be performed repetitively without morbidity (22); others feel the invasiveness and potential morbidity and mortality limits such an approach (23).

Treatment of the mother with steroids or IVIG is a less invasive approach but is not uniformly effective. The dose and duration of treatment with IVIG may well be one crit-

ical variable (24). Another is the ability of IVIG to cross the placenta. Studies with perfused human placental lobules demonstrated that when human IVIG and anti-Pl^A1 were simultaneously added to the maternal side of the placenta, there was no transfer of anti-Pl^A1, while anti-Pl^A1 alone did cross to the fetal circulation (25). Optimal management is still evolving (26, 27). High-risk patients, defined as those fetuses with a low fetal platelet count at an early stage of pregnancy and a previously clinically affected sibling, warrant platelet transfusions, particularly during the later part of pregnancy (28). High-dose IVIG and steroids, although less predictable, might also be given to the mother. When the platelet count is not dangerously low, IVIG and steroids alone may suffice until immediately predelivery. Predelivery platelet transfusion might then allow a vaginal delivery (29). Neonatal management should include preparation for the possible use of platelet-sepecific-antigen-negative platelets.

Case 4

An 11-year-old African male with sickle cell disease and a past history of transfusion in Nigeria presented for the first time to the hematology clinic with a history of pain in the extremities, joint swelling of the elbows and knees, deepening scleral icterus, and diffuse left upper quadrant abdominal pain. Chest, abdominal x-rays, and abdominal sonogram were compatible with a bilirubin stone in the common duct. The patient was admitted for hydration and further evaluation. He became febrile to 40.5°C and had a toxic appearance; the clinical diagnosis of acute cholecystitis was made. Blood and urine cultures were obtained, and antibiotics were begun.

The patient was group B, Rh negative, with a negative DAT, and 4+ positive IAT. An RBC panel and selected cell panel revealed anti-E, anti-C, and an unidentifiable antibody. Group B, Rh-negative, E-, c-antigen-negative units were crossmatch incompatible. Specimens were sent to a reference laboratory. Six days later, by using specialized selected cell panels and eluates of the patient's cells, an anti-Jk^b antibody was identified.

The hemoglobin concentration continued to fall, while his temperature decreased and abdominal pain improved. The surgeons elected to perform a cholestectomy after exchange transfusion. An order for 24 units of packed red cells was sent to the blood bank. The order could not be filled with compatible blood, and the surgery was postponed. The patient continued on oral analgesics and intravenous hydration. He was discharged home after 8 days, having been afebrile and without abdominal pain for 3 days. Two weeks later, he was readmitted for an isovolumetric exchange transfusion (erythrocytopheresis) performed on a cell separator, using frozen deglycerolized RBCs obtained through a rare-donor registry. They were group B, Rho(D) negative, and also negative for E, c, and Jk^b. Following this procedure, which took 15 units of blood, he underwent anesthesia induction and common bile duct exploration without incident and recovered uneventfully.

Transfusion Therapy in Sickle Cell Disease

Transfusion therapy is used in sickle cell disease (SCD) to relieve severe anemia by increasing the hemoglobin concentration or to reduce the likelihood of sickling by replacing the patient's cells with those from a hematologically normal donor. Examples of transfusion goals for the specific complications of sickle cell anemia are seen in Table 42.3.

With few exceptions, the kind of blood product chosen for the patient with SCD would be similar to that chosen for patients with other inherited or acquired anemias. One exception is that blood should be sickle hemoglobin tested and found negative by a solubility test. This is because the hemoglobin S from the donor with the trait may obscure the laboratory measurement of the proportions of hemoglobin belonging to the donor and the patient. Oxygen dissociation and 2,3-diphosphoglyceraldehyde characteristics of AS-donor blood and AA-donor blood do not differ.

Table 42.3. Transfusion Indications in Sickle Cell Disease

Short-term increase in hemoglobin
  Aplastic crisis
  Sequestration crisis
  Anemia with hemolysis
Short-term reduction in HbS concentration
  Acute transient ischemic attack, stroke
  Sepsis
  Priapism
  Acute chest syndrome or other cause of deoxygenation
  For general anesthesia
Long-term reduction in HbS concentration
  Prevention of recurrent stroke
  Prevention of recurrent sequestration crisis
  Prevention of severe disabling recurrent vaso-occlusion
  Pregnancy

The second distinctive feature is the need to identify the RBC-antigen profile of the SCD patient *before administration of the first transfusion.* This is because of the potential for the development of RBC alloantibodies in the patient. When such an antibody develops during the care of the patient, the antigen profile allows confirmation of the specificity of the alloantibody, distinguishes allo- from autoantibody, and distinguishes hemolytic transfusion reactions due to either auto- or alloantibodies. Rarely, particularly if plasma-containing products are transfused, passive antibody may be transferred to the donor and confuse the serologic picture. In these cases, the antibody needs to be identified.

The incidence of alloimmunization in SCD ranges between 3 and 26%. Rates of immunization vary; some individuals rarely become immunized despite repeated transfusions; others become immunized easily. The variability has not been well explored but may be due in part to previous immunization through pregnancy; number of transfusions administered; HLA A, B, or DR phenotype; and the presence of certain immune response genes. Giblett has theorized that African American recipients are at increased risk for alloimmunization if they are transfused with blood from donors who are not of African descent, and therefore, patients with SCD, most of whom are African Americans, may be at particular risk for alloimmunization. In SCD, several studies have demonstrated alloimmunization rates ranging from 7.5% to 36%, compared with rates of 5–21% for thalassemia (30, 31) and 0.8–1% in a transfused hospital-based population (32). Vichinsky et al. (33) compared rates of erythrocyte alloimmunization in 51 black patients with SCD with those of 19 nonblack patients with other chronic hemolytic anemias; they reported alloimmunization rates of 30% in SCD patients and 5% in the other group. Both clinically significant and clinically insignificant antibodies were detected and were included in the calculations of alloimmunization rates. Based on these differences in alloimmunization, Vichinsky et al. strongly recommended using antigen-matched blood, preferably from African American donors, for all patients with SCD, regardless of their alloimmunization status (33). This practice was hotly debated in editorials in both the *New England Journal of Medicine* (34) and *Transfusion* (35).

In the largest prospective study every performed, 3047 patients enrolled in the multiinstitutional Cooperative Study of Sickle Cell Disease were evaluated for several parameters related to alloimmunization (36). In toto, 13.1% of patients were found to be alloimmunized; a subgroup of 640 were evaluated more thoroughly. In this subgroup, patients with hemoglobin SS were alloimmunized more frequently than those with other sickle hemoglobinopathies, and those whose first transfusion was administered when they were 10 years of age or older were alloimmunized at a higher rate (20.7%) than those who had transfusions at age 10 or younger (9.6%) ($P < .001$), when number of transfusions administered was controlled. The most common antibodies were to C, E, Kell, and Lewis antigens.

This study showed alloimmunization rates more in keeping with those previously published and is validated by the large database. These authors are much less vehement in their recommendation for use of antigen-typed donor blood, but they do encourage an increase in the pool of African American donors. This can be accomplished by encouraging voluntary and community-based donations from African Americans or by more specific directed-donation programs targeted for SCD patients. Although no studies have yet proven the efficacy of these two approaches, such studies are under way.

The selection of blood for transfusion in SCD remains controversial, as it has been since the 1960s. Donor matching of units for the most common antigens other than ABO and D is time-consuming and costly and, more critically, could delay needed transfusion. Presurgical autologous blood donation and transfusion is not a viable alternative for most patients, because the purpose of transfusion is usually to lower the amount of hemoglobin S and replace it with hemoglobin A. For children with SCD, autologous transfusion is likely to be totally impractical because of the inability to collect and store volumes of blood that might be needed for any clinical indication. Directed donations, particularly from African American donors, would provide the necessary donor pool with which to antigen-match recipients, but this method is fraught with its own risks, including the potential for GVHD if the blood is from first- or second-degree relatives (37). Directed donations by their very nature are from donors coerced into donating; such donors carry a higher risk of transfusion-transmitted infections (36). The transfusion of volunteer blood known to come from an African American blood donor into an African American recipient raises emotional and ethical issues that demand an understanding of the science behind such practices. The scientific database needed to mandate such transfusion practices is not yet available. Patients with one or more clinically significant antibodies might well benefit from antigen matching for minor Rh and for K antigens, which account for 90% of antibodies detected in this population. It may well be that African patients require antigen-matched units once they develop an antibody, while African Americans do not, despite a similar antigen array (37). This may be based on the presence of an immune response gene in African patients with SCD. More effort should be placed on studying the immunobiology of alloimmunization (or its absence) and modifying the immune response to RBC antigens for all patients receiving transfusions.

By decreasing transfusion number and frequency, one might also be able to delay or even prevent alloimmunization. Recently, Vichinsky et al. (38) presented the results of a multiinstitutional study comparing a conservative transfusion regimen to a more aggressive one in adults and children undergoing more than 600 surgical procedures. The number of serious or life-threatening complications before and after surgery did not differ between groups. The more aggressively treated group had a higher incidence of new alloantibody formation (10 vs. 5%) and hemolytic transfusion reactions (6 vs. 1%), suggesting that a conservative approach (hemoglobin of 10 g/dL, regardless of the percentage of S hemoglobin) is advantageous for this population.

Delayed hemolytic transfusion reactions (DHTR) are defined as an accelerated destruction of transfused RBCs that occurs only when sufficient antibody has been produced as a result of an immune response induced by that transfusion. It classically occurs in patients who have been previously immunized but in whom the antibody is not detectable during pretransfusion testing. Three to seven days following a transfusion, the antibody titer begins to rise, and sensitized donor cells begin to lyse, resulting in fever, hyperbilirubinemia, anemia, or lack or adequate in vivo survival based on a calculated posttransfusion hemoglobin increment. Rarely, in vivo hemolysis results in disseminated intravascular coagulation (DIC) and renal failure (37). Serologically, the DAT is positive with a mixed-field pattern of agglutination. The serum or an eluate of the patient's red cells demonstrates an antibody, usually to the Rh (34%), Kidd (30%), Duffy (14%), Kell (13%), or MNS system (4%) (39). By 14 days posttransfusion, the DAT may become negative, and the eluate studies may fail to demonstrate an allo- or autoantibody. In some cases of DHTR, no antibody can be detected in vitro while the clinical presentation supports the diagnosis of DHTR. Usually, ^{51}Cr- or ^{99m}Tc-labeled survival studies are needed to confirm shortened survival. Such cases may be due to low concentrations of the antibody, another antibody class like IgA not detectable by current antiglobulin testing, or another cause of destruction such as antibody-mediated cytotoxicity in which there is a direct interaction between the antibody-sensitized cells and macrophages (40).

DHTR in SCD may mimic or incite a pain crisis and may be difficult to identify. While usually published as case reports, investigators report frequencies of 4% (40) and 11% (30), respectively, in transfused populations of patients with SCD followed over time with serologic studies designed to establish the diagnosis of DHTR (41, 42). Thus, DHTR is an important adverse reaction to transfusion in this patient population.

Summary

Knowledge of the natural role of blood group and other cell-based antigens is essential in the understanding of anemia and thrombocytopenia in maternal/fetal relationships and in acquired immunohematologic disorders and their management. No attempt has been made to cover the whole field of autoimmune disorders, and the use of blood group antigens in paternity testing, for example, has not been reviewed. Blood transfusion must be seen in the light of its immunologic background, and the risks and rewards of this form of therapy carefully considered.

REFERENCES

1. Issett PD. The Rh blood group system 1988. Transfus Med Rev 1989;3:1.

2. Wilkinson SL. Genetics and biochemistry of the Rh blood group system. In: Vengelen-Tyler V, Pierce S, eds. Blood group systems: Rh. Arlington, VA: American Association of Blood Banks, 1987.

3. Walker RH, ed. Technical manual. Arlington, VA: American Association of Blood Banks, 1990.

4. Zipursky A. Isoimmune hemolytic anemias. In: Nathan D, Oski F, eds. Hematology of infancy and children. Philadelphia: WB Sanders, 1987.

5. Ananth U, Queenan JD. Does midtrimester delta OD 450 of amniotic fluid reflect severity of Rh disease? Am J Obstet Gynecol 1989;161:47.

6. Boswell PJ, Selinger M, Ferguson J, et al. Antenatal fetal blood sampling for the management of alloimmunized pregnancies: effect upon maternal anti-D potency levels. Br J Obstet Gynaecol 1988;95:759.

7. Judd WJ, Luban NLC, Ness PM, et al. Prenatal and perinatal immunohematology recommendations for serological management of the fetus, newborn, infant and obstetrical patients. Transfusion 1990;30:175.

8. Bowman JM, Pollack JM. Amniotic fluid spectrophotometry and early delivery in the management of erythroblastosis fetalis. Pediatrics 1965;35:815.

9. Baumgart S, Kim HC. Exchange transfusion in the neonate. In: Stockman JA III, Pochedly C, eds. Developmental and neonatal hematology. New York: Raven Press, 1988.

10. Poissonnier MH, Brossard Y, Demedeiros N, et al. Two hundred intrauterine exchange transfusions in severe blood incompatibilities. Am J Obstet Gynecol 1989;161:709.

11. Bowman JM. Historical overview: hemolytic disease of the fetus & newborn. In: Kennedy MS, Wilson S, Kelton JG, eds. Perinatal transfusion medicine. Arlington, Va: American Association of Blood Banks, 1990.

12. Mueller-Eckhardt C, Kiefel V, Grubert A, et al. 348 cases of suspected neonatal alloimmune thrombocytopenia. Lancet 1989;2:363.

13. Kaplan C, Duffos F, Forestier F, et al. Current trends in neonatal alloimmune thrombocytopenia: diagnosis and therapy. In: Kaplan-Gouet C, Schlegel N, Salmon CH, McGregor J, eds. Platelet immunology: fundamental and clinical aspects. Paris: John Libby Qurotext, Colloque Inserm, 1991.

14. deWaal LP, van Dalen CM, Engelfriet CP, von dem Borne AEG. Alloimmunization against platelet-specific Zwᵃ antigen, resulting in neonatal alloimmune thrombocytopenia or post-transfusion purpura is associated with the supertypic DRw52 antigen including DR3 and DRw6. Hum Immunol 1990;17:45.

15. Blanchette VS. Neonatal alloimmune thrombocytopenia. In: Stockman JA, Pucedly C, eds. Developmental and neonatal hematology. New York: Raven Press, 1988.

16. Mueller-Eckhardt C, Kayser W, Förester C, et al. Improved assay for detection of platelet-specific Plᴬ¹ antibodies in neonatal alloimmune thrombocytopenia. Vox Sang 1982; 43:76.

17. McFarland JG, Frenzke M, Aster RH. Testing of maternal sera in pregnancies at risk for neonatal alloimmune thrombocytopenia. Transfusion 1989;29:128.

18. Sanders MR, Graber JE. Post-transfusion graft-versus-host disease in infancy. J Pediatr 1990;117:159.

19. Mueller-Eckhardt C, Kiefel V, Grobert A. High-dose treatment for neonatal alloimmune thrombocytopenia. Blut 1989; 59:145.

20. Ballin A, Andrew M, Ling E, et al. High-dose intravenous gammaglobulin therapy from neonatal autoimmune thrombocytopenia. J Pediatr 1988;112:789.

21. Bussel JB, MacFarland JG, Berkowitz RL. Antenatal management of fetal alloimmune and autoimmune thrombocytopenia. Transfus Med Rev 1990;4:149.

22. Daffos F, Forestier F, Kaplan C. Prenatal treatment of fetal alloimmune thrombocytopenia. Lancet 1988;2:910.

23. Nicolini V, Rodeck CH, Kochenour NK, et al. In utero platelet transfusion for alloimmune thromboctyopenia. Lancet 1988; 2:506.

24. Nicolini V, Tannirandorn Y, Gonzalez P, et al. Continuing controversy in alloimmune thrombocytopenia: fetal hyperimmune globulinemia fails to prevent thrombocytopenia. Am J Obstet Gynecol 1990;163:1174.

25. Morgan CL, Cannell GR, Addison R, et al. Intravenous gammaglobulin and platelet antibody transfer in the perfused human placental lobule. Transfus Med 1991;1:139.

26. Murphy MF, Metcalfe P, Waters AH, Ord J, Hambley H, Nicolaides K. Antenatal management of severe fetomaternal alloimmune thrombocytopenia: HLA compatibility may effect responses to fetal platelet transfusions. Blood 1993; 81:2174.

27. Kaplan C, Morel-Kopp MC, Clemenceau S, Daffos F, Forestier F, Tehernia G. Fetal and neonatal alloimmune thrombocytopenia: current trends in diagnosis and therapy. Transfus Med 1992;2:265.

28. Giblet ER. A critique of the theoretical hazard of inter- vs. intraracial transfusion. Transfusion 1961;1:233.

29. Waters A, Murphy M, Hambley H, Nicolaites K. Management of alloimmune thrombocytopenia in the fetus and neonate. In: Nance SJ, ed. Clinical and basic science aspect of immunohematology. Arlington, VA: American Association of Blood Banks, 1991.

30. Coles SM, Klein HG, Holland PV. Alloimmunization in two multitransfused patient populations. Transfusion 1981; 21:462.

31. Michail-Merianou V, Pamphili-Panouspoulou L, Piperi-Lowes L, Pelegrinis E, Karaklis S. Alloimmunization to red cell antigens in thalassemia: comparative study of usual versus better match transfusion programs. Vox Sang 1987;52:95.

32. Walker RH, Lin D-T, Hartrick MB. Alloimmunization following blood transfusion. Arch Pathol Lab Med 1989; 113:254.

33. Vichinsky EP, Earles A, Johnson RA, et al. Alloimmunization in sickle cell anemia and transfusion of racially unmatched blood. N Engl J Med 1990;322:1617.

34. Charache S. Problems in transfusion therapy [Editorial]. N Engl J Med 1990;332:1666.

35. Blumberg N. Beyond ABO and D antigen matching: how far and for whom? Transfusion 1990;30:482.

36. Rosse WF, Gallagher D, Kinney TR, et al. and the Cooperative Study of Sickle Cell Disease. Transfusion and alloimmunization in sickle cell disease. Blood 1990;76:1431.

37. Thaler M, Shamiss A, Orgad S, et al. The role of blood from HLA-homozygous donors in fatal transfusion-associated graft-versus-host disease after open heart surgery. N Engl J Med 1989;321:25.

38. Vichinsky E, Haberkern CM, Neumayr L, et al. A comparison of conservative and aggressive transfusion regimens in

the perioperative management of sickle cell disease. N Engl J Med 1995;333:206.

39. Starkey JM, MacPherson JL, Bolgiano DC, Simon ER, Zuck TF, Sayers MH. Markers for transfusion transmitted disease in different groups of blood donors. JAMA 1989;262:3452.

40. Luban NLC. Variability in rates of alloimmunization in different groups of children with sickle cell disease: effect of ethnic background. Am J Pediatr Hematol 1989;11:314.

41. Shirey RS, Ness PM. Delayed hemolytic transfusion reactions. In: Nance SJ, ed. Clinical & basic science aspects of immunohematology. Arlington, VA: American Association of Blood Banks, 1991.

42. Cox JV, Steane E, Cunningham G, Frenkel EP. Risk of alloimmunization and delayed hemolytic transfusion reaction in patients with sickle cell disease. Arch Intern Med 1988;148:2485.

Infection Control

CHAPTER 43

Infections in the Immunocompromised Host

PETER D. REUMAN, SAMUEL GROSS

In 1940 Waksman and Woodruff isolated actinomycin A, an antibiotic from *Streptomyces*, and, shortly thereafter, actinomycin D, an anti-cancer agent, appeared.
—Conference on Antibiotics, 1974.

General Factors to Consider

Evaluation of a patient for possible infectious disease demands that the clinician have optimal knowledge of the patient's immune status, the nature of possible or identified infecting pathogens, and the environment surrounding the patient from which the pathogen may have originated. In the immunocompromised patient, the first of these three, the host's immune status, becomes the overriding ingredient that directs patient management.

The population of immunocompromised patients has grown extensively over the last several years. This population has also changed from a relatively rare group of children with congenital immunodeficiencies to an increasingly larger population of children and adults with acquired immunodeficiencies. In all immunucompromised patients, the incidence and type of infection parallel alterations in components of the immune system.

Congenital immune deficiencies are usually very specific for malfunction of one component of the immune system. Such deficiencies lead to infections that are defined by the missing or nonfunctional immune component (table 43.1). Patients with recurrent abscesses should be evaluated for defects in granulocyte function. T-cell immunodeficiencies result in severe infections with intracellular microorganisms such as mycobacteria, fungi and viral agents. B-cell deficiencies are commonly identified by recurrent infections with polysaccharide-coated bacteria or persistent infections with viral or parasitic agents. Early complement deficiencies (complement components 1–3) commonly result in symptoms of autoimmune disease. Deficiencies late in the complement cascade result in recurrent infections with *Neisseria meningitidis*.

Acquired immunodeficiencies are associated with both immunosuppressive therapies and a number of infectious agents, the most classical being human immunodeficiency virus (HIV). In patients receiving cancer chemotherapy, profound alterations of normal host defenses can result from the malignancy, its treatment, or both. Neutropenia is the single most important factor predisposing these patients to infection. Although gram-negative infections predominate in this population, infections caused by gram-positive cocci have increased, probably related to the widespread use of intravenous catheters. Although the relationship of neutropenia to infection is clear, other risk factors also play a role in the cancer patient, such as damage to mucosal and skin barriers; the use of broad-spectrum antibiotics, indwelling central venous and urinary catheters; and exposure to hospital flora. Another acquired immunodeficiency is caused by HIV. Children and adults infected with HIV are compromised because of T4 helper-inducer cell deficiency and consequent B-lymphocyte dysfunction, which can result in infections, the severity of which depends on the degree of T4 deficiency.

The use of immunosuppressive drugs will result in infections causing significant morbidity and mortality. Infectious diseases associated with solid organ transplantation have changed from gram-negative infections with significant mortality to viral, fungal, and mycobacterial diseases. This change has occurred because of the use of less toxic immunosuppressives, effective screening of blood products, closer matching of donor and recipient, and selective antimicrobial prophylaxis (1). Viral infections occur in more than 50% of transplant recipients; bacterial infection accounts for 14%, and fungal for another 5% (2). In the recent past, cytomegalovirus (CMV) infection has been reported in 90% of CMV-seropositive patients and in as many as 60% of seronegative patients at some time following transplantation (3, 4). With the onset of aggressive gancyclovir prophylaxis in such CMV-positive patients and in CMV-negative recipients of stem cells (marrow, peripheral blood) from CMV-positive donors, the frequency of CMV disease has plummeted. Primary cytomegaloviremia is a predictor of significant illness 7 to 21 days after infection (5). Patients with pneumonia, obstructive airway disease, T-cell alterations, or impairment of renal function should be considered to have possible CMV-related disease (6–9). Other latent herpesviruses or papovaviruses can also be reactivated in the immunosuppressed host (4). Yeast and/or fungal infections, including systemic candidiasis, aspergillosis, cryp-

Table 43.1 Immunodeficiencies and Associated Infections

Primary Deficiency	Example	Infecting Agent
Phagocytic	Quant. deficiency:	*Staphylococous, Streptococcus, Neisseria*
	Cancer + chemotherapy	Gram-negative bacilli
	Asplenia	Fungi (*Candida, Aspergillus*, etc.)
	Functional defect:	
	Chronic granulocytic disease	*Plasmodium* spp.
T lymphocytes	Quant. deficiency:	Intracellular bacteria (*Listeria, Salmonella, Nocardia, Legionella*)
	HIV	Mycobacteria
	Functional defect:	Fungi (*Cryptococcus, Candida, Histoplasma, Coccidiodes*)
	SCID	Parasites (PCP, *Toxoplasma, Strongyloides, Cryptosporidium*)
	DeGeorge syndrome	Viral (HSV, CMV, VZV, measles, adenovirus)
B lymphocytes	Quant. deficiency:	Pyogenic/polysaccharide-coated bacteria:
	X-linked agammaglobulinemia	*S. pneumoniae* and *S. pyogenes*
	Functional defect:	*H. influenzae, N. meningitidis, P. aeruginosa*
	Dysgammaglobulinemia	Persistent viral/parasitic
		Enterovirus
		P. carinii
		Giardia lamblia
Complement	Quant. deficiency:	Pyogenic bacteria
	C′ consumption (SLE)	*Neisseria* spp.
	Functional defect:	
	C6, C7, C8 deficiency	

tococcosis, and mucormycosis, along with activation of *Pneumocystis* and *Toxoplasma* infections arev also well-described entities in the immunocompromised host (10).

Corticosteroid immunosuppression is multifaceted and includes depression of inflammatory responses, depletion of lymphatic tissue and inhibition of lymphatic function, and interference with polymorphonuclear leukocyte function (11-12). Immunosuppressives that act by interfering with the replication of cells (alkylating agents: nitrogen mustard, cyclophosphamide, busulfan, and chlorambucil; antimetabolites: cytosine arabinoside, 5-fluorouracil, azathioprine, 6-mercaptopurine, and 6-thioguanine; and the folic acid antagonist methotrexate) may suppress primary and secondary antibody responses and delayed hypersensitivity responses in some individuals.

The bone marrow transplant patient passes though successive stages of risk of infection that overlap, starting with granulocytopenia and mucosal damage, then cellular immunodeficiency, and finally humoral immunodeficiency (13). The median time to onset of most bacterial and fungal infections, 8–9 days after transplantation, corresponds to the period of most intense granulocytopenia. Two-thirds of these infections are attributable to organisms found in oral and stool cultures. Viral and protozoal infections (CMV and *Pneumocystis*) occur in the early postengraftment period, 2–3 months after transplantation, when cellular and humoral immune function is suppressed (14). Infections caused by encapsulated organisms like *Streptococcus pneumoniae* are more common a year or more following transplant, because of relative B-cell deficiency (15).

The choice of therapy for the immunocompromised patient requires identification of the immunodeficiency and recognition of the spectrum of infectious complications that can occur in association with this immunodeficiency. Although this knowledge allows definition of an empiric regimen for treatment and effective supportive care, appropriate antibiotic therapy should be based on culture results of blood and pus, tissue samples, or direct swabs from infected sites. The goal is to treat and prevent infections until immune components are replaced or supplemented.

Case 1

A 21-year-old white male, with a 2-week history of lethargy, malaise, pallor, poor appetite, petechiae, low-grade fever of 2 weeks duration, and a palpable spleen on examination had a presumptive diagnosis of acute leukemia. Blood counts revealed a hemoglobin of 66 g/L, hematocrit of 19.0%, white cell count of 17.2 × 10^9 cells/L with 1% polymorphonuclear leukocytes, 1% band forms, 97% lymphocytes, and 1% monocytes, and a platelet count of 9.6 × 10^9/L. A peripheral blood film revealed numerous lymphoblast-like cells. Bone marrow aspirate and biopsy established the diagnosis of acute (CD10+/CD19+, L2, hypodiploid) lymphocytic leukemia.

He received a platelet transfusion, and because of the fever, blood, throat, urine, and cerebrospinal fluid cultures and a chest radiograph were performed. All were noncontributory. Empiric broad spectrum antibiotic coverage with nafcillin and ceftazidine was initiated because of the low granulocyte count. He also received systemic antileukemic and prophylactic central nervous system therapy. His fever rapidly defervesced, his cultures remained negative, and 3 days later antibiotics were discontinued. He was discharged in stable condition on trimethoprim-sulfamethoxazole (TMP-SMC) and encouraged to avoid contact with patients with infectious diseases.

At the end of 4 weeks he was in clinical and hematologic remission. Shortly thereafter, while on consolidation chemotherapy, he developed a 0.5-cm suspected herpes simplex viral (HSV) lesion on his right cheek, which increased to 2 cm during therapy with topical acyclovir, but which resolved on oral acyclovir.

Eight months later he became anorectic, listless, and febrile. He had no other abnormal findings. He also had three small vesicles in his right cheek. His white blood cell count was 0.6×10^9/L. Bacterial cultures were negative before and during therapy with ceftazidime, vancomycin, and acyclovir. Fluorescent staining and culture of the vesicular lesions were negative for herpes simplex. After 5 days of therapy, his lesions and fever resolved. All cultures remained negative, and he was discharged home on oral dicloxacillin for another 10 days. The nature of the lesions was never resolved.

Three months later, with a minimally symptomatic upper respiratory infection, and following the appearance of extensive ecchymoses while playing basketball, he was seen in the emergency room and found to have low platelet and white blood cell counts (1.0×10^9 and 1×10^9/L, respectively). Blood and throat cultures were obtained; he received a platelet transfusion and outpatient therapy consisting of oral amoxicillin. He recovered fully in 1 week.

Sixteen months following diagnosis, he relapsed and received yet another course of induction therapy. Within 5 weeks he was once again in remission. A bone marrow transplant (BMT) was offered as the therapeutic option of choice. He refused and instead received maintenance therapy, consisting of modified induction therapy. Four months later, while in remission, he developed a fever of 105°F following a dose of interferon. Blood culture from his central venous catheter grew out gram-positive rods. Examination of the central line was unremarkable, and the remainder of his physical examination was normal. The lines were flushed with urokinase, and he was started on clindamycin after blood cultures were obtained from peripheral blood and both catheters. Forty-eight hours later the line cultures grew a Bacillus species sensitive to vancomycin and rifampin. The peripheral blood cultures remained negative. His antibiotics were readjusted, and the central line was removed. He became afebrile, antibiotics were discontinued after 14 days, and the central line was replaced.

He had a second marrow relapse 9 months later, at which time he accepted the BMT alternative. He was successfully reinduced with daunomycin and cytoxan, following which he received a BMT from his HLA-compatible brother after completing a preparative regimen of cytoxan and fractionated total body irradiation. Both his and his brother's pre-BMT CMV and HSV titers were positive. He received prophylactic acyclovir, trimethoprim sulfate, and antifungal troches. He also received a combination of short-course methotrexate and

long-course cyclosporine (CSA) for graft-versus-disease (GVHD) prophylaxis. Five days following the BMT, he developed a fever and received ceftazidime and vancomycin. Pretreatment blood culture grew Streptococcus viridans sensitive to vancomycin and ceftazoxime. Because of persistent fever on day 4 of therapy, he also received amphotericin B empirically. At day 15 he developed a maculopapular rash on 30% of his skin surface. One day later his granulocyte count rose from less than 0.1 to 0.5×10^9/L. A skin biopsy was consistent with GVHD. Apart from a low-grade fever and elevation in liver function, he had no other system involvement. High-dose steroid therapy was added to the cyclosporine regimen, and 24 hours later his fever defervesced. By 4 weeks he was in blatant remission, and after 6 weeks he was discharged to an outpatient domicile with ongoing dose reduction in steroids and CSA. His rash faded, and his liver function improved. He left the BMT outpatient service voluntarily and returned to his home city where he was sporadically followed by his local doctor. During that interval his rash reappeared and faded spontaneously on several different occasions. He also had an occasional cough. However, 2 months later the cough worsened and persisted in spite of oral Augmentin therapy. He was admitted when his chest radiograph showed a diffuse interstitial infiltrate. CMV was isolated from bronchoalveolar lavage as well as blood and urine. He received every-other-day high-dose gamma globulin (400 mg/kg) and gancyclovir (5 mg/kg every 12 hours) intravenously. He steadily worsened and required ever-increasing respiratory assist settings. After 2 months he developed irreversible multisystem failure and expired. During the course of therapy, the degree of viral involvement in the blood and urine had markedly decreased.

Autopsy results revealed pulmonary fibrosis with obliterative changes of the bronchioli consistent with CMV pneumonitis and pulmonary GVH.

This case history illustrates a number of points regarding the various manifestations of infection in the immunocompromised host. Vancomycin was not used during the first febrile episode because he had not yet been exposed to the hospital environment with its resistant organisms. His later experience with HSV required systemic therapy for adequate control of this disease because of the emergency of T-cell immunodeficiency. The vesicular skin lesions were treated empirically for both resistant staphylococcus and HSV for the same reason. When his immunosuppressive worsened, any simple infection would have mandated the use of broad-spectrum coverage. Bacterial contamination of the central venous catheter was not only treated with broad-spectrum antibiotics but also required removal of the catheter because of the characteristics of the bacterial isolate. Aggressive onset of therapy can also suppress serious sequelae in such patients. For example, bacteremia with Streptococcus viridans can produce severe disease, which was prevented in this pa-

tient because of the early use of empiric vancomycin. The final point is a tragic example of the difficulty in managing CMV disease.

Phagocytic Defects

The bone marrow normally produces 100 million polymorphonuclear leukocytes daily, about half of which adhere to small vessel endothelium. These cells can be reduced in quantity or their function can be impaired.

Quantitative Defects: Neutropenia

If the absolute neutrophil count is maintained at less than $1 \times 10^9/L^3$, there is increased susceptibility to infection. The infection rate is inversely proportional to the neutrophil count. An absolute count of $0.5 \times 10^9/L$ or fewer correlates with severity of infection. Neutropenia, regardless of whether it is primary or secondary to chemotherapy, radiotherapy, or the underlying cancer, is defined as fewer than 500 polymorphonuclear leukocytes and band forms per cubic millimeter (0.5×10^9 cells/L) (16).

The polymorphonuclear leukocyte is the principal component of the immune system that is responsible for production of symptoms and signs of infectious disease. Neutropenia impairs the acute inflammatory response. The usual local signs and symptoms of infection, such as redness (rubor), swelling (tumor), tenderness (dolor), heat (calor), and the ability to form abscesses, may be absent. Fever is often the only sign of infection in neutropenic patients (table 43.2).

Body temperature control is regulated in the preoptic region of the anterior hypothalamus (19). It is believed that there are discrete regions in the preoptic nucleus that are responsible for sensing and computing the core temperature (the "thermostat"), providing a reference point for normal temperature control (the "setpoint"), controlling heat production (the "heat gain center"), and dissipating heat (the "heat loss center") (19). Fever is defined as an oral temperature above 38.5°C on one occasion or above 38°C on three successive readings in a 24-hour pe-

riod. Fever should be clearly distinguished from heat illness (hyperthermia) as a centrally regulated rise in temperature in which the "set point" of the preoptic nucleus has been raised (20). The febrile response is mediated by interleukin 1 (IL-1) produced by polymorphonuclear leukocytes and other phagocytic cells (21). IL-1 acts directly on the preoptic nucleus to elevate the "set point." In any disease in which granulocytes and phagocytic cells are activated (infectious, autoimmune, or malignant), IL-1 plays the primary role in production of fever.

Fever produced by the action of phagocytes and the production of IL-1 should be distinguished from "heat illness." IL-1-initiated fevers rarely exceed 41.1°C (106°F) (22). Body temperatures above this generally suggest involvement of the central nervous system or other effects on heat regulation such as cardiac output or dehydration. There are no data to indicate that elevated body temperatures alone, in the range seen with IL-1-induced fevers, cause any permanent tissue damage. Temperatures seen with heat illness can have devastating permanent, or even lethal, effects on organs and tissues (23). Treatment of IL-1-associated fevers is debated but can be accomplished by use of antipyretic drugs such as aspirin and acetaminophen, which restore the "set point" to normal. In heat illness, the use of these agents is generally fruitless and possibly harmful because the thermoregulatory "set point" is already normal. Instead, the body must be externally cooled.

The febrile neutropenic patient should have a detailed physical examination including an oral and perianal evaluation. Only if signs of inflammation are noted should a digital rectal examination be performed. Preliminary laboratory studies should include a CBC, differential, and liver and renal evaluations to establish baseline values to follow response and drug toxicity. At least two blood cultures should be obtained. If an intravenous catheter is present, one culture should be obtained from each catheter lumen, and one should be obtained peripherally. It is also important to palpate a catheter's subcutaneous tunnel and culture any expressed pus. A urinalysis and culture should be performed. Localized lesions or any localized area of inflammation should be aspirated or biopsied, and material sent for cytology, cultures, and histology. A chest radiograph should be obtained, especially if pulmonary symptoms are present. On the other hand, radiologic signs of pneumonia may be delayed, and infiltrates may not appear until late in the course of disease. If neutropenia is not severe, autologous leukocytes labeled in vitro with indium-111 may permit localization of inflammation (23). Diagnostic procedures should be accomplished quickly, since empiric antibiotics should be initiated as soon as samples for these studies are drawn rather than waiting their return.

After empiric antibiotic therapy is initiated, the febrile patient should be monitored and reevaluated. If the causative organism is identified, empiric therapy

Table 43.2. Infection Sites from Two Recent Studies of Febrile Neutropenic Patients

Site	% of Cases	
	Granowetter (17) $n = 206$	Pizzo (18) $n = 550$
Not identified	63	72
Bacteremia	10	15
Respiratory tract	6	5
Head	—	2
Soft tissue/cellulitis	17	8
Gastrointestinal	—	0.7
Urinary tract	—	4
Other	4	0.4

may need to be optimized, but it should not be narrowed to cover only the isolated organism. Antibiotic toxicities should be considered. Physical examinations should be done twice daily, and cultures should be repeated every other day. Even if the patient becomes afebrile in less than 5 days after initiation of empiric antibiotics, the regimen should be continued for a full 10–14 days. The patient who remains febrile should undergo further evaluation. It is also arguable that antibiotics should be continued in the afebrile neutropenic patient until the WBC reaches and is maintained at 0.5×10^9/L.

Initial Empiric Therapy

Most febrile episodes in neutropenic patients have a bacterial etiology (tables 43.2 and 43.3). This fact is also illustrated by our case. Only after treatment with antibiotics and coincident modification of microbial flora does the risk of secondary or associated systemic fungal infection increase. The use of broad-spectrum antibiotics is the most important initial step in management. Early use of broad-spectrum antibiotics may help avoid complications of gram-negative infection.

The risk of bacteremia rises with the duration of granulocytopenia and the degree of neutropenia (28). Febrile neutropenic patients, with or without an identified cause, should be treated for both gram-negative rods and gram-positive cocci. The goals of choosing empiric antibiotics should be bactericidal activity, minimal toxicity, and cost. The choice of a specific antibiotic should be based on the institutional susceptibility patterns and on toxicities and cost analyses. Several factors that may help the choice of antibiotics include the patient's renal status, suspicion of staphylococcus, knowledge of former cultures, and the presence of an indwelling intravenous catheter. In patients with poor renal status, aminoglycosides should be avoided, and preference should be given to third-generation cephalosporins. If staphylococcus is suspected, however, third-generation cephalosporins should be avoided. Catheter-associated tenderness, drainage, or obstruction or symptoms temporally related to catheter care suggest the need for the addition of vancomycin or antifungal therapy. Once an organism is isolated, the antibiotic regimen can be revised to provide optimal coverage. Persistently culture-positive catheters must be removed, and broad-spectrum coverage should be maintained to prevent spread or occurrence of other bacterial infections (table 43.4).

Appropriate therapy for the patient with fever and neutropenia is administration of a combination antibiotic regimen. Aminoglycoside lactam combinations are widely used, as are combination aminoglycoside and a third-generation cephalosporin (with antipseudomonal activity: ceftazidime, cefoperazone), combination aminoglycoside and an antipseudomonal penicillin (ticarcillin-clavulanate or piperacillin). The latter has the advantages of broad-spectrum coverage, synergistic effects, and minimal emergence of resistant organisms (30, 31). All of the above regimens are variably nephrotoxic and ototoxic. Hypokalemia often results from excessive aminoglycoside usage (18).

Monotherapy using third-generation cephalosporins (especially ceftazidime because of its superior activity against *Pseudomonas aeruginosa*) or the carbapenems (especially imipenem against most gram-positives (including enterococcus) and most gram-negatives (except *Xanthomonas maltophilia*), and against anaerobes) compares favorably with combination therapy (18, 32). Drawbacks to the use of these regimens include the increase in gram-positive infections in patients given solely ceftazidime and a significantly higher incidence of *Clostridium difficile* colitis in subjects receiving imipenem. Imipenem has its own drawbacks, including the emergence of resistant pseudomonads, a low-

Table 43.3 Blood Culture Isolates from Febrile Neutropenic Patients at Time of Admission

| Organism | Percent Distribution of Isolates | | | | | Comment |
	Pizzo et al. 1986 (18)	EORTC 1987 (26)	Granowetter 1988 (17)	Shenep 1989 (219)	O'Hanley 1989 (27)	
S. aureus	17	11	21	22	0	Increased during 1980s
S. epidermidis	17	8	26	42	53	May be catheter related; center dependent
Streptococcus	15	17	11	23	5	Alpha-hemolytic: mucositis and respiratory distress syndrome; enterococcus: resistant to third-generation cephalosporins
E. coli	15	29	5	14	22	Predominant organisms in children with
K. pneumoniae	7	4	16	0	6	cancer
P. aeruginosa	12	16	11	0	6	Serious pathogen
Anaerobes	3	0	0	0	0	Mixed (oral, GI, perianal)
Fungi	2	0	0	0	0	*Candida*: most common; *Cryptococcus*: solitary pulmonary
Other	12	16	10	0	9	
No. of isolates	95	219	19	14	64	

From Hughes WT. Empiric antimicrobial therapy in the febrile granulocytopenic patient. Infect Control Hosp Epidemial 1990;3:151.

Table 43.4 Activity of Antibiotics against Predominant Pathogens in Pediatric Patients

Antibiotic	Enterc Gram −	Ps. Aerug.	Coagulase + Staphylococci	Coagulase − Staphylococci	Group D Streptococci	Non–group D Streptococci (+ α-hemolytic)	Anaerobes
Ceftazidime and cefoperazone	Good	Good	Mod (poor: MRSA)	Poor	Poor	Poor	Poor
Other third-generation cephalosporins	Good	Poor	Mod (poor: MRSA)	Poor	Poor	Good	Poor-Mod
Imipenemcilastatin	Good	Good	Good (poor: MRSA)	Poor	Good	Good	Good
Quinolones	Good	Good	Good (& MRSA)	Good	Poor-Mod	Poor-Mod	Poor
Aztreonam	Good	Good	Poor	Poor	Poor	Poor	Poor

From Pizzo PA, Rubin M, Freifeld A, Walsh TJ. The child with cancer and infection. I. Empiric therapy for fever and neutropenia and preventive strategies. J Pediatr 1991;119(5):679–694.

ering of the seizure threshold in susceptible patients, and frequent nausea and vomiting (32).

The routine use of vancomycin or teicoplanin results in fewer gram-positive infections (33). Empiric inclusion of vancomycin with the first dose of broad-spectrum antibiotics leads to rapid resolution of fever, fewer days of bacteremia, and fewer instances of treatment failure (33, 34). However, there is no unequivocal evidence that empiric use of these drugs improves survival (34, 35). Delaying the institution of these drugs until microbiologic or clinical indication occurs does not result in significantly higher morbidity in the early phases of immunosuppression (36). Infections from gram-positive organisms are subtle and rarely life-threatening, so cost and adverse effects can be avoided (17,18). Nonetheless, it is prudent to include vancomycin for those patients with evidence of infection at indwelling central venous catheter exit sites. *Staphylococcus epidermidis*, penicillin-resistant α-hemolytic streptococci, and methicillin-resistant *Staphylococcus aureus* have been shown to be important pathogens at some institutions. *Streptococcus viridans* can be a devastating pathogen in BMT recipients (37) if not covered empirically, as the above case demonstrates. In effect, the frequency and sensitivity profiles of infecting isolates should be used to formulate antibiotic use, and even severely immunosuppressed patients should receive aggressive multimoded therapy at the onset of fever (38).

Other agents, such as the monobactams (aztreonam) are best used in β-lactam-allergic patients who require empiric antipseudomonal treatment. β-Lactam inhibitors (clavulanic acid and sulfactam) may also have use in this regard (39). The quinolones, with limited activity against certain gram-positives (*Enterococcus* and *S. pneumoniae*) and little or no anaerobic use toward effects on weight-bearing joints in young experimental animals (40), should not be used alone but rather reserved for bacterial isolates that are not sensitive to other antibiotics.

Approach to Intravenous Catheter–Related Infections

Microbiologically documented infections related to central venous catheters are defined as (*a*) abscesses and cellulitis localized at the exit site, subcutaneous tunnel, or the entrance of the catheter into the blood vessel, (*b*) the presence of a positive blood culture from a catheter site but not from a simultaneous peripheral, noncatheter site, (*c*) the presence of the same organism at the catheter site and from other peripheral veins when simultaneous cultures are performed (it is important to culture all lumens of a multilumen catheter), and (*d*) clinical symptoms and signs synchronous with catheter manipulation. Quantitative cultures (e.g., using lysis-centrifugation systems) also help define a catheter-associated bacteremia more rapidly. These types of infections do not appear to correlate with the severity of neutropenia. Approximately 80% of these infections are caused by gram-positive organisms (especially coagulase-negative staphylococci, *S. aureus*, and *Streptococcus* spp.). Other species encountered include resistant corynebacteria (e.g., group CDC-JK), *Bacillus* species, atypical mycobacteria (*M. fortuitum* and *M. chelonia*), gram-negative organisms (especially *Acinetobacter* spp. and *Pseudomonas* spp.), and fungi (especially *Candida* spp., *Malassezia furfur*, and *Aspergillus flavus*) (40-43).

About 60% of catheter-related infections can be treated successfully without removing the catheter (table 43.5) (41-46). Fever in a neutropenic cancer patient with indwelling catheters should be treated empirically for the first 48–72 hours because of the risk of untreated catheter-associated gram-negative infection. Infection of a multilumen catheter should be treated by rotating antibiotics among the ports and lumens, as infection may be restricted to only one of the lumens. A catheter should be removed if there is evidence for a subcutaneous tunnel track infection, an obstructed lumen, septic emboli, inability to clear the organism from the

Table 43.5 Management of the Febrile Neutropenic Patient with an Indwelling Intravenous Catheter

No Evidence of Local Infection		Evidence for Local Infection			
Culture all ports and peripheral blood Begin empiric therapy Reassess at 48–72 hours		Exit site only Culture all ports, peripheral blood, and local site Begin oral antistaphylococcal coverage (diclox or first-generation cephalosporin)		Exit site with fever or bacteremia Culture all ports, peripheral blood, and local site Begin broad-spectrum i.v. antibiotics (plus vancomycin?)	Tunnel infection
Culture Negative	*Culture Positive*	*Reassess 48–72 Hours*		*Reassess 48–72 Hours*	
	Cultures remain + after 48 hours	Cultures become negative on Rx	Improved	Not improved	Culture negative and improved	Culture still positive
Continue Rx: see guide	Remove catheter	Complete 10–14 ds of Rx	Complete 10 to 14-day course of therapy	Trial of i.v. therapy	Continue therapy 10–14 days	Remove catheter	Remove catheter
Do not remove catheter	Continue Rx: see guide	Do not remove catheter		If not improved remove catheter	Do not remove catheter	ABics: see guide	ABics: see guide

bloodstream after 2–3 days of antibiotics, or documented hematogenous infection with *Bacillus* species, corynebacteriam of the JK group, mycobacteria (e.g., *M. chelonia* or *M. fortuitum*) or fungi (e.g., *Aspergillus* or *Candida* species) (42). The case at the beginning of this chapter illustrates the need for early removal of a catheter when *Bacillus* species are isolated from the catheter lumen. These organisms appear to produce a biofilm that enhances their attachment to catheters and impedes antibiotic killing.

The increase in the percentage of gram-positive catheter-related infections noted over the past 10 years (47, 48) is thought to be related to (*a*) the increasingly wide use of central venous catheters, which facilitates contamination with skin flora; (*b*) the antimicrobial action of cephalosporins, which has progressively shifted from gram-positive to gram-negative infection, (*c*) the use of prophylactic oral nonabsorbable antibiotics primarily directed at gram-negative organisms; and (*d*) the presence of gram-positive cocci in the upper airway.

The increasing role of gram-positive organisms and the frequent associated resistance to methicillin and oxacillin suggest a need to include vancomycin in early empiric antibiotic regimens. However, these gram-positive organisms do not appear to be as virulent as, and cause less mortality than, gram-negative organisms. Moreover, the use of vancomycin is often associated with side effects, which leaves initial empiric use of the drug in question (38). Recent evidence suggests that vancomycin is not needed in initial empiric regimens unless the microbial pattern of a particular hospital environment requires its use (48). If vancomycin is initiated, antibiotic therapy can be modified, depending on pretreatment culture results.

Approach to Pulmonary Infiltrates

Patients with neutropenia and a pulmonary infiltrate present a special diagnostic dilemma (table 43.6). The use of chest radiographs for the diagnosis of pulmonary disease in immunocompromised patients is of limited value (50). Any infection can present with several different patterns, and processes such as embolism, aspiration, edema, and hemorrhage may give appearances similar to that of infection. Because of this and the fact that most lung infiltrates in immunosuppressed patients are caused by bacteria, initial therapy for a pulmonary infiltrate in a neutropenic patient with fever is largely empiric.

If a patient with a pulmonary infiltrate has been neutropenic only briefly (≤1 week), a bacterial process is most likely. For such patients, blood and, if possible, sputum cultures should be obtained, (51) and broad-spectrum antibiotic therapy should be initiated. Depending on the degree of immunosuppression and the type of pulmonary infiltrate, consideration should also be given to treating for *Pneumocystis carinii*, mycoplasma, and *Legionella*. If a improvement follows, antibiotics should be continued for 10–14 days (TMP-SMX should be continued for 14 days, and erythromycin for 21 days). If a patient with a pulmonary infiltrate continues to deteriorate in the presence of negative culture results, early diagnostic bronchoalveolar lavage should be considered (52). *This is well illustrated in*

Table 43.6 Pulmonary Infiltrate in Neutropenic Patient

Patchy or Localized Infiltrate				Diffuse of Interstitial Infiltrate			
No Antibiotics Being Given		Antibiotics Being Given		No Antibiotics Being Given		Antibiotics Being Given	
Blood culture, sputum analysis, serologic study		Granulocyte count rising	Granulocyte count not rising				
Broad-spectrum antibiotics		Continue therapy expectantly		Broad-spectrum antibiotic and consider TMP-SMX plus erythromycin			
Reassess at 48–72 hr		Rx as per non-neutropenic infiltrate		Reassess at 72-96 hr			
Improved	Not improved	Can tolerate diagnostic procedure	Cannot tolerate Dx procedure	Improved or stable	No improvement	Can tolerate diagnostic procedure	Can not tolerate Dx
No further Dx	Continue Dx: bronchoscopy (lavage/Bx) and/or open lung biopsy	Dx: bronchoscopy (lavage/Bx) and/or open lung biopsy	Dx: blood culture	Continue Rx: broadspectrum ABic: 14 ds; TMP-SMX: 14ds; EES: 21 ds	Dx: bronchoscopy and/or open lung BX	Dx: bronchoscopy (lavage/Bx) and/or open lung Bx	
Rx for 10- to 14-day course	Rx according to findings	Rx according to findings	Add amphotericin 1–1.5, mg/kg/day		Rx by findings	Rx according to findings	Add: TMP-SMX; EES; amphotericin B

the case presentation. Further deterioration, without histologic diagnosis, may require an open lung biopsy, but the risks and benefits of this procedure must be weighed carefully (53). In a patient who is already being treated with broad-spectrum antibiotics, an infiltrate identified coincident with recovery of the neutrophil count may indicate development of inflammation at a previously unrecognized site of infection. In such circumstances, close observation of the patient's clinical course without any changes in therapy will allow determination of whether further diagnostic studies are necessary (54). If, on the other hand, a patient has been treated for more than 1 week and neutropenia persists, then fungal pneumonia should be considered, and amphotericin B should be added.

The decision about the performance and extent of diagnostic procedures hinges on the yield and risk of the procedure to the patient and on the duration of symptoms, signs, and therapy. A clinician must evaluate the underlying disease and its treatment, the rapidity of the clinical course, the physical examination, and the laboratory data. Invasive procedures for diagnostic proof of pulmonary disease result in changes in therapy in as few as 20% of patients. For low-risk procedures, the choice between empiric therapy and a diagnostic procedure is less controversial (55). For example, bronchoalveolar lavage or fiberoptic bronchoscopy with washings and brushings is a safe process. The choice is more complicated when weighing the risk of invasive procedures with the risk of toxicity from multiple empiric therapies (56, 57). Specimens obtained for diagnostic procedures should be submitted for newer techniques, including centrifugation cell culture coupled with immunofluorescent monoclonal antibody staining (58, 59) and PCR analysis.

Approach to Surface Infections

Although signs and symptoms of infection are often blunted in neutropenic patients, a complete investigation is always necessary. A thorough search for skin, oral, or anal abnormalities should be performed. Nonbacterial infections tend to have a more indolent course and demonstrate fewer signs of inflammation (60). Pain and the appearance of a lesion are not good indicators of the severity of an infection. Failure to recognize the potential for unusual pathogens can lead to delays in diagnosis and to tissue destruction unless appropriate cultures are requested.

Early skin biopsy and culture for bacterial, fungal, and mycobacterial and parasitic organisms are fundamental to the diagnosis of suspicious soft tissue infections (61). Less than 15% of disseminated infections produce cutaneous findings (62). In the case study, vesicular lesions require viral fluorescent staining, Tzanck testing, and culture, and any isolated organism should be seriously considered a potential pathogen.

Chemotherapy often causes severe mucositis that is moderately well controlled with cleansing solutions that decrease discomfort and control superinfection. The latter, however, may not be easily recognizable. Marginal or necrotizing gingivitis may be recognized by the appearance of erythematous periapical lines. Ideal antianaerobic treatment includes the use of clindamycin or metronidazole (63). In other cases, diagnosis may require direct staining for *Candida*, immunofluorescent staining for HSV, or viral cultures. Treatment of oral candidiasis is best carried out with oral clotrimazole troches or fluconazole. Oral HSV can be treated with oral acyclovir if the patient can reliably swallow medication.

Generalizations designed to orient an approach to likely pathogens include localized changes at the site of invasive devices and the fact that skin breaks are commonly caused by gram-positive organisms or *Candida*. Fulminant local infections are likely caused by gram-negative organisms and should be treated with antibiotics that cover pseudomonads. Nodular erythematous lesions are suggestive of fungal invasion (64). Perirectal pain and tenderness in the absence of erythema, induration, or fluctuance, once cultured, are best treated with (*a*) antibiotics for gram-negative enterics, anaerobic organisms, and group D streptococci, (*b*) sitz baths (when possible), (*c*) stool softeners, and (*d*) low-residue diets (65).

Guide to Empiric Therapy for Fever in the Patient with Prolonged Neutropenia

The duration of therapy in patients with granulocytopenia depends on the duration of neutropenia, localization of clinical findings, and bacterial isolation (table 43.7). If neutropenia resolves, the duration of therapy should correlate with that in the nonneutropenic host (66). Patients whose neutrophil counts are below 0.5 but above 0.1 × 10^9/L and who are free of infection may have antibiotics terminated after 5–7 afebrile days. In patients who have unexplained fever and prolonged neutropenia and who become afebrile in 5 days or less, antibiotics should be stopped after at least 14 days of therapy (67). The possibility of stopping intravenous therapy after 7 days and continuing oral antibiotics for another 7 days is arguably acceptable. If patients become febrile after antibiotics are discontinued, the same antibiotic regimen should be restarted. In patients who do not become afebrile by day 5, fungal infections should be suspected, and empiric amphotericin B at 0.5 mg/kg/day should be added at day 7 (68). Some investigations institute antifungal therapy at the onset of fever in all neutropenic hosts. Fluconazole is only minimally active against *Aspergillus* (69) and inconsistently active against other fungal infections (70). In patients in whom empiric antibiotics and amphotericin B have been started because of continued fever, a minimum of 2 weeks of amphotericin and 3 weeks of antibiotics is warranted, particularly in the BMT setting wherein neutropenia may be very prolonged. In patients with bacteriologically documented infections who become afebrile 7 days or less after the onset of treatment, antibiotic administration may be discontinued by 14 days unless clinical evidence for residual infection remains, (71) in which case antibiotic therapy should be continued until neutropenia resolves. Isolation of an organism should not initiate a change in antibiotics to a narrower spectrum (67).

Any patient with prolonged neutropenia and fever must be frequently reevaluated for new clinical and microbiologic findings (72). Evidence of catheter site infection or a gram-positive isolate would support the addition of vancomycin to cover coagulase-negative staphylococci and enterococci infections (34, 36). A new site of infection or progression at an old site may well require the addition of clindamycin or metronidazole for anaerobic coverage (71–73). Gastrointestinal or intraabdominal complaints should initiate evaluation for appendicitis, typhlitis, and (*C. difficile*) colitis (74). Documentation of *C. difficile* colitis requires therapy with oral vancomycin or metronidazole (75).

Infection at a new site while on broad-spectrum antibiotic coverage may warrant the addition of antifungal, antiviral, or antiparasitic therapy. Retrosternal pain is strongly suggestive of esophagitis, which is best treated empirically with amphotericin B for *Candida*, acyclovir for HSV, and antibiotics for gram-positive bacteria until a

Table 43.7 Management of Fever and Neutropenia after Preantibiotic Evaluation and Empiric Antibiotic Therapy for 7 Days

No Fever and No Neutropenia	Fever and No Neutropenia	No Fever but Neutropenia Continues	Continued Fever and Neutropenia
Source known or unknown	Infection clinically or microbiologically documented	Infection of unknown source	Start amphotericin B empirically
Duration of Rx depends on usual Rx for type of infection in nonneutropenic host	Rx for 10–14 days depending on disease; longer is residual, longer if TLC ≤100	Rx for full 14 days; longer if residual, longer if TLC ≤100	Min. Rx duration: amphotericin B: 2 weeks; ABics: 3 weeks or until fever or neutropenia resolves
If fever recurs after antibiotics discontinued: reculture and Rx with same antibiotics			

definitive diagnosis is established (76). Pulmonary infiltrates may be seen with neutrophil recovery and require no further therapy, or they may occur following prolonged neutropenia and indicate either fungal or *P. carinii* pneumonia and the attendant need for additional treatment (54). Overall, the choice between empiric therapy and diagnostic tests, including sputum evaluation, bronchiolar lavage, or open lung biopsy, depends on a clear assessment of the risks and benefits.

Functional Defects of Granulocytes (see also Chapter 21, Granulocyte Disorders)

Disorders of white cell function include those in which the chemotactic, migratory, phagocytic, and lysosomal components of the neutrophil killing are affected by inherited or acquired disorders.

Phagocytic and Lysosomal Disorders

Patients with phagocytic or mononuclear defects characterized by an inability to kill ingested organisms commonly present with abscesses. In chronic granulomatous disease, the prototype of these disorders, the patient experiences repeated episodes of severe infection associated with granulomas and leukocytosis. The patient may have lymphadenopathy, splenomegaly, pneumonitis, dermatitis, liver and perianal abscesses, and osteomyelitis of the small bones of the hands and feet (77).

The defect in the killing function of the mononuclear phagocytes of these patients concerns the oxygen-dependent mechanism for production of superoxide in the lysosome (78). Since the production of hydrogen peroxide is impaired, intralysosomal killing of bacteria occurs only if these bacteria generate their own hydrogen peroxide and do not break down this same hydrogen peroxide with catalase. These patients have problems with infections caused by catalase-positive organisms such as staphylococci and gram-negative enterics (79). Less commonly, organisms such as *Herellea, Chromobacterium, Nocardia, Candida,* and *Aspergillus* are isolated. Treatment of bacterial infections in these patients usually requires parenterally administered antibiotics (cephalosporin or semisynthetic penicillin combined with gentamicin or another aminoglycoside) after obtaining adequate cultures. Drainage of all abscesses is imperative, and antibiotics should be continued for an extended time, depending on the response of the patient. In patients with continued severe infections, prophylactic antibiotics have been recommended (80). Gamma interferon has also been found to be successful as a prophylactic agent because it improves superoxide generation and bacteriocidal activity (81). Other defects in phagocytic function that result in poor or insufficient killing by phagocytic cells (82) include Job's syndrome, (83) myeloperoxidase deficiency, (84) glucose-6-phosphate dehydrogenase deficiency, (82) and Chediak-Higashi syndrome (85).

Migratory and Chemotactic Disorders

Defective chemotaxis can occur with many humoral and cellular defects in the immune system. Such patients usually have increased numbers of circulating neutrophils, and their symptoms may include sinusitis, otitis, gingivitis, peritonitis, pneumonia, dermatitis, multiple cold abscesses, and delayed wound healing. Infecting organisms include *S. aureus, S. epidermidis, Haemophilus influenzae,* gram-negative enteric organisms, and fungi. Chemotactic disorders include C3b receptor deficiency, CD11/CD18 glycoprotein deficiency, and Kartagener syndrome (86).

Defective opsonization occurs in patients with asplenia. The spleen's normal function includes the rapid synthesis of opsonizing antibody designed to assist in phagocytosis early during bacteremia. Early phagocytosis results in limited multiplication of the circulating pathogen (87). Patients with functional asplenia or surgical splenectomy have an increased incidence of organisms such as *S. pneumoniae, H. influenzae* type b, *Salmonella, Shigella,* and *Mycoplasma* (88, 89). Patients whose splenic function is reduced early in life, including patients with Wiskott-Aldrich syndrome, thalassemia major, portal hypertension secondary to hepatitis, congenital asplenia, sickle cell disease, and related hemoglobinopathies resulting in obstruction of splenic sinusoids, do not produce opsonizing antibody and are at risk of dying from overwhelming sepsis. Such patients should receive prophylactic penicillin or ampicillin (90). For patients with elective splenectomy, pneumococcal, hemophilus, and meningococcal immunizations are absolute indications.

T-Cell Immunodeficiency

The prototype of a pure cellular immunodeficiency is the DiGeorge syndrome, a disorder characterized anatomically by failure of development of the third and fourth pharyngeal pouches (91). Such patients have normal B-cell regions in their lymph nodes, spleen, Peyer's patches, and appendix, have normal immunoglobulin levels, and respond normally to T-cell-independent antigens. Patients with this disorder are susceptible to intracellular organisms requiring cell-mediated immune recognition, such as the facultative intracellular organisms like *Mycobacterium tuberculosis* and *Listeria monocytogenes*; viruses such as CMV, measles, varicella-zoster, and vaccinia; and fungi such as *Candida albicans, Cryptococcus neoformans,* and *Histoplasma capsulatum.*

Patients presenting with infections suggestive of cell-mediated immune deficiencies may also have severe combined B- and T-cell deficiency (92) or acquired immunodeficiency. Such patients may present in infancy with failure to thrive, persistent oral thrush, intractable diarrhea, and/or fulminant pneumonia. An interstitial pneumonia with tachypnea and hyperinflation is commonly caused by *P. carinii* and can be treated with TMP-SMX or pentamidine (93). These infants are also susceptible to overwhelming infections with herpesviruses such as varicella,

CMV and HSV (94). If the immunodeficiency is congenital, BMT may be life saving (95).

B-Cell Immunodeficiency

B-cell production and function may be impaired in patients after recovery from BMT or during chemotherapy. Infections with encapsulated organisms are common in such patients, as are those with enteric gram-negatives and pseudomonads. Both quantitative and functional deficiencies of antibody can present with similar symptoms and signs.

Quantitative Deficiency of Antibody

X-linked agammaglobulinemia is the prototype of quantitative deficiencies of all classes of immunoglobulins. Antigenic stimulation does not result in antibody formation, and plasma cells are missing in lymphoid tissue (96). Quantitative deficiency of immunoglobulin results in inefficient phagocytosis and failure of agglutination and neutralization. Recurrent infection begins when maternal antibody declines to unprotective levels in later infancy. Typical infections are caused by encapsulated organisms such as *S. pneumoniae, S. aureus, H. influenzae, N. meningitidis,* and *P. aeruginosa* (97). Also seen with this disorder are chronic viral and parasitic diseases including vaccine-associated poliomyelitis (98), enterovirus encephalitis (99), and protein-losing diarrhea associated with rotavirus (100) or *Giardia lamblia* (101). Other immunoglobulin deficiencies include class-specific deficiencies and subclass deficiencies. Such patients have chronic histories of respiratory infection including multiple episodes of otitis media, sinusitis, and pneumonia; chronic gastrointestinal disease; and a higher incidence of autoimmune disease (102). Immunoglobulin replacement therapy is recommended for such patients.

Functional Deficiency of Antibody

Functional inability to produce specific immunoglobulin to antigenic stimulation is commonly associated with quantitative deficiencies. These disorders are recognized by the absence of specific response to antigenic stimulation in the presence of measurable amounts of antibody. These patients have clinical histories similar to those with the purely quantitative immunoglobulin deficiencies and are treated with replacement therapy, depending on the severity of their symptoms. Prophylactic antibiotics and close follow-up have been used in patients with milder symptoms and signs.

Complement Deficiency

The complement system plays an important role in chemotaxis, immune adherence, viral neutralization, phagocytosis, and antibody-mediated complement-dependent bacteriocidal activity. Such deficiencies may coexist with humoral and cellular deficiencies (103-105). Some splenectomized patients have deficient production of complement components, which contributes to increased susceptibility to, and death from, bacterial infections. In general, patients who have deficiencies in the earlier components of complement often experience lupuslike disorders, whereas patients with deficiencies in complement components C3 and later usually experience recurrent *Neisseria, S. pneumoniae, N. meningitidis,* or *Klebsiella aerogenes* (106). Patients with deficiencies of C5, C6, or properdin are often at increased risk of *N. meningitidis* infections, for which replacement therapy and prophylactic antibodies appear to be effective (107–109).

Fungi

Candida

Candidiasis, the most common nosocomial mycosis among patients with cancer (110), can involve the mucosa or present systemically. Contributing factors to the development of oropharyngeal candidiasis are chemotherapy with corticosteroids, defective T-cell immunity, herpes stomatitis, and broad-spectrum antibiotics (111, 112). Clinical oropharyngeal manifestations range from punctate foci to diffuse erythema, painful plaques, ulcers, or cheilitis. Scrapings often reveal blastoconidia or pseudohyphae. Hoarseness and stridor in an immunocompromised patient suggest epi- and/or infraglottic laryngeal candidiasis, which very likely will require aggressive airway support (113, 114). Therapy depends on the extent of invasiveness and systemic involvement. Oral administration of antifungals is the most effective treatment for mucosal lesions. Afebrile patients able to tolerate topical therapy are best treated with clotrimazole troches (115). Oral administration of ketoconazole or fluconazole has little or no value for the patients with systemic involvement, for whom intravenous administration of amphotericin B (0.5–1.0 mg/kg/day) is the treatment of choice.

As noted, patients with complaints of retrosternal pain, odynophagia, and dysphagia may have any variety of esophagitis (116). Antacids and H_2-receptor-blocking agents may increase the risk of esophageal candidiasis (117), and in the absence of systemic signs, empiric oral therapy with clotrimazole or ketoconozole and possibly acyclovir may suffice (118). Lack of response after 3–4 days should mandate a visualization approach (i.e., endoscopy, biopsy, etc.), depending upon the stability of the patient. For example, BMT recipients have 20% endoscopy-related bacteremia (119). Patients with continued granulocytopenia who fail to, or whose systems do not, respond to local therapy are best treated with amphotericin B (0.5–0.6 mg/kg/day) (120), for approximately 2 weeks (10 mg/kg/total dose) or until the resolution of neutropenia.

Candidal fungemia can occur with or without an intravenous device (121) and is particularly common in patients receiving vancomycin and imipenem (122). Patients with fever and positive fungal cultures should be treated promptly with amphotericin B with removal of involved catheters to minimize dissemination (123). All such patients should be examined carefully for eye, skin, liver, and splenic involvement initially and then after resolution of the granulocytopenia, i.e., at a time when the inflammatory process becomes visible (124). Hepatosplenic candidiasis is suggested by continued fever after recovery from granulocytopenia, fever unresponsive to antibacterial therapy accompanied with abdominal pain, leukocytosis, and elevated serum alkaline phosphatase activity (125). Definitive diagnosis requires laparoscopy and liver biopsy, but the characteristic "bull's eye" lesions seen on computed tomography or magnetic resonance imaging are strong presumptive evidence. Embolic skin lesions are more common with *Candida tropicalis*. Diffuse myalgias may indicate candidal myositis (126). Amphotericin B should be initiated at 1 mg/kg/day, followed by 0.5 mg/kg/day, since there is no evidence that stepwise escalation of the dose to the targeted daily dose decreases toxicity. *C. tropicalis* may require continuation of 1 mg/kg/day because of its greater resistance. Therapy should be continued until granulocytopenia resolves (118). Treatment of hepatosplenic candidiasis requires longer-term amphotericin therapy, averaging 5 g (80–90 mg/kg), with the likely addition of 5-fluorocytidine (5-FC) (127). Liposomal and lamellar preparations of amphotericin B may decrease toxicity and improve management of hepatosplenic candidiasis (128). The value of itraconozole in the treatment of fungal disease in the neutropenic host awaits further confirmation (129).

Aspergillus

Symptoms and signs associated with invasive pulmonary aspergillosis include nonproductive cough, pleuritic chest pain, pleural rub, hemoptysis, and occasionally adventitious breath sounds, the result of *Aspergillus*-induced tissue damage with associated vascular thrombosis, infarction, and tissue necrosis (130). Resultant broncho- or segmental pneumonia, lobar consolidation, multinodular lesions, or cavitation are best demonstrated by computed tomography (131). Pulmonary aspergillosis can lead to invasion of contiguous tissues or can metastasize to other areas of the body (1). Focal neurologic deficits, including seizures, hemiparesis, and cranial nerve palsies, combined with pulmonary infiltrates, are predictive of aspergillosis (133). *Aspergillus* sinusitis, identified by speculum examination of the nose and by computed tomography, can develop before or concomitantly with invasive pulmonary disease (134).

The isolation of *Aspergillus* from respiratory secretions of granulocytopenic patients with fever and pulmonary infiltrate correlates strongly with invasive disease (135). Absence of hyphal elements or lack of a positive culture does not exclude the diagnosis (136). A definitive diagnosis should be made with an open lung biopsy prior to initiation of antifungal therapy (137). This is especially important considering that therapy may require high doses of amphotericin B (1.5 mg/kg/day) with its associated nephrotoxicity (138). The risks of lung biopsy must be carefully weighed against the empiric use of high-dose therapy. Surgical resection is indicated for continued hemoptysis, continued progression, or infiltration into extrapulmonary tissue (139), with therapy continued to a cumulative dose of 40 mg/kg (118). Recurrent disease, unfortunately, is found in 50% of patients who continue intensive chemotherapy, unless antifungal therapy is continued (140).

Cryptococcus

Cryptococcal infection is found most frequently in those with lymphoid malignancy and AIDS and in patients receiving prolonged corticosteroids. The central nervous system and lungs are the most common sites of serious pathology (141). The onset of CNS symptoms is insidious, usually evolving over weeks to months; they include fevers, headaches, dizziness, somnolence, and signs of impaired cognition. Twenty percent of patients have cranial nerve abnormalities, and papilledema is found in 30%. Classical nuchal rigidity is rare. The characteristic cerebrospinal fluid (CSF) examination shows an elevated opening pressure, low glucose, elevated protein, and a mononuclear pleocytosis, usually of less than 500 cells. Cryptococcal-polysaccharide-antigen latex agglutination has 90% sensitivity and specificity and should be performed on both the CSF and serum. The treatment of choice for cryptococcal meningitis in AIDS patients is combination amphotericin B and 5-FC for 4–6 weeks, depending on the presence or absence of other risk factors (142). Maintenance therapy with fluconazole is recommended for patients with AIDS (143).

Other mycoses that are important in the febrile neutropenic host involve *Trichosporon* spp., *Zygomycetes*, *Pseudallescheria*, and *Fusarium*. Infections from *Trichosporon* spp. are found in hosts receiving corticosteroids and are characterized by refractory fungemia, funguria, renal dysfunction, cutaneous lesions, chorioretinitis, and pulmonary infiltrates that are inhibited but not safely killed by achievable levels of amphotericin B (144). Zygomycosis caused by the soil organisms *Rhizopus, Mucor, Rhizomucor, Absidia,* and *Cunninghamella*, invade blood vessels and cause extensive infarction in patients with neutropenia and organ transplant immunosuppression. Both amphotericin B and surgical debridement are important in the management of such infections (145). *Pseudallescheria* may cause the same constellation of symptoms as *Aspergillus* spp. and may be resistant to amphotericin B but respond to miconazole (146). *Fusarium* infection presents with pulmonary infiltrates, sinusitis, and cutaneous lesions and may also be refractory to amphotericin B (147). Dematiaceous fungi have a predilection for CNS invasion (148).

Virus

Herpes Simplex Virus

Herpes simplex virus, which also causes significant morbidity in immunocompromised patients, is primarily a localized pathogen because primary disease is rare and secondary disease rarely disseminates or causes death. Reactivation of HSV in immunocompromised patients most commonly occurs in and around the mouth, nose, and esophagus. Pain is the most important distinguishing symptom, and a prior history of recurrent lesions is not required for making the diagnosis. Esophagitis, with or without associated dysphagia, is recognized by chest pain and burning on swallowing. Bacterial and fungal pathogens can enter and disseminate from HSV lesions. Laboratory diagnosis is best made by using specific direct immunofluorescent staining and/or culture of lesions. Treatment of mild localized HSV is carried out with oral acyclovir (200 mg 5 times per day for 5–10 days), but localized severe HSV should be treated with intravenous acyclovir (250 mg/m² of 5 mg/kg given every 8 hours) for at least 1 week or until the lesions have crusted (149). *As was noted by the case presentation at the beginning of this chapter, topical acyclovir is not sufficient, and localized severe disease requires inpatient management.* The dose of acyclovir should be doubled for CNS or disseminated disease, and treatment should continue for at least 10 days. Persistence of HSV-positive lesions in spite of acyclovir treatment is most commonly recognized in AIDS or other patients treated previously for extended periods and should lead one to test for acyclovir resistance and to initiate vidarabine or foscarnet therapy (150).

Varicella-Zoster (VZV)

Primary VZV or chicken pox can cause significant mortality (7–20%) in the immunocompromised patient. Mortality usually occurs because of pulmonary involvement starting 3–7 days after the onset of skin lesions and is recognized by diffuse nodular infiltrates on chest radiographs. Hepatitis and meningoencephalitis are less frequent complications of primary infection in the immunocompromised host. The cutaneous lesions of chicken pox may not appear typical in immunosuppressed patients, and a direct fluorescent stain provides a more rapid and sensitive method for the diagnosis of VZV infection than the 10–14 days needed to identify this organism in culture (151). Early initiation of acyclovir in an immunocompromised patient with chicken pox (500 mg/m² of 10 mg/kg i.v. every 8 hours for a minimum of 7 days or until lesions are crusted) can significantly reduce complications from disseminated disease.

Herpes zoster, or shingles, reactivation of latent VZV, occurs more commonly in immunosuppressed patients, especially in patients with severe T-cell suppression (BMT recipients, AIDS patients, patients receiving intensive immunosuppression, and patients with lymphoma, especially Hodgkin's lymphoma) (152). Zoster occurs unilaterally in a dermatomal distribution at sites of stress (tumor damage or radiotherapy) and rarely disseminates viscerally or beyond the dermatome. High-risk patients (i.e., those at increased risk for dissemination of disease) should receive intravenous acyclovir (500 mg/m² every 8 hours for a minimum of 7 days or until all lesions are crusted) (153) as soon as possible, preferably within 72 hours after the appearance of lesions. Oral acyclovir should not be administered in high-risk patients because it has limited bioavailability and, along with the use of continuous low-level prophylaxis, leads to chronic resistant VZV. In these individuals the lesions appear hyperkeratotic, verrucous, or papular (154).

Cytomegalovirus

In any immunocompromised host CMV may cause severe morbidity leading to death. This was tragically illustrated in the foregoing case. This DNA virus can cause submucosal gastrointestinal ulcerations, hemorrhagic and explosive diarrhea, pancreatitis, cholecystitis and retinitis (which, if untreated, leads to blindness) (155). Pneumonitis is best diagnosed by direct pulmonary tree assessment. Diagnostic techniques include histologic evaluation for intranuclear inclusions, shell viral cultures, immunofluorescent staining, in situ nucleic acid hybridization, and polymerase chain reaction tests for antigenemia (156, 157). Possible other pathogens contributing to the overall process should not be overlooked. In the immunocompromised host, CMV pneumonitis is best treated with gancyclovir and hyperimmune gamma globulin (5 mg/kg every 12 hours and 400 mg/kg every 3–4 days, respectively (158, 159). The overall success rate with this therapy ranges from 24 to 85%. In refractory cases, foscarnet is rarely effective (160). For CMV infections involving other tissues, gancyclovir also is effective. Gancyclovir not only slows viral replication, it also suppresses cell replication and is almost as effective in inducing myelosuppression as CMV itself. In effect, the balance between disease and therapy is often precarious.

Had this CMV 21-year-old been diagnosed 1 or 2 years later, he would have received prophylactic gancyclovir alone; and if PCR analyses of blood samples (granulocytes) failed to reveal evidence of antigenemia, gancyclovir therapy might have been withheld in lieu of repeated surveillance. Gancyclovir prophylaxis has dramatically improved the outlook in CMV-positive transplants. PCR detection of preclinical disease followed by early and aggressive use of gancyclovir for previously asymptomatic seroconversion patients or in any PCR-identified newly infected patient may be more efficacious in that it reduces treatment-related toxicity. The use of white cell depletion procedures for CMV-positive transfused blood appears to be as effective as the use of CMV-negative blood products for CMV-negative recipients (161-170).

Parasites

P. carinii pneumonia (PCP) is characterized by fever, cough, tachypnea, and retractions in the absence of rales. Typical laboratory findings include a chest radiograph with a hazy bilateral perihilar infiltrate that spreads peripherally and blood gases with a low pO_2, normal pCO_2, and alkaline pH. The diagnosis requires demonstration of cysts or trophozoites in material obtained from the lung by induced sputum specimens, bronchoalveolar lavage, or open lung biopsy (171).

TMP-SMX is the preferred therapy for all patients because it is generally well tolerated, inexpensive, and available for oral and intravenous administration. Oral therapy can be used 60–80% of the time if a patient has mild-to-moderate disease and does not have evidence of altered gastrointestinal absorption or renal dysfunction. Parenteral therapy is best utilized at onset. However, patients with a pO_2 above 70 mm Hg on room air may well respond to therapy (171, 173). Parenteral pentamidine is the second most widely used therapy for PCP. It is as effective as TMP-SMX but is used less frequently because of toxicity associated with its intravenous administration. Aerosolized pentamidine is effective in mild disease, but relapse rates are higher than those with parenteral TMP-SMX and pentamidine (174). Trimethoprim-dapsone appears to be somewhat better tolerated than TMP-SMX but offers no other advantage (175). If PCP is clinically suspected and diagnostic material cannot be obtained, TMP-SMX and erythromycin (for *Legionella* infection) should be administered empirically. If such a patient continues to have fever, a depressed pO_2, and progressing infiltrates, pentamidine should be added. Other agents are being developed to treat *P. carinii* (176).

The natural history of therapy for PCP results in oxygen-induced preliminary deterioration, thought to be related to drug-induced death of *Pneumocystis* organisms and the consequent exacerbation of the inflammatory response. This decline in respiratory status can be avoided by administering corticosteroids within 72 hours after the initiation of anti-*Pneumocystis* therapy (177–179).

Preventive Modalities

Prophylaxis of immunocompromised patients against infectious agents requires simultaneous intervention on a number of fronts: reduction of colonization, especially in the hospital setting; suppression of potentially pathogenic organisms colonizing the patient; and enhancement of host defense functions. Patients who are to receive immunosuppressive therapy should have baseline studies performed to screen for past exposure and present carriage of a variety of pathogens. Serology should be performed for antibody to *Toxoplasma*, CMV, HSV, VZV, Epstein-Barr virus, and measles. Cultures of throat and nasal specimens need to be obtained for mycoplasma and fungi. The pa-

tient and family members should be skin tested with tuberculin and control antigens.

Severely immunocompromised patients should have indwelling catheters routinely monitored to provide a guide for therapy and prophylaxis. Periodic blood samples should be obtained from indwelling intravenous catheters and endotracheal tubes. Catheters that are removed should be tip cultured.

Decreasing Transmission

The hospital concentrates patients with infectious diseases in close proximity to susceptible patients so the potential for nosocomial infection is high. Eighty percent of the organisms causing infection in cancer patients are endogenous microbial flora, and since 50% of these are acquired during hospitalization, colonization is an important prerequisite to infection (180). A patient can be colonized from food (181), water (182), air (183,184), hospital personnel, hospital equipment, other patients (185), visiting family members, and improperly maintained soap dispensers.

Isolating the patient from those with primary or secondary VZV will prevent its spread. A singularly important technique for prevention of infection is careful hand-washing (186). Other components of reverse or protective isolation (single room requiring masks, gowns, and gloves) do not prevent infection because most agents causing infection come from the patient. VZV infection is spread primarily through contact with persons with primary or secondary disease. Other measures of protective isolation, such as a mask for the patient or the thorough cooking of all food, remain of unproven value. Laminar airflow combined with aggressive decontamination has been shown to reduce infections, especially pulmonary aspergillosis.

Although colonization often precedes infection (187), routine surveillance cultures are not cost effective or practical because of the difficulty of identifying the isolated organism(s) responsible for infection (188).

Prophylactic Use of Therapeutic Agents

Bacterial

Oral antibiotics have been used to attempt total decontamination of the gastrointestinal tract with nonabsorbable antibiotics and selective decontamination of gram-negative organisms with absorbable antibiotics (189, 190). A reduction in gram-negative infections has been demonstrated in studies using nonabsorbable antibiotics (191) and quinolones (192). However, total protective isolation is required with the former. Moreover, lack of infection-related mortality and development of drug resistance with the latter suggests that widespread use of antibiotic prophylaxis may be deleterious in the neutropenic patient (194, 195).

Fungal

Oral nonabsorbable antifungal agents have not shown clear benefit as prophylaxis against systemic fungal infections (198). Fluconazole, an absorbable agent, appears to be effective in hosts with neutropenia when used preventively (194–195).

Aspergillus, most commonly *A. fumigatus* and *A. flavus* (196, 197), infect the respiratory tract by inhalation of conidia into the lower respiratory tract where germination and invasion occur. Certain environmental conditions enhance infectivity, namely, contaminated air-conditioning units and construction sites (198, 199). Disseminated disease may also come from catheter sites. Any factors that compromise alveolar macrophage and granulocyte function damage the primary defense against *Aspergillus* (200, 201).

Viral

Acyclovir (250 mg/m² every 8 hr, p.o. or i.v) can decrease the incidence of recurrent HSV infection in severely immunosuppressed seropositive patients (202–204) and, as noted, has been shown to provide effective prophylaxis against CMV pneumonia (205) and HSV disease.

Parasitic

Clear prophylactic benefit has been shown with the use of TMP-SMX (75 mg/m² given twice a day on three consecutive days of each week (206)) to prevent PCP in patients undergoing antileukemic treatment, those in the BMT setting, or those with acquired immunodeficiency (207). Aerosolized pentamidine is effective in AIDS patients and other immunosuppressed patients (208, 209) These trials have been pivotal in revising the guidelines regarding the use of TMP-SMX for both primary and secondary prophylaxis. TMP-SMX may have the additional advantage of providing protection against toxoplasmosis (210).

Improving Host Defense

Passive Antibody

Studies to date on the use of pooled intravenous immunoglobulin administered weekly to those chemotherapy-introduced neutropenic patients show no effect on development of fever, time of its onset, or incidence of primary or secondary infections (211). In patients with humoral and combined immunodeficiencies, intravenous immunoglobulin has been shown to be beneficial (212).

Immunocompromised individuals known to be susceptible to chicken pox should avoid exposure to patients with this disease. If exposure occurs, specific VZIG should be given as soon after exposure as possible and preferably not more than 96 hours after exposure. Children given VZIG should remain in isolation for 1 week longer or from 10–28 days after exposure.

Bacterial. Specific antisera have been developed to common bacterial pathogens, but their prophylactic use is unclear (213). Monoclonal antibody against endotoxin did not appear to offer benefit unless a gram-negative organism was isolated from the blood (214). J-5 antiserum, collected from patients with high titers of antibody against the core glycolipid of *Enterobacteriaceae* (215), or human monoclonal antibody to J-5, may reduce morbidity in some patients with gram-negative sepsis, but the cost effectiveness and what role these antibody preparations should play in the neutropenic patient remain unclear (216).

Viral

When an immunosuppressed and seronegative patient is exposed to an active VZV infection, disease can occur from 7–10 days beyond the typical 21-day incubation period. VZIG should be administered as early as possible or within 96 hours. The use of CMV immunoglobulin or pooled immune globulin preparations may have value for renal transplantation patients, but its usefulness in BMT recipients is suspect (217). There is only anecdotal information to support its use in adenovirus pneumonia (218).

Active Immunization

The use of active immunization in the immunocompromised host depends on the degree of immunosuppression and the type of vaccine. In general, the inability to mount an immune response makes vaccination unsuccessful (219, 220), though some responses can be obtained in children receiving maintenance chemotherapy (221). Varicella vaccine has been shown to significantly reduce the incidence of varicella in children with acute lymphoblastic leukemia (222).

Cytokines and Lymphokines

Hematopoietic cytokines appear to play a favorable role in the treatment of both congenital and acquired immunodeficiencies. Both G- and GM-CSF stimulate dose-dependent increases in neutrophil numbers and variably shorten the duration of neutropenia when used in vivo or in vitro (223, 224). These factors are accompanied by a number of side effects, including fever, rash, malaise, myalgias, arthralgias, capillary leak syndrome, and large vessel venous thrombosis. Use of recombinant human G-CSF improves the likelihood of maintaining a timed chemotherapy course and appears to decrease both the need for empiric antibiotic therapy as well as the incidence of oral mucositis and to have fewer side effects than GM-CSF (225). Autoantibody has yet to be identified after administration of recombinant growth factors (226). Earlier concerns regarding possible stimulation of leukemic and other tumor cells in vitro are no longer apparent, and indeed, G-CSF is used in certain AML patients (227). Studies on the efficacy of combined human growth factors, (G-CSF, GM-CSF, M-CSF and others, including IL-3) are under way in an effort to determine the most effective means of enhancing stem cell recovery (228).

Adoptive Immune Therapy

Cloned CD8+ cells derived from CMV+ volunteers have been free of toxicity in early phase I trials. Should such an approach prove to be effective CMV control, it may well herald a new era of prophylaxis (229).

Conclusion

Infection continues to be the major cause of morbidity and mortality in the immunocompromised host. Those at greatest risk are patients with neutropenia and/or T-cell deficiencies. In all of these individuals, fever should be aggressively evaluated and treated as an infectious event. With the ability to improve the recovery of impaired immune function cells by intelligent use of cytokines along with promising initiatives of adaptive immunity, the heretofore tragic outcome in otherwise successful therapeutic ventures will be rendered inconsequential.

REFERENCES

1. Masur H, Cheigh JS, Stubenbord WT. Infection following renal transplantation: a changing pattern. Rev Infect Dis 1982;4:1208–1219.
2. Peterson PK, Balfour HH, Fryd DS, et al. Fever in the renal transplant recipient: causes, prognostic significance and changing patterns at the University of Minnesota Hospital. Am J Med 1981;71:345.
3. Braun WE, Nankervis G, Banowshy LH, et al. A prospective study of cytomegalovirus infections in 78 renal allograft recipients. Proc Clin Dial Transplant Forum 1976;6:8–11.
4. Ho M. Virus infections after transplantation in man. Brief review. Arch Virol 1977;55:1–24.
5. Meyers JD, Ljungman P Fisher LD. Cytomegalovirus excretion as a predictor of cytomegalovirus disease after marrow transplantation: importance of cytomegalovirus viremia. J Infect Dis 1990;162:378–380.
6. Meyers JD, Flournoy N, Thomas ED. Nonbacterial pneumonia after allogeneic marrow transplantation: a review of ten years' experience. Rev Infect Dis 1982;4:1119–1132.
7. Johnson FL, Stokes DC, Ruggiero M, et al. Chronic obstructive airways disease after bone marrow transplantation. J Pediatr 1984;105:370–376.
8. Verdonck LF, de Gast GC. Is cytomegalovirus infection a major cause of T cell alterations after "autologous" bone-marrow transplantation? Lancet 1984;1:932–935.
9. Richardson WP, Colvin RB, Cheeseman SH, et al. Glomerulopathy associated with cytomegalovirus viremia in renal allografts. N Engl J Med 1981;305:57–63.
10. Masur H, Cheigh JS, Stubenbord WT. Infection following renal transplantation: a changing pattern. Rev Infect Dis 1982;4:1208–1219.
11. Claman HN. Corticosteroids and lymphoid cells. N Engl J Med 1972;287:388–397.
12. Rinhart JJ, Sagone AL, Balcerzak SP, et al. Effects of corticosteroid therapy on human monocyte function. N Engl J Med 1975;292:236–241.
13. Pizzo PA, Schimpff SC. Strategies for the prevention of infection in the myelosuppressed or immunosuppressed cancer patient. Cancer Treat Rep 1983;67:223–234.
14. Winston DJ, Gale RP, Meyer DV, et al. Infectious complications of human bone marrow transplantation. Medicine 1979;58:1–31.
15. Meyers JD, Thomas ED. Infection complicating bone marrow transplantation. In: Rubin RH, Young LS, eds. Clinical approach to infection in the immunocompromised host. New York: Plenum Press, 1981:507–551.
16. Hughes WT, Armstrong D, Bodey GP, et al. Guidelines for the use of antimicrobial agents in neutropenic patients with unexplained fever: a statement by the Infectious Disease Society of America. J Infect Dis 1990;161:381–396.
17. Granowetter L, Wells H, Lange BJ. Ceftazidime with or without vancomycin vs cephalothin, carbenicillin and gentamicin as initial therapy of the febrile neutropenic pediatric cancer patient. Pediatr Infect Dis J 1988;7:165–170.
18. Pizzo PA, Hawthorn JW, Hiemenz J, et al. A randomized trial comparing combination antibiotic therapy to monotherapy in cancer patients with fever and neutropenia. N Engl J Med 1986;315:552–558.
19. Reaves TA, Hayward JN. Hypothalamic and extra-hypothalamic thermoregulatory centers. In: Lomax P, Schonbaum E, eds. Body temperature. New York: Marcel Dekker, 1979:58.
20. Lorin MI. The febrile child. Clinical management of fever and other types of pyrexia. New York: John Wiley & Sons, 1982:153,226–227.
21. Gander GW, Goodale F. The role of granulocyte and mononuclear leukocytes in fever. In: Lomax P, Schonbaum E, Jacob J,eds. Temperature regulation and drug action. Basel: S Karger, 1975:51–58.
22. DuBois EF. Why are fever temperatures over 106°F rare? Am J Med Sci 1949;217:361–368.
23. Stine RJ. Heat illness. J Am Coll Emerg Physicians 1979; 8:154–160.
24. Dutcher JP, Schiffer CA, Johnson GS. Rapid migration of indium labeled granulocytes to sites of infection. N Engl J Med 1981;304:586–589.
25. Hughes WT. Empiric antimicrobial therapy in the febrile granulocytopenic patient. Infect Control Hosp Epidemiol 1990;3:151.
26. EORTC International Antimicrobial Therapy Cooperative Groups. Ceftazidime combined with a short or long course of amikacin for empirical therapy of gram-negative bacteremia in cancer patients with granulocytopenia. N Engl J Med 1987;317:1692–1698.
27. O'Handley P, Easaw J, Rugo H, Easaw S. Infectious disease management of adult leukemic patients undergoing chemotherapy: 1982 to 1986 experience at Stanford University Hospital. Am J Med 1989;87:605–613.
28. Love LJ, Schimpff SC, Schiffer CA, et al. Improved prognosis for granulocytopenic patients with gram-negative bacteremia. Am J Med 1980;68:643–648.
29. Pizzo PA, Rubin M, Freifeld A, Walsh TJ. The child with cancer and infection. I. Empiric therapy for fever and neutropenia and preventive strategies. J Pediatr 1991;119(5):679–694.
30. Casali A, Ameglio, Gionfra T, et al. Amikacin plus ceftazidime versus amikacin plus piperacillin versus amikacin plus aztreonam in infections in neoplastic patients with granulocytopenia. Chemioterapia 1987;6:440–444.
31. Gucalp R, Lisa S, McKitrick JC, et al. Cefoperazone plus tobramycin venous ticarcillin plus tobramycin in febrile

granulocytopenic cancer patients. Am J Med 1988;85(Suppl 1A):31–35.

32. Huijgens PC, Ossenkoppele GJ, Weijers TF, et al. Imipenem cilastatin for empiric therapy in neutropenic patients with fever: an open study in patients with hematologic malignancies. Eur J Haematol 1991;46:42–46.

33. Karp JE, Dick JD, et al. Empiric use of vancomycin during prolonged treatment-induced granulocytopenia: randomized double-blind placebo-controlled trial in patients with severe leukemia. Am J Med 1986;81:237–242.

34. European Organization for Research and Treatment of Cancer (EORTC) International Antimicrobial Therapy Cooperative Group and National Cancer Institute of Canada-Clinical Trials Group. Vancomycin added to empirical combination therapy for fever in granulocytopenic cancer patients. J Infect Dis 1991;163: 951–958.

35. Novakova I, Donnelly JP, DePauw B. Ceftazidime as monotherapy or combined with teicoplanin for initial empiric treatment of presumed bacteremia in febrile granulocytopenic patients. J Antimicrobial Agents Chemother 1991; 35:672–678.

36. Rubin M, Hawthorn JW, Marshall D, Gress J, Steinberg S, Pizzo PA. Gram-positive infections and the use of vancomycin in 550 episodes of fever and neutropenia. Ann Intern Med 1988;108:88–100.

37. Villablanca JG, Steiner M, Kersey J, Ramsey NK, Ferrieri P, Haake R, Weisdorf D. The clinical spectrum of infections with viridans streptococci in bone marrow transplant patients. Bone Marrow Transplant 1990;5(6):387–393.

38. Recommendations for presenting the spread of vancomycin resistance. MMWR 1995;44:1–13.

39. Donowitz GR, Mandell GL. Beta-lactam antibiotics. N Engl J Med 1988;318:419–426,490–500.

40. Tatsumi H, Senda H, Yatera S, Takemoto Y, Yamayoshi M, Ohmishi K. Toxicological studies on pipemidic acid vs effect on diarthrodial joints of experimental animals. J Toxicol Sci 1978;3:357–367.

41. Heimenz J, Skelton J, Pizzo P. Perspective on the management of catheter-related infections in cancer patients. Pediatr Infect Dis 1986;5:6–11.

42. Viscoli C, Garavanta A, Boni L, et al. Role of Broviac catheters in infections in children with cancer. Pediatr Infect Dis J 1988;7:556–560.

43. Allo MD, Miller J, Townsend T, et al. Primary cutaneous aspergillosis associated with Hickman intravenous catheters. N Engl J Med 1987;317:1105.

44. Hoy JF, Rolston KVI, Hopfer RL, et al. *Mycobacterium fortuitum* bacteremia in patients with cancer and long term venous catheters. Am J Med 1987;83:213.

45. Benezra D, Kiehn TE, Gold JWM, et al. Prospective study of infections in indwelling central venous catheters using quantitative blood cultures. Am J Med 1988;85: 495–498.

46. Prince A, Heller B, Levy J, Heird W. Management of fever in patients with central vein catheters. Pediatr Infect Dis 1986;5:20–24.

47. Nachman JB, Honig GR. Fever and neutropenia in children with neoplastic disease. An analysis of 158 episodes. Cancer 1980;45:407–412.

48. Pizzo PA, Robichaud KJ, Wesley R, Commers JR. Fever in the pediatric and young adult patient with cancer. A prospective study of 1001 episodes. Medicine 1982;61: 153–165.

49. Rubin M, Todeschini G, Marshall D, et al. Does the presence of an indwelling venous catheter affect the type of infections in neutropenic cancer patients? An analysis of 505 episodes. Proceedings of the 27th Interscience Conference on Antimicrobial Agents and Chemotherapy, New York, 1987:264.

50. Ognibene FP, Pass HI, Roth JA, Shelhamer JH, Milne EN. Role of imaging and interventional techniques in the diagnosis of respiratory disease in the immunocompromised host. J Thorac Imaging 1988;3(2):1–20.

51. Foot AB, Caul EO, Roome AP, Oakhill A, Catterall JR. An assessment of sputum induction as an aid to diagnosis of respiratory infections in the immunocompromised child. J Infect 1992;24(1):49–54.

52. Pisani RJ, Wright AJ. Clinical utility of bronchoalveolar lavage in immunocompromised hosts. Mayo Clin Proc 1992;67(3):221–227.

53. Brown MJ, Potter D, Gress J, et al. A randomized trial of open lung biopsy versus empiric antimicrobial therapy in cancer patients with diffuse pulmonary infiltrates. J Clin Oncol 1990;8:222–229.

54. Commers JR, Robichaud KJ, Pizzo PA. New pulmonary infiltrates in granulocytopenic patients being treated with antibiotics. Pediatr Infect Dis 1984;3:423–428.

55. Ognibene FP, Gill VJ, Pizzo PA, et al. Induced sputum to diagnose *Pneumocystis carinii* pneumonia in immunosuppressed pediatric patients. J Pediatr 1989;115:430–433.

56. Heurlin N, Brattstrom C, Lonnqvist B, Westman L, Lidman C, Andersson J. Aetiology of pulmonary diseases in immunocompromised patients. Eur Respir J 1991;4(1):10–18.

57. Foglia RP, Shilyansky J, Fonkalsrud EW. Emergency lung biopsy in immunocompromised pediatric patients. Ann Surg 1989;210(1):90–92.

58. Gleaves CA, Smith TF, Shuster EA, et al. Comparison of standard tube and shell vial cell culture techniques for the detection of cytomegalovirus in clinical specimens. J Clin Microb 1985;21:217–221.

59. Martin WJ, Smith TF. Rapid detection of cytomegalovirus in bronchoalveolar specimens by monoclonal antibody method. 1986;23:1006–1008.

60. Fainstein V, Gilmore C, Hopfer RL, et al. Septic arthritis due to *Candida* species in patients with cancer: report of five cases and review of the literature. Rev Infect Dis 1982; 4(1):78–85.

61. Kingston ME, Mackey D. Skin clues in the diagnosis of life threatening infections. Rev Infect Dis 1986;8:1.

62. Pizzo PA. Infectious complications in the child with cancer. I. Pathophysiology of the compromised host and the initial evaluation and management of the febrile cancer patient. J Pediatr 1981;98:341.

63. Peterson DE, Minah GE, Overholser CD, et al. Microbiology of acute periodontal infection in myelosuppressed cancer patients. J Clin Oncol 1987;5:1461.

64. Walsh TJ, Pizzo PA. Nosocomial fungal infections: a classification for hospital acquired fungal infection and mycoses arising from endogenous flora or reactivation. Annu Rev Microbiol 1988;42:517.

65. Glenn J, Cotton D, Wesley R, et al. Anorectal infections in patients with malignant diseases. Rev Infect Dis 1988; 10:42.

66. Pizzo PA, Robichaud KJ, Gill FA, et al. Duration of empiric antibiotic therapy in granulocytopenic cancer patients. Am J Med 1979;67:194.

67. Pizzo PA, Commers J, Cotton D, et al. Approaching the controversies in the antibacterial management of cancer patients. Am J Med 1984;76:436–439.

68. Walsh TJ, Lee JW, Lecciones J, et al. Empiric amphotericin B in febrile granulocytopenic patients. Rev Infect Dis 1991;13:496–503.

69. Walsh TJ, Lee J, Aoki S, et al. Experimental basis for usage of fluconazole for prevention or early treatment of disseminated candidiasis in granulocytopenic hosts. Rev Infect Dis 1990;12:S307–317.

70. Navarro E, Lecciones J, Witebsky F, et al. Invasive aspergillosis developing during antifungal therapy. Proceedings of the 90th American Society for Microbiology (abstract F-71). Anaheim, CA: 1990;420.

71. Glenn J, Cotton D, Wesley R, Pizzo PA. Anorectal infections in patients with malignant diseases. Rev Infect Dis 1988;10:42–52.

72. Pizzo PA. After antibiotic therapy: what to do until the granulocyte count comes back. Rev Infect Dis 1987;9:214–219.

73. Fainstein V, Elting LS, Bodey GP. Bacteremia caused by non-sporulating anaerobes in cancer patients: a 12-year experience. Medicine 1989;68:151–162.

74. Skibber JM, Mather GH, Lotze MT, et al. Right lower quadrant complications in young patients with leukemia: a surgical perspective. Ann Surg 1987;206:711–716.

75. Gerding DN. Disease associated with *Clostridium difficile* infection. Ann Intern Med 1989;110:255–257.

76. McDonald GD, Sharma P, Hackman RC, et al. Esophageal infections in immunosuppressed patients after marrow transplantation. Gastroenterology 1985;88:1111–1117.

77. Johnson RB Jr, McMurray JS. Chronic familial granulomatosis: report of five cases and review of the literature. Am J Dis Child 1967;114:370–378.

78. Badley JA, Karnovsky ML. Active oxygen species and the functions of phagocytic leukocytes. Annu Rev Biochem 1980;49:695–726.

79. Klebanoff SJ, White LR. Iodination defect in the leukocytes of a patient with chronic granulomatous disease of childhood. N Engl J Med 1969;280:460–466.

80. Phillapart AI, Colodney AH, Baehner RJ. Continuous antibiotic therapy in chronic granulomatous disease. Pediatrics 1972;50:923–925.

81. Sechler JM, Malech HL, White CJ, et al. Recombinant human interferon-gamma reconstitutes defective phagocyte function in patients with chronic granulomatous disease of childhood. Proc Natl Acad Sci USA 1988;85:4874–4878.

82. Lomax KJ, Malech HL, Gallin JI. The molecular biology of selected phagocytic defects. Blood Rev 1989;3:94–104.

83. Donabedian H, Gallin JI. The hyperimmunoglobulin E recurrent (Job's) infection syndrome. Medicine 1983;62:195–208.

84. Lehrer RI, Cline MJ. Leukocyte myeloperoxidase deficiency and disseminated candidiasis; the role of myeloperoxidase in resistance to candida infection. J Clin Invest 1969;48:1478–1488.

85. Root RK, Rosenthal AS, Balestra DJ. Abnormal bacteriocidal metabolic and lysosomal functions of Chediak-Higashi syndrome leukocytes. J Clin Invest 1972;51:649–665.

86. Brown CC, Gallin JI. Chemotactic disorders. Hematol Oncol Clin North Am 1988;2:61–79.

87. Ellis EF, Smith RT. The role of the spleen in immunity. With special reference to the postsplenectomy problem in infants. Pediatrics 1966;37:111–119.

88. Barrett-Connor E. Bacterial infection and sickle cell anemia. An analysis of 250 infections in 166 patients and a review of the literature. Medicine 1971;50:96–112.

89. Shulman ST, Barlett J, Clyde WA Jr, et al. The unusual severity of mycoplasma pneumonia in children with sickle cell disease. N Engl J Med 1972;287:164–167.

90. Gaston MH, Verter JI, Woods G, et al. Prophylaxis with oral penicillin in children with sickle cell anemia. N Engl J Med 1986;314:1593–1599.

91. DiGeorge AM. Congenital absence of the thymus and its immunologic consequences: concurrence with congenital hypothyroidism. In: Bergsma D, Good RA, eds. Immunologic deficiency diseases in man. New York: The National Foundation, 1968:116–123.

92. Giblett ER, Anderson JE, Cohen F, et al. Adenosine-deaminase deficiency in two patients with severely impaired cellular immunity. Lancet 1972;2:1067–1069.

93. Waltzer PD, Schultz MG, Western KA, et al. *Pneumocystis carinii* pneumonia and primary immune deficiency diseases of infancy and childhood. J Pediatr 1973;82:416–422.

94. Lauson D, Delage G, Brochu P, et al. Pathogens in children with severe combined immune deficiency disease or AIDS. Can Med Assoc J 1986;135:33.

95. Reinherz EL, Geha R, Rappaport JM, et al. Reconstitution after transplantation with T-lymphocyte-depleted HLA haplotype-mismatched bone marrow for severe combined immune deficiency. Proc Natl Acad Sci USA 1982;79:6047–6051.

96. Pearl ER, Vogler LB, Okos AJ, et al. B lymphocyte precursors in human bone marrow. An analysis of normal individuals and patients with antibody-deficient states. J Immunol 1978;120:1169–1175.

97. Gitlin D, Janeway CA, Apt L, et al. Agammaglobulinemia. In: Lawrence HS, ed. Cellular and humoral aspects of the hypersensitive states. New York: Hoeber Medical Division, Harper & Row, 1959:375–441.

98. Wright PF, Hatch MH, Kasselberg AG, et al. Vaccine associated poliomyelitis in a child with sex-linked agammaglobulinemia. J Pediatr 1977;91:408–412.

99. Mease PJ, Ochs HD, Wedgwood RJ. Successful treatment of echovirus meningoencephalitis and myositis-fasciitis with intravenous immune globulin therapy in a patient with X-linked agammaglobulinemia. N Engl J Med 1981;304:1278–1281.

100. Saulsbury FT, Winklestein JA, Yolken RH. Chronic rotavirus infection in immunodeficiency. J Pediatr 1980;97:61–65.

101. Ochs HD, Ament ME, Davis SD. Giardiasis with malabsorption in X-linked agammaglobulinemia. N Engl J Med 1972;287:341–342.

102. South MA, Cooper MD, Wollheim FA, et al. The IgA system. II The clinical significance of IgA deficiency: studies in patients with agammaglobulinemia and ataxia-telangiectasia Am J Med 1968;44:168–178.

103. Berger M. Complement deficiency and neutrophil dysfunction as risk factors for bacterial infection in newborns and the role of granulocyte transfusion in therapy. Rev Infect Dis 1990;12(Suppl 4):S401-S409.

104. Agello V. Lupus diseases associated with hereditary and acquired deficiencies of complement. Springer Semin Immunopathol 1986;9:161.

105. Fries LF, O'Shea JJ, Frank MM. Inherited deficiencies of complement and complement-related proteins. Clin Immunol Immunopathol 1986;40:37.

106. Alper CA, Abramson N, Johnson RB Jr, et al. Increased risk of infection associated with abnormalities of complement-mediated functions and the third component of complement (C3). N Engl J Med 1970;282:350–354.

107. Fijen CA, Kuijper EJ, Lindeboom SF, et al. Two families with meningococcal infection and hereditary disorder of the 5th component of the complement system. Ned Tijdschr Geneeskd 1989;133:1796–1800.

108. Soderstrom C, Sjoholm AG, Svensson R, et al. Another Swedish family with complete properdin deficiency: association with fulminant meningococcal disease in one male family member. Scand J Infect Dis 1989;21:259–265.

109. Potter PC, Frasch CE, van der Sande WJ, et al. Prophylaxis against *Neisseria meningitidis* infections and antibody responses in patients with deficiency in the sixth component of complement. J Infect Dis 1990;161:932–937.

110. Wiley J, et al. Invasive fungal infections in children with cancer. J Clin Oncol 1990;8:280–286.

111. Dreizen S. Oral candidiasis. Am J Med 1984;77(Suppl 4D):28–33.

112. Leggott P, Robertson P, Greenspan D, Wara D, Greenspan J. Oral manifestations of primary and acquired immunodeficiency diseases in children. Pediatr Dent 1987;9:98–104.

113. Walsh T, Gray W. Candida esophagitis in immunocompromised patients. Chest 1987;91:482–485.

114. Hass A, Hyatt AC, Kattan M, Weiner M, Hodes DS. Hoarseness in immunocompromised children: association with invasive fungal infection. J Pediatr 1987;111:731–733.

115. Yeo E, Alvarado T, Fainstein V, Bodey G. Prophylaxis of oropharyngeal candidiasis with clotrimazole. J Clin Oncol 1985;3:1668–1671.

116. McDonald G, Sharma P, Hackman R, et al. Infectious esophagitis in immunosuppressed after marrow transplantation. Gastroenterology 1985;88:1111–1117.

117. Cipollini F, Altilia F. Candidiasis complicating cimetidine treatment. Lancet 1981;2:1047–1048.

118. Pizzo PA, Rubin M, Freifeld, Walsh TJ. The child with cancer and infection II. Nonbacterial infections. J Pediatr 1991;119:679–694.

119. Bianco J, et al. Prevalence of clinically relevant bacteremia after upper endoscopy in bone marrow transplant recipients. Am J Med 1990;89:134–136.

120. Ginsburg CH, Braden GL, Tauber AL, et al. Oral clotrimazole in the treatment of esophageal candidiasis. Am J Med 1981;71:891–895.

121. Bodey GP. Fungal infection and fever of unknown origin in neutropenic patients. Am J Med 1986;80(Suppl 5C):112–119.

122. Richet HM, Andremont A, Tancrede, Pico JL, Jarvis WR. Risk factors for candidemia in patients with acute lymphoblastic leukemia. Rev Infect Dis 1991;13:211–215.

123. Dato V, Dajani A. Candidemia in children with central venous catheters: role of catheter removal and amphotericin B therapy. Pediatr Infect Dis J 1990;9:309–314.

124. Edwards JE Jr, Foos RY, Montgomerie JZ, Guze L. Ocular manifestations of *Candida* septicemia: review of seventy-six cases of hematogenous *Candida* endophthalmitis. Medicine (Baltimore) 1974;53:47–75.

125. Thaler M, Pastakia B, Shawker TH, et al. Hepatic candidiasis in cancer patients: the evolving picture of the syndrome. Ann Intern Med 1988;108:98–100.

126. Arena FP, Perlin M, Brahman H, et al. Fever, rash, myalgias of disseminated candidiasis during antifungal therapy. Arch Intern Med 981;141:122–133.

127. Thaler M, Bacher J, O'Leary T, Pizzo PA. Evaluation of single-drug and combination antifungal therapy in an experimental model of candidiasis in rabbits with prolonged neutropenia. J Infect Dis 1988;158:80–88.

128. Tollemar J, Olle Ringden O, Tyden G. Liposomal amphotericin B (AmBisome) treatment in solid organ and bone marrow transplant recipients: efficacy and safety evaluation. Clin Transplant 1990;4:167–175.

129. Kauffman CA, Bradley SF, Ross SC, Weber DR, Band JD, Harrison DC. Successful treatment of hepatic candidiasis with fluconazole (abstract 577). Program and Abstracts of the 30th Interscience Conference on Antimicrobial Agents and Chemotherapy, Atlanta, 1990.

130. Panos R, Barr L, Walsh TJ, et al. Factors associated with fatal hemoptysis in cancer patients. Chest 1988;94:1008–1013.

131. Barloon TJ, Galvin JR, Mori M, Stanford W, Gingridr RD. High-resolution ultrafast chest CT in the clinical management of febrile bone marrow transplant patients with normal or nonspecific roentgenograms. Chest 1991;99:928–933.

132. Walsh TJ, Bulkley BH. *Aspergillus* pericarditis in the immunocompromised patient: a clinicopathology study. Cancer 1982;49:48–54.

133. Walsh TJ, Hier DB, Caplan LR. Fungal infections of the central nervous system: analysis of risk factors and clinical manifestations. Neurology 1985;35:1654–1657.

134. Talbot GH, Huong A, Provencher M. Invasive *Aspergillus* rhinosinusitis in patients with acute leukemia. Rev Infect Dis 1991;13:219–232.

135. Yu VL, Muder RR, Poorsattar A. Significance of isolation of *Aspergillus* from the respiratory tract in diagnosis of invasive pulmonary aspergillosis: results of a three-year prospective study. Am J Med 1986;81:2249–2254.

136. Treger TR, Visscher DW, Bartlett MS, et al. Diagnosis of pulmonary infection caused by *Aspergillus*: usefulness of respiratory cultures. J Infect Dis 1985;152:572–576.

137. McCabe RE, Brooks RG, Mark JBD, et al. Open lung biopsy in patients with acute leukemia. Am J Med 1985;78:609–616.

138. Karp JE, Burch PA, Merz WG. An approach to intensive antileukemia therapy in patients with previous invasive aspergillosis. Am J Med 1988;85:203–206.

139. Denning D, Stevens DA. Antifungal and surgical treatment of invasive aspergillosis: review of 2,121 published cases. Rev Infect Dis 1990;12:1147–1181.

140. Robertson MJ, Larson RA. Recurrent fungal pneumonias in patients with acute non-lymphocytic leukemia undergoing multiple courses of intensive chemotherapy. Am J Med 1988;84:233–239.

141. Perfect JR. Cryptococcosis. In: Moellering RC, Drutz DJ, eds. Systemic fungal infections. II. Diagnosis and treatment. Infect Dis Clin North Am 1989;3(1):777–802.

142. Dismukes WE, Cloud G, Gallis HA, et al. Treatment of cryptococcal meningitis with combinations of amphotericin B and flucytosine for four as compared with six weeks. N Engl J Med 1987;34:334–341.

143. Diamond RD. The growing problem of mycoses in patients infected with the human immunodeficiency virus. Rev Infect Dis 1991;13:480–486.

144. Walsh TJ. Trichosporinosis. Infect Dis Clin North Am 1989; 3:43–65.

145. Rinaldi M. Zygomycosis. Infect Dis Clin North Am 1989; 3:19–41.

146. Rippon J. Medical mycology: the pathogenic actinomycetes-pseudallescheriasis. Philadelphia: WB Saunders, 1988:651–680.

147. Merz W, Karp J, Hoagland M, et al. Diagnosis and successful treatment of fusarioses in the compromised host. J Infect Dis 1988;158:1046–1055.

148. Fader RC, McGinnis MR. Infections caused by dematiaceous fungi: chromoblastomycosis and phaeohyphomycosis. Infect Dis Clin North Am 1988;2(4):925–938.

149. Whitley RJ, Alford CA, Hirsch MS, et al. Vidarabine versus acyclovir therapy in herpes simplex encephalitis. N Engl J Med 1986;314:144–149.

150. Erlich KS, Jacobson MA, Koehler JE, et al. Foscarnet therapy for severe acyclovir-resistant herpes simplex virus type-2 infections in patients with the acquired immunodeficiency syndrome (AIDS): an uncontrolled trial. Ann Intern Med 1989;110:710–713.

151. Schmidt NJ, Gallo D, Delvin V, Woodie JD, Emmons RW. Direct immunofluorescence staining for detection of herpes simplex and varicella-zoster virus antigen in vesicular lesions and certain tissue specimens. J Clin Microbiol 1980;12:651–655.

152. Hirsch MS. Herpes group virus infections in the compromised host. In: Rubin RH, Young LS, eds. Clinical approach to infections in the immunocompromised host. New York: Plenum Medical, 1988 347–366.

153. Shepp DH, Dandliker PS, Meyers JD. Treatment of varicella-zoster virus infections in severely immunocompromised patients. N Engl J Med 1986;314:208–212.

154. Jacobsen MA, Berger TG, Fikrig S, et al. Acyclovir-resistant varicella zoster virus infection after chronic oral acyclovir therapy in patients with acquired immunodeficiency syndrome (AIDS). Ann Intern Med 1990;112:187–191.

155. Texidor HS, Hong CL, Norsoph E, et al. Cytomegalovirus infection of the alimentary canal: radiologic findings with pathologic correlation. Radiology 1987;163:317–323.

156. Crawford SW, Bowden RA, Hackman RC, et al. Rapid detection of cytomegalovirus pulmonary infection by bronchoalveolar lavage and centrifugation culture. Ann Intern Med 1988,108:180–185.

157. Einsele H, Ehnringer G, Hebart KM, et al. Polymerase chain reaction monitoring reduces the incidence of cytomegalovirus disease and the duration and side effects of antiviral therapy after bone marrow transplantation. Blood 1995;86:2815.

158. Reed EC, Bowden RA, Dandliker PS, et al. Treatment of cytomegalovirus pneumonia with gancyclovir and intravenous cytomegalovirus immunoglobulin in patients with bone marrow transplant. Ann Intern Med 1988;109: 783–788.

159. Emanuel D, Cunningham I, Jules-Elysee K, et al. Cytomegalovirus pneumonia after bone marrow transplantation successfully treated with the combination of ganciclovir and high-dose intravenous immune globulin. Ann Intern Med 1988;109:777–782.

160. Erica A, Chou S, Biron KK, Stanat SC, Balfour HH Jr, Jordan MC. Progressive disease due to ganciclovir-resistant cytomegalovirus in immunocompromised patients. N Engl J Med 1989;320:289–293.

161. Bratanow NC, Ash RC, Turner PA, et al. Successful treatment of serious CMV with gancyclovir and intravenous immunoglobulin in bone marrow transplant patients (abstract). Exp Hematol 1987;15:541.

162. Schmidt EM, Kovacs A, Zaia JA, et al. Gancyclovir/immunoglobulin combination for the treatment of human cytomegalovirus-associated interstitial pneumonia in bone marrow allograft recipients. Transplantation 1988;46:905.

163. Aulitsky WE, Tilg H. Niederweisser D, et al. Gancyclovir and hyperimmune globulin for treating cytomegalovirus infection in bone marrow transplant recipients. J Infect Dis 1988;158:488.

164. Schmidt GM, Horak DA, Nicano JC, et al. A randomized controlled trial of prophylactic gancyclovir for cytomegalovirus disease after allogeneic marrow transplantaion. N Engl J Med 1991;325:1601.

165. Goodrich JM, Mori M, Gleaves CA, et al. Early treatment with gancyclovir to prevent cytomegalovirus disease after allogeneic marrow transplantation. N Engl J Med 1991; 325:1601.

166. Ljungman P, Ashan J, Azinge JN, et al. Cytomegalovirus viraemia and specific T-helper responses as predictors of disease after allogeneic marrow transplantation. Blood J Haematol 1993;83:118.

167. Lucatelli F, Perncal E, Loundi P, et al. Human cytomegalovirus infection in pediatric patients after allogeneic bone marrow transplantation; role of early treatment of HCMC antigenemia in patients in time. Br J Haematol 1994;88:64.

168. Rice GPA, Schrier RD, Oldstone MBA, et al. Cytomegalovirus infects human lymphocytes and monocytes: virus expression is restricted to immediate-early gene products. Natl Acad Sci USA 1984;81:6134.

169. Zhang LJ, Hanff P, Rutherford C, et al. Detection of human cytomegalovirus DNA, RNA and antibody in normal donor blood. J Infect Dis 1995;171:1002.

170. Bowden LA, Slichter SJ, Sayers M, et al. A comparison of filtered leukocyte reduced and cytomegalovirus seronegative blood products for prevention of transfusion associated CMV infection after marrow transplantation. Blood 1885; 86:3598.

171. Kovacs JA, Hiemenz JW, Macher AM, et al. *Pneumocystis carinii* pneumonia: a comparison of clinical features in patients with the acquired immune deficiency syndrome and patients with other immune diseases. Ann Intern Med 1984;100:663–671.

172. Kovacs JA, Gill V, Swan JC, et al. Prospective evaluation of a monoclonal antibody in the diagnosis of *Pneumocystis carinii* pneumonia. Lancet 1986;2:1–4.

173. Garay SM, Greene J. Prognostic indicators in the initial presentation of *Pneumocystis carinii* pneumonia. Chest 1989;95:769–772.

174. Conte JE Jr, Chernoff D, Feigal DW Jr, Joseph P, McDonald C, Golden JA. Intravenous or inhaled pentamidine for treating *Pneumocystis carinii* pneumonia in AIDS: a randomized trial. Ann Intern Med 1990;113:203–209.

175. Lee BL, Medina I, Benowitz NL, Jacob P III, Wofsy CB, Mills JV. Dapsone, trimethoprim, and sulfamethoxazole plasma levels during treatment of *Pneumocystis* pneumonia in patients with the acquired immunodeficiency syndrome (AIDS): evidence of drug interactions. Ann Intern Med 1989;110:606–611.

176. Browne MJ, Potter D, Gress J, et al. A randomized trial of open lung biopsy versus empiric antimicrobial therapy in cancer patients with diffuse pulmonary infiltrates. J Clin Oncol 1990;8:222–229.

177. Masur H. Prevention and treatment of *Pneumocystis* pneumonia. N Engl J Med 1992;327(26):1853–1860.

178. Gagnon S, Boota AM, Fischl MA, Baier H, Kirksey OW, La Voie L. Corticosteroids as adjunctive therapy for severe *Pneumocystis carinii* pneumonia in the acquired immunodeficiency syndrome: a double-blind, placebo-controlled trial. N Engl J Med 1990;323:1444–1450.

179. The National Institutes of Health - University of California Expert Panel for Corticosteroids as Adjunctive Therapy for *Pneumocystis* Pneumonia. Consensus statement on the use of corticosteroids as adjunctive therapy for pneumocystis pneumonia in the acquired immunodeficiency syndrome. N Engl J Med 1990;323:1500–1504.

180. Schimpff SC, Young VM, Greene WH, et al. Origin of infection in acute non-lymphocytic leukemia: significance of hospital acquisition of potential pathogens. Ann Intern Med 1972;77:707–714.

181. Pizzo PA, Purvis DS, Waters C. Microbiological evaluation of food items for patients undergoing gastrointestinal decontamination and protected isolation. J Am Diet Assoc 1982;81:272–279.

182. Meyer RD. Legionnaires disease. Aspects of nosocomial infection. Am J Med 1984;76:657–663.

183. Aisner J, Schimpff SC, Bennett JE, et al. *Aspergillus* infection in cancer patients: association with fireproofing materials in new hospitals. JAMA 1976;235:411–412.

184. Leclair JM, Zaia JA, Levin MJ, et al. Airborne transmission of chickenpox in a hospital. N Engl J Med 1980;302:450–453.

185. Hughes WT, Townsend TR. Nosocomial infections in immunocompromised children Am J Med 1981;70:412–416.

186. Steere AC, Mallison GF. Handwashing practices for the prevention of nosocomial infections. Ann Intern Med 1975;83:683–690.

187. Fainstein V, Rodriguez V, Turk M, et al. Patterns of oropharyngeal and fecal flora in patients with leukemia. J Infect Dis 1981;144:10–18.

188. Kramer BJ, Pizzo PA, Robichaud KJ, et al. Role of serial microbiological surveillance and clinical evaluation in the management of cancer patients with fever and granulocytopenia. Am J Med 1982;72:561–568.

189. Hann IM, Prentice HG. Infection prophylaxis in the patient with bone marrow failure. Clin Haematol 1984;13:523–547.

190. Pizzo PA. Considerations for the prevention of infectious complications in patients with cancer. Rev Infect Dis 1989;11:S1551–1563.

191. Pizzo PA, Schimpff. Strategies for the prevention of infection in the myelosuppressed or immunosuppressed cancer patient. Cancer Treat Rep 1983;67:223–234.

192. Dekker AW, Rozenberg-Arska M, Verhoef J. Infection prophylaxis in acute leukemia: a comparison of ciprofloxacin with trimethoprim-sulfamethoxazole and colistin. Ann Intern Med 1987;106:7.

193. Trucksis M, Hooper DC, Wolfson JS. Emerging resistance to fluoroquinolones in staphylococci: an alert. Ann Intern Med 1991;114:424–426.

194. Meunier F. Prevention of mycoses in immunocompromised patients. Rev Infect Dis 1987;9:408.

195. Goodman JL, Winston DJ, Greenfield RA, Chandrasekar PH, Fox B, et al. A controlled trial of fluconazole to prevent fungal infections in patients undergoing bone marrow transplantation. N Engl J Med 1992;326(13):845–851.

196. Samonis G, Rolston K, Karl C, Miller P, Bodey GP. Prophylaxis of oropharyngeal candidiasis with fluconazole. Rev Infect Dis 1990; 12(Suppl 3):S369–373.

197. Saral R. *Candida* and *Aspergillus* infections in immunocompromised patients: an overview. Rev Infect Dis 1991;13:487–492.

198. Walsh TJ, Dixon DM. Nosocomial aspergillosis: environmental microbiology, hospital epidemiology, diagnosis, and treatment. Eur J Epidemiol 1989;5:131–142.

199. Dixon DM, Polak A, Walsh TJ. Fungus dose-dependent primary pulmonary aspergillosis in immunosuppressed mice. Infect Immun 1989;57:1452–1456.

200. Waldorf AR, Levitz SM, Diamond RD. In vivo bronchoalveolar macrophage defense against *Rhizopus oryzae* and *Aspergillus fumigatus*. J Infect Dis 1984;150:752–760.

201. Commers J, Robichaud KJ, Pizzo PA, et al. New pulmonary infiltrates in granulocytopenic patients being treated with antibiotics. Pediatr Infect Dis 1984;3:423–428.

202. Saral R, Ambinder RF, Burns WH, et al. Acyclovir prophylaxis against herpes simplex virus infection in patients with leukemia. Ann Intern Med 1983;99:773–776.

203. Wade JC, Newton B, Flournoy N, et al. Oral acyclovir for prevention of herpes simplex reactivation after marrow transplant. Ann Intern Med 1984;100:823–838.

204. Meyers JD, Reed EC, Shepp DH, et al. Acyclovir for prevention of cytomegalovirus infection and disease after allogeneic marrow transplantation. N Engl J Med 1988;318:70–75.

205. Schmidt GM, Horak DA, Niland JC, et al. A randomized controlled trial of prophylactic gancyclovir for cytomegalovirus pulmonary infection in recipients of allogeneic bone marrow transplants. N Engl J Med 1991;324:1005–1011.

206. Hughes WT, Rivera GK, Schell MJ, et al. Successful intermittent prophylaxis for *Pneumocystis carinii pneumonitis*. N Engl J Med 1987;316:1627–1632.

207. Recommendations for prophylaxis against *Pneumocystis carinii* pneumonia for adults and adolescents infected with human immunodeficiency virus. MMWR 1992;41(RR-4):1–11.

208. Schneider MME, Hoepelman AIM, Eeftinck Schattenkerk JKM, et al. A controlled trial of aerosolized pentamidine or trimethoprim-sulfamethoxazole as primary prophylaxis against *Pneumocystis carinii* pneumonia in patients with human immunodeficiency virus infection. N Engl J Med 1992;327:1836–1841

209. Hardy WD, Feinberg J, Finkelstein DM, et al. A controlled trial of trimethoprim-sulfamethoxazole of aerosolized pentamidine for secondary prophylaxis of *Pneumocystis carinii* pneumonia in patients with the acquired immunodeficiency syndrome: AIDS Clinical Trials Group, protocol 021. N Engl J Med 1992;327:1842–1848.

210. Carr A, Tindall B, Brew BJ, et al. Low-dose trimethoprim-sulfamethoxazole prophylaxis for toxoplasmic encephalitis in patient with AIDS. Ann Intern Med 1992;117:106–111.

211. Rubin M, Gress J, Marshall D, et al. Prophylaxis of infectious complications in neutropenic cancer patients with intravenous immunoglobulin (abstract 608). Twenty-eighth Interscience Conference on Antimicrobial Agents and Chemotherapy, American Society for Microbiology, Los Angeles, 1988.

212. Stiehm ER, Ashida E, Kim KS, et al. Intravenous immunoglobulins as therapeutic agents. Ann Intern Med 1987;107:367–382.

213. Young LS. Immunoprophylaxis and serotherapy of bacterial infections. Am J Med 1984;76:664–671.

214. Zeigler EJ, Fisher CJ, Sprung CL, et al. Treatment of gram-negative bacteremia and septic shock with HA-IA human monoclonal antibody against endotoxin: a randomized, double-blind, placebo-controlled trial. N Engl J Med 1991; 324:429–436.

215. Calandra T, Glauser MP, Schellekous J, Verhoef J, and the Swiss-Dutch J5 Immunoglobulin Study Group. Treatment of gram-negative septic shock with human IgG antibody to *Escherichia coli* J5: a prospective, double blind, randomized trial. J Infect Dis 1988;158:312–319.

216. Weeks JC, Tierney MR, Weinstein MC. Cost-effectiveness of prophylactic intravenous immunoglobulin in chronic lymphocytic leukemia. N Engl J Med 1991;325:81–86.

217. Winston DJ, Ho WG, Lin CH, et al. Intravenous immune globulin for prevention of cytomegalovirus infection and interstitial pneumonia after transplantation. Ann Intern Med 1987;106:12–18.

218. Dagan R, Schwartz RH, Insel RA, et al. Severe diffuse adenovirus 7a pneumonia in a child with combined immunodeficiency: possible therapeutic effect of human immune serum globulin containing specific neutralizing antibody. Pediatr Infect Dis 1984;3:246–251.

219. Hibberd PL, Rubin RH. Immunization strategies for the immunocompromised host: the need for immunoadjuvants. Ann Intern Med 1989;110:955–956.

220. Ljungman P, Fridell E, Lonnqvist B, et al. Efficacy and safety of vaccination of marrow transplant recipients with live attenuated measles, mumps and rubella vaccine. J Infect Dis 1989;159:610–615.

221. Kung FH, Ongd HA, Wallace UW, Hornberger RN. Antibody production following immunization with diphtheria and tetanus toxoids in children receiving chemotherapy during remission of malignant disease. Pediatrics 1989; 74:86.

222. Gershon AA, LaRussa P, Steinberg SP. Live attenuated varicella vaccine: current status and future uses. Semin Pediatr Infect Dis 1991;2(3):171–177.

223. Groopman J, Molina JM, Scadden D. Hematopoietic growth factors: biology and clinical applications. N Engl J Med 1989;321:1449–1459.

224. Nemunaitis J, Rabinowe SN, Singa JW, et al. Recombinant granulocyte-macrophage colony stimulating factor after autologous bone marrow transplantation for lymphoid cancer. N Engl J Med 1991;324:1773–1778.

225. Morstyn G, Souza L, Keech J, et al. Effect of granulocyte colony stimulating factor on neutropenia induced by cytotoxic chemotherapy. Lancet 1988;1:667–672.

226. Groopman J, Molina J-M, Scadden D. Hematopoietic growth factors: biology and clinical applications. N Engl J Med 1989;321:1449–1459.

227. Powles R, Smith C, Milan S, et al. Human recombinant GM-CSF in allogeneic bone marrow transplantation leukemia. A double-blind, placebo-controlled trial. Lancet 1990;336:1417.

228. Brugger W, Mocklin W, Heinfeld S, et al. Ex vivo expansion of enriched peripheral blood CD34+ progenitor cells by stem cell factor, interleukin-1B(IL-1B), IL-G, IL-3, interferon-gamma, and erythropoietin. Blood 1993;81:1883.

229. Riddell SR, Watanabe KS, Goodrich VII, et al. Restoration of viral immunity in immunodeficient humans by the adaptive transfer of T-cell clones. Science 1992;257:238.

EXERCISES AND TOOLS FOR INFECTION CONTROL

When to treat, how to treat, what to treat—or not to treat.

1. Prepare a schema that considers infectious processes, i.e., bacterial, viral, parasitic, fungal, etc., within various universes of inherited and acquired immune impairment. In the process, offer explanations for the different manifestations of immune deficient disorders.
2. Consider the role and the mechanisms of action of the various anti-infective agents and the manner by which these agents function within the aforementioned templates.
3. In developing these constructs, use the material derived from the chapters on white cell function and biological response controls.
4. Prepare a master protocol that addresses all possible experiences that could arise in the immune incompetent bone marrow transplant recipient.
5. Provide a construct of mechanisms designed to minimize infectious processes in the deliberately, immunologically paralyzed individual. Consider a 60-day period of hematopoietic failure in developing this construct.
6. Provide an operational process for the evaluation of the individual with frequent periods (approximately every three weeks) of granulocytopenia and lymphocytopenia secondary to anticancer therapy. Include in the evaluation those factors that play a major decision-making role.

Index

Entries followed by *t* refer to tables; those followed by *f* refer to figures.

for acute myeloid leukemia, 482–483
for aplastic anemia, 198
for chronic lymphocytic leukemia, 380
discharge planning, 736
donor and recipient preparation, 728
   antinausea control, 732
donor selection, 691–692, 692*t*, 727–728
engraftment, 732
exercises and tools for, 746
for follicular small cleaved cell lymphoma, 332
for Gaucher disease, 453
graft types, 704
graft-versus-host disease following
   acute form, 734*t*
   chronic form, 736–737, 737*t*
   development of, 734*t*
   in Gaucher disease, 454
   organ involvement, 733–735
   prophylactic measures, 733
   secondary malignancies and, 523
hematopoietic control, 735–736
   blood component support, 735
   cytokine support, 735–736
   platelet support, 735
hemoglobin SS disease and, 80
HLA typing and histocompatibility, 710–710, 710*f*
incidence (worldwide), 718*f*
infection following
   susceptibility, 766
   time sequences, 736*t*
late complications of, TBI correlation and, 685–686
marrow sources for, 727–728
minimal residual disease detection following, 737*t*
mismatches, outcomes for, 728
for multiple myeloma, 393
   outcome factors, 723–726, 725*t*
for myelodysplastic syndrome, 462–463
outcome factors
   in AIDS, 726
   in ALL, 720–721, 721*f*, 722*f*
   in AML, 721, 722*f*, 723*f*
   in lymphoma and chronic lymphocytic leukemia, 726, 726*f*
   in multiple myeloma, 723–724, 725*t*
      peripheral blood stem cells and, 725–726
   in myelodysplasia and myeloproliferative diseases, 721, 723, 724*f*, 724*t*
   in nonmalignant disorders of hematopoietic tissue, 726–727, 727*t*
pre-BMT induction and consolidation therapy, 719–720
predictive factors, 720
radiation therapy and, 679–686. *See also* Total body irradiation
reconstitution time, 736, 736*t*
relapsed acute lymphocytic leukemia and, 353
relapsed Hodgkin disease and, 319
secondary leukemia following, 524
for solitary plasmacytoma, 397
stem cells for, 725–726, 737
transplantation and environmental factors affecting, 720

with unmatched donor, 698
   unrelated donor marrow for, 727–728
Boyden apparatus, 424
Breast cancer
   M protein-associated, 392
   secondary leukemias and lymphomas and, 525
Breastfed infants, 36
Bulimia nervosa, folate deficiency in, 39
Burkitt lymphoma
   classification, 336
   clinical case presentation, 335
   diagnosis, 336
   differential diagnoses, 335
   epidemiology, 336
   high-grade B-cell lymphoma and, 335
   pathology, 335*f*, 335–336
   prognosis, 337
   staging, 336, 336*t*
   treatment, 336–337
Busulfan, for ACML management
   in chronic phase, 496, 497
   with αIFN, 498

C
C-abl gene, Philadelphia chromosome and, 287, 287*f*
Calcitonin gene
   in adult chronic myelogenous leukemia, 502–503
   myelodysplastic syndrome and, 461
Cancer
   blood. *See* Hematopoietic malignancies
   coagulopathies associated with, 602–603
   defined, 281
   immune-mediated thrombocytopenia in, 539, 539*f*
   secondary leukemias and lymphomas and, 525
Cancer chemotherapy. *See* Anticancer drugs; Chemotherapy
Cancer procoagulant, 622–623
Candida infection, in immunocompromised host, 775–776
Candidiasis, in immunocompromised host, 775–776
Carbapenems, for infection management in immunocompromised patient, 769
Cardiac toxicity, 731
   following chemotherapy
      agents implicated, 668
      clinical case presentation, 668
Cardiomegaly, hemoglobin SS disease, 89
Carrier testing, factor IX, 591
Cartilage hair hypoplasia, 415
Cataracts, glucose-6-phosphate dehydrogenase and, 166
Catheter-related infections, in immunocompromised patient, 770–771, 771*t*
CCR. *See* Complete cytogenetic remission
CD4, 223
   CD4/CD8 ratios in disease, 226
   subtypes, 223*t*, 223–224
CD8, 223
   CD4/CD8 ratios in disease, 226
   subtypes, 223*t*, 223–224
CD30, Reed-Sternberg cell lines and, 313
CD (cluster of differentiation) system, 265–266

Ceftazidime, for infection management in immunocompromised patient, 769
Celiac disease, 41
Cell death, induction of, 669
Cell divisions, adult chronic myelogenous leukemia and, 494–495
Cell expansion. *See* Clonal expansion of cells
Cell mutation, in chronic lymphocytic leukemia, 364–366, 367*f*
Cell surface markers, in acute myeloid leukemia prognosis, 483
Cellular assays, in bone marrow donor selection, 692
Cellular function, in adult chronic myelogenous leukemia, 493–494
Cellulose acetate electrophoresis, hemoglobinopathies, 74*f*
Cell volume, adult chronic myelogenous leukemia and, 491
Central nervous system
   involvement in acute lymphocytic leukemia, signs and symptoms, 351, 352*t*
   prophylactic therapy for, 671–672
   symptoms in ACML chronic phase, management of, 495–496
   toxicity scale for, 731
Cephalosporins, for infection management in immunocompromised patient, 769
Cerebral angiography, in hemoglobinopathies, 88*f*
Cerebrovascular accidents, 87–88
CFC. *See* Colony-forming cell
CFI. *See* Chemotactic factor inhibitor
CGD. *See* Chronic granulomatous disease
cGVHD. *See* Chronic graft-versus-host disease
Chediak-Higashi syndrome, 416, 416*t*
   in differential diagnosis of neutrophil defects, 419
Chelation therapy
   iron removal, 126–127
   β-thalassemia mutations and, 63
Chemotactic disorders, in immunocompromised host, 774
Chemotactic factor inhibitor, 424
Chemotaxis, defects in
   clinical case presentations, 418–425
   inherited and acquired disorders, 425*t*
Chemotherapeutic agents. *See* Anticancer drugs; Chemotherapy
Chemotherapy, 661–669. *See also* Anticancer drugs
   for acute lymphocytic leukemia
      agents, properties of, 353*t*
      guidelines, 353*t*
      historical induction data, 352*t*
      intensification stage, 352
      intrathecal, 353*t*
   adjuvant, 663–664
   for adult chronic myelogenous leukemia
      in chronic phase, 496
      with αIFN, 498
   in allo-BMT preparation, 729, 729*t*
   for AML, complications following, 481
   and auto-BMT compared
      for acute lymphocytic leukemia, 709

clinical case presentation, 445–446, 453–454. *See also* Splenomegaly
clinical manifestations, 448–449
demographics and expression, 449t
differential diagnosis, 447–448
epidemiology, 450
molecular biology, 450–451
pathology, 447–448, 448f
pathophysiology, 448f–450f, 449–450
therapy for, 451–453
G-CSF. *See* Granulocyte colony-stimulating factor
Gene mutations, in Gaucher disease, 451
Generic oligotyping, in HLA testing, 693t, 693–694
Gene therapy
for Gaucher disease, 453
for hemophilia B patients, 596
Genetic code, "universal," 298t
Genetic disorders, acute lymphocytic leukemia and, 347–349, 348t
Genetics, of hematopoietic malignancies, exercises and tools for, 407–408
Genitourinary tract, involvement in acute lymphocytic leukemia, 351
Genomes
human, 281
leukemia retrovirus, 284f
Genomic DNA
in aplastic anemia, 196
coding for plasminogen, 635, 635f
Germ cell tumors, secondary leukemias and lymphomas and, 525
Glanzmann's thrombasthenia
clinical case presentation, 561
diagnosis of, 561
features of, 561t
treatment of, 561
Globin synthesis, 107
Glucocerebrosidase, in Gaucher disease
molecular biology, 451
pathophysiology, 449–450
Glucocerebrosidase therapy, for Gaucher disease, 452
problems associated with, 452
Glucose-6-phosphate dehydrogenase, 107, 151–166. *See also* Naphthalene, and related compounds
activity and GSH stability test, 157f
cataracts and, 166
deficiency. *See* Glucose-6-phosphate dehydrogenase deficiency
enzyme polymorphisms and, 164
eyes and, 166
Fava beans and, 159–161
glutathione studies and, 153t
hematocrit and, pathogenetic mechanisms, 153
hemolysis. *See* Glucose-6-phosphate dehydrogenase hemolysis
henna and, 163f
lens and, 166
leukocytes and, 165
liver and, 165–166
naphthalene and. *See* Naphthalene, and related compounds
in newborns, pathogenetic mechanisms, 155, 161–163
pathogenetic mechanisms, 153–155

peripheral blood smears, 152f
population screening, 164
prematurity and, 155, 160f
red cells deficient in, factors hemolyzing, 158t
tissue distribution, 165
Glucose-6-phosphate dehydrogenase deficiency, 422
clinical case presentation, 151–153
drugs and infections implicated in, 161
genetics, 163–164
hemolytic anemia secondary to, identification of patient with, 156t
hemolytic factors, 157–158
Lyon hypothesis, 164–165
management, 166
neonatal hyperbilirubinemia and, 161–163
neonatal jaundice and, 161
Glucose-6-phosphate dehydrogenase hemolysis, 155–157
detection, 155–157
red cells and, 158t
screening tests, 156
Glutathione peroxidase, autosomal recessive inheritance of, 423
Glutathione reductase deficiencies, autosomal recessive inheritance of, 423
Glutathione synthetase, autosomal recessive inheritance of, 423
Glycogen storage disease, type IB, 416
Glycophorin C deficiency, hereditary elliptocytosis, 143
p-glycoprotein, and drug resistance in multiple myeloma treatment, 395
GM-CSF. *See* Granulocyte macrophage colony-stimulating factor
GM-CSF-IL-3 fusion protein (pixy321), 16
Gold-induced thrombocytopenia, 542–543
Golgi apparatus, granulocyte and, 414t
Grading scale, bone marrow transplantation and, 730–731
Graft-versus-host disease
acute form, 734t
in bone marrow transplantation with acute myeloid leukemia, 482
chronic form, 736–737, 737t
development of, 734t
in Gaucher disease, 454
induced, in allo-BMT, 711
organ involvement, 733–735
predictors, 692
prophylaxis, 733
secondary malignancies and, 523
Graft-versus-leukemia, in allo-BMT, 711
Granulocyte colony-stimulating factor, 10
use of, clinical case presentation, 9
Granulocyte disorders, bone marrow transplantation outcomes, 727, 727t
Granulocyte macrophage colony-stimulating factor, 10
juvenile chronic myelogenous leukemia, 507
Granulocyte macrophage colony-stimulating factor, juvenile chronic myelogenous leukemia and, 510
Granulocytes
compartments and production times, 414t

constituents, 414t
development, 413–414
functional defects, in immunocompromised host, 774
quantitative and qualitative disorders. *See* Neutrophil defects; *specific conditions and syndromes*
selectin and integrin families, 415t
Granuloma, 435
formation, 421
Granulopoiesis, ineffective, nutritional disorders and, 416
Growth factors
hematopoietic/hemopoietic. *See* Hematopoietic growth factors
in myelodysplastic syndrome
as etiologic agents, 461–462
as therapy, 463
Growth failure, in HIV-infected children, 595
Growth receptors, in myelodysplastic syndrome, 461–462
GVHD. *See* Graft-versus-host disease
GVL. *See* Graft-versus-leukemia

H

Haemophilus influenzae, disseminated intravascular coagulation and, 601
Hairy cell leukemia, 370
interferons in treatment of, 12
Ham-Dacie test, 188, 189, 190
Haploidy, acute lymphocytic leukemia and, 348, 348t
Haplotypes, in unrelated marrow donor testing, 695–696, 696t
HbE, as α-thalassemia determinant, 67–69
HbH disease, 55–65
HbH/retardation syndrome, 66
HC II deficiency. *See* Heparin cofactor II deficiency
HDN. *See* Hemolytic disease, of the newborn
Head trauma, as DIC cause, 604
Heart
involvement in acute lymphocytic leukemia, 351
toxicity scale for, 731
Heat illness, versus phagocyte-induced fever, 768
Heavy chain disease, multiple myeloma and, 392
Hemangioma, in neonatal thrombocytopenia, 565
Hemarthrosis, in hemophilia, 592
Hematocrit
algorithm for studying, 210f
blood viscosity and, 206–207, 207f
Hematologic disorders, bone marrow transplantation outcomes, 726–727, 727t
Hematologic malignancies, radiation therapy and, 671–676
Hematopoiesis
acute myeloid leukemia and, 472f, 472–473
and BMT practice, 703
colony-stimulating factors in, 432
of monocytes from pluripotent stem cell, 431–432, 433f
normal, 180–192, 190f, 191f